Clinical Neurology of the Older Adult

Clinical Neurology of the Older Adult

Edited by

Joseph I. Sirven, M.D.
Associate Professor of Neurology
Director, Electroencephalography Laboratory
Department of Neurology
Mayo Clinic
Scottsdale, Arizona

Barbara L. Malamut, Ph.D.
Adjunct Professor
Department of Psychology
Drexel University
Philadelphia, Pennsylvania

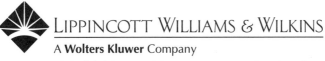

LIPPINCOTT WILLIAMS & WILKINS
A **Wolters Kluwer** Company
Philadelphia · Baltimore · New York · London
Buenos Aires · Hong Kong · Sydney · Tokyo

Acquisitions Editor: Charles W. Mitchell
Developmental Editor: Jenny Kim
Production Editor: Emily Lerman
Manufacturing Manager: Tim Reynolds
Cover Designer: Karen Quigley
Compositor: Lippincott Williams & Wilkins Desktop Division
Printer: Edwards Brothers

© 2002 by LIPPINCOTT WILLIAMS & WILKINS
530 Walnut Street
Philadelphia, PA 19106 USA
LWW.com

All rights reserved. This book is protected by copyright. No part of this book may be reproduced in any form or by any means, including photocopying, or utilized by any information storage and retrieval system without written permission from the copyright owner, except for brief quotations embodied in critical articles and reviews. Materials appearing in this book prepared by individuals as part of their official duties as U.S. government employees are not covered by the above-mentioned copyright.

Printed in the USA

Library of Congress Cataloging-in-Publication Data

Clinical neurology of the older adult / edited by Joseph I. Sirven, Barbara L. Malamut.
     p.;   cm.
   Includes bibliographical references and index.
   ISBN 0-7817-2789-8 (alk. paper)
   1. Geriatric neurology.   I. Sirven, Joseph I.   II. Malamut, Barbara L.
   [DNLM: 1. Nervous System Diseases—Aged. WL 140 C6407 2002]
   RC346.C543 2002
   618.97′68—dc21   2001038759

Care has been taken to confirm the accuracy of the information presented and to describe generally accepted practices. However, the authors, editors, and publisher are not responsible for errors or omissions or for any consequences from application of the information in this book and make no warranty, expressed or implied, with respect to the currency, completeness, or accuracy of the contents of the publication. Application of this information in a particular situation remains the professional responsibility of the practitioner.

The authors, editors, and publisher have exerted every effort to ensure that drug selection and dosage set forth in this text are in accordance with current recommendations and practice at the time of publication. However, in view of ongoing research, changes in government regulations, and the constant flow of information relating to drug therapy and drug reactions, the reader is urged to check the package insert for each drug for any change in indications and dosage and for added warnings and precautions. This is particularly important when the recommended agent is a new or infrequently employed drug.

Some drugs and medical devices presented in this publication have Food and Drug Administration (FDA) clearance for limited use in restricted research settings. It is the responsibility of the health care provider to ascertain the FDA status of each drug or device planned for use in their clinical practice.

10 9 8 7 6 5 4 3 2 1

And in the end, it's not the years in your life that count. It's the life in your years.
Abraham Lincoln

Youth is the gift of nature, but age is a work of art.
Garson Kanin

In memory of Barbara Bell, M.D., a wife, mother, teacher, and friend.
(1954–1998)

To Joan—For your steadfast presence and always believing that all is possible.

To Larry—For always sharing my dreams.

Contents

Contributing Authors

Neil B. Alexander, M.D. *Associate Professor, Department of Internal Medicine—Geriatrics, University of Michigan; Attending Physician, Department of Internal Medicine—Geriatrics, University of Michigan Health System, Ann Arbor, Michigan*

Enrica Arnaudo, M.D. *Assistant Professor, Department of Neurology, Thomas Jefferson University; Director of EMG Laboratory, Department of Neurology, Thomas Jefferson University Hospital, Philadelphia, Pennsylvania*

Alon Y. Avidan, M.D., M.P.H. *Clinical Assistant Professor, Department of Neurology, The University of Michigan Medical Center, Sleep Disorders Center, Ann Arbor, Michigan*

Kevin M. Biglan, M.D. *Instructor, Department of Neurology, University of Rochester; Instructor, Department of Neurology, Strong Memorial Hospital, Rochester, New York*

Jennifer J. Bortz, Ph.D. *Clinical Neuropsychologist, Department of Psychiatry/ Psychology, Mayo Clinic Hospital, Scottsdale, Arizona*

Orest B. Boyko, M.D., Ph.D. *Professor and Chair, Department of Diagnostic Imaging, Temple University Hospital, Philadelphia, Pennsylvania*

David J. Capobianco, M.D. *Assistant Professor, Department of Neurology, Mayo Clinic; Consultant, Department of Neurology, St. Lukes Hospital, Jacksonville, Florida*

Julio A. Chalela, M.D. *Staff Clinician, National Institute of Neurological Disorders and Stroke, National Institutes of Health, Bethesda, Maryland*

James C. Cloyd, Pharm.D. *Professor and Director, Epilepsy Research and Education Program, College of Pharmacy, University of Minnesota, Minneapolis, Minnesota*

Jeannine M. Conway, Pharm.D. *Assistant Professor, Department of Experimental and Clinical Pharmacology, University of Minnesota, Minneapolis, Minnesota*

John R. Corboy, M.D. *Associate Professor and Vice Chairman, Department of Neurology, University of Colorado School of Medicine; Staff Neurologist, Department of Neurology, University of Colorado Hospital, Denver, Colorado*

M. Cornelia Cremens, M.D., M.P.H. *Instructor, Departments of Psychiatry and Medicine, Harvard Medical School; Assistant, Departments of Psychiatry and Medicine, Massachusetts General Hospital, Boston, Massachusetts*

H. Gordon Deen, Jr., M.D. *Associate Professor, Department of Neurosurgery, Mayo Medical School, Rochester, Minnesota; Consultant, Department of Neurosurgery, Mayo Clinic, Jacksonville, Florida*

David W. Dodick, M.D. *Associate Professor, Department of Neurology, Mayo Clinic, Scottsdale, Arizona*

Ivo Drury, M.D. *Clinical Professor, Department of Neurology, University of Michigan, Ann Arbor; Chairman, Department of Neurology, Henry Ford Health System, Detroit, Michigan*

Jeffrey S. Durmer, M.D., Ph.D.   *Fellow, Department of Neurology, University of Pennsylvania; Fellow, Department of Neurology, Hospital of the University of Pennsylvania, Philadelphia, Pennsylvania*

James M. Ellison, M.D., M.P.H.   *Associate Clinical Professor, Psychiatry Department, Harvard Medical School, Boston; Clinical Director, Geriatric Psychiatry Program, McLean Hospital, Belmont, Massachusetts*

Jonathan L. Fellus, M.D.   *Clinical Assistant Professor, Department of Neurosciences, UMDNJ–NJ Medical School, Newark; Director, Brain Injury Services, Kessler Institute for Rehabilitation, East Orange, New Jersey*

Adam E. Flanders, M.D.   *Professor, Department of Radiology, Thomas Jefferson University; Department of Radiology/Neuroradiology, Thomas Jefferson University Hospital, Philadelphia, Pennsylvania*

Laura A. Flashman, Ph.D.   *Assistant Professor, Department of Psychiatry, Dartmouth Medical School, Lebanon; Co-Director, Neuropsychology Service, New Hampshire Hospital, Concord, New Hampshire*

Rod Foroozan, M.D.   *Fellow, Department of Neuro-ophthalmology, Wills Eye Hospital, Philadelphia, Pennsylvania*

Deborah W. Frazer, Ph.D.   *Director of Behavioral Health, Genesis ElderCare, Kennett Square, Pennsylvania*

Elliot M. Frohman, M.D., Ph.D.   *Associate Professor, Department of Neurology, University of Texas, Southwestern Medical Center, Dallas, Texas*

Gary L. Gottlieb, M.D., M.B.A.   *Professor, Department of Psychiatry, Harvard Medical School; Chairman, Partners Psychiatry and Mental Health System, Partners HealthCare System, Inc., Boston, Massachusetts*

Amparo Gutierrez, M.D.   *Co-Director, Neuromuscular Fellowship and Assistant Professor, Department of Neurology, Louisiana State University School of Medicine, New Orleans, Louisiana*

Julie E. Hammack, M.D.   *Assistant Professor, Department of Neurology, Mayo Clinic and Hospitals, Rochester, Minnesota*

Kathleen Hawker, M.D.   *Assistant Professor, Department of Neurology, University of Texas, Southwestern Medical Center, Dallas, Texas*

Susan L. Hickenbottom, M.D., M.S.   *Clinical Assistant Professor, Department of Neurology, University of Michigan; Director, Stroke Program, Department of Neurology, University of Michigan Health System, Ann Arbor, Michigan*

Reginald T. Ho, M.D.   *Assistant Professor, Department of Medicine, Division of Cardiology, Thomas Jefferson University Hospital, Philadelphia, Pennsylvania*

Michael D. Hollander, M.D.   *Assistant Professor, Department of Diagnostic Imaging, Temple University Hospital, Philadelphia, Pennsylvania; Deparment of Radiology, Carilion Roanoke Memorial Hospital, Roanoke, Virginia*

Howard I. Hurtig, M.D.   *Professor, Department of Neurology, University of Pennsylvania; Chairman, Department of Neurology, Pennsylvania Hospital/University of Pennsylvania Health System, Philadelphia, Pennsylvania*

Ricardo F. Izurieta, M.D. *Attending Physician, Department of Critical Care and Pulmonary Medicine, St. Vincent's Hospital, Jacksonville, Florida*

Bryan D. James, M. Bioethics *Research Coordinator, Department of Medicine, University of Pennsylvania, Institute on Aging, Philadelphia, Pennsylvania*

Uday S. Kanamalla, M.D. *Fellow, Department of Diagnostic Imaging, Temple University Hospital, Philadelphia, Pennsylvania*

Jason H.T. Karlawish, M.D. *Assistant Professor, Department of Medicine, University of Pennsylvania, Institute on Aging, Philadelphia, Pennsylvania*

Scott E. Kasner, M.D. *Assistant Professor, Department of Neurology, and Director, Comprehensive Stroke Program, University of Pennsylvania, Philadelphia, Pennsylvania*

Howard S. Kirshner, M.D. *Professor and Vice Chair, Department of Neurology, Vanderbilt University School of Medicine; Director, Stroke Service, Department of Neurology, Vanderbilt University Hospital, Nashville, Tennessee*

David S. Knopman, M.D. *Professor, Department of Neurology, Mayo Medical School; Senior Associate Consultant, Department of Neurology, Mayo Clinic, Rochester, Minnesota*

Joyce Liporace, M.D. *Assistant Professor, Department of Neurology, Jefferson Medical College; Residency Director, Department of Neurology, Thomas Jefferson University Hospital, Philadelphia, Pennsylvania*

Barbara L. Malamut, Ph.D. *Adjunct Professor, Department of Psychology, Drexel University, Philadelphia, Pennsylvania*

Elliot Mancall, M.D. *Professor, Department of Neurology and Interim Chair, Jefferson Medical College, Thomas Jefferson University, Philadelphia, Pennsylvania*

Robert E. Morales, M.D. *Assistant Professor, Department of Radiology, George Washington University; Staff Radiologist, Department of Radiology, George Washington University Hospital, Washington, DC*

Mark L. Moster, M.D. *Professor, Department of Neurology, Jefferson Medical College; Chairman, Department of Neurosensory Sciences, Albert Einstein Medical Center, Philadelphia, Pennsylvania*

Maromi Nei, M.D. *Assistant Professor, Department of Neurology, Thomas Jefferson University Hospital; Attending Physician, Department of Neurology, Jefferson Comprehensive Epilepsy Center, Philadelphia, Pennsylvania*

Enrique Noé, M.D., Ph.D. *Associate Professor, Department of Head Injury and Cognitive Rehabilitation, Hospital Valencia al Mar, Valencia, Spain*

Judith R. O'Jile, Ph.D. *Assistant Professor, Department of Psychiatry and Human Behavior, University of Mississippi; Neuropsychologist, Department of Psychiatry and Human Behavior, University of Mississippi Medical Center, Jackson, Mississippi*

Julie L. Pickholtz, Ph.D. *Staff Psychologist, Department of Psychiatry, University of Pennsylvania Health System, Philadelphia, Pennsylvania*

Carissa C. Pineda, M.D *Resident, Department of Neurology, Thomas Jefferson University Hosptial, Philadelphia, Pennsylvania*

Bernard M. Ravina, M.D. *Investigator, Neurogenetics Branch and Program Director, Clinical Trials Cluster, National Institute of Neurological Disorders and Stroke, Bethesda, Maryland*

Henry J. Riordan, Ph.D. *Director of Scientific Affairs, Ingenix Pharmaceutical Services, Chadd Ford; Assistant Professor, Department of Neurology, Thomas Jefferson University/Jefferson Medical College, Philadelphia, Pennsylvania*

Karen L. Roos, M.D. *John and Nancy Nelson Professor, Department of Neurology, Indiana University, Indianapolis, Indiana*

Laurie M. Ryan, Ph.D. *Assistant Professor, Department of Neurology, Uniformed Services University of the Health Sciences, Bethesda, Maryland; Neuropsychologist, Department of Neurology, Defense and Veterans Head Injury Program, Walter Reed Army Medical Center, Washington, DC*

Robert W. Schabbing, M.D. *Clinical Assistant Professor, Department of Neurology, University of Colorado Health Sciences Center; Department of Neurology, Colorado Kaiser-Permanente, Skyline Medical Center, Denver, Colorado*

Amy S. Schultz, M.A. *Department of Psychology, Arizona State University, Tempe, Arizona*

Vicki Shanker, M.D. *Deparment of Neurology, Montefiore Medical Center, Albert Eisntein College of Medicine, Bronx, New York*

Tanya Simuni, M.D. *Assistant Professor, Department of Neurology, Northwestern University Medical School; Staff Neurologist, Department of Neurology, Northwestern Memorial Hospital, Chicago, Illinois*

Joseph I. Sirven, M.D. *Assistant Professor of Neurology, and Director, Electroencephalography Laboratory, Department of Neurology, Mayo Clinic, Scottsdale, Arizona*

David Solomon, M.D., Ph.D. *Assistant Professor, Department of Neurology, University of Pennsylvania School of Medicine, Philadelphia, Pennsylvania*

Yaakov Stern, Ph.D. *Professor of Clinical Neuropsychology, Departments of Neurology and Psychiatry, Gertrude H. Sergievsky Center and The Taub Institute, Columbia University College of Physicians and Surgeons, New York, New York*

Austin J. Sumner, M.Med.Sc., M.B., F.R.A.C.P. *Professor and Head, Department of Neurology, Louisiana State University Health Sciences Center, New Orleans, Louisiana*

Lori H. Travis, M.D. *Chief Resident, Department of Neurology, Mayo Clinic, Rochester, Minnesota*

Jay D. Varrato, D.O. *Neuromuscular Fellow, Thomas Jefferson University, Philadelphia, Pennsylvania*

Naomi Wasserman, B.S. *Clinical Research Coordinator, Department of Neurology, Thomas Jefferson University, Philadelphia, Pennsylvania*

Eelco F.M. Wijdicks, M.D. *Professor, Department of Neurology, Mayo Clinic; Medical Director, Neurologic Neurosurgery Intensive Care Unit, Saint Mary's Hospital, Rochester, Minnesota*

Preface

Neurological illness is a major cause of disability and dependence in the elderly. It accounts for a disproportionate number of patients treated in neurological office and hospital settings. Thus, with the growth of the aging population there has been an increased demand for information regarding the course of normal aging and its impact on the nervous system, diseases that effect the elderly, and their treatment. In both medical and psychological settings, it has become abundantly clear that the approach to diagnosis and treatment of disorders in the aged can be quite different and markedly more complicated than in younger adults. It is not uncommon for the elderly patient to have a complex array of neurological and medical problems so that the usual treatment for one illness is prohibited due to complications from a second disease. These patients often take multiple medications, each with its own side effects, and the interactions of the various drugs can lead to adverse reactions that can resemble a new disorder. Thus, understanding of many areas of neurology is needed to make an accurate diagnosis and implement a well-integrated treatment plan. Yet there are few books that survey the field of geriatric neurology.

It is the purpose of this book to serve as a practical guide to all physicians, psychologists, medical students and others who serve the geriatric population. It also reflects the multidisciplinary nature of geriatric neurology by including chapters on the neuropsychology of various diseases, such as Parkinson's disease and dementia, as well as important psychosocial and ethical considerations that confront most clinicians in their day-to-day practice. The scope of this book is broad, to include the major categories of neurological illness in the peripheral and central nervous systems affecting the elderly. In the first section, diagnostic tests commonly used in the elderly are discussed. The second section includes common neurological problems based on signs and symptoms, such as mood or gait disorders. The third section discusses specific disease entities such as epilepsy or dementia, and the fourth section involves psychosocial issues. It is hoped that approaching this topic from two viewpoints, such as signs and symptoms and specific disease states, will prove to be a useful tool to clinicians because a disease can be referenced based by the symptom(s) it presents, or looked up by the disease entity itself. Moreover, many medication charts and diagnostic algorithms are provided so that beneficial information can be quickly obtained. In this way, *Clinical Neurology of the Older Adult* will assist all practitioners in helping people enjoy healthy, productive lives as they age.

Acknowledgments

The preparation of this text reflects research findings as well as day-to-day clinical issues in treating the elderly patient. In this regard, we thank all of our patients for providing an invaluable resource by teaching us many life lessons. We also thank our families, Joan, Larry, Robbie, Lucky, and Annie: without their support and understanding, this book would never have come to fruition.

1

Neurologic Examination of the Older Adult

Joseph I. Sirven and Elliott Mancall

The neurologic examination, for the most part, is an exercise in detailed observation, consisting of two tasks: (*a*) localizing the part of the nervous system that is malfunctioning, and (*b*) identifying the cause for that malfunction. Every aspect of the patient's behavior, including the way he or she sits, speaks, and responds, tells the physician about nervous system function. However, in older adults, the parameters of a normal neurologic examination require redefining and the results from a neurologic examination must be considered within the context of known age-related changes. Thus, findings in older patients that suggest pathology may not be pertinent if such findings occur frequently at advanced ages. Table 1-1 describes the normal morphologic and physiologic changes in the aging nervous system.

In his seminal papers on the neurologic changes in the aged, Critchley (1931; 1956) identified several changes that occur in the neurologic examination. These were subsequently confirmed by other reviews (Benassi et al., 1990; Kokmen et al., 1977). Changes tend to affect the visual, auditory, olfactory, motor, and sensory nervous systems. The most consistent of the neurologic signs of aging are shown in Table 1-2.

MENTAL STATUS EXAMINATION

Changes in mental status functioning that occur with aging may be apparent on formal standardized tests of mental status but they are difficult to detect clinically. Older patients are generally alert and have normal levels of consciousness. It is abnormal for an older patient not to maintain orientation to time, place, and situation. Judgment is expected to be normal and calculations and thought content are equally unaffected unless a pathologic process is present. Remote and recent memory is usually normal; however, the speed of processing and retrieving information slows. Thus, when abnormalities of speech or language are noted, an underlying brain lesion must be considered. For a detailed discussion regarding mental functioning, see Chapter 5.

CRANIAL NERVE CHANGES

Cranial nerve abnormalities are rarely associated with normal aging, yet important exceptions are seen. Changes in hearing, particularly progressive hearing loss (presbycusis), especially for high tones is commonly observed as well as a decline in speech discrimination. These changes are secondary to a reduction in the number of hair cells in Corti's organ. Similarly, olfaction generally declines symmetrically with age; the key to a pathologic process is finding asymmetric loss. Changes in visual acuity are almost always related to abnormalities in the eye and do not reflect changes in visual neural circuits. Pathologic conditions (e.g., cataracts, glaucoma, and other causes) must be sought in patients complaining of diminished vision and not be attributed to normal aging. Aging does not cause a change in the appearance of the retina. Thus, funduscopic changes should be considered abnormal and consideration given to systemic causes such as diabetes.

Older adults have smaller pupils than those seen in younger adults as well as sluggish light and accommodation reactions. These changes, which occur symmetrically, result from aging changes in the muscles of the sphincter pupillae. Thus, unilateral abnormalities need to be investigated. The aged also have abnormalities in eye movement, including restriction of upward gaze, failure to dissociate head movements from eye movements, and gaze nystagmus, which is generally associated with medications. For a more detailed discussion on the visual changes associated with aging, see Chapter 12.

MOTOR EXAMINATION

Muscle tone can alter with aging, with rigidity and paratonia (increased tone) being the most common manifestation. The increased tone can cause diminished agility. Motor strength is well preserved except for a mild reduction in muscle power, especially proximally, with advancing age. The reduction in power is

TABLE 1-1. *Age-related nervous system changes*

Neuroanatomic location	Change
Anterior horn cells, sensory ganglion	Decline of 25%
Brain weight	Weight decline of 233 g from third decade to sixth to seventh decade
Hippocampus	Neuronal loss and gliosis by 27%
Neuronal cytoplasm	Increased accumulation of lipofuscin granules
Nerve roots	Accumulation of amyloid
Blood vessels and flow	Hyalinization of the walls of small blood vessels
	Cerebral flow declines with age with an increase in cerebrovascular resistance
Neurotransmitters	Decline in the concentrations of acetylcholine, norepinephrine, dopamine, and gamma-aminobutyric acid
Muscles and peripheral nerves	Skeletal muscle fiber loss with concomitant atrophy
	Myelin changes occur with a decrease in conduction velocity
	Loss of motor and sensory axons

related to a decrease in the number of muscle fibers and the bulk of each fiber. The strength of handgrip lessens 20% to 30% from age 20 onward, with an equal decline on both sides of the body, but this is only apparent if an older adult is compared with a younger adult.

Aging is also associated with a decline in coordination when older adults are compared with young controls. This change is almost undetectable, but caution should be taken in assuming that ataxia is secondary to aging as well. Action tremors often occur in older adults. However, tremor should not be considered a normal sign of aging but rather a symptom aggravated by age that can be treated. Motor reaction time is decreased with older age. Common functions (e.g., donning trousers, rising from a chair, or climb-ing stairs) can require more time for an older adult as compared with a younger individual. A decrease in coordination occurs, with a possible increase of dysmetria on finger-to-nose testing, as well as dysdiadochokinesia. At times, a mild, unexplained ataxia is encountered.

Gait can slow with age and signs such as a reduced arm swing and a stooped posture is present. A shuffling gait should not be considered a normal sign of aging. If slowness is extreme with regard to these functions, then extrapyramidal pathology should be considered (i.e., Parkinson's disease). Although aged patients may have gaits that appear unsteady, they do not necessarily have repeated falls or trouble with tandem walking. For further information regarding gait and movements disorders, see Chapters 5 and 22, respectively.

TABLE 1-2. *Age-related changes in the neurologic examination*

Modality	Change
Auditory	Perceptive hearing loss for higher tones
Gait	Attitude of general flexion
	Decreased fluidity of movement
Motor	Diminished reaction time
	Impaired agility and coordination
	Reduced muscle bulk and power
Ophthalmic	Decreased pupillary size
	Delayed pupillary reaction to light and accommodation
	Diminished upward gaze
Olfactory	Diminishment in olfaction
Reflexes	Reduced or absent ankle reflex
Sensory	Impairment of vibratory sensation, but preservation of proprioception

REFLEXES

Deep tendon reflexes are generally preserved in the elderly, and their absence or asymmetry usually indicates disease. Loss of ankle jerks is considered common and may be a consequence of the inelasticity of the Achilles tendon rather than changes within the nerve or the reflex arc. In most instances, however, loss of a reflex is considered a sign of disease rather than a normal consequence of aging. Snout, glabellar (inability to inhibit blinking), and palmomental reflexes are a frequent finding in the elderly. However, the suck and grasp reflex are indicative of frontal lobe disease. Superficial reflexes (e.g., the abdominal responses) are frequently not obtainable. Flexor plantar responses can be difficult to attain because of withdrawal, but a positive response must be regarded as indicating a lesion in the corticospinal tract.

THE SENSORY EXAMINATION

One of the most common manifestations of aging seen on the neurologic examination is the change in sensation. Impairment or loss of vibratory sense in the toes and ankles is a well-known finding, with a decrease in function of 50% to 60% in the feet of persons over 80 years of age, whereas proprioception is well preserved. Thresholds for the perception of cutaneous stimuli increase with age but can be difficult to detect. The changes in cutaneous sensation correlate with a loss of sensory fibers on sural nerve biopsy, as well as reduced amplitude of sensory nerve action potentials and loss of dorsal root ganglion cells. Decreases in both two-point discrimination and stereognosis have been reported, but are not well characterized in the context of the neurologic examination.

AUTONOMIC NERVOUS SYSTEM

Autonomic function is impaired with aging. Autonomic control of heart and peripheral vasculature may be impaired and lead to orthostatic hypotension. Orthostatic hypotension accounts for a small but significant number of falls by older patients. This hypotension may be related to dysfunction of several anatomic loci, including the hypothalamus, brainstem, spinal cord, or peripheral nerve. Temperature control mechanisms can also be reduced, with hypothermia or hyperthemia a possible consequence. For a more detailed discussion, see Chapter 7.

EFFECT OF AGING ON THE ACTIVITIES OF DAILY LIVING IN THE HEALTHY ELDERLY

When multiple illnesses are superimposed on normal aging, physical reserves used to perform the complex motor activities required for daily living are compromised. Table 1-3 shows the result from the Bronx aging study, which consisted of healthy, ambulatory, community-living volunteers, aged 74 to 85 years, studied over time (Wolfson and Katzman, 1983). The study helped to define the effects of normal aging with regard to activities of daily living. For the most part, function is well preserved but, clearly, decrements in motor strength take their toll as evidenced by the difficulties in getting out of bed and climbing stairs.

It is the loss of functional ability that is most important to understand, as this is what frequently leads to a request for neurologic, psychological, and psychiatric consultation. Detailed discussions of the normal changes of aging with respect to various aspects of the central and peripheral nervous system are found throughout this text.

SUMMARY

Healthcare practitioners who care for the older adult must first understand the neurologic changes that occur with age and how they affect function. The aging process in essentially healthy, disease-free persons is associated with decrements in many aspects of motor and sensory function. It is important to comprehend these changes and understand their impact on function in order to accurately diagnose, treat, and care for the older adult with neurologic disease.

REFERENCES

Benassi G, D'Alessandro RD, Gallassi R, et al. Neurological examination in subjects over 65 years: an epidemiological survey. *Neuroepidemiology* 1990;9:27–38.
Critchley M. The neurology of old age. *Lancet* 1931;1: 1119–1127.

TABLE 1-3. *Age-related changes in activities of daily living*

Function	No difficulty (%)	With difficulty, but does not need help (%)	Needs help (%)
Getting in and out of bed	78	21	1
Sitting or standing from a chair	69	29	2
Continence	68	31	1
Eating, cutting food	96	4	0
Preparing own meals	92	1	7
Dressing	82	17	1
Climbing stairs	50	45	5
Shopping	83	9	8
Handling finances	88	8	4

From Katzman R, Terry R, eds. *The neurology of aging,* 1983, with permission.

Critchley M. Neurological changes in the aged. *Journal of Chronic Diseases* 1955;3(5):459–477.

Jenkyn LR, Reeves AG. Neurologic signs in uncomplicated aging. *Semin Neurol* 1981;1(1):21–30.

Kokmen E, Bossemeyer RW, Barney J, et al. Neurological manifestations of aging. *J Gerontol* 1977;32(4):411–419.

Potvin AR, Syndulko K, Tourtellotte W, et. al. Human neurologic function and the aging process. *J Am Geriatr Soc* 1980;28(1):1–9.

Wolfson LI, Katzman R. The neurologic consultation at age 80. In: Katzman R, Terry RD, eds. The neurology of aging. Philadelphia: FA Davis, 1983:221–244.

2.1

Imaging of the Aging Brain

Michael D. Hollander, Robert E. Morales, Uday S. Kanamalla,
Adam E Flanders, and Orest B. Boyko

Alterations in the brain with aging have been the focus of many investigations. With the advances in radiologic techniques and the ever-expanding aged population, an understanding of both normal and pathologic imaging findings in the elderly is vital. Elderly people have a far greater percentage of neurologic disease when compared with the young; therefore, the need to understand the normal alterations in brain structure and function is important.

Computed tomography (CT), magnetic resonance imaging (MRI), single photon emission computed tomography (SPECT), and positron emission tomography (PET) are the primary imaging techniques currently being used to evaluate the brain. CT and MRI allow for an easy, safe, noninvasive way to study the brain. CT is essentially limited by single plane imaging and poor visualization of the temporal lobe and posterior fossa structures from skull base artifacts. MRI has the advantage of being multiplanar and, therefore, the temporal lobe can be evaluated in the coronal plane with little or no artifact from the skull base. SPECT and PET imaging allow for a physiologic evaluation of the brain and for physiologic comparison of different regions of the brain. These two techniques require the intravenous injection of a radiopharmaceutical and give less information about the morphologic appearance of the brain. Therefore, for the complete evaluation of the aging brain, most studies suggest using both an imaging study and a nuclear medicine study to allow for a morphologic and functional assessment of the brain.

Various pitfalls must be recognized when analyzing elderly people, whether healthy or diseased (Drayer, 1988). From the third decade of life to the beginning of the tenth decade, the weight of the average male brain declines from 1,394 to 1,161 g, a loss of 233 g, presumably caused by degeneration of neurons and replacement gliosis (Critchley, 1956; Ball, 1997). This change is slow initially, but accelerates with advancing age, beginning usually by the seventh decade. Changes involve both the cerebrum and the cerebellum (Lemay,

1984). The neuronal population in the neocortex is progressively depleted in the seventh, eighth, and ninth decades. The greatest loss appears to be among the small neurons of the second and fourth layers (external and internal granular laminae) in the frontal and superior temporal regions, approaching a 50% loss by the ninth decade. Neuronal loss and replacement gliosis, which represent the primary aging process, proceed without a relationship to the development of neurofibrillary changes seen in Alzheimer's disease (AD) and senile plaques (Critchley 1956; Ball 1997).

NORMAL AGING

Ventricular Enlargement

The median and paramedian parts of the brain show regression early, and the third ventricle slowly begins to widen (Lemay, 1984). Yakovlev studied the growth and maturation of the nervous system and noted the regression of the median nuclei of the thalamus and widening of the third ventricle beginning by the fifth decade (Lemay, 1984). In addition, he saw a progressive shrinkage in the massa intermedia (Lemay, 1984). In a different study, Morel and Wildi measured the ventricular volume in cadaveric specimens ranging in age from 55 to 99 years and noted an increase in the size of the ventricles up to the ninth decade (Lemay, 1984). The ventricles were larger in the men than in the women, and the left lateral ventricle was usually larger than the right (Lemay, 1984). In addition to the ventricles becoming larger, Knudson found that the temporal lobes, particularly the hippocampus, uncus, parahippocampal, and fusiform gyri, and area around the insula involutes (Lemay, 1984). The progression in size of the lateral ventricles with age is more variable than that of the third ventricle (Lemay, 1984).

Studies using CT have been performed to assess the limits of normalcy seen in aging. Various measurements and ratios, including the Evans, frontal horn, bi-

TABLE 2-1. *Computed tomography ratios*

Evans: Frontal horn span or internal diameter of skull (Gawler et al., 1976)
    <0.29 in patients <60 yr
    >0.50 obstructive hydrocephalus (LeMay, 1984)
Bicaudate: width of ventricles between caudate or internal diameter of skull (Pelicci, 1979)
    <0.17 normal
    >0.20 abnormal (Hahn and Rim, 1976)
Third ventricle: sum of distance lateral margin of third and sylvian fissure/internal diameter of skull
    <0.59 demented patients (Brinkman et al., 1981)
Gray matter to white matter (normal values):
    1.13 (20 yr) 1.28 (50 yr) 1.55 (100 yr) (Miller et al., 1980)

caudate, and third ventricle-Sylvian fissure methods have been reported (Table 2-1). These studies all appear to find progressive enlargement of the ventricles and cortical sulci (Fig. 2-1). In fact, Nagata et al. reported that the cerebrospinal fluid (CSF)-to-brain ratio remains constant for the first six decades and then becomes variable with increasing age (Drayer, 1988). Ratios of the width of the ventricles to the width of the skull or brain are most easily made and reproducible.

Sulcal Enlargement

Enlargement of the superficial sulci, particularly in the frontal parasagittal region and in the parietal and temporal lobes, is commonly described as a normal

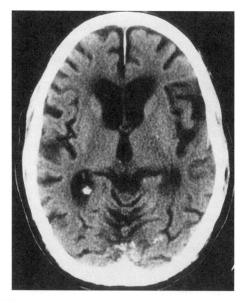

FIG. 2-1. A 92-year-old man with atrophy. Non-contrast axial-computed tomography imaging demonstrates diffuse ventricular and sulcal widening.

feature of aging. The reason for this is not certain, but may be related to a decrease in volume of subcortical structures rather than to a change in width of the cortex (LeMay, 1984). Miller et al. reported that the ratio of gray matter versus white matter was 1.13 at age 20, 1.28 at age 50, and 1.55 at age 100, which suggests that white matter atrophy exceeds that of gray matter (Miller et al., 1991). Most authors feel that this physiologic atrophy commences at the age of 50. However, CT studies on postmortem and living patients do show a wide variation in the CSF-space size, ranging between 30% and 50% the size of healthy young adults. A widening is also seen of the interhemispheric fissure, extending posteriorly to or beyond the callosomarginal sulci. Progressive widening of the sulci occurs in the frontal lobes and cerebellar vermis, beginning in the teenaged years (Cala et al., 1982). Widening of the superficial sulci seen with normal aging is often termed *cortical* atrophy by radiologists; however, in fact, this should be referred to as *gyral* or *superficial* atrophy. Sulcal enlargement in aging is diffuse; however, changes are best seen in specific locations (e.g., the median nuclei of the thalamus) after 50 years of age (Brody, 1955). Only mild enlargement of the temporal horns of the lateral ventricles is seen, with the left being larger than the right. Widening of the superficial cortical sulci is seen first in the frontal and parietal parasagittal regions (Tomlinson, 1968). The anterior interhemispheric fissure and the CSF spaces around the cerebellar vermis also widen with age (Huag, 1977). The sulci around the central, precentral, postcentral and superior frontal gyri widen later (Kido et al., 1980, Valentine et al.,1980).

Cerebral White Matter

Most recent studies have shown that 30% to 80% of elderly individuals without neurologic deficits have focal abnormalities in the white matter (Bradley et al., 1984). These foci are seen as areas of bright signal in the periventricular, subcortical white matter, and capping the lateral ventricular margins on long TR-weighted images. On electron microscopy, atrophy of axons and myelin with associated gliosis, tortuous, thickened vessels, and increased intracellular water (Drayer, 1988) can be seen. Some of these changes histologically are thought to be secondary to ectasia of the arterioles, with enlargement of the surrounding perivascular spaces (Drayer, 1988). These findings were first described by Durand-Fardel in 1843 (Drayer, 1988) and are termed *e`tat crible*. In addition to the white matter changes, an increase is seen in the deposition of iron in the brain, specifically in the corpus striatum (Awad et al., 1986). This increased iron is thought to be related to a decrease in oligodendroglial function and dopamine production and an increase in the free radical formation (Awald et al., 1986). Iron is also deposited in the walls of blood vessels. Iron is best seen on T2-weighted images as low signal secondary to field heterogeneity and magnetic susceptibility (Drayer, 1986).

Skull Changes with Aging

Finby and Kraft (LeMay, 1984) found that most skull films taken of the same individuals over time indicated an increase in the size of the skull vault, facial bones, paranasal sinuses, and the skull thickness, which is thought to be secondary to continuous resorption and regrowth of the skull and facial bones.

(1H) Proton Magnetic Resonance Spectroscopy

Magnetic resonance spectroscopy (MRS) is showing great promise in adding to the understanding of the physiologic processes that affect the aging brain. Spectroscopy is interpreted in terms of the identity of a chemical and its concentration (Ross et al., 1998). MRS provides a noninvasive way to identify tissue markers, which can aid in differentiating disease states. The major peaks of the MR spectrum are N-acetylaspartate (NAA), total creatine (Cr), total choline (Cho), myoinositol (mI), and glutamate plus glutamine (Glx). The current approach to differential diagnosis is to determine whether a metabolite is elevated, reduced, or unchanged with respect to a reference, typically Cr (Ross et al.,1998).

The basic function of the four principal metabolites in the MR spectrum is as follows:

NAA is a marker of neuronal or axonal content.
Cr is an indicator of energy.
Cho marks membrane changes
mI can indicate astrocyte (or glial) disease (Ross et al., 1999).

TABLE 2-2. *Magnetic resonance changes in aging*

Age range	NAA/Cr	Cho/Cr	mI/Cr
Gray matter			
16–25	1.40	0.56	0.60
26–37	1.36	0.61	0.60
40–78	1.26	0.60	0.59
White matter			
16–25	1.54	0.77	0.59
26–37	1.49	0.78	0.60
40–78	1.41	0.82	0.63

Cho, total choline; Cr, total creatine; mI, myoinositol; NAA, N-acetylaspartate.
From Ross BD, Bluml S, Cowan R, et al. In vivo MR spectroscopy of human dementia. *Neuroimaging Clin N Am* 1998;8(4):809–822, with permission.

As seen in Table 2-2, in the normal aging brain are very small but definite changes in the MR spectrum as compared with a young adult. The NAA has been shown to decrease in the occipital gray matter, the Cho/Cr is higher, and the mI/Cr is lower. Ross has shown that none of these changes exceed 10%.

Imaging and Radiopharmaceuticals

The complex but close relationship between brain physiologic activity and brain blood flow is the basis for nuclear medicine imaging protocols for the brain. The development of scintillation multiprobe systems provided a technique to quantify regional cerebral blood flow (rCBF), or perfusion, within individual regions of the cortex, and ultimately to compare the rCBF with regional brain function. SPECT and PET systems, with their ability for rapid three-dimensional imaging, have revolutionized physiologic brain imaging. This has now become particularly important in geriatric brain imaging, especially in the differentiation of various causes of dementia.

Radiopharmaceuticals currently used (Alavi and Hirsch, 1991) to evaluate brain physiology by rCBF SPECT include 99mTc-hexamethyl propylene amine oxime (HMPAO, exametazime, ceretec, Amersham Inc.), 123I-inosine monophosphate (which is intermittently available), 133Xe gas (General Electric Corp.), and 99mTc-ethyl cysteinate (ECD, Merck Du Pont Inc.).

The most commonly used radiopharmaceuticals for PET imaging (Diksic and Reba, 1991) of the brain are 18F-fluorodeoxyflucose (18F-FDG), which measures the cerebral metabolic rate for glucose (CMR-GIc), and 15O H_2O, which measures rCBF.

Radiopharmaceuticals in Normal Aging

Normal, age-related atrophy could significantly influence qualitative and quantitative analyses of 18F-FDG-PET studies. Several reports have appeared that deal with normal aging and brain volume on MRI and found that the best correlation was seen between age and ventricular volumes and total brain volumes (Fig. 2-1). Sulcal volumes correlated less well with age (Tanna et al., 1991). Age correlated with decreasing brain and increasing CSF volumes, with steeper regression slopes in men compared with women, suggesting more atrophy with age in men.

The 18F-FDG-PET findings in normally aging brain, as reported in the literature, have been inconsistent. A number of investigators have described diminished regional glucose metabolism in the temporal, parietal, somatosensory, and, especially, the frontal regions. Others have described more prominent decreases in the frontal and somatosensory cortices in comparison with young controls (Chawluk et al., 1987; Kuhl et al., 1987; Yoshii et al., 1988). When brain atrophy was not considered, mean CMRGlc values were lower in older patients, particularly in the frontal, parietal, and temporal regions. Also, women had significantly higher mean CMRGlc than men. Cerebrovascular risk factors in the population were also seen not to have any effect on CMRGlc (Yoshii et al., 1988).

PATHOLOGIC CONDITIONS

Most dementing illnesses are typically irreversible and progressive (Foster et al., 1999). It is therefore, of the utmost importance to exclude systemic causes such as infection, electrolyte or chemical imbalance, heart disease, or nutritional disorders. The major role of imaging is to detect treatable structural disorders such as hemorrhage, malignancy, posttraumatic lesions, infection, and hydrocephalus (Larson et al., 1986). CT and MRI have greatly improved our ability to detect these treatable conditions. In addition, physiologic imaging procedures (e.g., MRS, SPECT, and PET) are leading the advances in early diagnosis of such debilitating diseases such as AD.

Alzheimer's Disease

Although it is possible to make an accurate clinical diagnosis of dementia in most patients with severe disease, it is very difficult to differentiate between AD and other dementing disorders in patients with mild disease (Tierney et al., 1988). With functional imaging studies such as SPECT and PET, it is be-

TABLE 2-3. *Value of imaging techniques in Alzheimer's disease*

CT	Of limited value (bone artifact inhibits evaluation of the medial temporal lobe)
MRI	Allows for volumetric measurements of the temporal lobe with significant reduction seen in Alzheimer's disease (AD) as compared with depression and other dementias
MRS	Myoinositol is elevated in AD and decreased in other dementias
SPECT	Bilateral hypoperfusion of the temporal and parietal lobes using HMPAO or inosine 5′-monophosphate
PET	Decrease in whole brain CMRGlc values, especially in the temporal and parietal lobes

CMAGlc, cerebral metabolic rate for glucose; CT, computed tomography; HMPAO, ^{99m}Tc-hexamethyl-propyleneamine oxime; MRI, magnetic resonance imaging; MRS, magnetic resonance spectroscopy; PET, positron emission tomography; SPECT, single photon emission computed tomography.

lieved possible to make an early diagnosis of AD and possibly help in elucidating the mechanisms underlying the disorder. Thus, neuroimaging studies have focused their attention on detection of early structural changes in the hippocampal formation and parahippocampal gyrus because memory loss is a prominent feature of AD. Table 2-3 summarizes the benefits and disadvantages of various imaging techniques.

Computed Tomography

CT is diagnostically limited because of skull base artifacts and a limited view of the hippocampus. However, studies using angled CT scan to measure the minimal width of the medial temporal lobe (MTL) have shown this measurement to be a useful marker for AD versus depression (O'Brien et al., 2000). A significant reduction is seen in the MTL in patients with AD when compared with patients with depression. O'Brien et al. showed that the mean MTL for patients with AD was 10.8 mm and 14.0 mm for patients with depression (O'Brien et al., 2000).

Magnetic Resonance Imaging

The best visualization of the MTLs is provided by MRI (Fig. 2-2). High resolution imaging in the coronal plane, using a fluid attenuated inversion recovery (FLAIR) sequence as well as a three-dimensional volume gradient echo sequence, is useful to image the temporal lobe, allowing for both morphologic and

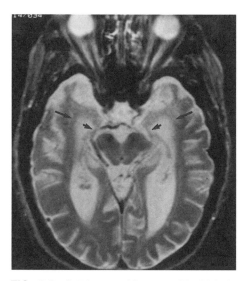

FIG. 2-2. A 76-year-old man with Alzheimer's disease. Axial T₂-weighted magnetic resonance imaging demonstrates bilateral hippocampal (*short arrows*) and temporal lobe atrophy with resulting compensatory widening of the temporal horns (*long arrows*).

volumetric analysis to be done. Volumetric evaluation of the temporal lobes can be performed and compared with normative data published by Bhatia et al. (Scheltens, 1999). In patients with AD, volumetric measurements reveal significantly lower measurements as compared with a group of controls (Kesslak, 1991). A more recent study by Cuenod et al. (1993) has shown that atrophy of the amygdala can occur earlier than hippocampal atrophy.

Magnetic Resonance Spectroscopy

Using proton (¹H) MRS (Lazeyras et al., 1998) in the evaluation of AD has shown a loss of NAA and an increase in mI/Cr (Fig. 2-3), which suggests a loss of neuronal content. The elevation in mI has been used to distinguish patients with AD from normal patients or those with other causes of dementia. This elevation is thought to result secondary to an astrocytic reaction to the presence of neurofibrillary tangles. Elevation of Cho/Cr has been neither reproducible nor specific to AD (Ross et al., 1999). Ross et al. have shown that MRS can distinguish AD with a specificity of 95% (Ross et al., 1998).

Single Photon Emission Computed Tomography

Several studies report that tracers (e.g., HMPAO or IMP) have high sensitivity (64% to 100%) and a similar specificity in the diagnosis of AD (Holman et al., 1992; Claus et al., 1994; Messa et al., 1994). Many of these studies emphasize that bilateral hypoperfusion of the temporal and parietal lobes is the most common and, diagnostically, the most specific finding in AD. Also seen is infrequent involvement of the frontal lobes, generally in association with the temporoparietal hypoperfusion and in the more advanced cases of the disease. In actual practice, however, almost 30% of patients will present with a unilateral posterior perfusion defect, when first seen, more commonly on the patient's left, whereas bilateral defects are often asymmetric. Frontal flow defects can appear later in the course of the disease (Bonte et al., 1986; Jagust et al., 1987; Perani et al., 1988; Testa et al., 1988). Some observers have related left posterior perfusion defects to short-term memory deficits, and

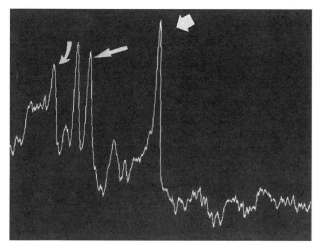

FIG. 2-3. A 71-year-old woman with Alzheimer's disease. Magnetic resonance spectroscopy demonstrates decreased *N*-acetylaspartate (*short arrow*) and an increase in myoinositol (*curved arrow*) related to creatine (*long arrow*).

right posterior defects to visual spatial abnormalities, whereas a left frontal perfusion defect is often accompanied by a degree of aphasia (Bonte et al., 1986; Jagust et al., 1987; Perani et al., 1988; Testa et al., 1988).

Positron Emission Tomography

Initial 18F-FDG-PET studies reported a decrease in whole brain CMRGlc values, with particular reduction in the bilateral temporal and parietal lobes, in patients with AD when compared with healthy, age-matched controls (Duara et al., 1986; Jamieson et al., 1987; Bonte et al., 1990; Friedland, 1983). Also, in patients with AD of varying severity, the magnitude and extent of hypometabolism on PET correlate with the severity of the dementia symptoms (Duara et al., 1986; Jamieson et al., 1987; Frackowiak et al., 1981). Studies indicate no significant CMRGlc changes or only minor decreases in the parietal lobes with early AD. Moderately affected patients show significantly decreased metabolism in the midfrontal lobes, bilateral parietal lobes, and superior temporal regions. In patients with severe AD, the same regions are affected, but the hypometabolism is more pronounced. In all patients with AD, the parietal lobes show the greatest changes, with a 38% decrease in patients with moderate disease and a 53% decrease in patients with severe disease; other areas (sensorimotor and visual cortices, subcortical nuclei, brainstem, and cerebellum) have relatively preserved CMRGlc (Alavi and Hirsch, 1991; Kushner et al., 1987).

The temporoparietal defects have been found to be the best discriminant between normal and Alzheimer's patients. In mild AD, the sensitivity was 42%, whereas in moderate and severe disease, it was 56% and 79%, respectively (Claus et al., 1994). In assessing the sensitivity of FDG studies versus HMPAO studies to detect AD, it appears that FDG-PET may be a more sensitive tracer.

Whereas the bilateral temporoparietal pattern is highly predictive of AD, it is not pathognomonic for it (Miller et al., 1991; Kuwabara et al., 1990; Friedland et al., 1984; Friedland 1989; Bonte et al., 1993). Therefore, in evaluating a patient with perfusion abnormalities in the temporoparietal regions, it is important to exclude stroke and a comparison with MRI or CT studies is required. In patients with predominant frontal hypoperfusion, also consider Pick's disease, dementia of the frontal type, and progressive supranuclear palsy (PSP). PSP can be differentiated by clinical findings (e.g., parkinsonian symptoms and ocular findings). Also note, patients with Parkinson disease with dementia have patterns that appear to be indistinguishable from those seen in AD. Other entities that can produce a similar pattern to that seen in AD include Creutzfeldt-Jakob disease, vascular dementia, dementia in association with Down's syndrome, carbon monoxide poisoning, and occasionally, normal pressure hydrocephalus (Bonte et al., 1993).

Stroke

Multiinfarct Dementia

Computed Tomography and Magnetic Resonance Imaging

Multiinfarct dementia (MID) is characterized by separate episodes of infarction. In the presence of diffuse cerebral atrophy, multiple old and new cortical infarcts are seen on CT scan and MRI, with none involving an entire vascular territory.

Single Photon Emission Computed Tomography And Positron Emission Tomography

Either SPECT or PET imaging is performed on occasion, especially when the evolution of vascular dementia is subtle and can simulate AD. This disease entity exists as a spectrum of imaging abnormalities, which, in its most severe form, results in subcortical hyperintensities characteristic of Binswanger microangiopathic leukoencephalopathy (Drayer, 1988). A relative sparing is seen of the subcortical arcuate fibers in the peripheral white matter and also associated lacunar infarctions in the basal ganglia, thalamus, and pons. Lastly, abnormally decreased signal intensity is seen in the putamen secondary to iron deposition.

Multiinfarct Dementia

In MID, SPECT or FDG-PET imaging demonstrates multiple scattered areas of hypoperfusion or hypometabolism throughout the brain (both gray and white matter) corresponding to areas of infarctions seen on CT or MR (Benson et al., 1983; Duara et al., 1989). Often, involvement is seen of the sensory-motor cortex, which is almost invariably spared in AD.

Binswanger's Disease

Computed Tomography and Magnetic Resonance Imaging

Binswanger disease is characterized by severe, bilaterally symmetric, confluent regions of increased

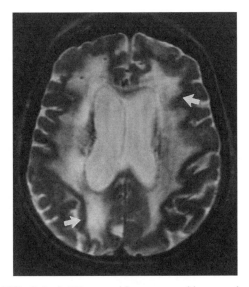

FIG. 2-4. A 75-year-old woman with vascular dementia. Axial T₂-weighted magnetic resonance imaging demonstrates marked, confluent hyperintensity in the periventricular white matter bilaterally that extends subcortically (*arrows*).

signal intensity in the cerebral white matter as seen on long T2-weighted images (Fig. 2-4). The presence of a marked degree of periventricular white matter lucency or hyperintensity is thought to be secondary to athero- and arteriosclerosis of the cerebral vessels. In addition, small infarcts are seen in the basal ganglia and thalamus. The corpus callosum is not involved and the cerebral cortex is preserved in contradistinction to MID.

Magnetic Resonance Spectroscopy

The spectroscopic signature has not been characterized, but a decrease in NAA and mI would be expected.

Single Photon Emission Computed Tomography and Positron Emission Tomography

Patient's with Binswanger's disease (or chronic progressive subcortical encephalopathy) have been found to have decreased rCBF and regional cerebral metabolism rate for oxygen on PET in the white matter and in the frontal, temporal, and parietal cortices, despite normal CT or MRI scans (Yao et al., 1990; Babikian, 1987). The occipital cortex and striatum are less affected. It is suggested that the decrease in rCBF and regional cerebral metabolic rate for oxygen

(rCMRO2) in the white matter is caused by the primarily damage sites from ischemia, whereas similar decreases in the cortex likely represent disconnection between cortical and subcortical structures. Benson et al. (1983) suggested that PET scanning could distinguish between AD and MID because in AD the primary motor and sensory cortex are spared, whereas in MID multifocal, asymmetric irregular areas of hypometabolism are seen.

Vascular Dementia

Vascular diseases of the brain (e.g., stroke) can be of varying severity and result in derangement of higher mental function. Vascular dementia can be regarded as a syndrome of various cerebrovascular diseases, which are heterogeneous in both morphology and clinical manifestations (Kalashnikova et al., 1999). Dementia can result from single infarcts that are located in strategically important areas of the brain.

Imaging Studies

A *CT* scan of the brain reveals small hypodensities, although MRI is more sensitive to ischemic lesions because of its better contrast discrimination (Larson, *1999). MRI* shows hyperintense foci on long T2-weighted images in the corresponding regions of the *brain. MRS* shows elevation in lactate and decrease in NAA. *SPECT* demonstrates reductions in perfusion in the frontal lobe of the brain on the side of small infarcts in the dorsomedial part of the optic region and lower parts of the internal capsule. (Kalashnikova et al., 1999). *PET* demonstrates ipsilateral reductions in hemisphere metabolism, especially in the frontal lobe in patients with single small infarcts in the optic region.

Frontal Dementia

The appearance of frontal dementia includes severe frontal atrophy evident as wide separation of the hemispheres on imaging. A pronounced reduction is seen in cortical flow and metabolism in the frontal regions compared with the posterior temporoparietal—areas best evident on the sagittal sections, clearly differing from the pattern of AD (Neary et al., 1988; Jagust et al., 1989).

Pick's Disease

The neuropathologic markers for Pick's disease are Pick bodies, which are round cytoplasmic inclusions

(Osborne, 1994). Pick's disease is a neurodegenerative dementia with a predilection for the frontal and temporal lobes where Pick bodies are seen on histopathologic examination.

Computed Tomography and Magnetic Resonance Imaging

Frontal and temporal lobe atrophy is seen on CT scan and MRI. The parietal and occipital lobes are commonly spared. Osborne described the changes seen on MRI as markedly shrunken gyri, which have a knifelike appearance (Osborne, 1994).

Magnetic Resonance Spectrography

With the spectra taken in the frontal lobes, MRS shows a marked reduction in NAA (by as much as 30%), indicating neuronal loss, an increase in mI, and the presence of lactate. In contrast, in AD, with the spectra collected in the frontal lobes, no lactate is present and the NAA is not reduced to the same degree as seen in Pick's disease. However, an increase is seen in mI as seen in patients with Pick's disease (Ross et al., 1998).

Single Photon Emission Computed Tomography and Positron Emission Tomography

The most common finding on HMPAO-SPECT and FDG-PET images is hypoperfusion and hypometabolism, respectively, in the frontal and anterior temporal lobes bilaterally (Bonte et al., 1993; Kamo et al., 1987; Salmon et al., 1988). This pattern of anterior hypometabolism is consistent with the findings on histopathologic examination. Although the pattern of anterior hypoperfusion or hypometabolism is easily distinguishable from that of AD, it is not characteristic of any particular entity. Various disorders, including multiple system atrophy, PSP, nonspecific frontal gliosis, adult polyglucosan body disease (a storage disorder), neurosyphilis, and chronic alcohol-related dementia, can all demonstrate a similar pattern (Bonte et al., 1993).

Parkinson's Disease

Parkinson's disease (PD) is an affliction of the dopamine system, centered in the basal ganglia. The neuropathologic marker of PD is loss of the neuromilin-containing neurons in the substantia nigra, the locus ceruleus, and the dorsal vagal nucleus (Osborne, 1994). Approximately 25% of patients with PD have more severe symptoms and respond poorly to dopamine replacement; these are then grouped into the plus syndromes. This group of disorders includes Shy-Drager (SD) PSP, and olivopontocerebellar degeneration (OPCD).

Computed Tomography

In general, CT imaging has not been helpful in the differential diagnosis of PD, except it can exclude other causes of dementia (e.g., normal pressure hydrocephalus or subcortical arteriosclerotic encephalopathy) (Paulus and Trenkwalder, 1998). Imaging studies are nonspecific, showing generalized atrophy with large, supratentorial sulci and posterior fossa cisterns (Osborne, 1994).

Magnetic Resonance Imaging

Patients with SD syndrome can demonstrate low signal in the putamen as seen on T_2-weighted images. PSP is characterized by midbrain and tectal atrophy. OPCD typically reveals atrophy of the pons and cerebellum, with a bright signal seen in the transverse pontine fibers and brachium pontis (the tiger sign) as seen on T_2-weighted images.

Magnetic Resonance Spectrography

Currently, MRS has not been useful in diagnosing PD or its plus syndromes. However, severe dementia in PD can be indistinguishable from AD on PET images, both showing significant bilateral parietal hypometabolism (Rougemont et al., 1984; Peppard et al., 1990). Patients with PD and dementia differed from those without dementia in that the former had hypometabolic perirolandic and angular gyrus regions (Peppard et al., 1990).

However, patients with PD and dementia did not have significantly different CMRGIc values than patients with AD, indicating that patients with PD and dementia may suffer from an underlying Alzheimer's-type process. In fact, histopathologic studies have shown findings of true AD, in conjunction with those of Parkinsonism.

Huntington's Disease (HD)

Computed Tomography and Magnetic Resonance Imaging

CT scans and MRI often show no changes early in the course of Huntington's disease and reveal atrophy of the head of the caudate and frontal cortex in the later stages of the disease (Simmons et al., 1986; Starkstein et al., 1989). PET studies have consistently revealed hypometabolism in the caudate and the putamen nuclei, which often precedes the atrophy seen on CT or MRI (Phelps et al., 1985; Kuwert et al., 1989; Kuhl et al., 1982). It has been postulated that cortical changes in glucose metabolism, especially in the frontoparietal and temporooccipital areas, may correlate with the severity of dementia in patients with Huntington's disease (Kuwert et al., 1990).

Normal Pressure Hydrocephalus

Normal pressure hydrocephalus (NPH), a chronic communicating hydrocephalus, is a clinical condition associated with the triad of dementia, incontinence, and ataxia in conjunction with enlarged ventricles and normal CSF pressure (Peterson et al., 1985).

Computed Tomography and Magnetic Resonance Imaging

CT scans and MRI often demonstrate ventricular enlargement that is out of proportion to the degree of sulcal enlargement, possibly with a prominent flow void at the level of the third ventricle, aqueduct of Sylvius, or both (Fig. 2-5). Some investigators suggest CSF flow patterns and velocity are important, not only in diagnosing this disease, but in predicting the results of surgical intervention. White matter lucency might be seen on CT scans and marked hyperintensity on the MRI T_2-weighted images.

Single Photon Emission Computed Tomography and Positron Emission Tomography

Questionable cases of NPH could be evaluated with radionuclide cisternogram, which is performed using a lumbar intrathecal injection of 111In-DTPA (Datz et al., 1992). Head imaging is performed at 4, 24, and 48 hours in the anterior, left lateral, and posterior projections. In normal adults, tracer activity enters the basal cisterns and extends into the interhemispheric and sylvian fissures by 3 to 4 hours, with subsequent activity over the convexities by 24 hours.

Normally, no reflux of activity occurs into the lateral ventricles. The "classic" diagnostic finding of NPH is early entry of pharmaceutical into the lateral ventricles, which persists at 24 and 48 hours with impairment of flow over the convexities of the brain (Bannister et al., 1967; Patten and Benson, 1968). The procedure helps in the diagnosis of NPH, but it cannot predict which patients would benefit from diversionary ventriculoperitoneal (VP) surgery (James et al., 1972). Later investigations have proved this pattern is not specific and results in several false-positive findings, with no improved outcome from VP shunting (Greenberg et al., 1977).

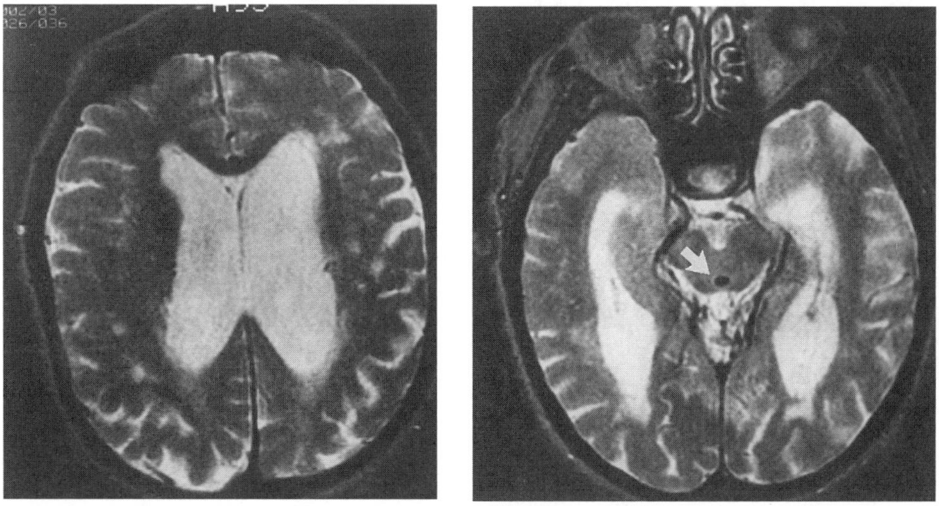

FIG. 2-5. A. A 74-year-old man with normal pressure hydrocephalus. Axial T_2-weighted magnetic resonance imaging (MRI) demonstrates marked widening of the lateral ventricles, out of proportion to the sulcal widening. **B.** Axial T_2-weighted MRI demonstrates widening of the temporal horns out of proportion to the sulcal widening of the temporal lobes. A prominent flow void from cerebrospinal fluid pulsation is seen within the aqueduct (*arrow*).

Brain Tumors

Brain tumors, a rare cause of dementia, account for 1% to 4% of cases. Most brain tumors are either metastatic or malignant primary tumors (Foster et al., 1999) (Fig. 2-6).

Computed Tomography

With noncontrast CT, a region of white matter hypodensity is seen representing vasogenic edema caused by the tumor. With the administration of intravenous contrast, the neoplasm will be identified.

Magnetic Resonance Imaging

MRI allows for more complete evaluation of the size of the lesion and the extent of the vasogenic edema. Mass effect, midline shift, and possibly other small lesions can also be identified to aid in the differentiation between primary and metastatic neoplasm.

Magnetic Resonance Spectroscopy

The spectroscopic signature of tumor is elevation of Cho and the presence of lipid, both equating with

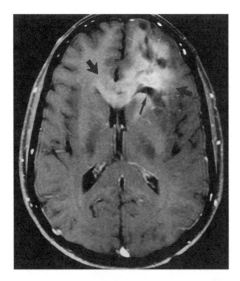

FIG. 2-6. A 45-year-old man with a mixed oligoastrocytoma. Axial postcontrast T₁-weighted magnetic resonance imaging demonstrates a heterogeneously enhancing lesion within the left frontal lobe crossing the corpus callosum (*large arrows*). Note some of the markedly hypointense signal represented calcification (*small arrow*).

cell membrane turnover, and a reduction in the NAA, which represents neuronal death.

Single Photon Emission Computed Tomography and Positron Emission Tomography

Thallium-201 (201Tl) SPECT and FDG-PET are not used for primary diagnosis of brain neoplasms. Their main role is to help in the differentiation of low-grade (1 and 2) from high-grade (3 and 4) gliomas and thereby determine the prognosis in these patients. A thallium SPECT and FDG-PET index have often been used to distinguish low- from high-grade gliomas. The index compares tumor uptake normalized to the homologous contralateral hemisphere and corrected for tissue attenuation. With 201Tl, a threshold index of 1.5 helps distinguish low- versus high-grade gliomas with an accuracy of 89%, with high-grade gliomas showing greater values (Kim et al., 1990; Black et al., 1989). The studies had also noted that low-grade gliomas with an index higher than 1.5 acted biologically more like high-grade tumors with decreased median patient survival time (Black et al., 1989). Similarly, with FDG-PET, a tumor-to-white matter ratio of more than 1.5 was indicative of a high-grade tumor, with a sensitivity and specificity of 94% and 77%, respectively (Delbeke et al., 1995).

Tumor Versus Radiation Necrosis

Conventional imaging techniques, including CT and MRI, are often unreliable in distinguishing between recurrent glioma and radiation necrosis in patients who are symptomatic after high-dose radiotherapy. It is well known that therapeutic doses of radiation can produce necrosis of the irradiated brain. The associated clinical syndrome is usually one of worsening of the already existing neurologic signs and symptoms. Both 201Tl SPECT and FDG-PET have been shown to be effective in differentiating glioma from radiation necrosis (Schwartz et al., 1992; Patronas et al., 1982). Regions of increased thallium uptake (i.e., greater than the scalp uptake) suggests active tumor, whereas regions of low to no uptake is suggestive of radiation necrosis.

Ample evidence indicates that radiation affects the glucose metabolism of tumor cells in tissue cultures. More specifically, it has been shown that glycolysis of tumor cells is severely reduced by radiation. Thus, using the PET technique, areas of radiation necrosis, where the rate of glucose utilization is markedly reduced compared with normal brain parenchyma, can be distinguished from tumor areas, where the rate of

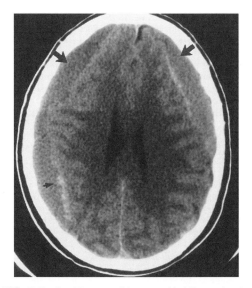

FIG. 2-7. An 80-year-old man with bilateral subdural hematomas. Axial noncontrast computed tomography imaging demonstrates bilateral iso-hypodense subdural hematomas (*large arrows*) resulting in no significant midline shift. The hyperdense component represents more recent hemorrhage (*small arrow*).

glucose utilization will be increased in comparison with normal brain parenchyma.

Subdural Hematomas

Computed Tomography

On CT scan, an acute subdural hematoma is crescentic and hyperdense and will often span the convexity. Chronic subdurals will become more like CSF density and may become more difficult to diagnose (Fig. 2-7).

Magnetic Resonance Imaging

On MRI, the chronic subdural hematoma is often loculated and of a mixed signal intensity, differing from CSF. Nuclear medicine scans are not typically done to diagnose subdural hematoma.

CONCLUSION

Subdural hematomas, brain tumors, and infarcts are typically not diagnostic dilemmas when imaging the demented patient. However, distinguishing between the various conditions that result in widening of the CSF spaces, because of normal aging, pathologic atrophy, or hydrocephalus, can often be challenging. A few key imaging features are helpful. Whereas normal aging and Parkinson's disease result in generalized atrophy, other diseases lead to more focal volume loss. AD results in atrophy of the MTLs (including the amygdala and hippocampus), Pick's disease the frontal and temporal lobes, and Huntington's disease the caudate, putamen, and frontal cortex. Further evaluation with physiologic studies (e.g., SPECT and PET) may be necessary. In normal pressure hydrocephalus, the widened CSF spaces are not caused by atrophy, but by obstruction that leads to diffuse widening of the ventricular system, out of proportion to the sulci.

Imaging can be helpful in diagnosing numerous diseases in the geriatric patient. Structural and physiological imaging, as well as spectroscopy, has specific functions. The main role of imaging, however, is to determine if a surgically correctable, structural lesion is present.

REFERENCES

Alavi A, Hirsch LJ. Studies of central nervous system disorders with single photon emission computed tomography and positron emission tomography. Evolution over the past 2 decades. *Semin Nucl Med* 1991;21:58–81.

Awad IA, Johnson PC, Spetzler RF, et al. Incidental subcortical lesions identified on magnetic resonance imaging in the elderly. II. Postmortem pathological correlations. *Stroke* 1986;17(6):1090–1097.

Babikian V, Ropper A. Binswanger disease. A review. *Stroke* 1987;18:2–12.

Ball MJ. Neuronal loss, neurofibrillary tangles and granulovacuolar degeneration in the hippocampus with aging and dementia. *Acta Neuropathol (Berl)* 1997;111:27.

Bannister R, Gilford E, Kocen R. Isotope encephalography in the diagnosis of dementia due to communicating hydrocephalus. *Lancet* 1967;2:1014–1017.

Benson DF, Kuhl DE, Hawkins RA, et al. The fluorodeoxyglucose 18F scan in Alzheimer's disease and multiinfarct dementia. *Arch Neurol* 1983;40:711–714.

Black KL, Hawkins RA, Kim KT, et al. Use of thallium-201 SPECT to quantitate malignancy grade of gliomas. *J Neurosurg*1989;71:342–346.

Bonte FJ, Hom J, Tinter R, et al. Single photon tomography in Alzheimer's disease and the dementias. *Semin Nucl Med* 1990;20:342–352.

Bonte FJ, Ross ED, Chehabi HH, et al. SPECT study of regional cerebral blood flow in Alzheimer's disease. *J Comput Assist Tomogr* 1986;10:579–583.

Bonte FJ, Tintner R, Weiner MF, et al. Brain blood flow in the dementias: SPECT with histopathologic correlation. *Radiology* 1993;186:361–365.

Bradley WG, Waluch V, Brant-Zawadzki M, et al. Patchy, periventricular white matter lesions in the elderly: a common observation during NMR imaging. *Noninvasive Medical Imaging* 1984;1(1):35–41.

Brody H. Organization of cerebral cortex. Study of aging in human cortex. *J Comput Neurol* 1955;102:511–556.

Cala LA, Thickbroom GW, Black JL, et al. Brain density and cerebrospinal fluid space size: CT of normal volunteers. *AJNR* 1982;2:41–47.

Chawluk JB, Alavi A, Dann R, et al. Positron emission tomography in aging and dementia: effect of cerebral atrophy. *J Nucl Med* 1987;28:431–437.

Claus JJ, Harskamp VF, Bretler MMB, et al. The diagnostic value of SPECT with Tc-99m HMPAO in Alzheimer's disease: a population-based study. *Neurology* 1994;44:454–461.

Critchley M. Neurologic changes in the aged. *J Chronic Dis* 1956;3:459.

Cuenod CA, Denys A, Michot JL, et al. Amygdala atrophy in Alzheimer's disease. An in vivo magnetic resonance imaging study. *Arch Neurol* 1993;50:941–945.

Datz FL, Patch CG, Arias JM, et al., eds. *Nuclear medicine: a teaching file*. St. Louis: CV Mosby, 1992:240–243.

Delbeke D, Meyerowitz C, Lapidus RL, et al. Optimal cutoff levels of F-18 fluorodeoxyglucose uptake in the differentiation of low-grade from high-grade brain tumors with PET. *Radiology* 1995;195:47–52.

Diksic M, Reba RC, eds. *Radiopharmaceuticals and brain pathology studied with PET and SPECT*. Boca Raton: CRC Press, 1991.

Drayer B, Burger P, Darwin R, et al. Magnetic resonance imaging of brain iron. *AJNR* 1986;7:373–380.

Drayer B. Imaging of the aging brain. Part II: Pathologic conditions. *Radiology* 1988;166:797–806.

Drayer B. Imaging of the aging brain. Part I: Normal findings. *Radiology* 1988;166:785–796.

Duara R, Barker W, Loewenstein D, et al. Sensitivity and specificity of positron emission tomography and magnetic resonance imaging studies in Alzheimer's disease and multi-infarct dementia. *Eur Neurol* 1989;29:9–15.

Duara R, Grady C, Haxby J, et al. Positron emission tomography in Alzheimer's disease. *Neurology* 1986;36:879–887.

Durand-Fardel M. *Traite du ramollissement du cerveau*. Paris: Bailliere, 1843.

Foster G, Scott D, Payne S. The use of CT scanning in dementia. A systematic review. *Int J Technol Assess Health Care* 1999;15(2):406–425.

Frackowiak R, Poizilli C, Legg N, et al. Regional cerebral oxygen supply and utilization in dementia. A clinical and physiologic study with oxygen-15 and positron emission tomography. *Brain* 1981;104:753–788.

Friedland RP, Prusiner SB, Jagust WJ, et al. Bitemporal hypometabolism in Creutzfeldt-Jakob disease measured by positron emission tomography with 18F-2-fluorodeoxyglucose. *J Comput Assist Tomogr* 1984;8:978–981.

Friedland RP. "Normal"-pressure hydrocephalus and the saga of treatable dementia. *JAMA* 1989;262:2577–2581.

Friedland RP. Positron emission tomography in dementia. *Semin Neurol* 1989;9:338–344.

Greenberg JO, Shenkin HA, Adam R. Idiopathic normal pressure hydrocephalus—a report of 73 patients. *J Neurol Neurosurgery Psychiatry* 1977;40:336–341.

Holman BL, Johnson KA, Gerada B, et al. The scintigraphic appearance of Alzheimer's disease: a prospective study using technitium-99m-HMPAO SPECT. *J Nucl Med* 1992;33:181–185.

Jagust WJ, Budinger TF, Reed BR. The diagnosis of dementia with single photon emission computed tomography. *Arch Neurol* 1987;44:258–262.

Jagust WJ, Reed BR, Seab JP, et al. Clinical-physiological correlates of Alzheimer's disease and frontal lobe dementia. *Am J Physiol Imaging* 1989;4:89–96.

James AE, DeBlanc HJ, DeLand FH, et al. Refinements in cerebrospinal fluid diversionary shunt evaluation by cisternography. *AJR* 1972;115:766–773.

Jamieson DG, Chawluck JB, Alavi A, et al. The effect of disease severity on local cerebral glucose metabolism in Alzheimer's disease. *J Cereb Blood Flow Metab* 1987;7:S410.

Kalashnikova, LA, Gulevskaya TS, Kashina EM. Disorders of higher mental function due to single infarctions in the thalamus and in the area of the thalamofrontal tracts. *Neurosci Behav Physiol* 1999;29(4):397–403.

Kamo H, Mcgeer R, Haroop R, et al. Positron emission tomography and histopathology in Pick's disease. *Neurology* 1987;37:439.

Kido DK, LeMay M, Levinson AW, et al. Computed tomographic localization of the precentral gyrus. *Radiology* 1980;135:373–377.

Kim KT, Black KL, Marciano D, et al. Thallium-201 SPECT imaging of brain tumors: methods and results. *J Nucl Med* 1990;31:965–969.

Kuhl DE, Metter EJ, Reiger WH, et al. Effects of human aging on patterns of local cerebral glucose utilization determined by the 18-F fluorodeoxyglucose method. *J Cereb Blood Flow Metab* 1987;7:411.

Kuhl DE, Phelps ME, Markham CH, et al. Cerebral metabolism and atrophy in Huntington's disease determined by 18-F-FDG and computed tomography scan. *Ann Neurol* 1982;12:425–434.

Kushner M, Tobin M, Alavi A, et al. Cerebral glucose consumption in normal and pathological states using fluorine-FDG and PET. *J Nucl Med* 1987;28:1667–1670.

Kuwabara Y, Ichiya Y, Otuska M, et al. Differential diagnosis of bilateral parietal abnormalities in I-123 IMP SPECT imaging. *Clin Nucl Med* 1990;15:893–899.

Kuwert T, Lange HW, Langen KJ, et al. Cortical and subcortical consumption measured by PET in patients with Huntington's disease. *Brain* 1990;113:1405–1423.

Kuwert T, Lange HW, Langin KJ, et al. Cerebral glucose consumption measured by PET in patients with and without psychiatric symptoms of Huntington's disease. *Psychiatry Res* 1989;29:361–362.

Larson EB. Must dementia remain a silent epidemic? [Review] *Hosp Pract* (off ED) 1999;34(11):137–141.

Larson EB, Reifler BV, Sumi SM, et al. Diagnostic tests in the evaluation of dementia: a prospective study of 200 elderly outpatients. *Arch Intern Med* 1986;146:1917–1922.

Lazeyras F, Charles HC, Tupler LA, et al. Metabolic brain mapping in Alzheimer's disease using proton magnetic resonance spectroscopy. *Psychiatry Res* 1998;82:95–106.

LeMay M. Radiologic changes of the aging brain and skull. [Review] *AJR* 1984;143(2):383–389.

Messa C, Perani D, Luciganani G, et al. High-resolution technitiun-99m-HMPAO SPECT in patients with probable Alzheimer's disease: comparison with fluorine-18-FDG PET. *J Nucl Med* 1994;35:210–216.

Miller BL, Cummings JL, Villaneuva-Meyer J, et al. Frontal lobe degeneration: clinical, neuropsychological, and SPECT characteristics. *Neurology* 1991;41:1374–1382.

Neary D, Snowden JS, Northen B, et al. Dementia of the frontal lobe type. *J Neurol Neurosurg Psychiatry* 1988;51:353–361.

O'Brien JT, Metcalfe S, Swann A, et al. Medial temporal lobe width on CT scanning in Alzheimer's disease: comparison with vascular dementia, depression and dementia with Lewy bodies. *Dement Geriatr Cogn Disord* 2000;11:114–118.

Osborn A. *Diagnostic neuroradiology*. Philadelphia: Mosby, 1994.

Patronas NJ, Chiro GD, Brooks RA, et al. Work in progress: fluorodeoxyglucose and positron emission tomography in the evaluation of radiation necrosis of the brain. *Radiology* 1982;144:885–889.

Patten DH, Benson DF. Diagnosis of normal-pressure hydrocephalus by RISA cisternography. *J Nucl Med* 1968; 9:457–461.

Paulus W, Trenkwalder C. Imaging of nonmotor symptoms in Parkinson syndromes. *Clin Neurosci* 1998;5:115–120.

Peppard RF, Martin WF, Clark CM, et al. Cortical glucose metabolism in Parkinson's and Alzheimer's disease. *J Neurosci Res* 1990;27:561–568.

Perani D, DiPiero V, Vallar G, et al. Technetium-99m-HM-PAO SPECT study of regional cerebral perfusion in early Alzheimer's disease. *J Nucl Med* 1988;29:1507–1514.

Peterson RC, Modri B, Laws E. Surgical treatment of idiopathic hydrocephalus in elderly patients. *Neurology* 1985; 35:307–311.

Phelps ME, Mazziota JC, Wapenski J, et al. Cerebral glucose utilization and blood flow in Huntington's disease. *J Nucl Med* 1985;26:47.

Ross BD, Bluml S, Cowan R, et al. In vivo MR spectroscopy of human dementia. *Neuroimaging Clin N Am* 1998;8(4): 809–822.

Rougemont D, Baron JC, Collard P, et al. Local cerebral glucose utilization in treated and untreated patients with Parkinson's disease. *J Neurol Neurosurg Psychiatry* 1984; 47:824–830.

Salmon E, Maquet P, Sadzot B, et al. Positron emission tomography in Alzheimer's and Pick's disease. *J Neurol* 1988;235:S1.

Scheltens P. Early Diagnosis of dementia: Neuroimaging. *J Neurol* 246: 16–20 1999.

Schwartz RB, Carvalho PA, Alexander E, et al. Radiation necrosis vs high-grade recurrent glioma: differentiation by using dual-isotope SPECT with ^{201}Tl and ^{99m}Tc-HM-PAO. *AJNR* 1992;12:1187–1192.

Simmons JT, Pastakea B, Chase TN, et al. Magnetic resonance imaging in Huntington's disease. *Am J Neuroradiol* 1986;7:25–28.

Starkstein SE, Folstein SE, Brandt J, et al. Brain atrophy in Huntington's disease. A CT-scan study. *Neuroradiology* 1989;31:156–159.

Tanna NK, Kohn MI, Horwich DN, et al. Analysis of brain and cerebrospinal fluid volumes with MR imaging. Impact on PET data, correction for atrophy. *Radiology* 1991; 178:123–130.

Testa HJ, Snowden JS, Neary D, et al. The use of Tc-99m HMPAO in the diagnosis of primary degenerative dementia. *J Cereb Blood Flow Metab* 1988;8:S123–S126.

Tierney MC, Gisher RH, Lewis AJ, et al. The NINCDS-ADRDA Workgroup criteria for the clinical diagnosis of probable Alzheimer's disease. A clinical pathological study of 57 cases. *Neurology* 1988;38:359–364.

Tomlinson BE, Blessed G, Roth M. Observations on the brains of non-demented old people. *J Neurol Sci* 1968; 7(2):331–356.

Valentine AR, Moseley IF, Kendall BE. White matter abnormality in cerebral atrophy: clinicoradiological correlations. *J Neurol Neurosurg Psychiatry* 1980;43: 139–142.

Yao H, Sadoshima S, Kuwabara Y, et al. Cerebral blood flow and oxygen metabolism in patients with vascular dementia of the Binswanger type. *Stroke* 1990;21:1694–1699.

Yoshii F, Barker WW, Chang JY, et al. Sensitivity of cerebral glucose metabolism to age, gender, brain volume, brain atrophy, and cerebrovascular risk factors. *J Cereb Blood Flow Metab* 1988;8:654–661.

SUGGESTED READING

Banna M. The ventriculo-cephalic ratio on computed tomography. *Can Assoc Radiol J* 1977;28:208–210.

Bottino C, Almeida O. Can neuroimaging techniques identify individuals at risk of developing Alzheimer's disease? *Int Psychogeriatr* 1997;9(4):389–403.

Brinkman SD, Sarwar M, Levin H, et al. Quantitative indexes of computed tomography in dementia and normal aging. *Radiology* 1981;138:89–92.

Chase TN, Fedio P, Foster NL, et al. Wescher adult intelligence scale performance. *Arch Neurol* 1984;16:649–654.

Cutler NR, Haxby J, Duara R, et al. Clinical history, brain metabolism, and neurophysiological function in Alzheimer's disease. *Ann Neurol* 1985;18:298–309.

De Leon MJ, George AE, Golomb J, et al. Frequency of hippocampal formation atrophy in normal aging and Alzheimer's disease. *Neurobiol Aging* 1997;18(1):1–11.

Erkinjunitti T, Bowler J, DeCarli C. Imaging of static brain lesions in vascular dementia: implications for clinical trials. *Alzheimer Dis Assoc Disord* 1999;13(Suppl 3): 581–590.

Faulstich ME. Brain imaging in dementia of the Alzheimer type. *Int J Neurosci* 1991;57:39–49.

Fayad PB, Brass LM. Single photon emission computed tomography in cerebrovascular disease. *Stroke* 1991;22: 950–954.

Fieschi C, Argentino C, Lenzi GL, et al. Clinical and instrumental evaluation of patients with ischemic stroke during the first six hours. *J Neurol Neurosurg Psychiatry* 1989; 91:311–322.

Foster NL, Chase TN, Mansi L, et al. Cortical abnormalities in Alzheimer's disease. *Ann Neurol* 1984;16:649–654.

Foundas A, Zipin D, Browning C. Age-related changes of the insular cortex and lateral ventricles: conventional MRI volumetric measures. *J Neuroimaging* 1998;8(4):216–221.

Friedland RP, Budinger TF, Ganz E, et al. Regional cerebral metabolism in dementia of the Alzheimer's type. Positron emission tomography with (18F) fluorodeoxyglucose. *J Comput Assist Tomogr* 1983;7:590–598.

Gawler J, duBoulay GH, Bull JHD, et al. Computerized tomography: a comparison with pneumoencephalography and ventriculography. *J Neurol Neurosurg Psychiatry* 1976;39:203–211.

Golomb J, Kluger A, deLeon M, et al. Hippocampal formation size in normal human aging: a correlate of delayed secondary memory performance. *Learning and Memory* 1994;1:45–54.

Granado JM, Diaz F, Alday R. Evaluation of brain SPECT in the diagnosis and prognosis of normal pressure hydrocephalus syndrome. *Acta Neurochir* 1991;112:88–91.

Hahn FJY, Rim K. Frontal ventricular dimensions on normal computed tomography. *AJR* 1976;126:492–496.

Hanyu H, Imon Y, Sakurai H, et al. Regional differences in diffusion abnormality in cerebral white matter lesions in patients with vascular dementia of the Binswanger type and Alzheimer's disease. *Eur J Neurol* 1999;6:195–203.

Haug G. Age and sex dependence of the size of normal ventricles on computed tomography. *Neuroradiology* 1977; 14:201–204.

Haxby JC, Grady CL, Koss E, et al. Heterogeneous anterior-posterior metabolic patterns in dementia of the Alzheimer's disease. *Neurology* 1988;38:1853–1863.

Hilker R, Thiel A, Geisen C, et al. Cerebral blood flow and glucose metabolism in multi-infarct-dementia related to primary antiphospholipid antibody syndrome. *Lupus* 2000;9:311–316.

Jelic V, Nordberg A. Early diagnosis of Alzheimer disease with positron emission tomography. *Alzheimer Dis Assoc Disord* 2000;14(Suppl 1):S109–S113.

Jobst KA, Hindley NJ, King E, et al. The diagnosis of Alzheimer's disease: a question of image? *J Clin Psychiatry* 1994;55(Suppl 11):22–31.

Katzman R, Saitoh T. Advances in Alzheimer's disease. *FASEB J* 1991;5:278–286.

Khujneri R, DeSousa JA. Magnetic resonance imaging of the ageing brain. *East Afr Med J* 1997;October: 656–659.

Kinkel WR, Jacobs L, Polachini I, et al. Subcortical arteriosclerotic encephalopathy (Binswanger's disease). Computed tomographic, nuclear magnetic resonance, and clinical correlations. *Arch Neurol* 1985;42:951–959.

Larseen A, Moonen M, Bergh AC, et al. Predictive value of quantitative cisternography in normal pressure hydrocephalus. *Acta Neurol Scand* 1990;81:327–332.

Mann DMA, South PW. The topographic distribution of brain atrophy in frontal lobe dementia. *Acta Neuropathol* 1993;85:334–340.

Moretti J, Defer G, Sinotti L, et al. "Luxury perfusion" with [Tc99m] HMPAO and [I-123] IMPSPECT imaging during the subacute phase of stroke. *Eur J Nucl Med* 1990; 16:17–22.

Nagy ZS, Hindley NJ, Braak H, et al. The progression of Alzheimer's disease from limbic regions to the neocortex: clinical, radiological and pathological relationships. *Dement Geriatr Cogn Disord* 1999;10:115–120.

Pantono P, Baron JC, Samson Y, et al. Crossed cerebellar diaschisis. Further studies. *Brain* 1986;109:677–694.

Rhinehart DL, Cox LA, Long BW. MR spectroscopy of Alzheimer disease. *Radiol Technol* 1998;70(1):23–28.

Sandson TA, Daffner KR, Carvalho PA, et al. Frontal lobe dysfunction following infarction of the left-sided medial thalamus. *Arch Neurol* 1991;48:1300–1303.

Terry RD, Katzman R. Senile dementia of the Alzheimer type. *Ann Neurol* 1983;14(5):497–506.

Van Gijn J. Leukoaraiosis and vascular dementia. *Neurology* 1998;51(3 Suppl 3):S3–S8.

Vermersch P, Leys D, Pruvo JP, et al. Parkinson's disease and basal ganglia calcifications: prevalence and clinico-radiological correlations. *Clin Neurol Neurosurg* 1992;94: 213–217.

2.2

Diagnostic Tests in the Older Adult: EEG

Ivo Drury

Electroencephalography (EEG) is a technique that measures temporal changes in summated postsynaptic potentials from the superficial layers of the cerebral cortex. Currently, EEG is used principally in two major areas of clinical practice: seizure disorders and alterations in mental status. Technicians record EEGs and physicians interpret them. Interpretation is usually performed after the study is completed; in emergency situations, however, the EEG should be viewed while it is being recorded. The technician places a series of electrodes in symmetric locations over the scalp and connects them to a specialized recording device. Typically, a routine EEG recording takes 30 minutes. While the EEG is being recorded, the technologist documents the patient's behavioral state (i.e., awake, drowsy, stuporous), asks the patient to perform certain tasks to judge his or her level of alertness, has the patient open and close his or her eyes,

and performs activation procedures such as hyperventilation and photic stimulation. The technologist observes the patient closely and indicates on the record any alteration in responsiveness, seizurelike activity, or responses to noxious or auditory stimuli. In certain clinical circumstances (e.g., status epilepticus), a physician may administer antiepileptic drugs (AEDs) intravenously during the study. An EEG can also be recorded for a longer duration, either with concurrent video monitoring or in the ambulatory setting, the latter akin to Holter monitoring of cardiac rhythms. Concurrent video-EEG recording allows optimal matching of electrographic and behavioral features and is especially useful where epilepsy is one consideration in a differential diagnosis, or in the workup for epilepsy surgery of a patient with medically refractory partial seizures. Most ambulatory EEG (AEEG) techniques do not allow a concurrent matching of behavior and EEG other than by the patient or family members keeping a log of symptoms that they may experience. It does, however, allow physicians to study patients who may have events happen in home environments or in whom an attempt is being made to document the amount of seizures or interictal EEG activity.

NORMAL ELECTROENCEPHALOGRAM

The appearance of the normal EEG changes from birth through the teenage years, then it remains relatively unchanged until at least age 80 years. The EEG also changes markedly with the behavioral state of the patient. In interpreting EEG studies, it is important to be familiar with changes that may be explained by age and behavioral state. EEG rhythms are divided into four normal-frequency bands: delta (<4 Hz), theta (4 to 7 Hz), alpha (8 to 13 Hz), and beta (>13 Hz). The potentials are small; most scalp-derived EEG activity is between 10 and 100 μV. In the normal awake adult whose eyes are closed, the most prominent background rhythm consists of sinusoidal 30 to 60 μV, 9 to 10 Hz alpha activity over the parietooccipital region that attenuates when the eyes are open. A mixture of faster and slower frequencies predominates over the more anterior head regions and is relatively unaffected by eye opening or closure. In younger children, the rhythms are somewhat slower and less organized. In advanced age (>80 years), some slowing of this dominant posterior rhythm and a greater amount of intermittent, more focal slowing may be seen.

Hyperventilation provokes physiologic slowing of the background rhythm and further intermittent slowing in many normal subjects. These changes are most pronounced in young children and commonly absent in the elderly. Intermittent photic stimulation can evoke a repetitive, time-locked occipital rhythm at the frequency or a harmonic of the frequency of the photic stimulus in normal subjects. Characteristic changes in the EEG background occur in drowsiness, each stage of nonrapid eye movement (NREM) sleep, and REM sleep itself. In many patients with seizures, it is particularly valuable to record the EEG in sleep or after sleep deprivation because abnormal waveforms may be seen more commonly in these recording conditions than in well-rested, awake subjects.

NORMAL EEG CHANGES IN THE ELDERLY

Extensive literature describes normal EEG changes in the elderly. Some variation in what is considered normal exists, chiefly because of the care involved in case selection. Recent studies indicate that truly normal people—even at very advanced years—show remarkably well-formed EEG rhythms.

Dominant Background Frequency

Hubbard et al. (1976) reported EEG findings in 10 centenarians. Seven of the 10 were living in the community and were considered generally healthy. Six of these 7 had a background alpha frequency of 8 Hz or faster. In four separate studies of patients aged 60 to 80 years (Katz and Horowitz, 1982; Torres et al., 1983; Arenas et al., 1986; Giaquinto and Nolfe, 1986), the mean alpha frequency was approximately 9.5 Hz. Thus, it seems clear that to at least age 80 and probably beyond, an alpha frequency of 9 Hz should be the normal finding in healthy subjects (Fig. 2-8).

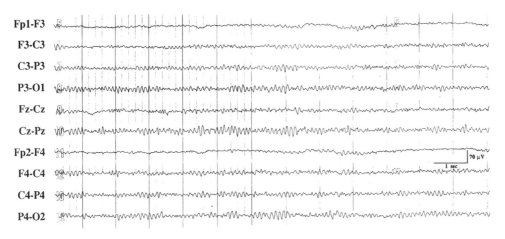

FIG. 2-8. Well-regulated, symmetric 8–9 Hz alpha activity in a normal 89-year-old man.

After age 50, alpha frequency activity may appear in either temporal region, especially the left. It is often higher in voltage than occipital alpha. Fragments can appear as wicket spikes, one of the benign epileptiform variants seen in older adults and the elderly to be discussed later.

Intermittent Focal Slowing

Intermittent focal slowing, especially in the left temporal region (Fig. 2-9), was considered a normal finding from middle life on in early reports (Silverman et al., 1955). However, recent studies in which patients have been rigorously screened suggest that this finding, when present, should be infrequent. Katz and Horowitz (1982) found intermittent focal slowing in 17% of 52 normal septuagenarians, but in no patient did it occupy more than 1% of the total record. Arenas et al. (1986) found slowing in 18 (36%) of 50 subjects. Theta activity was present in all 18 subjects, but delta in only 6 (12%). The combined theta and delta activity occupied less than 1.8% of the total recording in all but one subject. Maximal temporal slowing was left-sided in 72% of these patients. Intermittent slowing was best displayed on the transverse bipolar montage.

Visser et al. (1987) correlated EEG, neuroimaging, and neuropsychologic data in 27 "normal" subjects aged 65 to 83 years (mean 78). They divided patients into those with left frontotemporal slowing and those without. Patients with focal slowing into the delta range showed a statistically significant decrease in performance on tests of verbal fluency and increased

ventricular dilatation on head computed tomography. Therefore, the frequency of intermittent focal slowing and the proportion of the record occupied by the slowing are the most important factors in deciding whether a finding is normal or not.

Substantial variation remains between electroencephalographers in interpretation of this phenomenon. Figure 2-9 is an example of a baseline EEG from a patient 73 years of age with new onset complex partial seizures. It displays a normal phenomenon in the sharply contoured alpha transient seen in the third second in the right temporal region, highlighted with a narrow arrowhead. The abnormal feature of this patient's EEG was the high amplitude, sharply contoured slowing seen over the left temporal region, highlighted with the large arrowhead. At no stage of this patient's record was clear interictal epileptiform activity (IEA) seen.

Changes in Sleep or Drowsiness

Katz and Horowitz (1983) reported the abrupt onset of drowsiness or sleep in healthy normal septuagenarians with frontally dominant rhythmic delta activity of 1 to 4 Hz and 40 to 150 μV for at least 3 seconds at a time. Morphologically, this was indistinguishable from pathologic frontal intermittent rhythmic delta activity. Some changes also occur in sleep features and sleep cycles. K-complexes and spindles of stage II sleep are decreased in amplitude, number, and duration compared with younger adults (Guazelli et al., 1986) and the delta activity of stages III and IV is low in voltage (Katzmann and Terry, 1983). Older

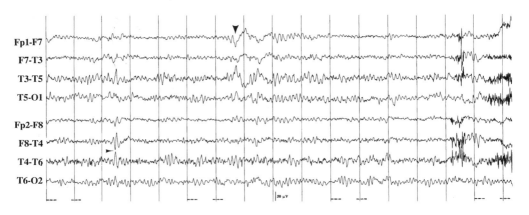

FIG. 2-9. Sharply contoured left temporal slowing (*large arrowhead*) in a 73-year-old patient with new onset of partial seizures. The *narrow arrowhead* points to a higher amplitude alpha wave in the right temporal region (an isolated wicket spike) that is part of the normal background at this age and is not epileptiform.

subjects spend less time in delta sleep compared with younger subjects.

Benign Epileptiform Variants

Two benign variants occur with much greater frequency in middle-aged and older subjects than in younger subjects. Wicket spikes, seen in wakefulness and sleep in adults, consist of monophasic, arciform waves with a temporal emphasis, a predominant frequency of 6 to 8 Hz, and a tendency to recur in brief trains of about 1 second (Fig. 2-10) (Reiher and Lebel, 1977). Although these wicket spikes occur in wakefulness, they are often masked by normal background activities. Occasionally, they appear singly when they retain the morphology of the individual waves in a train. They usually appear in a bilateral, independent fashion, with approximately equal frequency over both hemispheres. Wicket spikes need to be distinguished from anterior or middle temporal focal spikes but have no correlation with epilepsy or any particular symptom complex.

Subclinical rhythmic EEG discharge of adults (SCREDA) (Westmoreland and Klass, 1981) consists of repetitive discharges of abrupt onset and termination without any clinical accompaniment. Typically, it has a bilateral temporoparietal emphasis and occurs primarily in wakefulness in older adults. The most common EEG manifestation is the appearance of bilateral, sharply contoured, monophasic waves of up to 300 milliseconds. A gradual acceleration of frequency usually reaches 4 to 7 Hz before termination, sometimes ending in long-duration, monophasic wave forms again. The average duration is 40 to 80 seconds. SCREDA occurs in patients with diverse clinical complaints and does not have an association with a clinical history of seizures. In some patients, it can be triggered by hyperventilation.

EEG IN THE ELDERLY WITH EPILEPSY

Definition of Interictal and Ictal Activity

IEA encompasses spikes, sharp waves, or spike-wave complexes that are isolated or repeat in brief trains; they are either focal or generalized, and are not associated with an alteration in awareness or behavior.

Ictal activity usually consists of a rhythmic discharge that is distinct from the interictal pattern in at least duration (especially in the generalized epilepsies) but usually also in morphology and topography. An EEG may be diagnostic of a seizure only when a behavioral change occurs in conjunction with an electrical change, but so-called "subclinical" or "electrographic" seizures can occur without observable clinical change.

APPROACH TO EEG ANALYSIS

An orderly approach to the analysis of EEG activity is crucial. EEG analysis must always begin with an assessment of background activities that are judged against the age and behavioral state of the patient.

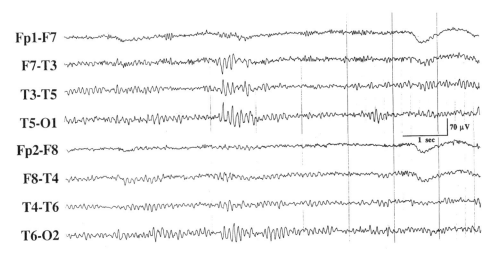

FIG. 2-10. A 1-second train of left temporal wicket spikes from a middle-aged patient without a history of seizures.

Those transients that are potentially epileptiform must satisfy the following criteria: *a*) they are of cerebral and not artifactual origin; *b*) they are abnormal for the age and the state of the patient, recognizing that many features that are normal at one age may be abnormal at another; *c*) they have a significant epileptiform character (i.e., they are not one of the benign epileptiform variants).

Interictal EEG

Although EEG findings in the appropriate clinical setting can be extremely useful in establishing the diagnosis in a patient with seizures, the test has inherent limitations. Some normal members of the population can have abnormal EEGs and, certainly, some patients with epilepsy have repeatedly normal studies. Of 1,824 EEG records from 308 patients with a reasonably certain diagnosis of epilepsy (average six records per patient), 30% had consistently "positive" EEG, 52% had some "positive" and some "negative" studies, and 17.5% had consistently "negative" EEG. Only 8% of 79 patients with a follow-up of at least 1 year had consistently "negative" EEG. "Positive" findings in the first examination were obtained in 55.5% of the patients. Generally, the type of seizure disorder was unrelated to "positivity" or "negativity" of the records. The only exception was a group of patients with partial complex seizures of temporal lobe origin in whom only 2% had exclusively "negative" records (Ajmone-Marson and Zivin, 1970).

A clear relationship exists between the presence of IEA and the individual patient's seizure frequency. In the study of Ajmone-Marsan and Zivin (1970), patients with one or more seizures per month had 60.2% positive records. Patients with less than one seizure per year had 37.6% positive records. EEG records were significantly more likely to be positive when obtained on the same day as a clinical seizure.

Interictal activities rarely occur in individuals who will never have an epileptic condition. In Zivin and Ajmone-Marsan's study (1968) of 6,497 unselected, nonepileptic patients receiving EEG examinations, 142 (2.2%) had epileptiform discharges. With clinical and EEG follow-up ranging from a few months to more than 10 years, 20 of these patients (14.1%) ultimately developed seizures.

Relatively few data are found in the literature about the frequency of IEA in the elderly. Most of the relevant studies concern the presence of epileptiform activity in patients after stroke (Gupta et al., 1998; Luhdorf et al., 1986) and, therefore, are not representative of most elderly patients with unprovoked seizures seen in the outpatient setting. We have recently completed an analysis of 125 ambulatory patients aged 60 years or older in whom a confident diagnosis of epilepsy was made by a board-certified neurologist (Drury and Beydoun, 1998). Seventy of these patients had the onset of their epilepsy after age 60. The waking background EEG in these 70 patients was normal in 8, showed generalized slowing in 13, and focal slowing with or without additional generalized slowing in 49. IEA was present on the first EEG in 35% of 55 patients (mean age, 65 years) with preexisting epilepsy, and 26% of 70 patients (mean age 70) with seizure onset after age 60 years. No significant differences were seen in the frequency of IEA in patients with late onset epilepsy in the seventh or eighth decade of life. Most IEA was focal. Of the 18 patients with onset of epilepsy above 60 years of age, IEA was generalized in 3 and focal in 15. Of those 15 patients with focal IEA, discharge was in the temporal region in 14. Activation procedures added little additional information. Patients with at least one seizure per month were significantly more likely to have IEA present ($P = 0.016$). No differences were found in the presence of IEA, depending on the underlying cause of the seizures. No correlation was found between the presence or absence of IEA and the type of seizures seen in patients, nor was any relationship seen between the detection of IEA and whether patients were taking no, one, or more than one AED.

In 308 patients with epilepsy (Ajmone-Marsan and Zivin, 1970), the frequency of IEA on the first EEG in the first four decades of life was 77%, 60%, 56%, and 51%, respectively. In 51 patients aged 40 years or more, the frequency of IEA was 39%, but this group was not further divided. The frequency of IEA we found in elderly patients (Drury and Beydoun, 1998) appears consistent with an overall trend toward a lower frequency with advancing age. Age-related epileptogenesis has been little studied (Dichter and Weinberger, 1997). It is tempting to speculate that the decreased number and complexity of synaptic connections with age may contribute to less synchronized neuronal discharges and, therefore, less frequent IEA detected on scalp EEG.

Diagnostic Closed Circuit Television-EEG

The clinical manifestations of epilepsy, which are more diverse in the elderly than in younger patients, are more easily confused with other common medical problems (e.g., cardiac arrhythmias, transient ischemic attacks, or dizziness). Elderly patients with epilepsy are more likely to be seen by primary care providers or specialists in other disciplines who may be unfamiliar with the fact that EEG can be normal or abnormal only in a nonspecific way. A low rate of definitively abnormal EEGs in the elderly patient with epilepsy increases the likelihood of the diagnosis being missed.

Prolonged inpatient closed circuit television (CCTV)-EEG monitoring, an extremely useful diagnostic tool in patients with possible epilepsy, is used rarely in the elderly. Only 1.4% of such studies at a major epilepsy referral center was performed on elderly patients (Lancman et al., 1996). We have recently reviewed our experience with admissions to an inpatient adult epilepsy monitoring unit (Drury et al., 1999). Over a consecutive 6-year period ending December 31, 1997, 976 admissions were for monitoring, 419 as part of presurgical assessment and 557 for diagnostic purposes. Of the 557 patients, 26 (4.6%) admitted for diagnostic monitoring were above the age of 60 years. Of these, 8 were critically ill with known or suspected status epilepticus, and 18 were patients whose primary reason for hospitalization was the monitoring itself. Of the 18 patients admitted for monitoring only, mean age was 69.5 years (range, 60–90 years). The mean length of stay was 4.3 days (range, 2–9). Five patients had complex partial seizures recorded. Three patients, all treated with AEDs, had no spells recorded, and no additional diagnostic information was gained from the admission. The other 10 patients, 8 of whom had been treated with AEDs, were symptomatic during their admissions, leading to a variety of neurologic but not epileptic, psychiatric, or other medical disorders, and allowing tapering of AEDs. Thus, 15 of the 18 patients received a conclusive diagnosis of the nature of their spells during admission. Our results indicate that inpatient CCTV-EEG monitoring is useful in elderly patients in whom the diagnosis of epilepsy is being considered. More conclusive diagnosis of epilepsy, primary psychiatric illnesses, or other neurologic or medical conditions will diminish inappropriate use of AEDs in a patient population in which side effects of treatment and drug-interactions may be problematic, and help direct other more appropriate therapeutic approaches. Follow-up information in those patients for whom such data were available suggests sustained benefit from establishing the correct diagnosis in many patients.

Although seizures are a likely explanation for a current neurologic event seen in patients with a history of seizures, we found that only four of our eight patients with a prior history of seizures proved to have epileptic events as the underlying cause for their apparent episodes. Even in those patients, the ictal semiology was distinct from that reported as occurring earlier in life, supporting the observation that ictal semiology can change with age (Tinuper, 1997). Our results are similar to those of Lancman, et al. (1996). The 20 patients in their report represented 1.5% of all patients who had CCTV-EEG recording at a major epilepsy center. Monitoring in their nine diagnostic cases led to diagnoses such as sleep apnea in two, epilepsy in two, nonepileptic events of psychogenic origin in two, syncope in one, and was not diagnostic in two, results comparable to ours.

Short-term (2–6 hour) diagnostic CCTV-EEG is also underused in the elderly in our experience. At the University of Michigan Epilepsy Program, over a consecutive 5-year period, 26 of 375 (6.9%) patients who had this procedure were more than 60 years of age (Drury, unpublished data). In summary, given how common epilepsy is in the elderly and the extensive differential diagnosis that must be considered, CCTV-EEG is a valuable and underutilized diagnostic tool in this population. The ictal appearances on scalp EEG in the elderly are no different than those seen in younger patients with epilepsy and will not be discussed in further detail here.

AMBULATORY EEG

Electroencephalograms can be recorded outside of the hospital environment with AEEG. These techniques are akin to Holter cardiac monitoring. They permit recording in more "real life" circumstances. Patients are instructed to keep a diary of their activities and any episodes that they experience. It is common, but especially important in the elderly, that one channel is dedicated to ECG, as the differential diagnosis between intermittent episodes of cardiac or neurologic origin is sometimes difficult. AEEG recording devices have improved significantly in recent years and are comfortable for the patient to wear. They now include the capability of concurrent video recording to allow home video-EEG, and incorporate spike and seizure detection software in the analysis phase, all increasing their diagnostic capabilities.

EEG IN ENCEPHALOPATHIES AND DEMENTIA

Abnormalities on EEG that are slower than expected for the age and behavioral state of the patient are termed "slow-wave abnormalities." These can be generalized or focal, and intermittent or persistent, the latter defined as present for >80% of an EEG

TABLE 2-4. *Electroencephalogram findings of patients with dementia, stupor, or coma*

Diagnosis	EEG findings
Stupor (i.e., renal or hepatic)	Moderate degree of background slowing with intermittent further slowing. Stimulation of the patient accelerates the background frequency.
Coma (i.e., posthypoxic-ischemic injury)	Marked and persistent slowing that does not react to stimulation.
Brain death	Isoelectric EEG.
Focal brain lesions	Focal slowing. Periodic lateralized epileptiform discharges (PLEDs), if acute.
Encephalitis	PLEDs or Bi-PLEDs; generalized or multifocal slowing.
Creutzfeldt-Jakob disease	Generalized periodic sharp wave complexes.
Alzheimer's disease	Mild to moderate generalized background slowing.

EEG, electroencephalogram.

recording. Slow-wave abnormalities can be seen in patients with epilepsy, but when they occur without other associated abnormalities, they are nonspecific. Focal slow-wave abnormalities imply a local disturbance of cortical and sometimes adjacent subcortical structures in the focal epilepsies, but they also can occur in other conditions (e.g., stroke, brain tumors, severe migraine) or in localized brain injury after head trauma. Generalized, intermittent slowing occurs most commonly in diverse encephalopathies. The frequency of the slowing and the percent to which it is present in the EEG correlate with the severity of the encephalopathy. Stuporous patients will show a moderate degree of slowing of background rhythms and brief trains of even slower waveforms intermittently. Stimulation of the patient accelerates the background frequency. Comatose patients show a more marked and persistent degree of slowing that typically does

not change with stimulation. Occasionally, comatose patients have EEG findings highly suggestive of a particular cause (Table 2-4). A combination of unreactive delta rhythms with superimposed widespread beta activity should lead to a suspicion of overdose with barbiturates or benzodiazepines. In heavily sedated patients or patients who are paralyzed with neuromuscular blocking agents, EEG recordings are an extremely useful bedside measure of the integrity of brain function. EEG is one of the confirmatory tests that can be useful in establishing a diagnosis of brain death. EEG should be used to confirm brain death only when the patient has met all clinical criteria for the absence of any brain function from a known and irreversible cause (American Clinical Neurophysiology Society Guidelines, 1994).

In patients with well-defined focal brain lesions such as tumors or stroke, no indication exists for the

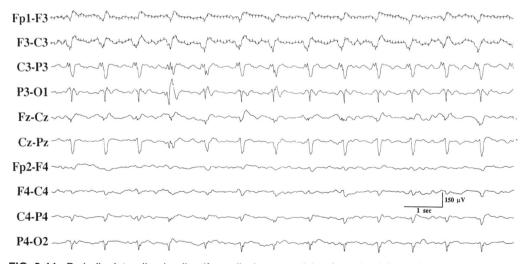

FIG. 2-11. Periodic, lateralized epileptiform discharges arising from the left hemisphere with a posterior maximum after acute posterior cerebral territory ischemic infarction in an elderly patient.

routine use of EEG. A characteristic EEG pattern seen in severe focal encephalitis or other acute focal brain lesions such as stroke is known as "periodic lateralized epileptiform discharges "(PLEDs). PLEDs are high-amplitude, regularly recurring sharp waves on a background of marked voltage and frequency attenuation (Fig. 2-11). Focal seizures, secondarily generalized tonic-clonic seizures, and signs of more generalized cerebral dysfunction with altered levels of alertness may all be seen. Typically, the EEG and behavioral features are transient. Later, a localization-related epilepsy with associated focal slowing and IEA may be seen.

The EEG has no particular utility in the investigation of patients with degenerative disorders of the nervous system with one notable exception. Patients with the acute or subacute presentation of a dementing illness should have one or more EEG recordings performed to search for the generalized periodic sharp wave complexes (PSWC) of Creutzfeldt-Jakob disease. This illness is characterized by rapidly progressive dementia, myoclonus, and cerebellar and visual dysfunction. EEGs may be useful in establishing a diagnosis in those suspected of having the illness. Typical features are the 1 to 2 Hz PSWC, which may be present as early as early as 3 weeks after onset and has been seen in 88% of EEGs after the twelfth week of illness (Levy et al., 1986). Myoclonic jerks often occur in association with PSWC but no consistent temporal relationship exists between the jerks and the complexes.

CONCLUSION

EEG has a limited but important role as a diagnostic test in the older adult. It is a critically important study in patients with known or suspected seizure disorders and should be used more with concurrent video monitoring in cases where epilepsy is one consideration in the differential diagnosis. A valuable role continues to be seen for using EEG in acute encephalopathies and dementing illnesses where characteristic patterns may occur.

REFERENCES

Ajmone-Marsan C, Zivin LS. Factors related to the occurrence of typical paroxysmal abnormalities in the EEG records of epileptic patients. *Epilepsia* 1970;11:361–381.

American Clinical Neurophysiology Society Guidelines. Minimum technical standards for EEG recording in suspected cerebral death. *J Clin Neurophysiol* 1994;11: 10–13.

Arenas AM, Brenner RP, Reynolds CF. Temporal slowing in the elderly revisited. *American Journal of EEG Technology* 1986;26:105–114.

Dichter MA, Weinberger LM. Epileptogenesis and the aging brain. In: Rown AJ, Ramsay RE, eds. *Seizures and epilepsy in the elderly.* Boston: Butterworth-Heinemann, 1997:21–27.

Drury I, Beydoun A. Interictal epileptiform activity in elderly patients with epilepsy. *Electroencephalogr Clin Neurophysiol* 1998;106:369–373.

Drury I, Selwa LN, Schuh LA, et al. Value of inpatient diagnostic CCTV-EEG monitoring in the elderly. *Epilepsia* 1999;40:1100–1102.

Giaquinto S, Nolfe G. The EEG in the normal elderly: a contribution to the interpretation of aging and dementia. *Electroencephalogr Clin Neurophysiol* 1986;3:540–546.

Guazelli M, Feinberg I, Aminoff M, et.al. Sleep spindles in normal elderly: comparison with young adult patterns and relation to nocturnal awakening, cognitive function and brain atrophy. *Electroencephalogr Clin Neurophysiol* 1986;63:526–539.

Gupta SR, Naheedy MH, Elias D, et al. Postinfarction seizures: a clinical study. *Stroke* 1998;19:1477–1481.

Hubbard O, Sunde D, Goldensohn ES. The EEG in centenarians. *Electroencephalogr Clin Neurophysiol* 1976;40: 407–417.

Katz RI, Horowitz GR. Electroencephalogram in the septuagenarian: studies in a normal geriatric population. *J Am Geriatr Soc* 1982;3:272–275.

Katz RI, Horowitz GR. Sleep-onset frontal rhythmic slowing in a normal geriatric population. *Electroenccephalogr Clin Neurophysiol* 1983;56:27P.

Katzmann R, Terry R. *The neurology of aging.* Philadelphia: FA Davis, 1983:1–249.

Lancman ME, O'Donovan C, Dinner D, et al. Usefulness of prolonged video-EEG monitoring in the elderly. *J Neurol Sci* 1996;142:54–58.

Levy SR, Chiappa KH, Burke CJ, et al. Early evolution and evidence of electroencephalographic abnormality in Creutzfeldt-Jakob disease. *J Clin Neurophysiol* 1986;3: 1–21.

Luhdorf K, Jensen LK, Plesner AM. The value of EEG in the investigation of postapoplectic epilepsy. *Acta Neurol Scand* 1986;74:279–283.

Reiher J, Lebel M. Wicket spikes: clinical correlates of a previously undescribed EEG pattern. *Can J Neurol Sci* 1977;4:39–47.

Silverman AJ, Busse EW, Barnes RH. Studies in the processes of aging: electroencephalographic findings in 400 elderly subjects. *Electroencephalogr Clin Neurophysiol* 1955;7:67–74.

Tinuper T. The altered presentation of seizures in the elderly. In: Rowan AJ, Ramsay RE, eds. *Seizures and epilepsy in the elderly.* Boston: Butterworth-Heinemann, 1997: 123–127.

Torres F, Faoro A, Loewenson R, et al. The electroencephalogram of elderly subjects revisited. *Electroencephalogr Clin Neurophysiol* 1983;56:391–398.

Visser SL, Hooijer C, Jonker C, et.al. Anterior temporal focal abnormalities in EEG in normal aged subjects; correlations with psychopathological and CT brain scan findings. *Electroencephalogr Clin Neurophysiol* 1987;66:1–7.

Westmoreland BF, Klass DW. A distinctive rhythmic EEG discharge of adults. *Electroencephalogr Clin Neurophysiol* 1981;51:186–191.

Zivin L, Ajmone-Marsan C. Incidence and prognostic significance of "epileptiform" activity in the EEG of nonepileptic subjects. *Brain* 1968;91:751–778.

SUGGESTED READING

Rowan AJ, Ramsay RE, eds. *Seizures and epilepsy in the elderly*. Boston: Butterworth-Heinemann, 1997.

Daly DD, Pedley TA, eds. *Current practice of clinical electroencephalography*, 2nd ed. New York: Raven Press, 1990.

GLOSSARY OF TERMS

Benign epileptiform variants: One of a number EEG patterns that has epileptiform features but occurs in the normal population and has no known association with epilepsy.

Ictal: That which occurs during a seizure.

Ictal epileptiform activity: EEG feature of a rhythmic discharge that is distinct from the interictal pattern in at least duration (especially in the generalized epilepsies) but usually also in morphology and topography.

Interictal: The periods between seizures.

Interictal epileptiform activity: EEG feature of spikes, sharp waves or spike-wave complexes that are isolated or repeat in brief trains, are either focal or generalized, and are not associated with an alteration in awareness or behavior.

Montage: In EEG, the manner in which electrodes are linked together to examine the EEG, hence transverse bipolar when scalp electrodes are linked in chains going transversely across the scalp.

PLED: Periodic lateralized epileptiform discharges. EEG feature seen in acute focal insults to the brain. When bilateral and independent, known as BiPLED.

SCREDA: Subclinical rhythmic electroencephalographic discharge of adults. A benign EEG phenomenon consisting of repetitive discharges of abrupt onset and termination without any clinical accompaniment. Superficially resembles an ictal EEG discharge.

Semiology: The behavioral manifestations and experiences of the patient during an epileptic seizure.

2.3

Diagnostic Tests in the Older Adult: EMG

Amparo Gutierrez and Austin J. Sumner

Nerve conductions and electromyography (EMG), which are commonly performed in the evaluation of suspected neuromuscular disease, provide an objective measure of pathophysiology. Nerve conductions are considered the "gold standard" for the noninvasive evaluation of large, myelinated nerve fiber function. Several physiologic factors have a known direct effect on nerve conduction studies: height, anomalous innervation, temperature, and age. The aging process affects nerve conductions and EMG study findings in both extremes of life—in the very young and in the older adult. We will review these changes as they pertain to the older adult.

HISTOLOGIC CHANGES AND AGING

Morphologic changes of the peripheral nervous system occur with aging and bear directly on the changes seen in electrophysiologic testing. It is widely accepted that the volume of the peripheral nervous system is reduced with aging. This is secondary to a loss of nerve cells and axons. Less often considered are the important changes occurring in the Schwann cells and their myelin sheaths. It has been shown that the density of large myelinated fibers in the distal portions of the sural sensory nerve progressively decline after the second decade of life (Jacob and Love, 1985). Only about half of these sensory myelinated fibers innervating the distal portions of the lower extremities survive the aging process (Dumitru, 1995). Above 65 years of age, the relationship between the distances separating the nodes of Ranvier (internodal length) and the diameter of myelinated fibers undergoes changes. A progressive shortening occurs of the internodal length and thinning of the fibers, which are believed to result from demyelination and remyelination, particularly after the sixth decade (Lascelles and Thomas, 1966).

Histochemical studies of limb muscles from elderly individuals without evidence of neuromuscular disease reveal fiber size variation, hyaline or granular degeneration, loss of striations, clumps of pyknotic nuclei, increased fat and connective tissue, and significant neurogenic fiber type grouping (Jennekens et al., 1971).

NERVE CONDUCTION STUDIES AND AGING

Sensory and motor nerve conduction studies are performed to evaluate the speed of conduction along a particular nerve and to assess the number of functioning nerve fibers. The results of aging on conduction velocity, distal latency, and duration have been studied in a number of nerves. Sensory nerve conduction velocities (NCV) demonstrate a consistent decline, approximating 1 to 2 M/sec/decade beginning with the second decade (Dumitru, 1995). Some authors feel that this decline is nonlinear in respect to age and that the maximal effect is not seen until the sixth to eighth decade (Norris et al., 1953). Motor nerve conduction studies reveal changes similar to sensory nerves. The distal latency in motor conductions is mildly prolonged with age. In the median nerve, the distal latency was prolonged by 20% in subjects aged 75 to 89 years compared with those aged 15 to 24 years (Rigshospitalet Laboratory of Clinical Neurophysiology, 1975). In older individuals, Buchthal et al. (1975) also observed increased temporal dispersion (Dyck et al., 1975). They reported that the duration of the sensory compound action potential (CNAP) was 20% to 25% longer in older than in young individuals.

Summarizing the above findings, in patients over the age of 60, there is slowing of motor NCV by 1 M/decade and 2 M/decade for the sensory NCV when using surface electrodes (Oh, 1993). Slight increases in distal latency and duration should be anticipated when interpreting nerve conductions in the older adult.

The amplitude of the compound motor action potential (CMAP) is also shows a gradual decline with aging. This change does not seem to be important in practice because of the wider range of CMAP amplitudes found in normal individuals. Lafratta reported that the amplitude of the sensory (CNAP) also decreases with age (Lafratta, 1966). Using surface electrodes, he found that by the age of 60 years, the sensory CNAP amplitude drops by 36 %.

The nerve conduction findings seen in older adults are explained in part by considering the histologic changes associated with the aging of the peripheral nervous system. The aging nervous system experiences a loss of the large myelinated fibers as well as ongoing demyelination and remyelination.

ELECTROMYOGRAPHY AND AGING

Motor unit potentials (MUAP) are routinely assessed by EMG in the electrophysiologic evaluation of patients. The shape properties (amplitude, duration, complexity) of MUAP reflect the spatial and temporal organization of the motor units in muscle. Studies have demonstrated an age-related effect on the MUAP. In older adults are found an increase in duration, complexity, and amplitude (Bischoff et al., 1991). Motor unit populations are also found to decrease significantly with age in distal muscles (Galea, 1996).

Of the three parameters—shape, duration, and amplitude—the total duration is of special importance, because it best distinguishes between myopathy and neuropathy (Buchthal, 1977). The duration of the MUAP depends mainly on the total number of fibers around the sensitive side of the recording electrode. Other contributing factors in determining duration of the MUAP are the position of the recording electrode in the muscle and the neuromuscular transmission. Changes in the number of muscle fibers per motor unit are correlated with changes in total duration. A common reason for an increased MUAP duration is an increase in fiber density caused by neurogenic disorders. The reinnervation following a neurogenic disorder causes an increase in the fiber density of the motor unit because of sprouting. Some controversy exists concerning when the MUAP duration begins to increase with age. Current theory suggests that MUAP durations do not obviously change between the ages of 20 and 60 years; after the age of 60, however, a clear age-dependent lengthening of the MUAP duration appears to occur. It has been thought that the age-related changes in MUAP duration may be a result of neurogenic processes that do not reach pathologic significance. These changes in MUAP are more prominent when examining distal muscles.

The MUAP amplitude, which is mainly determined by the number and size of fibers in the vicinity of the recording electrode, provides information only about the fibers closest to the needle (Chu-Andrews and Johnson, 1987). Howard et al., using automatic decomposition EMG, demonstrated that a highly significant, progressive increase occurs in the mean MUAP amplitude and complexity (number of turns) with age (Howard et al., 1988). The complexity of the MUAP reflects the temporal dispersion of the individual muscle fiber action potentials, which is influenced by variability in fiber diameter and by fiber density per motor unit (Nandedkar et al., 1988). Therefore, the complexity of the MUAP increases in reinnervated motor units.

Together, the progressive increase in all three properties (amplitude, duration, complexity) and age strongly suggest increasing average motor unit size. This could reflect either selective loss of small motor units or progressive expansion of all motor units from an ongoing, age-related process of gradual muscle denervation with compensatory reinnervation. The evaluating clinician must be aware of the changes found in the EMG of the older adult to draw accurate conclusions.

REGENERATION AND AGING

One of the tasks that the EMG clinician is frequently asked to perform is to evaluate peripheral nerve injury and the extent of regeneration. Although human studies have been limited, observations in animal models have consistently shown age as an important variable in nerve regrowth. The results of these studies show a decline on peripheral nerve regeneration with age. Reduced axonal transport and sprouting appear to occur along with impaired reoccupation of sites for motor nerve terminals in older subjects (Kerezoodi and Thomas, 1999). Clinically, a slower rate of nerve regrowth is seen in the older adult as compared with the younger adult.

REFERENCES

Bischoff C, Machetanz J, Conrad B. Is there an age-dependent continuous increase in the duration of the motor unit action potential? *Electrencephalogr Clin Neurophysiol* 1991;81:304–311.

Buchthal F. Electrophysiological signs of myopathy as related with muscle biopsy. *Acta Neurol Scand* 1977;32: 1–29.

Buchthal F, Rosenfalck A, Behse F. Sensory potentials of normal and diseased nerves. In: Dyck PJ,Thomas PK, Lambert EH, eds. *Peripheral neuropathy*. Philadelphia: WB Saunders, 1975:442–464.

Chu-Andrews J, Johnson RJ. *Electrodiagnosis*. Philadelphia: JB Lippincott, 1987.

Dumitru D. *Electrodiagnostic medicine*. Philadelphia: Hanley & Belfus, 1995.

Galea V. Changes in motor unit estimates with aging. *J Clin Neurophysiol* 1996;13(3):253–260.

Howard JE, McGill KC, Dorfman LJ. Age effects on properties of motor unit action potentials: ADEMG analysis. *Ann Neurol* 1988;24:207–213.

Jacob JM, Love S. Qualitative and quantitative morphology of human sural nerve at different ages. *Brain* 1985; 108:897.

Jennekens FGI, Tomlinson BE, Walton JN. Histochemical aspects of five limb muscles in old age: an autopsy study. *J Neurol Sci* 1971;14:259–276.

Kerezoodi E, Thomas PK. Influence of age on regeneration in the peripheral nervous system. *Gerontology* 1999;45 (6):301–306.

Lafratta CW. A comparison of sensory and motor NCV as related with age. *Arch Phys Med Rehabil* 1966;47: 2286–2290.

Lascelles RG, Thomas PK. Changes due to age in internodal length in the sural nerve in man. *J Neurol Neurosurg Psychiatry* 1966;29:40–44.

Nandedkar SD, Sanders DB, Stalberg EV, et al. Simulation of concentric needle EMG motor unit action potentials. *Muscle Nerve* 1988;70:177–184.

Norris AH, Shock NW, Wagman IH. Age changes in the maximum conduction velocity of motor fibers of human ulnar nerves. *J Appl Physiol* 1953;5:589.

Oh SJ. *Clinical electromyography: nerve conduction studies*, 2nd ed. Baltimore, Williams & Wilkins, 1993.

Rigshospitalet Laboratory of Clinical Neurophysiology. EMG-sensory and motor conduction. Findings in normal subjects. Copenhagen: RLCN, 1975.

3

Age-Related Changes in Pharmacokinetics, Drug Interactions, and Adverse Effects

James C. Cloyd and Jeannine M. Conway

Older adults (65 years of age) comprise 13% of the population, account for 35% of all prescription expenditures ($12.7 to $14.3 billion in 1991) and more than 69% of the elderly have more than one chronic medical condition (Soumerai and Ross-Degnan, 1999; Hoffman et al., 1996). Community-dwelling older adults are reported to take, on average, 3.1 to 7.9 prescription and nonprescription medications, whereas nursing home residents have an average of 7.2 medication orders (Stewart, 2001; Beers et al., 1993). An estimated one of six older hospitalized adults are admitted secondary to an adverse drug reaction (ADR) (Mannesse et al., 1997). Neuropsychiatric medications are among the most common causes of ADRs (Larson et al., 1987; Schor et al., 1992). Age alone does not appear to be a risk factor for ADRs, but the older adult is at greater risk because of the larger number of medications taken and multiple disease states (Hanlon et al., 2001; Carbonin et al., 1991; Grymonpre et al., 1988). Alterations in pharmacokinetics and pharmacodynamics can also increase the susceptibility to ADRs in older adults, but no well-controlled studies have evaluated their influence on ADRs (Hanlon et al., 2001). Problems associated with drug therapy in the elderly will likely become even more pronounced with the rapid rise in population of the oldest old (≥85 years of age). Individuals ≥85 years are projected to increase in size by 2050, representing 5% of the US population (Taeuber, 1992). Age-related changes in parameters necessitate a different approach to drug therapy in the elderly and place the older patient at greater risk for serious drug interactions and adverse events than would occur in younger adults. An understanding of the effects of advancing age on disposition and response, and the mechanisms by which interactions occur, permits the clinician to rationally prescribe and more effectively manage neuropsychiatric drug therapy in the older patient.

AGE-RELATED CHANGES IN PHYSIOLOGY: EFFECT ON PHARMACODYNAMICS AND PHARMACOKINETICS

The marked alterations in physiology that occur with advancing age affect both the pharmacokinetics and pharmacodynamics of drugs used to treat neuropsychiatric disorders. Changes in pharmacokinetics result in either higher or lower drug concentrations, depending on the variable contributions of absorption and elimination. Response, either beneficial or adverse, can be exaggerated or diminished even when plasma drug concentration is unchanged. Physiologic changes affecting all aspects of drug disposition—absorption, distribution, metabolism, and elimination—occur as a person ages (Table 3-1). Aging also alters the number and function of central nervous system (CNS) receptors that determine the nature and intensity of response to drugs (Roberts and Tumer, 1988). Many diseases common to the elderly alter pharmacokinetics, pharmacodynamics, or both.

TABLE 3-1. *Age-related changes in physiology*

Absorption	
Gastrointestinal blood flow	↓
Absorption	↔
Gastric pH	↓
Gastric emptying	↓
Intestinal motility	↓
Distribution	
Lean body mass	↓
Body fat	↑
Plasma albumin	↓↔
Metabolism	
Liver mass	↓
Hepatic blood flow	↓
Excretion	
Kidney mass	↓
Renal blood flow	↓
Glomerular filtration	↓
Filtration fraction	↓

Absorption

Drug absorption is influenced by several anatomic and physiologic factors, including gastric emptying, gastric and intestinal pH, quantity and quality of bile secretions, intestinal motility, condition and the number of the absorptive cells, enterocyte efflux, metabolizing enzymes, and intestinal blood flow (Bender, 1968; Zhang et al., 1999). Absorption is also dependent on a drug's physical and chemical properties, such as release from the dosage form, dissolution, and lipophilicity (Fleisher et al., 1999).

No significant age-related change appears to exist in the anatomic features of the small intestine (Lovat, 1996). In contrast, important changes do occur in gastrointestinal physiology. Approximately one fourth of the elderly (>70 years) have lost the ability to secrete acid, or they are taking medications that increase gastric pH (Saltzman et al., 1994; Krasinski et al., 1986; Vanzant et al., 1932). Gastric pH is important for drugs, including iron salts, ketoconazole, and ampicillin, that require an acidic pH for absorption (Iber et al., 1994). Gastric emptying can be decreased by half in 25% of the elderly above 70 years of age (Evans et al., 1981). Reduced motility will result in a longer residual time for medications and can affect absorption, depending on a drug's chemical properties. If a medication is rapidly absorbed because it readily dissolves and easily diffuses across luminal membranes into systemic circulation, changes in motility are unlikely to affect absorption. Drugs that are slowly absorbed because of poor aqueous solubility or decreased diffusion rate will exhibit increased bioavailability because of a longer resident time in the absorptive segment of the small intestine (Fleisher et al., 1999). Blood flow to the gastrointestinal tract is reduced with age; theoretically, this could result in decreased absorption of some drugs, but insufficient evidence is found to determine if this is clinically important (Bender, 1968).

Until recently, it was assumed that the mechanism for drug absorption across the intestinal mucosa was passive diffusion. Active influx and efflux transport enzymes are now known to play a role in both the rate and extent of absorption. Gabapentin bioavailability is primarily mediated by an l-amino acid transport system that becomes saturated at clinically relevant doses (Stewart et al., 1993). P-glycoprotein (PGP), an efflux transporter located in intestinal enterocytes, pumps medications out of the cell and into the intestinal lumen, thereby decreasing drug absorption (Watkins, 1997). PGP is expressed in many tissues, including the adrenal cortex, brush border of the proximal renal tubule epithelium, pancreatic ductules, luminal surface of biliary hepatocytes, immunomodulation cells, blood–brain barrier, and the mucosa of the small and large intestines (Yu, 1999; Gupta, 1995). PGP is responsible for excreting 16% of an intravenous dose of digoxin into the gut lumen in mice, whereas only 2% of the dose was excreted in a PGP knock-out mouse (Mayer et al., 1996). Drugs can either induce or inhibit PGP, resulting in a decrease or increase in the bioavailability of the affected medication (Fromm, 2000). Finally, drug absorption is affected by the presence of drug metabolizing enzymes in the gastrointestinal mucosa. Cytochrome P-450 (CYP) enzymes, which are located in intestinal enterocytes (Watkins et al., 1987), can have a substantial impact on absorption. Midazolam, a CYP 3A4 substrate, has a bioavailability of >90% following intramuscular administration, but approximately 36% when given by mouth [Versed (midazolam), 1998]. The difference is largely attributable to metabolism in the gut wall. It is not known if either the amount or function of PGP or CYP enzymes in the gut changes with age.

Age-related changes in gastrointestinal physiology do not have a predictable effect on drug absorption. Intrapatient alterations in gastrointestinal motility, which are common in the elderly, will also alter the bioavailability of slowly absorbed drugs and should be considered when changes in response occur.

Distribution

Drug distribution has two components: the extent to which the drug distributes throughout the body and the percentage bound to plasma proteins. Both are altered in old age. The distribution of a drug is partially dependent on its polarity. Highly polar compounds are hydrophilic and tend to distribute mainly into extracellular water. Lipophilic drugs tend to distribute mainly into the tissue compartment, particularly muscle and adipose tissue (Parker et al., 1995). Age-related changes in body disposition will alter volume of distribution (Vd). The percent of body fat increases and lean body mass decreases with age (Shock et al., 1963; Forbes and Reina, 1970; Edelman and Leibman, 1959). This shift in body composition may cause an increase in the Vd for lipophilic drugs and a decrease in the Vd for hydrophilic drugs.

Distribution volume is the key parameter in calculating loading doses as is shown in the following equation:

Loading dose = (Concentration desired − baseline concentration) · wt in kg · Vd (L/kg)

Distribution volume is usually estimated in younger adults. The elderly may have an unexpected response to a medication because their Vd deviates from the average younger adult values, resulting in a subtherapeutic or toxic plasma drug concentration.

Advancing age affects the extent to which CNS drugs bind to plasma proteins. Medications may bind to albumin, alpha₁-acid glycoprotein, globulins, and lipoproteins (Pike et al., 1984). Some drugs (e.g., zonisamide and topiramate) may also bind to erythrocytes (Nishiguchi et al., 1992; Gidal and Lensmeyer, 1999; Jusko and Gretch, 1976). In the older adult, albumin, on average, declines slightly with age (Campion et al., 1988; Greenblatt, 1979). Other conditions common in the elderly such as renal insufficiency, rheumatoid arthritis, and malnutrition also reduce albumin concentrations (Greenblatt, 1979; Wallace and Verbeeck, 1987). Alpha₁-acid glycoprotein, which binds alkaline drugs, increases with age and further elevations can occur from physiologic stressors such as stroke, heart failure, infection, trauma, myocardial infarction, arthritis, surgery, and chronic obstructive pulmonary disease (Wallace and Verbeeck, 1987).

Only drugs protein-bound 90% or more are significantly affected by alterations in plasma proteins (Table 3-2). Most disruptions in binding are clinically unimportant but can cause a misinterpretation of drug concentrations. As shown in Figure 3-1, a decrease in protein binding results in lower total but not unbound concentrations for low hepatic extraction drugs. This occurs because only unbound drug in plasma diffuses into the hepatocyte or renal cell where it is either metabolized or excreted. At steady state, the dose and the clearance of unbound drug determine the unbound concentration in plasma. Drug freed from protein binding sites (e.g., because of decreased albumin) becomes available for elimination. Because neither daily dose nor unbound clearance changes, unbound drug concentrations remain the same. Alterations in plasma proteins can complicate interpretation of laboratory values of highly bound drugs such as phenytoin (PHT). PHT is normally 90% bound to albumin. At a total PHT concentration of 15 mg/mL, the unbound concentration is 1.5 mg/L. This relationship can change over time as an elderly patient experiences a decline in plasma albumin. In such a patient, binding can decline to 80%, resulting in a total concentration of 7.5 mg/L, whereas the unbound concentration remains at 1.5 mg/L. In this situation, an increase in dose is not indicated.

Metabolism

The two most important age-related physiologic changes that occur in the liver are decreased mass and reduced blood flow (Fig. 3-2). Wynne et al. examined changes in liver mass (as assessed by ultrasound) and liver blood flow (indocyanine green clearance) with respect to age in men (Wynne et al., 1989). Sixty-five

TABLE 3-2. *Neurologic drugs highly bound to plasma proteins*

Medication	Protein bound (%)	References
Donepezil (Aricept)	96	Tiseo et al., 1998
Phenytoin (Dilantin)	88 to 93	Herun, 1995
Valproate (Depakote)	90	Marty et al., 1984
Tiagabine (Gabitril)	96	Brodie, 1995
Fluoxetine (Prozac)	94.5	Aronoff et al., 1984
Sertraline (Zoloft)	99	van Harten, 1993
Paroxetine (Paxil)	95	Kaye et al., 1989
Nefazodone (Serzone)	99	Prod Info Serzone, 1998
Diazepam (Valium)	94 to 99	Hallstrom et al., 1980
Lorazepam (Ativan)	85 to 91	Kyriakopoulos, 1978
Tolcapone (Tasmar)	99.9	Prod Info Tasmar, 1998
Pergolide (Permax)	>90	Rubin et al., 1981
Bromocriptine (Parlodel)	90 to 96	Schran, 1980
Ibuprofen (Advil, Motrin)	99	Lookwood, 1983
Celecoxib (Celebrex)	97	Davies, 2000
Haloperidol (Haldol)	>90	Forsman and Ohman, 1977
Risperidone (Risperdal)	90	Prod Info Risperdal, 2000
Clozapine (Clozaril)	97	Schaber, 1998
Olanzapine (Zyprexa)	93	Prod Info Zyprexa, 2000
Ziprasidone (Geodon)	>99	Geodon (ziprasidone, 2001)
Midazolam (Versed)	95	Versed (midazolam), 1998

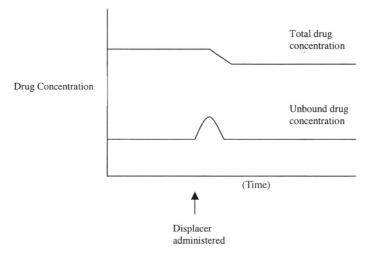

FIG. 3-1. Effect of changes in protein binding and clearance on total concentration and unbound concentrations.

subjects were divided into three groups (<40, 40–64, >65 years) with 20 patients over the age of 65. A 21% decrease in liver volume (in relation to body weight) was observed in the elderly male population. A 28% reduction in liver blood flow was also observed. The impact of advancing age on drug metabolism has

been primarily studied in healthy, ambulatory subjects aged 65 to 75 years. No information is found regarding hepatic changes in the oldest old (≥85 years), nor in frail older patients. Both groups are likely to have diminished drug-metabolizing capacity relative to younger, healthier elderly adults.

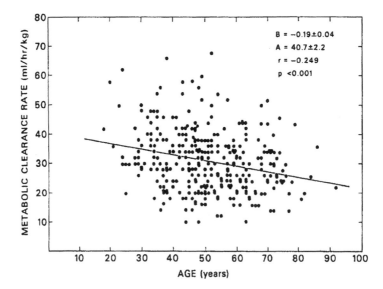

FIG. 3-2. Effect of advancing age on antipyrine clearance. From Vestal RE, Norris AH, Tobin JD, et al. Antipyrine metabolism in man: influence of age, alcohol, caffeine, and smoking. *Clin Pharmacol Ther* 1975;18(4):425–432.

Hepatic metabolism is divided into two phases. Phase I consists of oxidative, reduction, and hydroxylation reactions. The CYP family of enzymes generally catalyzes the oxidative reactions. Phase II reactions are conjugation reactions involving glucuronic acid or sulfates in which conjugated product is made more polar, which allows it to be excreted into the urine or bile. Conjugation reactions can involve either the drug (primary conjugation) or the metabolite of a phase I reaction. (Woodhouse and Wynne, 1992).

The CYP system consists of a family of closely related enzymes known as isoenzymes, each of which catalyzes the metabolism of a unique set of substrates. Table 3-3 lists the major isoenzymes that catalyze the metabolism of numerous neurologic drugs. Available evidence indicates that CYP metabolizing activity declines approximately 1% a year beginning at age 40, although substantial intrasubject variability is seen (Sotaniemi et al., 1997). Antipyrine metabolism is associated with CYP metabolism and clearance of antipyrine declines with age as shown in Figure 3-2.

Many CNS drugs that undergo either primary or secondary metabolism via conjugation reactions with glucuronic acid are mediated by uridine glucuronyl transferases (Tephly et al., 1988; Anderson, 1998). This system is also composed of isoenzymes with specific drug substrates. (Radominska-Pandya et al., 1999). The effect of age on glucuronidation is less well understood than the CYP system. Greenblatt et al. studied the pharmacokinetics of several benzodiazepines that undergo extensive glucuronidation (Greenblatt et al., 1991; Greenblatt et al., 1980; Divoll et al., 1981). Oxazepam, temazepam, and lorazepam have been studied in elderly subjects, most of whom ranged in age from 65 to 75 years. Drug clearance was similar in elderly and younger subjects. The studies gave rise to the view that glucuronidation activity is spared in the elderly. The validity of this assumption has been questioned in recent years, as additional studies with drugs undergoing glucuronidation show age-related changes in clearance comparable to the CYP system.

Excretion

Many drugs and their metabolites are eliminated completely or partly by the kidney. Age-related changes in renal function are well established. (Nyengaard and Bendtsen, 1992; Meyer, 1989; Lindeman, 1990; Roxe, 1991). Anatomic changes result in decreased renal size, decreased renal blood flow, a loss

of glomeruli, and renal tubular changes (Nyengaard and Bendtsen, 1992; Meyer, 1989). Functional changes include a decrease in glomerular filtration, decreased creatinine clearance, and increased serum creatinine concentrations (Rowe, 1976). Renal function decreases begin at age 40, resulting in a 40% decline in renal function by age 70 as compared with age 30 (Lindeman et al., 1985).

Reductions in renal function will result in a decrease of drug clearance eliminated by the kidney. Serum creatinine is not a reliable marker of renal function in the elderly. Creatinine is a byproduct of muscle and as individuals age, lean body mass and serum creatinine declines (Muhlberg and Platt, 1999). A serum creatinine level (Scr) of 1.0 mg/dL, which is within the normal laboratory range for a 41-kg woman 80 years of age, is not a reliable indicator of renal function. An estimated creatinine clearance adjusted for age, gender, and weight (when a patient is within 30% of his or her ideal body weight) provides a better indicator of renal function in the elderly. In most patients, an estimate of creatinine clearance can be used to adjust dosage. One such method is the Cockcroft-Gault equation:

$$Ccr = \frac{(wt \text{ in kg})(140-age) \cdot (0.85 \text{ if patient is female})}{72 \cdot Scr}$$

Using this equation, a woman 80 years of age would have a creatinine clearance of 35 mL/min, necessitating a substantial change in dose for drugs such as gabapentin, which is virtually 100% renally eliminated. In contrast a 65-kg woman 30 years of age with a serum creatinine of 1.0 mg/dL, would have a creatinine clearance of 100 mL/min. There are limitations to this equation, particularly if the patient has significant muscle wasting that might have occurred because of stroke or head injury, and it may not always be appropriate for the frail elderly (Cockcroft and Gault, 1976).

Evidence supports the conclusion that drug elimination via renal excretion or metabolism by either phase I or phase II declines with advancing age. As a general rule, elderly patients should initiate therapy at a dose 30% to 50% less than younger adults and dosing intervals can be extended as the elimination half-life is prolonged.

Pharmacodynamics

Pharmacodynamics is the major source of variation in drug response (Levy, 1998). Age-related changes in pharmacodynamics are drug specific and can result in greater or diminished responses (Chapron, 2001). Studies indicate that the elderly are more sensitive to CNS depressants than younger adults. Following administration of the same dose of diazepam, elderly patients experienced more pronounced sedative effects, although unbound serum concentrations were comparable to those observed in younger adults (Cook et al., 1984). Older adults also exhibited exaggerated sedative effects after administration of midazolam, although the dose was reduced for the elderly study group and both groups had similar plasma concentrations (Platten et al., 1998). Little information is found about altered pharmacodynamics of other CNS drugs with age. It is reasonable to conclude that CNS depressants are likely to produce a greater effect in the elderly than in younger adults, even when doses are adjusted.

DRUG INTERACTIONS

The probability of a drug interaction increases significantly with the number of medications a person takes (Nolan and O'Malley, 1989). The elderly have an increased risk of an unintended drug interaction because of the larger number of medications they take, age-related reductions in clearance, and greater sensitivity to drug effects. Drug interactions fall into two categories: pharmacokinetic and pharmacodynamic. In the former, one or both drugs affect the concentration of the other. In the latter, a drug combination can produce an additive (or supraadditive) effect in which the desired or toxic response is exaggerated or an antagonistic effect in which one drug diminishes the desired effect of another. Advances in clinical pharmacology now provide clinicians with a better understanding of the underlying mechanisms and probability of drug interactions.

Knowledge of a drug's metabolic pathway and its activity as an inhibitor or inducer of metabolizing enzymes permits the prediction of drug combinations that are likely to interact. This allows the clinician to either select drugs without interaction potential or implement a plan to manage an interaction through patient education, monitoring, and dosage adjustment.

Pharmacokinetic Drug Interactions

Absorption

Most medications are prescribed as oral dosage forms, which makes them susceptible to absorption interactions. Interactions can affect both the rate and extent of absorption. Changes in the rate of absorption will either increase or decrease the maximal plasma concentration (C_{max}) depending on the effect of the interacting drug. Such interactions are important for medications, such as analgesics or sedatives, in which C_{max} is an important contributor to response. Interactions resulting in either an increase or decrease in the extent of absorption (bioavailability) affect the total drug exposure. Changes in bioavailability are known to alter the response to antiepileptic drugs. Several different mechanisms reduce the absorption of drug from the gastrointestinal tract. Absorption will be hindered if the active medication binds to a cation to form an insoluble chelate. This interaction occurs when phenytoin is taken in combination with calcium-containing antacids (Kulshrestha et al., 1978). This can be a particularly relevant drug interaction because the older adult is more likely to use antacids to treat dyspepsia. Medications, disease, or aging can induce alterations in gastrointestinal tract motility. Anticholinergic medications (amitriptyline) and opioids decrease gastrointestinal motility, whereas prokinetic medications (metoclopramide) have the opposite effect (Fleisher et al., 1999). The bioavailability of drugs that are slowly absorbed (e.g., phenytoin and carbamazepine) or are given as controlled release formulations can decrease with prokinetic medications. The bioavailability of drugs that are incompletely and slowly absorbed can increase in the presence of reduced gastrointestinal motility.

Inhibition or induction of PGP can affect drug response. The best characterized interaction is PGP inhibition by quinidine, which results in digoxin toxicity. (Fromm et al., 1999). As of yet, no reports have documented an inhibition of intestinal PGP transport of CNS medications. Conversely, induction of PGP will result in decreased bioavailability of susceptible drugs, although little is known about the importance of this transporter enzyme in the absorption of neurologic drugs. Rifampin is an inducer of PGP as well as CYP isoenzymes (Greiner et al., 1999; Teunissen et al., 1984). Serum concentrations of neurologic drugs that are substrates for both PGP and CYP enzymes can be significantly reduced in the presence of rifampin or other inducers affecting both systems. Additional research is necessary to determine which neurologic drugs are transported by PGP and how PGP inhibition and induction affects the absorption of these drugs.

Protein Binding

Certain drugs can displace others from protein binding sites. As discussed earlier in this chapter, the net result of such an interaction is a decrease in total but not unbound steady-state drug concentration. This interaction is only apparent for drugs in which plasma concentrations are measured. In most cases, protein-binding interactions do not require any adjustment in dosage.

Metabolism

The most clinically important drug interactions involve inhibition or induction of metabolism. Drug-drug interactions can be unilateral (i.e., one drug affects the other) or bilateral (each drug affects the other). Interactions can produce significant increases or decreases in the concentration of the affected drugs. The most common form of inhibition is the competitive type in which the inhibitor binds at or near the site where the affected drug is metabolized. Drugs that are metabolized by the same isoenzyme are more likely to interact; however, an inhibitor can bind to isoenzymes other than the one that mediates its metabolism. For example, fluoxetine is primarily metabolized by CYP 2D6, but is an intermediate inhibitor of 3A4 *in vitro* (Ring et al., 1995). The extent of an inhibition interaction is determined by the fraction of the affected drug metabolized by the inhibited pathway and the concentration of the inhibitor relative to its inhibitory constant (Ki).

Inhibition of a CYP enzyme occurs via three mechanisms: reversible inhibition, quasi-irreversible, and irreversible inhibition (Lin and Lu, 1998). The most common mechanism is reversible inhibition that results from competition at the enzyme site. The time course for inhibition is dependent on the half-lives and the time to steady state of the interacting drugs (Michalets, 1998). As the inhibitor concentration approaches its Ki, the clearance of the affected drug decreases and the plasma level rises. This can occur with the first dose of the inhibitor. The full effect of an inhibition reaction can take several days or longer, as it is dependent on the new, prolonged half-life of the affected drug.

The most complex drug interactions are those that alter protein binding and metabolism simultaneously. As shown in Figure 3-3, valproate displaces phenytoin from protein-binding sites, thus lowering total plasma PHT levels. At clinically relevant concentrations, valproate modestly inhibits phenytoin metabolism, resulting in an increase in unbound PHT levels. Depending on the extent of each interaction, a patient may present with symptoms of blurred vision and ataxia with total PHT concentrations that are unchanged or decreased.

Deinhibition of the enzyme is dependent on the elimination half-life of the inhibiting drug (Michalets,

1998). The time for the affected drug to adjust to deinhibition is determined by its half-life to reach a new steady state.

Induction of metabolic enzymes occurs when a stimulus causes more enzyme to be synthesized. Time course for induction is dependent on the rate of degradation of enzyme and the formation of new enzyme (Okey, 1990). It appears the half-life of a drug that triggers induction may partially account for the rate of induction. Rifampin has a half-life of 3 to 4 hours and shows induction at 2 to 3 days, whereas phenobarbital has a half-life up to 140 hours and takes several weeks to exert its effect (Michalets, 1998).

The implication of enzyme inhibition and induction interactions is that the drug interaction may not be immediately clinically evident. It can take days to weeks for a patient to become dizzy and unsteady on a dose that had been changed 2 weeks previous. If the medication that causes the enzyme induction or inhibition is discontinued, the patient might begin to experience toxicity or the drug may lose efficacy (Table 3-3).

Renal Elimination

Drug interactions involving elimination can occur. A few medications can inhibit tubular secretion and cause the clearance of affected drugs to decrease. The most common example of this interaction is the concomitant administration of probenecid with penicillin. Probenecid inhibits the secretion of penicillin into the urine, thereby decreasing its clearance (Gibaldi and Schwartz, 1968).

Many medications and their metabolites are eliminated via glomerular filtration. The elderly have decreased renal function and may take medications that acutely alter their renal function. Nonsteriodal anti-inflammatory drugs (NSAID) can inhibit prostaglandins that are necessary to maintain the proper blood flow to the kidney. Acutely administered NSAIDs can cause decreased blood flow to the kidney, thereby decreasing glomerular filtration and the clearance of the medication or active metabolite. Generally, renal function is restored when the drug is discontinued (Blackshear et al., 1983; Whelton et al., 2000).

Pharmacodynamics

Understanding pharmacology helps predict possible drug interactions caused by pharmacodynamics. Medications that exert their effect on similar recep-

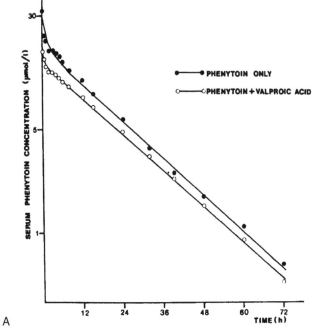

FIG. 3-3A. Effect of valproic acid on phenytoin total and unbound drug.

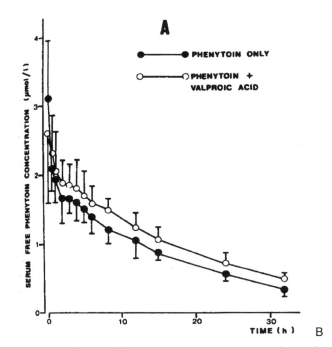

FIG. 3-3B. Perucca E, Hebdige S, Frigo GM, et al. Interaction between phenytoin and valproic acid: plasma protein binding and metabolic effects. *Clin Pharmacol Ther* 1980;28(6):779–789.

TABLE 3-3. *Cytochrome P-450 enzymes responsible for neurologic drug metabolism and their induction and inhibition*

1A2	2C9	2C19	2D6	3A4
		Drugs metabolized by CYP isoenzymes		
Tacrine	Fluoxetine	Phenytoin (minor)	Donepezil	Donepezil
Fluvoxamine	Phenytoin	Felbamate	Galantamine	Galantamine
Mirtazapine (minor)	Valproic Acid	Sertraline (minor)	Amitriptyline	Carbamazepine
Ropinirole	(Minor)	Imipramine	Desipramine	Tiagabine
Clozapine		Clomipramine	Fluoxetine (minor)	Zonisamide
Olanzapine		Citalopram	Sertraline	Midazolam
Carbamazepine		Diazepam	Paroxetine	Sertraline (major)
Caffeine		Phenobarbital	Fluvoxamine	Triazolam
			Venlafaxine	Citalopram
			Mirtazapine (minor)	Mirtazapine
			Risperidone	Nefazodone
			Haloperidol	Alprazolam
			Imipramine	Clonazepam
			Nortriptyline	Ropinirole (minor)
			Clozapine	Haloperidol
			Thioridazine	Clozapine
			Desipramine	Ziprasidone
			Perphenazine	Zolpidem
		Inducers		
Lansoprazole	Rifampin	Rifampin		Rifampin
Omeprazole	Phenobarbital	Phenytoin		Phenobarbital
	Carbamazepine	Carbamazepine		Phenytoin
				Carbamazepine
				Primidone
		Inhibitors		
Ciprofloxacin	Fluconazole	Fluvoxamine	Fluoxetine	Clarithromycin
Fluvoxamine	Cimetidine	Fluconazole	Paroxetine	Erythromycin
Cimetidine	Fluvoxamine	Ticlopidine	Ticlopidine	Fluoxetine
	(moderate)			(moderate)
Tacrine	Nicardipine	Omeprazole		Fluvoxamine
				(moderate)
Mexiletine		Fluoxetine		Grapefruit juice
				substances
				Itraconazole
				Ketoconazole
				Fluconazole
				Nefazodone
				Sertraline (weak)

Adapted from Michalets EL. Update: clinically significant cytochrome P-450 drug interactions. *Pharmacotherapy* 1998;18(1):84–112.

http://www.georgetown.edu/departments/pharmacology/clinlist.html; http://gentest.com/human p450 database/index.html.

tors can create an interaction. For example, administering haloperidol to a patient on levodopa may result in blocking the effects of the levodopa on dopamine receptors (Wright, 2000). Another interaction is the additive effect two medications may have on a patient (e.g., amitriptyline and diphenhydramine). Amitriptyline has a high incidence of anticholinergic side effects when administered alone. When a patient adds diphenhydramine (an over-the-counter antihistamine), the patient increases his or her chance of having an additional anticholinergic side effect (Blazer et al., 1983). Also, a risk exists of a medication with an unknown mechanism or multiple mechanisms of action creating a pharmacodynamic effect that was not intuitively predictable, hence requiring the practitioner to be further vigilant. Although consideration of the above factors improve the ability to prevent or manage drug interactions, they remain difficult to predict because of inter-patient variability in pharmacokinetics and pharmacodynamics.

ADVERSE DRUG REACTIONS

ADRs are defined by the World Health Organization to be "any response to a drug that is noxious or unintended, and which occurs at doses used in man for prophylaxis, diagnosis, or therapy" (Venulet and ten Ham, 1996). ADR have been estimated to account for 7.9% to 24% of all hospitalizations of elderly patients (Hallas et al., 1992; Mannesse et al., 1997). In a recent study by Hanlon et al., an examination of veteran outpatients taking at least five medications demonstrated that the second most common cause of adverse reactions were CNS drugs (Hanlon et al., 1997).

Minimizing the number of medications is the key to reducing the risk of ADRs in the elderly. Assessing all medications a patient takes, including over-the-counter products, prescription drugs, and dietary supplements, is essential to prevent or to manage predictable adverse reactions before they occur (Cunningham, 1997).

Drugs that are not benefiting the patient should be discontinued. In some situations, a less toxic drug can be substituted for one causing side effects without loss of therapeutic effect. ADRs associated with CNS drugs can also result from changes in health status such as the onset of dementia or the development of tremor. The clinician should ascertain if the ADR is a symptom of a medical problem or is exacerbated by that problem. Dosage requirements for older adults are generally reduced. The initial main-

tenance dose should be lower than that used in younger adults and dose titration should proceed more slowly. Ensuring medication adherence, implementing therapeutic drug monitoring strategies, and periodically checking laboratory tests are other important steps associated with reducing the risk of ADR.

Discontinuing medications also puts the patient at risk for ADR (Graves et al., 1997). Benzodiazepines can cause withdrawal symptoms and need to be slowly tapered. Medications that inhibit or induce drug metabolizing enzymes can cause ADR due to alterations in the concentration of the affected drug while they are being discontinued, as the liver returns to its baseline metabolic activity. See *Drug Interactions* section above for further discussion.

ADRs can be divided into two classes: intrinsic and idiosyncratic. Intrinsic drug effects are adverse effects that tend to be an exaggeration of a medication's pharmacology; they are predictable and dose related. Examples of intrinsic ADR include drowsiness, headache, and nausea, which account for 70% to 80% of all side effects, most of which are preventable (Bates and Leape, 2000). Idiosyncratic drug effects occur unpredictably and can be severe reactions that are occasionally associated with significant morbidity and mortality such as Stevens-Johnson rash, acute organ failure, and blood dyscrasias. Some of the more commonly prescribed neurologic drugs have adverse reactions that can be particularly troublesome for older adults.

Antiepileptic Drugs

All of the older antiepileptic drugs (AED)—phenobarbital, phenytoin, carbamazepine, and valproic acid—are associated with numerous ADRs, including concentration-dependent CNS effects resulting in dizziness, unsteadiness, nystagmus, and diplopia. Carbamazepine-induced hyponatremia is more prevalent in the elderly (Miller, 1997). A major disadvantage to phenobarbital therapy is sedation, particularly in a population that may already have decreased mentation. All of the older AED medications have been associated with an increased risk of syncope and fall in the elderly (Hanlon et al., 2001).

The newer AEDs (felbamate, gabapentin, topiramate, tiagabine, lamotrigine, oxcarbazepine, levetiracetam, and zonisamide) also cause CNS adverse reactions including dizziness, headache, and somnolence similar to the older AEDs. Felbamate is rarely used because of the risk of aplastic anemia and hepatic failure. Lamotrigine is associated with a 7% occurrence of nonserious rash and a 1% occurrence of serious rash (i.e., Stevens-Johnson syndrome) (Wong et al., 1999). It should be dosed and monitored carefully when given concomitantly with valproic acid, as the latter inhibits lamotrigine's metabolism and greatly increases the risk of rash (Messenheimer et al., 1998). Oxcarbazepine can cause hyponatremia, which requires medication discontinuation (Pendlebury et al., 1989; Nielsen et al., 1988). Tiagabine may cause dizziness, nervousness, tremor, and depression. Topiramate can cause significant cognitive impairment in the younger adults and should be titrated carefully in the older adult (Aldenkamp et al., 2000). It can also cause weight loss (Rosenfeld et al., 1997) and renal calculi (Wasserstein et al., 1995), which can be problematic with the frail older adult. Zonisamide can also cause CNS side effects and renal calculi (Leppik et al., 1993). Levetiracetam has been shown to have an increased incidence of dizziness and somnolence in a younger adult population, which may be magnified when it is administered to an older population (Cereghino et al., 2000).

Antidepressants

Antidepressants are used in the geriatric population for various reasons, including pain, headache, and depression. ADRs commonly occur with both tricyclic antidepressants (TCA) and selective serotonin reuptake inhibitors (SSRI). TCAs are noted for their anticholinergic effects that result in dry mouth, blurred vision, tachycardia, constipation, urinary retention, and confusion, all of which can be problematic in an elderly patient. Tricyclics can also cause orthostatic hypotension, seizures, and cardiac arrhythmias that may be magnified in the elderly (Naranjo et al., 1995). SSRIs and the newer antidepressants lack the cardiac side effects of tricyclic antidepressants, making them the preferred medications for initial treatment of depression in the elderly (Gutierrez and Stimmel, 2001). The most frequent adverse reactions associated with SSRIs are insomnia, nausea, loose stools, and sexual dysfunction (Menting et al., 1996). Weight changes can also occur (Rigler et al., 2001). The most common adverse reactions to bupropion are insomnia and headache, although it can cause seizures if the dose is increased quickly or exceeds 450 mg/d (Davidson, 1989). It is not clear if elderly patients are more likely to have seizures than younger adults. Venlafaxine, in a small

percentage of older adults, caused a dose-related increase in blood pressure, which should be recognized as a potential adverse reaction and, therefore, reduce the addition of potentially unnecessary treatment for hypertension (Staab and Evans, 2000). Nefazodone causes dose-related sedation, somnolence, dizziness, lightheadedness, blurred vision, and asthenia (Robinson et al., 1996). Mirtazapine has been associated with transient somnolence (Fawcett and Barkin, 1998).

Although adverse reactions to antidepressants can occur at any age, it is clear that the risk for cognitive impairment is greater when administering TCAs in elderly patients (Moore and O'Keefe, 1999). Adverse reactions to which younger adults can adjust may have a greater impact on an older adult's ability to function.

Benzodiazepines

Benzodiazepines are frequently used in the elderly. Of the prescriptions written for benzodiazepines, 40% are for patients older than 65 years (Reynolds et al., 1985). Benzodiazepines, one of the most common causes of adverse events in the older adult, can result in side effects and falls. Medications with an extremely long half-life can cause daytime somnolence, confusion, and increased risk of falls (Sorock and Shimkin, 1988). Although the older adult may have a similar plasma concentration of drug as their younger counterparts, they have significantly more CNS depression (Castleden et al., 1977; Swift et al., 1985).

Parkinson's Medications

Patients with Parkinson's disease are a challenge to dose and monitor because the disease has many symptoms that mirror the common adverse reactions to medications, including lethargy, cognitive impairment, falls, and sedation (Berchou, 2000). Medications are classified as presynaptic drugs (e.g., carbidopa or levodopa, tolcapone, selegiline, and amantadine) and postsynaptic drugs (e.g., pergolide, bromocriptine, pramipexole, and ropinirole). The most common adverse reactions associated with these medications are abdominal discomfort and nausea, at the initiation of therapy (Koller, 2000). Increased peripheral dopamine levels are associated with hypotension, nausea, and vomiting. These effects are decreased by an adequate carbidopa dose (Koller and Pahwa, 1994).

Alzheimer Drugs

Pharmacotherapy for Alzheimer's disease is limited. All of the approved medications presumably exert their therapeutic effect by increasing acetylcholine concentrations. This mechanism is also the underlying cause for most adverse effects of these drugs. Tacrine has been available for the past 8 years; however, its use is limited by a high incidence of nausea, vomiting, diarrhea, dyspepsia, and myalgias (Gracon et al., 1998). Donepezil has an adverse effect profile similar to tacrine (Rogers and Friedhoff, 1996). The Food and Drug Administration recently approved rivastigmine and galantamine. Rivastigmine's adverse reactions are also gastrointestinal; they are usually short lived, occurring while the dose is being titrated upward, requiring initiation of therapy to be gradual (Rosler et al., 1999). Galantamine has also demonstrated similar gastrointestinal adverse reactions (Fulton and Benfield, 1996). Patients may overcome the gastrointestinal adverse reactions if therapy is initiated at the lowest dose available and gradually titrated up to the desired level.

Antipsychotics

Some conditions that occur in the elderly (e.g., Alzheimer's and Parkinson's diseases), have symptoms of dementia. Adverse reactions associated with all of the antipsychotic drugs can be serious and irreversible. Older antipsychotics (i.e., haloperidol) can cause drug-induced parkinsonism in the older adult (Sweet and Pollock, 1995). The risk of developing tardive dyskinesia is greater in the elderly and the risk is increased after as few as 3 months of antipsychotic drug (Jeste et al., 1995; Glazer et al., 1993; Sweet et al., 1995). Atypical antipsychotics have equal efficacy compared with the older drugs with fewer extra pyramidal side effects (Meltzer, 1993). Clozapine causes orthostatic hypotension and requires a slow titration to overcome this adverse effect (Masand, 2000). Blood counts should be monitored weekly for the first 6 months, or until stable, and then biweekly indefinitely during clozapine treatment because of the possible development of agranulocytosis, for which age is thought to be a risk factor (Alvir et al., 1993). Risperidone can cause extrapyramidal symptoms at higher doses, therefore, therapy should begin with a low dose (Marder and Meibach, 1994). Olanzapine appears to be well tolerated in the older adult, with somnolence and abnormal gait occurring at a rate greater than placebo (Street et al., 2000). Quetiapine also appears to be tolerated, with the most common adverse reactions being somnolence, dizziness, postural hypotension, and agitation. Extrapyramidal adverse effects can also occur (McManus et al., 1999). The Food and Drug Administration recently approved ziprasidone and no published literature is found on the adverse effects in the older adult. The package insert states there were no age-related differences in pharmacokinetics. A risk exists for QT prolongation and caution is warranted in the elderly patient, particularly for those with an underlying cardiac arrhythmia [Geodon (ziprasidone), 2001].

CONCLUSIONS

Neurologic drug therapy in the elderly presents formidable challenges for the clinician. Alterations in pharmacokinetics and pharmacodynamics because of aging and disease affect response and increase the risk of adverse reactions. Although drug elimination declines with advancing age, substantial interpatient variability is seen, which complicates dose estimation. The use of multiple prescription and over-the-counter drugs, vitamins, and natural products significantly increases the likelihood of drug interactions. Minimizing the number of drugs, maintaining up-to-date records on medication use, ensuring good compliance, and starting with low doses and slowly titrating a drug are important factors in providing safe and effective therapy. Patients need to be told to advise their physicians when they are starting or discontinuing a medication or natural product. Application of basic principles will result in improved outcomes, a lower risk of adverse reactions, and the ability to prevent or manage interactions.

REFERENCES

Aldenkamp AP, Baker G, Mulder OG, et al. A multicenter, randomized clinical study to evaluate the effect on cognitive function of topiramate compared with valproate as add-on therapy to carbamazepine in patients with partial-onset seizures *Epilepsia* 2000;41(9):1167–1178.

Alvir JM, Lieberman JA, Safferman AZ, et al. Clozapine-induced agranulocytosis. Incidence and risk factors in the United States. *N Engl J Med* 1993;329(3):162–167.

Anderson GD. A mechanistic approach to antiepileptic drug interactions. *Ann Pharmacother* 1998;32(5):554–563.

Aronoff GR, Bergstrom RF, Pottratz ST, et al. Fluoxetine kinetics and protein binding in normal and impaired renal function. *Clin Pharmacol Ther* 1984;36(1):138–144.

Bates D, Leape L. Adverse drug reactions. In: Carruthers S, Hoffman B, Melmon K, et al., eds. *Melmon and Morrelli's clinical pharmacology*, 4th ed. New York: McGraw-Hill, 2000:1223–1256.

Beers MH, Fingold SF, Ouslander JG, et al. Characteristics and quality of prescribing by doctors practicing in nursing homes. *J Am Geriatr Soc* 1993;41(8):802–807.

Bender A. Effect of age on intestinal absorption: implications for drug absorption in the elderly. *J Am Geriatr Soc* 1968;16(12):1331–1339.

Berchou RC. Maximizing the benefit of pharmacotherapy in Parkinson's disease *Pharmacotherapy* 2000;20(1 Pt 2):33S–42S.

Blackshear JL, Davidman M, Stillman MT. Identification of risk for renal insufficiency from nonsteroidal anti-inflammatory drugs. *Arch Intern Med* 1983;143(6):1130–1134.

Blazer DGD, Federspiel CF, Ray WA, et al. The risk of anticholinergic toxicity in the elderly: a study of prescribing practices in two populations. *J Gerontol* 1983;38(1):31–35.

Brodie MJ. Tiagabine pharmacology in profile. *Epilepsia* 1995;36(Suppl 6):S7–S9.

Campion EW, deLabry LO, Glynn RJ. The effect of age on serum albumin in healthy males: report from the Normative Aging Study. *J Gerontol* 1988;43(1):M18–M20.

Carbonin P, Pahor M, Bernabei R, et al. Is age an independent risk factor of adverse drug reactions in hospitalized medical patients? *J Am Geriatr Soc* 1991;39(11):1093–1099.

Castleden CM, George CF, Marcer D, et al. Increased sensitivity to nitrazepam in old age. *BMJ* 1977;1(6052):10–12.

Cereghino JJ, Biton V, Abou-Khalil B, et al. Levetiracetam for partial seizures: results of a double-blind, randomized clinical trial. *Neurology* 2000;55(2):236–242.

Chapron D. Drug disposition and response. In: Delafuente J, Stewart R, eds. *Therapeutics in the elderly*, 3rd ed. Cincinnati: Harvey Whitney Books Company, 2001:257–288.

Cockcroft DW, Gault MH. Prediction of creatinine clearance from serum creatinine. *Nephron* 1976;16(1):31–41

Cook PJ, Flanagan R, James IM. Diazepam tolerance: effect of age, regular sedation, and alcohol. *BMJ* 1984;289(6441):351–353.

Cunningham G. Adverse drug reactions in the elderly and their prevention. *Scott Med J* 1997;42(5):136–137.

Davidson J. Seizures and bupropion: a review. *J Clin Psychiatry* 1989;50(7):256–261.

Davies NM, McLachlan AJ, Day RO, et al. Clinical pharmacokinetics and pharmacodynamics of celecoxib: a selective cyclo-oxygenase-2 inhibitor. *Clin Pharmacokinet* 2000;38(3):225–242.

Divoll M, Greenblatt DJ, Harmatz JS, et al. Effect of age and gender on disposition of temazepam. *J Pharm Sci* 1981;70(10):1104–1107.

Edelman I, Leibman J. Anatomy of body water and electrolytes. *Am J Med* 1959;27:256–277.

Evans M, Triggs E, Cheung M, et al. Gastric emptying rate in the elderly: implications for drug therapy. *J Am Geriatr Soc* 1981;29(5):201–205.

Fawcett J, Barkin RL. Review of the results from clinical studies on the efficacy, safety and tolerability of mirtazapine for the treatment of patients with major depression. *J Affect Disord* 1998;51(3):267–285.

Fleisher D, Li C, Zhou Y, et al. Drug, meal and formulation interactions influencing drug absorption after oral admin-

istration. Clinical implications. *Clin Pharmacokinet* 1999;36(3):233–254.

Forbes G, Reina J. Adult lean body mass declines with age: some longitudinal observations. *Metabolism* 1970;19(9):653–663.

Forsman A, Ohman R. Studies on serum protein binding of haloperidol. *Current Therapeutic Research, Clinical & Experimental* 1977;21(2):245–255.

Fromm MF. P-glycoprotein: a defense mechanism limiting oral bioavailability and CNS accumulation of drugs International. *J Clin Pharmacol Ther* 2000;38(2):69–74.

Fromm MF, Kim RB, Stein CM, et al. Inhibition of P-glycoprotein-mediated drug transport: a unifying mechanism to explain the interaction between digoxin and quinidine [see comments]. *Circulation* 1999;99(4):552–557.

Fulton B, Benfield P. Galanthamine. *Drugs Aging* 1996;9(1):60–67.

Geodon (ziprasidone). Package insert. Pfizer, New York, 2001.

Gibaldi M, Schwartz MA. Apparent effect of probenecid on the distribution of penicillins in man. *Clin Pharmacol Ther* 1968;9(3):345–349.

Gidal BE, Lensmeyer GL. Therapeutic monitoring of topiramate: evaluation of the saturable distribution between erythrocytes and plasma of whole blood using an optimized high-pressure liquid chromatography method. *Ther Drug Monit* 1999;21(5):567–576.

Glazer WM, Morgenstern H, Doucette JT. Predicting the long-term risk of tardive dyskinesia in outpatients maintained on neuroleptic medications. *J Clin Psychiatry* 1993;54(4):133–139.

Gracon SI, Knapp MJ, Berghoff WG, et al. Safety of tacrine: clinical trials, treatment IND, and postmarketing experience. *Alzheimer Dis Assoc Disord* 1998;12(2):93–101.

Graves T, Hanlon JT, Schmader KE, et al. Adverse events after discontinuing medications in elderly outpatients *Arch Intern Med* 1997;157(19):2205–2210.

Greenblatt D. Reduced serum albumin concentration in the elderly: a report for the Boston Collaborative Drug Surveillance program. *J Am Geriatr Soc* 1979;27(1):20–22.

Greenblatt DJ, Divoll M, Harmatz JS, et al. Oxazepam kinetics: effects of age and sex. *J Pharmacol Exp Ther* 1980;215(1):86–91.

Greenblatt DJ, Harmatz JS, Shader RI. Clinical pharmacokinetics of anxiolytics and hypnotics in the elderly. Part I. Therapeutic considerations. *Clin Pharmacokinet* 1991;21(3):165–177.

Greiner B, Eichelbaum M, Fritz P, et al. The role of intestinal P-glycoprotein in the interaction of digoxin and rifampin. *J Clin Invest* 1999;104(2):147–153.

Grymonpre RE, Mitenko PA, Sitar DS, et al. Drug-associated hospital admissions in older medical patients *J Am Geriatr Soc* 1988;36(12):1092–1098.

Gupta S. P-glycoprotein expression and regulation. Age-related changes and potential effects on drug therapy. *Drugs Aging* 1995;7(1):19–29.

Gutierrez M, Stimmel G. Psychiatric disorders. In: Delafuente J, Stewart R, eds. *Therapeutics in the elderly*, 3rd ed. Cincinnati; Harvey Whitney Books Company, 2001:471–490.

Hallas J, Gram LF, Grodum E, et al. Drug related admissions to medical wards: a population based survey. *Br J Clin Pharmacol* 1992;33(1):61–68.

Hallstrom C, Lader MH. Diazepam and *N*-desmethyldiazepam concentrations in saliva, plasma and CSF. *Br J Clin Pharmacol* 1980;9(4):333–339.

Hanlon J, Gray S, Schmader K. Adverse drug reactions. In: Delafuente J, Stewart R, eds. *Therapeutics in the elderly*, 3rd ed. Cincinnati. Harvey Whitney Books Company, 2001:289–314.

Hanlon JT, Schmader KE, Koronkowski MJ, et al. Adverse drug events in high risk older outpatients. *J Am Geriatr Soc* 1997;45(8):945–894.

Henn K. Phenytoin interactions with other drugs: clinical aspects. In: Levy R, Mattson RH, Meldrum BS, eds. *Antiepileptic drugs*, 4th ed. New York: Raven Press, 1995: 315–328.

Hoffman C, Rice D, Sung HY. Persons with chronic conditions. Their prevalence and costs *JAMA* 1996;276(18): 1473–1479.

Iber FL, Murphy PA, Connor ES. Age-related changes in the gastrointestinal system. Effects on drug therapy. *Drugs Aging* 1994;5(1):34–48.

Jeste DV, Caligiuri MP, Paulsen JS, et al. Risk of tardive dyskinesia in older patients. A prospective longitudinal study of 266 outpatients. *Arch Gen Psychiatry* 1995;52 (9):756–765.

Jusko WJ, Gretch M. Plasma and tissue protein binding of drugs in pharmacokinetics. *Drug Metab Rev* 1976;1: 43–140.

Kaye CM, Haddock RE, Langley PF, et al. A review of the metabolism and pharmacokinetics of paroxetine in man. *Acta Psychiatr Scand Suppl* 1989;350(2):60–75.

Koller WC. Levodopa in the treatment of Parkinson's disease. *Neurology* 2000;55(11):S2–S12.

Koller WC, Pahwa R. Treating motor fluctuations with controlled-release levodopa preparations. *Neurology* 1994;44 (7 Suppl 6):S23–S28.

Krasinski SD, Russell RM, Samloff IM, et al. Fundic atrophic gastritis in an elderly population. Effect on hemoglobin and several serum nutritional indicators. *J Am Geriatr Soc* 1986;34(11):800–806.

Kulshrestha VK, Thomas M, Wadsworth J, et al. Interaction between phenytoin and antacids. *Br J Clin Pharmacol* 1978;6(2):177–179.

Kyriakopoulos AA, Greenblatt DJ, Shader RI. Clinical pharmacokinetics of lorazepam: a review. *J Clin Psychiatry* 1978;39(10 Pt 2):16–23.

Larson EB, Kukull WA, Buchner D, et al. Adverse drug reactions associated with global cognitive impairment in elderly persons. *Ann Intern Med* 1987;107(2):169–173.

Leppik IE, Willmore LJ, Homan RW, et al. Efficacy and safety of zonisamide: results of a multicenter study. *Epilepsy Res* 1993;14(2):165–173.

Levy G. Predicting effective drug concentrations for individual patients. Determinants of pharmacodynamic variability. *Clin Pharmacokinet* 1998;34(4):323–333.

Lin JH, Lu AY. Inhibition and induction of cytochrome P450 and the clinical implications *Clin Pharmacokinet* 1998;35 (5):361–390.

Lindeman RD. Overview: renal physiology and pathophysiology of aging. *Am J Kidney Dis* 1990;16(4): 275–82.

Lindeman RD, Tobin J, Shock NW. Longitudinal studies on the rate of decline in renal function with age. *J Am Geriatr Soc* 1985;33(4):278–285.

Lockwood GF, Albert KS, Szpunar GJ, et al. Pharmacokinetics of ibuprofen in man. III: Plasma protein binding. *J Pharmacokinet Biopharm* 1983;11(5):469–482.

Lovat LB. Age related changes in gut physiology and nutritional status. *Gut* 1996;38(3):306–309.

Mannesse CK, Derkx FH, de Ridder MA, et al. Adverse drug reactions in elderly patients as contributing factor for hospital admission: cross sectional study. *BMJ* 1997;315(7115):1057–1058.

Marder SR, Meibach RC. Risperidone in the treatment of schizophrenia. *Am J Psychiatry* 1994;151(6):825–835.

Marty JJ, Kilpatrick CJ, Moulds RF. Intra-dose variation in plasma protein binding of sodium valproate in epileptic patients. *Br J Clin Pharmacol* 1982;14(3): 399–404.

Masand PS. Side effects of antipsychotics in the elderly. *J Clin Psychiatry* 2000;61(3; Suppl 8):43–51.

Mayer U, Wagenaar E, Beijnen JH, et al. Substantial excretion of digoxin via the intestinal mucosa and prevention of long-term digoxin accumulation in the brain by the mdr 1a P-glycoprotein. *Br J Pharmacol* 1996;119(5): 1038–1044.

McManus DQ, Arvanitis LA, Kowalcyk BB. Quetiapine, a novel antipsychotic: experience in elderly patients with psychotic disorders. Seroquel Trial 48 Study Group. *J Clin Psychiatry* 1999;60(5):292-298.

Meltzer HY. Serotonin receptors and antipsychotic drug action. *Psychopharmacol Ser* 1993;10:70–81.

Menting JE, Honig A, Verhey FR, et al. Selective serotonin reuptake inhibitors (SSRIs) in the treatment of elderly depressed patients: a qualitative analysis of the literature on their efficacy and side-effects. *Int Clin Psychopharmacol* 1996;11(3):165–175.

Messenheimer J, Mullens EL, Giorgi L, et al. Safety review of adult clinical trial experience with lamotrigine. *Drug Saf* 1998;18(4):281–296.

Meyer BR. Renal function in aging. *J Am Geriatr Soc* 1989;37(8):791–800.

Michalets EL. Update: clinically significant cytochrome P-450 drug interactions. *Pharmacotherapy* 1998;18(1): 84–112.

Miller M. Renal and hormonal changes affecting fluid and electrolyte balance in the elderly. In: Rowan AJ, Ramsay RE, eds. *Seizures and epilepsy in the elderly*. Boston: Butterworth-Heinemann, 1997:29–43.

Moore AR, O'Keeffe ST. Drug-induced cognitive impairment in the elderly. *Drugs Aging* 1999;15(1):15–28.

Muhlberg W, Platt D. Age-dependent changes of the kidneys: pharmacological implications *Gerontology* 1999;45 (5):243–253.

Naranjo CA, Herrmann N, Mittmann N, et al. Recent advances in geriatric psychopharmacology. *Drugs Aging* 1995;7(3):184–202.

Nielsen OA, Johannessen AC, Bardrum B. Oxcarbazepine-induced hyponatremia, a cross-sectional study. *Epilepsy Res* 1988;2(4):269–271.

Nishiguchi K, Ohnishi N, Iwakawa S, et al. Pharmacokinetics of zonisamide: saturable distribution into human and rat erythrocytes and into rat brain. *J Pharmacobiodyn* 1992;15(8):409–415.

Nolan L, O'Malley K. Adverse drug reactions in the elderly. *British Journal of Hospital Medicine* 1989;41(5):446, 448,452–457.

Nyengaard JR, Bendtsen TF. Glomerular number and size in relation to age, kidney weight, and body surface in normal man. *Anat Rec* 1992;232(2):194–201.

Okey AB. Enzyme induction in the cytochrome P-450 system. *Pharmacol Ther* 1990;45(2):241–298.

Parker BM, Cusack BJ, Vestal RE. Pharmacokinetic optimisation of drug therapy in elderly patients. *Drugs Aging* 1995;7(1):10–18.

Pendlebury SC, Moses DK, Eadie MJ. Hyponatraemia during oxcarbazepine therapy. *Hum Toxicol* 1989;8(5):337–344.

Pike E, Skuterud B, Kierulf P. The relative importance of albumin, lipoproteins and orosomucoid for drug serum binding. *Clin Pharmacokinet* 1984;9(Suppl 1):84–101.

Platten HP, Schweizer E, Dilger K, et al. Pharmacokinetics and the pharmacodynamic action of midazolam in young and elderly patients undergoing tooth extraction. *Clin Pharmacol Ther* 1998;63(5):552–560.

Radominska-Pandya A, Czernik PJ, Little JM, et al. Structural and functional studies of UDP-glucuronosyltransferases. *Drug Metab Rev* 1999;31(4):817–899.

Reynolds CF 3rd, Kupfer DJ, Hoch CC, et al. Sleeping pills for the elderly: are they ever justified? *J Clin Psychiatry* 1985;46(2 Pt 2):9–12.

Rigler SK, Webb MJ, Redford L, et al. Weight outcomes among antidepressant users in nursing facilities. *J Am Geriatr Soc* 2001;49(1):49–55.

Ring BJ, Binkley SN, Roskos L, et al. Effect of fluoxetine, norfluoxetine, sertraline and desmethyl sertraline on human CYP3A catalyzed 1'-hydroxy midazolam formation in vitro. *J Pharmacol Exp Ther* 1995;275(3): 1131–1135.

Risperidal (risperidone). Package Insert. Janssen Pharmaceutica, Titusville, NJ, 1999.

Roberts J, Tumer N. Pharmacodynamic basis for altered drug action in the elderly. *Clin Geriatr Med* 1988;4(1): 127–149.

Robinson DS, Roberts DL, Smith JM, et al. The safety profile of nefazodone. *J Clin Psychiatry* 1996;57(Suppl 2): 31–38.

Rogers SL, Friedhoff LT. The efficacy and safety of donepezil in patients with Alzheimer's disease: results of a US multicentre, randomized, double-blind, placebo-controlled trial. The Donepezil Study Group. *Dementia* 1996; 7(6):293–303.

Rosenfeld W, Schaefer P, Pace K. Weight loss patterns with topiramate therapy [abstract]. *Epilepsia* 1997;38(Suppl 3):58.

Rosler M, Anand R, Cicin-Sain A, et al. Efficacy and safety of rivastigmine in patients with Alzheimer's disease: international randomised controlled trial. *BMJ* 1999;318 (7184):633–638.

Roxe DM. Aging and renal function. *Compr Ther* 1991;17 (2):13–19.

Rubin A, Lemberger L, Dhahir P. Physiologic disposition of pergolide. *Clin Pharmacol Ther* 1981;30(2):258–265.

Saltzman JR, Kowdley KV, Pedrosa MC, et al. Bacterial overgrowth without clinical malabsorption in elderly hypochlorhydric subjects [see comments]. *Gastroenterology* 1994;106(3):615–623.

Schaber G, Stevens I, Gaertner HJ, et al. Pharmacokinetics of clozapine and its metabolites in psychiatric patients: plasma protein binding and renal clearance. *Br J Clin Pharmacol* 1998;46(5):453–459.

Schor JD, Levkoff SE, Lipsitz LA, et al. Risk factors for delirium in hospitalized elderly *JAMA* 1992;267(6): 827–831.

Schran HF, Bhuta SI, Schwarz HJ, et al. The pharmacokinetics of bromocriptine in man *Adv Biochem Psychopharmacol* 1980;23(4):125–139.

Serzone (nefazodone). Package Insert. Bristol-Myers Squibb, Princeton, NJ, 2001.

Shock N, Watkin D, Yiengst M, et al. Age difference in the water content of the body as related to basal oxygen consumption in males. *J Gerontol* 1963;18:1–8.

Sorock GS, Shimkin EE. Benzodiazepine sedatives and the risk of falling in a community-dwelling elderly cohort. *Arch Intern Med* 1988;148(11):2441–2444.

Sotaniemi EA, Arranto AJ, Pelkonen O, et al. Age and cytochrome P450-linked drug metabolism in humans: an analysis of 226 subjects with equal histopathologic conditions. *Clin Pharmacol Ther* 1997;61(3):331–339.

Soumerai SB, Ross-Degnan D. Inadequate prescription-drug coverage for Medicare enrollees—a call to action [published erratum appears in *N Engl J Med* 1999;340(12): 976] *N Engl J Med* 1999;340(9):722–728.

Staab JP, Evans DL. Efficacy of venlafaxine in geriatric depression. *Depress Anxiety* 2000;12(Suppl 1):63–68.

Stewart BH, Kugler AR, Thompson PR, et al. A saturable transport mechanism in the intestinal absorption of gabapentin is the underlying cause of the lack of proportionality between increasing dose and drug levels in plasma. *Pharm Res* 1993;10(2):276–281.

Stewart RB. Drug use in the elderly. In: Delafuente J, Stewart R, eds. *Therapeutics in the elderly*, 3rd ed. Cincinnati: Harvey Whitney Books Company, 2001:235–256.

Street JS, Clark WS, Gannon KS, et al. Olanzapine treatment of psychotic and behavioral symptoms in patients with Alzheimer disease in nursing care facilities: a double-blind, randomized, placebo-controlled trial. The HGEU Study Group. *Arch Gen Psychiatry* 2000;57(10): 968–976.

Sweet RA, Mulsant BH, Gupta B, et al. Duration of neuroleptic treatment and prevalence of tardive dyskinesia in late life. *Arch Gen Psychiatry* 1995;52(6):478–486.

Sweet RA, Pollock BG. Neuroleptics in the elderly: guidelines for monitoring. *Harv Rev Psychiatry* 1995;2(6): 327–335.

Swift CG, Swift MR, Ankier SI, et al. Single dose pharmacokinetics and pharmacodynamics of oral loprazolam in the elderly. *Br J Clin Pharmacol* 1985;20(2): 119–128.

Taeuber CM. Numerical growth. In: *Current population reports sixty-five plus in America*. 1992;Chapter 2.

Tasmar (tolcapone). Package insert. Roche Laboratories, Nutley, New Jersey, 1998.

Tephly T, Green M, Puig J, et al. Endogenous substrates for UDP-glucuronosyltransferases. *Xenobiotica* 1988; 18(11):1201–1210.

Teunissen MW, Bakker W, Meerburg-Van der Torren JE, et al. Influence of rifampicin treatment on antipyrine clearance and metabolite formation in patients with tuberculosis. *Br J Clin Pharmacol* 1984;18(5):701–706.

Tiseo PJ, Rogers SL, Friedhoff LT. Pharmacokinetic and pharmacodynamic profile of donepezil HCl following evening administration. *Br J Clin Pharmacol* 1998;46 (Suppl 1):13–18.

van Harten J. Clinical pharmacokinetics of selective serotonin reuptake inhibitors. *Clin Pharmacokinet* 1993;24 (3):203–220.

Vanzant F, Alvarez W, Eusterman G, et al. The normal range of gastric acidity from youth to old age. *Arch Intern Med* 1932;49(3):345–359.

Venulet J, ten Ham M. Methods for monitoring and documenting adverse drug reactions. *Int J Clin Pharmacol Ther* 1996;34(3):112–129.

Versed (midazolam). Package Insert. Roche Laboratories Inc., Nutley, New Jersey, 1998.

Wallace SM, Verbeeck RK. Plasma protein binding of drugs in the elderly. *Clin Pharmacokinet* 1987;12(1): 41–72.

Wasserstein A, Rak I, Reife R. Nephrolithiasis during treatment with topiramate [abstract]. *Epilepsia* 1995;36(Suppl 3):S153

Watkins PB. The barrier function of CYP3A4 and P-glycoprotein in the small bowel. *Adv Drug Deliv Rev* 1997;27 (2-3):161–170.

Watkins PB, Wrighton SA, Schuetz EG, et al. Identification of glucocorticoid-inducible cytochromes P-450 in the intestinal mucosa of rats and man. *J Clin Invest* 1987;80(4): 1029–1036.

Whelton A, Schulman G, Wallemark C, et al. Effects of celecoxib and naproxen on renal function in the elderly. *Arch Intern Med* 2000;160(10):1465–1470.

Wong IC, Mawer GE, Sander JW. Factors influencing the incidence of lamotrigine-related skin rash. *Ann Pharmacother* 1999;33(10):1037–1042.

Woodhouse K, Wynne HA. Age-related changes in hepatic function. Implications for drug therapy. *Drugs Aging* 1992;2(3):243–255.

Wright J. Drug interactions. In: Carruthers S, Hoffman B, Melmon K, et al., eds. *Melmon and Morrelli's clinical pharmacology*, 4th ed. New York: McGraw-Hill, 2000: 1257–1266.

Wynne HA, Cope LH, Mutch E, et al. The effect of age upon liver volume and apparent liver blood flow in healthy man. *Hepatology* 1989;9(2):297–301.

Yu DK. The contribution of P-glycoprotein to pharmacokinetic drug-drug interactions. *J Clin Pharmacol* 1999;39 (12):1203–1211.

Zhang QY, Dunbar D, Ostrowska A, et al. Characterization of human small intestinal cytochromes P-450. *Drug Metab Dispos* 1999;27(7):804–809.

Zyprexa (olanzapine). Package Insert. Eli Lilly and Company, Indianapolis, IN, 2000.

4

Neurologic Considerations in the Postmenopausal Woman

Joyce Liporace, Carissa C. Pineda, and Naomi Wasserman

Hormones play a critical role in the regulation and maintenance of normal health and in the expression of neurologic disorders. In women, cyclic alterations in steroid hormones during reproductive life and the subsequent marked decline of hormones with ovarian failure can have specific influences on disease. Today, women are aging successfully and living longer. They typically spend one third of their lives after menopause. In the United States, there are 35 million women over the age of 65 and 5 million women over the age of 85. These numbers will double by the year 2040 (Lobo, 1999). A woman at age 50 has an average life expectancy of 82.8 years. Her lifetime risk of developing stroke is 20% and of dying from it 8%. For Alzheimer's dementia, her risk of disease increases rapidly after age 65, with a 50% risk after age 85. For epilepsy, she faces a second peak in incidence after age 60. Endogenous and supplemental steroid hormones alter the expression of these as well as other neurologic disorders. This has led to an increased interest in understanding the link between hormones and neurologic disease.

This chapter addresses special neurologic concerns for postmenopausal women and provides a rationale for strategies to improve healthcare for the mature woman. An overview of menopause and the interactions of steroid hormones and the brain are discussed, followed by discussion of specific diseases.

MENOPAUSE

Menopause is the permanent cessation of menstruation after the loss of ovarian function. The median age at menopause in the United States is 50 to 52 years, with 1% of women experiencing menopause before age 40 (Lobo, 1999). Menopause is a process, derived from the Greek word, *meno* or month and *pausis* or cessation, which can only be defined retrospectively after 12 months of amenorrhea. The phase from the onset of irregular menses to menopause is called "perimenopause," which has an average duration of 5 years. It includes the year after cessation of menses. This time is also referred to as the "climacteric," which is the transition from reproductive to nonreproductive life. A woman is perimenopausal if serial follicle-stimulating hormone (FSH) levels are >20 IU/L and estradiol is <60 pg/mL. During perimenopause, ovarian function is variable with a shortened follicular phase and an increase in defective ovulation and anovulation. Other symptoms (e.g., hot flashes and night sweats) also occur. Hyperestrogenemia can be an early feature of perimenopause, but decreased estrogen levels mark the immediate premenopausal period (Lobo, 1999). It is not a time of steady decline; instead, it is marked by peaks and valleys. This feature can be clinically frustrating because it can lead to fluctuating symptoms (e.g., changes in seizure and headache frequency).

The hypothalamic-pituitary axis changes dramatically during and before menopause. The most marked change is the increased secretion of FSH, by the pituitary. Luteinizing hormone (LH) levels remain in the normal range, despite a rise in FSH before menopause. With menopause, LH levels rise and plateau. The increased levels of FSH and LH are secondary to loss of negative feedback from lower circulating estrogen levels. Additionally, ovarian follicles no longer release inhibin, which normally suppresses FSH.

With cessation of menstruation, a decline occurs in estradiol concentration that is dramatic for the first 12 months and then declines only gradually. The concentration of estrone, a weaker estrogen, also falls after menopause. Peripheral aromatization of adrenal androgens in adipose tissue, muscle, and skin becomes the major source of estrogens after menopause. Obese postmenopausal women have higher levels of circulating estrogen because of increased aromatization in adipose tissues.

Progesterone levels in perimenopausal women can be normal, but luteal phase progesterone typically declines. Women can go through long phases of amenorrhea with absent progesterone secretion. With menopause, levels decline to approximately 30% of the concentration present in young women during the follicular phase of the menstrual cycle. The main source of progesterone becomes the adrenal gland. Peripheral conversion of steroids to progesterone is not seen in nonpregnant women.

With aging, ovarian androgen secretion declines. A shift in the pattern of androgen secretion occurs with the maintenance of testosterone at the expense of androstenedione. With the fall in androstenedione, a major source of testosterone, circulating levels of testosterone cannot be maintained and serum levels decline. Typically, the decline in circulating androgens begins before menopause.

STEROID HORMONES AND THE BRAIN

Steroid hormones exert powerful effects on the brain, beginning shortly after conception and continuing throughout life. Sex steroids are highly lipophilic and readily cross the blood–brain barrier. The brain is well known as a target site of peripheral steroid hormones; however, it is also the site of *de novo* synthesis of steroid hormones from cholesterol (Tsutsui et al., 2000). Steroid hormones influence function by immediate membrane effects and by genomic effects. Genomic effects are delayed, taking days to occur, and their effects are sustained for days to weeks after hormone exposure. Steroid hormones bind intranuclear receptors and act as transcription factors that regulate gene expression. Their diversity and magnitude suggest that hormonal therapy may be helpful to treat or prevent neurologic conditions that are sensitive to hor-

mones. A review of the sex steroid hormones and their physiologic effects follow.

Estrogen

The ovary converts acetate to cholesterol and subsequently to other steroids (Fig. 4-1). FSH regulates the formation of estrogen by the ovarian follicle. Additionally, peripheral tissues including liver, fat, skeletal muscle, and hair follicles can convert adrenal androstenedione and testosterone to estrogen. This is the major source of estrogen in men and in postmenopausal women.

During reproductive years, the dominant follicle and the corpus luteum it forms are the main sources of estrogen. Natural estrogens include estradiol, estrone, estriol, and their conjugates. Of the three main human estrogens, estradiol-17 *B* is the most potent. Estradiol is the principal estrogen produced in menstruating women. Estrone, the second major estrogen and the main estrogen in postmenopausal women, is metabolized from estradiol and from peripheral aromatization.

All estrogens circulate in blood, either free or bound to sex hormone-binding globulin (SHBG) or nonspecifically to albumin. Changes in SHBG occur secondary to some medications, for example, enzyme-inducing antiepileptic drugs. Alterations in SHBG alter the concentration of free estradiol and affect bioavailability.

Estrogen has both direct and inductive effects on neurons, glia, and microglia. Neurons contain nuclear receptors for estrogen, predominantly in the pituitary, hypothalamus, amygdala, hippocampus, raphe nuclei, and cerebral cortex. As transcriptional regulators, activated estrogen receptors direct or modulate synthesis of many neurotransmitters and neuropeptides. Estrogen increases acetylcholine (Ach) by inducing choline acetyltransferase, the rate-limiting step of

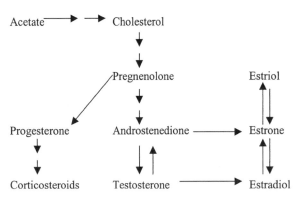

FIG. 4-1. Steroid hormone production.

production. In the hippocampus, estrogen up-regulates N-methyl D-aspartic acid (NMDA) glutamate receptor subtype. It down-regulates gamma-aminobutyric acid (GABA)-A receptor subunits and the synthesis of GABA. Neuronal excitability is further increased by induction of synaptic sprouting. Morphologic studies have shown that estrogen and progesterone induce anatomic changes in neurons of the CA1 region of the hippocampus, a structure critical in memory processing and learning, which has implications for aging, Alzheimer's disease (AD), and epilepsy. Within 12 to 24 hours after estrogen exposure in animals, hippocampal neurons form new dendritic spines and increase synaptic connections (Wooley and McEwen, 1993). The increase in dendritic spine density is reversed with progesterone.

Progesterone

A progestin is a substance that binds to the progesterone receptor and has progestational activity. The most widely recognized progestational activity is transformation of proliferative to secretory endometrium in an estrogen-primed uterus. Progestins can be divided into two groups: natural (the only one is progesterone) and synthetic. All synthetic progesterones are not equal; some are derived from progesterone, whereas others are an alteration of testosterone with greater androgenic properties. Natural progesterone is secreted by the ovary mainly from the corpus luteum during the second half of the menstrual cycle. LH controls progesterone secretion. Progesterone circulates primarily bound to albumin and is extensively metabolized. Its half-life in blood is just a few minutes, although its actions on tissues continue after it has disappeared from serum.

Progesterone receptors are found in the hypothalamus and hippocampus, and diffusely throughout the cerebral cortex, a distribution similar to estrogen, although progesterone receptors are more widespread throughout the neocortex. Progesterone and several of its metabolites induce sedation and decrease neuronal excitability. Its anxiolytic and hypnotic effects are partly mediated by enhancement of the inhibitory action of the neurotransmitter GABA. Additionally, progesterone reduces glutamate excitation. Genomic effects include up-regulation of GABA and GABA-A receptor subunits.

Androgens

Traditionally, androgens are thought of as male hormones. However they clearly are important in women, playing a role in sexual drive, enhancement

of insulin effect, cognition, bone health, sexual hair development, muscle mass, stature, and development of the immune system.

Women have androgen receptors in the brain, as do men. As with estrogen and progesterone, androgens can modify nervous system structures, cognition, and mood. The major sources for circulating androgens during the reproductive period are the ovary, the adrenal cortex, and peripheral conversion of dehydroepiandrosterone and androstenedione. After menopause, the main source of circulating testosterone is peripheral conversion of adrenal androstanedione. Decreased adrenal androgen production is noted with age but is independent of menopause. Adrenal and ovarian production of androgens declines beginning at age 20, and serum androgen levels are decreased by half at age 40. Smaller changes are seen after age 60 (Lobo, 1999).

STROKE

Stroke, one of the leading causes of death in the United States, is a primary cause of adult disability. Although stroke is more common in men, the overall mortality rate is higher in postmenopausal women (60.6% versus 39.4%) (Kaplan, 1998).

Stroke risk factors are identical in men and women, although women carry the added burden of risks associated with pregnancy, hormonal contraception, and the effects of hormonal decline after ovarian failure. Estrogen is considered to be an endogenous neuroprotective agent. Vascular endothelium and smooth muscle bind estrogen with high affinity. Estrogen promotes vasodilatation and alters both short-term and long-term vasomotor tone. Its actions depend on changes in renin, angiotensin-converting enzyme, nitric oxide, and prostaglandins (Mendelsohn and Karas, 1998). Estrogen favorably alters serum lipid concentrations through mediation of hepatic apoprotein genes. It decreases serum cholesterol, lowers low-density lipoprotein (LDL) cholesterol, and increases serum high-density lipoprotein (HDL) cholesterol. Coadministration of progesterone blunts these lipid effects because progesterone alone tends to raise LDL and lower HDL cholesterol.

Sex steroids may play a role during ischemic stress (Table 4-1). It is hypothesized that estrogen decreases oxygen free radical induced brain injury by preserving endogenous antioxidants. Additionally, estrogen and testosterone are associated with a greater potential for fibrinolysis.

Reports evaluating hormone replacement therapy (HRT) and the risk of stroke in the postmenopausal

TABLE 4-1. *Sex steroid effects on the brain related to stroke*

Estrogen	Increased vasodilatation
	Decreased total and LDL cholesterol
	Increased HDL cholesterol
	Decreased fibrinogen, antithrombin III
	Increased nitric oxide
	Antioxidant effects
Progesterone	Increased LDL cholesterol
	Decreased HDL cholesterol
	Decreased vasodilatation
Testosterone	Decreased plasminogen activator inhibitor
	Decreased lipoprotein
	Enhanced fibrinolysis

HDL, high-density lipoprotein; LDL, low-density lipoprotein.

population are inconsistent. The Framingham Heart Study showed that postmenopausal use of HRT resulted in an increased risk of stroke (Kaplan, 1998). However, others report a reduced risk or no effect on stroke incidence (Pettiti et al., 1998). HRT may benefit a subpopulation of women at greater risk for disease, that is, women with risk factors of smoking and elevated cholesterol. Additionally, HRT has been found to reduce the risk of subarachnoid hemorrhage, particularly in postmenopausal smokers (Longstreth et al., 1994).

It is important to recognize the secondary effects of hormone therapy on cardiovascular disease because this is a critical stroke risk factor. Women with menopause at a younger age who never used hormonal therapy have a higher risk of cardiovascular disease and stroke (Hu et al., 1999). Prospective and retrospective studies demonstrate that estrogen replacement reduces the primary risk of cardiovascular disease in previously healthy postmenopausal women by 35% to 50% (Mendelsohn and Karas, 1998).

Estrogen in women with established cardiac disease shows little benefit. In a study of 309 nurses with heart disease, neither estrogen alone nor estrogen and progesterone affected progression of coronary atherosclerosis measured by angiography (Herrington et al., 2000). In one randomized study of elderly postmenopausal women with many cardiac risk factors, estrogen replacement increased the risk of coronary disease in the first year but decreased coronary events in years 4 to 5 (Hulley et al., 1998). The Women's Health Initiative trial, which is enrolling 8,000 women, will provide additional information on this topic in 2005. There are ongoing trials studying the

effects of selective estrogen receptor modulators (SERM) on the secondary prevention of heart disease.

MEMORY AND DEMENTIA

Women and men perform similarly on most cognitive tests; however, on average, men score better on visuospatial and mathematical reasoning, whereas women score higher on verbal memory and verbal fluency. Such differences may be mediated by both long-term and short-term exposure to steroid hormones.

Evidence indicates that specific aspects of memory co-vary with sex steroids in healthy men and women. Alterations in performance are noted across the menstrual cycle in normal women, with higher estradiol levels linked to better verbal memory (Phillips and Sherwin, 1992). In postmenopausal women, estrogen users attained higher scores on specific cognitive tasks of immediate and delayed paragraph recall. No changes were found in other cognitive tasks or in tests of spatial memory (Kampen and Sherwin, 1994). This suggests a specific—not global—effect in some women. In contrast, progesterone can reduce cognitive performance. In one study, oral progesterone given to healthy young women resulted in impaired symbol copying, fatigue, and confusion, along with reduced immediate verbal recall scores (Freeman et al., 1993).

AD is the most common form of dementia characterized by memory loss that ultimately interferes with occupational and social functioning. Beginning at age 65, the prevalence of AD doubles every 5 years. Independent of age, women are two to three times more likely than men to have AD. Language is more severely affected in women, independent of disease severity. A growing number of studies support the concept that supplemental estrogen may delay the onset of cognitive decline.

A number of estrogen effects may be relevant to AD (Table 4-2). Estrogen modulates growth factors, reduces oxidative stress, and promotes the formation of synaptic connections. It influences several neurotransmitters, including Ach, which plays a critical role in AD. Additionally, estrogen increases the expression of apolipoprotein E and may reduce the formation of B amyloid protein.

A metaanalysis of 10 studies (8 case-control) suggested that neurologically normal estrogen users had a 29% lower rate of developing AD (Yaffe et al., 1998). Two large, prospective, community-based studies investigated the association of estrogen re-

TABLE 4-2. *Sex steroid effects on the brain related to Alzheimer's disease*

Estrogen
  Increased cholinergic transmission
  Antioxidant effect
  Increased apolipoprotein E
  Decreased beta amyloid protein
  Stimulation of synaptic density in hippocampal
    neurons
  Modulation of growth factors
Progesterone
  Reduction of synaptic density in hippocampal
    neurons

TABLE 4-3. *Sex steroid effects on the brain related to epilepsy*

	Estrogen	Progesterone
GABA-A chloride conductance	Decreased	Increased
GABA synthesis	Increased	Decreased
Excitatory response to glutamate	Increased	Decreased
Hippocampal dendritic synapses	Increased	Decreased
GABA-A receptor subunit mRNA	Decreased	Increased

GABA, gamma-aminobutyric acid.

placement therapy (ERT) and the risk of developing AD (Tang et al., 1996; Kawas et al, 1997). They provide additional clinical support for a protective role of estrogen. In these studies, oral estrogen used during the postmenopausal period delayed the development of AD and lowered the risk of the disease by 60%. This risk reduction remained significant after adjusting for age, education, ethnicity, and apolipoprotein E genotype.

In contrast to these positive studies, others have found no effect of conjugated estrogen on the treatment of women with mild to moderate AD (Wang et al., 2000; Mulnard et al., 2000; Henderson et al., 2000). Low dose estrogen had no effect on mood, behavior, cognitive performance, or cerebral perfusion in Wang's 12-week study of 50 women. Currently, results of clinical trials do not support the use of estrogen in the treatment of women with AD. Additional long-term studies evaluating the effects of earlier treatment on disease are needed.

No studies have been published on the effect of progesterone or androgens on AD prevention or treatment in either sex.

EPILEPSY

Sex hormones influence the electrical activity of the brain through immediate membrane effects and genomic mechanisms (Table 4-3). Both estrogen and progesterone exert membrane effects, in part, at the GABA-A receptor complex. Animal models of epilepsy demonstrate that estrogen lowers the threshold for seizures. Topical application of estradiol to the brains of rabbits produces paroxysmal epileptiform discharges (Logothesis and Harner, 1960). Estradiol acts as an agonist at the NMDA receptor, which increases excitation. It also binds the GABA-A receptor, alters chloride conductance, and reduces GABA-mediated inhibition. Genomic effects of estrogen include reduction of GABA concentration and a re-

duction in GABA-A receptor subunits. Exposure to estrogen affects neuronal morphology, which promotes synaptogenesis (see Steroid Hormones and the Brain, page 46). Progesterone has the opposite effect and protects against seizures. It enhances GABA-mediated neuronal inhibition and reduces glutamate excitation. In humans, intravenous progesterone diminishes epileptic discharges (Backstrom et al., 1984). Little is known about the association of testosterone with neuronal excitability and the effect appears to vary with age and gender.

Seizures linked to the menstrual cycle are termed "catamenial epilepsy." With ovulatory cycles, the relatively high estrogen-to-progesterone ratio at ovulation and the rapid progesterone withdrawal just before menses are linked with seizure exacerbation. With anovulatory cycles, seizures are noted throughout the entire luteal phase because of the unopposed action of estrogen. Supplemental natural progesterone has been reported to reduce seizures in women with partial epilepsy (Herzog, 1999), although double-blind placebo trials are needed.

Limited information is available concerning the effects of menopause on epilepsy. Because menopause is a complex process, it is difficult to study and, thus, good prospective studies are lacking. Early in menopause, an increase occurs in anovulatory cycles and in the estrogen-to-progesterone ratio. This would be expected to promote seizures. At the end of menopause, estrogen declines, which may reduce seizures. It can also be predicted that ERT might worsen seizure control.

In a retrospective study based on self-report, most women with epilepsy noted a change in their seizure pattern with menopause: 41% noted worsening, whereas 29% experienced improved seizure control. Additionally, it was suggested that menopause may be a risk factor for seizures: 20% of women in that study had new-onset seizures coincident with menopause (Abassi, 1999). In another self-reported study, 68% of women with catamenial epilepsy reported increased seizures during perimenopause and a subsequent decline in seizures after menopause. This study also found that menopausal women given HRT were at increased risk for seizure exacerbation (63% versus 12% not receiving HRT). The numbers were too small to determine if a differential effect existed for estrogen alone versus combined estrogen and progesterone therapy (Harden et al., 1999). It would be predicted that the addition of progesterone to estrogen might reduce the seizure risk. Epilepsy is not a contraindication to HRT. Instead, women with epilepsy who are prescribed hormones should be monitored carefully for a change in seizure pattern. Safety of HRT in women with epilepsy needs to be evaluated by a large, prospective, randomized trial. The role and safety of SERM is unknown.

HEADACHE

No gender differences are seen in migraine prevalence before puberty. However, after puberty, more women (17.6%) than men (6%) have migraine (Lipton and Stewart, 1993). Peak incidence in women occurs at menarche. Migraines commonly occur in association with menses, with 60% of women experiencing catamenial headaches. The primary trigger appears to be estrogen withdrawal; however, fluctuations in estrogen play a key role. Although prevalence decreases with age, migraine can either improve or worsen with menopause. Typically, migraine without aura increases in frequency and severity with perimenopause; however, after natural menopause, two thirds of women note substantial improvement in their headaches. For migraine with aura, postmenopausal women often note the aura without the headache. Surgical menopause can exacerbate migraine, probably because of the abrupt decline in estradiol. The favorable response of migraine in the postmenopausal period is attributed to the lack of variation in sex hormones.

Women with hormonal responsive migraines may experience headache exacerbation with initiation of cyclic HRT. Reducing the estrogen dose or continuous administration instead of interrupted estrogen replacement may be effective in treating headaches (Fig. 4-2). Androgens may also be useful for treatment of headache (Silberstein and Merrian, 1991). No evidence supports hysterectomy or oophorectomy to treat refractory migraine at any age.

PARKINSON'S DISEASE

Deficits in dopaminergic activity underlie the movement disorder of Parkinson's disease. Estrogen modulates dopaminergic activity in the nigrostriatal system and may influence disease (Table 4-4). It has a direct stimulatory effect on the synthesis of dopamine by activation of tyrosine hydroxylase, the rate-limiting enzyme. Additionally, physiologic levels of estrogen can increase dopamine by reducing catechol-O-methyltransferase (COMT) transcription by as much as 50%, resulting in reduced dopamine degradation (Tsang et al., 2000).

Most studies find that Parkinson's disease is more common in men than women, however the course of disease is not identical in both sexes. The mortality rate is higher in women (Diamond et al., 1990). Conflicting studies exist regarding the effects of estrogen on clinical signs. Some report motor fluctuations linked to the menstrual cycle consistent with a dopaminergic effect. Dyskinesias are increased midcycle while estrogen levels are high, and parkinsonism is increased just before menses when estrogen levels decline (Strijks et al., 1999). Additionally, pregnancy can induce chorea in susceptible women. In one study, low-dose estrogen replacement alone in postmenopausal women with Parkinson's disease significantly reduced motor fluctuation compared with placebo, improving both "on" time and "off," time, based on patient's diaries (Tsang et al., 2000). However, other reports suggest that estrogen has the opposite effect. During the luteal phase of the menstrual

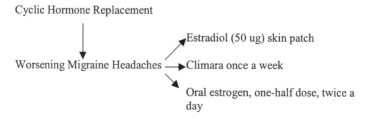

FIG. 4-2. Treatment options for continuous estrogen replacement in women with migraine headache.

TABLE 4-4. *Sex steroid effects on the brain important in Parkinson's disease*

Estrogen
    Increased dopamine synthesis
    Increased dopamine release
    Increased D_1 and D_2 receptors
    Decreased catechol-O-methyltransferase

cycle when both estrogen and progesterone levels are high, some women need an increased dose of levodopa therapy. This indirect sign has been interpreted as an antidopaminergic effect of estrogen (Giladi and Honigman, 1995); however, it may represent a progesterone effect. A double blind, placebo-controlled study in postmenopausal women with Parkinson's disease found no effect on symptoms when estradiol was given but did note that progesterone worsened both objective motor scores and subjective reports (Strijks et al., 1999).

Supplemental estrogen does not seem to reduce disease risk. ERT did not affect the development of Parkinson's disease in 989 healthy postmenopausal women, but it was found to protect against dementia in women with established disease, after adjusting for age, education, and ethnicity (Marder et al., 1998). The effects of combined estrogen and progesterone therapy as well as estrogen replacement alone needs to be evaluated in a large, prospective, controlled trial to determine if progesterone has antagonistic effects on estrogen in Parkinson's disease.

SLEEP

Hypothalamic nuclei and periaqueductal gray are brain areas involved in the regulation of sleep. Because these regions have a high content of estrogen and progesterone receptors, sex steroids can influence sleep architecture. Loss of these hormones with menopause interrupts sleep. The two significant sleep problems affecting menopausal women are insomnia and obstructive sleep apnea, which both have an impact on daytime fatigue, tiredness, and cognitive functioning. Although obstructive sleep apnea is usually more common in men, its incidence increases in postmenopausal women, suggesting a link to hormonal changes (Empson and Purdie, 1999). The mechanism is poorly understood. One possible explanation may be related to decreased respiratory drive and upper airway muscular tone (Ware et al., 2000). It is also thought that premenopausal women are protected from sleep apnea because progesterone stimulates breathing (Shaver and Zenk, 2000).

Furthermore, hot flashes can disturb sleep, causing decreased sleep efficiency and increased rapid eye movement latency (Lobo, 1999). Hot flashes are a vasomotor change that correlates with bursts of activity in hypothalamic pacemaker cells, which trigger release of LH. They are accompanied by short-lived tachycardia, cortical arousal, and awakenings.

Hormonal therapy has been shown to be beneficial in cases of both insomnia and sleep apnea. Effects were seen after 1 month of either estrogen alone or estrogen and progestin in patients with sleep apnea syndrome (Keefe et al., 1999). Healthy postmenopausal women who took estrogen indicated subjective alleviation of sleep complaints (Polo-Kantola et al., 1998), as well as a restoration of normal sleep based on electroencephalographic patterns (Antonijevic et al., 2000).

MULTIPLE SCLEROSIS

Multiple sclerosis, a progressively disabling disease, has a strong gender preference that affects twice as many women as men. The exception to this preference is primary progressive disease, which occurs equally in men and women. Onset of symptoms typically begins between 15 and 40 years of age, with a steep decline in frequency after age 45 to 50. Disease onset is often within a few years of puberty. Because of the strong gender link, there is speculation that a relationship exists between sex hormones and disease prevalence.

The cause of multiple sclerosis remains unknown, but autoimmune processes are critical in development of the disease. Research supports the concept that gender and sex hormones influence autoimmune reactions. Much of the data come from *in vitro* studies, which may not necessarily apply to *in vivo* functioning. Nevertheless, the following observations can be made. Estrogens as a group have both immunosuppressive and immunostimulatory properties, whereas progesterone and androgens tend to suppress the immune system. *In vitro* studies show that progesterone and androgens down-regulate T-cell proliferative response to mitogens. *In vivo*, the number of CD8+ T cells increases after administration of progesterone (Vollenhoven and McGuire, 1994). Additionally, androgens interfere with the *in vitro* maturation processes of B cells.

Clinical data concerning the hormonal effects of multiple sclerosis during pregnancy, suggest that menopause may also modulate multiple sclerosis. High estrogen levels found in the third trimester of pregnancy bring about a reduction in the rate of multiple sclerosis relapse, whereas the sudden withdrawal of estrogen characterizing the postpartum period is associated with a two- to threefold increase in relapse rate (Smith and Studd, 1992). In a self-report study of 149 women with multiple sclerosis, many (60%) noted increased symptoms 1 week before the onset of menses (Kaplan, 1998). These reports, along with the observation that young women with multiple sclerosis seemed less disabled when taking oral contraception, suggest that estrogen exerts a stabilizing or protective effect on the clinical manifestations of multiple sclerosis (Bauer and Hanefeld, 1993). A pilot study involving HRT for pre- and postmenopausal women with multiple sclerosis showed a beneficial effect. Of the postmenopausal women, 54% reported a worsening of symptoms with menopause and 75% of those who had tried HRT reported an improvement (Smith and Studd, 1992).

The protective role of estrogens in the general health of women with multiple sclerosis is further supported by improvement in cognition and bone health with supplementation. Although osteoporosis is linked to menopause and age, patients with multiple sclerosis compound their risk for even greater bone loss as a result of common steroid treatments and immobility. HRT provides a logical treatment choice for those with multiple sclerosis. Further studies to clarify the role of combined estrogen and progesterone in multiple sclerosis are needed.

NEUROONCOLOGIC DISEASES

The scope of neurooncologic disease in mature women includes primary as well as metastatic tumors of the central nervous system (CNS). Although the incidence of primary brain tumors is greater in men than in women (9.2/100,000 versus 8.7/100,000), meningiomas occur most commonly in women (Cudlowicz and Irizarry, 1997).

Meningiomas contain hormonal receptors; consequently, they can become more aggressive during pregnancy or during the luteal phase of the menstrual cycle. High proportions of progesterone and androgen receptors are found in meningiomas. Interestingly, normal adult meninges express very low levels of progesterone receptors. Progesterone may be responsible for meningioma growth (Carroll et al., 1993), although additional studies to clarify the effects of estrogen are needed with the discovery of a second estrogen receptor (Carroll et al., 1999). Interruption of hormone therapy in postmenopausal women with small or asymptomatic meningiomas does not seem warranted; instead, serial imaging is needed (Boullot et al., 1994).

For women, breast tumors account for 27% of all cancers and are the leading cause of brain metastases. Prevalence increases with age. Notably, postmenopausal obesity, which is associated with higher estrogen levels, is associated with a higher risk of breast cancer. Transition to menopause does not affect survival for those diagnosed with cancer early in life; however, HRT increases the risk of developing breast cancer as discussed in the following section.

RISKS AND BENEFITS OF HORMONE REPLACEMENT THERAPY

Menopause is an event in a woman's life that should trigger a risk assessment for chronic disease and initiation of preventive health strategies, including consideration of HRT. Risk assessment begins with a detailed history and physical examination focusing on genitourinary, neuroendocrine, skeletal, and cardiovascular systems. This can be followed by a variety of screening tests for chronic disease (Table 4-5).

Women who use postmenopausal hormones have a lower mortality rate than nonusers. The benefit in survival is greatest for women with high risk of cardiovascular disease (Grodstein et al., 1997), although not in women with established disease (see Stroke section). This survival benefit is lost 5 years after discontinued use and becomes attenuated among long-term hormonal users.

Short-term benefits of HRT include reduction of hot flashes, emotional lability, and vaginal dryness, along with improved sleep. Long-term benefits include reduction in risks for osteoporosis, coronary artery disease, and dementia. The decision to initiate hormonal supplements should take into account each woman's risk for potential benefit as well as potential harm (Fig. 4-3).

Cardiovascular disease is the number one killer of women in the United States. Estrogen can modify disease with its beneficial effects on serum lipids, vascular tone, antioxidant systems, and prostaglandins.

TABLE 4-5. *Screening tests for chronic disease in menopausal women*

12-hour fasting lipid panel
Thyroid function tests
Electrocardiogram
Mini-mental status examination
Papanicolaou smear
Mammogram
Bone density scan

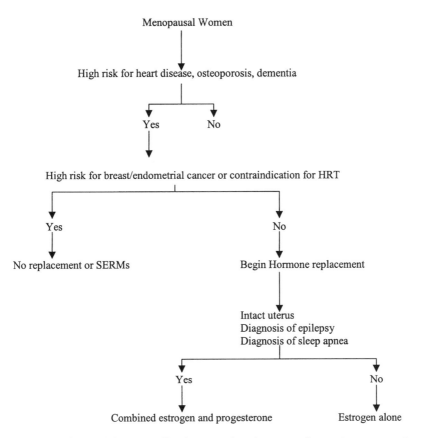

FIG. 4-3. Algorithm for decision regarding hormonal replacement for postmenopausal women.

The presence of cardiovascular risk factors should promote the consideration of ERT.

Osteoporosis is a disease characterized by low bone mass and the consequent increase in fracture risk. It is one of the most common disabling diseases of older women. The National Osteoporosis Foundation recommends bone density screening for all women >65 years of age. Women with one or more risk factors should be screened earlier (Table 4-6). Healthy bone requires adequate attainment of bone matrix formation in childhood and bone remodeling throughout adult life. Peak bone mass is attained by age 20 years followed by gradual decline. Bone loss is accelerated by estrogen deficiency, averaging 2% to 3% per year after menopause. The presence of an abnormal bone scan in postmenopausal women should support the consideration of supplemental estrogen. Both oral and transdermal estrogen decrease bone loss and reduce the incidence of fracture.

Absolute contraindications to ERT include undiagnosed vaginal bleeding, acute liver disease, acute thrombosis or emboli, and current breast or endometrial cancer. Estrogen can induce tumors of the breast, uterus, bone, and kidney. ERT increases the risk of endometrial cancer 5 to 15 times. The risk of breast cancer increases after 5 years of ERT, although 5 years after withdrawal of estrogen this risk is gone (Lobo, 1999). In women at low risk for cardiovascular disease, dementia, and osteoporosis but at high risk for breast or endometrial cancer, the risks of hor-

TABLE 4-6. *Risk factors for osteoporosis*

Genetic: Caucasian race, female sex, familial prevalence
Nutritional: low calcium or vitamin D intake, alcoholism, high caffeine, high sodium, high animal protein
Lifestyle: smoking, low physical activity
Endocrine: early age of menopause (<45 yr), low body weight (<127 pounds)
Medications: corticosteroids, thyroid, antiepileptic drugs

monal replacement outweigh the benefits. A history of breast cancer is a contraindication to traditional estrogens but not to SERM such as raloxifene.

The SERM class of drugs has mixed agonist or antagonist activities at the estrogen receptor, yet they are structurally distinct from estrogen. Although SERM have beneficial effects on lipids and bone health, they do not increase the risk of breast cancer. Unlike estrogen, they do not provide relief from hot flashes or urogenital atrophy. Their effect on CNS estrogen receptors is unknown.

SUMMARY

Gender-based differences in health and disease need to be considered by healthcare providers. We still face the challenge of fully understanding the complex interaction of sex hormones and the brain, along with their relationship to expression of disease. Menopause is a time in a woman's life when hormonal changes cause clinical symptoms and can alter the expression of neurologic disease. It represents an ideal time for assessment of risk for chronic disease and initiation of health maintenance to improve quality of life.

As research continues, promising strategies to reduce the risk of disease and novel hormonal therapies to treat neurologic disorders may be discovered.

REFERENCES

Abbasi F, Krumholz A, Kittner S, et al. Effects of menopause on seizures in women with epilepsy. *Epilepsia* 1999;40(2):205–210.

Antonijevic I, Stalla G, Steiger A. Modulation of the sleep electroencephalogram by estrogen replacement in postmenopausal women. *Am J Obstet Gynecol* 2000;182(2):277–282.

Backstrom T, Zetterlund B, Blom S, et al. Effects of intravenous progesterone infusions on the epileptic discharge frequency in women with partial epilepsy. *Acta Neurol Scand* 1984;69:240–248.

Bauer H, Hanefeld F. *Multiple sclerosis. Its impact from childhood to old age.* London: WB Saunders Company, Ltd, 1993.

Boullot P, Pellissier JF, Devictor B. Quantitative imaging of estrogen and progesterone receptors, estrogen-related protein, and growth fraction: immunocytochemical assays in 52 meningiomas. Correlation with clinical and morphological data. *J Neurosurg* 1994;81:765.

Carroll RS, Glowacka D, Dashner K. Progesterone receptor expression in meningiomas. *Cancer Res* 1993;53:1312.

Carroll RS, Zhang J, Black PM. Expression of estrogen receptors alpha and beta in human meningiomas. *J Neurooncol* 1999;42(2):109–116.

Cudlowicz M, Irizarry M., eds. *Neurologic disorders in women.* Boston: Butterworth-Heinemann, 1997.

Diamond SG, Markham CH, Hoehn MM, et al. An examination of male-female differences in progression and mortality of Parkinson's disease. *Neurology* 1990;40:763–766.

Empson JA, Purdie DW. Effects of sex steroids on sleep. *Ann Med* 1999;31(2):141–145.

Freeman E, Purdy R, Coutifaris C, et al. Anxiolytic metabolites of progesterone: correlation with mood and performance measures following oral progesterone administration to healthy female volunteers. *Clinical Neuroendocrinology* 1993;58:478–484.

Giladi N, Honigman S. Hormones and Parkinson's disease. *Neurology* 1995;45:1028.

Grodstein F, Stampfer M, Colditz G, et al. Postmenopausal hormone therapy and mortality. *N Engl J Med* 1997;236:1769–1775.

Harden C, Pulver M, Ravdin L, et al. The effect of menopause and perimenopause on the course of epilepsy. *Epilepsia* 1999;40(10):1402–1407.

Henderson VW, Paganini-Hill A, Miller BL, et al. Estrogen for Alzheimer's disease in women: randomized, double-blind, placebo-controlled trial. *Neurology* 2000;54:295–301.

Herrington D, Reboussin D, Brosnihan B, et al. Effects of estrogen replacement on the progression of coronary artery atherosclerosis. *N Engl J Med* 2000;343(8):522–529.

Herzog A. Progesterone therapy in women with epilepsy: a 3-year follow-up. *Neurology* 1999;52:1917–1918.

Hu F, Grodstein F, Henneckens C, et al. Age at natural menopause and risk of cardiovascular disease. *Arch Intern Med* 1999;159:1061–1066.

Hulley S, Grady D, Bush T, et al. Randomized trial of estrogen plus progestin for secondary prevention of coronary heart disease in postmenopausal women. Heart and Estrogen/Progestin Replacement Study (HERS) Research Group. *JAMA* 1998;280:605–613.

Kampen D, Sherwin B. Estrogen use and verbal memory in healthy postmenopausal women. *Obstet Gynecol* 1994;83:979–983.

Kaplan P. *Neurologic disease in women*, 1st ed. New York: Demos Medical Publishing, 1998.

Kawas C, Resnick S, Morrison, et al. A prospective study of estrogen replacement therapy and the risk of developing Alzheimer's disease: the Baltimore Longitudinal Study of Aging. *Neurology* 1997; 48:1517–1521.

Keefe DL, Watson R, Naftolin F. Hormone replacement therapy may alleviate sleep apnea in menopausal women: a pilot study. *Menopause* 1999;6(3):196–200.

Lipton R, Stewart W. Migraine in the United States: a review of epidemiology and health care use. *Neurology* 1993;43 (S3): S6–S10.

Lobo RA. *Treatment of the postmenopausal woman: basic and clinical aspects*, 2nd ed. Philadelphia: Lippincott Williams & Wilkins, 1999.

Logothesis J, Harner R. Electrocortical activation by estrogens. *Arch Neurol* 1960;9:352–360.

Longstreth WT Jr, Nelson LM, Koepsall TD. Subarachnoid hemorrhage and hormonal factors in women: a population based case-control study. *Arch Intern Med* 1994;150:2557–2562.

Marder K, Tang M-X, Alfaro B, et al. Postmenopausal estrogen use and Parkinson's disease with and without dementia. *Neurology* 1998;50:1141–1143.

Mendelsohn M, Karas R. The protective effects of estrogen on the cardiovascular system. *N Engl J Med* 1998; 340: 1801–1811.

Mulnard R, Cotman CW, Kawas C, et al. Estrogen replacement therapy for treatment of mild to moderate Alzheimer's Disease: a 1-year randomized controlled trial. *JAMA* 2000;283:1007–1015.

Petitti B, Sidney S, Quesenberry C, et al. Ischemic stroke and use of estrogen and estrogen/progesterone as hormone replacement therapy. *Stroke* 1998;29:23–28.

Phillips S, Sherwin B. Variations in memory function and sex steroid hormones across the menstrual cycle. *Psychoneuroendocrinology* 1992;17(5):497–506.

Polo-Kantola P, Erkkola R, Helenius H, et al. When does estrogen replacement therapy improve sleep quality? *Am J Obstet Gynecol* 1998;178:1002–1009.

Shaver J, Zenk S. Sleep disturbance in menopause. *Journal of Women's Health & Gender-Based Medicine* 2000;9(2): 109–118.

Silberstein S, Merriam G. Estrogens, progestins, and headache. *Neurology* 1991;41:786–793.

Smith R, Studd J. A pilot study of the effect upon multiple sclerosis of the menopause, hormone replacement therapy, and the cycle. *J R Soc Med* 1992;85:612–613.

Strijks E, Kremer J, Horstink M. Effects of female sex steroids on Parkinson's disease in postmenopausal women. *Clin Neuropharmacol* 1999;22(2):93–97.

Tang M-X, Jacobs D, Stern Y, et al. Effect of oestrogen during menopause on the risk and age at onset of Alzheimer's disease: a population-based study in Rochester, Minnesota. *Lancet* 1996;348:429–432.

Tsang K, Ho S, Lo S. Estrogen improves motor disability in parkinsonian postmenopausal women with motor fluctuations. *Neurology* 2000;54:2292–2298.

Tsutsui K, Ukena K, Usui M, et al. Novel brain function: biosynthesis and actions of neurosteroids in neurons. *Neurosci Res* 2000;36(4):261–273.

Vollenhoven R, McGuire J. Estrogen, progesterone, and testosterone: can they be used to treat autoimmune diseases? *Cleve Clin J Med* 1994;61(4):276–284.

Wang PN, Liao SQ, Liu R, et al. Effects of estrogen on cognition, mood, and cerebral blood flow in AD. *Neurology* 2000;54:2062–2066.

Ware JC, McBrayer R, Scott JA. Influence of sex and age on duration and frequency of sleep apnea events. *Sleep* 2000; 23(2):165–170.

Wooley C, McEwen B. Roles of estradiol and progesterone in regulation of hippocampal dendritic spine density during the estrus cycle in the rat. *J Comp Neurol* 1993;336: 293–306.

Yaffe K, Sawaya G, Lieberburg I, et al. Estrogen therapy in postmenopausal women: effects on cognitive function and dementia. *JAMA* 1998;279:688–695.

WEB SITES OF NATIONAL SUPPORT GROUPS

American College of Obstetricians and Gynecologists *http://www.acog.org*

American Epilepsy Society *http://www.aesnet.org*

American Medical Women's Association *http://amwa-doc.org*

Association of Reproductive Health Professionals *http://www.arhp.org*

National Institutes of Health, Women's Health Initiative *http://www.healthtouch.com*

National Osteoporosis Foundation *http://www.nof.org*

Chat rooms: *www.DrKoop.com*; *www.ivillage.com*; *www.webMD.com*

5

Cognitive Changes Associated with Normal Aging

Julie L. Pickholtz and Barbara L. Malamut

With advances in healthcare in the United States and other industrialized countries, the number of healthy adults living beyond age 65 years has risen over the past few decades. As these individuals have been able to sustain their health status, fewer cognitive changes have been noted. Thus, the significant mental decline that was once thought to be an inevitable part of the aging process may not be characteristic of normal healthy aging. Although cognitive stability seems to be greater than was once expected, specific age-related cognitive changes occur, even in healthy individuals. It is estimated that two of three intact elderly individuals exhibit some degree of performance decrement on neuropsychologic testing (Keefover, 1998). Longitudinal studies indicate an acceleration of memory and cognitive decline after age 70 years. These changes affect certain areas of cognitive functioning and are not synonymous with dementia. Although the focus of this chapter is on the neuropsychologic, rather than biological aspects of aging, a short discussion of normal age-related changes in the brain is included because these neuropathologic events are thought to play a role in the cognitive changes.

NEUROPATHOLOGY

With aging, it is generally accepted that a number of cerebral changes occur universally, which are considered normal and are independent of disease processes (Ritchie et al., 2000). For example, computed tomography (CT) and magnetic resonance imaging (MRI) studies have shown that aging is associated with enlargement of the cerebral ventricles and sulci, and a decline in gray and white matter volumes (Blatter et al., 1995; Raz et al., 2000). Gray matter loss is more pronounced than white matter loss in the overall brain. The age at which brain changes occur has been found to differ between men and women. A precipitous increase in ventricular volume begins in the fifth decade in men and the sixth decade in women, with an approximate 20% increase in ventricular volume per decade for both sexes (Kaye et al., 1992).

Longitudinal MRI studies looking at regional differences indicate that age-specific volume changes do not appear to be uniform across brain areas. For both men and women, age differences are greatest in the parietal region compared with the frontal, temporal and occipital areas. However, men show a greater loss of brain volume in all cortical regions (Coffey et al., 1998; Resnick et al., 2000; Murphy et al., 1996). Loss of hippocampal volume has also been found to be greater for men than for women (Coffey et al., 1998, Resnick et al., 2000). In fact, volume decline in the hippocampus was found to begin as early as the third decade in men (Pruessner, 2001). With regard to gender-specific differences among brain regions, the greatest difference between the sexes appears to be in the volumes of the frontal and temporal regions.

The relationship between these age-related structural changes and functional decrements is less clear. Because normal aging affects some brain areas more than others, a decline would be expected in the cognitive functions supported by those regions. However, in one study, variations in total and limbic brain volumes were not predictive of memory test performance when the effects of age were controlled (Tisserand et al., 2000). Similarly, increase in ventricle volume independent of age did not explain normal age-related declines seen in intelligence scores (Kay et al., 1992). Functional imaging studies have raised the issue that aging may involve a functional plasticity or reallocation of brain network operations when performing a cognitive task. For example, when old and young subjects were compared using positron emission tomography (PET) during a verbal memory task, hypometabolism in the frontal region and greater activation in the occipital region was associated with age-related decline (Hazlett et al., 1998). Similarly, results from another PET study comparing young and old subjects who were matched for level of performance suggested that a different hippocampal network was activated during a visual memory test in the older subjects (Della-Maggiore et al., 2000). Thus, these studies provide evidence that when older subjects perform at the same level as younger individuals, they go about the task using different brain pathways.

AREAS OF COGNITIVE DECLINE IN NORMAL AGING

Intellectual Abilities

General intelligence can be divided into eight cognitive factors: fluid reasoning (i.e., involves processing and manipulating information in a novel way); comprehensive knowledge (i.e., involves retrieval of well-learned factual or semantic information); processing speed; short-term memory; long-term retrieval; quantitative ability; auditory processing; and visual processing. The basic trend in general intellectual abilities over time is for slight improvement in these abilities in early adulthood, stability in the middle years, and decline in later years (La Rue, 1992). However, the decline is not uniform across cognitive areas. Evidence suggests that fluid reasoning, processing speed, and short-term memory are particularly vulnerable to the effects of aging, whereas quantitative ability, long-term retrieval, and comprehensive knowledge do not appear to be adversely affected by the aging process (Compton et al., 2000). In general, spared abilities tend to be overlearned, well-practiced, and familiar skills that are influenced by educational and cultural opportunities.

Many of these age-related changes are reflected on standardized intellectual testing. On the Wechsler Adult Intelligence Scale (WAIS), decline on performance scales occurs at about the age of 60, whereas decline on the verbal scales occurs at around age 80 (Albert and Moss, 1988; Wechsler, 1981).

Performance Speed

Aging is associated with slowing of many motor and cognitive behaviors and is most readily seen on timed tests. Speed of motor performance is inversely related to age on measures of walking speed and finger-tapping (Ruff and Parker, 1993). However, performance decrements noted on many timed measures

are not caused simply by motor slowing, but involve slowing of higher level integrative processes as well (Gilmore, 1995). Thus, any task that involves initiation, redirection, or decision-making may be slowed, as measured by reaction time, because of slowed mental processing speed. An even more direct measure of cognitive slowing that assesses central processing time (i.e., event-related P300 and other evoked potentials, demonstrates a positive relationship between increasing age and longer latency intervals). These age-related changes in motor and cognitive speed are reflected in lower scores on the performance subtests of the WAIS, because many of the subtests are timed (Keefover, 1998).

Memory

The most common cognitive complaint among elderly people is a change in memory, although complaints about declining memory do not always correlate with poor performance on tests of memory (Williams et al., 1987). As seen in Table 5-1 and discussed below, memory can be divided into several components (i.e., immediate, declarative, nondeclarative, and remote) and studies have shown that different aspects of memory are sensitive to aging in various degrees.

Immediate Memory Span

Immediate memory is the ability to retain small amounts of information that remains untransformed for a very short period of time. Immediate memory span is usually measured with the number of digits one can repeat in correct sequential order immedi-

TABLE 5-1. *Changes in memory functioning with normal aging*

Immediate memory	Unchanged
Short-term memory	Reduced
Long-term memory	Variable
Declarative	
Semantic	Unchanged up to age 70 years
Episodic	Reduced
Free recall	Reduced
Cued recall	Large benefit
Recognition	Unchanged
Acquisition	Reduced
Retrieval	Reduced
Percent retention	Unchanged
Source memory	Reduced
Nondeclarative	Mild decline
Remote memory	Unchanged

ately after presentation (i.e., Digit Span). Older adults perform more poorly on tests of immediate memory than younger adults (Zacks et al., 2000), although recent studies have suggested that the reduction of performance on traditional immediate memory tests may be related to factors other than memory. For example, some evidence indicates that the slower articulation rate of older adults contributes to their reduced span measures and, when the rate of presentation is slowed, older adults perform equivalent to younger adults (Multhaup et al., 1996). Furthermore, items from early trials involving digit span have been found to interfere with performance on later trials. Because older adults are susceptible to interference, they are at a disadvantage on later trials, which are used to measure higher levels of memory span (McDowd and Shaw, 2000).

Short-Term Memory

Short-term memory refers to the ability to retain larger amounts of new information very shortly after it is presented. Studies have shown significant age-related declines in the immediate recall of stories, word lists, and designs. As with immediate memory, age-related effects can be attenuated when information is presented at a slower pace, cuing is provided, and rehearsal is allowed (Multhaup et al., 1996).

Long-Term Memory

Long-term memory refers to the ability to retain large amounts of newly learned information over a substantial period of time. It involves manipulating and transforming the material. It can be subdivided into declarative and nondeclarative memory.

Declarative Memory

Declarative memory, which is also known as "explicit memory," refers to conscious learning and remembering of events and facts, and is tested by measures of recall and recognition. Many studies have shown that declarative or explicit memory declines with age but the degree of change depends on the testing method. In general, older people perform significantly worse on free recall than recognition tests. Furthermore, age-related decline is not uniform across all of its components (Keefover, 1998). Declarative memory can be further subdivided into *semantic* and *episodic* memory. Semantic memory, which refers to memory for factual information or general word knowledge, is relatively spared until age

70 and then declines precipitously (LaBarge et al., 1986; Tulving, 1983). Episodic memory, which involves memories for personally experienced events that occur at a specific place and time, has also been shown to decline with age.

The ability to acquire episodic memory appears to decline progressively after the age of 70 years, as measured by recall and recognition tests of newly learned information (Small et al., 1999; Celsis, 2000). The age-related changes are not limited to performance on standard memory tests, but also occur on batteries of tasks that are designed to emulate memory in everyday life (Prull et al., 2000). This memory decline primarily affects *initial* learning of information rather than *retention* of the material once it has been acquired. One explanation for the decrease in initial learning is that older people demonstrate a reduction in the use of encoding strategies that enhances new learning. Another explanation could be related to the decline in *source memory* (i.e., attributing the source—time and place—where information was learned that is associated with aging) (Wegesin et al., 2000).

Although a reduction in the acquisition of new information can occur, healthy aging individuals do not tend to forget information that has been learned. However, difficulty in retrieving that information has been observed. Some evidence indicates that the ability for strategic retrieval of newly learned information appears to be at least partially responsible for the decline in episodic memory. First, memory performance of older adults improves when cues are provided (Petersen et al., 1992). Second, older adults have a lowered tendency for spontaneous organization of the information that they are trying to learn, which can affect learning efficiency (Stuss et al., 1996). Third, older adults perform more favorably on tests of recognition than on tests of recall (Craik and McDowd, 1987), which require more strategic functions.

In clinical settings, it is often difficult to detect declines in memory because elderly individuals are sometimes able to provide elaborate autobiographic information about their remote history. Evidence suggests that in old age, personal experiences from early in life are remembered more easily than experiences from later in life. In contrast, younger adults show the reverse pattern, remembering recent events more easily than more remote events (Prull et al., 2000).

Nondeclarative Memory

Nondeclarative memory, also known as "implicit memory," refers to learning as a result of prior experience without conscious reference to that experience. It has been noted that implicit memory declines less dramatically with age than explicit memory (Keefover, 1998; Prull et al., 2000). One measure of nondeclarative memory is skill learning, in which improvement in speed or accuracy on a challenging task is measured. Some of the limited studies that have been performed with respect to aging have generally suggested that, relative to younger adults, the rate of skill learning in older adults is slower (Wright and Payne, 1985).

To summarize, aging is associated with a decline in declarative short-term and long-term memory, particularly for new episodic information. This memory decline is most pronounced when strategies are required for new learning. Aged individuals perform most favorably when asked to recognize rather than recall information. Furthermore, semantic information is remembered more easily than episodic information. Some evidence also suggests that certain types of nondeclarative memory decline with aging, although to a lesser extent than declarative memory.

Attention

Attention is composed of a complex set of functions responsible for maintaining focus and selecting and processing certain aspects of experience. As is the case with memory, different aspects of attention are affected in aging to varying degrees.

Selective Attention

The ability to attend selectively to specific aspects of the environment is important for everyday behaviors that require an individual to ignore irrelevant information. Selective attention is important for such tasks as driving an automobile and conversing in noisy environments. Studies have demonstrated that older adults are more negatively affected by the presence of distracting information when engaged in a task (Earles et al., 1997; Carlson et al., 1995). Relative to younger adults, they tend to have greater difficulty ignoring irrelevant information (McDowd and Shaw, 2000).

Divided Attention

It has been noted that older subjects are more penalized than younger subjects when they must divide their attention between two sources (Craik, 1977). Although experimental findings have varied, task difficulty and task novelty have been found to mediate the degree to which age differences in divided attention are demonstrated (Salthouse et al., 1995; Tun and Wingfield, 1995). Thus, declines in divided attention are most apparent in aging adults when the task is novel or at a high level of difficulty.

Sustained Attention

Sustained attention, also known as "vigilance," refers to the ability to maintain concentration or focus over time. The studies that have investigated age differences in vigilance task performance have generally demonstrated little evidence for age-related declines (McDowd and Shaw, 2000). However, some evidence indicates that under conditions when task difficulty is increased, sustained attention performance declines with age (Mouloua and Parasuraman, 1995).

Executive

Executive functions encompass a broad range of cognitive skills that rely on the functions of the prefrontal cortex, including monitoring of behavior, generating goals, memory of temporal sequences, inhibiting overlearned responses, and alternating behavioral responses in response to feedback. Because executive functions are composed of a number of heterogeneous skills, it is not surprising that some tasks of executive functioning have been found to decline with age, whereas other tasks appear to be more resilient to the effects of aging.

A classic example of an executive task is the Wisconsin Card Sorting Test (WCST) that involves problem solving and the ability to shift mental set when provided feedback (WCST; Heaton et al., 1993). Aged individuals have been shown to make more perseverative errors on this task (i.e., persist in using a failed strategy) than their younger counterparts (Raz, 2000). Older individuals also make more perseverative errors on a variety of other cognitive tasks (Daigneault et al., 1999), suggesting a decline in mental flexibility.

Abstract reasoning ability is another skill that relies on executive functions (e.g., flexible thinking) that has been found to decline with old age. Older people often approach reasoning tasks in a rigid (i.e., concrete) way. For example, older people are more likely than young adults to give concrete responses to proverb interpretation (La Rue, 1992). Aging has also been found to have a negative effect on a person's ability to inhibit a usual response in a situation in favor of producing a novel response (Wecker et al., 2000).

Aging has been associated with a decline in the ability to judge the order in which new information is presented. Studies have shown a decreased ability to judge the relative recency of presentation, for both pictures and words, with age (Mittenberg et al., 1989).

Working Memory

Working memory refers to an individual's ability to momentarily hold information in mind and simultaneously manipulate that information. For example, digit span backward requires working memory because a person must hold all the numbers in abeyance to recall them in reverse. Age-related changes have been demonstrated in working memory and are thought to be related to disruption in executive functions, as well as encoding and retrieval systems in the brain (Keefover, 1998). Many studies have demonstrated that older people show moderate deficits on a variety of working memory tasks (Salthouse, 1994). Event-related potential studies suggest that age-associated disturbances in frontal lobe function contribute to these declines (Chao and Knight, 1997). Furthermore, PET studies comparing young and old subjects have reported increased metabolism in several frontal lobe regions during working memory tasks in older subjects, which is thought to be caused by their need for compensatory strategies (Furey et al., 1997).

Language

Normal aging is associated with a decline in specific language skills. Reading abilities (Rubin et al., 1998) and functional knowledge of syntax and grammar (La Rue, 1992) are essentially preserved, whereas semantic knowledge changes significantly with age. The most frequent language complaint of older individuals involves difficulty in naming. Indeed, studies have shown that problems in accessing words (also known as lexical retrieval or the "tip-of-the-tongue" phenomenon) are greater for older than younger adults (Bowles and Poon, 1985). Performance on confrontational naming tests tends to remain stable between the ages of 30 and 50 years, decline slightly in the 60s, and clearly decrease among people aged 70 years or older (Borod et al., 1980; LaBarge et al., 1986). Qualitative changes in errors made on naming tests are also seen. These errors include (*a*) circumlocutions, or using more words than necessary to provide accurate information; (*b*) nominalizations, or words describing the function of the pictured object (e.g., "mouth organ" for harmonica); (*c*) visual-perceptual errors, or misidentifications of the stimulus (e.g., "mouse" for beaver); and (*d*) semantic association errors, or responses that name a conative associate of the pictured object (e.g., "dice" for dominoes). These errors indicate that older people are familiar with information about the objects that they are asked to name, but they may have difficulty retrieving specific words. Thus, they "know" an item, but cannot think of its name (La Rue, 1992). In addition, lowered performance in rate of verbal output (i.e., fluency) has been found to be affected from the age of 70 onward (Ritchie et al., 1997; Obler and Albert, 1985). Comprehension of spoken language has been found to be affected at an older age than naming and does not begin to decline until around the age of 80 years (Ritchie et al., 1997).

OTHER FACTORS AFFECTING COGNITION IN THE ELDERLY

Growing evidence indicates that many factors besides changes in brain functioning influence cognitive functioning in aging. The next section includes a discussion of some of the variables shown to be related to decline in cognition.

General Health and Wellness

Even in the absence of medical illness, subtle changes in health status among intact older adults can be associated with cognitive changes. Research suggests that aerobic fitness can improve certain aspects of attention and memory performance (Kramer et al., 1998; Bunce et al., 1996; Hawkins et al., 1992) and reaction time (Clarkson-Smith and Hartley, 1989). For example, fitness level has been shown to affect performance on sustained attention tasks in the elderly (Bunce et al., 1993), whereas fitness is unrelated to sustained attention in young adults. In addition, chronic smokers have been found to show lower scores than nonsmokers on tests of fluid intelligence (Zacks et al., 2000).

Diminished gastrointestinal absorption associated with aging can compromise nutritional status (Keefover, 1998) and, therefore, affect cognitive functioning. Because low vitamin levels are more prevalent in old age (Backman et al., 2000), vitamin status should be considered when an older individual complains of cognitive changes. An inverse relationship exists between levels of vitamin B12 and folic acid and performance on various tests of visual spatial functioning, attention, and memory (Riggs et al., 1996).

Medications

Given increasing health complaints in the elderly, it is not surprising that aging adults take medication more frequently than younger adults. Diminished medication metabolism in older people can result in lowered tolerance, which often has negative effects on cognitive function (Keefover, 1998). In particular, several studies have found that benzodiazepines can cause decline in cognitive performance among elderly individuals (Taylor et al., 1987). For example, use of benzodiazepines are associated with decreases in episodic memory performance (Pomara et al., 1991; Kruse, 1990). In Chapter 3, the actions of specific medications are discussed in detail. When a change in cognition is presented, it is important to consider the possibility of medication change. Over-the-counter medications also need to be considered, as they can also cause significant cognitive problems.

Estrogen Replacement Therapy

Results from studies linking estrogen levels and cognitive performance in women have yielded conflicting results. Several studies have demonstrated that hormone replacement therapy (HRT) in postmenopausal women may have a protective effect on cognitive performance compared with women not using HRT (Kampen and Sherwin, 1994; Resnick, 1995). It has also been suggested that HRT enhances verbal and visual memory in women and may forestall deterioration in short- and long-term memory that occurs with normal aging (Resnick, 1997; Sherwin, 1999). Verbal fluency has also been shown to benefit from HRT (Grodstein et al., 2000). However, other studies have not found any relationship between estrogen levels and memory performance (Barret-Connor et al. 1993).

Depression

Because depression has been associated with declines in overall cognitive performance, particularly attention and memory, elderly individuals can often appear as if they have a dementia when they are actually depressed. This misdiagnosis is common because it is more difficult to detect depression in the elderly because depression in old age is more chronic in nature than that which occurs in younger adults. The lengthy development of depression in elderly adults, in contrast with the short clinical onset of depression in younger adults, can lead to undiagnosed depressive symptoms in the earlier stages of the disorder in older individuals (American Psychiatric Association, 1994). Some studies have found reduced levels of memory performance in depressed older adults in cases of high demands on effortful encoding of infor-

mation. Additionally, depressed older adults tend to benefit less from being provided with an inherent organizational structure when learning new material (Backman and Forsell, 1994). Subjective memory complaints are more common among depressed than nondepressed older adults, even in the absence of memory deficits (Williams et al., 1987).

Education

In general, level of education has been found to have significant associations with performance on neuropsychological measures (Plassman et al., 1993). Studies among healthy elderly individuals suggest that those with higher levels of education tend to have better cognitive functioning and that this functioning is less likely to decline over time (Inouye et al., 1993; Schaie, 1990). In particular, highly educated individuals appear to have an advantage on tests that depend on the use of previously learned materials (e.g., tests of language and conceptualization). Education appears to be strongly related to abstraction and naming and less related to recognition and some recall memory measures (Inouye et al., 1993). However, lower education is also associated with larger age-related differences in memory for word lists (Verhaeghen et al., 1993).

Many plausible explanations are seen for the relationship between education and cognitive performance. For example, education is positively related to nutritional habits and health behaviors and, thus, may serve as a marker for better health, resulting in superior cognitive performance. Moreover, education increases exposure to general experiences and knowledge, which provides a larger context for problem-solving and reasoning. These experiences may enable elderly educated individuals to develop compensatory strategies and adapt to cognitive losses more effectively (Compton et al., 2000). Level of education also appears to be directly related to changes in brain structure. In nonclinical, elderly individuals, higher educational attainment was inversely related to cerebral atrophy (Coffey et al., 1998). It is hypothesized that education results in increased synaptic connections in the brain, preventing greater loss over time.

Living Environment

In old age, a significant interaction occurs between psychosocial and neuropsychological factors. The living environment of older people has been shown to have a tremendous impact on the level of cognitive functioning. For example, in comparing older individuals living in a community with their counterparts living in institutions (e.g., senior citizen residents), those in the former group significantly out-performed the institutional group on tests of cognitive functioning, despite being matched for age, education, IQ, and health status (Winocur et al., 1987). Although marked variability existed within both elderly groups, people living in institutions demonstrated greater cognitive variability, particularly in memory and functions associated with the frontal lobes than those living in the community. No clear explanation is found for this difference between groups, but longitudinal studies of aging adults have shown that the level of cognitive functioning within an individual is not necessarily stable and will vary in parallel with variations in some psychosocial variables. In particular, two psychosocial variables—optimism and locus of control (i.e., belief in whether a person controls his or her own life or whether it is controlled by external forces)—best predicted level of cognitive functioning for both community or institutional-dwelling individuals over time (Winocur et al., 1990). It is possible, therefore, that older people living in institutions may experience greater difficulties in relation to their environments that affects their optimism and feelings of control.

SUMMARY

Cognition in healthy aging people is a complex process that, at the very least, involves an interaction between psychosocial adjustment, premorbid cognitive functioning, level of education, nutritional and health status, environmental factors, and changes in the brain itself. Although many cognitive changes are associated with aging, the decline is not necessarily a linear process and, depending on the situation, can be reversed. Lastly, most healthy elderly people have the cognitive resources to function well in their own environments and to make appropriate accommodations when necessary.

REFERENCES

Albert MS, Moss MB. *Geriatric neuropsychology.* New York: Guilford Press, 1988.

American Psychiatric Association. *Diagnostic and statistical manual of mental disorders*, 4th ed. Washington, DC: American Psychiatric Association, 1994.

Backman L, Forsell Y. Episodic memory functioning in a community-based sample of old adults with major depression: utilization of cognitive support. *J Abnorm Psychol* 1994;103:361–370.

Backman L, Small BJ, Wahling A. Cognitive functioning in very old age. In: Craik FI, Salthouse TA, eds. *The hand-book of aging and cognition*, 2nd ed. Mahwah, NJ: Lawrence Erlbaum Associates, 2000.

Barret-Connor E. Hormone replacement. *Am J Geriatr Cardiol* 1993;2(5):36–37.

Blatter DD, Bigler ED, Gade SD, et al. Quantitative volumetric analysis of brain MR: normative database spanning 5 decades of life. *Am J Neuroradiol* 1995;16:241–251.

Borod JD, Goodglass H, Kaplan E. Normative data on the Boston Diagnostic Aphasia Examinations. *J Clin Neuropsychol* 1980;2:209–215.

Bowles NL, Poon LW. Aging and retrieval of words in semantic memory. *J Gerontol* 1985; 40:71–77.

Bunce DJ, Warr PB, Cochrane T. Blocks in choice responding as a function of age and physical fitness. *Psychol Aging* 1993;8:26–33.

Carlson MC, Hasher L, Connelly SL, et al. Aging, distraction, and the benefits of predictable location. *Psychol Aging* 1995;10:427–436.

Celsis P. Age-related cognitive decline, mild cognitive impairment or preclinical Alzheimer's disease. *Ann Med* 2000;32:6–14.

Chao LL, Knight RT. Age-related prefrontal alterations during auditory memory. *Neurobiol Aging* 1997;18:87.

Clarkson-Smith L, Hartley AA. Relationships between physical exercise and cognitive abilities in older adults. *Psychol Aging* 1989;4:183–189.

Coffey CE, Lucke JF, Saxton JA, et al. Sex differences in brain aging: a quantitative magnetic resonance imaging study. *Arch Neurol* 1998:55(5):169–179.

Compton DM, Bachman LD, Brand D, et al. Age-associated changes in cognitive function in highly educated adults: emerging myths and realities. *Int J Geriatr Psychiatry* 2000;15:75–85.

Craik FIM. Age differences in human memory. In: Birren JE, Schaie KW, eds. *Handbook of the psychology of aging.* New York: Van Nostrand Reinhold, 1977.

Craik FIM, McDowd JM. Age differences in recall and recognition. *J Exp Psychol Learn Mem Cogn* 1987;13: 474–479.

Daignealt S, Braun CMJ, Whitaker HA. Early effects of normal aging on perseverative and non-perseverative prefrontal measures. *Dev Neuropsychol* 1999;8(1):99–114.

Della-Maggiore V, Sekuler AB, Grady CL, et al. Corticolimbic interactions associated with performance on a short-term memory task are modified by age. *J Neuroscience* 2000;20(22):8410–8416.

Earles JL, Connor LT, Frieske D, et al. Age differences in inhibition: possible causes and consequences. *Aging, Neuropsychology, and Cognition* 1997;4:45–57.

Furey ML, Pietrini P, Haxby JV. Cholinergic stimulation alters performance and task-specific regional cerebral blood flow during working memory. *Proc Natl Acad Sci USA* 1997;94:6512.

Gilmore R. Evoked potentials in the elderly. *J Clin Neurophysiol* 1995;12:132.

Grodstein F, Chen J, Pollen DA, et al. Postmenopausal hormone therapy and cognitive function in healthy older women. *J Am Geriatr Soc* 2000;48:746–752.

Hawkins HL, Kramer AF, Capaldi D. Aging, exercise and attention. *Psychol Aging* 1992;7:643–653.

Hazlett EA, Buchsbaum MS, Mohs RC, et al. Age-related shift in brain region activity during successful memory performance. *Neurobiol Aging* 1998;19(5):437–445.

Heaton RK, Chelune GJ, Talley JL, et al. *Wisconsin card sorting test manual: revised and expanded* Odessa, FL: Psychological Assessment Resources, 1993.

Inouye SK, Albert MS, Mohs R, et al. Cognitive performance in a high-functioning community-dwelling elderly population. *J Gerontol* 1993;48(4):M146– M151.

Kampen D, Sherwin BB. Estrogen use and verbal memory in healthy postmenopausal women. *Obstet Gynecol* 1994;83:979–983.

Kaye JA, DeCarli C, Luxenberg JS, et al. The significance of age-related enlargement of the cerebral ventricles in healthy men and women measured by quantitative computed x-ray tomography. *J Am Geriatric Soc* 1992;40(3): 225–231.

Keefover RW. Aging and cognition. *Neurol Clin* 1998;16(3): 635–648.

Kramer A, Hahn S, Banich M, et al. *Influence of aerobic fitness on the neurocognitive function of sedentary older adults.* Poster session presented at the Cognitive Aging conference, Atlanta, GA, 1998.

Kruse WH. Problems and pitfalls in the use of benzodiazepines in the elderly. *Drug Saf* 1990;7:328–344.

LaBarge E, Edwards D, Knesevich JW. Performance of normal elderly on the Boston Naming Test. *Brain Lang* 1986; 27:380–384.

La Rue A. *Aging and neuropsychological assessment.* New York: Plenum Press, 1992.

McDowd JM, Shaw RJ. Attention and aging: a functional perspective. In: Craik FI, Salthouse TA, eds. *The handbook of aging and cognition, 2nd ed.* Mahwah NJ: Lawrence Erlbaum, 2000.

Mittenberg W, Seidenberg M, O'Learly DS, et al. Changes in cerebral functioning associated with normal aging. *J Clin Exp Neuropsychol* 1989;11(6):918–932.

Mouloua M, Parasuraman R. Aging and cognitive vigilance: effects of spatial uncertainty and event rate. *Exp Aging Res* 1995;21:17–32.

Multhaup KS, Balota DA, Cowan, N. Implications of aging lexicality, and item length for the mechanisms underlying memory span. *Psychon Bull Rev* 1996;3(1):112–120.

Murphy DG, DeCarli C, McIntosh AR, et al. Sex differences in human brain morphometry and metabolism: an *in vivo* quantitative magnetic resonance imaging and positron emission tomography study on the effect of aging. *Arch Gen Psychiatry* 1996;53(7):585–594.

Obler LK, Albert ML. Language skills across adulthood. In: Birren JE, Schaie KW, eds. *Handbook of the psychology of aging,* 2nd ed. New York: Van Nostrand Reinhold, 1985:463–473.

Petersen R, Smith G, Kokmen E, et al. Memory function in normal aging. *Neurology* 1992;42:396–401.

Plassman BL, Welsh KA, Helms BS, et al. Intelligence and education as predictors of cognitive state in life. *Neurology* 1995;45:1446–1450.

Pomara N, Deptula D, Singh R, et al. Cognitive toxicity of benzodiazepines in the elderly. In: Salzman CL, Liebowitz B, eds. *Anxiety disorders and the elderly.* New York: Springer, 1991:175–196.

Pruessner JC, Collins DL, Pruessner M, et al. Age and gender predict volume decline int eh anterior and posterior hippocampus in early adulthood. *J Neurosci* 2001;21 (1):194–200.

Prull MW, Gabrieli DE, Bunge SA. In: Craik FI, Salthouse TA, eds. *The handbook of aging and cognition,* 2nd ed. Mahwah, NJ: Lawrence Erlbaum Associates, 2000.

Rapp SR. Postmenopausal estrogen-replacement therapy and dementia. *Journal SOGC* 2000:22:39–43.

Raz N. Aging of the brain and its impact on cognitive performance: integration of structural and functional findings. In: Craik FI, Salthouse TA, eds. *The handbook of aging and cognition,* 2nd ed. Mahwah, NJ: Lawrence Erlbaum Associates, 2000.

Raz N, Gunning-Dixon FM, Head D, et al. Neuroanatomical correlates of cognitive aging: evidence from structural magnetic resonance imaging. *Neuropyshcology* 1998;12 (1):95–114.

Resnick SM. Estrogen replacement therapy and cognitive aging. In: Keenan PA, Chairman. *Neuroendocrinological influences on cognition.* Symposium conducted at the American Psychological Association Convention, New York, NY, 1995. *The Clinical Neuropsychologist* 1995;9:3.

Resnick SM, Goldszal AF, Davatzikos C, et al. One-year age changes in MRI brain volumes in older adults. *Cereb Cortex* 2000;10:464–472.

Resnick SM, Metter J, Zonderman AB. Estrogen replacement therapy and longitudinal decline in visual memory: a possible protective effect? *Neurology* 1997:49:1491–1497.

Riggs KM, Spiro A, Tucker K, et al. Relations of vitamin B-12, vitamin B-6, folate, and homocysteine to cognitive performance in the Normative Aging Study. *Am J Clin Nutr* 1996; 63:306–314.

Ritchie K, Touchon J, Ledesert B, et al. Establishing the limits and characteristics of normal age-related cognitive decline. *Rev Epidemiol Sante Publique* 1997;45:373–381.

Ritchie K, Ledesert B, Touchon J. Subclinical cognitive impairment: epidemiology and clinical characteristics. *Compr Psychiatry* 2000;41(2):61–65.

Rubin E, Storandt M, Miller J, et al. A prospective study of cognitive function and onset of dementia in cognitively healthy elders. *Arch Neurol* 1998;55:395–401.

Ruff RM, Parker SB. Gender and age-specific changes in motor speed and eye-hand coordination in adults: normative values for the Finger Tapping and Grooved Pegboard tests. *Percept Mot Skills* 1993;76:1219.

Salthouse TA. The aging of working memory. *Neuropsychology* 1994;8:535–543.

Salthouse TA, Fristoe NM, Lineweaver TT, et al. Aging of attention: does the ability to divide decline? *Mem Cognit* 1995;23:59–71.

Schaie KW. The optimization of cognitive functioning in old age; predictions based on cohort-sequential and longitudinal data. In: Baltes PB, Baltes MM, eds. *Successful aging: perspectives from the behavioral sciences.* Cambridge, UK: Cambridge University Press, 1990:94–117.

Sherwin BB. Can estrogen keep you smart? Evidence from clinical studies. *J Psychiatry Neurosci* 1999;24(4):315–321.

Small S, Stern Y, Tang M, et al. Selective decline in memory function among healthy elderly. *Neurology* 1999;52: 1392–1396.

Stuss DT, Craik FIM, Sayer L, et al. Comparison of older people and patients with frontal lesions: evidence of wordlist learning. *Psychol Aging* 1996;11:387–395.

Taylor JL, Tinklenberg JR. Cognitive impairment and benzodiazepines. In: Melzer HY, ed. *Psychopharmacology: the third generation of progress.* New York: Raven Press, 1987:1449–1454.

Tisserand DJ, Visser PJ, van Boxtel MP, et al. The relation between global and limbic brain volumes on MRI and cognitive performance in healthy individuals across the age range. *Neurobiol Aging* 2000;21(4):569–76.

Tulving E. *Elements of episodic memory.* New York: Oxford University Press, 1983.

Tun PA, Wingfield A. Does dividing attention become harder with age? Findings from the Divided Attention questionnaire. *Aging and Cognition* 1995;2:39–66.

Verhaeghen P, Marcoen A, Goossens L. Facts and fiction about memory aging: a quantitative integration of research findings. *J Gerontol*, 1993;48(4):157–171.

Wechsler D. *WAIS-R manual*. New York: The Psychological Corporation, 1981.

Wecker NA, Kramer JH, Wisniewski A, et al. Age effects on executive ability. *Neuropsychology* 2000;14(3):409–414.

Wegesin DJ, Jacobs DM, Zubin NR, et al. Source memory and encoding strategy in normal aging. *J Clin Exp Neuropsychol* 2000;22(4):455–464.

Williams JMG, Little MM, Scates S, et al. Memory complaints and abilities among depressed older adults. *J Consult Clin Psychol* 1987;55:595–598.

Winocur G, Moscovitch M. A comparison of cognitive function in institutionalized and community-dwelling old people of normal intelligence. *Canadian Journal of Psychology* 1990;44:435–444.

Winocur G, Moscovitch M, Freedman J. An investigation of cognitive function in relation to psychosocial variables in institutionalized old people. *Canadian Journal of Psychology* 1987;41(2):257–269.

Wright BM, Payne RB. Effects of aging on sex differences in psychomotor reminiscence and tracking proficiency. *J Gerontol* 1985;40:179–184.

Zacks RT, Hasher L, Li KZH. Human memory. In: Craik FI, Salthouse TA, eds. *The handbook of aging and cognition*, 2nd ed. Mahwah, NJ: Lawrence Erlbaum Associates, 2000.

SUGGESTED WEB SITES

http://www.nih.gov/nia/health
http://www.healthandage.com

6

Acute Confusional State: Delirium, Encephalopathy

M. Cornelia Cremens and Gary L. Gottlieb

Delirium, acute confusional state and encephalopathy, are they all the same syndrome?

Confusion is a state of reduced coherence, clarity, comprehension, and reasoning. When a patient has the aforementioned symptoms of confusion and is sleepy or drowsy, the diagnosis of *encephalopathy* is applied. In *acute confusional states*, agitation and hallucinations are prominent. Systemic metabolic changes or brain lesions typically manifest symptoms of both drowsiness and confusion. These changes are a result of the dysfunction of the central nervous system (CNS) caused by failure of neuronal or glial metabolism. Brain metabolism is dependent on both oxygen and glucose, and brain damage results if either is lacking.

Psychiatrists use *delirium* interchangeably with acute confusion or encephalopathy, whereas neurologists reserve the term "delirium" for the hyperactive, agitated, hallucinating state caused by withdrawal or intoxication. Delirium is in the broad differential diagnosis for psychotic disorders according to the *Diagnostic and Statistical Manual of Mental Disorders*, edition IV-TR (DSM-IV). (American Psychiatric Association [APA]). The nosology of this syndrome is important to clarify to allow standardization and comparison of various studies (Gottlieb, 1998). The DSM-IV-TR definition of delirium divides the diagnosis into four divisions:

1. Delirium due to general medical condition,
2. Substance induced delirium,
3. Delirium due to multiple etiologies, and
4. Delirium not otherwise specified (APA 2000).

The DSM-IV-TR describes an abrupt disturbance of consciousness with a change in cognition not explained by preexisting or evolving dementia as the cardinal feature of delirium (APA, 2000). The change in consciousness can be either reduced or increased with impaired ability to focus, attend, sustain, or shift attention. Altered cognition can include memory disturbance, disorientation, language disturbance, and perceptual disturbance. Perceptual disturbances or psychotic symptoms include delusions, misperceptions, illusions, or hallucinations. Sleep-wake cycle and psychomotor behavioral disturbances accompany these symptoms, compounding the confusion, disorientation and psychosis (Lipowski, 1990). Symptoms develop abruptly over a short period of time and fluctuate throughout the day. The syndrome is transient, although some longstanding symptoms may be present because of possible brain damage related to lack of oxygen or glucose from the acute insult (APA 2000; Tzrepacz 1996).

Delirium is underrecognized, underreported, and inadequately documented by physicians because of the subtle presentation and varying types of delirium. As with any illness, diagnosis depends on its recognition. However, many studies suggest that delirium goes undetected in up to half of the patients who develop the syndrome. Signs and symptoms of delirium are documented in only 30% to 50% of cases (Francis et al., 1990). The epidemiology is not well reported. Even when delirium is recognized and accurately diagnosed, it remains undocumented in the medical record (Glick et al.,1996). Approximately 10% to 20% of all hospitalized patients manifests some degree of delirium at admission or during their hospital stay, with a higher percentage of delirium seen in the elderly (Francis et al.,1990; Marcantonio et al., 2000). Symptoms can be confused with medical, neurologic, affective, psychotic, and personality disorders (Meagher and Trzepacz, 1998). Premorbid dementia places the patient at greater risk for delirium and impaired outcome (Rahkonen et al., 2000). Although delirium is acute, it can proceed unrecognized for a period of time because of its mild subsyndromal symptoms and, thus, appear chronic (Levkoff et al., 1992). Elderly patients are at highest risk for delirium from multiple comorbid illness and age-associated sensitivity to medications (Kraemer et al., 1997). Drug-induced delirium can be precipitated by any medication and a close scrutiny of all medications is essential in the initial evaluation of a patient with delirium (Brown 2000). The fluctuating status of illness and multiple changes in medications during the initial stages of hospitalization increase the risk of delirium in older patients. Medical illness is often the culprit and medications used to treat the illness can add another order of magnitude to the delirium. In the elderly, delirium is a harbinger of significant morbidity and mortality (Levkoff et al., 1992; Rothchild et al., 2000). Many patients require nursing home placement after the incident hospitalization and statistics related to death after an episode of delirium hover around 50% within 2 years after discharge (Rahkonen et al., 2000; Rockwood et al., 1999).

EPIDEMIOLOGY

Delirium is one of the most frequent symptoms of disease in the older patient. A large variation of incidence and prevalence exists because of the different patient populations, inconsistent diagnostic criteria, and failure to diagnose and document (Sanders, 1992). In medical and surgical patients, studies report a prevalence rate of approximately 10% to 30% (Fann, 2000; Levkoff et al.,1992). In hospitalized elderly patients, the incidence and prevalence of delirium varies greatly, depending on patient population and clinical setting (Lipowski, 1990). Approximately 10% to 15% of elderly patients exhibit delirium on admission and another 10% to 40% are diagnosed during the hospitalization (Fann, 2000; Lipowski, 1989). In nursing home patients, the prevalence is even higher, up to 60%, and often confounded by comorbid dementia (Cole et al., 1998). Statistical data support that delirium is most often found in medically ill, hospitalized older patients and, with the rising numbers of older patients in hospitals, the prevalence and incidence of delirium can be expected to increase (Francis et al., 1992). Not surprisingly, the incidence is greatest among subjects who are older and sicker (Francis et al., 1992).

Prevalence of delirium in the terminally ill is approximately 85%, notably occurring in the last few weeks of life (Breitbart and Strout, 2000). The presence of delirium results in increased morbidity and interferes with pain control and comfort at the end of life. The cause is multifactorial and usually cannot be determined or reversed in the dying patients. In ap-

proximately one third of patients, delirium can be managed successfully only by providing sedation (Brietbart and Strout, 2000).

Cognitive impairment is often cited as one of the primary risk factors for delirium. One study followed patients admitted with a diagnosis of acute delirium without severe underlying illness for 2 years after discharge from the hospital. More than one half of these patients were diagnosed with dementia by a neuropsychologist after resolution of the delirium within that 2-year follow-up period (Rahkonen et al., 2000). The additional risk is increased morbidity while in the hospital of older delirious patients who have a significantly diminished physiologic reserve, with comorbidities and functional status important predictors of adverse events (Rothchild et al., 2000).

Pathogenesis

Delirium is a nonspecific neuropsychiatric presentation of a global disorder of central nervous system metabolism and neurotransmission. A final common pathway described by Trzepacz involves a variety of neural pathways and neurotransmitters, and the magnitude of effect, either increased or decreased, results in an altered mental state (Trzepacz 2000, 1996). The common medical causes of delirium are listed in Table 6-1. They can be associated with a variety of metabolic derangements of neurons and astrocytes. The reversible toxic effects of these conditions on the brain are not understood but, in different cases, can impair energy supplies, change ion fluxes across neuronal membranes, and cause neurotransmitter abnormalities temporarily (van der Mast, 1998). Numerous causes are implicated, including long lists of both medical illness and pharmacologic agents. Reversible conditions that require immediate diagnosis and treatment because of the danger of permanent brain damage are Wernicke's, hypoxia, hypoglycemia, hypertensive encephalopathy, intracerebral hemorrhage, meningitis or encephalitis, and poisoning (Cassem and Murray, 1997).

TABLE 6-1. *Common medical causes of delirium*

Hyponatremia,
Hyperosmolarity
Hypercapnia
Hyercalcemia
Encephalopathies of hepatic and renal failure

Dopamine and Acetylcholine

When increased, dopamine and acetylcholine contribute to the range of symptoms identified in DSM-IV-TR criteria for delirium and the interaction can be explained at the neurotransmitter, receptor or neural pathway level (Trzepacz, 1996). Trzepacz proposes that delirium involves specific neural pathways, with lateralization to the right. Prefrontal cortices, right basilar mesial temporoparietal cortex, and anterior and right thalamus are indicated in the theory of a neural pathway. Dopamine is involved in motor activity, stereotypy, motivation, perception, attention, memory, mood, and thought. It can contribute to the alteration in the level of consciousness that is diagnostic in delirium. A relative excess of dopamine implicated in the cause of delirium may explain why dopamine blockers such as haloperidol and the newer atypical antipsychotics are helpful in providing symptomatic benefit. The mesocortical dopaminergic system primarily innervates the frontal cortex and is probably not involved in general cortical arousal. This system selectively regulates the frontal cortex role in maintaining and shifting attention (Trzepacz, 2000). The effectiveness of antipsychotics in controlling the hallucinations and delusions of delirium suggests the involvement of dopamine largely in the development of these symptoms.

Dopaminergic activity is located in the hypothalamic-pituitary, nigrostriatal, and ventral tegmentum. Abnormalities in cholinergic neurotransmission precipitates the delirium commonly seen in the elderly when, with the use of anticholinergic drugs, symptoms of delirium are produced (Tune, 2000). Memory impairment can be associated with basal forebrain cholinergic pathways, and changes in level of consciousness can be associated with pontine cholinergic pathways projecting to frontal cortices and brainstem (Trzepacz, 2000).

Gamma Aminobutyric Acid

Gamma aminobutyric acid (GABA), the predominant inhibitory neurotransmitter in the central nervous system, is implicated in hepatic encephalopathy. Elevated serum ammonia levels contribute to increased glutamate and glutamine levels being precursors to GABA. An endogenous benzodiazepinelike toxin can be produced in liver failure, causing encephalopathy, by binding to benzodiazepine receptors in the hypothalamus. Overstimulation of these GABA benzodiazepine postsynaptic receptors results in the somnolence seen in hepatic encephalopathy. Withdrawal from benzodiazepines or alcohol understimulates these receptors, precipitating a hyperactive form of delirium.

Serotonin

Other neurotransmitters, including serotonin, are implicated as pathophysiologic factors in the development of delirium. Serotonin is either increased or decreased in different types of delirium. It is increased in hepatic encephalopathy, sepsis, and serotoninergic syndrome and decreased in postcardiotomy. Serotonin can contribute to dopamine regulation in various neural pathways, including the striatum and limbic system. This is a possible explanation for the benefit of antipsychotic drugs with multiple receptor sites, as is seen in the newer atypical antipsychotic agents.

However, some forms of delirium are caused by drugs or toxins acting on specific brain neurochemical systems or, as with cytokines, can affect a global disturbance in cerebral function, such as a reduction of serum albumin, disruption of the integrity of the blood–brain barrier, implication of large neutral amino acids, and electrophysiologic changes (van der Mast and Fekkes, 2000; Tune, 2000). The term "delirium" refers to an acute, reversible state of confusion, but this state can proceed to a chronic state of impairment, which may be explained at the molecular level with regard to the large neutral amino acids and neurotransmitters (van der Mast et al., 2000). The permanent decline in cognition may be related to the impact of these large amino acids, cytokines, and the electrophysiologic changes.

ETIOLOGY

Common causes of delirium in the elderly can be found in Table 6-2. When the medical problem (e.g., known drug ingestion, hypoxia, stroke, trauma, or liver or kidney failure) is obvious, attention then focuses on the primary illness. Infections are most commonly pneumonia or urinary tract infection. Cerebrovascular disease may be obvious, as in stroke, or subtle with multiple transient ischemic attacks. Dementia may or may not have been diagnosed before the diagnosis of delirium. A complete listing of all diseases, drugs, or substances that cause delirium would serve little purpose, because it would not aid diagnosis. Predisposing factors in the older patient include chronic illness, aging or injured brain, impaired drug metabolism, substance use and abuse, and sensory impairments (Rummans et al., 1995). The addi-

TABLE 6-2. *Common causes of delirium in the elderly*

Infections
Medications
Metabolic abnormalities
Dementia
Cerebrovascular disease
Cardiovascular disease
Substance intoxication or withdrawal

tional risk is increased morbidity in older, hospitalized delirious patients who have a significantly diminished physiologic reserve. Comorbidities and functional status are important predictors of adverse events (Rothchild et al., 2000). Rothchild noted that older patients were at greater risk for adverse drug events, falls, nosocomial infections, pressure sores, delirium, and surgical and perioperative complications. In each category, the older patient's risk ranged from a 2.2 times increase for perioperative complications to a 10 times increase for falling. Age alone is a less important predictor of adverse events than comorbidities and functional status. Serum albumin declines in delirious patients, probably because of the underlying cause of the delirium. However, low serum albumin level is a risk factor for mortality in older persons (Corti et al., 1994). A combined measure of albumin and disability reveals a strong gradient in mortality risk and may serve as a simple but useful index of frailty that can identify a group of older men and women at high risk who could be targeted for preventive and treatment efforts. Delirium is an important marker of risk for dementia and death, even in older patients without prior cognitive or functional deficits (Rockwood et al., 1999).

CLINICAL FEATURES OF DELIRIUM

Clinical features of delirium include prodrome, abrupt onset, rapid fluctuating course, decreased attention, altered mental status, disturbed sleep wake cycle, impaired memory, disorganized thinking, disorganized speech, language alterations, disorientation, altered perceptions, hallucinations, delusions, and, possibly, an identified underlying medical or physical cause (Lipowski, 1989) (Fig. 6-1). Other symptoms of delirium are often mistakenly attributed to an underlying neurologic or psychiatric disorders. Neurologic features of delirium that are often confused with other diagnoses include dysphagia, con-

structional apraxia, dysnomic aphasia, motor abnormalities, and an abnormal electroencephalogram (EEG) study. Although nonspecific, EEG changes reveal prominent slowing, with diffuse bilateral slowing, and can be useful in confirming a puzzling presentation (Leuchter et al., 1993). Emotional disturbances can be prominent: intense anger or fear, mania, irritability, depression, euphoria, sadness, rage, apathy, anxiety, and panic (Lipowski, 1989). All of the above symptoms can represent a neuropsychiatric state of altered and fluctuating consciousness that develops from a generalized cerebral impairment or dysfunction related to an illness, substance intoxication, or substance withdrawal. Hyperactive, hypoactive, or mixed clinical subtypes of delirium are widely accepted as a common method of categorization, with the hyperactive type more frequently reported (Camus et al., 2000). Motor subtypes are perplexing. Patients with increased agitation or hyperactive subtype are more often diagnosed with delirium, whereas those with hypoactive or mixed subtype are at great risk for adverse outcome from delirium not yet diagnosed (Meagher and Trzepacz, 2000). No significant difference is found in terms of cause or outcome profile between clinical subtype groups. The variety of delirium presentations further confuses the diagnosis; hence, the discrepancy among neurologists' and psychiatrists' criteria for delirium.

The symptoms of delirium develop over hours to days and, rarely, weeks. The abrupt development of symptoms is the distinguishing feature of delirium versus dementia. Patients with dementia can exhibit paranoia, irrational suspiciousness, and mistrust of those caring for them, even close family members (Jacobson, 1997). Delusions are common in dementia, presenting as fixed, false ideas or beliefs even when given evidence to the contrary. For example, a person may complain that something has been stolen, food poisoned, or someone who is deceased has visited them. Hallucinations are often visual, with a range from a dreamlike state to terrifying visions. In addition, auditory, olfactory, tactile, and gustatory hallucinations are reported, but with less frequency.

Prodromal symptoms can last up to several days before the diagnosis of delirium is made. Symptoms tend to fluctuate in intensity, with periods of relative clarity interspersed with periods of severe impairment. Delirium can resolve within hours to days or last up to weeks, months, or a year in some cases, especially in the older population (Franco et al., 2001). Elderly individuals with better premorbid cognition

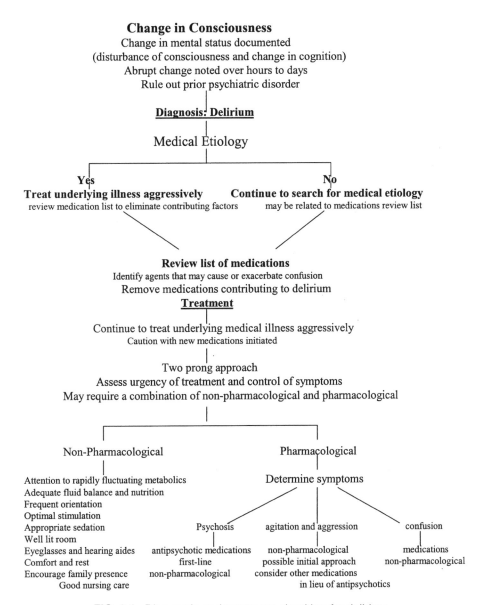

FIG. 6-1. Diagnostic and treatment algorithm for delirium.

and physical functioning often have a more rapid recovery (Cole et al., 1998).

DIFFERENTIAL DIAGNOSIS

The multiple confounding factors involved in the diagnosis of delirium result in the inability to accurately diagnose, determine the etiology, and provide appropriate treatment promptly (Table 6-3). The complex nature of delirium contributes to the task of defining the offending agents, medical illness, and complicating factors that contribute to the intensity of this state. Drug-induced delirium is the most common cause of delirium especially in the elderly. Older pa-

TABLE 6-3. *Differential diagnosis of delirium*

	Delirium	Dementia	Depression
Symptom onset	Abrupt	Insidious	Slow
Orientation	Fluctuates	Poor	Normal
Duration	Hours to months	Years	Weeks to months
Consciousness	Fluctuates	Normal	Normal
Attention	Impaired	Varies	Usually intact
Memory	Impaired	Poor	Normal or impaired
Thought	Disordered	Poor	Impaired
Speech	Incoherent	Mild errors	Normal, slowed
Perceptions	Altered	Altered, normal	Normal
Hallucinations	Often	Intermittently	Not usually
Delusions	Often	Intermittently	Not usually

tients are on multiple combinations of prescribed drugs; however, often overlooked are over-the-counter drugs, more frequently herbal and alternative remedies, and alcohol or illicit drugs. Pharmacokinetic and pharmacodynamics are altered in older patients, thereby making them more susceptible to drug-induced delirium. The integrity of the blood–brain barrier with aging is altered and predisposes to dementia. Common risk factors for delirium in the elderly are listed in Table 6-4.

Initial assessment and establishment of cognitive impairment are documented with the use of a screening instrument. The Folstein Mini-Mental State Examination (MMSE) remains the easiest to administer and is fine as a screen (Folstein et al., 1975). The other screening tools are used more in research and, although they might be helpful in tracking the development and resolution numerically, that is not necessary for patient care. Among the screening instruments specific for delirium are (*a*) the Delirium Rating scale (DRS), an eight-item linear scale (Trzepacz et al., 1988); (*b*) Memorial Delirium Assessment Scale (MDAS), a ten-item,

four-point scale (Breitbart et al., 1997); and (*c*) Confusion Assessment Method (CAM), a nine-item, four-point scale (Inouye et al., 1990). Although not used routinely in clinical practice, these scales may add more continuity and comparability to the diagnosis (Trzepacz 1996; Breitbart et al., 1996; Inouye et al., 1999).

Drug-induced delirium had higher DRS scores than both the anticholinergic and infectious or electrolyte group for changes in sleep-wake cycle and fluctuation of symptoms. Those from the anticholinergic group were more likely to fit the hypoactive, motoric subtype (Meagher and Trzepacz, 1998). Six categories of patients at high risk for delirium are in Table 6-5. Disagreement exists over the relationship between delirium and dementia. Underlying dementia is a risk factor for the development of delirium, and the evolution from delirium to dementia is thought to be infrequent. However, prolonged and permanent memory impairment in subjects who have experienced delirium can persist in 50% of patients permanently. Delirium can herald the onset of dementia and not be the cause. The diagnosis of dementia cannot be made during an episode of delirium or recovery. It is best to reevaluate the patient after an appropriate recovery period (e.g., 3 to 6 months or a year). before concluding the patient has a dementia.

TABLE 6-4. *Common risk factors for delirium in the elderly*

Low serum albumin
Multiple, severe, or unstable medical problems
Dementia or cognitive impairment
Polypharmacy
Metabolic disturbances
Isolation
Advanced age (especially >80 yrs)
Infection (especially urinary tract or pneumonia)
Fractures
Visual impairment
Fever or hypothermia
Psychoactive drug use

TABLE 6-5. *Patients at high risk for delirium*

Elderly
Brain damage (including dementia and strokes)
Burn
Postcardiotomy
Drug withdrawal
Acquired immunodeficiency syndrome

MANAGEMENT AND TREATMENT OF DELIRIUM

Delirium management and treatment are complex. Accurate diagnosis is paramount and treatment of the underlying cause imperative. Eliminate any contributing factors and structure the environment for the patient to avoid worsening of the delirium.

In addition to medication, supportive care and adequate fluid balance, other factors contributing to the control of symptoms include adequate nutrition, sedation, rest, comfort; attention to rapidly fluctuating metabolic rate; good nursing care, family presence, frequent orientation, optimal stimulation, a well-lit room; and eyeglasses and hearing aides in place (Inouye and Carpenter, 1996; Inouye et al., 1999).

Establishing the diagnosis of delirium is the benchmark of appropriate management; identifying the underlying cause and aggressive treatment comprise the initial step. Elimination of factors contributing to the clinical features (e.g., medications, environmental impediments or stimuli) will enhance recovery for the patient (Inouye et al., 1999).

Pharmacologic treatments are the most common initial interventions in delirium while treating the underlying cause. Because of potency and rapid onset of action, intravenous medications are the mainstay of the pharmacopoeia. In acutely agitated delirious patients, intravenous medication affords better access to administration of medications. For many years, haloperidol has been the drug of choice and it is well documented in the literature. However, with the advent of newer atypical antipsychotic agents and after reviewing complex data on neurotransmitters and neural pathways, the choice for treatment of the psychotic symptoms has been widened.

Decision to give medications begins with the identification of specific symptoms: agitation, aggression, hallucinations, delusions, risk of injury to patient or to those caring for the patient. Then, review the side effects of medications with reference to the patient's medical or surgical problem.

MEDICATIONS

Medications to treat delirium have traditionally been high potency neuroleptics (Cassem and Murray, 1997). Haloperidol has been the drug of choice, but the newer atypical agents are being used more frequently with fewer side effects (Marsand, 2000). The atypical antipsychotics do not have a parenteral formula; therefore, in emergencies or intensive care units, haloperidol or droperidol would remain the drug of choice. Atypical antipsychotics have not been systematically tested against the typical antipsychotics but numerous case reports have confirmed their efficacy. Starting dose with any drug is always the lowest possible level (Table 6-6). Intravenous haloperidol has the most rapid effect; start with a low dose and titrate until the desired effect is attained with the least side effects (Tesar and Stern, 1988). Haloperidol also can be given orally or intra-

TABLE 6-6. *Cost of medications*

Drug	Dose (mg every day)	Risks	Cost/month ($)
Haloperidol (Haldol)	0.25–10	EPS, TD	10–27
Best given IV for acute agitation	IV dosing	Arrhythmia	4 (2 mg/mL 4 mL)
Droperidol (Inapsine)	IV dosing	Hypotension	10 (2 mg/mL 4 mL)
Perphenazine (Trilafon)	2–16	EPS, TD	58–70
Available IV for acute agitation	IV dosing	Arrhythmia	25 (2.5 mg/mL 4 mL)
Fluphenazine (Prolixin)	2.5–10	EPS, TD	34–62
Olanzapine (Zyprexa)	2.5–15	Weight gain	122–216
Risperidone (Risperdal)	0.25–2.0	EPS at higher doses	69–133
Clozapine (Clozaril)	12.5–200	Sedation, hypersalivation	38–95
Quetiapine (Seroquel)	12.5–300	Sedation, mild hypotension	36–120
Lorazepam (Ativan)	0.25–3.0	Sedation, confusion	20–35
Available IV for acute agitation	IV dosing	Sedation confusion	38 (2 mg/mL 4 mL)
Alprazolam (Xanax)	0.25–2.0	Sedation, confusion	17–43
Diazepam (Valium)	1.0–30.0	Long half-life, active metabolites	5–8
Clonazepam (Klonopin)	0.25–3.0	Long half-life, sedation, confusion	20–30
Donepezil (Aricept)	2.5–10	Diarrhea, confusion	160

EPS, extrapyramidal symptoms; IV, intravenous; TD, tardive dyskinesia.

muscularly. It has minimal effects on hemodynamic, neurologic, and respiratory function and does not cause or aggravate delirium (Menza et al., 1987). Haloperidol is not approved by the Food and Drug Administration for intravenous use but the numerous reports in the literature support its use. The potency of intravenous drugs is twice that of oral medications, with a faster onset of action (minutes), and a faster elimination half-life (hours), thus, providing expeditious treatment of this life-threatening syndrome. Bolus dosing is usually started at a low dose (0.5–2.0 mg) as an initial dose. For mild delirium, the range is from 0.5 to 20 mg (Tesar and Stern, 1988). In difficult cases, haloperidol can be administered by continuous intravenous infusion (Stern, 1994; Riker, 1994). It has a relatively safe side-effect profile when used in the seriously medically ill, including congestive heart failure, chronic obstructive pulmonary disease, epilepsy, and renal insufficiency. It does not cause significant hypotension. Unlike orally or intramuscularly administered drug, intravenous haloperidol has rare extrapyramidal side effects (Menza et al., 1987). Prolonged QTc interval on electrocardiogram (ECG) and torsades de pointes arrhythmia (multifocal ventricular tachycardia) have been attributed to intravenous haloperidol (Hunt and Stern, 1995). Medical conditions that can heighten the risk of torsades de pointes are cardiomyopathy, metabolic abnormalities (low magnesium or potassium), ethanol abuse, sympathomimetic and antiarrhythmic drugs, status asthmaticus, hypothyroidism, and bradyarrhythmias. Cardiac monitoring is used, especially with higher doses or continuous infusion. Intravenous haloperidol is often combined with intravenous lorazepam, which is thought to have a synergism that potentiates their effectiveness. Benzodiazepines have mixed benefit in that they can disinhibit the patient or cause paradoxical reactions in older patients. However, in patients who require more sedation, the combination is advantageous. Extrapyramidal symptoms (EPS) are more severe in older patients with Parkinson's disease, acquired immunodeficiency syndrome (AIDS) dementia, or Lewy body dementia (Klatka et al., 1996; Schneider, 1999). Fernandez reports the increased EPS sensitivity is likely caused by the subcortical nature in AIDS dementia (Fernandez and Levy, 1994). Intravenous droperidol provides more sedation and may have a faster onset of action. It has similar antidopaminergic potency to haloperidol but may have less antipsychotic activity. Droperidol is a potent alpha$_1$-adrenergic antagonist and hypotension can be a significant problem (Cassem and Murray, 1997). In critically ill patients, paralysis and ventilation may be required, whereby the intensive care physician can use neuromuscular blocking agents (curare), sedative-hypnotics (e.g., propofol), and benzodiazepines (Shapiro et al., 1995; Cassem and Murray, 1997).

Benzodiazepines

Benzodiazepines are first-line treatment for delirium associated with seizures or withdrawal from alcohol or sedatives. Lorazepam is advantageous because of its sedative properties and rapid onset and short duration of action. Its bioavailability is more predictable when it is given intramuscularly, but a low risk exists of accumulation and no major active metabolites. Lower doses are recommended in elderly patients, hepatic disease, and with compounds that undergo extensive hepatic oxidative metabolism. Benzodiazepines can both protect against delirium and be a risk factor for delirium in older patients. This highlights the need for judicious use in older patients dependent on alcohol or benzodiazepines. Conversely, the patient may require a large dose of benzodiazepines to forestall delirium tremens (Kraemer et al., 1997).

Atypical Antipsychotics

Atypical antipsychotics are indicated for elderly patients with neurodegenerative disorders and medical conditions because of the low side effect profile. Basic science research indicates the use of these novel agents in delirium is favorable with the research implication of acetylcholine, dopamine, and serotonin in the pathophysiology of delirium (van der Mast et al., 2000; Trzepacz, 2000). Newer atypical antipsychotics are more selective for specific dopamine and serotonin receptors. *Clozapine* was the first atypical antipsychotic on the market. Clozapine is a tricyclic dibenzodiazepine derivative with a high potency in treating psychosis, with minimal central dopaminergic antagonism. Clozapine appears to be more active at the limbic dopamine receptors than at the striatal receptors and does not induce parkinsonian symptoms or tardive dyskinesias and, therefore, is the drug of choice for patients with Parkinson's disease. Clozapine continues to require weekly-monthly white blood cell count because of the risk of agranulocytosis.

Olanzapine, a newer atypical neuroleptic, like risperidone, blocks 5HT$_2$ as well as D$_2$ receptors and has been shown to have a better side-effect profile than haloperidol in terms of EPS (Sipahimalani and

Masand, 1998). Patients with Parkinson's disease with drug-induced hallucinations caused by the dopaminergic medications were randomized in a trial of clozapine versus olanzapine. Olanzapine exacerbated the parkinsonism, bradykinesia, and gait, in comparison with clozapine, which reduced the hallucinations and improved behavior (Goetz et al., 2000).

Riperidone binds with high affinity to dopamine D2, serotonin $5HT_2$, and alpha$_1$-adrenergic receptors with a lower affinity to an alpha$_2$-adrenergic and H_1 receptors and has proved to be relatively safe for use in elderly with comorbid disease (Zarate et al., 1997).

Quetiapine interacts with a broader range of neurotransmitters, including dopamine D_1 and D_2, and serotonin $5HT_2$ and $5HT_{1a}$; the higher selectivity for $5HT_2$ relative to D_2 is probably what contributes to the antipsychotic properties and low EPS. The sedation associated with quetiapine is an advantageous side effect in a patient with a hyperactive type of delirium (Jeste et al., 1999).

Cholinesterase Inhibitors

Cummings (1997) reports success with cholinergic therapies used to treat symptoms commonly associated with Alzheimer's disease: apathy, agitation, mood disturbances, irritability, disinhibition, delusions, aberrant motor behavior, and abnormalities of sleep and eating. Changes in neuropsychiatric symptoms suggest these abnormalities may respond to cholinergic therapy. The symptoms are based on brain dysfunction similar to delirium, which in turn results in poor recovery from illness and adverse consequences for those caring for the patient. Cholinomimetic therapy ameliorates the behavioral and emotional disturbances of Alzheimer's disease and exhibits disease specificity. The use of cholinesterase inhibitors has been reported with great success in patients with Lewy body disease. Wengel et al. (1999) report a case of an older man, with dementia, complicated by delirium after surgery; the patient's symptoms responded rapidly to a cholinesterase inhibitor.

ENVIRONMENTAL

Inouye studied interventions to prevent delirium by addressing the management of cognitive impairment, sleep deprivation, immobility, visual impairment, hearing impairment, and dehydration. When comparing the intervention group with the usual care group, the incidence of delirium was 9.9% versus 15%. The average length of hospital stay was unchanged, but in the intervention group the total number of days of

TABLE 6-7. *Simple interventions to prevent delirium*

Attention to rapidly fluctuating metabolics
Adequate fluid balance and nutrition
Frequent orientation
Optimal stimulation
Appropriate sedation
Well-lit room
Eyeglasses and hearing aides
Comfort and rest
Encourage family presence
Good nursing care

delirium and episodes of delirium were reduced (Inouye, 1998). Simple interventions such as those listed in Table 6-7 also result in a significant impact on outcome.

COURSE AND PROGNOSIS OF DELIRIUM

The course of delirium waxes and wanes; it fluctuates and is variable, with endpoints of slow recovery, residual cognitive impairment, or a downward spiral to stupor, coma, and death. Mortality rate depends on the setting and the rates vary widely in the elderly population (17% to 75%). Whenever possible, engage family members in discussions about current, predicted, or resolving delirium. An explanation of the biologic basis of this syndrome helps the family members understand that the words and actions of the delirious patient are not necessarily accurate and that they are not intended to be hurtful. Family members who are aware of the memory impairment in delirium can assist the hospital staff in reorienting the patient and may find it easier to handle the frequent repetition that is necessary for this task. Family members also need to understand that the onset of delirium does not mean that the patient has "lost his or her mind" or become demented. In particular, decisions regarding long-term placement should be postponed until the delirium has cleared. Otherwise, many patients with delirium would inappropriately or prematurely be considered for nursing home placement.

Delirium, a serious and potentially life-threatening syndrome, requires early diagnosis and aggressive treatment. It presents challenges to the physicians managing elderly patients who are at greatest risk for adverse outcomes. Outcome studies and hospital follow-up after hospitalization comprise the direction for future studies, in hope of preparing patients at risk before hospitalization, which may reduce both the incidence of delirium and length of stay if a delirium develops.

PREVENTION

Paramount in prevention is early diagnosis of underlying causes, judicious use of medications, and aggressive treatment of cause and symptoms to prevent greater morbidity. Preexisting cognitive impairment is a risk factor for the development of delirium (Wengel et al., 1999). Cholinergic dysfunction may have a role in the development of delirium with dementia, especially of the Alzheimer's disease type. Using a cholinesterase inhibitor, either before surgery in susceptible patients or to treat delirium in a subgroup of patients at risk, may be indicated.

SUMMARY

Greater longevity certainly brings with it an increase in frailty and morbidity. The aging process and physiologic deterioration, in addition to the impact of age-related diseases and lifestyle, put elderly at greater risk for delirium. Efforts to define symptoms and identify risk factors are paramount. The use of standardized measures will enhance the establishment of reliable measures to clarify the identification and outcome of this disorder. The etiology, aggressive treatment, and course of delirium require greater investigation in order to implement effective diagnosis and treatment to reduce the morbidity and prolonged hospitalizations of the elderly (Gottlieb, 1998). As is known, the longer an older patient remains in the hospital and immobilized by illness, the more prolonged the recovery. Newer medications, more expeditious assessments, and increased attention to prevention will reduce the burden of this disorder.

REFERENCES

American Psychiatric Association. *Diagnostic and statistical manual of mental disorder*, 4th ed., text revision. Washington, DC: American Psychiatric Association 2000:136–147.

American Psychiatric Association. Practice guideline for the treatment of patients with delirium. *Am J Psychiatry* 1999;156(Suppl):1–20.

Breitbart W, Marotta R, Platt MM, et al. A double blind trial of haloperidol, chlorpromazine, and lorazepam in the treatment of delirium in hospitalized AIDS patients. *Am J Psychiatry* 1996;153:231–237.

Breitbart W, Rosenfeld B, Roth A, et al. The memorial delirium assessment scale. *J Pain Symptom Manage* 1997;13 (3):128–137.

Breitbart W, Strout D. Delirium in the terminally ill. *Clin Geriatr Med* 2000;16:357–372.

Brown TM. Drug-induced delirium. *Seminars in Clinical Neuropsychiatry* 2000;5:113–124.

Camus V, Gonthier R, Dubos G, et al. Etiologic outcomes in hypoactive and hyperactive subtypes of delirium. *J Geriatr Psychiatry Neurol* 2000;13:38–42.

Camus V, Burton B, Simeone I, et al. Factor analysis supports the evidence of existing hyperactive and hypoactive subtypes of delirium. *Int J Geriatr Psychiatry* 2000;15:313–316.

Cassem NH, Murray GB. Delirious patients. In: Cassem NH, ed. *Massachusetts General Hospital handbook of general hospital psychiatry*. St. Louis: Mosby, 1997.

Cole MG, Primeau FJ, Elie LM. Delirium: prevention, treatment, and outcome studies. *J Geriatr Psychiatry Neurol* 1998;11:126–137.

Corti MC, Guralnick JM, Salive ME, et al. Serum albumin level and physical disability as predictors of mortality in older persons. *JAMA* 1994;272:1036–1042.

Cummings JL. Changes in neuropsychiatric symptoms as outcome measures in clinical trials with cholinergic therapies for Alzheimer disease. *Alzheimer Dis Assoc Disord* 1997;11(Suppl 4):S1–S9).

Fann JR. The epidemiology of delirium: a review of studies and methodological issues. *Semin Clin Neuropsychiatry* 2000;5:64–74.

Fernandez F, Levy JK. Psychopharmacology in HIV spectrum disorders. *Psychiatric Clin North Am* 1994;17:135–148.

Folstein MF, Folstein SE, McHugh PR. "Mini-mental state": a practical method for grading the cognitive state of patients for the clinician. *J Psychiatr Res* 1975;2:189–198.

Francis J, Martin D, Kapoor WN. A prospective study of delirium in hospitalized elderly. *JAMA* 1990;263:1097–1101.

Francis J, Martin D, Kapoor WN. Prognosis after hospital discharge of older medical patients with delirium. *J Am Geriatr Soc* 1992;40:601–606.

Franco K, Litaker D, Joseph Locala J, et al. The cost of delirium in the surgical patient. *Psychosomatics* 2001;42:68–73.

Glick RE, Sanders KM, Stern TA. Failure to record delirium as a complication of intra-aortic balloon pump treatment: a retrospective study. *J Geriatr Psychiatry Neurol* 1996;9:97–99.

Goetz CG, Blasucci LM, Leurgans S, et al. Olanzapine and clozapine: comparative effects on motor function in hallucinating PD patients. *Neurology* 2000;55:789–794.

Gottlieb GL, Johnson J, Wanich C, et al. Delirium in the medically ill elderly: operationalizing the DSM-III criteria. *Int Psychogeriatr* 1991; 2:181–196.

Gottlieb GL. The future of delirium research. *J Geriatr Psychiatry Neurol* 1998;11:146–149.

Hunt N, Stern TA. The association between intravenous haloperidol and torsades de pointes: three cases and a literature review. *Psychosomatics* 1995;36:541–549.

Inouye SK, Van Dyck CH, Alessi CA, et al. Clarifying confusion: the confusion assessment method—a new method for detection of delirium. *Ann Intern Med* 1990;113:941–948.

Inouye SK. Delirium in hospitalized older patients: recognition and risk factors. *J Geriatr Psychiatry Neurol* 1998;11:118–125.

Inouye SK, Viscoli CM, Horwitz RI. A predictive model for delirium in hospitalized elderly medical patients based on admission characteristics. *Ann Intern Med* 1993;119:474–481.

Inouye SK, Chapentier PA. Precipitating factors for delirium in hospitalized elderly persons. *JAMA* 1996;275:852–857.

Inouye SK, Bogardus ST, Charpentier PA, et al. A multi-component intervention to prevent delirium in hospitalized older patients. *N Engl J Med* 1999;340:669–676.

Jacobson SA. Delirium in the elderly. *Psychiatr Clin North Am* 1997;20:91–110.

Jeste DV, Rockwell E, Harris MJ, et al. Conventional vs newer antipsychotics in elderly patients. *Am J Geriatr Psychiatry* 1999;7:70–76.

Klatka LA, Louis ED, Schiffer RB. Psychiatric features of Lewy body disease: a clinicopathologic study using Alzheimer's disease and Parkinson's disease comparison groups. *Neurology* 1996;47:148–1152.

Kraemer KL, Mayo-Smith MF, Calkins DR. Impact of age on the severity, course, and complications of alcohol withdrawal. *Arch Intern Med* 1997;157:2234–2241.

Leuchter AF, Daly KA, Rosenberg-Thompson S, et al. Prevalence and significance of electroencephalographic abnormalities in patients with suspected organic mental syndromes. *J Am Geriatr Soc* 1993;41:605–611.

Levkoff SE, Evans DA, Liptzin B, et al. Delirium: The occurrence and persistence of symptoms among elderly hospitalized patients. *Arch Intern Med* 1992;152:334–340.

Lipowski ZJ. Delirium in the elderly patient. *N Engl J Med* 1989;320:578–583.

Lipowski ZJ. *Delirium: acute confusional states.* New York: Oxford University Press, 1990.

Marcantonio ER, Flacker JM, Michaels M, et al. Delirium is independently associated with poor functional recovery after hip fracture. *J Am Geriatr Soc* 2000;48:618–624.

Marcantonio ER, Goldman L, Mangione CM, et al. A clinical prediction rule for delirium after elective noncardiac surgery. *JAMA* 1994;271:134–139.

Marsand P. Atypical antipsychotics for elderly patients with neurodegenerative disorders and medical conditions. *Psychiatric Annals* 2000;30:202–208.

Meagher DJ, O'Hanlon D, O'Mahony E, et al. Relationship between etiology and phenomenologic profile in delirium. *J Geriatr Psychiatry Neurol* 1998; 11:146–149.

Meagher DJ, Trzepacz PT. Delirium phenomenology illuminates pathophysiology, management, and course. *J Geriatr Psychiatry Neurol* 1998;11:150–156.

Meagher DJ, Trzepacz PT. Motoric subtypes of delirium. *Seminars in Clinical Neuropsychiatry* 2000;5:76–85.

Menza MA, Murray GB, Holmes VF, et al. Decreased extrapyramidal symptoms with intravenous haloperidol. *J Clin Psychiatry* 1987;48:278–280.

Mesulam MM. *Principles of behavioral and cognitive neurology.* New York: Oxford University Press, 2000: 177–182, 238.

Rahkonen T, Luukkainen-Markkula R, Paanila S, et al. Delirium episode as a sign of undetected dementia among community dwelling elderly subjects: a two-year follow-up. *J Neurol Neurosurg Psychiatry* 2000;69:519–521.

Riker RR, Fraser GL, Cox PM. Continuous infusion of haloperidol controls agitation in critically ill patients. *Crit Care Med* 1994;22:433–440.

Rockwood K, Cosway S, Carver D, et al. The risk of dementia and death after delirium. *Age Ageing* 1999;28: 551–556.

Rothschild JM, Bates D,W Leape LL. Preventable medical injuries in older patients. *Arch Intern Med* 2000;160: 2717–2728.

Rummans TA, Evans JM, Krahn LE, et al. Delirium in elderly patients: evaluation and management. *Mayo Clin Proc* 1995;70:989–998.

Sanders KM, Stern TA, O'Gara PT, et al. Delirium induced intra-aortic balloon pump therapy. *Psychosomatics* 1992; 33:35–44.

Schneider LS. Pharmacologic management of psychosis in dementia. *J Clin Psychiatry* 1999;60(Suppl):54–60.

Shapiro BA, Warren J, Egol AB, et al. Practice parameters for intravenous analgesia and sedation for adult patients in the intensive care unit: an executive summary. Society of Critical Care Medicine. *Crit Care Med* 1995;23: 1596–1600.

Sipahimalani A, Masand PS. Olanzapine in the treatment of delirium. *Psychosomatics* 1998;39:422–430.

Stern TA. Continuous infusion of haloperidol in agitated, critically ill patients. *Crit Care Med* 1994;22:378–379.

Tesar GE, Stern TA. Rapid tranquilization of the agitated intensive care unit patient. *Journal of Intensive Care Medicine* 1988; 3:195–201.

Trzepacz PT. Is there a final common neural pathway in delirium? *Seminars in Clinical Neuropsychiatry* 2000;5: 132–148.

Trzepacz PT. Delirium: Advances in diagnosis, pathophysiology, and treatment. *Psychiatric Clin North Am* 1996;19: 429–448.

Trzepacz PT, Baker RW, Greenhouse J. A symptom rating scale for delirium. *Psychiatry Res* 1988;23:89–97.

Tune LE. Serum anticholinergic activity levels and delirium in the elderly. *Seminars in Clinical Neuropsychiatry* 2000; 5:149–153.

van der Mast RC. Pathophysiology of delirium. *J Geriatr Psychiatry Neurol* 1998; 11:138–145.

van der Mast RC, Fekkes D. Serotonin and amino acids: partners in delirium and pathophysiology? *Seminars in Clinical Neuropsychiatry* 2000;5:125–131.

van der Mast RC, van den Broek WW, Fekkes D, et al. Is delirium after cardiac surgery related to plasma amino acids and physical condition? *J Neuropsychiatry Clin Neurosci* 2000;12:57–63.

Wengel SP, Burke WJ, Roccaforte WH. Donepezil for postoperative delirium associated with Alzheimer's disease. *J Am Geriatr Soc* 1999;47:379–380.

Zarate CA, Baldessarini RJ, Siegel AJ, et al. Risperidone in the elderly: a pharmacoepidemiologic study. *J Clin Psychiatry* 1997;58:311–317.

SUGGESTED READINGS

Inouye SK, Bogardus ST, Charpentier PA, et al. A multi-component intervention to prevent delirium in hospitalized older patients. *N Engl J Med* 1999;340:669–676.

Kamholz B. Introduction: the puzzles of delirium. *J Geriatr Psychiatry Neurol* 1998;11(3):115–117.

Lipowski ZJ. *Delirium: acute confusional states.* New York: Oxford University Press, 1990.

Trzepacz PT, guest editor. Is there a final common neural pathway in delirium? Focus on acetylcholine and dopamine. *Seminars in Clinical Neuropsychiatry* 2000;5(2):132–148.

Trzepacz, PT. Delirium: advances in diagnosis, pathophysiology, and treatment. *Psychiatr Clin North Am* 1996;19: 429–448.

7

Transient Loss of Consciousness: Syncope and Seizure

Maromi Nei and Reginald T. Ho

INTRODUCTION

Transient loss of consciousness in the elderly often presents one of the most difficult diagnostic challenges, particularly because of the high incidence of chronic medical conditions and associated medication usage.

The major differential diagnoses include neurologic and cardiovascular causes, with seizures and syncope leading the list. Seizures, which often present for the first time in the elderly, frequently are related to vascular and degenerative conditions. Cardiovascular disease and medication use also increases with age, as does the incidence of syncope (Kapoor et al., 1986; Savage et al., 1985).

PRESENTATION AND DIFFERENTIAL DIAGNOSIS

Details regarding the symptoms preceding and following the event are critical to determining the cause for loss of consciousness (Benbadis et al., 1995; Hoefnagels et al., 1991; Kapoor, 1990). A history regarding specific symptoms preceding loss of consciousness, particularly the duration and quality, should be elicited, and any triggering events should be identified (Tables 7-1 and 7-2).

Seizures

Seizures generally present as stereotyped spells, which follow a specific and consistent progression of symptoms during each event. In partial onset seizures, a specific aura can occur before the onset of alteration in level of consciousness. A clue may be a specific aura occurring in isolation as well as at the onset of a complex partial (those associated with alteration in level of consciousness but without generalization) or secondarily as a generalized tonic-clonic seizure. The duration of seizures is brief, generally less than 2 minutes. However, in those seizures asso-

ciated with an alteration in level of consciousness, patients are often amnestic for the seizure itself and may not recall events immediately preceding or following the seizure. Postictal confusion can last for several minutes to hours.

Focal Cerebral Ischemia

Focal cerebral ischemia resulting in transient alteration in level of consciousness is not common. Nor-

TABLE 7-1. *Spells in the elderly: differential diagnosis*

Neurologic
  Seizure
    Complex partial
    Secondarily generalized tonic-clonic
    Absence
    Nonconvulsive status epilepticus
  Transient ischemic attack
    Basilar artery ischemia
  Transient global amnesia
  Migraine
  Sleep disorder
  Nonepileptic psychogenic seizure
Cardiac
  Obstruction to outflow (aortic stenosis, idiopathic hypertrophic subaortic stenosis, pulmonary embolus)
  Loss of effective pump function (myocardial infarction, tamponade)
  Arrhythmias (bradyarrhythmias, tachyarrhythmias)
Reflexogenic
  Vasovagal syncope
  Situational syncope (cough, micturition, swallowing)
  Carotid sinus hypersensitivity
Orthostatic hypotension
  Medication effect
  Hypovolemic
  Neurogenic
Metabolic
  Hypoglycemia
  Hyperventilation

TABLE 7-2. *Variables that distinguish common spells in the elderly*

Variable	Seizure	Syncope	TIA	TGA
Premonitory symptoms	None vs. aura	None vs. N/V, lightheadedness Diaphoresis	None	None
Posture effect	None	Often erect	None	None
Onset	Acute	Variable	Acute	Acute
Bystander observations				
Duration	1–2 minutes	Seconds to minutes	Minutes to hours	Hours
Movements	Variable tonic-clonic movements	Loss of tone Clonic jerks	Deficits along vascular pattern	None
Incontinence	Variable	None	None	None
Heart rate	Increased or decreased	Variable	Normal	Normal
Electroencephalogram during ictus	Epileptiform pattern	Diffuse Slowing	Focal Slowing or normal	Rare Slowing
Trauma	Tongue laceration or ecchymoses	Ecchymoses or fracture	None	None
Offset	Confusion Sleep	Alert or mild confusion	Alert	Alert

N/V, nausea and vomiting; TGA, transient global amnesia; TIA, transient ischemic attack.

mal consciousness depends on the functioning of both cerebral hemispheres, the reticular formation, other upper brainstem structures, the thalamus, and hypothalamus (Plum and Posner, 1980). Thus, focal cerebral ischemia, as during a transient ischemic attack or stroke, must involve either both cerebral hemispheres or the brainstem and other deeper structures to result in alteration in level of consciousness. Posterior circulation ischemia or massive hemisphere infarction with shift can present with alteration in level of consciousness. Posterior circulation ischemia generally results in focal signs and symptoms (e.g., diplopia, eye movement abnormalities, other cranial nerve abnormalities, cerebellar dysfunction, motor and sensory dysfunction), which aid in the diagnosis. Massive infarction, of course, results in a sustained alteration in level of consciousness.

Transient Global Amnesia

Transient global amnesia (TGA) presents with marked anterograde amnesia that generally persists for hours, as well as retrograde amnesia. Although patients may be disoriented to time and place, they retain knowledge of their identity. The patient often repeatedly asks the same questions and has difficulty encoding new memories during this event. No focal neurologic deficits are seen, and the patient is fully conscious throughout the episode, unlike during a complex partial seizure. The pathophysiology is debated, but may be related to either cerebral ischemia or seizure. The incidence of TGA has been estimated to be approximately 5/100,000. Less than 25% of pa-

tients experience recurrent episodes (Adams et al., 1997; Miller et al., 1987).

Sleep Disorders

Sleep disorders (e.g., sleep apnea or narcolepsy) present with other symptoms that suggest a sleep disorder, particularly excessive daytime sleepiness, which results in lapses in consciousness. However, a history of sedation and concomitant symptoms (e.g., snoring or apnea) clearly differentiates the diagnosis of sleep disorders from others.

Nonepileptic Psychogenic Seizures

Nonepileptic psychogenic seizures are more common in younger individuals; however, they also occur in the elderly. A variety of different types of presentations are seen. Although slumping and sudden apparent loss of consciousness can occur, shaking and other movements can occur as well. Common features include (*a*) nonstereotyped spells; (*b*) irregular, nonrhythmic movements; (*c*) eye closure during the event; (*d*) waxing and waning of symptoms; (*e*) prolonged symptoms over several minutes to hours; (*f*) no history of spells arising directly from sleep; and (*g*) no history of severe injury (e.g., fracture, burn) during the spells. The patient may have a history of sexual or physical abuse, lack of response to anticonvulsant medication, and history of a psychiatric disorder. Video-electroencephalographic (EEG) monitoring or EEG and observation of the episode are helpful in establishing the diagnosis.

Cardiovascular Syncope

Cardiovascular syncope should be considered in any patient with a history of significant cardiovascular disease or cardiac surgery. Tachyarrhythmias (particularly ventricular tachycardia) need to be considered in any patient with reduced left ventricular function. Of particular concern is traumatic syncope occurring in a patient with a prior myocardial infarction. Such instances should raise a high index of suspicion for an arrhythmia. Bradyarrhythmias should be considered in those with significant conduction abnormalities on a baseline ECG (e.g., atrioventricular block, bundle branch block) or telemetry monitoring.

Reflexogenic Syncope

Reflexogenic syncope refers to vasovagal, viscerovagal, and situational syncope or carotid sinus hypersensitivity; it is caused by excessive vagal tone or sympathetic withdrawal often related to a triggering event. Such episodes are accompanied by hypotension, bradycardia, or both. Vasovagal syncope often has a prodrome of lightheadedness, warmth, nausea, and diaphoresis, although abrupt syncopal episodes can also occur (malignant vasovagal syncope). Situational syncope is easily identified by precipitating events, as may carotid sinus hypersensitivity.

Orthostatic Syncope

Orthostatic syncope is a transient loss of consciousness caused by an abrupt drop in blood pressure while assuming an erect posture. Primary autonomic failure can be caused by multiple system atrophy, which is generally associated with brainstem dysfunction or Parkinsonism. The Shy-Drager or Bradbury-Eggleston types of autonomic failure are associated with other evidence of autonomic dysfunction, including sexual and bladder dysfunction and anhidrosis. Secondary autonomic dysfunction can result from an autonomic neuropathy, often associated with a peripheral neuropathy, which may be seen in diabetes mellitus, chronic inflammatory demyelinating neuropathy, amyloidosis, and other types of neuropathy.

Metabolic Derangements

Syncope triggered by metabolic causes is uncommon. Acute hyperventilation with a reduction in P_{CO_2} can cause cerebral vasoconstriction but rarely syncope. Although hypoglycemia can cause syncope, episodic weakness is more common.

SEIZURES

Seizures are among the most common causes of transient loss of consciousness in the elderly. The incidence of both acute symptomatic and unprovoked seizures increases with age. The incidence of acute symptomatic seizures is approximately 100/100,000 population in those above 60 years of age (Annegers et al., 1995 Loiseau et al., 1990). These seizures may be caused by acute cerebrovascular ischemia (40% to 50%), metabolic derangements (10% to 15%), drug withdrawal, central nervous system (CNS) infection, acute trauma, or toxic insults (Annegers et al., 1995 Loiseau et al., 1990). The incidence of unprovoked seizures exceeds 100/100,000 in this same age group (Hauser et al., 1993). Unprovoked seizures can occur as the result of a prior stroke or head trauma, or in association with degenerative diseases, such as Alzheimer's disease. However, a definitive cause for epilepsy (having two or more unprovoked seizures) is identified only in the minority of patients (30% to 50%) (Annegers et al., 1995 Loiseau et al., 1990).

Risk factors for the development of epilepsy include a history of stroke, associated with more than a twenty times increase in risk of epilepsy; brain neoplasm; neurodegenerative disease; drug or alcohol withdrawal; CNS infection, associated with a threefold increase in risk; and head trauma, associated with a threefold increase in risk (Holt-Seitz et al., 1999; Rowan and Ramsay, 1997). Alzheimer's disease is associated with a five- to tenfold increase in risk for epilepsy (Dichter and Weinberger, 1997; Hauser et al., 1986; Hesdorffer et al., 1996; McAreavey et al., 1992; Romanelli et al., 1990). Major depression may also be a risk factor for seizures in the elderly (Hesdorffer et al., 2000).

Multiple seizure types may be seen. Partial onset seizures, often related to degenerative, vascular, or neoplastic causes, are most common. However, generalized seizures, related to toxic-metabolic encephalopathies and, perhaps, to genetic predisposition, also occur.

Temporal Lobe

Temporal lobe seizures are the most common type of seizures in the adult population, although extratemporal seizures may be more common in the elderly than in other age groups. Temporal lobe seizures can begin with an aura, such as a feeling of epigastric discomfort, an indescribable sensation, *déjà vu*, fear, or tinnitus. Although seizures are typically associated with positive phenomena, rather than the absence of normal function, both types of symptoms can be seen. During the seizure, speech arrest can occur, particularly in seizures originating in the left hemisphere. Complex partial seizures (those associated with an alteration in level of consciousness) arising from the temporal lobe may be manifested by automatisms, lip-smacking, teeth grinding, chewing, and the utterance of phrases or sentences that can be unintelligible or repetitive. Staring without automatisms is a common presentation in this age group, and head or eye deviation or dystonic posturing can occur. Postictally, confusion can last for several minutes to hours and the patient may be amnestic for the seizure. Because the temporal lobes are important for memory, patients with seizures arising from this area often complain of memory difficulty interictally as well.

Because of connections to the hypothalamus, temporal lobe seizures can be associated with autonomic changes. These include pupillary dilatation, apnea, hyperventilation, flushing, diaphoresis, urinary urgency or incontinence, and heart rate and rhythm changes. Both ictal tachycardia and bradycardia can occur during seizures arising from the temporal lobes. Most temporal lobe seizures are associated with an increase in heart rate, but supraventricular tachycardia, sinus arrest, atrial fibrillation, and frequent premature atrial and ventricular depolarizations can occur (Blumhardt et al., 1986; Nei et al., 2000). This association is particularly important to keep in mind when interpreting electrocardiographic (ECG) telemetry data during a typical spell. The ECG data alone without concomitant EEG during the spell may suggest that the event is primarily arrhythmic in origin, when in reality, the seizure is the primary event. Thus, simultaneous EEG-ECG monitoring is important in these cases.

Extratemporal Seizures

Partial seizures arising from other areas of the brain can also produce characteristic symptoms. Frontal lobe seizures are typically brief; they often occur in clusters (particularly nocturnally) and are often mistaken for nonepileptic events because of the irregular limb movements that are sometimes seen. Violent movements of the extremities, at times accompanied by vocalizations, are seen, as are focal clonic movements, forced eye and head deviation, and rapid secondary generalization. Other seizures, such as those arising from the supplementary motor cortex unilaterally, can result in complex movements of the limbs bilaterally or in asymmetric posturing. The diagnosis can be difficult, particularly because the EEG may be normal both interictally and during the seizure. An EEG revealing frontal spikes or neuroimaging demonstrating a frontal lobe lesion may suggest the diagnosis. Additionally, a history of symptoms arising directly from sleep is helpful. Although the individual can be confused postictally, he or she may regain full consciousness quickly after the seizure.

Seizures can also arise from the parietal or occipital lobes, and seizures arising from these areas may be more common in the elderly than in younger populations. Parietal lobe seizures can present with numbness, tingling, or other sensation on the side contralateral to the seizure focus. Both occipital and parietal lobe seizures can present with visual symptoms as well. Nystagmus or eye deviation can occur during occipital lobe seizures as well.

Alteration of level of consciousness can also occur in the setting of nonconvulsive status epilepticus. Patients may present with waxing and waning confusion, oftentimes accompanied by subtle facial twitching, nystagmus, or other focal twitching. The diffuse encephalopathy that can accompany this entity can be erroneously attributed solely to a toxic-metabolic derangement or medication effect, rather than to seizures. An EEG is invaluable in the diagnosis of this entity.

SYNCOPE

Syncope is defined as transient loss of consciousness, usually accompanied by concomitant loss of postural tone. Syncope results from a diffuse reduction in cerebral blood flow. Loss of consciousness occurs approximately 6 to 7 seconds after complete cessation of cerebral blood flow and is confirmed by the development of concomitant diffuse slowing on EEG (Fig. 7-1). A wide variety of disorders can cause syncope. A useful framework by which to classify these disorders is to consider four separate categories: (*a*) cardiovascular, (*b*) reflexogenic, (*c*) orthostatic, and (*d*) metabolic. Such a working classification is important because the diagnostic evaluation and prognosis in each category differs. The incidence of syncope increases with age. Cardiovascular diseases are more common in older individuals, who are also particularly susceptible to drug effects and overmedication. It is estimated that syncope accounts for 1% of hospital admissions and 3% of emergency room visits (Kapoor, 1992).

Vital information is provided by the patient's underlying medical conditions, the context of prior syn-

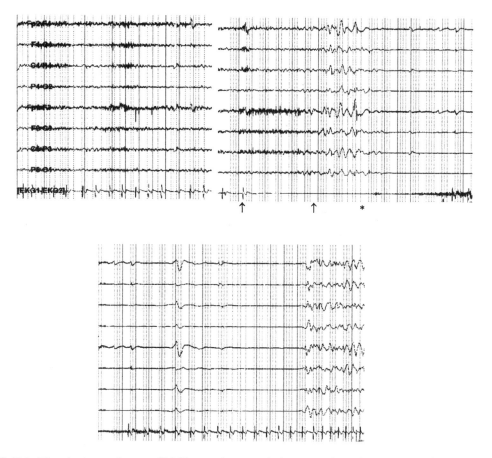

FIG. 7-1. The electrocardiogram (ECG) reveals asystole for approximately 15.5 seconds, beginning at the *bold arrow*. Diffuse slowing of the electroencephalogram (EEG) follows 6 seconds later and suppression of cerebral activity 10 seconds later. The suppression continues for approximately 18 seconds, including 12 seconds after return of the cardiac rhythm. This is again followed by diffuse slowing of the EEG, which is later followed by return of the EEG to a normal waking pattern (not shown).

copal episodes, medication use, use of alcohol or illicit drugs, and a family history of syncope. Important historical clues about the episode include (*a*) triggering events, (*b*) prodromal and associated symptoms, (*c*) body position, (*d*) onset and offset of syncope, and (*e*) bystander observations.

Triggering events can provide essential information to the underlying mechanism of syncope, particularly reflexogenic or orthostatic syncope. Exercise can precipitate syncope in individuals with severe aortic stenosis or hypertrophic cardiomyopathy as a result of peripheral vasodilation with left ventricular outflow obstruction or in patients with exercise-induced bradyarrhythmias or tachyarrhythmias. Prodromal symptoms (e.g., rapid palpitations before syn-

cope) suggest the presence of a tachycardia, whereas chest pain and shortness of breath should raise suspicion of a myocardial infarction or pulmonary embolus. Lightheadedness, nausea, yawning, and diaphoresis are symptoms of a vagal reaction.

Body position at the time of syncope provides important information. Prolonged standing can result in vasovagal syncope. Loss of consciousness associated with standing abruptly is seen with orthostatic syncope. Atrial myxomas can cause syncope with bending over. Abrupt onset syncope suggests acute cessation of cerebral blood flow, as occurs in arrhythmic syncope, but can also be seen in other causes of cardiovascular syncope, carotid sinus hypersensitivity, and malignant vasovagal syncope. Traumatic or catastrophic syncope is particularly concerning and suggests that the loss of consciousness is so abrupt that the patient was unable to protect him- or herself from the fall. Ventricular tachycardia should be considered in any elderly patient with left ventricle (LV) dysfunction who presents with traumatic syncope of unknown origin. Nonabrupt syncope is more common in vasovagal or orthostatic syncope. A patient with convulsive syncope demonstrates clonic movements caused by cerebral hypoperfusion and can be mistakenly diagnosed as having seizures (Aminoff et al., 1988; Zaidi et al., 2000).

Orientation after syncope (offset) is another important historical detail. Offset confusion can occur with hypoglycemia or seizures, whereas preserved orientation is more common with arrhythmic syncope. Patients suffering a vagal reaction may feel tired afterward. Retrograde amnesia after a syncopal episode is common in elderly patients and, therefore, bystander observations of the patient are important. Furthermore, medically trained bystanders might provide critical information on the blood pressure and pulse of the patient.

Cardiovascular Syncope

Cardiovascular syncope is important to identify because the 1-year mortality rate approaches 30% (Kapoor et al., 1983). Important causes include (*a*) obstruction to right or left ventricular outflow (aortic stenosis, hypertrophic obstructive cardiomyopathy, pulmonary embolus, pulmonary hypertension); (*b*) loss of effective pump function (e.g., myocardial infarction, tamponade); and (*c*) arrhythmias (i.e., brady- and tachyarrhythmias).

Specific causes of cardiovascular syncope are worth noting. Aortic stenosis presenting with syncope is associated with a poor long-term prognosis, if untreated, with an average survival of 3 years (Ross et al., 1968). It should be considered in any patient with a late-peaking, harsh systolic murmur in the second left intercostal space with low amplitude, delayed carotid upstrokes. The diagnosis can be confirmed by echocardiography, especially with an aortic valve area <1 cm^2. Generally, an aortic valve area >1.2 cm^2 is not hemodynamically significant.

Ventricular tachycardia is a serious but potentially treatable cause of syncope. The most common underlying cardiac substrate is a prior myocardial infarction. However, any patient with LV dysfunction is susceptible to ventricular tachyarrhythmias, which should be considered in those with a history of significant cardiovascular disease, infarction, bundle branch pattern on ECG, or LV dysfunction on echocardiography.

Supraventricular tachycardias (e.g., atrial fibrillation) rarely causes syncope with rapid ventricular rates in elderly patients who have stiff, noncompliant ventricles (e.g., LV hypertrophy) and require effective atrial transport function to maintain cardiac output.

Bradyarrhythmias (sick sinus syndrome, atrioventricular [AV] block) increase in the elderly because of sclerodegenerative changes and progressive calcification of the conduction system. Negatively dromotropic medications (beta-blockers, calcium channel blockers, digoxin) can aggravate symptoms.

Sick sinus syndrome-induced syncope should be considered in any elderly patient who presents with (*a*) atrial fibrillation with slow ventricular rates or ventricular pauses; (*b*) atrial fibrillation or flutter alternating with sinus bradycardia (tachy-brady syndrome) with prolonged pauses after conversion to sinus rhythm; and (*c*) extreme sinus bradycardia, sinus pauses, or arrest. AV block-induced syncope (Stokes-Adams-Morgagni syncope) should be considered in cases of atrioventricular or bifascicular block on ECG. Syncope is an uncommon but potentially lethal manifestation of acute myocardial infarction and pulmonary embolus. A detailed history, physical examination, and ECG study provide important clues to their diagnosis.

Reflexogenic Syncope

Reflexogenic syncope is caused by excessive bradycardia or hypotension resulting from exaggerated neural reflexes. Various receptors (e.g., LV mechanoreceptors [C fibers] in vasovagal syncope, carotid baroreceptors in carotid sinus hypersensitivity) send afferent inputs to the nucleus *tractus solitarius* (vasodepressor region of the medulla) resulting in efferent output (excessive parasympathetic tone or sympathetic withdrawal) and, therefore, bradycardia and/or hypotension. Although the prognosis is generally good, recurrent syncopal episodes can be a source of alarming symptoms and morbidity. Vagal tone decreases with age; thus, vasovagal syncope is not common in the elderly. Triggering events include prolonged standing (e.g., standing in church, kitchen), which decreases venous return and therefore increases cardiac contractility, leading to C-fiber activation. Prodromal symptoms include "vagal reactions" (i.e., lightheadedness, warmth, nausea, and diaphoresis). Loss of consciousness is brief and resolves with assuming a supine position. The diagnosis is considered with a compatible history and a normal ECG and echocardiogram.

Carotid Sinus Hypersensitivity

Carotid sinus hypersensitivity is a disease of older patients that is associated with atherosclerotic carotid disease and prior neck surgery (e.g., carotid endarterectomy). Triggering events include shaving (syncope at a barber's shop) or putting on a tie. The diagnosis can be confirmed by gentle carotid massage (first to the right carotid sinus, then the left) provided that significant atherosclerotic disease is not present. Carotid sinus massage can result in a cardioinhibitory response (asystole), vasodepressor response (hypotension), or both. Situational syncope should be diagnosed by identifiable triggers that result in abnormal viscerovagal reflexes (e.g., swallowing [deglutition syncope], urination [postmicturition] syncope).

Orthostatic Hypotension

Orthostatic syncope refers to transient loss of consciousness resulting from an abrupt drop in blood pressure associated with assuming an erect posture. In such instances, the body is unable to compensate rapidly enough to the demands of gravitational stress, either because of excessive volume depletion or inad-

equate vasoconstrictor mechanisms. Hypovolemia can be caused by excessive diuretic use. Also, medications (particularly antihypertensive medications), and autonomic neuropathies can cause inadequate peripheral vasoconstriction.

DIAGNOSTIC EVALUATION

Seizure Likely

Initial Evaluation

Based on the clinical presentation, the diagnosis of either seizure or syncope may be more likely. When the most likely diagnosis is seizure (Fig. 7-2), the initial workup should include an evaluation for possible metabolic derangements that may account for an acute seizure. Measurements of blood chemistry, including glucose, sodium, urea nitrogen, calcium, and magnesium, as well as an assessment of oxygenation status, are vital in the acute setting. If a CNS infection is suspected, a lumbar puncture should be performed. Medications should be carefully evaluated, and the evaluation of the past medical history should include any alcohol or illicit drug usage. Toxicologic tests should be performed as clinically indicated.

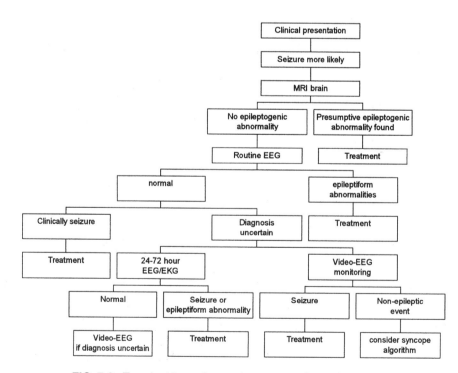

FIG. 7-2. Transient loss of consciousness: seizure more likely.

Seek a history of head trauma, which may not necessarily immediately precede the seizure. The elderly are at increased risk for subdural hematomas, which can develop even after relatively mild head trauma. Oftentimes, subtle or no obvious neurologic deficits are seen in such cases. If the history includes recent head trauma, focal neurologic deficits, or a postictal Todd's paralysis, computed tomography (CT) scan or magnetic resonance imaging (MRI) of the head should be done in the acute setting to exclude a contusion, mass lesion, stroke, or hemorrhage. An EEG may be helpful in the acute setting to rule out possible non-convulsive status epilepticus, if clinically indicated.

Neuroimaging

All adults who present with a probable epileptic seizure should have an MRI of the brain performed, barring no contraindications. In the acute setting, a CT of the head may be adequate; however, a head CT does not adequately assess for the possibility of a neoplastic lesion.

Electroencephalography and Long-Term Monitoring

If uncertain whether a spell may have represented a seizure, additional tests may be helpful in making the diagnosis. A routine EEG, particularly if sleep is captured (the frequency of epileptiform abnormalities generally increase during sleep), may reveal epileptiform abnormalities. Although nonspecific, epileptiform abnormalities (sharp waves or spikes) in the EEG support the diagnosis of epilepsy. However, a normal EEG or one that reveals focal or generalized nonepileptogenic abnormalities, does not exclude the diagnosis of epilepsy. In the elderly, it has been estimated that the frequency of interictal epileptiform activity is 26% to 35% on an initial EEG and lower than in the general population of patients with epilepsy, in whom 51% to 56% have interictal epileptiform abnormalities on an initial EEG (Ajmone-Marsan and Zivin, 1970; Drury and Beydoun, 1998).

If a routine EEG does not reveal interictal epileptiform abnormalities and the diagnosis is still uncertain, prolonged EEG monitoring is helpful, particularly if the spells are recurrent and frequent. Ambulatory EEG-ECG monitoring over a 24- to 72-hour period has three major advantages over the routine EEG: (a) increased likelihood of detecting interictal epileptiform abnormalities because of the lengthy recording duration, particularly during sleep; (b) increased likelihood of recording the EEG during a typical spell; and (c) an evaluation for possible subclinical or nocturnal seizures. It is particularly helpful when the spells are frequent and it is unclear whether the spell is related to a seizure or an arrhythmia.

Another option in uncertain cases is video-EEG monitoring performed in the inpatient setting over several days. Advantages over ambulatory EEG monitoring include (a) decreased likelihood of artifact, which often arises during long-term outpatient EEG-ECG recording, and (b) visual characterization of the spells in question and the ability to correlate EEG changes with clinical observation. This type of monitoring is particularly useful in the diagnosis of nonepileptic psychogenic seizures, during which seizurelike activity may be observed without accompanying ictal changes on the EEG. However, some caution should be used in making this diagnosis because simple, partial seizures and some types of complex, partial seizures (particularly those of frontal origin) can have a normal EEG during the event in question.

Syncope Likely

Initial Evaluation

The initial evaluation (history, physical examination, 12-lead electrocardiogram) provides a presumptive diagnosis in 50% to 60% of cases of syncope (Fig. 7-3). Given the poor prognosis for cardiovascular syncope, the initial evaluation should attempt to identify a cardiovascular cause.

In the acute setting, the physical examination should focus on the patient's vital signs, clues that may provide a cause of syncope, and areas of trauma that require medical attention. A complete neurologic and cardiovascular examination is therefore crucial, as are orthostatic measurements of blood pressure. The history and physical examination should include a search for offending medications, evidence of volume loss, and autonomic failure.

Electrocardiogram

The 12-lead electrocardiogram is a simple, inexpensive test that should be a part of every initial evaluation of the patient with syncope. Specific clues of a potential bradyarrhythmic etiology include sinus node dysfunction (extreme sinus bradycardia or sinus exit block), atrioventricular node dysfunction (particularly second and third degree heart block), and His-Purkinje dysfunction (bundle branch block). Clues to possible ventricular tachycardia include infarct patterns, bundle branch block, and a prolonged QT in-

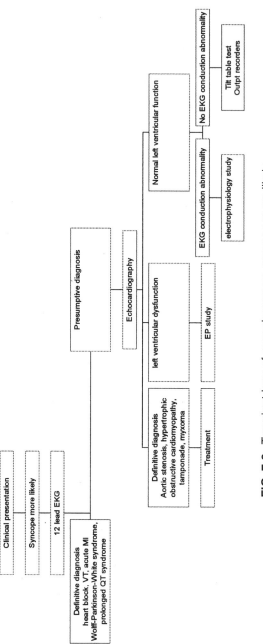

FIG. 7-3. Transient loss of consciousness: syncope more likely.

terval. A Wolff-Parkinson-White pattern should raise suspicion of a supraventricular tachycardia.

Outpatient recording devices can provide syncope-arrhythmia correlation that is often absent with admission ECG or inpatient telemetry recordings. When an arrhythmic cause is suspected but undiagnosed after a complete cardiac evaluation, outpatient recorders can be rewarding, provided that syncope occurs during the recording period (Fogel et al., 1997). It is important to keep in mind that if a serious arrhythmic event (e.g., ventricular tachycardia) is a realistic cause of syncope, every attempt should be made to establish its diagnosis during the initial hospitalization. Attempts to record such an arrhythmic event as an outpatient can be fatal. If syncope occurs several times a month, a 30-day event monitor can capture an event. However, most episodes of syncope are sporadic and unpredictable and, therefore, difficult to capture. An implantable loop recorder (Medtronic REVEAL, Minneapolis, MN) is now available (Krahn et al., 1999). This device is implanted subcutaneously for 14 months and can provide symptom-arrhythmia correlation.

Echocardiography

The transthoracic echocardiogram is a noninvasive tool that should be used in every elderly patient who presents with syncope when the initial evaluation does not provide the diagnosis or to confirm a diagnosis made by the initial evaluation (e.g., aortic stenosis). The principal value of the echocardiogram is to exclude significant structural heart disease, but it can rarely establish a diagnosis (e.g., aortic stenosis, hypertrophic obstructive cardiomyopathy, left atrial myxoma, tamponade, pulmonary embolus in transit).

Electrophysiologic Testing

The electrophysiologic study attempts to identify an arrhythmic cause of syncope. Although syncope-arrhythmia correlation may be uncertain after the initial evaluation, the electrophysiologic study provides a presumptive arrhythmic cause of the patient's symptoms by identifying patients at high risk for a particular arrhythmia. Of particular concern are (*a*) ventricular tachycardia in patients with a prior myocardial infarction or LV dysfunction; and (*b*) intermittent AV block in patients with ECG-documented bundle branch block, particularly bifascicular block. The electrophysiologic study can also identify patients with syncope presumptively caused by sinus node dysfunction, carotid sinus hypersensitivity, and

supraventricular tachycardia. Electrophysiologic studies are indicated in any elderly patient when the initial evaluation does not provide a diagnosis and an arrhythmic cause is suspected (e.g., bundle branch block on ECG, LV dysfunction on echocardiography) (Zipes et al., 1995).

Tilt-Table Testing

Head-up tilt table testing identifies patients who are susceptible to vasovagal syncope (Benditt et al., 1996; Grubb et al., 1992). It can confirm the diagnosis of vasovagal syncope in the elderly, especially because the specificity of the test increases with age. Vasovagal syncope can be confirmed with head-up tilt testing, which has an overall specificity of approximately 90%. It is important to note, however, that given the lethality of cardiac syncope, tilt-table testing should be reserved for patients with both normal electrocardiograms and echocardiograms or those in whom the diagnosis is still unclear after complete cardiac evaluation.

The Signal-Averaged Electrocardiogram

The signal averaged ECG (SAECG), by detecting areas of slow conduction (i.e., late potentials) within the heart, identifies the cardiac substrate susceptible to ventricular tachyarrhythmias (Berbari et al., 2000; Steinberg et al., 1994). Although less widely used than the electrophysiologic study, the principal value of the SAECG lies in its high negative predictive value (>90%). The absence of late potentials identifies a group of patients at low risk for ventricular tachycardia. The presence of late potentials in syncopal patients with structural heart disease identifies those who should have an electrophysiologic study.

Exercise Testing

Exercise testing, although not routinely helpful, can suggest a cause of undiagnosed exercise-induced syncope (e.g., exercise-induced AV block or ischemic-induced ventricular tachycardia).

TREATMENT

Seizure and Epilepsy

When the diagnosis, based on the clinical evaluation, is of seizure, the decision must be made whether the patient should be treated with prophylactic medication. If the seizure is an acute symptomatic seizure related to a specific precipitating factor not associated with recurrent seizures, then treatment should be directed at eliminating the offending agent. When a specific precipitant cannot be found, other factors must be considered. Overall, approximately 33% to 50% of patients who experience one seizure will have a second seizure (Berg and Shinnar, 1991; Hauser and Hesdorffer, 1990). Specific factors can increase the likelihood that someone will experience recurrent seizures. MRI of the brain revealing a focal cortical abnormality, a history of a previous neurologic insult, history of Todd's paresis, status epilepticus, and an abnormal EEG increase the likelihood of recurrent seizures. In these cases, treatment with prophylactic medication may be considered. In cases of brain neoplasms, the likelihood of recurrent seizures is particularly high; thus, anticonvulsant medication is generally begun after an initial seizure. If a second seizure occurs, approximately three fourths of patients will experience recurrent seizures and most would opt to treat at this point (Hauser et al., 1998). Many personal factors can also affect the decision to treat a single seizure, including the need to drive again and employment concerns. Before beginning an anticonvulsant medication, discuss the pros and cons of medication, including the patient's individual likelihood of having recurrent seizures, based on the clinical data, efficacy of the drugs, and potential side effects.

Medication Selection

When the decision is made to treat with an anticonvulsant medication, any concomitant medical conditions and current medications (including over-the-counter and nontraditional medications and supplements) should be evaluated carefully. Additional factors that can affect the medication choice include cost, dosing schedule, need for blood monitoring, potential side effects of the medications, history of drug allergies, and preferred route and form of drug administration.

Most patients' seizures can be controlled with the use of antiepileptic drugs (AED). The likelihood of control with medication should be discussed with the patient. It should be clear that the first medication may not result in complete control. In the general population, approximately 35% will be refractory to medications. However, the longer a patient is seizure-free on medication, the less likely recurrent seizures will occur.

Certain side effects are possible with most of the currently available AED, including sedation, diplopia, nausea, and ataxia, particularly at higher levels

(Brodie et al., 1999; Craig and Tallis, 1994; Moshe, 2000; Ramsay and Pryor, 1990; Rowan and Ramsay, 1997). Slow medication titration and careful monitoring of serum drug levels can help prevent many of these side effects. Monitoring of drug levels is also helpful in the assessment of medication compliance, which can be difficult in the elderly because of the greater likelihood of memory difficulties and concomitant use of multiple other medications.

Among the older AED, carbamazepine (Tegretol), phenytoin (Dilantin), and valproic acid (Depakote, Depakene) appear to be equally efficacious in the treatment of partial seizures. Because carbamazepine, phenytoin, and valproic acid are highly protein-bound, measurement of free levels is more helpful than total AED levels in this population. Carbamazepine is generally well tolerated, but can cause ataxia or adverse cognitive effects at higher levels, as can phenytoin. Valproic acid often causes a tremor at therapeutic levels and can result in a tremor resembling that seen in Parkinson's disease. Phenobarbital and primidone (Mysoline), although effective, are more likely to result in significant cognitive side effects, and are generally considered to be second-line medications.

As seen in Table 7-3, many of the newer anticonvulsant medications have favorable side-effect profiles and pharmacokinetics, making them attractive for use in this age group (Brodie et al., 1996, 1999; Haria and Balfour, 1997; Moshe, 2000).

Syncope

Treatment of syncope depends on its underlying cause. Cardiac syncope requires a detailed cardiac evaluation and treatment of any correctable lesions (e.g., aortic valve replacement). Permanent pacemaker implantation effectively treats bradyarrhythmic syncope and can be indicated for syncopal patients with bifascicular block on ECG where syncope is not proved to be caused by AV block, but other likely causes of syncope have been excluded (Gregoratos et al., 1998). Implantable cardioverter-defibrillators are the treatment of choice for syncopal ventricular tachycardia, and may also be indicated for those with LV dysfunction and inducible ventricular arrhythmias at electrophysiologic study where other causes of syncope have been excluded (Gregoratos et al., 1998).

Avoidance of triggering events is important in reflexogenic syncope. Initial pharmacologic therapy for vasovagal syncope is a beta-blocker. Beta-blockers reduce cardiac contractility and, therefore, mechanoreceptor (C fiber) activation, which forms the afferent

TABLE 7-3. *Medication chart: epilepsy, syncope, and orthostatic hypotension*

Drug	Typical dose	Side effects/risks	Cost/month ($)
Phenytoin (Dilantin)	300–500 mg/d	Sedation, ataxia, gingival-hyperplasia, diplopia, hirsutism	<50
Carbamazepine (Tegretol)	400–800 mg/d	Sedation, nausea, ataxia, rash, diplopia, hyponatremia	<50
Valproic acid (Depakote)	750–3,000 mg/d	Sedation, pancreatitis, hepatitis, weight gain, tremor	>50
Tiagabine (Gabitril)	32–52 mg/d	Sedation, cognitive side effects	>50
Gabapentin (Neurontin)	900–3,600 mg/d	Sedation, weight gain, edema	>50
Lamotrigine (Lamictal)	300–800 mg/d	Rash, sedation, ataxia	>50
Topiramate (Topamax)	100–500 mg/d	Sedation, cognitive problems, nephrolithiasis	>50
Zonisamide (Zonegran)	200–600 mg/d	Sedation, nephrolithiasis, rash	>50
Oxcarbazepine (Trileptal)	600–2,400 mg/d	Sedation, rash, hyponatremia	>50
Levetiracetam (Keppra)	1,000–3,000 mg/d	Sedation	>50
Fludrocortisone (Florinef)	0.3–1 mg/d	CHF, edema, headache, HTN hypokalemia, weight gain	<50
Indomethacin (Indocin)	25–50 mg t.i.d.	Interstitial nephritis, gastrointestinal upset, liver toxicity	<50
Ephedrine	12.5–25 mg t.i.d.	Anxiety, tachycardia, tremor	<50
Methylphenidate (Ritalin)	5–10 mg t.i.d.	Anxiety, tachycardia, tremor	>50
Midodrine (ProAmitine)	2.5–5 mg t.i.d. NTE 30 mg/d	Hypertension, piloerection, pruritis	>50
Phenylpropanolamine	25–75 mg b.i.d.	Hypertension	<50
Atenolol (Tenormin)	25–100 mg q.d.	CHF, hypotension, bradycardia, fatigue, exercise intolerance	<50
Metoprolol (Lopressor)	25–50 mg b.i.d.	CHF, hypotension, bradycardia, fatigue, exercise intolerance	<50
Theophylline (Theo-Dur)	200–300 mg q.d.	Nausea, vomiting, tremors Overdose: arrhythmia, seizure	<50
Scopolamine	1 patch q3d	Anticholinergic side effects: dry mouth, blurry vision, urinary retention	>50
Disopyramide (Norpace)	600 mg/d (dosing b.i.d. or q.i.d.)	CHF, anticholinergic side effects: dry mouth, blurry vision, urinary retention	>50

b.i.d., two times per day; CHF, congestive heart failure; HTN, hypertension; NTE, not to exceed; q, every; q.d., every day; q.i.d., four times per day; t.i.d., three times per day.

limb of the reflex arc. Other medications include theophylline (adenosine receptor antagonist), midodrine (alpha agonist), scopolamine (anticholinergic), disopyramide (anticholinergic and negatively inotropic), and sertraline (serotonin reuptake inhibitor). Nonpharmacologic therapy includes permanent pacemaker implantation in selected individuals who have cardioinhibitory vasovagal syncope. Patients with the hypersensitive carotid sinus syndrome can also be effectively treated with permanent pacemaker implantation, as can patients with recurrent, unprovoked syncope who have a hypersensitive cardioinhibitory response to carotid sinus stimulation. Avoiding abrupt changes in posture and withdrawing offending medications help to prevent orthostatic syncopal episodes. Nonpharmacologic therapy includes tight fitting leg stockings (to increase venous return) and salt tablets (to increase volume). Pharmacologic therapy includes volume expanders (e.g., Florinef (mineralocorticoid)) and vasoconstrictors (e.g., ephedrine).

SUMMARY AND ADVICE

A careful clinical evaluation with appropriately guided tests will reveal a likely cause for transient loss of consciousness in most patients. However, the diagnosis can remain elusive, despite a thorough evaluation, particularly with sporadic episodes. In these patients reevaluation may be necessary. Therapeutic trials can be useful in selected patients. Lack of response to therapy may also indicate that the true cause remains undiagnosed. Fortunately, the cause for transient loss of consciousness can be determined for most individuals.

REFERENCES

Adams RD, Victor M, Ropper AH. *Principles of neurology*, 6th ed. New York: McGraw-Hill, 1997.

Ajmone-Marsan C, Zivin LS. Factors related to the occurrence of typical paroxysmal abnormalities in the EEG records of epileptic patients. *Epilepsia* 1970;11: 361–381.

Aminoff MJ, Scheinman MM, Griffin JC, et al. Electrocerebral accompaniments of syncope associated with malignant ventricular arrhythmias. *Ann Intern Med* 1988;108: 791–796.

Annegers JF, Hauser WA, Lee JR-J, Rocca WA. Acute symptomatic seizures in Rochester, Minnesota, 1935–1984. *Epilepsia* 1995;36:327–333.

Benbadis SR, Wolfamuth BR, Goren H, et al. Value of tongue biting in the diagnosis of seizures. *Arch Intern Med* 1995;155:2346–2349.

Benditt D. Head-up tilt table testing: rationale, methodology; and applications. In: Zipes DP, Jalife J, eds. *Cardiac Electrophysiology from Cell to Bedside*, 3rd ed. Philadelphia: WB Saunders, 2000:746–753.

Benditt DG, Ferguson DW, Grubb BP, et al. Tilt-table testing for assessing syncope. An American College of Cardiology expert consensus document. *J Am Coll Cardiol* 1996;28(1):263–275.

Berbari EJ. High-resolution electrocardiography. In: Zipes DP, Jalife J, eds. *Cardiac electrophysiology from cell to bedside*, 3rd ed. Philadelphia: WB Saunders, 2000:730–737.

Berg AT, Shinnar S. The risk of seizure recurrence following a first unprovoked seizure: a quantitative review. *Neurology* 1991;41:965–972.

Blumhardt LD, Smith PE, Owen L. Electrocardiographic accompaniments of temporal lobe epileptic seizures, *Lancet* 1986;1(8489):1051–1056.

Brodie MJ, Richens A, Yuen AWC. Double-blind comparison of lamotrigine and carbamazepine in newly diagnosed epilepsy. *Lancet* 1996;346: 476–479.

Brodie MJ, Overstall PW, Giorgi L. Multicentre, double-blind, randomised comparison between lamotrigine and carbamazepine in elderly patients with newly diagnosed epilepsy. *Epilepsy Res* 1999;37(1):81–87.

Craig I, Tallis R. Impact of valproate and phenytoin on cognitive function in elderly patients: results of a single-blind randomized comparative study. *Epilepsia* 1994;35(2):381–390.

Dichter M, Weinberger LM. Epileptogenesis and the aging brain. In: Rowan AJ, Ramsay RE, eds. *Seizures and epilepsy in the elderly*. Boston: Butterworth-Heinemann, 1997.

Drury I, Beydoun A. Interictal epileptiform activity in elderly patients with epilepsy. *Electroencephalogr Clin Neurophysiol* 1998;106:369–373.

Eagle KA, Black HR, Cook EF, et al. Evaluation of prognostic classifications for patients with syncope. *Am J Med* 1985;79:455–460.

Fisher CM. Syncope of obscure nature. *Can J Neurol Sci* 1979;6(1):7–20.

Fogel RI, Evans JJ, Prystowsky EN. Utility and cost of event recorders in the diagnosis of palpitations, presyncope, and syncope. *Am J Cardiol* 1997;79:207–208.

Gregoratos G, Cheitlin MD, Conill A, et al. ACC/AHA guidelines for implantation of cardiac pacemakers and antiarrhythmia devices. A report of the ACC/AHA Task Force on Practice Guidelines. *J Am Coll Cardiol* 1998;37:1175–1206.

Grubb BP, Wolfe D, Samiol D, et al. Recurrent unexplained syncope in the elderly: the use of head-upright tilt table testing in evaluation and management. *J Am Geriatr Soc* 1992;40:1123–1128.

Haria M, Balfour JA. Levetiracetam. *Drugs* 1997;7(2): 159–164.

Hauser WA, Anneger JF, Kurland LT. Incidence of epilepsy and unprovoked seizures in Rochester, Minnesota: 1935–1984. *Epilepsia* 1993;34(3):453–468.

Hauser WA, Rich SS, Lee JRJ, et al. Risk of recurrent seizures after two unprovoked seizures. *N Engl J Med* 1998;338(7):429–434.

Hauser WA, Morris ML, Hewton LL, et al. Seizures and myoclonus in patients with Alzheimer's disease. *Neurology* 1986;36:1226–1230.

Hesdorffer DC, Hauser WA, Annegers JF, et al. Dementia and adult onset unprovoked seizures. *Neurology* 1996; 46:727–730.

Hesdorffer DC, Hauser WA, Annegers JF, et al. Major depression in a risk factor for seizures in older adults. *Ann Neurol* 2000;47(2):246–249.

Hoefnagels WAJ, Padberg GW, Overweg J, et al. Transient loss of consciousness: the value of the history for distinguishing seizure from syncope. *J Neurol* 1991;238: 39–43.

Holt-Seitz A, Wirrell EC, Sundaram MB. Seizures in the elderly: etiology and prognosis. Can J Neurol Sci 1999;26: 110–114.

Kapoor WN, Karpf M, Wieand S, et al. A prospective evaluation and follow-up of patients with syncope. *N Engl J Med* 1983;309:197–204.

Kapoor WN. Evaluation and outcome of patients with syncope. *Medicine* 1990;69:160–175.

Kapoor W, Snustad D, Peterson J, et al. Syncope in the elderly. *Am J Med* 1986;80:419–428.

Krahn AD, Klein GJ, Yee R, et al., for the Reveal Investigators. Use of an extended monitoring strategy in patients with problematic syncope. *Circulation* 1999;99: 406–410.

Loiseau J, Loiseau P, Duche B, et al. A survey of epileptic disorders in southwest France: seizures in elderly patients. *Ann Neurol* 1990;27:232–237.

Miller JW, Petersen RD, Metter EJ, et al. Transient global amnesia: clinical characteristics and prognosis. *Neurology* 1987;37:733–737.

Moshe SL. Mechanisms of action of anticonvulsant agents. *Neurology* 2000;(Suppl 1):32–40.

McAreavey MJ, Ballinger BR, Fenton GW. Epileptic seizures in elderly patients with dementia. *Epilepsia* 1992;33(4):657–660.

Nei M, Ho RT, Sperling MR. EKG abnormalities during partial seizures in refractory epilepsy. *Epilepsia* 2000; 41:542–548.

Plum F, Posner JB. The pathologic physiology of signs and symptoms of coma. In: *The diagnosis of stupor and coma*, 3rd ed. Philadelphia: FA Davis, 1980.

Ramsay RE. Seizures and epilepsy in the elderly. Boston: Butterworth-Heinemann, 1997.

Ramsay RE, Pryor F. Epilepsy in the elderly. *Neurology* 2000;55(Suppl 1):9–14.

Romanelli MF, Morris JC, Ashkin K, et al. Advanced Alzheimer's disease is a risk factor for late onset seizures. *Arch Neurol* 1990;47:847–850.

Ross J Jr, Braunwald E. Aortic stenosis. *Circulation* 1968;38 (Suppl 5):61–67.

Savage DD, Corwin L, Mcgee DL, et al. Epidemiologic features of isolated syncope: the Framingham study. *Stroke* 1985;16:626–629.

Sharief MK, Singh P, Sander JWAS, et al. Efficacy and tolerability study of ucb L059 in patients with refractory epilepsy. *J Epilepsy*1996;9(2):106–112.

Sirven JI, Malamut B, O'Connor MJ, et al. Temporal lobectomy in older versus younger adults. *Neurology* 2000;54 (11):2166–2170.

Steinberg JS, Prystowsky E, Freedman RA, et al. Use of the signal-averaged electrocardiogram for predicting inducible ventricular tachycardia in patients with unexplained syncope: relation to clinical variables in a multivariate analysis. *J Am Coll Cardiol* 1994;23:99–106.

Zaidi A, Clough P, Cooper P, et al. Misdiagnosis of epilepsy: many seizure-like attacks have a cardiovascular cause. *J Am Coll Cardiol* 2000;36(1):181–184.

Zipes DP, DiMarco JP, Gillette PC, et al. Guidelines for clinical intracardiac electrophysiological and catheter ablation procedures. *J Am Coll Cardiol,* 1995;26:555–573.

SUGGESTED READINGS:

Calkins H. Syncope. In: Zipes DP, Jalife J. *Cardiac electrophysiology from cell to bedside*, 3rd ed. Philadelphia: WB Saunders, 2000:873–881.

Martin JB, Ruskin J. Faintness, syncope, and seizures. In: Wilson JD, Braunwald E, Isselbacher KJ, et al. *Harrison's principles of internal medicine*, 12th ed. New York: McGraw-Hill, 1991:134–142.

Rowan AJ, Ramsay RE, eds. Seizures and epilepsy in the elderly. Boston: Butterworth-Heinemann, 1997.

Stein B, Roberts R. Syncope, presyncope, palpitations, and sudden death. In: Schlant RC, Alexander RW, eds. *Hurst's the heart*, 8th ed. New York: McGraw-Hill, 1994:475–479.

8

Dizziness and Vertigo in Older Adults

Jeffrey S. Durmer and David Solomon

INTRODUCTION

In this chapter, is presented the epidemiology, causes, pathogenesis, diagnosis, and treatment strategies for the most frequently encountered causes of dizziness in the elderly patient. Although a complaint of dizziness might seem enigmatic at first, rational way exists to evaluate this sensation and establish a cause based on a number of well-recognized health problems that affect many elderly patients (i.e.; cardiovascular disease, depression, cervical spondylosis, polypharmacy, deconditioning). Dizziness, the number one complaint of all medical patients over 75 years of age, has been referred to as a geriatric "syndrome," similar to falling and delirium (Tinetti et al., 2000). By understanding the symptom of dizziness as a common final pathway, the syndrome of dizziness may be more clearly seen as a number of defined and undefined entities. Because of the multitude of underlying health conditions and situations that can cause it, many different physicians and healthcare professionals treat dizziness. Internists, geriatricians, family care physicians, neurologists, otorhinolaryngologists, psychiatrists, physiatrists, emergency physicians, and physical therapists all have the opportunity to diagnose and treat many patients with dizziness. This chapter is intended to help organize the approach to the elderly dizzy patient, given the latest clinical and basic research on the causes and treatments of dizziness.

EPIDEMIOLOGY OF DIZZINESS

Dizziness is reported in approximately 30% of all people over the age of 65 (Colledge, 1994; Sloane and Baloh, 1989). In the United States, it is the most common presenting complaint to office practices among patients over the age of 75 (Koch and Smith, 1980; 1981; 1985). The physician consultation rate in 1981 for the symptom of dizziness in the United Kingdom was approximately 54/1,000 for people aged 65 to 74 years and 76/1000 for those aged 75 years or older (Royal College of General Practitioners, 1981–1982). One of the most serious consequences of dizziness is falls. The National Health Interview Survey Supplement on Aging in 1986 determined that more than 18% of all persons 65 to 74 year of age and more than 25% of all those 75 years of age or older had fallen in the previous year. In these groups, 15% to 23% fell because of dizziness alone (Havlik, 1984; 1986). The same survey reported that a staggering 34% and 37% of persons 65 to 74 year of age and those older than 75 years, respectively, had limited their activity because of dizziness. Smaller studies using more select populations of older people find between 20% and 30% of falls are caused by dizziness (Baloh, 1992; Weindruch et al., 1989). Some of these studies also suggest that patients who are older than 60 years have an increased incidence of potentially treatable diseases as a cause for their dizziness (Baloh, 1992; Lawson et al., 1999).

Another sequel of falling is the subsequent deterioration of function after the fall. Many elderly people who fall develop a fear of falling that limits their daily activity. This, in turn, leads to more deconditioning, which increases the risk of falling. Dynamic posturography studies of elderly people with dizziness and without dizziness show that a fear of falling is associated with an increased sway velocity and risk for fall, regardless of dizziness status (Baloh et al., 1998). Clearly, with advancing age, dizziness is more common, and it represents an increasing risk for falls, as well as for syncope, functional disability, nursing home placement, stroke, and death (Sloane and Baloh, 1989; Boult et al., 1991; Grimby and Rosenhall, 1995; Kroenke et al., 1992; Tilvis et al., 1996).

The characteristics of dizziness in older people are different than they are in younger people. In 1992, Kroenke et al., studied 185 consecutive outpatients with a chief complaint of dizziness. They found within a subgroup of 85 younger patients (average age 49 years), that the symptoms of dizziness differed from the 100 older remaining patients (average age 61 years). The older group was significantly more likely to have daily dizziness, limitation of function because of dizziness, fear of underlying illness, and increased use of medications for dizziness (Kroenke et al., 1992). These findings may mean that older individuals who experience dizziness are either less able to compensate for the dizziness, have more severe dizziness, or report dizziness more often.

The differential diagnosis of dizziness in elderly patients is extensive. Studies designed to determine the cause of dizziness in geriatric patients have returned highly variable results, partly because of the different populations, criteria, and study designs used. Alternatively, dizziness is a highly variable symptom, with a number of conditions that predispose to it. Tinetti et al. (2000), using Drachman's categorization of dizziness symptoms, determined the prevalence of dizziness subtypes and associated treatable factors in a population of 1,087 independent people 72 years of age and older. The study, conducted over an 11-year period, showed that 29% of individuals experienced dizziness. No single cause for dizziness was found in this study, although many factors were related to its development. The authors suggest that dizziness can occur with either severe impairment of a single system (vision, vestibular, sensory, motor, or cerebellar) or with mild to moderate impairment of several systems. They conclude that dizziness should be considered a geriatric syndrome so that physicians will regard the symptom as a complex of interrelated systems which, when perturbed, result in the disorienting sensation (Tinetti et al., 2000).

DEFINITION OF TERMS

When a patient complains of being dizzy, the subjective experience can be described with a perplexing number of seemingly equally nebulous terms: swimming, floating, light-headedness, whirling, fainting, disorientation, unsteadiness, rocking, giddiness, dissociation, imbalance, or spinning.

The description and history given by the patient determine much of what the subsequent interview, examination, and testing are based. In fact, some researchers have reported that, for chronically dizzy geriatric patients, a careful history of the dizziness can predict the eventual diagnosis in 70% of cases (Sloane et al., 1989; Sloane and Baloh, 1989). Thus, the term "dizziness" must be elaborated and subcategories established. Clinical studies of dizziness in the elderly often divide the symptom into the four cate-

gories initially proposed by Drachman and Hart (Drachman and Hart, 1972). These dizziness subtypes include:

- Vertigo: a sensation of rotational, spinning movement
- Presyncope: a sensation of fainting or "passing-out"
- Dysequilibrium: a sensation of imbalance while standing or walking with no abnormal sensation in the head
- Other sensations: loosely defined as nonspecific dizziness, floating, giddiness, or other descriptions that fall outside of the previous categories (Table 8-1)

Although nearly 50% to 60% of individuals fall into more than one symptom category (Tinetti et al., 2000; Kroenke et al., 1992; Sloane and Baloh, 1989, Colledge et al., 1996), it is important to determine the dizziness type by episode to establish a possible cause. For example, a patient 75 years of age with Parkinson's disease experiences a fainting type of dizziness after taking his antidepressant medications and also has a feeling of a dysequilibrium type of dizziness if he does not take his dopaminergic medications.

Vertigo, defined as the perception of motion, has a prevalence of 25% to 54% in elderly persons complaining of dizziness (Tinetti et al., 2000; Kroenke et al., 1992; Sloane and Baloh, 1989; Colledge et al., 1996). A careful history of dizziness has been shown to be 87% sensitive for vertigo (Kroenke et al., 1992). Other symptoms often associated with vertigo include nausea, vomiting, unsteadiness, and sometimes hearing loss. The underlying mechanisms implicated include disorders of the peripheral or vestibular, and cerebellar systems. Specific diseases are discussed below.

In elderly patients complaining of dizziness, *presyncope*, defined as a feeling of fainting, has a prevalence of 11% to 42% (Tinetti et al., 2000; Sloane and Baloh, 1989). History alone carries a sensitivity of 74% for presyncope (Kroenke et al., 1992). Associated symptoms include pallor, perspiration, palpitations, and syncope. The underlying mechanisms of presyncope stem from decreased cerebral perfusion caused by cardiovascular disease, hypovolemia, overmedication, orthostatic intolerance, dysautonomia, and hypercapnia.

Dysequilibrium, as a category of dizziness, includes people with a sensation of imbalance while on their feet. The symptom of dizziness is not directly referred to as a sensation in the head, and is usually dependent on standing, movement, or both. Therefore, this type of dizziness can include people suffering from gait ab-

TABLE 8-1. *Characteristics that distinguish common dizziness subtypes in elderly patients*

Subtype	Onset/duration	Primary symptoms	Associated symptoms or findings
Vertigo			
Peripheral			
Benign paroxysmal vertigo	Acute with movement/<60 sec	Multiepisodic environmental rotation, nausea, oscillopsia	Sweating, fear, nystagmus, ability to walk preserved
Meniere's disease	Subacute/hr	Constant rotation, fullness in ear	Hearing loss, tinnitus, recurrent episodes of same symptoms
Labyrinthitis	Subacute/days	Constant rotation, viral prodrome	Hearing loss, vesicular rash
Vestibular neuritis	Subacute/days	Constant rotation, viral prodrome	No hearing loss, vesicular rash
Central			
Transient ischemic attack	Acute/<60 min	Single episode rotation, nausea, vomiting	Weakness, numb, hearing loss, dysarthriaphagia-metria, diplopia
Stroke	Acute/days	Moderate rotation, brainstem signs, symptoms worse at onset	Headache, hiccups, mental status change, inability to walk
Presyncope			
Hyperventilation	Acute to chronic/situational to constant	Floating, lightheaded	Fear, anxiety, depression
Orthostatic hypotension	Acute with standing/sec	Faint, lightheaded, syncope	Tachycardia, pallor, nausea, tremor
Vasovagal	Acute with stress/sec	Faint, lightheaded, syncope	Tachycardia, pallor, nausea, tremor
Cardiac	Variable	Constant or postural faintness, syncope	Palpitations, chest pain, shortness of breath, pallor, sweating
Dysequilibrium			
Visual	Subacute/constant	Imbalance—in light or dark	Blurred vision, monocular diplopia
Vestibular	Subacute/constant	Imabalance with head movements	Oscillopsia, nausea, hearing loss
Cerebellar	Variable/constant	Ataxia, dysmetria, worse in dark	Oscillopsia, nystagmus
Sensory	Subacute-chronic/constant	Imbalance worse in dark	Sensory examination abnormal, hand/foot wounds
Motor	Subacute-chronic/constant	Imbalance worse with speed	Motor examination abnormalities
Nonspecific			
Anxiety/panic	Acute with situation/variable	Internal rotation, floating, lightheaded, presyncope	Sweating, palpitation, shortness of breath, perioral numbness, paresthesias
Depression	Subacute-chronic/variable	Depersonalization, floating	Paresthesias, fatigue, insomnia, weight loss, anxiety
Medications	Subacute with medication use/variable	Constant rotation, presyncope, or dysequilibrium	Associated with time of medication

normalities (e.g., dysequilibrium syndrome, presbyastasis, or senile gait). In clinical studies of geriatric patients who complain of dizziness, 28% to 78% are diagnosed with dysequilibrium (Tinetti et al., 2000; Kroenke et al., 1992; Sloane and Baloh, 1989; Colledge et al., 1996). Extreme variability in the prevalence of this problem primarily results from the different patient populations under consideration. For example, some investigations that study nursing home residents show significantly higher numbers of a dysequilibrium type of dizziness than similar outpatient community-based studies. The higher rate of dysequilibrium in the nursing home populations is likely because of the fact that placement in a nursing home environment is often predicated on mobility problems. Also, independent elderly outpatients with a gait abnormality are less likely to remain in the general community. A retrospective study of 116 neurootology clinic patients, average age of 75 years, with the presenting complaint of dizziness, showed that dysequilibrium was the dizziness type most frequently reported to occur in combination with other types (55% of cases). As a primary cause, it was seen in 28% of cases (Sloane and Baloh, 1989).

Because studies show that up to 50% to 60% of people with dizziness above the age of 65 years experience more than one dizziness symptom (Tinetti et al., 2000; Sloane and Baloh, 1989; Colledge et al., 1996; Sloane, 1996), dysequilibrium is likely a part of many geriatric causes of dizziness. The underlying mechanisms for dysequilibrium vary, but disorders of the visual, vestibulospinal, proprioceptive, somatosensory, cerebellar, pyramidal and extrapyramidal motor systems can all cause this type of dizziness. A more detailed discussion of gait disorders can be found in Chapter 9.

In most studies of older people, the category *nonspecific dizziness* comprises 17% to 33% of the study samples (Tinetti et al., 2000; Kroenke et al., 1992; Sloane and Baloh, 1989; Colledge et al., 1996; Sloane et al., 1994; Fife and Baloh, 1993). An important reason for this variability in prevalence is the difference in how each study accounts for various psychiatric problems (e.g., panic disorders, anxiety, and obsessive-compulsive and mood disorders). It is also likely that cognitive decline in some older people makes reporting of symptoms, especially in large epidemiologic surveys, inaccurate or vague.

ANATOMY AND PHYSIOLOGY OF DIZZINESS

Before a discussion of the multiple causes of dizziness can begin, it is important to appreciate some of the anatomic and physiologic changes that occur with age in the nervous system. Age-related degeneration of the vestibular, cerebellar, visual, somatosensory, and proprioceptive systems can all have important implications for the development of different types of dizziness. Dysequilibrium can result from the accumulation of mild to moderate deficits in multiple systems, or more severe deficits in one sensory system. Presyncope usually results from vascular or cardiac causes, and nonspecific lightheadedness can have many causes without a clear pathophysiology. In particular, vertigo is attributable to processes that affect the peripheral and central vestibular systems. To appreciate the effects of age-related degeneration on the systems that are known to result in symptoms of vertigo and imbalance, requires a familiarity with the normal anatomy and physiology of the vestibular system. Furthermore, central nervous system, visual and somatosensory signals are as important as labyrinthine input in processing vestibular information. The sense of motion, therefore, is truly multimodal.

Peripheral Vestibular System

The human vestibular system is composed of peripheral and central components. Both components function to maintain visual and postural stability during movement and provide sensory input to a perceptual mechanism subserving spatial orientation and navigation. The peripheral system begins with the end organs that transform angular and linear accelerations of the head into neural signals. These transformations occur in two endolymph-filled, paired membranous labyrinths in the petrous portion of each temporal bone. Within each labyrinth, is a specialized sensory neuroepithelium arranged in two types of unique sensory receptors: (*a*) the three semicircular canals (SCC)—posterior, anterior, and lateral—and (*b*) the two otolith organs— utricle and saccule. The three SCC are oriented orthogonally to transduce head rotation about any axis. These function in pairs with a contralateral canal that lies in the same plane (e.g., the lateral SCC pair, the left anterior and the right posterior SCC pair). The otolith organs sense linear acceleration caused by gravity or translation, with the utricular maculae roughly in the same horizontal plane and the saccular maculae close to the midsagittal plane.

Mechanical transduction occurs at specialized projections at the apices of the hair cells. Each SCC has a patch of neuroepithelium at a widening of the canal termed the "ampulla," where hair cells can be deflected by movement of the *cupula*, a structure that spans the inner diameter of each canal. When the head is at rest, primary vestibular afferents in the VIIIth nerve have a spontaneous discharge rate, so input from each side is balanced. When the head is about an axis that lies perpendicular to the plane containing a SCC pair, the cupula is pushed into the column of fluid (endolymph) contained within the canal. The cupula is deflected, exciting hair cells innervating the canal toward which the head is rotating, and inhibiting the afferents from the contralateral canal in a push-pull manner. For example, rotation of the head to the right increases the firing rate of VIIIth nerve fibers on the right and decreases in the firing rate of primary vestibular afferents on the left. The brain receives more neural activity from the right compared to the left and correctly interprets this information as rightward head turning in space. This generates leftward slow phase eye velocity and rightward quick phases of nystagmus. This is the basis for the vestibular ocular reflex (VOR), which provides stable gaze, despite head movements during locomotion. The absence of the VOR leads to oscillopsia (i.e., movement of the visual image on the retina).

The hair cell processes of the otolith organs are in contact with the *otoconial membrane*, a structure imbedded with calcium carbonate crystals. These "ear stones" are subjected to linear accelerations when the head is tilted with respect to gravity or with changes in linear velocity, generating a shear force that deflects the hair cells. While a normal constituent of the labyrinth, otoconia may become dislodged from an otolith organ and migrate into a SCC, making the canal sensitive to gravity when it normally only responds to head rotation. This is the mechanism of *benign paroxysmal positional vertigo* (BPPV), discussed below.

Additional peripheral vestibular structures include the cell bodies of primary vestibular afferent neurons in Scarpa's ganglion, with their peripheral process innervating the hair cells and their central processes, which are the Schwann cell-myelinated axons of the vestibular nerve. The VIIIth nerve travels through the internal auditory canal along with the facial nerve, traverses the subarachnoid space and enters the lateral brainstem at the pontomedullary level. Vestibular nerve axons terminate within the vestibular nuclei and the flocculonodular lobe of the cerebellum.

Central Vestibular System

The central vestibular system is composed of projections from the four vestibular nuclei (superior, inferior, medial, and lateral) and the vestibulocerebellum (flocculonodular lobe and posterior vermis).

These nuclei project to brainstem, thalamic, and spinal cord targets involved in orienting and reflexive righting movements of the eyes (vestibulo-ocular system), head and neck (vestibulocolic system), and body (vestibulospinal system). The cerebellum is crucial for adaptation through inhibition of the brainstem vestibular neurons via direct Purkinje cell projections, and it influences ocular motor function via fibers from the fastigial nucleus. The nodulus of the cerebellum and commissural brainstem connections play a role in the central velocity storage mechanism, which is responsible for the duration of nystagmus following labyrinthine stimulation. To summarize the activity of the central vestibular system is well beyond the scope of this chapter, and the reader is referred to texts devoted to this topic (Leigh and Zee, 1999). However, central vestibular structures involved in the generation of horizontal and vertical VOR eye movements are important for clinicians caring for dizziness patients to understand, because nystagmus is a compelling and informative examination finding in many of these people.

Movement of the head about the long axis of the body (as if saying "no-no") stimulates the lateral SCC, as mentioned above. To maintain fixation on a salient visual target, such as an oncoming car, the eyes are moved in a lateral conjugate fashion away from the direction of head movement. The distance and speed that the eyes move is dictated by the neural activity initiated by the magnitude and velocity of the response from the lateral SCC. Many pathways are shared with the saccadic system, which organizes a coordinated burst of activity required to move the eyes and shift gaze onto a target. The paramedian pontine reticular formation (PPRF) is the burst generator for horizontal rapid eye movements (saccades and quick phases of nystagmus), whereas another pontine nucleus, the nucleus prepositus hypoglossi (NPH), integrates the burst signal to an eye position signal. This latter function maintains final eye position achieved by the burst, and allows for stabilization of the eyes in an eccentric position in the orbit. A similar midbrain system initiates and maintains eye movements in response to head movements about the pitch axis (as if saying yes-yes). The PPRF counterpart in the vertical system is the rostral interstitial nucleus of the medial longitudinal fasciculus (riMLF), and the corresponding integrator is the interstitial nucleus of Cajal (INC). Deficits in gaze holding, caused by structural or toxic metabolic damage compromise these neural integrators and result in damage direction-changing nystagmus, with quick phases in the direction of attempted gaze. Cerebellar dysfunction also causes an ipsilateral deficit in gaze holding and a gaze-evoked nystagmus. This should be distinguished from nystagmus that occurs following a unilateral vestibular loss, which is a direction-fixed spontaneous nystagmus that may be observed with the eyes in the straight-ahead position (especially with fixation removed).

One important anatomic fact allows for the rapid excitation of the proper eye muscles via vestibular ocular motor pathways. Individual SCC excite only the specific oculomotor nuclei necessary to move the eyes in the opposite direction of the head movement responsible for the activation of that SCC. In other words, the VOR acts to maintain stable gaze by activating the eye muscles needed to precisely counteract any three-dimensional head movement. Thus, pathologic nystagmus can reveal its vestibular origins when it occurs in a direction predicted by dysfunction of one or more SCC. All of these reflexive movements of the eye are under the influence of the cerebellum, cortex, and sensory systems. A loss of vestibulocerebellar function alone can lead to inaccurate eye movements, nystagmus, and sensations of vertigo. A loss of cortical activity leads to a lack of saccadic eye movement necessary for rapid fixation of a visual target. A loss of visual sensation often leads to a spontaneous horizontal and vertical nystagmus and drift.

Two additional basic principles are worth mentioning. First, the central vestibular system has the ability to adapt to changes in peripheral sensitivity with time. After an acute unilateral loss of labyrinthine function, for instance, the initial response to the altered input is nausea, ataxia, and a sensation of vertigo, with nystagmus beating toward the intact side. Many days later, the vertigo and associated symptoms dissipate and only careful examination may reveal the imbalance between the two ears. This adaptive response to an acute change requires an intact central vestibular system and cerebellum, and this capacity for plasticity is reduced with age (Paige, 1992). Second, the central vestibular system works with cortical structures to maintain posture and a sense of position in space. This can be important in conditions that mainly affect the cortex and deep white matter projections such as multiinfarct dementia, normal pressure hydrocephalus, and frontotemporal atrophy.

AGE-RELATED CHANGES IN THE ANATOMY AND PHYSIOLOGY OF DIZZINESS

Peripheral and central vestibular structures degenerate with age (Table 8-2). The functional implications that are suggested by the loss of these structures

TABLE 8-2. *Age-dependent changes in the vestibular system*

Labyrinths	Deformation of walls, abnormal endolymphatic flow
Cupula	Deposition of debris, inaccurate response to movements
Otoconia	Fragmentation, formation of endolymphatic debris
Hair cells	Apices accumulate lipofuscin
	Cilial derrangement, fusion, formation of giant cilia
	Loss in cristae (40%), loss in maculae(20% to 30%)
Scarpa's ganglion	Large decrease in number of neurons over 60 years
Saccular nerve	Degeneration of small and large fibers
Utricular nerve	Degeneration of small and large fibers
Vestibular nerve	Decrease in number of myelinated fibers over 40 years
	Slower conduction times with age
Vestibular nucleus	Loss of neurons (3*% per decade) between ages 40 and 90 years
Cerebellum	Dramatic decrease in Purkinje's cell number over 60 years

are multiple. Loss of peripheral vestibular components such as hair cells (up to 40% in crista ampullaris and 30% in the maculae), Scarpa's ganglion cells (especially over 60 years of age), and saccular and utricular nerve degeneration can all lead to increased neural response times (Rosenhall, 1972; Richter, 1980). After the age of 40, a selective loss of large fiber vestibular axons also results in increased conduction times (Bergstrom, 1973). Within the labyrinths, otoconia fragmentation and deposition on the cupula have been demonstrated to occur with aging (Ross et al., 1976). The increased incidence of benign paroxysmal positional vertigo as a function of age may be related to this anatomic change (Oghalai et al., 2000). Others claim that changes such as deformation of the labyrinthine walls that occur with age can lead to altered endolymphatic flow and symptoms of vertigo (Schuknecht and Merchant, 1988).

Central vestibular structures also undergo changes with age. It is estimated that a 3% decrease occurs per decade in the number of neurons in the vestibular nuclear complex in humans (Lopez et al., 1997). Age-induced loss of cerebellar Purkinje cells can decrease the coordination of movements and visual-vestibular adaptability (discussed below) (Torvik et al., 1986; Hall et al., 1975). In a study of 90 healthy people of widely varying ages, a 2.5% per decade decrease in Purkinje cell number from ages 0 to 100 years was found. The relationship between age and cell loss was curvilinear and showed no profound difference until the fifth or sixth decade, when a precipitous drop in cell number was noted (Hall et al., 1975). It is thought that the age-dependent atrophy of the cerebellar vermis, especially lobes 6 and 7, may also play a role in disorders of the visual-vestibular system that result in sensations of dizziness (Raz et al., 1992).

Impairment of distal somatosensory function and proprioception also occurs with age and can lead to feelings of dysequilibrium or "spindle vertigo" (Fife and Baloh, 1993; Lord et al., 1991; Skinner et al., 1984). As vestibular degeneration accumulates with age, reliance on somatosensory systems for balance is increased. In a study of 30 healthy people aged 20 to 81 years, the subjective sensation of straight-ahead was demonstrated using a subject-controlled laser pointer on a blank screen. The head-fixed measurement was made with and without unilateral neck vibratory stimulation. Both young and old subjects showed that subjective straight-ahead moved toward the side of vibratory stimulation (presumably because of compensation secondary to the illusion of movement away from the side being vibrated). However, older subjects showed significantly greater changes from true straight-ahead than the younger subjects (Strupp et al., 1999). This implies that compensatory systems are part of a normal sensory substitution process in the course of aging. It is already known that an increase in the gain of the cervico-ocular reflex occurs after bilateral vestibular lesions in humans (Sawyer et al., 1994). Thus, even a mild to moderate deficiency in visual or somatosensory systems can be an important predisposing risk factor for the development of dizziness or unsteadiness.

Degenerative changes in the vestibular system attributable to age are well known; however, the functional implications of these changes are less well understood. Vestibulo-ocular movements can be tested in humans using electronystagmography (ENG), in which eye movements are recorded using electrooculography (EOG) or video-oculography during caloric irrigation of each ear and positional testing. Rotational chair studies provide quantitative assessment of VOR gain and phase. The clinical applications of these tests are discussed later in this chapter. Vestibulospinal and vestibulocolic reflexes are also testable in humans with posturography. The normative data for elderly subjects in vestibulo-ocular testing are limited, but appear to demonstrate a clear decline in function with age. In a 5-year longitudinal study of 110 healthy people aged 75 or older, a decrease in central vestibulo-ocular motor pathway responses was demonstrated as a function of age. ENG and rotary chair data demonstrated that gain (or the size of response) of the VOR was decreased and the phase lead of the VOR was increased with age (Enrietto et al., 1999). Additionally, a significant drop was noted in the average gain of visual-vestibular reflexes and optokinetic nystagmus (OKN). The basis for this may be related to the rapid drop-off in Purkinje cell number after the sixth decade as previously discussed (Hall et al., 1975). However, the neural systems responsible for OKN and visual-vestibular responses include many different structures such as the primary visual cortex, frontal and parietal visual motor centers, thalamic and brainstem nuclei, and cerebellum. The authors of this study pointed out that the abnormal visual-vestibular responses they observed could lead to deficits in VOR function with normal head movements, resulting in sensations of dizziness. Plasticity in these pathways is required with changes in spectacle correction or while using bifocals, as many elderly do, which challenges the system even more. Other studies of the VOR and visual-vestibular responses in healthy elderly volunteers show age-related functional changes such as an amplitude-dependent decrease in VOR gain, and a shorter dominant VOR time constant (increased phase lead) (Fife and Baloh, 1993; Paige, 1992; Paterka et al., 1990; Baloh et al., 1993). Thus, as evidence supporting the natural aging process as a predisposing factor for dizziness develops, it is important to view *normal* in the elderly population as distinct from *normal* in younger groups.

Colledge et al. (1996) reported such a high prevalence of asymptomatic abnormalities in healthy control subjects over the age of 65 years with routine ENG, electrocardiogram (ECG), and magnetic resonance imaging (MRI) testing that these tests had no value in screening for causes of dizziness in the elderly. They did find that posturography was sensitive for dizziness but it lacked specificity. In a separate study, a significant difference in dynamic posturography testing was seen between younger and older healthy people (Baloh et al., 1998). A significant increase was seen in sway velocity for older people with dizziness and imbalance than for older people who were healthy. Increased sway velocity also correlated with an increased chance of falling (Baloh et al., 1998). Other studies find similar results with increased sway velocity and dysequilibrium (Fife and Baloh, 1993). Thus, even if it lacks specificity, abnormal sway velocities and dynamic posturography studies may help determine the elderly at risk for falling.

The caloric test, which has also been shown to be of little value in discerning age-dependent changes in healthy individuals (Strupp et al., 1999; Enrietto et al., 1999; Paterka et al., 1990), is generally useful in indicating an asymmetry between the two lateral SCC, but not in quantifying the overall level of vestibular function. The exception would be in a patient with a significant bilateral peripheral weakness, which is seen following aminoglycoside (usually gentamicin) ototoxicity or with neurofibromatosis type II. Normal caloric responses have been reported in persons with up to 25% reduction in crista ampullaris hair cells (Nadol and Schuknecht, 1989; Bruner and Norris, 1971). It seems that a loss of *some* vestibular function as a process of aging is not enough to cause sensations of dizziness in most people. More likely, the reason for age-associated dizziness is the simultaneous loss of compensatory sensory (vision and somatosensory) and motor (pyramidal and extrapyramidal) systems. This seems relatively clear, given the large number of medical conditions that affect these compensatory systems and present with dizziness as a primary symptom.

SPECIFIC CAUSES OF DIZZINESS IN THE ELDERLY

Dizziness has many causes in older people. Chronic medical problems, medications, deconditioning, depression, and degenerative diseases are just a few of the factors that play a role in producing dizziness. In elderly patients, the fact that they may be taking multiple medications and have multiple medical, neurologic, or psychiatric problems makes the task of organizing the possibilities more difficult. One way to approach the cause for dizziness in an individual is to begin with a description of the symptoms. Although only about 50% of elderly individuals will have a single type of dizziness symptom (Sloane and Baloh, 1989; Sloane, 1996), it is worth defining them to establish the causes. Thus, the following discussion of the major causes of dizziness is divided into the four types of dizziness: vertigo, presyncope, dysequilibrium, and nonspecific dizziness. In addition, a separate section on medications is included because the effects of drugs can exacerbate symptoms of any type.

Vertigo

Vertigo is often caused by peripheral vestibular and central vestibular disease. Diseases that affect the peripheral vestibular system cause vertigo of exquisite intensity, termed "peripheral" (or "true" spinning) vertigo. The intense nature of this vertigo usually remits over days because of central vestibular compensation; however, this is not always the case with purely episodic peripheral vertigo. In some studies of chronic dizziness, the symptom of vertigo is found in up to 50% of persons over the age of 66 years (Kroenke et al., 1992). Benign paroxysmal positional vertigo (BPPV) is by far the most common cause for peripheral vertigo in elderly patients (Bloom and Katsarkas, 1989). BPPV occurs in women twice as often as in men. A peak incidence for idiopathic BPPV occurs in the sixth decade. Viral-related cases peak in the fourth and fifth decades, and traumatic BPPV is seen with equal frequency across all ages (Baloh, 1992). Studies of chronically dizzy geriatric patients report BPPV is the primary cause in 16% to 23% of cases (Lawson et al., 1999; Kroenke et al., 1992; Sloane and Baloh, 1989). In a study of 100 healthy elderly patients, 9% were diagnosed with unrecognized BPPV (Oghalai et al., 2000). The pathophysiology of BPPV is related to the effects of free-floating debris (usually degenerating or damaged otoconia) in the posterior semicircular canal (Parnes and McClure, 1992). A sudden change in position of the head causes debris to slowly settle within the labyrinth by the force of gravity causing a sense of rotation. The symptoms have a latency of 2 to 10 seconds before onset and can last up to 45 seconds. Other medical conditions that can cause positional vertigo include alcohol intoxication and, rarely, macroglobulinemia (Brandt, 1990).

Labyrinthitis (vestibular and auditory loss) and, especially, vestibular neuritis are also common causes for peripheral vertigo. The symptoms, which are acute in onset and last for days to weeks, usually are preceded by an upper respiratory tract infection. A predilection is seen for the spring and early summer months (Baloh, 1992), and herpes simplex virus is thought to play a disproportionate role in the pathogenesis of these disorders (Strupp and Brandt, 1999). Ménière's disease infrequently develops in the elderly. It is characterized by recurrent bouts of peripheral vertigo lasting hours, associated with unilateral, low frequency fluctuating hearing loss, and preceded by a sensation of fullness in the ear and tinnitus. Some investigators suggest that in older people ischemia of the inner ear is a more common cause for vertigo than infection (Sloane, 1996). Labyrinthine infarction caused by isolated occlusion of the internal auditory artery (IAA) is rare, but can be associated with a severe peripheral vertigo and hearing loss and occur with ischemia in the posterior cerebral circulation.

Recurrent symptoms consistent with a Meniere-like presentation but without the aural and auditory symptoms are often referred to as "recurrent vestibulopathy" or "vestibular Ménière's." This is usually associated with a diagnosis of migraine, although the link is often overlooked. Patients with migrainous vertigo generally do not have vertigo temporally associated with their headaches (Cutrer and Baloh, 1992), and onset of vertigo symptoms is frequently later than onset of headache, with vestibular complaints beginning in some patients as late as the seventh decade of life (Neuhauser et al., 2001).

The most common presenting symptom of vertebrobasilar transient ischemic attacks (VBTIA) is episodic vertigo. In fact, rotatory dizziness is considered to be a risk factor for stroke, whereas nonrotatory dizziness is not (Sloane, 1996). Although vertigo can be a symptom of VBTIA, it usually occurs with other posterior fossa symptoms such as visual loss, dysarthria, dysmetria, diplopia, or dysphagia (Grad and Baloh, 1989). Although recurrent, isolated episodic vertigo is usually not cardiovascular in origin, elderly patients with associated risk factors for stroke or myocardial infarction may be at higher risk for impending stroke. Patients with arteriosclerosis, postural hypotension, cervical spondylosis, arteritis, thromboembolic disease, polycythemia, and hypercoagulable states may experience vertigo caused by VBTIA. Basilar migraine has similar symptoms to VBTIA but is less common. It usually occurs in young women, but can also affect the elderly. Symptoms can include headache and marching paresthesias, but radiologic and serum examination are routinely normal.

Stroke is associated with persistent mild to moderate (central) vertigo of acute onset. Central vertigo is continuous because vestibular adaptation relies on intact brainstem and cerebellar systems. This sensation of vertigo is usually less severe than with peripheral vertigo, and recognizable stroke syndromes can occur simultaneously. Vertebral artery occlusion or, less often, posterior inferior cerebellar artery (PICA) occlusion, causes the lateral medullary, or Wallenberg syndrome. Vertigo is associated with ipsilateral facial numbness and Horner's syndrome, contralateral loss of pain and temperature sensation on the body, ipsipulsion of the eyes and body, dysarthria, dysphagia, nausea, hiccups, and oscillopsia. Anterior inferior cerebellar artery (AICA) infarct, or the lateral pontomedullary syndrome, causes hearing loss and continuous vertigo that can be as severe as peripheral vertigo because it damages the labyrinths within the IAA territory. In addition, the inferolateral cerebellum and dorsolateral pons are damaged, causing ataxia, dysmetria, and facial paralysis. Isolated cerebellar infarcts caused by superior cerebellar artery (SCA), vertebral artery, PICA or AICA occlusion initially can look similar to acute labyrinthitis with vertigo, nausea, vomiting, and ataxia. After swelling begins to compress the fourth ventricle, brainstem structures in the dorsal pons, such as the facial colliculi, can become involved. Thus, it is crucial to be able to distinguish between vertigo caused by cerebellar infarction, which causes a spontaneous purely vertical or direction-changing gaze-evoked nystagmus, with a more benign peripheral process that causes a unilateral vestibular loss and a direction fixed nystagmus. Other processes that can cause central vertigo include tumors of the posterior fossa.

Presyncope

Sensations of near fainting, especially on standing, are associated with medical conditions that affect blood flow to the brain or decreased oxygen delivery to the brain. Problems of the cardiovascular system are sometimes treated with medications that can increase dizziness symptoms. Some of these are discussed in the medication section below. Studies that delineate presyncope from other types of dizziness have generally evaluated orthostatic blood pressure changes in relationship to symptoms. Comparing recumbent to standing systolic or diastolic blood pressures and using the criteria of a drop in systolic blood pressure of 20 mmHg or more, or a 10-mmHg drop in diastolic blood pressure after standing for 2 minutes are typical endpoints. Studies such as this in healthy elderly populations indicate that presyncope is associated with recurrent episodes of orthostatic blood pressure changes, higher mean supine blood pressures, and lower body mass indexes (Puisieux et al., 1999). In the Cardiovascular Health Study, 14.8% of those aged 65 to 69 years were diagnosed with orthostatic hypotension, and the numbers jumped to 26% in persons over the age of 85 years (Rutan et al., 1992). Thus, presyncopal dizziness increases with age.

The actual numbers of elderly people with presyncope caused by orthostatic hypotension may be falsely low (Sloane and Baloh, 1989). In many studies, systolic blood pressure changes within a 2-minute period of standing are used as criteria for orthostatic hypotension (Lawson et al., 1999). An entity termed "postural dizziness" without postural hypotension is used to explain the symptoms of dizziness in persons with these symptoms. Recently researchers have shown that mean arterial pressure (MAP) is a more sensitive measure for orthostatic hypotension because it is a better indicator of cerebral perfusion pressure (Tinetti et al., 2000). Some older individuals with postural dizziness without postural hypotension may be able to pool enough blood in their lower extremities to affect cerebral perfusion, but not lower their systemic blood pressure (by the strict systolic and diastolic criteria) to be considered hypotensive (Hargreaves and Muir, 1992; Hackel et al., 1991). Also, a number of older people do not become immediately hypotensive on standing, but rather have delayed orthostatic hypotension (sometimes up to 30 minutes later) (Streeten, 1992).

Conditions that predispose to presyncope include physical deconditioning, depression, autonomic dysfunction such as parasympathetic hyperactivity and vasovagal reactions to emotions; neurodegenerative diseases (e.g., Shy-Drager syndrome); progressive supranuclear palsy; Parkinson's disease; Alzheimer's disease; cardiovascular disease; and hyperventilation. Because the causes for presyncope are so broad in scope, individuals can have multiple problems that contribute to their symptoms, and sometimes multiple professionals are required for successful treatment.

Dysequilibrium

Of all the subcategories of dizziness, dysequilibrium is the most pervasive in elderly people. As discussed, the multifactorial nature of this symptom leads to it being a component of dizziness in many older people. Degenerative changes that occur with age and disease in the visual, vestibular somatosensory, motor, and cerebellar systems can lead to dysequilibrium. In terms of causes, visual loss and vestibular loss can often be the most incapacitating and result in the most severe disturbances of balance and gait. Visual disturbances caused by cataracts, anterior chamber diseases, and retinal degeneration can all have a dramatic effect on equilibrium in older people. Vision is also extremely important as a compensatory sensory input for balance and orientation. This is why imbalance problems in the elderly are often worse when it is dark. Bilateral vestibular loss caused by ototoxic medications result in symptoms of continuous unsteadiness and oscillopsia, because of loss of VOR, and is usually worse in the dark (Baloh, 1992). Gentamicin-induced ototoxicity is not uncommon, and as a rule occurs *without vertigo or hearing loss*, and need not be associated with abnormal peak or trough levels or renal failure (Halmagyi et al., 1994). Unilateral vestibular dysfunction usually re-

sults in vertigo, but slow growing tumors (e.g., acoustic neuromas) can cause imbalance and unilateral slowness that is less dramatic.

Severe problems with balance and orientation can be caused by central nervous system disorders, such as frontal atrophy (e.g., Pick's disease), diffuse white matter degeneration, Parkinson's disease, Binswanger's disease, cerebral autosomal dominant arteriopathy with subcortical infarct and leukoencephalopathy (CADASIL), hydrocephalus, and other neurodegenerative diseases (Baloh, 1992; Weindruch et al., 1989; Sloane, 1996; Fife and Baloh, 1993; Kerber et al., 1998; Baloh and Vinters, 1995; Baloh et al., 1995; Whitman et al., 1999). In studies designed to determine the neuropathology of dysequilibrium, four common factors were found on postmortem analysis of patients with undiagnosed dysequilibrium: (*a*) prominent frontal atrophy; (*b*) ventriculomegaly; (*c*) reactive astrocytes in the periventricular white matter; and (*d*) increased arteriolar wall thickness (Whitman et al., 1999). These findings correspond well with MRI findings of ventriculomegaly and frontal atrophy in similar patients (Baloh and Vinters, 1995; Baloh et al., 1995; Masdeu et al., 1989). The presumed mechanism of dysequilibrium in these patients is disruption of long-loop reflex fibers traversing the deep periventricular white matter (Masdeu et al., 1989). A slowing of righting reflexes in the lower extremities would result and sensory-motor integration delayed. Evidence indicates slowed reaction times in older healthy individuals (Shaw, 1992). In addition, central-processing time, which is needed to decide between two responses, increases with age (Grabiner and Jahnigen, 1992). Thus, systemic conditions and behavioral risk factors that might predispose to subcortical strokes (e.g., hypertension, diabetes, hyperlipidemia, hypercholesterolemia, hypercoagulable states, sleep apnea, smoking, and illicit drug use) must be sought by physicians caring for patients with dysequilibrium.

Cerebellar and motor system dysfunction can also precipitate dysequilibrium. As mentioned, Parkinson's disease and other neuromuscular diseases can lead to dysequilibrium. Leg weakness is often seen with deconditioning in older people, and can add to a feeling of imbalance and dizziness when standing. Primary cerebellar disorders can affect motor system coordination and modulation of vestibular-initiated righting reflexes. These disorders include Chiari malformations, spinocerebellar atrophy, paraneoplastic syndromes, vitamin E deficiency (Bassen-Kornzweig syndrome), medication or toxin exposure (alcohol, anticonvulsants, lithium and organic solvents), and infections (Solomon, 2000). Many of these disorders will have associated cerebellar findings such as ataxia, dysmetria, impaired smooth pursuit eye movements, and OKN, and reduced ability to suppress VOR with fixation. Sensory abnormalities, often seen with toxin exposures and vitamin deficiencies, can also be associated with cerebellar disease.

Somatosensory deficits occur with age and disease and alter the perception of body position with regard to space. Often referred to as "multi-neurosensory impairment," the loss of proprioception in combination with any of the other sensory systems can lead to a pervasive dysequilibrium. The symptoms of dysequilibrium are often worse in the dark, and are readily quantifiable by electrodiagnostic criteria and physical examination. Some conditions that predispose to sensory loss and dysequilibrium include diabetes, renal disease, liver disease, cervical osteoarthritis, toxin exposures (i.e., acrylamide, thallium, arsenic, pyridoxine, diptheria, and dimethylaminopropionitrile), vitamin deficiencies (i.e., E, thiamine, pyridoxine, folate, and pantothenic acid), and medication exposures (i.e., neoplastic agents, amiodarone, almitrine, dapsone, disulfuram, isoniazid, metronidazole, phenytoin, and hydralazine). A thorough review of this topic can be found in a number of neurology textbooks.

Nonspecific Dizziness

When patients do not fit into a diagnostic category the term "idiopathic" or "nonspecific" seems to suffice. Most studies that attempt to divide dizziness into subtypes report between 17% and 33% of dizzy patients fall into this designation. Many of these people may have psychiatric diagnoses in the realm of anxiety and panic disorders, mood disorders, or personality disorders. Studies indicate that psychiatric causes of dizziness in older individuals account for between 5% and 37% of cases (Tinetti et al., 2000; Sloane et al., 1989; Lawson et al., 1999; Kroenke et al., 1992; Sloane and Baloh, 1989; Drachman and Hart, 1972; Colledge et al., 1996; Sloane et al., 1994; Kanton, 1984; McRae, 1960; Nedzelski et al., 1986; Simpson et al., 1988). People with anxiety and panic disorders present with complaints of dizziness in 18% of cases (Kanton, 1984). In one study of patients attending a dizziness clinic, 20% met the criteria for the diagnosis of panic disorder (Clark et al., 1994). Psychiatric causes for dizziness can create symptoms reminiscent of any of the other three categories, however, symptoms that occur in specific situations or environments

or that occur continuously without evidence of systemic medical or neurologic disease, suggest a psychiatric etiology. Some researchers have suggested that psychiatric causes of dizziness are not as prevalent in the elderly as in younger groups (Lawson et al., 1999; Sloane and Baloh, 1989). Other studies illustrate a strong link between depression, anxiety, somatoform disorders, and dizziness in geriatric patients (Tinetti et al., 2000; Baloh et al., 1998; Kroenke et al., 1992; Sloane et al., 1994; Kroenke et al., 1993). In a study of 56 chronically dizzy elderly patients, 37% had psychiatric diagnoses contributing to their dizziness, including anxiety disorders, depression, and adjustment disorders (Sloane et al., 1994). Only 5% had primary psychiatric disorders, including panic disorder, obsessive-compulsive disorder, and conversion disorder, as the primary reason for their dizziness.

A common problem in all persons with dizziness is the subsequent increase in psychological stress (Sloane et al., 1994). The presence of dizziness and the debilitating effect that it has on daily activities account for more than 25% of dizzy people reporting symptoms of agoraphobia and panic (Yardley et al., 1998; 2000). Patients with mixed physical and psychiatric symptoms also tend to have the highest level of handicap from dizziness. In longitudinal studies of dizziness in both primary care and community-based populations, patients with the most severe, persistent, and numerous physical and psychiatric symptoms remained symptomatic and handicapped the longest (Yardley, 1998; Bailey et al., 1993). Thus, psychiatric disorders can cause (or more frequently be caused by) either an episode of dizziness or fear of future episodes of dizziness. In any case, it is clear that an increase in the chronicity of symptoms occurs by erosion of the physical and psychological state of the individual. This seems especially pertinent to elderly patients with dizziness who may be more likely to suffer from other physical ailments and degenerative diseases that increase the incidence of depression, anxiety, and panic disorder.

Patients have been seen who complain of vague dizziness following unilateral cataract extraction with intraocular lens implantation. This frequently results in spectacle correction being used only for the nonoperated eye. This presents a problem to the vestibular system; although both the spectacle and intraocular lenses magnify or shrink the visual surround, one moves with the eyes and one is fixed to the head, necessitating nonconjugate eye movements for perfect gaze stability.

Medications

Approximately 13% of the US population is over the age of 65 years and accounts for more than 30% of all medications prescribed (Montamat et al., 1989). Dizziness is listed as an adverse side effect for 90% of all oral medications in the *Physicians Desk Reference*. National health expenditures for drugs in the United States have increased from $10 billion in 1965, to $20 billion in 1980, to $60 billion in 1995 (Avron, 1995). The classes of medications most often associated with dizziness are antiarrhythmics, anticonvulsants, antidepressants, anxiolytics, antipsychotics, sedatives or hypnotics, muscle relaxants, and nonsteroidal anti-inflammatory drugs (NSAID) (Tinetti et al., 2000; Sloane, 1996; Monane and Avorn, 1996). A clear medication effect alone is difficult to ascertain, given that most of the conditions being treated with these types of medications are known to cause dizziness themselves. Depression, anxiety, panic disorders, dementia, arthritis, cardiovascular disease, and stroke are all conditions that can cause dizziness or are treated with medications that can cause dizziness.

The mechanisms by which medications cause symptoms differ, but a few factors make older people more vulnerable to medication effects than younger people. With age comes an increase in body fat percentage (up to 35%) between the ages of 20 and 70 years and a small decrease in plasma volume (lower by 8%) (Shader et al., 1977). An age-dependent decrease has been demonstrated in cytochrome P-450 system efficiency in the liver (Vestal et al., 1992). Also, a decline in renal clearance by 30% to 50% between the ages of 30 and 80 years has been shown (Rowe et al., 1976). Thus, elderly people are more likely to suffer the unwanted effects of any drug. Because falls are a primary outcome that is measurable in elderly populations using medications, many studies are designed to measure falls rather than dizziness in relationship to medications. In a study of 1,358 community-dwelling persons 65 years of age or older, benzodiazepines, digoxin, laxatives, diuretics, and diltiazem were shown to be associated with presyncope, syncope, and falls (Cumming et al., 1991). A prospective study of older people on medications showed an odds ratio risk of fall while on sedatives of 28.3 (Tinneti et al., 1988). A prospective cohort study of people aged above 65 years living in nursing homes demonstrated that patients using benzodiazepines, tricyclic antidepressants, or multiple psychotropic medications more than doubled their risk

for recurrent falls (Thapa et al., 1995). In the same study, 36% of all falls were directly attributed to medications. In a cross-sectional investigation of 1,087 people aged 72 years or older, antidepressant medication use, depression, and use of five or more medications were significantly associated with dizziness (Tinetti et al., 2000). In summary, studies concerned with the association of medication use with dizziness and risk of falls in older people support the following: (*a*) shorter-acting medications, especially sedatives and anxiolytics, are preferable; (*b*) care in the prescription of blood pressure lowering agents is advisable because of the risk of orthostatic hypotension; (*c*) antidepressants and depression itself can contribute to dizziness and falls; and (*d*) any medication, especially those psychoactive in nature, can have prolonged or enhanced effects because of the reduced metabolic processes in older people.

Characteristics Associated With Dizziness Of Any Type

Risk factors associated with developing dizziness in old age include angina, hypertension, myocardial infarction (MI), stroke, Parkinson's disease, arthritis, diabetes, syncope, neurosensory impairment, alcohol use, smoking, nervousness, and medication use. In terms of medication use, antihypertensive agents, anticonvulsants, anxiolytics, antidepressants, and antipsychotics carry the highest risk for causing dizziness. In a 2000 study by Tinneti et al., 1,087 independent healthy people above 72 years of age were analyzed for complaints of dizziness and associated risk factors. They identified seven associated characteristics and the following relative risks (Tinetti et al., 2000):

1. Anxiety, 1.69
2. Depression, 1.36
3. Impaired balance, 1.34
4. Past MI, 1.31
5. Postural hypotension, 1.31
6. Five or more medications, 1.30
7. Impaired hearing, 1.27

When they compared the 29% of the study population who reported dizziness with those who were not dizzy, each of the four types of dizziness were associated with a significantly higher number of these characteristics (2.0–2.5 on average) than the nondizzy group (1.5 on average). Therefore, when assessing a geriatric patient even without a primary complaint of dizziness, recognition of one or more of these characteristics may help in uncovering an unreported problem. Also, recognition of the "syndrome" should not preclude a search for a specific cause (Drachman, 2000).

INITIAL DIAGNOSIS AND MANAGEMENT OF THE DIZZY PATIENT

In taking the patient's history, attempt to distinguish the nature of the symptoms (e.g., vertigo versus presyncope), the actual duration of any vertigo, whether any brainstem or cerebellar symptoms are also present (indicating a central or vascular cause), or whether unilateral hearing or aural symptoms indicate the side of peripheral involvement (Fig. 8-1). Determine if symptoms are truly spontaneous and episodic (migraine, Ménière's, VBTIA), provoked by rolling over in bed (BPPV), or elicited by rich visual motion environments (e.g., supermarket aisles) noncompensated or fluctuating vestibular dysfunction,

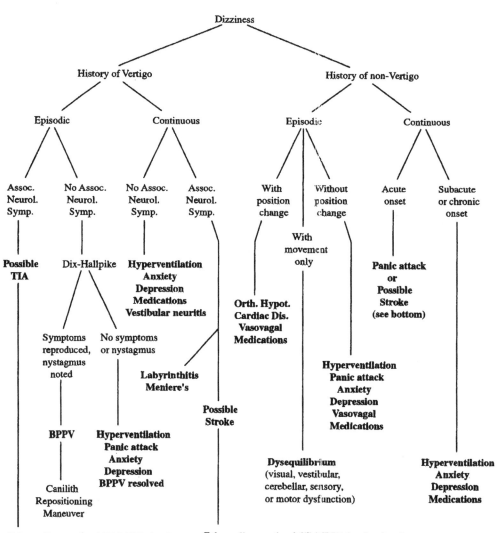

FIG 8-1. Algorithm for dizziness in elderly patients.

anxiety disorders. Ask whether patients are avoiding any activities, locations, or head movements, and if symptoms are chronically elicited by these activities; encourage a vestibular rehabilitation evaluation (Herdman, 1992), habituation exercises or tai chi (Hain et al., 1999).

An excellent description of the bedside vestibular and ocular motor examination is recommended for a more complete treatment of this topic (Walker and Zee, 2000). Spontaneous peripheral vestibular nystagmus is direction fixed, present in straight-ahead gaze, suppressed with visual fixation, and is mixed horizontal torsional with quick phases beating toward the more active ear. It can be brought out by removing fixation with the use of Frenzel lenses or by performing occlusive ophthalmoscopy (look for systematic drift of the nerve head while covering the fellow eye). Nystagmus caused by brainstem or cerebellar disease is direction-changing, gaze-evoked, and often associated with misalignment (skew deviation); it is not suppressed with vision and can be disconjugate (as with an internuclear ophthalmoplegia). A purely vertical or torsional nystagmus should prompt evaluation for central disease (Table 8-3).

Diagnostic Tests

Basic laboratory tests in a neuro-otologic workup include an audiogram and electronystagmography (ocular motor studies and caloric testing). An audiogram would be expected to show symmetric, high-frequency sensorineural hearing loss (SNHL) that is consistent with normal aging. Any asymmetry in pure-tone thresholds unexplained by a conductive

hearing loss or other known etiology should prompt an imaging study to rule out a schwannoma of the VIIIth nerve. The ideal study is a gadolinium-enhanced MRI, with attention to the internal auditory canals (IAC). A unilateral, low-frequency SNHL is consistent with Ménière's disease, especially if fluctuations can be documented.

Emergent imaging is recommended when transient vertigo is associated with unilateral or asymmetric hearing loss; brainstem or cerebellar symptoms other than vertigo (diplopia, dysarthria, appendicular dysmetria, dysphagia, downbeat or direction-changing nystagmus, Horner's syndrome, face or body sensory or motor changes); stroke risk factors (diabetes, hypertension, history of MI); acute onset neck pain (magnetic resonance angiography to rule out dissection); new onset severe headache; or the inability to stand or walk.

Ocular motor studies typically include tests of the smooth pursuit, fixation, and saccadic systems. Smooth pursuit deficits are normally seen in the aging population; responses that are asymmetric, however, should prompt concern about cerebellar pathology. An excess number of square wave jerks during visual fixation (0.5 to 5 degree saccades made away and back to fixation, at a frequency no greater than two per second) may be associated with progressive supranuclear palsy. Any spontaneous nystagmus recorded with the eyes straight ahead is abnormal; purely vertical nystagmus is indicative of brainstem or cerebellar pathology, but can be seen with medication toxicity (lithium). Gaze-evoked (direction changing) nystagmus recorded when upright similarly suggests cerebellar dysfunction or a toxic or metabolic

TABLE 8-3. *Common medications used for dizziness symptoms: mechanisms and costs*

Medication (Dose)	Indication	Risks	Cost
Acetazolamide (250–1,000 mg/d)	Meniere's disease	Nephrolithiasis, electrolyte disturbance, parasthsias	$29 (60 tabs, 250 mg) $71 (500 mg sequel caps)
Promethazine (12.5–25 mg q6h)	Acute nausea, vomiting[a]	Extrapyramidal side effects, warning with glaucoma, sedation	$9 (30 tabs, 25 mg)
Meclizine (12.5–50 mg q.d.)	Acute nausea, vomiting[a]	Sedation, confusion, xerostomia, hypotension	$5 (30 tabs, 25 mg)
Root of ginger, ginger tea	Chronic nausea	Unknown	Variable
Clonazepam (0.25 mg b.i.d. or t.i.d.)	Vestibular suppressant, anxiety[a]	Sedation, confusion	$60 (30 tabs, 0.5 mg)
Diazepam (2–5 mg t.i.d., p.r.n.)	Vestibular suppressant, anxiety[a]	Sedation, confusion	$5 (30 tabs, 2 or 5 mg)

[a]For short-term treatment of acute vestibular crises only. Benzodiazepines may be used to treat associated anxiety disorders.

b.i.d., twice daily; caps, capsules; p.r.n., when needed; q.d., every day; tabs, tablets; t.i.d., three times daily.

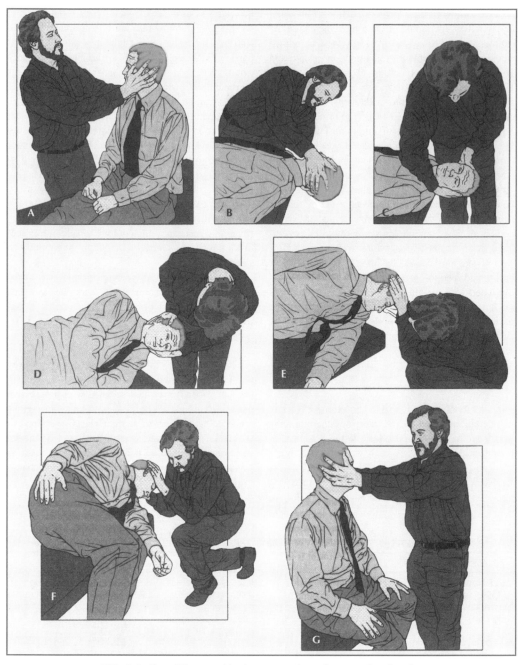

FIG. 8-2. Canalith repositioning procedure. See text for details.

derangement. A direction-fixed, mixed horizontal-torsional nystagmus seen in primary gaze, which increases when fixation is removed, and with gaze in the quick phase direction is consistent with an acute unilateral vestibular loss. Caloric studies should confirm a peripheral weakness in the ear contralateral to the nystagmus quick phase direction. This can also be confirmed at the bedside using the head impulse test (Halmagyi and Curthoys, 1988). Positional nystagmus is elicited both in static head orientations (supine, head turned left and right) as well as with the Dix-Hallpike maneuver, which is used to diagnose BPPV.

Benign Paroxysmal Positional Vertigo

Benign paroxysmal positional vertigo is vertigo that is provoked by movement of the head with respect to gravity (rolling over or getting in and out of bed, looking up, bending over). Typically, vertigo emanates from a single posterior SCC, lasts less than 60 seconds, and may be worse in the morning (matutinal vertigo). It is diagnosed by performing the Dix-Hallpike maneuver to each side, with the patient returning to the upright position between each maneuver. The first two panels in Figure 8-2 demonstrate this maneuver for the right posterior SCC. When positive, a mixed vertical-torsional nystagmus is observed, with slow phases downward (with respect to the head) and the top of the eyes rolling away from the dependent ear. The nystagmus can appear more vertical when looking toward the up ear, and more torsional when looking toward the undermost ear. After being placed in the Dix-Hallpike position, nystagmus and vertigo should have a latency of several seconds (rarely up to 45 seconds), and is transient (usually less than 30 seconds). On returning to the upright position, the nystagmus may reverse direction and have a downbeating component.

More than 90% of BPPV cases can be treated successfully with a particle repositioning maneuver (for review, see Furman and Cass and Lanska and Remlar [Furman and Cass, 1999; Lanska and Remler, 1997]). The maneuver shown in Figure 8-2 is based on Epley's description (Epley, 1992). While seated, rotate the head 45° toward the affected ear. Lay the patient back to the supine position, and maintain this position until the nystagmus decays completely. While supine, rotate the head 90° toward the unaffected side, and hold this position for the same duration. Rotate the whole body 90° with the patient in the lateral decubitus position and again maintain this position. Sit the patient upright, keeping the head turned and chin

down. The maneuver is best repeated to ensure that it was successful, and treatment can be repeated as often as necessary. Posttreatment, patients are instructed to keep their heads upright for at least the remainder of the day.

Other Treatments

Treatment for Ménière's disease includes use of the carbonic anhydrase inhibitor acetylzolamide, reduction of salt intake and judicious use of vestibular suppressants as noted in Table 8-3. Additionally, surgical procedures are used to reduce the endolymphatic pressure within the inner ear, or to eliminate symptoms by vestibular nerve transection.

Because the causes of presyncopal and dysequilibrium dizziness are multifactorial, the specific treatments depend on a clear understanding of their causes.

REFERENCES

Avron J. Medication use and the elderly: current status and opportunities. *Health Affairs* 1995;14:276–286.

Bailey KE, Sloane PD, Mitchell M, et al. Which primary care patients with dizziness will develop persistent impairment? *Arch Fam Med* 1993;2:847–852.

Baloh RW, Vinters HV. White matter lesions and disequilibrium in older people. II. Clinicopathologic correlation. *Arch Neurol* 1995;52:975–981.

Baloh RW. Dizziness in older people. *J Am Geriatr Soc* 1992;40:713–721.

Baloh RW, Jacobson KM, Enrietto JA, et al. Balance disorders in older persons: quantification with posturography. *Otolaryngol Head Neck Surg* 1998;119:89–92.

Baloh RW, et al. White matter lesions and disequilibrium in older people. I. Case-controlled comparison. *Arch Neurol* 1995;52:970–974.

Baloh RW, Jacobson KM, Socotch TM. The effect of aging on visual-vestibuloocular responses. *Exp Brain Res* 1993; 95:509–516.

Bergstrom B. Morphology of the vestibular nerve. III. Analysis of the calibers of the myelinated vestibular nerve fibers in man at various ages. *Acta Otolaryngol (Stockh)* 1973;76:331–338.

Bergstrom B. Morphology of the vestibular nerve. II. The number of myelinated vestibular nerve fibers in man at various ages. *Acta Otolaryngol (Stockh)* 1973;76: 173–179.

Bloom J, Katsarkas A. Paroxysmal positional vertigo in the elderly. *J Otolaryngol*, 1989;18:96–98.

Boult C, Murphy J, Sloane P, et al. The relation of dizziness to functional decline. *J Am Geriatr Soc* 1991;39:858–861.

Brandt T. Positional and positioning vertigo and nystagmus. *J Neurol Sci* 1990;95:3–28.

Bruner A, Norris TW. Age-related changes in caloric nystagmus. *Acta Otolaryngol (Stockh)* 1971;(Suppl 282):1–24.

Clark DB, Hirsch BE, Smith MG, et al. Panic in otolaryngology patients presenting with dizziness or hearing loss. *Am J Psychiatry* 1994;151:1223–1225.

Colledge NR, Barr-Hamilton RM, Lewis SJ, et al. Evaluation of investigations to diagnose the cause of dizziness in elderly people: a community based controlled study. *BMJ* 1996;313:788–792.

Colledge NR, Wilson JA, Macintyre CC, et al. The prevalence and characteristics of dizziness in an elderly community. *Age Ageing* 1994;23:117–120.

Cumming RG, Miller JP, Kelsey JL, et al. Medications and multiple falls in elderly people: the St. Louis OASIS Study. *Age Ageing* 1991;20:455–461.

Cutrer FM, Baloh RW. Migraine associated dizziness. *Headache* 1992;32:300–304.

Drachman DA, Hart CW. An approach to the dizzy patient. *Neurology* 1972;22:323–334.

Drachman DA. Occam's razor, geriatric syndromes, and the dizzy patient. *Ann Intern Med* 2000;132(5):403–404.

Enrietto JA, Jacobson KM, Baloh RW. Aging effects on auditory and vestibular responses: a longitudinal study. *Am J Otolaryngol* 1999;20:371–378.

Epley JM. The canalith repositioning procedure for treatment of benign paroxysmal positional vertigo. *Otolaryngol Head Neck Surg* 1992;107:399–404.

Fife TD, Baloh RW. Disequilibrium of unknown cause in older people. *Ann Neurol* 1993;34:694–702.

Furman JM, Cass S. Benign paroxysmal positional vertigo. *N Engl J Med* 1999;341(21):1590–1596.

Grabiner MD, Jahnigen DW. Modeling recovery from stumbles: preliminary data on variable selection and classification efficiency. *J Am Geriatr Soc* 1992;40:910–913.

Grad A, Baloh RW. Vertigo of vascular origin. Clinical and electronystagmographic features in 84 cases. *Arch Neurol* 1989;46:281–284.

Grimby A, Rosenhall U. Health-related quality of life and dizziness in old age. *Gerontology* 1995;41:286–298.

Hackel A, Linzer M, Anderson N. Cardiovascular and catecholamine responses to head-up tilt in the diagnosis of recurrent unexplained syncope in elderly patients. *J Am Geriatr Soc* 1991;39:663–668.

Hain TC, Fuller L, Weil L, et al. Effects of tai chi on balance. *Arch Otolaryngol Head Neck Surg* 1999;125(11):1191–1195.

Hall TC, Miller KH, Corsallis JAN. Variations in the human Purkinje cell population according to age and sex. *Neuropathol Appl Neurobiol* 1975;1:267–292.

Halmagyi GM, Curthoys IS. A clinical sign of canal paresis. *Arch Neurol* 1988;45(7):737–739.

Halmagyi GM, Fattore CM, Curthoys IS, et al. Gentamicin vestibulotoxicity. *Otolaryngol Head Neck Surg* 1994;111(5):571–574.

Hargreaves A, Muir A. Lack of variation in venous tone potentiates vasovagal syncope. *Br Heart J* 1992;67:486–490.

Havlik RJ. Aging in the eighties, impaired senses for sound and light in persons age 65 and over. Preliminary data from the Supplement on Aging to the National Health Interview Survey, United States January–June 1984, 1986. Hyattsville, MD: National Center for Health Care Statistics. Public Health Service.

Herdman SJ. Physical therapy management of vestibular disorders in older patients. *Physical Therapy Practice* 1992;1:77–87.

Kanton W. Panic disorder and somatization. *Am J Med* 1984;77:101–106.

Kerber KA, Enrietto JA, Jacobson KM, et al. Disequilibrium in older people; a prospective study. *Neurology* 1998;51:574–580.

Koch H, Smith MC. Office-based ambulatory care for patients 75 years and over. National Ambulatory Medical Care Survey, 1980 and 1981; 1985. Hyattsville, MD: National Center for Health Statistics, Public Health Service.

Kroenke K, Lucas CA, Rosenberg ML, et al. Causes of persistent dizziness: a prospective study of 100 patients in ambulatory care. *Ann Intern Med* 1992;117:898–904.

Kroenke K, Lucas CA, Rosenberg ML, et al. Psychiatric disorders and functional impairment in patients with persistent dizziness. *J Gen Intern Med* 1993;8:530–535.

Lanska DJ, Remler B. Benign paroxysmal positioning vertigo: classic descriptions, origins of the provacative positioning technique, and conceptual developments. *Neurology* 1997;48(5):1167–1177.

Lawson J, Fitzgerald J, Birchall J, et al. Diagnosis of geriatric patients with severe dizziness. *J Am Geriatr Soc* 1999;47:12–17.

Leigh RJ, Zee DW, eds. *The neurology of eye movements*, 3rd ed. Philadelphia: FA Davis, 1999.

Lopez I, Honrubia V, Baloh RW. Aging and the human vestibular nucleus. *J Vestib Res* 1997;7:77–85.

Lord SR, Clark RD, Webster IW. Postural stability and associated physiological factors in a population of aged persons. *J Gerontol* 1991;46:M69–M76.

Masdeu JC, Wolfson L, Lantos G, et al. Brain white-matter changes in the elderly prone to falling. *Arch Neurol* 1989;46:1292–1296.

McRae D. The neurologic aspects of vertigo. *California Medicine* 1960;92:255–259.

Monane M, Avorn J. Medications and falls: causation, correlation and prevention. *Clin Geriatr Med* 1996;12:847–858.

Montamat SC, Cusack BJ, Vestal RE. Management of drug therapy in the elderly. *N Engl J Med* 1989;321:303–309.

Nadol JB, Schuknecht HF. The pathology of peripheral vestibular disorders in the elderly. *Ear, Nose Throat J* 1989;68:930–933.

Nedzelski JM, Barber HO, McIlmoyl L. Diagnoses in a dizziness unit. *J Otolaryngol* 1986;15:101–104.

Neuhauser H, Leopold M, von Brevern M, et al. The interrelations of migraine, vertigo, and migrainous vertigo. *Neurology* 2001;56(4):436–441.

Oghalai JS, Manolidis S, Barth JL, et al. Unrecognized benign paroxysmal positional vertigo in elderly patients. *Otolaryngol Head Neck Surg* 2000;122:630–634.

Paige GD. Senescence of human visual-vestibular interactions. 1. Vestibulo-ocular reflex and adaptive plasticity with aging. *Exp Brain Res* 1992;2:133–151.

Parnes LS, McClure JA. Free-floating endolymph particles: a new operative finding during posterior semicircular canal occlusion. *Laryngoscope* 1992;102(9):988–992.

Paterka RJ, Black FO, Schoenhoff MB. Age-related changes in human vestibulo-ocular reflexes: sinusoidal rotation and caloric tests. *J Vestib Res* 1990;1:49–59.

Puisieux F, Boumbar Y, Bulckaen H, et al. Intraindividual variability in orthostatic blood pressure changes among older adults: the influence of meals. *J Am Geriatr Soc* 1999;47:1332–1336.

Raz N, Torres IJ, Spencer WD. Age-related regional differences in cerebellar vermis observed in vivo. *Arch Neurol* 1992;49:412–416.

Richter E. Quantitative study of human Scarpa's ganglion and vestibular sensory epithelium. *Acta Otolaryngol (Stockh)* 1980;90:199–208.

Rosenhall U. Mapping of the crista ampullares in man. *Ann Otol Rhinol Laryngol* 1972;81:882–889.

Rosenhall U. Vestibular macular mapping in man. *Ann Otol Rhinol Laryngol* 1972;81:339–351.

Ross MD, Peacor D, Johnson LG. Observations on normal and degenerating human otoconia. *Ann Otol Rhinol Laryngol* 1976;85:310–326.

Rowe JW, Andres R, Tobin JD, et al. The effect of age on creatinine clearance in man: a cross-sectional and longitudinal study. *J Gerontol* 1976;31:155–163.

Royal College of General Practitioners, OoCaS. Morbidity statistics from general practice. Table 13, 1981–1982. Third National Study.

Rutan GH, Hermanson B, Bild DE. Orthostatic hypotension in older adults: the Cardiovascular Health study. *Hypertension* 1992;19:508–519.

Sawyer RN Jr, Thurston SE, Becker KR, et al. The cervicoocular reflex of normal human subjects in response to transient and sinusoidal trunk rotations. *J Vestib Res* 1994;4:245–249.

Schuknecht HF, Merchant SN. Vestibular atelectasis. *Ann Otol Rhinol Laryngol* 1988;97:565–576.

Shader RI, Greenblatt DJ, Harmatz JS, et al. Absorption and disposition of chlordiazepoxide in young and elderly male volunteers. *J Clin Pharmacol* 1977;17:709–718.

Shaw NA. Age-dependent changes in central somatosensory conduction time. *Cin Electroencephalogr* 1992;23:105–110.

Simpson RB, Nedzelski JM, Barber HO, et al. Psychiatric diagnoses in patients with psychogenic dizziness or severe tinnitus. *J Otolaryngol* 1988;17:325–330.

Skinner HB, Barrack RL, Cook SD, et al. Joint position sense in total knee arthroplasty. *J Orthop Res* 1984;1:276–283.

Sloane D, Baloh RW. Persistent dizziness in geriatric patients. *J Am Geriatr Soc* 1989;37:1031–1038.

Sloane D, Blazer D, George LK. Dizziness in a community elderly population. *J Am Geriatr Soc* 1989;37:101–108.

Sloane D. Evaluation and management of dizziness in the older patient. *Clin Geriatr Med* 1996;12:785–801.

Sloane D, Hartman M, Mitchell M. Psychological factors associated with chronic dizziness in patients aged 60 and older. *J Am Geriatr Soc* 1994;42:847–852.

Solomon D. Distinguishing and treating causes of central vertigo. *Otolaryngol Clin North Am* 2000;33:579–601.

Streeten D. Delayed orthostatic intolerance. *Arch Intern Med* 1992;152:1066–1072.

Strupp M, Brandt T. Vestibular neuritis. *Adv Otorhinolaryngol* 1999;55:111–136.

Strupp M, Arbusow V, Borges Pereira C, et al. Subjective straight-ahead during neck muscle vibration: effects of ageing. *Neuroreport* 1999;10:3191–3194.

Thapa PB, Gideon P, Fought RL, et al. Psychotropic drugs and risk of recurrent falls in ambulatory nursing home residents. *Am J Epidemiol* 1995;142:202–211.

Tilvis RS, Hakala SM, Valvanne J, et al. Postural hypotension and dizziness in a general aged population: a four-year follow-up of the Helsinki Aging Study. *J Am Geriatr Soc* 1996;44:809–814.

Tinetti ME, Williams CS, Gill TM. Dizziness among older adults: a possible geriatric syndrome. *Ann Intern Med* 2000;132:337–344.

Tinetti ME, Speechley M, Ginter SF. Risk factors for falls among elderly persons living in the community. *N Engl J Med* 1988;319:1701–1707.

Torvik A, Torp S, Lindboe CF. Atrophy of the cerebellar vermis in ageing: a morphometric and histologic study. *J Neurol Sci* 1986;76:283–294.

Vestal RE, Montamat SC, Nielson C. Drugs in special patient groups: the elderly. In: Melmon KL, et al., eds. *Clinical pharmacology.* New York: McGraw Hill, 1992:851–874.

Walker MF, Zee DS. Bedside vestibular examination. In: Shepard NT, Solomon D, eds. *Practical issues in the management of the dizzy and balance patient.* Philadelphia: WB Saunders, 2000:495–506.

Weindruch R, Korper S, Hadley E. The prevalence of dysequilibrium and related disorders in older persons. *Ear Nose Throat J* 1989;68:925–929.

Whitman GT, DiPatre PL, Lopez IA, et al. Neuropathology in older people with disequilibrium of unknown cause. *Neurology* 1999;53:375–382.

Yardley L, Owen N, Nazareth I, et al. Prevalence and presentation of dizziness in a general practice community sample of working age people. *Br J Gen Pract* 1998;48:1131–1135.

Yardley L. Overview of psychologic effects of chronic dizziness and balance disorders. *Otolaryngol Clin North Am* 2000;33:603–616.

SUGGESTED READINGS

Baloh RW. Dizziness in older people. *Progress in Geriatrics* 1992;40:713–721.

Hotson JR, Baloh RW. Acute vestibular syndrome. *N Engl J Med* 1998;339:680–685.

Leigh RJ, Zee DS. The neurology of eye movements, 3rd ed. In: Plum F, editor-in-chief. *Contemporary neurology series.* Philadelphia: FA Davis, 1999.

Shepard NT, Solomon D. Functional operation of the balance system in daily activities. *Otolaryngol Clin North Am* 2000;33(3):455–469.

Tinetti ME, Williams CS, Gill TM. Dizziness among older adults: a possible geriatric syndrome. *Ann Intern Med* 2000;132:337–344.

9

Definition and Epidemiology of Falls and Gait Disorders

Neil B. Alexander

INTRODUCTION

Falls

A fall is a sudden, unintentional change in position causing an individual to land at a lower level, on an object, or the ground. Because most falls are not associated with syncope, most investigators exclude falls associated with loss of consciousness (e.g., as from a seizure), although loss of consciousness can occur after the fall. Other overwhelming events (e.g., sustaining a violent blow or sudden onset of paralysis) are also not as common as nonsyncopal falls. Annually, falls occur in approximately one third of community-dwelling older adults and one half of nursing home residents. The nursing home resident rate, 1.5 falls per bed annually, is likely caused by the increased frailty of these residents and the increased reporting in this setting (Rubinstein et al., 1994). Depending on the published series, although up to 2% of falls result in hip fractures, other fractures can occur in up to 5% and other serious injuries (e.g., head injury) can occur in up to 10%. Often more than 50% of persons who fall sustain at least some minor injury (e.g., a laceration); more importantly, however, these and others who fall can develop fear of falling and restrict their activity. Those who fall, particularly repeat fallers, tend to have activities of daily living (ADL) and instrumental ADL disability, and are at high risk for subsequent hospitalization, further disability, institutionalization, and death (King and Tinetti, 1995; Tinetti and Williams, 1997; Tinetti and Williams, 1998).

Gait Disorders

Determining that a gait is "disordered" is difficult because no clearly accepted standards are generally seen for "normal" gait in older adults. Some believe that slowed gait speed suggests a disorder, whereas others believe that deviations in smoothness, symme-try, and synchrony of movement patterns suggest a disorder. However, a slowed and aesthetically abnormal gait, in fact, can provide the older adult with a safe, independent gait pattern. Self-reports of difficulty walking are common. At least 20% of noninstitutionalized older adults admit to having difficulty walking or require the assistance of another person or special equipment to walk (Oschiega et al., 2000). Limitations in walking also increase with age. In some samples of noninstitutionalized older adults aged 85 years and older, the incidence of limitation in walking can be more than 54% (Oschiega et al., 2000). Although age-related gait changes (e.g., in speed) are most apparent past age 75 or 80, most gait disorders appear in connection with underlying diseases, particularly as disease severity increases. Attributing a gait disorder to one disease cause in older adults is particularly difficult because similar gait abnormalities are common to many diseases (Alexander, 1996a).

CAUSES, RISK FACTORS AND CLINICAL MANIFESTATIONS

Multiple factors frequently contribute to falls, fall-related injury, and gait disorders. In falls, often a complex interaction occurs between individual impairments (intrinsic factors), situational factors (aspects related to the ADL task being performed), and extrinsic factors (environmental demand and hazards). In terms of intrinsic factors, the diseases and impairments that are implicated in gait disorders are similar to those that place an older adult at risk for falls and fall-related injury. At least seven major intrinsic factors or conditions can be implicated and, although age-related changes can be present (such as in reduction of leg strength), the major contributors to risk of fall and gait disorders are the diseases that influence each factor (Table 9-1). These functions in-

TABLE 9-1. *Intrinsic factors contributing to risk of falls, fall-related injury, and gait disorders*

Factor	Typical diseases involved
Central processing	Dementia
Neuromotor	Parkinson's disease, stroke, myelopathy (such as from cervical or lumbar spondylosis), cerebellar degeneration, carotid sinus hypersensitivity, peripheral neuropathy, vertebrobasilar insufficiency
Vision	Cataracts, glaucoma, age-related macular degeneration
Vestibular	Acute labyrinthitis, Ménière's disease, paroxysmal positional vertigo
Proprioception	Peripheral neuropathy (such as from diabetes mellitus), B_{12} deficiency
Musculoskeletal	Arthritis, foot disorders
Systemic	Postural hypotension, metabolic disease (e.g., thyroid), cardiopulmonary disease, other acute illness (e.g., sepsis)

clude vestibular, proprioceptive, and visual function; cognition; and musculoskeletal factors. For example, patients with leg arthritis (with associated pain and limited range of motion and strength) and dementia (with associated lack of judgment, inattention, and confusion) are at risk for falls. Medications are also major risk factors and are categorized according to their major mechanism of effect (Table 9-2). Extrinsic and situational factors (Table 9-3) contribute to the risk of falls and fall-related injury when (*a*) environmental hazards are present; (*b*) the environment or tasks performed demand greater postural control and mobility; and (*c*) situations require changing positions (such as transferring and turning). For example, a patient with Parkinson's disease (intrinsic factor) may trip over a rug (extrinsic factor), but only under certain situations, such as walking to the bathroom at night (situational factor). Situational factors are particularly important when an injury results from a fall

(Tinetti et al., 1995). For example, major injuries are more likely when falling from an upright position (with greater potential energy to be dissipated) and when falling laterally, with direct impact on the hip. Other environmental factors (e.g., hardness of impact surface) and other intrinsic factors (e.g., low femoral bone mineral density and body mass index) also contribute to increased risk of fall-related injury (Cummings and Nevitt, 1989; Greenspan et al., 1994).

The relative contribution of intrinsic, extrinsic, and situational factors also depends on the person falling and the environment in which that person is living. Community-dwelling fallers tend to be exposed to greater environmental demand and hazards and tend to be less physically impaired; thus, extrinsic factors make more contributions to fall and fall injury risk (King and Tinetti, 1995). Nursing home fallers are usually more physically impaired and are exposed to fewer environmental hazards and demand; thus, intrinsic factors such as weakness and balance disorders contribute more to falls and fall injury risk (Rubinstein et al., 1994).

TABLE 9-2. *Medications contributing to risk of falls, fall-related injury, and gait disorders*

Medication category	Typical medications
Reduce alertness or retard central processing	Analgesics (especially narcotics)
	Psychotropics (especially tricyclics, long-acting benzodiazepines, phenothiazines)
Impair cerebral perfusion	Antihypertensives (especially vasodilators)
	Antiarrythmics
	Diuretics (especially when dehydration occurs)
Direct vestibular toxicity	Aminoglycosides
	High dose loop diuretics
Extrapyramidal syndromes	Phenothiazines

TABLE 9-3. *Extrinsic and situational factors contributing to risk of falls and fall-related injury*

Factor	Examples
Environmental hazard	Slippery or uneven walking surface, poor lighting
Increased environmental demand	Using stairs, rising from low chair
Situational	Changing position, risk-taking behavior, recent relocation to new nursing home

From author's own original work and adapted from King MB, Tinetti ME. Falls in community-dwelling older persons. *J Am Geriatr Soc* 1995;43:1146–1154.

ASSESSMENT OF GAIT DISORDERS AND FALL RISK

Diagnoses Contributing to Falls and Gait Disorders

Disordered gait may not be an inevitable consequence of aging, but rather a reflection of the increased prevalence and severity of age-associated diseases. These underlying diseases, both neurologic and non-neurologic, are the major contributors to disordered gait. In a primary care setting, patients consider pain, stiffness, dizziness, numbness, weakness, and sensations of abnormal movement to be the most common contributors to their walking difficulties (Hough et al., 1987). The most common diagnoses found in a primary care setting thought to contribute to gait disorders include degenerative joint disease, acquired musculoskeletal deformities, intermittent claudication, postorthopedic surgery and poststroke impairments, and postural hypotension (Hough et al., 1987). Usually, more than one contributing diagnosis is found. Factors such as dementia and fear of falling also contribute to gait disorders. The diagnoses found in a neurologic referral population are primarily neurologically oriented (e.g. Sudarsky and Rontal, 1983; Fuh et al., 1994): frontal gait disorders [usually related to normal pressure hydrocephalus (NPH) and cerebrovascular processes]; sensory disorders (also involving vestibular and visual function); myelopathy; previously undiagnosed Parkinson's disease or Parkinsonian syndromes; and cerebellar disease. Known conditions causing severe impairment (e.g., hemiplegia and severe hip or knee disease) are frequently not referred to a neurologist. Thus, many gait disorders, particularly those that are classical and discrete (e.g., related to stroke and osteoarthritis) and those that are mild or may relate to irreversible disease (e.g., multiinfarct dementia), are presumably diagnosed in a primary care setting and treated without a referral to a neurologist. Other less common contributors to gait disorders include metabolic disorders (related to renal or hepatic disease), central nervous system (CNS) tumors or subdural hematoma, depression, and psychotropic medications. Case reports also document reversible gait disorders caused by clinically overt hypo- or hyperthyroidism and B12 and folate deficiency (for detailed review, see Alexander 1996a).

A potentially useful classification system (based on Nutt et al., 1993 and elaborated in Alexander, 1996b) (Table 9-4) categorizes these diseases according to the sensorimotor levels that are affected. Diseases considered part of the low sensorimotor level can be divided into peripheral sensory and peripheral motor dysfunction, including musculoskeletal (arthritic) and myopathic or neuropathic disorders that cause weakness. These disorders are generally distal to the CNS. With peripheral sensory impairment, vestibular disorders, peripheral neuropathy, posterior column (proprioceptive) deficits, or visual impairment commonly cause unsteady and tentative gait. With peripheral motor impairment, a number of classical gait patterns emerge, including obvious compensatory maneuvers. These conditions involve extremity (both body segment and joint) deformities, painful weightbearing, and focal myopathic and neuropathic weakness. Note that if the gait disorder is limited to this low sensorimotor level (i.e., the CNS is intact), the person adapts well to the gait disorder, compensating with an assistive device or learning to negotiate the environment safely. At the middle level, the execution of centrally selected postural and locomotor responses is faulty, and the sensory and motor modulation of gait is disrupted. Gait can be initiated normally but stepping patterns are abnormal. Examples include diseases causing spasticity (e.g., related to myelopathy, B_{12} deficiency, and stroke), Parkinsonism (idiopathic as well as drug-induced), and cerebellar disease (e.g., alcohol-induced). Classical gait patterns appear when the spasticity is sufficient to cause leg circumduction and fixed deformities (e.g., equinovarus), the Parkinson's produces shuffling steps and reduced arm swing, and the cerebellar ataxia increases trunk sway sufficiently to require a broad base of gait support. At the high level, the gait characteristics become more nonspecific and cognitive dysfunction and slowed cognitive processing become more prominent. Behavioral aspects such as fear of falling are also important, particularly in cautious gait. Frontal-related gait disorders often have a cerebrovascular component, and are not merely the result of frontal masses and NPH. The severity of the frontal-related disorders runs a spectrum from gait ignition failure (i.e., difficulty with initiation) to frontal dysequilibrium, where unsupported stance is not possible. Cognitive, pyramidal, and urinary disturbances can also accompany a gait disorder. Gait disorders that might fall in this category have been given a number of overlapping descriptions, including gait apraxia, marche' a petits pas, and arteriosclerotic parkinsonism.

Note that more than one disease or impairment is likely present that contributes to a gait disorder; one example could be the long-standing diabetic with peripheral neuropathy and a recent stroke who is now very fearful of falls. Certain disorders can actually in-

TABLE 9-4. *Gait disorders classified by sensorimotor level, with a description of the specific pathologic condition and associated gait findings**

Sensorimotor level	Within level classification	Condition (pathology, symptoms, signs)	Typical gait findings
Low	Peripheral sensory	Sensory ataxia (posterior column, peripheral nerves)	Unsteady, uncoordinated
		Vestibular ataxia	Unsteady, weaving (*drunken*)
		Visual ataxia	Tentative, uncertain
	Peripheral motor	Arthritic (antalgic; joint deformity)	Avoids weight bearing on affected side, shorten stance phase. Painful hip may produce *Trendelenberg* (trunk shift over affected side). Painful knee is flexed. Painful spine produces short, slow steps and decreased lumbar lordosis. Other nonantalgic features: contractures, deformity-limited motion, buckling with weight bearing. Kyphosis and ankylosing spondylosis produce stooped posture. Unequal leg length can produce trunk and pelvic motion abnormalities (including *Trendelenberg*).
		Myopathic and neuropathic (weakness)	Pelvic girdle weakness produces exaggerated lumbar lordosis and lateral trunk flexion (*Trendelenberg* and *waddling* gait). Proximal motor neuropathy produces *waddling* and *foot slap*. Distal motor neuropathy produces distal weakness (especially ankle dorsiflexion, *foot drop*), which may lead to exaggerated hip flexion/foot lifting (*steppage gait*) and *foot slap*.
Middle	Spasticity	Hemiplegia/paresis	Leg swings outward and in semicircle from hip (*circumduction*). Knee may hyperextend (*genu recurvatum*), and ankle may excessively plantar flex and invert (*equinovarus*). With less paresis, some may only lose arms swing and only drag or scrape the foot.
		Paraplegia/paresis	Both legs circumduct, steps are short shuffling and scraping, and when severe, hip adducts so that knees cross in front of each other (*scissoring*).
	Parkinsonism		Small shuffling steps, hesitation, acceleration (*festination*), falling forward (*propulsion*), falling backward (*retropulsion*), moving the whole body while turning (*turning en bloc*), absent arm swing.
High	Cerebellar ataxia		Wide-based with increased trunk sway, irregular stepping, especially on turns.
	Cautious gait		Fear of falling with appropriate postural responses, normal to widened base, shortened stride, decreased velocity, and *en bloc* turns.
	Frontal-related gait disorders, other white matter lesions	Cerebrovascular, normal pressure hydrocephalus	Proposed spectrum ranges from gait ignition failure, to frontal gait disorder, to frontal dysequilibrium. May also have cognitive, pyramidal, and urinary disturbances. Gait ignition failure: difficulty initiating gait, short shuffling gait, may freeze with diversion of attention or turning. Frontal gait disorder: similar to Parkinson's but wider base, upright posture, preservation of arm swing. Frontal dysequilibrium: cannot stand unsupported.

*See text for additional details.
Adapted from Alexander NB. Differential diagnosis of gait disorders in older adults. *Clin Geriatr Med* 1996;12:697–698.

volve multiple levels, such as Parkinson's disease affecting high (cortical) and middle (subcortical) structures. Drug-metabolic causes (e.g., from sedatives, tranquilizers, and anticonvulsants) can involve more than one level: phenothiazines, for example, can cause high (sedation) and middle (extrapyramidal) level effects.

Other factors that contribute to gait disorders are frequently disease-associated (e.g., related to cardiopulmonary disease) but are often assessed separately include marked reductions in activity and aerobic fitness, reductions in joint strength and range of motion, and previous falls.

Although older adults may maintain a relatively normal gait pattern well into their 80s, some slowing occurs, and decreased stride length becomes a common feature described in older adult gait disorders (reviewed by Alexander, 1996a). Some authors have proposed the emergence of an age-related gait disorder without accompanying clinical abnormalities (i.e. essential "senile" gait disorder) (Koller et al., 1983). This gait pattern is described as broad-based with small steps, diminished arm swing, stooped posture, flexion of the hips and knees, uncertainty and stiffness in turning, occasional difficulty initiating steps, and a tendency toward falling. These and other nonspecific findings (e.g., inability to perform tandem gait) are similar to gait patterns found in a number of other diseases and yet the clinical abnormalities are insufficient to make a specific diagnosis. This "disorder" may be a precursor to an as-yet-asymptomatic disease (e.g., related to subtle extrapyramidal signs) and is likely to be a manifestation of concurrent, progressive cognitive impairment (e.g., Alzheimer's disease or vascular dementia) (Elble et al., 1992). "Senile" gait disorder, thus, potentially reflects a number of potential disease causes and is generally not useful in labeling gait disorders in older adults.

History and Physical Examination

Emphasis should be placed on assessing the cardiovascular, visual, vestibular, musculoskeletal, and neurologic systems, as well as assessing medication use. A history of the fall and the circumstances surrounding it, including associated symptoms and associated movements or activities that may have elicited the fall, are useful. Subject reports of premonitory or associated symptoms (e.g., palpitations, shortness of breath, chest pain, vertigo, light-headedness, and associated activities) help determine contributing medical conditions. Of particular importance is the determination of syncope or near-syncope, which leads to

a different differential diagnosis and workup, including Holter monitor, tilt table, and carotid massage. Recent data from selected populations suggest underrecognition of near-syncope, as caused by carotid sinus hypersensitivity (CSH) (Ward et al., 1999; Allcock and O'Shea, 2000), but the contribution of CSH to an actual fall is not completely clear. Symptoms that are postprandial or postmicturition can help better define accompanying risk. The vestibular or cardiovascular origin of dizziness or light-headedness, particularly when positional, is sometimes difficult to differentiate (see examination discussed below). A careful medical history and a review of the factors given in Table 9-1 will help elucidate the multiple factors contributing to the fall. A brief systemic evaluation for evidence of subacute metabolic disease (e.g., thyroid disorders), acute cardiopulmonary disorders (e.g., myocardial infarction), or other acute illness (e.g., sepsis) is warranted because falling may be the presenting feature of acute and subacute systemic decompensation in an older adult. An assessment of mobility is also indicated, to include ADL function and ambulation (i.e., wheelchair use, distance ambulated, and the extent of human or device assistance required; see below).

Using the factors given in Table 9-1, the physical examination should include an attempt to identify motion-related factors, such as by provoking both objective and subjective responses to the Hallpike-Dix maneuver and to supine and standing blood pressure and pulse measurements. In the Hallpike-Dix maneuver, while the patient is seated on an examination table, the examiner holds the patient's head, turns the head to one side, and lowers the head to the level of the table, classically 30 degrees below the table level. The patients then sits up and the maneuver is repeated again to the other side. Blood pressure should be measured with the patient both supine and standing to rule out orthostatic hypotension. Vision screening, at least for acuity, is essential. Examining the cardiovascular system helps exclude arrhythmia, valvular heart disease, and heart failure. The neck, spine, extremities, and feet should be evaluated for deformities, and pain or limitations in range of motion. A formal neurologic assessment is critical, to include assessment of strength and tone, sensation (including proprioception), coordination (including cerebellar function), and station and gait. In regard to the latter, the Romberg test screens for simple postural control and whether the proprioceptive and vestibular systems are functional. Some investigators have proposed one-legged stance time less than 5 seconds as a risk factor for injurious falls (Vellas et al., 1997), although even relatively healthy older adults aged 70 can have difficulty with one-legged stance (Rossiter-Fornoff et al., 1995). Given the importance of cognition as a risk factor, screening for mental status is also indicated.

Performance-Based Functional Assessment

Technologically oriented assessments involving formal kinematic and kinetic analyses have not been applied widely in clinical assessments of older adult balance and gait disorders. Using a functional gait and balance battery, which includes aspects such as turning while standing, has been proposed as a means to detect and quantify abnormalities and direct interventions. Fall risk, for example, can be increased with more abnormal gait and balance scale scores (Tinetti et al., 1988). Clinical gait assessments use a battery of items, either timed or scored semiquantitatively, usually based on whether a subject is able to perform the task and, if able, how normal or abnormal the performance was. Batteries that focus primarily on gait include

- Functional Ambulation Classification scale (Holden et al., 1986), rating the use of assistive devices, the degree of human assistance (either manual or verbal), the distance the patient can walk, and the types of surfaces the patient can negotiate.
- Performance Oriented Balance and Mobility Assessment (POMA) gait subsection (Tinetti, 1986), a rating of gait initiation, turning, step length and height, step symmetry and continuity, path deviation, and trunk sway.
- Get Up and Go Test (Posiadlo and Richardson, 1991), a timed sequence of rising from a chair, walking 3 M, turning, and returning to the chair.
- Dynamic Gait Index (Shumway-Cook and Woollacott, 1995), a rating of a series of tasks, including turning, walking while turning the head, clearing obstacles and using stairs.
- Functional Obstacle Course (Means et al., 1998), a timed test of negotiating different floor textures, graded surfaces, stairs, and simultaneous functional activities while walking (e.g., opening and closing doors).
- Gait Abnormality Rating Scale (Van Swearingen et al., 1998), modified to score gait variability, guardedness, staggering, foot contact, hip range of motion, shoulder extension, and arm-heel synchrony.
- Emory Functional Ambulation Profile (Wolf et al., 1999), a battery of timed tasks, including walking on a hard floor, on a carpeted surface, stepping over an obstacle, and up and down four stairs.

These scales were used reliably in smaller, selected published samples, although perhaps less reliably in larger epidemiologic settings (e.g., see Rockwood et al., 2000 for critique of Get Up and Go Test).

Comfortable gait speed has become a powerful assessment and outcome measure. Measured as part of a timed short distance (e.g., 8 feet) walk or as measured in terms of distance walked over time (such as 6 minutes), gait speed predicts disease activity, (e.g., arthritis), cardiac and pulmonary function (particularly in congestive heart failure), and ultimately mobility and ADL disability, institutionalization, and mortality (for review, see Alexander 1996a).

Laboratory and Diagnostic Tests

Depending on the history and physical examination, further laboratory and diagnostic evaluation may be warranted. Tests such as electrocardiograms, Holter monitors, cardiac enzymes, and echocardiograms are not routinely recommended unless a cardiac source is suspected. Similarly, complete blood count, chemistries, and stool for occult blood are useful only where acute systemic disease is suspected. Head or spine imaging, including x-ray study, computed tomography (CT), or magnetic resonance imaging (MRI) are of unclear use unless the history and physical examination suggest neurologic abnormalities, either preceding or of recent onset, related to the gait disorder. A possible exception relates to cerebral white matter changes on CT scan, considered to be ischemic in nature (termed "leukoaraiosis"), which can cause nonspecific gait disorders. Recently, periventricular high signal measurements on MRI as well as increased ventricular volume, even in apparently healthy older adults (Camicoli et al., 1999, see discussion for review of previous studies) are associated with gait slowing. Age-specific guidelines, sensitivity, specificity, and cost-effectiveness of these workups remain to be determined.

INTERVENTIONS TO REDUCE FALLS, FALL-RELATED INJURY AND GAIT DISORDERS

Falls

Interventions to reduce falls, fall-related injury, and gait disorders attempt to improve functional capacity, decrease falls, and decrease injuries, but sometimes patterns of independence are altered as well (i.e., for safety reasons, ambulating in inclement weather conditions is discouraged). Interventions can be divided into at least four categories (Table 9-5). In-

TABLE 9-5. *Interventions to reduce falls, fall-related injury, and gait disorders*

Intrinsic
  Treat the underlying disease
  Eliminate drugs or reduce dosages
  Initiate physical therapy program
    Balance and gait training (including training with
      an assistive device)
    Vestibular rehabilitation and habituation training
  Initiate exercise program
    Tai chi
    Resistive (strength) training
    Other balance training
Extrinsic
  Reduce environmental hazards
  Reduce active restraints
  Improve fall surveillance
    Identify those at risk
    Increase staff proximity and ratio
    Improve motion detection
  Decrease or dissipate impact force
    Protective pads and flooring

terventions that deal directly with intrinsic factors focus on decreasing disease-related impairment and providing therapy. Extrinsic factor interventions have thus far focused primarily on decreasing hazards and environmental demand. Examples of these extrinsic interventions include improving lighting, adding grab bars, raising the toilet seat, finding an appropriate bed height, and providing an appropriately structured environment for those who are cognitively impaired. Because restraint use may be associated with more falls and injuries (Capezuti et al., 1998), reducing active mechanical restraints (e.g., vests) may not necessarily increase falls or fall-related injury. More passive alternatives, such as wheelchair adaptations, removable belts, and wedge seating, can apparently provide adequate fall protection with less mobility limitation. Few controlled studies have addressed situational factors, although caregiver or nurse surveillance, particularly with those who are considered for restraint, may be useful. Use of motion detectors has a mixed benefit because a staff person still needs to be present to respond to the triggered alarm. Finally, protective padding worn over the hip can be a useful alternative for fallers at risk for hip injury. A recent randomized, community-based study found a reduction in hip fractures (relative hazard 0.4) in those wearing hip protector pads (Kannus et al., 2000). In this study, most hip fractures in the hip pad group occurred in those who were not wearing the pad at the time of the fall. Note, however, as in previous hip pad studies, compliance was still a problem; 31% of those randomized to the hip pad group refused to wear the pad. Alternatively, flooring materials exist that will help dissipate the impact force, although a floor that is too compliant may be destabilizing by itself.

A multifactorial approach seems most appropriate, individualizing a combination of medical, rehabilitative, environmental, and intervention strategies for each faller or potential faller (Feder et al., 2000). In a multifactorial approach (Tinetti et al., 1994) for nonsyncopal falls, in-home interventions were performed in community-dwelling older adults with at least one of the following risk factors: postural hypotension; use of benzodiazepines or hypnotic-sedatives; use of four or more prescription medications; inability to transfer safely to a bathtub or toilet; environmental hazards for falls or tripping; gait impairment; balance impairment; and arm and leg strength or range of motion impairment. Although 47% of the controls fell during 1-year follow-up, only 35% of the intervention group fell (Tinetti et al., 1994). Reductions in postural blood pressure changes (and medication use), and in balance, gait, and transfer problems contributed the most to reducing falls (Tinetti et al., 1996). The intervention group had a lower incidence of injurious falls and hospitalizations but the difference did not reach statistical significance. However, given the financial costs of the injuries and medical care required, average costs for the controls exceeded that of those in the intervention group (Rizzo et al., 1996). A bidisciplinary intervention (medical and single occupational therapy home visit) also showed a reduction in falls (odds ratio 0.39 versus controls) in community-dwelling emergency room patients seen for nonsyncopal and syncopal falls (Close et al., 1999). A randomized trial of a fall reduction consultation service used in 14 nursing homes showed a decline in the proportion of recurrent fallers (44% in intervention homes versus 54% in control homes) and a trend toward a lower incidence of injurious falls (Ray et al., 1997). The consultation service made a series of recommendations according to domains (in order of most to least commonly recommended) related to wheelchairs, the environment, transferring and ambulation, and psychotropic medication use.

Other controlled studies provide more caveats about the effect of interventions on fall reduction. No fall prevention study has had sufficient power to show a reduction in serious fall injuries, such as hip fracture (Gardner et al., 2000), although a reduction in hip fracture was recently noted with the use of hip pads (see above). Some studies demonstrate no change in falls but, because of the multidisciplinary evaluation, other comorbid conditions are identified that might lead to improved overall health and decreased hospitalizations (Rubinstein et al., 1990). Some studies suggest that environmental hazards relate poorly to fall occurrence (Sattin et al, 1998) and even home modification interventions may reduce falls by mechanisms unrelated to the modifications themselves (Cumming et al., 1999 and accompanying editorial by Gill, 1999). Also of note is the success of fall reduction with the withdrawal of psychotropic medications (66% reduction in falls) and yet by 1 month following study completion, 47% restarted their psychotropic medications (Campbell et al., 1999). Studies that focus on low intensity exercise or behavioral interventions find small and transient, if any, effects on fall reduction, with the greatest effects in targeted high risk groups who are given individually tailored exercise programs (Feder et al., 2000). A recent meta-analysis of seven independent, randomized clinical studies suggests that intervention programs that include exercise and balance training, in particular, can reduce falls by 10% (Province et al., 1995). Moreover, one recent controlled study found that a 15-week program of tai chi reduced the risk of falls by 48% (Wolf et al., 1996).

Gait Disorders

Even if a diagnosable condition is found on evaluation, many conditions causing a gait disorder, at best, are only partially treatable (for a more extensive review of the studies below, see Alexander, 1996a). The patient is often left with at least some residual disability. However, other functional outcomes (e.g., reduction in weight-bearing pain) can be equally important in justifying treatment. Achievement of premorbid gait patterns may be unrealistic, and improvement in measures such as gait speed, is reasonable as long as gait remains safe. Comorbidity, disease severity, and overall health status tend to strongly influence treatment outcome.

Many of the reports dealing with treatment and rehabilitation of gait disorders in older adults are retrospective chart reviews and case studies. Gait disorders presumably secondary to B_{12} deficiency, folate deficiency, hypothyroidism, hyperthyroidism, knee osteoarthritis, Parkinson's disease, and inflammatory polyneuropathy show improvement in ambulation as a result of medical therapy. A variety of modes of physical therapy for diseases such as Parkinson's disease, knee osteoarthritis, and stroke also result in modest improvements but continued residual disability. Recent studies suggest the use of a special apparatus and techniques for gait rehabilitation of patients with specific diseases and impairments (e.g., body weight support and a treadmill) to enhance poststroke gait retraining (Visintin et al., 1998).

Modest improvement and residual disability are also the result of surgical treatment for compressive cervical myelopathy, lumbar stenosis, and NPH. Few controlled prospective studies and randomized studies address the outcome of surgical treatment for compressive cervical myelopathy, lumbar stenosis, and NPH. A number of problems plague the available series: outcomes (e.g., pain and walking disability) are not reported separately; the source of the outcome rating is not clearly identified or blinded; the criteria for classifying outcomes differ; the follow-up intervals are variable; the selection factors for conservative versus surgical treatment between studies differ or are unspecified; and publication bias exists (only positive results are published). Most of the surgical series include all ages, although the mean age is usually above 60 years. Many older adults have reduced pain and increased maximal walking distance following laminectomies and lumbar fusion surgery, although they have continued residual disability. A few studies document equivalent surgical outcomes with conservative, nonsurgical treatment. Finally, it is unclear how many of the initial postoperative gains are maintained long term, particularly in NPH.

Outcomes for hip and knee replacement surgery for osteoarthritis are better, although some of the same methodologic problems exist with these studies. Other than pain relief, sizable gains in gait speed and joint motion occur, although residual walking disability continues for a number of reasons, including residual pathology on the operated side and symptoms on the nonoperated side.

REFERENCES

Alexander NB. Gait disorders in older adults. *J Am Geriatr Soc* 1996a;44:434–451.

Alexander NB. Differential diagnosis of gait disorders in older adults. *Clin Geriatr Med* 1996b;12:697–698.

Allcock LM, O'Shea D. Diagnostic yield and development of a neurocardiovascular investigation unit for older adults in a district hospital. *J Gerontol* 2000;55A:M458–M462.

Camicoli R, Moore MM, Sexton G, et al. Age-related changes associated with motor function in healthy older people. *J Am Geriatr Soc* 1999;47:330–334.

Campbell AJ, Robertson MC, Gardner MM, et al. Psychotropic medication withdrawal and a home-based exercise program to prevent falls: a randomized controlled trial. *J Am Geriatr Soc* 1999;47:850–853.

Capezuti E, Strumpf NE, Evans LK, et al. The relationship between physical restraint removal and falls and injuries among nursing home residents. *J Gerontol* 1998;3A:M47–M52.

Close J, Ellis M, Hooper R, et al. Prevention of falls in the elderly (PROFET): a randomized controlled trial. *Lancet* 1999;353:93–97.

Cumming RG, Thomas M, Szonyi G, et al. Home visits by occupational therapists for assessment and modification of environmental hazards: a randomized trial of falls prevention. *J Am Geriatr Soc* 1999;47:1397–1402.

Cummings SR, Nevitt MC. A hypothesis: the causes of hip fractures. *J Gerontol* 1989;44:M107–M111.

Elble RJ, Hughes L, Higgins C. The syndrome of senile gait. *J Neurol* 1992;239:71–75.

Feder G, Cryer C Donovan S, et al. Guidelines for the prevention of falls in people over 65. *BMJ* 2000;321:1007–1011.

Fuh JL, Lin KN, Wang SJ, et al. Neurologic diseases presenting with gait impairment in the elderly. *J Geriatr Psychiatry Neurol* 1994;7:89–92.

Gardner MM, Robertson MC, Campbell AJ. Exercise in preventing falls and fall related injuries in older people: a review of randomized controlled trials. *Br J Sports Med* 2000;34:7–17.

Gill TM. Preventing falls: to modify the environment or the individual? *J Am Geriatr Soc* 1999;47:1471–1472

Greenspan SL, Myers ER, Maitland LA, et al. Fall severity and bone mineral density as risk factors for hip fracture in ambulatory elderly. *JAMA* 1994;271:128–133.

Holden MK, Gill KM, Magliozzi MR. Gait assessment for neurologically impaired patients: standards for outcome assessment. *Phys Ther* 1986;66:1530–1539.

Hough JC, McHenry MP, Kammer LM. Gait disorders in the elderly. *Am Fam Pract* 1987;30:191–196.

Kannus P, Parkkari J, Niemi S, et al. Prevention of hip fracture in elderly people with use of a hip protector. *N Engl J Med* 2000;343:1506–1513.

King MB, Tinetti ME. Falls in community-dwelling older persons. *J Am Geriatr Soc* 1995;43:1146–1154.

Koller WC, Wilson RS, Glatt SL, et al. Senile gait: correlation with computed tomographic scans. *Ann Neurol* 1983; 13:343–344.

Means KM, Rodell DE, O'Sullivan PS, et al. Comparison of a functional obstacle course with an index of clinical gait and balance and postural sway. *J Gerontol* 1998;53A: M331–M335.

Nutt JG, Marsden CD, Thompson PD. Human walking and higher-level gait disorders, particularly in the elderly. *Neurology* 1993;43:268–279.

Oschiega Y, Harris TB, Hirsch R, et al. The prevalence of functional limitations and disability in older persons in the US: data from the National Health and Nutrition Examination survey III. *J Am Geriatr Soc* 2000;48:1132–1135.

Posiadlo D, Richardson S. The timed "Up & Go": a test of basic functional mobility for frail elderly persons. *J Am Geriatr Soc* 1991;39:142–148

Province MA, Hadley EC, Hornbrook MC, et al. The effects of exercise on falls in elderly persons: a population-based randomized trial. *JAMA* 1995;273:1341–1347.

Ray WA, Taylor JA, Meador KG, et al. A randomized trial of a consultation service to reduce falls in nursing homes. *JAMA* 1997;278:557–562.

Rizzo JA, Baker DI, McAvay G, et al. The cost-effectiveness of a multifactorial targeted prevention program for falls among community elderly persons. *Med Care* 1996;34 (9):954–69.

Rockwood K, Awalt E, Carver D, et al. Feasibility and measurement properties of the functional reach and timed up and go tests in the Canadian Study of Health and Aging. *J Gerontol* 2000;55A:M70–M73.

Rossiter-Fornoff JE, Wolf SL, Wolfson LI, et al. A cross-validation study of the FICSIT common data base static balance measures. *J Gerontol* 1995;50A:M291–M297.

Rubinstein LZ, Ribbins A, Josephson K, et al. The value of assessing falls in the elderly population: a randomized clinical trial. *Ann Intern Med* 1990;113:308–316.

Rubinstein LZ, Josephson KR, Robins AS. Falls in the nursing home. *Ann Intern Med* 1994;121:442–451.

Sattin RW, Rodriguez JG, DeVito CA, et al. Home environmental hazards and the risk of falling injury events among community-dwelling older persons. *J Am Geriatr Soc* 1998;46:669–676.

Shumway-Cook A, Woollacott MH. Assessment and treatment of the patient with mobility disorders. In: *Motor control: theory and practical applications*, 1st ed. Baltimore: Williams & Wilkins, 1995.

Sudarsky L, Rontal M. Gait disorders among elderly patients: a survey study of 50 patients. *Arch Neurol* 1983;40: 740–743.

Tinetti ME. Performance-oriented assessment of mobility problems in elderly patients. *J Am Geriatr Soc* 1986;34: 119–126.

Tinetti ME, Baker DI, McAvay G, et al. A multifactorial intervention to reduce the risk of falling among elderly people living in the community. *N Engl J Med* 1994;331: 821–827.

Tinetti ME, Speechley M, Ginter SF. Risk factors for falls among elderly persons living in the community. *N Engl J Med* 1988;319:1701–1707.

Tinetti ME, McAvay G, Claus E. Does multiple risk factor reduction explain the reduction in fall rate in the Yale FICSIT trial? *Am J Epidemiol* 1996;144:389–399.

Tinetti ME, Douchette JT, Claus EB. The contribution of predisposing and situational risk factors to serious fall injuries. *J Am Geriatr Soc* 1995;43:1207–1213.

Tinetti ME, Williams CS. Falls, injuries due to falls, and the risk of admission to a nursing home. *N Engl J Med* 1997; 337:1279–1284.

Tinetti ME, Williams CS. The effect of falls and fall injuries on functioning in community-dwelling older persons. *J Gerontol* 1998;53A:M112–M119.

Van Swearingen JM, Paschall KA, Bonino P, et al. Assessing recurrent fall risk of community-dwelling frail older veterans using specific tests of mobility and the physical performance test of function. *J Gerontol* 1998;53A:M457–M464.

Vellas BJ, Wayne SJ, Romero L, et al. One-leg balance is an important predictor of injurious falls in older persons. *J Am Geriatr Soc* 1997;45:735–738.

Visintin M, Barbeau H, Korner-Bitensky N, et al. A new approach to retrain gait in stroke patients through body weight support and treadmill stimulation. *Stroke* 1998;29: 1122–1128.

Ward CR, McIntosh S, Kenny RA. Carotid sinus hypersensitivity—a modifiable risk factor for fractured neck of the femur. *Age Ageing* 1999;28:127–133.

Wolf SL, Catlin PA, Gage K, et al. Establishing the reliability and validity of measurements of walking time using the Emory Functional Ambulation Profile. *Phys Ther* 1999;79:1122–1133.

Wolf DSL, Barnhart HX, Kutner NG, et al. Reducing frailty and falls in older persons: an investigation of tai chi and computerized balance training. *J Am Geriatr Soc* 1996; 44:489–497.

10

Disorders of Speech and Language in Older Adults

Howard S. Kirshner

Language is one of the higher functions most commonly affected by aging and dementia. Discussed in this chapter are changes in speech and language function that occur in normal aging, in dementing diseases such as Alzheimer's disease, and in the rarer, focal diseases, primary progressive aphasia (PPA) and frontotemporal dementia. A discussion of speech and language disorders in general provides background information.

MOTOR SPEECH DISORDERS

Motor speech disorders are abnormalities of articulation, the motor production of speech. Language production in a patient with a motor speech disorder should be normal in the written modality, and language comprehension for both spoken and written language, likewise, should be intact. Motor speech disorders include dysarthrias, disorders of speech articulation, and apraxia of speech, a motor programming disorder for speech.

Dysarthrias

Dysarthrias involve the abnormal articulation of sounds or phonemes, especially distortions of consonant sounds. The Mayo Clinic classification of dysarthria (Duffy, 1995), widely used in the United States, includes six categories:

1. Flaccid
2. Spastic and "unilateral upper motor neuron"
3. Ataxic
4. Hypokinetic
5. Hyperkinetic
6. Mixed dysarthria

Flaccid dysarthria is associated with disorders involving lower motor neuron weakness of the bulbar muscles, such as polymyositis, myasthenia gravis, and bulbar poliomyelitis. The speech pattern is breathy and nasal, with mispronounced consonants. *Spastic* dysarthria occurs in patients with bilateral lesions of the motor cortex or corticobulbar tracts, such as bilateral strokes. The speech is harsh or "strain-strangle" in vocal quality, with reduced rate, low pitch, and consonant errors. A milder variant of spastic dysarthria, *unilateral upper motor neuron* dysarthria, is associated with unilateral upper motor neuron lesions such as stroke. *Ataxic* dysarthria or "scanning speech," associated with cerebellar disorders, is characterized by irregular or slow cadence of speech, with pauses and abnormal or excessively equal stress on every syllable. *Hypokinetic* dysarthria, the typical speech pattern in Parkinson's disease, is notable for decreased and monotonous loudness and pitch, rapid rate, and occasional consonant errors. *Hyperkinetic* dysarthria, in movement disorders such as Huntington's disease and dystonia musculorum deformans, is characterized by marked variation in rate, loudness, and timing, with distortion of vowels. The final category, *mixed* dysarthria, involves combinations of the other five types; in multiple sclerosis, for example, speech may be both spastic and ataxic, and in amyotrophic lateral sclerosis, speech contains both spastic and flaccid elements.

Apraxia of Speech

Apraxia of speech is a disorder of the programming of articulation of sequences of phonemes, especially consonants. Consonants are substituted rather than distorted, as in dysarthria. Patients have special difficulty with multisyllabic words and consonant shifts, but they also have trouble initiating articulation of a word, groping for initial sounds. Errors are inconsistent from one attempt to the next, in contrast with the consistent distortion of phonemes in dysarthria.

Apraxia of speech is rare in isolated form, but it frequently contributes to the aphasic deficit of Broca's aphasia. A patient with apraxia of speech, in addition to aphasia, often writes better than he or she can speak, and comprehension is relatively preserved. Dronkers (1996) has presented evidence that links lesions of the insula to apraxia of speech.

APHASIA

Aphasias are language disorders, defined as abnormalities of symbolic communication acquired as a result of brain disease. This definition distinguishes aphasias from motor speech disorders, from congenital or developmental language disorders (often called "dysphasias"), and from psychiatric thought disorders.

Aphasia is diagnosed by a six-part bedside language evaluation (Table 10-1). More detailed examination of language function can be obtained by consultation with a speech/language pathologist or neuropsychologist.

Classification and Diagnosis

Aphasias are traditionally classified into eight syndromes: Broca's, Wernicke's, global, conduction, anomic, and three transcortical aphasias. A brief discussion of the syndromes of aphemia, pure word deafness, the "subcortical" aphasias, and the two syndromes of abnormal reading, alexia with and without agraphia are discussed. Readers wishing more detailed discussion and references regarding the aphasias are referred to Kirshner et al., 1999 or Kirshner, 1995.

Broca's Aphasia

Broca's aphasia is a nonfluent aphasia, varying from mutism to hesitant, struggling efforts to speak (Table 10-2). The patient may be able to utter meaningful nouns and verbs but omits small grammatical

TABLE 10-2. *Features of Broca's aphasia*

Spontaneous speech	Nonfluent: hesitant, agrammatic, often dysarthric
Naming	Impaired (*tip-of-the-tongue*)
Auditory comprehension	Intact for simple material, impaired for complex syntax
Repetition	Impaired
Reading	Difficulty reading aloud, reading comprehension often worse than auditory comprehension
Writing	Difficulty writing, even with left hand
Associated signs	Right hemiparesis, right hemisensory loss, apraxia of left limbs
Behavior	Frustrated, depressed, but appropriate

words, producing a "telegraphic" speech pattern, also referred to as "agrammatism." In naming, the patient has difficulty but can often produce the first letter or initial phoneme of the word, a phenomenon referred to in both aphasic and normal speech as a "tip-of-the-tongue" experience. Repetition is effortful and slow; auditory comprehension is adequate for simple conversations and commands but breaks down on complex grammatical constructions. Reading is often more impaired than auditory comprehension. Writing is abnormal, even with the nonparalyzed left hand. Patients with Broca's aphasia are aware of their deficits, often acting frustrated or depressed.

The lesion of Broca's aphasia involves the posterior portion of the left inferior frontal gyrus. Small lesions of Broca's area permit nearly complete recovery, whereas larger left frontoparietal lesions produce an early global aphasia that evolves gradually into Broca's aphasia. According to Naeser et al. (1987), damage to the subcortical and periventricular white matter results in lasting loss of expressive speech.

Aphemia is a transitory syndrome of muteness or nonfluent speech, with preserved writing and comprehension. Aphemia overlaps with apraxia of speech. The lesion involves the face area of the motor strip, sometimes with extension into the inferior frontal gyrus and underlying white matter.

Wernicke's Aphasia

Wernicke's aphasia may be thought of as somewhat opposite to Broca's aphasia, in that the speech is fluent, rather than nonfluent, with empty phrases, circumlocutions, and paraphasic errors (Table 10-3). When asked to name, the patient often utters bizarre, paraphasic substitutions instead of hesitating like a Broca's aphasic. Auditory comprehension is severely

TABLE 10-1. *Bedside language examination*

1. Spontaneous speech: fluent versus nonfluent? Errors
2. Naming
3. Auditory comprehension
4. Repetition
5. Reading: aloud, for comprehension
6. Writing: copying, to dictation, spontaneously

TABLE 10-3. *Characteristics of Wernicke's aphasia*

Spontaneous speech	Fluent, with paraphasic errors
Naming	Impaired, often paraphasic
Auditory comprehension	Impaired, often for even simple material
Repetition	Impaired
Reading	Usually impaired
Writing	Well-formed but paragraphic
Associated signs	± right hemianopia, usually no motor or sensory abnormalities
Behavior	Often unaware of deficits, may be inappropriately happy, later sometimes angry, suspicious

TABLE 10-4. *Characteristics of global aphasia*

Spontaneous speech	Nonfluent, mute, or stereotyped
Naming	Impaired
Auditory comprehension	Impaired
Repetition	Impaired
Reading	Impaired
Writing	Impaired
Associated deficits	Most have right hemianopia, right hemiparesis, right hemisensory loss, often apraxia
Behavior	Often depressed

impaired. Reading is affected similarly to auditory comprehension, but some patients are better in one modality than the other. The patient with Wernicke's aphasia can write easily but produces errors of spelling and incorrect word selection. These patients are usually not depressed, but they may be unaware of their deficits and become angry when not understood. Motor and sensory functions are usually normal, although some patients have a right hemianopia. The lesion typically involves Wernicke's area, the posterior two thirds of the left superior temporal gyrus. Destruction of most of Wernicke's area appears necessary for lasting loss of comprehension, but often associated damage is seen in the supramarginal and angular gyri (Naeser et al., 1989).

Pure word deafness is a rare syndrome in which the patient appears deaf to language but can hear pure tones and nonverbal sounds. The patient cannot repeat or comprehend spoken language but performs normally in expressive speech. Traditionally, pure word deafness results from bilateral temporal lesions that disconnect Wernicke's area from the auditory cortex in both temporal lobes, although the syndrome has been reported with unilateral, left temporal lesions.

Global Aphasia

Global aphasia may be thought of as the sum of both Broca's and Wernicke's aphasia. It involves the loss of all six major language functions (Table 10-4). Spontaneous speech is nonfluent, as in Broca's aphasia, but comprehension is poor, as in Wernicke's aphasia, and the patient cannot name, repeat, read, or write. Most patients have extensive left hemisphere lesions and severe neurologic deficits of right hemiplegia, right hemisensory loss, and right hemianopia.

Conduction Aphasia

Conduction aphasia is a less common language syndrome, involving deficits in repetition out of proportion to other language difficulties (Table 10-5). Speech is fluent but often contains phoneme substitutions ("literal paraphasic errors"), and the patient may pause to correct these errors. Auditory comprehension is intact. Conduction aphasia was traditionally explained as a disconnection between Wernicke's and Broca's areas. The lesions of conduction aphasia involve either the left temporal lobe, without destruction of Wernicke's area, or the inferior parietal lobule.

Anomic Aphasia

Anomic aphasia is a selective deficit of naming. Speech is fluent, except for word-finding pauses and circumlocutions, and the other language modalities are intact (Table 10-6). This syndrome is less localizing than other types of aphasia. Anomic aphasia occurs with focal lesions of the left temporal or inferior parietal region, and it is frequently the last stage in recovery from any type of aphasia. Anomia is common

TABLE 10-5. *Characteristics of conduction aphasia*

Spontaneous speech	Fluent, with literal paraphasic errors
Naming	Variable
Auditory comprehension	Intact
Repetition	Poor
Reading	Variable aloud, comprehension intact
Writing	Variable
Associated deficits	Right hemiparesis, right hemisensory loss, visual field defect, apraxia
Behavior	No characteristic pattern

TABLE 10-6. *Characteristics of anomic aphasia*

Spontaneous speech	Fluent, with word-finding pauses and circumlocutions
Naming	Impaired
Auditory comprehension	Intact
Repetition	Intact
Reading	Intact
Writing	Intact, except for word-finding difficulty
Associated signs	Variable, often absent
Behavior	No characteristic features

in delirium and dementia and, to some extent, even in normal aging.

Transcortical Aphasias

The transcortical aphasias have in common preserved repetition (Table 10-7). Lichtheim (1885) originally coined the word "transcortical" to refer to lesions outside the perisylvian language circuit, rather than damage to the language cortex itself. Three transcortical aphasias are seen. *Transcortical motor aphasia* (TCMA) resembles Broca's aphasia, with very hesitant speech, but repetition is normal. The lesions of TCMA spare Broca's area but involve the adjacent left frontal cortex, medial frontal cortex, or subcortical white matter. Strokes associated with TCMA are generally within the territory of the anterior cerebral artery and, hence, the syndrome is distinct from the previous aphasias—Broca's, Wernicke's, global, and conduction—all of which involve the middle cerebral artery territory. *Transcortical sensory aphasia* (TCSA) resembles Wernicke's aphasia, but again, repetition is spared. The lesions involve the posterior left temporooccipital region. This syndrome also occurs in Alzheimer's disease. *Mixed transcortical aphasia*, also referred to as the "syn-

drome of the isolation of the speech area," involves a severe loss of language functions as in global aphasia, except that repetition is not only spared but may be excessive or palilalic. Reported cases have had large, watershed infarctions sparing the perisylvian language area or advanced dementia.

Subcortical Aphasias

In contrast with the other aphasia syndromes, subcortical aphasias are diagnosed by the location of the brain lesion rather than by language features. Aphasia syndromes have increasingly been reported in patients with subcortical lesions. First, patients with lesions of the left putamen, anterior limb of internal capsule, and caudate nucleus often have dysarthria and nonfluent speech, with less disruption of repetition than Broca's aphasia. This syndrome, in effect is an atypical, Broca-like aphasia, is sometimes called the "anterior subcortical aphasia syndrome." Lesions extending into the deep temporal white matter or "temporal isthmus" can impair comprehension, producing subcortical equivalents of Wernicke's and global aphasia.

The second subcortical aphasia syndrome occurs in patients with lesions of the left thalamus. These patients have fluent aphasia, usually with better comprehension and repetition as compared with Wernicke's aphasia. Some patients show a fluctuation between periods of drowsiness, during which they are severely aphasic, and periods of alertness, with improved speech and language.

Alexias and Agraphias

Alexias are acquired disorders of reading. Only the two classical syndromes, alexia with and without agraphia, are discussed here. Neurolinguistic researchers have also divided the alexias into a number of other classifications (Kirshner et al. 1999; Kirshner 1995).

TABLE 10-7. *Characteristics of transcortical aphasias*

Feature	Transcortical motor aphasia	Transcortical sensory aphasia	Mixed transcortical aphasia
Speech	Nonfluent	Fluent	Nonfluent
Naming	Impaired	Impaired	Impaired
Repetition	Preserved	Echolalic	Echolalic
Comprehension	Preserved	Impaired	Impaired
Reading	Preserved	Impaired	Impaired
Writing	Reduced	Paragraphic	Poor
Associated signs	Right leg > arm weakness, abulia	Variable, often none	Right or bilateral hemiparesis

Alexia with Agraphia

Alexia with agraphia is an acquired illiteracy, with intact spoken language modalities, although many patients do exhibit anomia and mild fluent, paraphasic speech (Table 10-8). The syndrome is associated with lesions in the left parietal lobe, often involving the left angular gyrus. Associated deficits include the "Gerstmann syndrome" of agraphia, inability to calculate, right-left confusion, and "finger agnosia," an inability to name or point to specific fingers on the patient's or examiner's hand.

Pure Alexia without Agraphia

Pure alexia without agraphia, summarized in Table 10-9, is an isolated inability to read. The lesions involve the left posterior cerebral artery territory, including the left medial occipital and medial temporal lobes and the splenium of the corpus callosum. Patients often have difficulty naming colors. Most have a partial or complete right hemianopia. Another feature of the alexia without agraphia syndrome is short-term memory loss, likely related to damage to the hippocampus and adjacent medial temporal structures. Pure alexia has traditionally been explained as a disconnection between the intact right occipital visual cortex and the left hemisphere centers for decoding of visual language symbols.

Agraphias

Just as some language disorders predominantly affect reading, some "agraphias" reflect abnormal writing out of proportion to other language deficits. Pure agraphia is a rare disorder, seen in patients with left frontal lesions. As in reading disorders, complex neurolinguistic classifications of the agraphias have been presented (Kirshner et al., 1999; Kirshner, 1995).

TABLE 10-8. *Characteristics of pure alexia with agraphia*

Spontaneous speech	Fluent, often paraphasic
Naming	Often impaired
Auditory comprehension	Intact
Repetition	Intact
Reading	Impaired
Writing	Impaired
Associated signs	Gerstmann's syndrome, right visual field defect

TABLE 10-9. *Characteristics of pure alexia without agraphia*

Spontaneous speech	Normal
Naming	Color naming difficulty
Auditory comprehension	Intact
Repetition	Intact
Reading	Impaired
Writing	Intact
Associated signs	Right hemianopsia, short-term memory loss, occasional motor, sensory signs

LANGUAGE IN AGING

Most discussions of the cognitive deterioration of both normal aging and dementia emphasize memory loss, rather than loss of speech or language ability. Descriptions of altered speech and language with aging, however, have appeared since ancient times. Ecclesiastes, as quoted by Critchley (1984), contains a description of the deterioration of speech with aging: "And all the daughters of musick shall be brought low." Shakespeare also depicted alterations in voice and in articulation in the "seven ages of man" oration from *As You Like It*: ". . . and his big manly voice turning again toward childish treble pipes, and whistles in his sound."

Recent studies of speech and language function in normal aging have generally found only modest changes. In fact, tests of vocabulary and reading aloud have been used as estimates of premorbid intelligence in demented patients, because these functions tend to be resistant to the ravages of dementing illness. Although vocal quality can change, the articulation of speech sounds and even complex phoneme sequences remain largely intact with normal aging.

Language functions do change with normal aging, although these changes are relatively mild in most cases. The mechanics of language production and comprehension remain relatively intact; the production of syntactically correct sentences and the comprehension of language tend to be preserved late into senescence (Bayles, 1995). Other, specific linguistic patterns change with normal aging. The patterns of spontaneous speech become simplified, especially syntax. The utterances of older people tend to be simple clauses, with a decrease in compound phrases and sentences. Abstract or metaphorical linguistic content tends to diminish or to disappear entirely (Burke and McKay, 1997). Comprehension or repetition of long, complex sentences can break down, perhaps because they tax the memory system excessively. Naming declines with age, as most normal people can attest from their own difficulty in recalling the proper names of former friends and classmates, such as at college reunions. In most cases, however, these changes remain mild until the 70s (Borod et al., 1980). A related age-sensitive function is the generation of lists, such as the animal-naming subtest of the Boston Diagnostic Aphasia Examination. Normal, young subjects name in excess of 20 animals in 1 minute, whereas older adults tend to name 10 to 20 (Borod et al. 1980; Albert et al., 1987). Another, recently studied aspect of language that declines with age is the production of discourse (Bayles 1995; Glosser and Deser, 1992). Spontaneous discourse in elderly people tends to become less organized, sometimes reduced in total numbers of words but, even so, less concise and coherent (Glosser and Deser, 1992). In general, despite these language changes, even very aged individuals continue to communicate effectively.

LANGUAGE IN DEMENTIA

As in normal aging, language is less emphasized than memory in accounts of the cognitive deficit of dementia. Alzheimer's seminal case report (Critchley, 1984), however, contains a clear description of fluent aphasia, along with other cognitive and memory deficits.

Recent, systematic studies of language functions in patients with Alzheimer's disease document nearly universal involvement of language (Bayles, 1995; Burke and McKay, 1997). As in normal aging, the mechanical aspects of speech and language (e.g., articulation, repetition, and reading aloud) tend to be preserved late into the illness. Spoken language remains fluent, although devoid of the richness of vocabulary, abstraction, and metaphor that characterizes normal expressive language. Naming is affected prominently in Alzheimer's disease, and tests of naming are likely to be abnormal, even early in the disease (Bayles 1995; Burke and McKay, 1997; Borod, 1980). Williams et al. (Borod et al., 1980) reported that a simple naming test reliably separated normal elderly people from those with Alzheimer's disease. Although some studies have suggested that faulty visual perception of the item to be named accounts for some of the deficit, linguistic factors involved in word search appear more important (Albert et al., 1987). As in aging, generation of lists is especially sensitive in detecting the naming difficulty in Alzheimer's disease (Dronkers, 1996; Bayles, 1995). Patients with Alzheimer's disease frequently fail to produce even 10 animal names in 1 minute. Comprehension of spoken language is usually preserved, in

terms of receptive vocabulary and comprehension of spoken commands, unless the length or complexity of the material overburdens the immediate memory store. Late in the illness, auditory comprehension also declines. Reading and writing are generally more affected in patients with Alzheimer's disease than are speech and auditory comprehension (Bayles 1995; Burke and McKay, 1997). Reading for meaning becomes more deficient than reading aloud (Bayles 1995; Glosser and Deser, 1992), but even word recognition and reading aloud of word lists eventually deteriorate. Agraphia, or decreased ability to produce written language, is a regular feature of Alzheimer's disease (1977). Writing of single, irregularly spelled words can be deficient in patients with Alzheimer's disease, a writing disorder referred to as "lexical agraphia."

One way of summarizing the extensive research on language in dementia is to epitomize the course of language involvement in a "typical" patient with dementia. The earliest stage often begins with memory loss, including deficient memory for names. Aphasia testing in early dementia often shows anomic aphasia (Appell et al., 1982). As the disease progresses, speech becomes progressively impoverished in both discourse elements and abstract content. In linguistic terms, syntax and articulation are preserved long after semantics and discourse fail. In the middle stages of the disease, aphasia testing may diagnose a transcortical sensory or Wernicke's aphasia (Appell et al., 1982). Nonfluent aphasias such as Broca's or TCMA are rare in Alzheimer's disease (Appell et al., 1982; Price et al., 1993). In the final phase of the disease, patients can become almost mute, uttering only expressions of biological need. By this point, most patients are bedridden and require custodial care.

PRIMARY PROGRESSIVE APHASIA

PPA is a syndrome resembling a focal lesion with aphasia, except that the language disorder is slowly progressive. In contrast to the pattern of Alzheimer's disease, in PPA language deteriorates selectively, without generalized dementia. Mesulam (1982) reported six patients with progressive language dysfunction, without impairment of memory, visual-spatial functions, social graces, or reasoning. Mesulam proposed that PPA is a selective neuronal degeneration of the left perisylvian language cortex.

The PPA syndrome is defined as a progressive disorder of language, with preservation of other mental functions and of activities of daily living for at least 2 years (Weintraub et al., 1990). Most patients with progressive aphasia do not appear demented, often maintaining the ability to take care of themselves, pursue hobbies, and even remain employed.

The pattern of language deterioration in PPA differs from that of Alzheimer's disease, but considerable variability in language profile is seen. Whereas patients with Alzheimer's disease usually have fluent aphasias such as anomic, Wernicke's, or TCSA, patients with PPA usually have nonfluent aphasias such as Broca's and TCMA (Weintraub et al., 1990). Literal (phonemic) rather than verbal (semantic) errors in naming characterize PPA. In linguistic terms, the syntactic, morphologic, and phonologic aspects of language, which are typically preserved in Alzheimer's disease, become affected in PPA, whereas the lexical and semantic aspects are more typically affected in Alzheimer's disease. Karbe et al. (1993), in a report of language testing in 10 patients with PPA, found anomia, reduced fluency, and mild agrammatism most commonly, with relative preservation of comprehension. Not all patients with PPA, however, follow the pattern of reduced fluency and agrammatism. A number of cases have been reported with fluent aphasia (Williams et al., 1987; Bayles and Tomoeda, 1983; Cummings et al., 1986; Henderson et al., 1992) and with selective auditory comprehension difficulty resembling pure word deafness (Kirshner et al., 1987; Holland et al., 1985). In the series of Caselli and Jack (1992) 7 of 12 patients with progressive aphasia were dysfluent, whereas 5 were fluent.

A subtype of progressive aphasia is the syndrome of "semantic dementia" (Hodges et al., 1992), or progressive fluent aphasia with severe anomia, poor auditory comprehension, and poor semantic memory. These patients have intact phonology, spoken syntax, and comprehension of syntactic commands. Some show the reading disorder called "surface dyslexia," in which patients can slavishly read by translating printed syllables into sounds but cannot read a word at a glance.

Brain imaging studies have confirmed the focal, selective pattern of loss of cortical areas related to language in PPA. Brain imaging studies such as computed tomography and magnetic resonance imaging scans show either focal left perisylvian or generalized atrophy. Functional brain imaging with positron emission tomographic (PET) or single photon emission computed tomographic (SPECT) scanning, on the other hand, has been helpful in progressive aphasia. Areas of focal hypometabolism in the left hemisphere have been reported by several groups (Kempler et al., 1990; Chawluk et al., 1986; Tyrell et al., 1990). Tyrrell et al. (1990) reported that early cases of

PPA had isolated, left temporal hypometabolism, whereas more advanced cases showed additional frontotemporal involvement. They suggested that the disease begins in the left temporal lobe and then spreads to adjacent cortical areas. Other patients have shown isolated left frontal hypometabolism. These PET changes are distinct from those of Alzheimer's disease, in which reduced blood flow and metabolism characteristically begin in both temporoparietal regions. Similar findings have been reported with single photon emission computed tomography (SPECT) scanning (Grossman et al., 1998; Abe et al., 1997).

Controversy has persisted as to whether progressive aphasia is truly separate from Alzheimer's disease. Several authors (Kirshner et al., 1984; Poeck and Luzzatti, 1988; Green et al., 1990) have reported patients in whom aphasia was a presenting or disproportionate symptom, but in whom a generalized dementia was either evident at onset or developed later. Recent neuropathologic studies have discovered a variety of pathologic substrates underlying progressive aphasia.

Pick's disease is a neurodegenerative disease first described in 1893 (Rottenberg and Hochberg, 1977); the patient had prominent language deterioration along with dementia. Pick anticipated contemporary studies in noting that the aphasia was similar to the syndrome of TCSA. He also addressed the issue of focal versus diffuse disease: "simple progressive brain atrophy can lead to symptoms of local disturbance through local accentuation of the diffuse process." Several pathologically proved cases of Pick's disease have presented with progressive aphasia (Graff-Radford et al., 1990; Holland et al., 1985; Wechsler et al., 1982). These cases have had varied language profiles, including anomia (Graff-Radford et al., 1990), pure word deafness (Holland et al., 1985), and fluent aphasia (Wechsler et al., 1982).

Closely related to Pick's disease is the familial disorder termed "hereditary dysphasic dementia" (Morris et al., 1984). Multiple members of this family, following an autosomal dominant genetic distribution, have had anomia, fluent aphasia, and dementia. At autopsy, frontal and temporal lobe atrophy were seen, without Pick bodies, and the pathology included elements of Alzheimer's disease, nonspecific neuronal loss with gliosis, and even Parkinson's disease.

Kirshner et al. (1987) reported autopsy findings of two patients with progressive aphasia. The first had a 10-year history beginning with word deafness and logoclonia (prefixing and suffixing extra syllables to words), later giving way to jargon speech and finally to muteness. Reading, writing, deportment, and memory remained intact for more than 5 years. The second patient had a mixed aphasia with anomia and paraphasic errors, progressive over 3 years. This patient also developed muscle atrophy and fasciculations suggesting motor neuron disease. At autopsy, both patients had focal atrophy of the left frontal and temporal lobes, with microscopic changes of neuronal loss, gliosis, and spongiform change, or vacuolation of the neuropil, present principally in the second cortical layer. Changes of Alzheimer's disease and Pick bodies were absent. This pathologic pattern of neuronal loss, gliosis, and microvacuolation, or a "nonspecific" pathology, has been the most common finding in more recent cases reported with PPA (Kempler et al., 1990; Tyrrell et al., 1990; Green et al., 1990; Scheltens et al., 1994).

Another neurodegenerative disease associated with PPA is corticobasal degeneration, with neuronal achromasia. Lippa et al. (1991) described a man aged 69 years with a 3-year history of progressive TCMA, associated with posturing of the right arm, decreased right arm swing, and a right upgoing toe. At autopsy, focal cortical degeneration was found in the left frontal lobe. Remaining neurons showed swollen cytoplasm and loss of Nissl substance ("achromasia"), a pattern seen in patients with a combination of motor and cognitive deficits referred to as "corticobasal degeneration." Other cases of corticobasal degeneration have presented with isolated aphasia or prominent, progressive dysarthria (Lang, 1992; Broussolle et al., 1992; Kertesz et al., 1994; Chapman et al., 1997; Sakurai et al., 1996). A patient of the author with progressive dysarthria leading to complete muteness was diagnosed in life with corticobasal degeneration, but at autopsy features of multisystem atrophy were seen.

Kertesz et al. (1994; 2000) suggested that Pick's disease, neuronal achromasia, and nonspecific dementing pathology all share the common findings of neuronal loss, gliosis, and vacuolation of the neuropil, and that these disorders may all be variants of Pick's disease. Others have preferred to consider those cases without Pick bodies as "nonspecific" dementias (Kirshner et al., 1987; Scheltens et al., 1994). In the absence of a neurochemical or genetic marker for these diseases, the distinctions between them are somewhat arbitrary. Whatever terminology is used, however, these non-Alzheimer's disease pathologies do fulfill Mesulam's postulate (1982) of a neurodegenerative process affecting the perisylvian language cortex. Tau mutations have been found in PPA and in frontotemporal dementia (see Chapter 21.1).

Creutzfeldt-Jakob disease (CJD), or transmissible prion encephalopathy, rarely presents with aphasia.

Mandell et al. (1989) reported a patient with pathologically proved CJD who presented with fluent aphasia but developed dementia and fatal seizures within 1 year of onset. The rapid course and characteristic symptoms of CJD usually distinguish it from PPA; this patient did not meet the criteria of an isolated, progressive language disorder for 2 years.

Alzheimer's disease, the most common dementing disease, might be expected to be the most common cause of progressive aphasia. In addition, Alzheimer clearly described aphasia in his original patient (1907) with the disease. Few cases of pathologically proved Alzheimer's disease have been documented to have isolated, progressive aphasia (Kempler et al., 1990; Green et al., 1990; Pogacar and Williams, 1984). The syndrome of "semantic dementia" described by Hodges et al. (1992) has included Alzheimer's disease pathology. In general, patients reported with progressive aphasia secondary to Alzheimer's disease have had fluent aphasia; progressive nonfluent aphasia remains outside the behavioral spectrum of Alzheimer's disease.

FRONTOTEMPORAL DEMENTIA

At the same time authors in the United States were delineating the syndrome of PPA, British and European authors described a complementary group of focal dementing illnesses, under the term "frontotemporal dementia" (Neary and Snowden, 1996). Case descriptions of frontotemporal dementia have included focal aphasias when the disease process affected the left frontal or temporal lobe, but other behavioral presentations are also common and can predate the language disturbance (Neary and Snowden, 1996; Neary et al., 1998). Table 10-10 shows the language characteristics included in the criteria for frontotemporal dementia published by Neary et al. (1998).

TABLE 10-10. *Language features of frontotemporal dementia*

Speech and language
    Altered speech output
        Aspontaneity and economy of speech
        Press of speech
    Stereotypy of speech
    Echolalia
    Perseveration
    Mutism

From Neary D, Snowden JS, Gustafson L, et al. Frontotemporal lobar degeneration. A consensus on clinical diagnostic criteria. *Neurology* 1998;51:1546–1554.

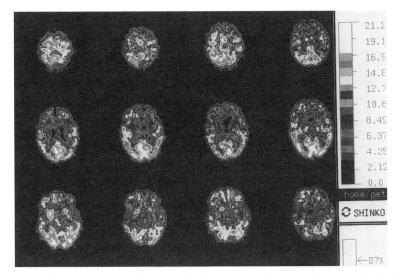

FIG 10-1. 18 Fluorodeoxyglucose positron emission tomography scan from a patient with progressive aphasia followed by behavioral change; note the reduced metabolism in both frontal lobes.

Within frontotemporal dementia, patients with predominantly frontal or temporal (Edwards-Lee et al., 1997) variants have been distinguished. In the temporal cases (Edwards-Lee et al., 1997), aphasia was a predominant symptom when the left hemisphere was predominantly involved, whereas right hemisphere patients had impulsive behavior, bizarre changes in dress, or religious preoccupation. Progressive aphasia has also been described in association with frontotemporal dementia (Snowden et al., 1992; Neary et al., 1993). The phenomena of the progressive aphasia are variable from case to case and, in general, not distinguishable from cases of PPA. Figure 10-1 is a PET scan from a patient who presented initially with nonfluent language deficits, then developed a behavioral disturbance with disinhibition, aggressive outbursts, and personality change. The scan shows bifrontal hypometabolism.

SUMMARY AND CONCLUSIONS

The language deterioration of aging, dementia, and the syndrome of PPA have been reviewed in this chapter. Language deterioration is generally mild in normal aging but is a universal accompaniment of dementing diseases. Isolated, progressive language disturbance, especially nonfluent aphasia, is the hallmark of the syndrome called "primary progressive aphasia." The language findings in these patients illustrate that distinctions between "focal" and "generalized" brain disease are difficult. Much remains to be learned about the spectrum of diseases that can produce progressive aphasia. The discovery of biological or genetic markers for these diseases is likely to lead to a better understanding of their behavioral characteristics.

REFERENCES

Abe K, Ukita H, Yanagihara T. Imaging in primary progressive aphasia. *Neuroradiology* 1997;39:556–559.

Albert MS, Heller HS, Milberg W. Changes in naming ability with age. *Psychol Aging* 1987;41:141–157.

Alzheimer A. Uber eine eigenartige erkrankung der hirnrinde. Allg. *Zeitschrift fur Psychiatrie und Psychisch-Gerichliche Med* 1907;64:146–148. English translation in Rottenberg DA, Hochberg FH. *Neurological classics in modern translation.* New York: Hafner Press, 1977:41–43.

Appell J, Kertesz A, Fisman M. A study of language functioning in Alzheimer patients. *Brain Lang* 1982;17:73–91.

Bayles KA, Tomoeda CK. Confrontation naming impairment in dementia. *Brain Lang* 1983;19:98–114.

Bayles KA. Language in aging and dementia. In: Kirshner HS, ed. *Handbook of neurological speech and language disorders.* New York: Marcel Dekker, 1995:351–372.

Borod J, Goodglass H, Kaplan E. Normative data of the Boston Diagnostic Aphasia examination, parietal lobe battery, and Boston Naming test. *J Clin Neuropsychol* 1980;2:209–215.

Broussolle E, Tommasi M, Mauguiere F, et al. Progressive anarthria with secondary Parkinsonism: a clinico-pathological case report. *J Neurol Neurosurg Psychiatry* 1992;55:577–580.

Burke DM, McKay DG. Memory, language, and aging. *Philos Trans R Soc London B Biol Sci* 1997;352:1845–1856.

Caselli R, Jack CR. Asymmetric cortical degeneration syndromes. A proposed clinical classification. *Arch Neurol* 1992;49:770–780.

Chapman SB, Rosenberg RN, Weiner MF, et al. Autosomal-dominant progressive syndrome of motor-speech loss without dementia. *Neurology* 1997;49:1298–1306.

Chawluk JB, Mesulam M-M, Hurtig H, et al. Slowly progressive aphasia without generalized dementia: studies with positron emission tomography. *Ann Neurol* 1986;19:68–74.

Critchley M. And all the daughters of musick shall be brought low. Language function in the elderly. *Arch Neurol* 1984;41:1135–1139.

Cummings JC, Houlihan JP, Hill MA. The pattern of reading deterioration in dementia of the Alzheimer type: observations and implications. *Brain Lang* 1986;29:315–323.

Dronkers NF. A new brain region for coordinating speech articulation. *Nature* 1996;384:159–161.

Duffy JR. *Motor speech disorders: substrates, differential diagnosis, and management.* St. Louis: Mosby, 1995.

Edwards-Lee T, Miller BL, Benson DF, et al. The temporal variant of frontotemporal dementia. *Brain* 1997;120: 1027–1040.

Glosser G, Deser T. A comparison of changes in macrolinguistic and microlinguistic aspects of discourse production in normal aging. *J Gerontol Psychol Sci* 1992;47:266–272.

Graff-Radford NR, Damasio AR, Hyman BT, et al. Progressive aphasia in a patient with Pick's disease: a neuropsychological, radiologic, and anatomic study. *Neurology* 1990; 40:620–626.

Green J, Morris JC, Sandson J, et al. Progressive aphasia; a precursor of global dementia? *Neurology* 1990;40:423–429.

Grossman M, Payer F, Onishi K, et al. Language comprehension and regional cerebral defects in frontotemporal degeneration and Alzheimer's disease. *Neurology* 1998; 50:157–163.

Henderson VW, Buckwalter JG, Soble E, et al. The agraphia of Alzheimer's disease. *Neurology* 1992;42: 776–784.

Hodges JR, Patterson K, Oxbury S, et al. Semantic dementia. Progressive fluent aphasia with temporal lobe atrophy. *Brain* 1992;115:1783–1806.

Holland AL, McBurney DH, Moossy J, et al. The dissolution of language in Pick's disease with neurofibrillary tangles: a case study. *Brain Lang* 1985;24:36–58.

Karbe H, Kertesz A, Polk M. Profiles of language impairment in primary progressive aphasia. *Arch Neurol* 1993; 50:193–201.

Kempler D, Metter EJ, Riege WH, et al. Slowly progressive aphasia: three cases with language, memory, CT and PET data. *J Neurol Neurosurg Psychiatry* 1990;53:987–993.

Kertesz A, Hudson L, Mackenzie IRA, et al. The pathology and nosology of primary progressive aphasia. *Neurology* 1994;44:2065–2072.

Kertesz A, Martinez-Lage P, Davidson W, et al. The corticobasal degeneration syndrome overlaps progressive aphasia and frontotemporal dementia. *Neurology* 2000; 55:1368–1375.

Kirshner HS, Alexander M, Lorch MP, et al. Disorders of speech and language. *Continuum* 1999;5:1–237.

Kirshner HS, Tanridag O, Thurman L, et al. Progressive aphasia without dementia: two cases with focal spongiform degeneration. *Ann Neurol* 1987;22:527–532.

Kirshner HS, Webb WG, Kelly MP, et al. Language disturbance. An initial symptom of cortical degenerations and dementia. *Arch Neurol* 1984;41:491–496.

Kirshner HS. *Handbook of neurological speech and language disorders.* New York: Marcel Dekker, 1995:1–532.

Lang AE. Cortical basal ganglionic degeneration presenting with "progressive loss of speech output and orofacial dyspraxia." *J Neurol Neurosurg Psychiatry* 1992;55:1101.

Lichtheim L. On aphasia. *Brain* 1885;7:433–484.

Lippa CF, Cohen R, Smith TW, et al. Primary progressive aphasia with focal neuronal achromasia. *Neurology* 1991; 41:882–886.

Mandell AM, Alexander MP, Carpenter S. Creutzfeldt-Jakob disease presenting as isolated aphasia. *Neurology* 1989; 39:55–58.

Mesulam M-M. Slowly progressive aphasia without generalized dementia. *Ann Neurol* 1982;11:592–598.

Morris JC, Cole M, Banker BQ, et al. Hereditary dysphasic dementia and the Pick-Alzheimer spectrum. *Ann Neurol* 1984;16:455–466.

Naeser MA, Helm-Estabrooks N, Haas G, et al. Relationship between lesion extent in "Wernicke's area" on CT scan and predicting recovery of comprehension in Wernicke's aphasia. *Arch Neurol* 1987;44:73–82.

Naeser MA, Palumbo CL, Helm-Estabrooks N, et al. Role of the medial subcallosal fasciculus and other white matter pathways in recovery of spontaneous speech. *Brain* 1989; 112:1–38.

Neary D, Snowden J. Fronto-temporal dementia: nosology, neuropsychology, and neuropathology. *Brain Cogn* 1996; 31:176–187.

Neary D, Snowden JS, Gustafson L, et al. Frontotemporal lobar degeneration. A consensus on clinical diagnostic criteria. *Neurology* 1998;51:1546–1554.

Neary D, Snowden JS, Mann DMA. Familial progressive aphasia: its relationship to other forms of lobar atrophy. *J Neurol Neurosurg Psychiatry* 1993;56; 1122–1125.

Pick A. 1892. Uber die beziehungen der senilen hirnatrophie zur aphasie. *Prager Med Wochenschrift* 1892;17:165–167. Translated in Rottenberg DA, Hochberg FH, eds. *Neurological classics in modern translation.* New York: Hafner Press, 1977:35–40.

Poeck K, Luzzatti C. Slowly progressive aphasia in three patients. *Brain* 1988;111:151–168.

Pogacar S, Williams RS. Alzheimer's disease presenting as slowly progressive aphasia. *R I Med J* 1984;67:181–185.

Price BH, Gurvit H, Weintraub S, et al. Neuropsychological patterns and language deficits in 20 consecutive cases of autopsy-confirmed Alzheimer's disease. *Arch Neurol* 1993;50:931–937.

Rahman S, Sahakian BJ, Hodges JR, et al. Specific cognitive deficits in mild frontal variant frontotemporal dementia. *Brain* 1999;122:1469–1493.

Sakurai Y, Hashida H, Uesugi H, et al. A clinical profile of corticobasal degeneration presenting as primary progressive aphasia. *Eur Neurol* 1996;36:134–137.

Scheltens P, Ravid R, Kamphorst W. Pathologic findings in a case of primary progressive aphasia. *Neurology* 1994; 44:279–282.

Snowden JS, Neary D, Mann DMA, et al. Progressive language disorder due to lobar atrophy. *Ann Neurol* 1992;31:174–183.

Tyrrell PJ, Warrington EK, Frackowiak RSJ, et al. Heterogeneity in progressive aphasia due to focal cortical atrophy. *Brain* 1990;113:1321–1336.

Wechsler AF, Verity A, Rosenschein S, et al. Pick's disease. A clinical, computed tomographic, and histologic study with Golgi impregnation observations. *Arch Neurol* 1982; 39:287–290.

Weintraub S, Rubin NP, Mesulam M-M. Primary progressive aphasia: longitudinal course, neuropsychological profile, and language features. *Arch Neurol* 1990;47:1329–1335.

Williams BW, Mack W, Henderson VW. Boston Naming Test in Alzheimer's disease. *Neuropsychologia* 1989;27: 1073–1079.

11

Tremor

Tanya Simuni

INTRODUCTION AND DEFINITIONS

Tremor is defined as a rhythmic involuntary oscillatory movement of a body part (Deuschl et al., 1998). The visibility and unique characteristics of tremor make it easy to recognize, however, defining the type of tremor can be more challenging. Classification of tremor is based on its clinical characteristics. Agreement between the observers on the terms is essential for correct classification, which ultimately will lead to accurate diagnosis and treatment. As seen below, tremor is described according to the behavioral circumstances in which it occurs.

I. *Rest tremor* occurs in a body part that is not voluntarily activated, and is completely supported against gravity (e.g., as when resting on a couch or arm rest).
II. *Action tremor* occurs during any voluntary contraction of skeletal muscle and can be a combination of postural, kinetic, and isometric tremor.
   A. *Postural tremor* occurs in an attempt to hold a body part motionless against gravity (e.g., outstretched arms).
   B. *Kinetic tremor* occurs during a voluntary movement and can be of three types:
      1. *Isometric tremor* occurs during a muscle contraction against a stationary rigid object (pushing against a wall)
      2. *Intention tremor* with which tremor amplitude increases as the limb approaches the target during a visually guided movement (finger-to-nose testing).
      3. *Task-specific tremor* appears or becomes exacerbated during specific tasks (e.g., primary writing tremor or occupational tremors).

TREMOR EPIDEMIOLOGY

Tremor is the most common type of all movement disorders, the incidence of which increases with age independent of the cause. Considering that tremor can be a manifestation of a variety of neurologic conditions, prevalence data are available only with respect to the most common diagnostic entities, specifically, essential tremor (ET), which is a monosymptomatic disorder with no neurologic signs other than postural or action tremor, and parkinsonian tremor. Even in those settings, the numbers are inconsistent. Reported ET prevalence varies from 0.0005% to 5.5% (Aiyesimoju et al., 1984; Rautakorpi et al., 1982), depending on the study methodology and the population age. Despite such a wide range, unanimous agreement exists between investigators of the increasing prevalence of ET with age. Larrson and Sjogren (1960) reported a twofold increase of tremor prevalence rate in the population over the age of 40 years, compared with the general population. Another study reported a tenfold increase in prevalence of ET in those 70 to 79 years of age compared with those 40 to 69 years of age (Haerer et al., 1982). It is estimated that about 5 million individuals above the age of 40 are affected by ET in the United States, making it undoubtedly the most common movement disorder (Koller, 1997).

Similar to ET, a clear age-dependent increase is seen in the prevalence of parkinsonian tremors. It is estimated that Parkinson's disease affects 1% of the population above the age of 65 (Tanner and Aston, 2000). Generally, tremor is present in 75% of patients with Parkinson's disease, making Parkinson's disease tremor (PDT) the second most common cause of tremor. Prevalence of tremor in the setting of various metabolic derangements (e.g., renal, hepatic encephalopathy, hypoglycemia, hyperthyroidism) is unknown; however, the incidence of these conditions is clearly age-dependent. The same is true for drug-induced tremor, considering the exponential increase of medications intake with age.

TREMOR PATHOPHYSIOLOGY

Despite the high prevalence of tremor, knowledge of its pathophysiology and anatomic generators is limited. Central versus peripheral nervous system origin of tremor is still debated. It remains unclear if tremor generators are disease specific or if a common final pathway exists that is independent of tremor cause. Four mechanisms have been postulated (Hallett, 1998; Rothwell, 1998):

1. Mechanical oscillations of the extremity, which is based on simple mechanical properties of any mass-spring system: extremity attached to a stiff joint oscillates after a mechanical perturbation. The resonance frequency is inversely related to the mass of the body part, and it can be measured by a sensitive accelerometer attached to the outstretched limb. This mechanism can potentially explain physiologic tremor, but doubtfully represents a solo mechanism of pathologic tremors.
2. Reflex activation of tremor. This mechanism is based on the muscle stretch reflex. The oscillation of a limb activates muscle spindle receptors, which via the Ia afferents monosynaptically connect to the motor neuron, and through the motor axon back to the extrafusal muscle fibers. That creates a reflex loop. These reflex loops, if appropriately timed, can produce rhythmic bursts of muscle activity, consistent with tremor.
3. Central oscillators. Specific cell populations within the central nervous system have the capacity to fire repetitively because of the unique properties of their membrane potential. Single-cell oscillation is insufficient to produce a visible tremor in the periphery. However, if cell activity is synchronized, the synchronized volley can cause sufficient motor neuron pool activation to produce a visible tremor. Two regions within the central motor pathways demonstrate oscillatory behavior under certain conditions: the inferior olive and the relay nuclei of the thalamus. It is believed that the pattern of tremor produced is oscillator dependent. Essential type tremor has been linked to the inferior olive, whereas parkinsonian tremor to the basal ganglia region, with the thalamus being the potential cortical projection relay nuclei for both. That hypothesis would explain the effectiveness of thalamic target for surgical treatment of both types of tremor.
4. Cerebellum. Cerebellar lesions can be associated with tremor. It is unlikely that the cerebellum has its independent tremor oscillator region, but it can participate in tremor generation by altering feed-forward and feedback loops. Based on positron emission tomography (PET) data, cerebellar blood flow is increased in almost all types of tremor (Boecker and Brooks, 1998). Such non-

selective activation supports the hypothesis that the cerebellum is likely a relay site for tremor rather than the primary generator, although the data are inconclusive.

It is still unclear whether one mechanism plays a leading role in a particular tremor generation versus occurring in parallel, or whether it might be additive. It seems, at least in the setting of ET and Parkinson's disease, that a central tremor generator exists, whose activity can be augmented or modified by the peripheral input.

TREMOR CAUSE

Table 11-1 summarizes multiple potential causes of tremor. It is beyond the scope of this chapter to discuss each of them. From a clinical standpoint, it is useful to define the tremor syndrome, which will narrow the causative differential diagnosis and guide in the choice of therapeutic intervention (Deuschl et al., 1998).

Physiologic Tremor

In every healthy subject, physiologic tremor is present in the joint or muscle that is free to oscillate. It has a low amplitude and high frequency. Usually, it is not visible, but for intermittent fingers tremor.

Enhanced Physiologic Tremor

Enhanced physiologic tremor (EPT) has the same frequency characteristics as physiologic tremor but is easily visible. It is mainly postural. The diagnosis should not be made in the presence of an underlying neurologic pathology. This form of tremor overlaps the category of drug- or toxin-induced tremor. Screening for potential metabolic derangements associated with tremor should be performed (Table 11-2). Distinction between EPT and mild forms of ET is arbitrary, and usually is based on the presence of functional disability with the latter.

Essential Tremor

The diagnosis of ET is based on the presence of bilateral, largely symmetric postural or kinetic tremor, involving hands and forearms, which is visible and persistent (Deuschl et al., 1998). Tremor can involve head and voice; however, chin or leg involvement is atypical. In cases of severe ET, resting tremor can be present, however, the possibility of coexisting Parkinson's disease has to be ruled out. Tremor frequency is

TABLE 11-1. *Tremor: etiologic classification*

Physiologic tremor
  Enhanced physiologic tremor
Pathologic tremors
  Hereditary, degenerative, and idiopathic disease
    Essential tremor
      Definite essential tremor (ET)
        (monosymptomatic ET)
      Probable ET (ET with atypical distribution of
        tremor)
      Possible ET (ET + other neurologic findings)
    Parkinsonian tremor
      Parkinson's disease
      Other parkinsonian syndromes (e.g., multiple
        system atrophy, progressive supranuclear
        palsy, Wilson's disease)
    Task-specific tremor (e.g., writers tremor,
      voice tremor)
    Dystonic tremor syndromes (generalized or focal
      dystonia + tremor in the affected body part)
    Cerebellar tremor syndromes (e.g.,
      spinocerebellar degenerations,
      olivopontocerebellar atrophy)
  Cerebral diseases of various etiologies
    Central nervous system infections (e.g.,
      neurosyphilis, neuroborreliosis, HIV, smallpox)
    Inflammatory conditions (multiple sclerosis)
    Space occupying lesions (e.g., tumors,
      cerebrovascular insults, atrioventricular
      malformation)
    Posttraumatic tremor
  Metabolic diseases
    Hyper/hypothyroidism
    Hyperparathyroidism
    Hypocalcemia
    Hypomagnesimia
    Hypoglycemia
    Hepatic encephalopathy
    Renal encephalopathy
  Drug-induced
    Centrally acting substances (e.g., neuroleptics,
      antidepressants—especially tricyclics, lithium,
      cocaine, alcohol, caffeine)
    Sympathomimetics (bronchodilators)
    Steroids
    Miscellaneous (valproate, perhexiline,
      amiodarone, mexilitine, vincristine, cyclosporin
      A)
  Toxin-induced (mercury, lead, manganese, cyanide,
    carbon monoxide, nicotine, arsenic, alcohol)
  Peripheral neuropathies
    Roussy—Levy syndrome
    Other hereditary neuropathies
    Polyneuropathy of various origin (diabetes,
      uremia, porphyria)
  Other disorders with tremor symptoms
    Emotions, fatigue, cooling
    Drug withdrawal
    Psychogenic tremor

Modified from Deuschl G, Bain P, Brin M. Consensus statement of the Movement Disorder Society on Tremor. Ad Hoc Scientific Committee. *Mov Disord* 1998;13(Suppl 3):2–23, with permission.

TABLE 11-2. *Screening for potential symptomatic causes of tremor*

1. Thyroid function (thyroid-stimulating hormone, T_3, T_4)
2. Metabolic screen (Na, K, Cl, Ca, Mg, creatinin, blood urea nitrogen, glucose)
3. Liver function tests (alanine aminotransferase, aspartate aminotransferase)
4. Ceruloplasmin, serum and urine copper[a]
5. Cortisol, parathyroid hormone[a]
6. Toxicology test[a]

[a]To be performed only when clinically indicated.

4 to 12 Hz. Some patients, especially women, can present with head tremor as an isolated manifestation of ET. Caution should be taken to rule out an underlying cervical dystonia with a prominent tremor component. The possibility of underlying symptomatic cause (drugs, toxins, metabolic abnormalities) should be excluded before making the diagnosis of ET. A distinction should be made between ET as the causative entity, also referred to as "benign familial essential tremor," versus ET as a clinical syndrome, which defines tremor of a particular type that potentially can be associated with other neurologic findings (Bain et al., 2000). The former is labeled as definite ET in the Tremor Investigation Group (TRIG) nomenclature, whereas the latter is labeled as probable versus possible, depending on the type of associated neurologic findings (Bain et al., 2000). Definite ET is a monosymptomatic disease, meaning that no other abnormal neurologic findings should be present. It has strong familial predisposition, with about 50% of patients having a positive family history for tremor, pointing to likely autosomal-dominant inheritance, although the gene has yet to be identified (Findley, 2000). Conversely, lack of family history does not preclude the diagnosis of ET. Symptoms have an insidious onset with a variable rate of progression. The most disabling feature of ET is action or kinetic tremor of the arms, which interferes with the patient's ability to perform the simplest daily activities (e.g., eating, drinking, writing). Patients with severe ET can be completely disabled, so the label *benign* is a misnomer. A number of patients have a combination of ET and other movement disorders (dystonia, parkinsonism, myoclonus, or restless legs syndrome). Those patients are classified as possible ET according to TRIG criteria (Bain et al., 2000).

Primary Orthostatic Tremor

Primary orthostatic tremor is a unique syndrome, characterized by the presence of high frequency

(13–18 Hz) tremor of the trunk and legs that occurs only with stance (Britton and Thompson, 1995). The patients are asymptomatic when lying down or sitting. Rarely, symptoms persist with walking. Subjectively, patients report a feeling of unsteadiness when standing up. Constant change of the position of the feet relieves the symptoms, thus, patients quickly learn to march in one spot. The clinical examination finding is benign, except for minimally visible and sometimes only palpable fine amplitude rippling of the leg muscles. The diagnosis can be confirmed by an electromyographic (EMG) study of the quadriceps muscles, which records a typical tremor patter of 13 to 18 Hz. Symptoms respond to low dose clonazepam.

Task- and Position-Specific Tremor

Tremors that are task- and position-specific comprise a group of tremor syndromes that share a common feature of tremor activation when engaged in a specific task. The most common type is primary writing tremor, when symptoms appear only or predominantly with that particular activity. Use of the limb with other activities (e.g., eating, weight-lifting) is not associated with tremor. The other examples include task-specific tremors of musicians and athletes, as well as isolated voice tremor. Some of these patients have dystonic posturing of the limb in conjunction with tremor. Those cases should be classified as focal dystonia with dystonic tremor.

Dystonic Tremor Syndromes

Tremor in a body part affected by dystonia is a well-known phenomenon, although its mechanism is unknown. The pattern of tremor differs from ET: it is localized to the dystonic body part, has an irregular pattern with variable frequency, and usually resolves with complete rest. *Gestes antagonistes*, a sensory trick used by a lot of patients to overcome dystonic movement by touching the involved body part, such as placing the hand on the cheek in cases of cervical dystonia, frequently reduces tremor. This type of tremor responds to botulinum toxin injections. Sometimes patients with dystonia (e.g. patients with cervical dystonia and upper limbs postural tremor) may have an ET type of tremor in the body part not affected by dystonia. These patients should not be classified as having dystonic tremor. They likely have an ET–dystonia overlap syndrome.

Parkinsonian Tremor Syndromes

Parkinsonism is a clinical syndrome, not a disease entity. However, parkinsonian tremor has unique characteristics, believed to be stigmata of striatonigral dysfunction. Classic parkinsonian tremor occurs in a resting limb, has a pill-rolling pattern, and low (4–6 Hz) frequency. It characteristically diminishes with activity of the affected limb. Tremor can be accelerated with mental activity, stress, or when movement of another body part is performed. As noted earlier, parkinsonian tremor is not an obligatory sign of Parkinson's disease; however, it is present in 75% of patients with Parkinson's disease. Alternatively, rest tremor is unusual in patients with atypical parkinsonian syndromes (e.g., multiple systems atrophy, progressive supranuclear palsy). Tremor in Parkinson's disease typically involves distal arms, but also legs and chin; head or voice tremor are atypical in these patients. Parkinson's disease tremor is asymmetric, or at least initially starts on one side of the body. Tremor usually is not the major cause of disability, as it abates when the limb is involved in action. Aside from classic resting tremor, patients with Parkinson's disease can have various degrees of postural and action tremor. That tremor component can be either at the same frequency as a resting one or it can be faster, and nonharmonically related to the rest tremor. The former type is believed to be the continuation of rest tremor under postural or kinetic conditions, whereas the mechanism of the latter is unknown. Few patients with Parkinson's disease have pure postural or kinetic tremor with no rest tremor component. Some, however, will have that type of tremor at the onset of the disease, developing the classical rest tremor pattern later on.

Generally, distinction between classic ET and a parkinsonian-type tremor is straightforward, based on the distinct tremor characteristics. In some cases, however, distinction can be difficult, especially at the early stages of the disease. It is estimated that about 20% of patients with ET are misdiagnosed for Parkinson's disease and vice versa (Findley and Koller, 1987). The differential diagnosis criteria are summarized in Table 11-3.

Monosymptomatic Rest Tremor

Some patients exhibit isolated rest tremor without evidence of associated parkinsonian signs (bradykinesia, rigidity). According to the brain bank Parkinson's disease diagnostic criteria, the diagnosis of Parkinson's disease should not be made in absence of bradykinesia, although PET data in some of these patients provide evidence of dopaminergic dysfunction to the degree similar to otherwise typical Parkinson's disease (Brooks et al., 1992). However, for clinical purposes, these patients should be labeled as having

TABLE 11-3. *Differential diagnosis of essential tremor and Parkinsonian tremor*

	Essential tremor[a]	Parkinson's disease
Resting tremor	+	+++
Postural or action tremor	+++	+
Tremor asymmetry	+	+++
Rigidity	±	+++
Bradykinesia	–	+++
Chin tremor	–	++
Leg tremor	±	+++
Voice tremor	+++	–
Head tremor	+++	–
Hereditary tremor	+++	–
Response to alcohol	+++	–
Response to dopaminergic (+/–)	–	+++

[a]± indicate presence versus absence and the severity of the symptoms on the scale from one to three, with three being most severe.
Adapted from Deuschl G, Krack P. Tremors: differential diagnosis, neurophysiology, and pharmacology. In: Jankovic J, Tolosa E, eds. *Parkinson's disease and movement disorders.* Baltimore: Williams & Wilkins, 1998: 419–452.

"monosymptomatic rest tremor," unless they develop other clinical signs of Parkinson's disease.

Cerebellar Tremor Syndromes

Various types of tremor have been described in cerebellar disorders, however, the most common type, considered to be the stigmata of cerebellar dysfunction, is intentional tremor. As discussed, it is a kinetic tremor, the amplitude of which increases during a visually guided movement toward a target. It frequently is irregular and unilateral, having a frequency below 5 Hz and no rest tremor component. It typically involves the limbs and is elicited on the finger-to-nose or heel-to-chin tests. The pathophysiologic basis of cerebellar tremor is unknown, although anatomically it is associated with the damage of either superior cerebellar peduncles or dentate nuclei. Another pattern of tremor associated with cerebellar pathology is slow-frequency oscillation of the body trunk or head, the amplitude of which increases with movement. That pattern is known as titubation.

Holmes' Tremor

Holmes' tremor, also known as midbrain, rubral tremor, or myorhythmia, is a unique tremor syndrome usually of symptomatic origin, caused by a lesion of the central nervous system. Originally, it was believed to be associated with the lesions in red nuclei or midbrain, hence the name. Recently, however, more and more cases have been reported in which the lesion was located outside the midbrain. The pattern of tremor is a combination of resting and intention. It

frequently is irregular and has slow frequency (<4.5 Hz). The proximal muscles can be involved more than distal muscles, unlike other tremor types. Tremor frequently is unilateral. In cases of cerebrovascular events as the cause of the structural lesion, a delay is seen to the time of tremor onset, which can be up to 2 years (Krack et al., 1994). Pathophysiology of this type of tremor is unknown, but PET data suggest that it is caused by a combined lesion of cerebellothalamic and nigrostriatal pathways (Remy et al., 1995).

Palatal Tremor Syndromes

Palatal tremor was formally classified as palatal myoclonus, however, rhythmicity of movement is consistent with the tremor pattern. Palatal tremor can be either symptomatic or essential (Deuschl et al., 1994). Symptomatic causes of tremor include preceding brainstem or cerebellum lesion, with subsequent inferior olivary hypertrophy, which can be demonstrated on MRI scan. Rhythmic movement may not be limited to the soft palate, but can also involve other brainstem innervated muscles (frequently, extraocular musculature). In essential cases, by definition, no identifiable underlying structural lesion exists and the MRI scan is normal. Clinically, signs are limited to the soft palate, and the patients usually have an ear click, a rhythmic sound in the ears.

Drug-Induced and Toxic Tremor Syndromes

The incidence of toxin- or drug-induced tremor is unknown; however, potentially it can be the most common cause of tremor, exceeding ET and those of

Parkinson's disease, specifically in the elderly. The pattern of tremor can be variable, depending on the agent and individual predisposition. The most common pattern is enhanced physiologic tremor that occurs when using tremorogenic drugs. The list of the potential offending agents is extensive, however, the most frequently cited ones are sympathomimetics, stimulants, steroids, and antidepressants (Deuschl et al., 1998). For patients with an acute onset of tremor, medication lists must be carefully reviewed for a potential causative relationship to the symptoms. Tremorogenic effects might not be limited to the pharmaceutic agent, but can be associated with certain food and beverages (caffeinated drinks). Another common pattern of drug-induced tremor is parkinsonian tremor with the use of dopamine-blocking agents (Llau et al., 1994). The best recognized offending agents are neuroleptics because of their ability to block postsynaptic dopamine receptors. However, less well-known and less-utilized presynaptic dopamine-depleting agents (e.g., reserpine and tetrabenazine) can cause the same syndrome (Lorenc-Koci et al., 1995). The effect of dopamine-blocking agents is not limited to tremor; they cause the full triad of parkinsonian symptoms. Withdrawal of the offending agent should lead to resolution of tremor and other symptoms within 3 weeks to 6 months. Rare cases of persistent symptoms have been reported, despite withdrawal of the offending agents (Klawans et al., 1973). Such cases raise the possibility of underlying Parkinson's disease in those individuals that was clinically unveiled by neuroleptic exposure.

The association of tremor with toxin exposure has been known for some time, and the list of potential offending agents is long (Manyam, 1998). A detailed history, especially in the setting of acute onset of tremor, will help to isolate the potential toxin or drug and proceed with the appropriate investigation.

Tremor Syndromes in Peripheral Neuropathy

Tremor has been described with various kinds of peripheral neuropathies, however, most commonly with the demyelinating ones (Thomas, 1999). The pattern of tremor is usually postural or kinetic. Roussy-Lévy is the syndrome characterized by the presence of demyelinating hereditary motor sensory neuropathy (HSMN type I) and essential type tremor (Plante-Bordeneuve et al., 1999). In some patients, tremor responds to alcohol and propranolol. The pathophysiology of tremor in neuropathies is unclear, but it is believed to involve both peripheral and central mechanisms.

Psychogenic Tremor

Generally, the diagnosis of psychogenic movement disorder is the most challenging, even for an experienced movement disorders neurologist. Clues to the diagnosis have been established and include (Koller and Lang 1989; Lang et al., 1995; Deuschl et al., 1998) the following:

- Acute onset of the symptoms or spontaneous remissions
- Pattern of tremor inconsistent with any known syndrome
- Distractibility of symptoms
- Ability to provoke symptoms with suggestion
- History of somatization in the past
- Additional nonphysiologic signs found on neurological examination
- Presence of secondary gain

These are only clues to the diagnosis. Careful examination by an experienced professional allows the correct diagnosis to be made in most cases, while avoiding unnecessary testing and pharmacologic exposure. Nonconfrontational counseling and referral to a psychologist are essential, however, they do not always guarantee a good recovery.

DIFFERENTIAL DIAGNOSIS OF TREMOR

In most cases, tremor is easy to recognize and distinguish from other types of movement disorders, based on its clinical characteristics. Rhythmicity of the movement differentiates it from chorea and hemiballism. Oscillatory pattern of movement distinguish tremor from dystonia or myoclonus, even in cases when the latter carry pseudoperiodic pattern. Tics can be rhythmic but their rapid speed and stereotypy allow separating them from tremor. Rhythmicity and oscillating pattern of movement differentiate tremor from asterixis, which is a negative myoclonus, usually seen in the setting of metabolic encephalopathy. *Epilepsia partialis continua* is rarely misinterpreted as tremor because of the presence of rhythmic jerks. However, acute onset of symptoms, lack of prior history of tremor, localization of symptoms to one limb, and electroencephalogram data allow differentiation of the syndromes. Clonus can be rhythmic; however, localization of the symptoms around the joint and presence of other pyramidal findings make it an unlikely cause of confusion with tremor. Despite unique characteristics of tremor that distinguish it from other movements, differentiating the type of tremor can be more challenging. Differential diagnosis of tremor syndromes, discussed above, is

TABLE 11-4. *Tremor syndromes: differential diagnosis*

Tremor diagnosis	Distribution	Activation by [a]			Frequency (Hz)
		Rest	Posture	Action[a]	
Physiologic	Arms	−	+	+	8–12
Enhanced physiologic	Arms	−	+	+	8–12
Essential	Arms, head, voice	−	++	++	4–12
Dystonic	Part of body with dystonia	−	+	++	<7
Primary writing	Arm	−	+	+++	5–10
Orthostatic	Legs, trunk	−	+++	+	13–18
Parkinson's	Arms, legs, chin	+++	+	+	4–6
Cerebellar	Arms, head trunk	−	+	+++ Intention	<5
Holmes' (rubral)	Arm, leg; usually unilateral	++	+	+++	<4.5
Neuropathic	Limbs	−	++	+	3–10
Drug-induced	Limbs[a]	++	++	++	[b]
Psychogenic	Any body part	Any combination, inconsistent pattern			

[a]± indicate presence versus absence and the severity of the symptoms on the scale from one to three, with three being most severe.
[b]Depending on the type of medication, can be predominantly essential or parkinsonian type.

summarized in Table 11-4. The major source of confusion is distinguishing ET and tremor of Parkinson's disease, especially at the early stages. Table 11-3 summarizes criteria for differentiating tremor in these two common entities.

APPROACH TO THE DIAGNOSIS AND MANAGEMENT OF TREMOR

When a clinician evaluates a patient with any kind of involuntary movement, the first step is to define the type of movement disorder. The following is the suggested stepwise approach to evaluation of patients with tremor (Fig. 11-1):

Step 1. Does patient have a tremor?
Step 2. What is the pattern of tremor (resting, postural, kinetic, goal-directed)?
Step 3. What is the distribution of tremor (head, chin, voice, upper or lower limbs, trunk)?
Step 4. What is the tremor frequency (fast >7 Hz, medium 4–7 Hz, low < 4 Hz)?
Step 5. Are there any other positive findings on the neurologic examination (bradykinesia, rigidity, gait abnormality, pyramidal findings, cerebellar signs, dystonia, neuropathic signs)?
Step 6. Based on the above data, define the tremor syndrome:
   1. Physiologic
   2. Parkinsonian
   3. Essential
   4. Other

Step 7. Review medical history for:
   1. Mode of tremor onset (acute versus insidious)
   2. Family history of neurologic disease (specifically tremor)
   3. Alcohol sensitivity
   4. History of medication exposure
   5. History of toxin exposure
Step 8. Determine the cause of the tremor syndrome based on the above data (not always possible).
Step 9. Decide if additional testing is necessary
Step 10. Evaluate treatment options based on the type of the tremor syndrome (essential versus parkinsonian).
Step 11. Treat only if symptoms produce functional compromise and no reversible cause is identified.
Step 12. Reevaluate the diagnosis, if necessary, based on the treatment response and the cause of the disease (appearance of new neurologic findings).

DIAGNOSTIC STUDIES

The diagnosis of tremor is a clinical one, based on the history and examination. Diagnostic studies to confirm tremor as the type of movement disorder are rarely necessary. Surface electromyography can be performed to clarify tremor frequency, and is most useful to confirm the diagnosis of orthostatic tremor (high frequency tremor) (McManis and Sharbrough, 1993). EMG can also be a useful tool when psychogenic tremor is suspected as it will reveal an inconsistent muscle-firing pattern (McAuley et al., 1998). Nerve conduction study in conjunction with

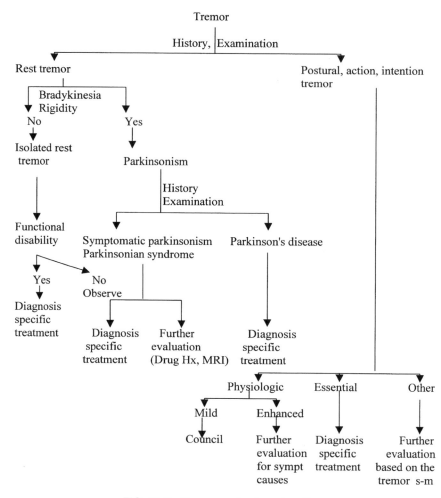

FIG. 11-1. Tremor evaluation algorithm.

EMG should be performed if neurogenic cause (peripheral neuropathy) of tremor is suspected.

Screening for potential symptomatic causes of tremor should be performed in all cases of acute onset of symptoms. The suggested evaluation panel is presented in Table 11-2. The extent of testing should be geared to each particular case. Thyroid studies should be performed in all patients with the syndrome of enhanced physiologic tremor.

Patients with tremor and an otherwise normal neurologic examination do not require neuroimaging. Neuroimaging, preferably MRI, should be performed in the presence of other positive focal findings on examination (e.g., pyramidal or cerebellar signs) to rule out an underlying structural lesion.

TREATMENT OPTIONS

Choice of tremor therapy is based on the tremor syndrome (Wasielewski et al., 1998). The major distinction is between essential and parkinsonian type tremor. Physiologic tremor does not require pharmacologic therapy. In the setting of enhanced physiologic tremor, the primary objective is to find and correct the potential underlying symptomatic cause. Treatment should be attempted only if the investigation is not revealing, and symptoms produce a functional compromise. The choice of therapy is the same as for ET, however, the treatment should be started with a long-acting benzodiazepine (clonazepam). Some patients benefit from use of propranolol (10

TABLE 11-5. *Medication chart: tremor*

Medication	Dose	Risks	Cost/month ($)
Parkinson's tremor			
Levodopa/carbidopa	25/100 mg 3–6/d	Orthostasis, confusion, nausea, hallucinations	>50.00
Dopamine agonists			much more expensive than 50.00
Pramipexole	0.75–3.0 mg/d	Orthostasis, confusion, nausea, hallucinations, somnolence	
Ropinirole	3–16 mg/d		
Pergolide	0.75–3 mg/d		
Bromocriptine	7.5–30 mg/d		
Amantadine	100–300 mg/d	Confusion, LE edema	>50.00
Trihexyphenidyl	1–2 mg three times daily	Confusion, dry mouth, urinary retention; should not be used in patients with glaucoma	<50.00
Clozapine	25–50 mg/d	Neutropenia, sedation	much more expensive than 50.00
Essential tremor			
Propranolol	60–320 mg/d	Orthostasis, sleep disturbance, depression; contraindicated in asthma, diabetes, heart block	<50.00
Primidone	50–250 mg/d	Sedation, confusion	<50.00
Clonazepam	0.5–3.0 mg/d	Sedation	<50.00
Enhanced physiologic tremor			
Propranolol	10 mg as needed		<50.00
Clonazepam	0.5 mg at bedtime		<50.00
Cerebellar tremor	No effective therapy, essential tremor (ET) medications can be tried		
Holme's tremor	No effective therapy, parkinsonian and ET medications can be tried		

LE, lower extremities.

mg) on as needed basis. The major groups of medications used for treatment of parkinsonian and ET tremor are presented in Table 11-5.

SUMMARY

Tremor is a common neurologic sign, especially in the elderly. It can be a symptom of a variety of underlying medical and neurologic conditions. A complete history, careful examination, and stepwise approach to defining the type of tremor are essential for correct diagnosis and appropriate management.

REFERENCES

Aiyesimoju AB, Osuntokun BO, Bademosi O, et al. Hereditary neurodegenerative disorders in Nigerian Africans. *Neurology* 1984;34:361–362.

Bain P, Brin M, Deuschl G, et al. Criteria for the diagnosis of essential tremor. *Neurology* 2000;54(11 Suppl 4):S7–S7.

Boecker H, Brooks DJ. Functional imaging of tremor. *Mov Disord* 1998;13(Suppl 3):64–72.

Britton TC, Thompson PD. Primary orthostatic tremor [editorial]. *BMJ* 1995;310:143–144.

Brooks DJ, Playford ED, Ibanez V, et al. Isolated tremor and disruption of the nigrostriatal dopaminergic system: an 18F-dopa PET study. *Neurology* 1992;42:1554–1560.

Deuschl G, Bain P, Brin M. Consensus statement of the Movement Disorder Society on Tremor. Ad Hoc Scientific Committee. *Mov Disord* 1998;13(Suppl 3):2–23.

Deuschl G, Toro C, Hallett M. Symptomatic and essential palatal tremor. 2. Differences of palatal movements. *Mov Disord* 1994;9:676–678.

Findley LJ. Epidemiology and genetics of essential tremor. *Neurology* 2000;54(11 Suppl 4):S8.–S13.

Findley LJ, Koller WC. Essential tremor: a review. *Neurology* 1987;37:1194–1197.

Haerer AF, Anderson DW, Schoenberg BS. Prevalence of essential tremor. Results from the Copiah County study. *Arch Neurol* 1982;39:750–751.

Hallett M. Overview of human tremor physiology. *Mov Disord* 1998;(13 Suppl 3):43–48.

Klawans HLJ, Bergen D, Bruyn GW. Prolonged drug-induced Parkinsonism. *Confin Neurol* 1973;35:368–377.

Koller W, Lang A, Vetere-Overfield B, et al. Psychogenic tremors. *Neurology* 1989;39:1094–1099.

Koller WC. Essential tremor: the beginning of a new era [editorial; comment]. *Mov Disord* 1997;12:841

Krack P, Deuschl G, Kaps M, et al. Delayed onset of "rubral tremor" 23 years after brainstem trauma [letter]. *Mov Disord* 1994;9:240–242.

Lang AE, Koller WC, Fahn S. Psychogenic parkinsonism. *Arch Neurol* 1995;52:802–810.

Larson T, Sjogren T. Essential tremor: a clinical and genetic population study. *Acta Psychiatr Neurol Scand* 1960; 44:36.

Llau ME, Nguyen L, Senard JM, et al. [Drug-induced parkinsonian syndromes: a 10-year experience at a regional center of pharmaco-vigilance.] Syndromes parkinsoniens d'origine medicamenteuse: experience d'un centre regional de pharmacovigilance sur dix ans. *Rev Neurol (Paris)* 1994;150:757–762.

Lorenc-Koci E, Ossowska K, Wardas J, et al. Does reserpine induce parkinsonian rigidity? *J Neural Transm Park Dis Dement Sect* 1995;9:211–223.

Manyam BV. Uncommon forms of tremor. In: Jankovic J, Tolosa E, eds. *Parkinson's disease and movement disorders.* Baltimore: Williams & Wilkins, 1998:387–403.

McAuley JH, Rothwell JC, Marsden CD, et al. Electrophysiological aids in distinguishing organic from psychogenic tremor. *Neurology* 1998;50:1882–1884.

McManis PG, Sharbrough FW. Orthostatic tremor: clinical and electrophysiologic characteristics. *Muscle Nerve* 1993;16:1254–1260.

Plante-Bordeneuve V, Guiochon-Mantel A, Lacroix C, Lapresle J, Said G. The Roussy-Levy family: from the original description to the gene. *Ann Neurol* 1999;46:770–773.

Rautakorpi I, Takala J, Marttila RJ, et al. Essential tremor in a Finnish population. *Acta Neurol Scand* 1982;66:58–67.

Remy P, de Recondo A, defer G, et al. Peduncular "rubral" tremor and dopaminergic denervation: a PET study. *Neurology* 1995; 45: 472–477.

Rothwell JC. Physiology and anatomy of possible oscillators in the central nervous system. *Mov Disord* 1998;13 (Suppl 3):24–28.

Tanner CM, Aston DA. Epidemiology of Parkinson's disease and akinetic syndromes [In Process Citation]. *Curr Opin Neurol* 2000;13.(4.):427–430.

Thomas PK. Overview of Charcot-Marie-Tooth disease type 1A. *Ann NY Acad Sci* 1999;883:1–5.

Wasielewski PG, Burns JM, Koller WC. Pharmacologic treatment of tremor. *Mov Disord* 1998;13(Suppl 3):90–100.

SUGGESTED READING

Deuschl G, ed. Tremor: basic mechanisms and clinical aspects. *Mov Disord* 1998;13(Suppl 3).

Deuschl G, Krack P. Tremors: differential diagnosis, neurophysiology, and pharmacology. In: Jankovic J, Tolosa E, eds. *Parkinson's disease and movement disorders.* Baltimore: Williams & Wilkins, 1998: 419–452.

Koller WC, ed. Essential tremor. *Neurology* 2000;54(11 Suppl 4).

12

Neuro-Ophthalmology

Rod Foroozan and Mark L. Moster

INTRODUCTION

In this chapter we discuss the common neuro-ophthalmic disorders that occur in the elderly, including causes of visual loss from vascular occlusive disease (including giant cell arteritis), optic disc swelling, orbital disease (including thyroid eye disease), disorders of ocular motility (including myasthenia gravis), and disorders of the face and eyelid.

Many neuro-ophthalmic disorders can be diagnosed solely by a complete ocular history. A thorough ocular history should include the onset and severity of visual dysfunction, the timing and progression of the visual disturbance, the presence of pain, and exacerbating and relieving factors. Specific attention should be paid to establishing whether the ocular complaint is unilateral or bilateral. A prior ocular history, including a history of strabismus, surgery, and trauma, should be sought, and any family history of ocular disease should be noted. The use of medications, both systemic and topical preparations, should be recorded in a general review of the medical history. During the examination, both eyes must be assessed, even if the patient believes that the problem is unilateral.

An important assessment of central visual function can be made by testing the best corrected visual acuity, and each eye should be tested separately. Although most measures of visual acuity depend on subjective responses, electrophysiologic testing can be used to gain some objective measure of visual function.

Pupillary reactivity should be assessed in the dark by instructing the patient to view a distant target, eliminating the miosis that occurs with accommodation and the near response. The response depends on the intensity of light projected and the efficiency of transmission through the afferent visual pathway (Fig. 12-1). This response is dependent on a difference between the conduction of the two afferent pupillary pathways, hence, the designation "relative afferent pupillary defect" (RAPD), also known as a Marcus Gunn pupil (Thompson et al., 1981). Patients with symmetric deficits in the afferent pupillary pathway may not have a RAPD. Instead, they show a pattern similar to that seen with a less intense light source because the conduction of the afferent pathway is less efficient.

Assessment of the afferent visual system must include confrontation visual field testing. Each eye is tested separately by fully occluding the opposite eye (Fig. 12-2). The superior visual field is tested by asking the patient to count the number of fingers seen on each hand of the examiner. An impairment of either the nasal or temporal portion of the superior visual field can be confirmed by retesting each quadrant individually. Similarly, test the inferior visual field by presenting fingers just below the level of the patient's chin, and then test the fellow eye in a similar fashion.

Electrophysiologic testing is generally not required in the evaluation of the afferent visual system, but can be helpful in cases of unexplained visual loss (Carr and Siegel, 1990). The electroretinogram (ERG) represents the sum of the response of retinal photoreceptors, and specific testing conditions can aid in differentiating the cone and rod responses. The visual-evoked potential (VEP) can assess the latency and amplitude of the afferent visual response, including the visual cortex, but typically is not specific enough to determine the site of visual dysfunction.

RETINAL DISORDERS

Retinal Arterial Occlusions

Acute visual loss from retinal disease is most commonly from vascular disease. Retinal arterial occlusion, both central retinal artery occlusion (CRAO) and branch retinal artery occlusion (BRAO), causes painless loss of vision that is acute and often catastrophic. Patients with retinal artery obstruction will have visual field loss consistent with the area of oc-

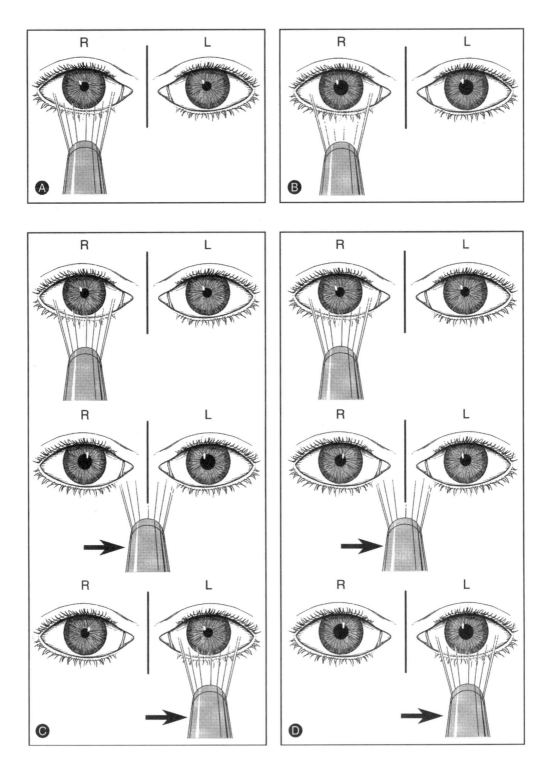

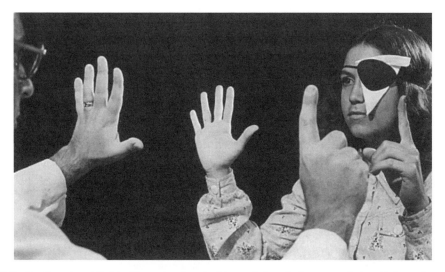

FIG. 12-2. Testing visual fields. The examiner holds each hand at one arm's length from the patient. The patient's left eye is occluded and the patient is then asked to count the number of fingers presented in the superior portion of the visual field. This should then be repeated in the inferior portion of the visual field. Alternatively, each quadrant of the visual field can be tested separately. From Skarf B, Glaser JS, Trick GL, et al. Neuro-ophthalmologic examination: the visual sensory system. In: Glaser JS, ed. *Neuro-ophthalmology*, 3rd ed. Philadelphia: Lippincott Williams & Wilkins, 1999.

clusion and those with central retinal artery occlusion will have a small RAPD and visual acuity of worse than 20/400 in most cases (Brown and Magargal, 1982). Funduscopy reveals retinal whitening (a marker of ischemia) in the area of obstruction (Fig. 12-3), which may enhance the darker appearance of the fovea ("cherry red spot"), as well as attenuation of the retinal arterioles and, occasionally, stagnant arterial blood flow ("box-carring"). The most common type of ocular arterial obstruction, CRAO, is thought to be caused by emboli, thrombosis, vasculitis, arterial spasm, and trauma.

Patients with retinal vascular arterial occlusions most commonly have vasculopathic risk factors (e.g., hypertension and diabetes), and an increase in mortality from cardiac disease and stroke, has been documented in patients with visible retinal arterial emboli (Savino et al., 1977, Klein et al., 1999). The evaluation of patients with retinal arterial occlusions remains controversial, but many authors suggest carotid ultrasonography and cardiac echocardiography as screening tests (Sharma, 1998). It is important to assess elderly patients with retinal vascular occlusions for signs and symptoms of giant cell arteritis (GCA), as this inflammatory disorder has been estimated to account for 1% of central retinal arterial occlusions. Hence, a careful funduscopic examination should document the presence of arterial emboli (Fig. 12-4), which would largely exclude GCA as a cause of arterial occlusion.

←

FIG. 12-1. The pupillary response. **A.** Light projected into the right eye causes constriction of both pupils. **B.** Light of lesser intensity than that in (A) causes pupillary constriction that is less brisk. **C.** Light first projected into the right eye is then moved to the other eye. As the light moves between the eyes, pupillary dilation occurs. This is followed by constriction when light is shown into the left eye (a normal pupillary response). **D.** Light first projected into the right eye causes constriction of both pupils. On swinging the light to the left eye, the pupils continue to dilate rather than constrict (a relative afferent pupillary defect of the left eye, also known as a "Marcus Gunn pupil"). From Foroozan R, Bailey RS. Essentials of the ophthalmologic examination. In: Maus M, Jeffers JB, Holleran DK, eds. *The clinics atlas of office procedures: essentials of ophthalmology*. Philadelphia: WB Saunders, June 2000, with permission.

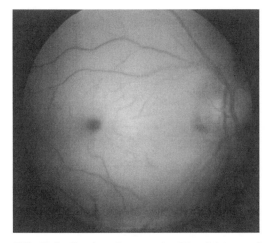

FIG. 12-3. Fundus photograph of the right eye of a patient with a central retinal arterial occlusion shows pallor within the macula and a cherry red spot. (Courtesy of the Resident Slide Collection of the Wills Eye Hospital.)

An improvement in visual outcome has been noted in anecdotal reports of CRAO with intraarterial thrombolytic therapy, hyperbaric oxygen, ocular massage, and anterior chamber paracentesis, but only early in the course (within the first 1–2 hours of symptoms) (Rumelt et al., 1999). Despite the many treatments which have been proposed for patients presenting acutely with retinal arterial occlusions, no

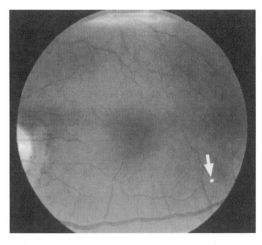

FIG. 12-4. Fundus photograph of the left eye of a patient with a retinal embolus (*arrow*). (Courtesy of the Resident Slide Collection of the Wills Eye Hospital.)

therapy has shown a definitive benefit when compared with observation.

AMAUROSIS FUGAX

Amaurosis fugax, or a temporary loss of vision, is thought to occur from a transient occlusion of the ophthalmic circulation and is a known risk factor for acute stroke. Patients often report a dimming of the vision that lasts 10 to 20 minutes before resolution. Funduscopy findings are most commonly normal, but can reveal evidence of prior retinal arterial emboli or arterial attenuation, both associated findings of hypertension. Elderly patients with amaurosis fugax should have carotid ultrasonography and cardiac echography in an attempt to find a source for the embolic phenomena (Biousse, 1997).

Amaurosis fugax was one of the three symptoms evaluated in the North American Symptomatic Carotid Endarterectomy Trial. Patients with carotid stenosis of 70% to 99% by ultrasonography who had endarterectomy had a reduced risk of subsequent stroke (9%) compared with those treated medically (26%) 2 years after treatment (North American Symptomatic Carotid Endarterectomy Trial Collaborators, 1991). In the absence of visible emboli, patients with amaurosis fugax should be evaluated for GCA with an erythrocyte sedimentation rate, because elderly patients with this disorder can present with transient episodes of visual loss. Although somewhat less common than in younger patients, elderly patients with a migraine equivalent may present with amaurosis secondary to vasospasm of the retinal circulation.

RETINAL VENOUS OBSTRUCTIONS

Acute painless loss of vision occurs with central retinal vein occlusion (CRVO). Risk factors for CRVO include hypertension, diabetes mellitus, and glaucoma (Central Vein Occlusion Study Group [CVOSG], 1993). Funduscopy reveals hemorrhagic optic disc swelling, with diffuse surrounding retinal hemorrhages and dilated and tortuous retinal veins (Fig. 12-5). Exudate and subretinal fluid within the macula—the most important prognostic factors in patients presenting with vein occlusions—is chiefly responsible for the decrease in vision at presentation. Bilateral vein occlusions are atypical and should prompt a hematologic assessment for severe anemia, hypertension, thrombocytopenia, and other blood dyscrasias.

Patients with CRVO typically have visual acuities of 20/40 or worse. Although no treatment has been

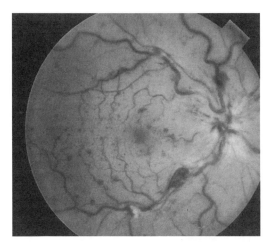

FIG. 12-5. Fundus photograph of the right eye of a patient with a central retinal vein occlusion shows hemorrhagic optic disc swelling, dilated and tortuous retinal veins, and scattered intraretinal hemorrhages. (Courtesy of the Resident Slide Collection of the Wills Eye Hospital.)

shown to result in visual improvement, ophthalmologic follow-up is essential, because as many as 30% of patients with CRVO can develop neovascularization of the iris, leading to an aggressive form of glaucoma, which requires retinal laser photocoagulation (CVOSG, 1993).

OCULAR ISCHEMIC SYNDROME

Similar fundus findings as seen in patients with CRVO can occur in patients with carotid occlusive disease. A 90% or greater occlusion of the carotid artery can lead to chronic ipsilateral diffuse retinal hemorrhages, mostly in the midperipheral retina, and dilated retinal veins, in the ocular ischemic syndrome (OIS) (Brown and Green., 1994). Patients often complain of photophobia, ocular pain, and decreased visual acuity with bright light, as the hypoxia caused by carotid insufficiency is believed to cause impairment in photoreceptor metabolism, which is accentuated in bright light. Patients can have mild corneal edema and inflammation within the anterior chamber that can cause the eye to appear red from conjunctival injection. Ocular ischemic syndrome is distinguished from CRVO by its chronic course, absence of optic nerve swelling, and absence of tortuous retinal veins. Patients with OIS should have close ophthalmologic follow-up, as chronic hypoxia of the retina predisposes to neovascularization of the iris and can cause neovascular glaucoma (Mizener et al., 1997).

ACQUIRED RETINAL DEGENERATION

Retinal dysfunction can occur in cases of cancer-associated retinopathy (CAR or MAR for melanoma-associated retinopathy). This is a paraneoplastic syndrome thought to be caused by antibodies to retinal photoreceptors, which cause photopsia (sensation of seeing lights), nyctalopia (difficulty seeing at night), and constricted visual fields associated with retinal degeneration (Keltner et al., 1992). No abnormality may be seen during funduscopy, especially early on in the disorder, and electrophysiologic studies with ERG may be required to document the reduced photoreceptor amplitudes.

OPTIC NEUROPATHY

The causes of optic neuropathy are extensive; however, optic nerve dysfunction, including a RAPD, visual field defect, acquired color vision deficit (dyschromatopsia), and impaired contrast sensitivity, are invariably present. The onset, duration, and progression of visual symptoms will help differentiate acute from chronic causes of optic nerve dysfunction. Funduscopy in optic neuropathy often shows optic disc swelling acutely; over time, however, all causes of optic neuropathy will cause the optic nerve to appear pale. In many cases (e.g., traumatic optic neuropathy and neuropathy from compressive lesions), disc swelling may not be noted because the site of pathology lies posterior to the optic nerve head.

OPTIC DISC SWELLING (DISC EDEMA)

The presence of bilateral disc edema requires immediate attention. Associated retinal hemorrhages and cotton wool spots, including cotton wool spots of the optic nerve, are suggestive of hypertensive retinopathy. Central nervous system tumors can cause bilateral disc swelling secondary to increased intracranial pressure. Thus, patients with bilateral disc edema should have their blood pressure taken and neuroimaging performed emergently to rule out a compressive lesion (see Fig. 12-6 for assessment of the elderly patient with optic disc swelling).

Unilateral disc swelling in elderly patients most commonly results from anterior ischemic optic neuropathy (AION). Nonarteritic ischemic optic neuropathy (NAION) occurs most commonly in vasculopathic patients in the fifth and sixth decades. Patients with NAION have an abrupt onset of painless visual loss (with visual acuities typically in the 20/60 to 20/200 range), often in the early morning hours, and

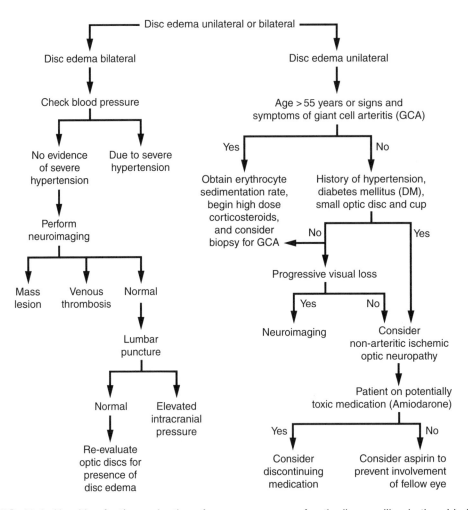

FIG. 12-6. Algorithm for the evaluation of common causes of optic disc swelling in the elderly.

an altitudinal visual field defect (Ischemic Optic Neuropathy Decompression Trial Study Group, 1996). Disc swelling, thought to be secondary to vascular insufficiency of the short posterior ciliary circulation that supplies the optic nerve head, is most often hyperemic and may be sectoral with splinter nerve fiber layer (NFL) hemorrhages. Examination of the uninvolved eye often reveals a small optic cup, suggesting a "disc at risk" for ischemia and crowding of the retinal blood vessels (Doro and Lessell, 1985). Because NAION has only rarely been associated with embolic phenomena, carotid and cardiac ultrasonography are not indicated in the evaluation of patients with typical NAION. Some risk factors for NAION have been identified, including diabetes mellitus, hypertension, smoking, and nocturnal hypotension. As

many as 10% to 40% of patients with NAION will have infarction of the fellow optic nerve (Beri et al., 1987). Although some patients with NAION may have an improvement in visual acuity over the ensuing months, most will be left with a significant visual deficit. No medical or surgical therapy has shown consistent benefit for patients with NAION. Some authors have suggested that aspirin may prevent infarction of the fellow eye (Beck et al., 1997) but long-term benefit has not been proven.

A number of patients using the antiarrhythmic amiodarone have been noted to have disc swelling that is virtually indistinguishable from that caused by NAION (Mantayjarvi et al., 1988). However, patients in some of these cases have shown a more progressive visual deficit, and bilateral involvement, which are uncommon in NAION. Amiodarone also causes crystalline deposits within the superficial cornea, in a whorl-like fashion, which are not visually disabling. Because the progression of visual loss has been halted in some patients after discontinuing this agent, patients on amiodarone with what appears to be NAION, should be carefully observed for progression and fellow eye involvement (Brazis and Lee., 1998).

Patients with diabetes mellitus, often with poorly controlled blood sugar levels, may present with hyperemic disc swelling and mild visual dysfunction (sometimes without visual complaints), which are consistent with diabetic papillopathy (Regillo et al., 1995). The disc swelling and visual deficit will typically resolve weeks to months after the onset of symptoms.

Anterior ischemic optic neuropathy from GCA occurs most commonly in patients in their sixth through eighth decades (mean age 75 years) and women are affected more commonly than men. Acute visual loss may occur after a history of brief episodes of transient visual loss. Visual acuities and visual field defects in AION caused by GCA are more commonly worse than those in patients with NAION. The disc edema of GCA is often noted to be "chalky white" in appearance because of the difffuse pallid swelling (Fig. 12-7). A history of headache, scalp tenderness, jaw claudication, fever, malaise, decreased appetite, weight loss, and symptoms of polymyalgia rheumatica should be sought (Ghanchi and Dutton., 1997). In addition to optic neuropathy from AION, other cranial nerves can be affected in GCA and diplopia, facial nerve palsy, and facial pain have been noted.

Patients suspected of having GCA should have an erythrocyte sedimentation rate (ESR) drawn and be placed on corticosteroids without delay to prevent visual loss in the fellow eye, as visual loss in the affected eye is typically irreversible. Although most patients with GCA will have an elevated ESR (up to 10% of biopsy-proved cases may not), those patients suspected of having GCA should have biopsy of the superficial temporal artery to confirm the diagnosis. An elevated C-reactive protein level may be helpful in suspicious cases with a normal ESR, and bilateral biopsy should be considered in cases with a high clinical suspicion because skip lesions can lead to a false-negative biopsy result. Most patients require high doses of corticosteroids (prednisone, 60–100 mg) for at least 6 months to 1 year and attempts to taper steroid therapy should be very gradual. Despite the differences outlined above, the disc swelling from NAION can be difficult to distinguish from that caused by GCA and an ESR study is warranted in all patients over the age of 55 years with optic disc edema.

Optic nerve tumors (e.g., malignant optic gliomas and meningiomas) can cause optic disc swelling; however, more commonly, optic atrophy is present with these lesions. Patients may present with findings suggestive of an acute optic neuropathy without evidence of optic disc swelling, the so-called "posterior ischemic optic neuropathy" (PION) thought to be caused by ischemia of the retrobulbar circulation of the optic nerve (Isayama et al., 1983). Optic neuropathy from PION has been noted after acute ischemic states, such as after cardiac bypass surgery, and in patients with GCA. Patients suspected of having PION, without a history of an acute ischemic event, should have an ESR drawn (Hayreh et al., 1998). Electrophysiologic testing showing a normal ERG and absent VEP is suggestive of PION and can confirm the diagnosis.

OPTIC ATROPHY

Glaucoma

Glaucomatous optic atrophy is characterized by optic nerve cupping and elevated intraocular pressure (IOP) in the presence of visual field defects. It is estimated that 1% to 2% of the population has glaucoma and 50% are thought to be unaware of the diagnosis (Quality of Care Committee, Glaucoma Panel, 1992). Hence, a screening fundus examination is paramount to the diagnosis. Elevated IOP, the only

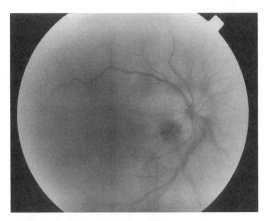

FIG. 12-7. Fundus photograph of the right eye of a patient with arteritic anterior ischemic optic neuropathy from giant cell arteritis shows pale swelling of the optic nerve head. (Courtesy of the Resident Slide Collection of the Wills Eye Hospital.)

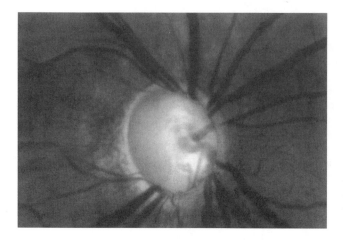

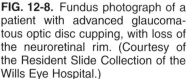

FIG. 12-8. Fundus photograph of a patient with advanced glaucomatous optic disc cupping, with loss of the neuroretinal rim. (Courtesy of the Resident Slide Collection of the Wills Eye Hospital.)

known modifiable risk factor, is not present in all cases of glaucomatous optic neuropathy. Typically, involvement is bilateral, but can be asymmetric. Older age is an important risk factor for glaucomatous optic atrophy and a family history of glaucoma is frequently present in first-degree relatives. Optic atrophy in glaucoma is typically associated with disc pallor, which coincides with the loss of the neuroretinal rim of the optic nerve head (Fig. 12-8), and pallor, which appears to be out of proportion to the degree of cupping, should prompt further investigation (American Academy of Ophthalmology [AAO], 1998). Visual loss in glaucoma is most often progressive, with loss of the peripheral visual field occurring before loss of central fixation. It is often difficult to make a diagnosis solely on one encounter, as IOP can fluctuate, and close follow-up, with quantitative visual field testing, of patients suspected of having glaucoma is paramount.

Although open angle glaucoma accounts for more than 90% of all patients with glaucoma in the United States, angle closure glaucoma can result in diffuse conjunctival injection, ocular pain, nausea, and vomiting from an extreme rise in intraocular pressure (AAO, 1998). However, some cases of chronic angle closure may not manifest the more acute findings noted above, and will require ophthalmologic examination to reveal the cause of visual dysfunction.

Optic Nerve Meningiomas

Meningiomas of the sphenoid wing and, less commonly, the optic nerve cause progressive visual loss, optic nerve pallor, and sometimes optic disc venous collaterals or "shunt vessels" (Dutton, 1992). Meningiomas are most commonly found in middle-aged

and elderly women, and an external examination may reveal a mass within the temporal fossa. Although surgical and hormonal therapies have been recommended, many patients have been sucessfully treated with radiation therapy (Lee et al., 1996).

Other Causes of Optic Atrophy

The finding of unexplained optic atrophy requires investigation. A family history of visual loss may suggest a hereditary optic neuropathy and a remote history of trauma may suggest traumatic optic neuropathy. Patients with a history of alcohol abuse and smokers are at risk for developing a form of toxic optic neuropathy characterized by visual field defects that involve fixation and the blind spot (cecocentral scotomas) (Rizzo and Lessell, 1993). In addition, a dietary history should be obtained because many of these patients are deficient in the essential B vitamins. A long list of medications is associated with optic neuropathy, which can first present acutely with disc swelling and show progressive disc pallor.

It is important to assess potentially treatable conditions that can cause unexplained optic atrophy; hence, neuroimaging with attention to the optic nerves is recommended. In addition, patients should be evaluated for syphilis, Lyme disease, and nutritional deficiency (B12 and folate).

Optic Chiasm and Optic Tracts

Vascular insufficiency and mass lesions most frequently cause disorders of the optic chiasm and optic tracts. Involvement of the optic chiasm or tracts causes similar signs and symptoms, as found in patients with optic neuropathy, but because of decussation of the nasal retinal ganglion cells, these more posterior lesions cause binocular visual field defects.

Pituitary adenomas are the most common cause of chiasmal dysfunction and, as these tumors enlarge superiorly, involvement of the chiasm progresses. Visual acuity may be normal and the only finding may be a bitemporal visual field defect because of the involvement of the crossing nasal fibers of each optic nerve. However, progression of the lesion will cause optic neuropathy and decreased vision, which can occur acutely if the tumor hemorrhages, as in pituitary apoplexy. Chronic compression of the optic chiasm will result in optic neuropathy, which can be bilateral. Hemorrhage of enlarging pituitary adenomas can cause compression within the cavernous sinus and multiple cranial nerve palsies. Pituitary apoplexy is an ophthalmic, endocrinologic, and, neurosurgical emergency because infarction can lead to both an acute cortisol insufficiency, requiring intravenous corticosteroids, and blindness from chiasmal compression (Glaser, 1999). Other lesions that can cause chiasmal dysfunction include craniopharyngiomas (a second peak of incidence occurs in the elderly), meningiomas, and arterial aneurysms.

Lesions of the optic tract result in homonymous hemianopias because they contain ipsilateral temporal retinal fibers and contralateral nasal retinal fibers. The cause of optic tract lesions is similar to that of chiasmal lesions and longstanding lesions result in optic atrophy.

Posterior Afferent Pathway

Unilateral involvement of the lateral geniculate nucleus (LGN), optic radiations, and occipital cortex, most commonly from cerebrovascular disease, results in binocular visual field defects without affecting visual acuity. The more posterior the lesion, the more congruous the visual field defect (Rizzo and Barton, 1999).

Patients with homonymous hemianopias from parietal lobe disease may have an associated disturbance of higher cortical function (e.g., agnosia, alexia, and dyscalculia). Visual loss from bilateral occipital disease results in a visual deficit with normal pupillary responses (Rizzo and Barton, 1999). Patients with cortical visual loss may not be aware of their deficit (Anton's syndrome) and claim that they can see, in the absence of dementia or delirium.

Bilateral involvement of the mesial anterior and mesial occipital lobes will result in cerebral dyschromatopsia, most commonly with an associated superior visual field defect. Loss of facial recognition,

prosopagnosia, is also thought to be caused by disorders of the medial occipitotemporal cortex. Cortical disconnection syndromes (e.g., alexia without agraphia), in which the patient can write but cannot read, because of involvement of the splenium of the corpus callosum and the dominant occipital cortex, demonstrate the complexity of higher cortical function.

Visual hallucinations associated with visual deficits (Charles Bonnet syndrome), especially in the elderly, have been well described. These hallucinations are commonly formed and occur in a lucid state, with patients commonly aware that what they are "seeing" is really not there. Most hallucinations are well tolerated, especially with reassurance (Teunisse et al., 1995).

Patients with neurodegenerative disorders may present with visual complaints, despite normal visual acuity and a normal ocular examination. Disturbances can include visual blurring, difficulty reaching for objects, and impaired depth perception. However, these rarely occur in isolation and are often associated with other disorders of higher cortical function. Late in the course, these patients may develop visual hallucinations (Rizzo and Barton, 1999).

EFFERENT VISUAL SYSTEM

Assessment of Ocular Alignment and Extraocular Motility

To assess ocular alignment and extraocular motility, the patient should fixate at a distant object, while the examiner occludes one eye. If the uncovered eye turns to achieve fixation, this implies that the eye was not previously in alignment. If the refixation movement is in the nasal direction, then the eye was initially temporal and the deviation is known as an "exodeviation." If the refixation movement is in the temporal direction, an esodeviation is present. Prisms can be used to quantitate the angle of deviation.

The actions of the six extraocular muscles (Table 12-1) should be tested by instructing the patient to look in the direction of the muscle's greatest action. Each muscle and its yoke-pair act to move the eyes in the same direction of gaze. In right gaze, for example, the right lateral rectus muscle abducts the right eye while the left medial rectus muscle adducts the left eye.

Diplopia

Patients with diplopia often report perceiving two images of a single object, with the image of the more dominant eye being clearer than that of the fellow

TABLE 12-1. *Primary functions of the extraocular muscles*

Muscle	Function	Innervation
Lateral rectus	Abduction	VI cranial nerve
Medial rectus	Adduction	III cranial nerve
Superior rectus	Elevation	III cranial nerve
Inferior rectus	Depression	III cranial nerve
Superior oblique	Intorsion	IV cranial nerve
Inferior oblique	Extorsion	III cranial nerve

eye. However, diplopia from a small ocular misalignment can produce "blurred" images as the brain attempts to fuse the two images. Hence, the evaluation of unexplained visual blurring should assess the oculomotor system.

In evaluating a patient with diplopia, establish whether the symptoms occur under monocular or binocular conditions. Diplopia that persists despite occlusion of the fellow eye is, with rare exception, secondary to an ocular media disturbance (e.g., corneal irregularity, cataract, subluxed lens). Patients with monocular diplopia often report that they see blurred, multiple, or "ghost" images rather than two images, and a pinhole (2–3 mm in diameter) placed in front of the eye will often eliminate the blurred images.

Diplopia that is relieved with occlusion of one eye is suggestive of ocular misalignment. By quantifying the deviation in primary gaze (straight gaze), left, right, up, downgaze, and on head tilt to the right and left, the examiner can determine whether the deviation is comitant (the same or similar in each position of gaze) or incomitant (different, depending on gaze direction). Comitant horizontal deviations should be measured with the patient fixing at a distant object and again at a near object.

Third Nerve Palsy

The oculomotor nerve is composed of parasympathetic fibers, from the Edinger-Westphal nucleus, and fibers of the subnuclei of motor neurons to each of the extraocular muscles. The nuclear centers for the third cranial nerve are in the midbrain, at the level of the red nuclei. The oculomotor nerves run anteriorly in the midbrain, adjacent to the cerebral peduncles, and into the subarachnoid space to lie between the superior cerebellar and the posterior cerebral arteries (Glaser and Siatkowski, 1999). The third nerve then courses into the wall of the cavernous sinus and enters the superior orbital fissure, branching into superior (supplying the levator palpebrae superioris and superior rectus muscles) and inferior (supplying the inferior oblique, medial rectus muscle, and the parasympathetic fibers to the ciliary ganglion, which innervate the iris sphincter) divisions. In addition to the iris sphincter, the ciliary ganglion also innervates the ciliary muscle, which stimulates accommodation of the lens. Only isolated third nerve palsy (TNP) will be discussed here, and any patient with evidence of dysfunction of more than a single cranial nerve requires further investigation. Patients with TNP may complain of pain, horizontal diplopia (in cases of incomplete ptosis), or ptosis (Glaser and Siatkowski, 1999).

Nuclear and fascicular lesions, which frequently have accompanying neurologic signs (tremor from involvement of the red nuclei [Benedikt syndrome], hemiparesis from involvement of the cerebral peduncles [Weber syndrome], and ataxia from involvement of the superior cerebellar peduncle [Nothnagel syndrome]), are most commonly caused by ischemic injury. Because of the anatomy of the third nerve nucleus, an isolated unilateral complete TNP is unlikely to be from a nuclear lesion.

In the subarachnoid space, the third nerve is vulnerable to mass lesions, the most common being cerebral arterial aneurysms. Because the parasympathetic fibers course in the periphery of the nerve compressive lesions causing complete TNP involve the pupil in addition to the extraocular muscles. However, in incomplete TNP the pupil may not be affected initially, hence, these patients should be followed daily for at least 1 week to confirm that the pupil does not dilate.

Vascular insufficiency is the most common cause of TNP in the elderly, with most patients having a history of diabetes mellitus or hypertension. GCA rarely causes TNP, and elderly patients with diplopia should be questioned for symptoms of GCA. Because the pupillary fibers course in the periphery of the nerve, collateral blood flow is thought to spare the parasympathetic fibers in cases of vascular TNP. Despite this, pupillary dysfunction indistinguishable from that caused by mass lesions can still occur in vascular TNP; thus, any patient with TNP who has pupillary involvement should have a neuroimaging study with magnetic resonance imaging (MRI) and magnetic resonance angiography (MRA) or routine angiography. The role of MRA versus routine angiography is controversial; however, angiography is currently the standard, because smaller aneurysms capable of causing a third nerve palsy may be missed with MRA.

Vascular TNP typically improves within 2 to 4 months after the onset of symptoms; thus, patients suspected of having a vascular TNP should have a neuroimaging study if progression of the TNP is noted or the symptoms fail to improve.

Lesions within the cavernous sinus, superior orbital fissure, and orbit rarely cause isolated TNP because of involvement of the surrounding structures. However, both isolated superior and inferior division TNP do occur. Because it is rare for the muscles innervated by the oculomotor nerve to be involved singly and in isolation, other conditions such as thyroid eye disease and myasthenia gravis should be considered in these cases.

Aberrant regeneration, an anomalous rewiring of damaged neurons, can occur months after the onset of TNP from compressive lesions. Neuronal misdirection can result in abnormal movements such as eyelid elevation on downgaze and pupillary constriction with adduction. Because this neuronal miss wiring occurs almost exclusively with compressive lesions, patients followed for presumed vascular TNP should have a neuroimaging study if aberrant regeneration is noted.

Fourth Nerve Palsy

The fourth nerve nuclei, which lie caudal to the third nerve nuclei within the midbrain, send crossed fibers that exit dorsally from the brainstem (Glaser and Siatkowski, 1999). These fibers run anteriorly to enter the wall of the cavernous sinus and then through the superior orbital fissure to innervate the superior oblique muscle. Trauma, in which patients often have bilateral involvement, and ischemic injury are the most common causes of fourth nerve paresis.

Patients with fourth nerve palsies typically complain of vertical diplopia because the superior oblique muscle acts to infraduct the eye, and they may adopt a compensatory head tilt, which can diminish the vertical deviation. The superior rectus and superior oblique muscles act to intort the eye (rotate the 12 o'-clock meridian inward, toward the patient's nose), whereas the inferior rectus and oblique muscles act to extort the eye. Thus, fourth nerve palsies will result in extorsion as well as supraduction of the affected eye.

The diagnosis should be made using the three-step test for vertical diplopia described elsewhere (Glaser and Siatkowski, 1999).

Vasculopathic patients with isolated acquired fourth nerve palsies may be observed (see discussion of third nerve palsy above). If the fourth nerve palsy is progressive or if symptoms do not improve after several months, neuroimaging should be performed.

Sixth Nerve Palsy

The sixth cranial nerves arise in the pons and exit the brainstem anteriorly to rise up the clivus (where the two nerves are closest together) and pierce the dura at Dorello's canal, which bridges the petrous portion of the temporal bone (Glaser and Siatkowski, 1999). The sixth nerve travels in the cavernous sinus under the internal carotid artery (where it can be compressed by an aneurysm of the carotid artery) and anteriorly to enter the superior orbital fissure and innervate the lateral rectus muscle. Patients with sixth nerve palsies will present with esotropia, which increases with gaze toward the affected side. Patients may adopt a head turn toward the involved side to put the affected eye in an adducted position and minimize the diplopia.

Within the brainstem, the sixth nerve nucleus lies adjacent to the horizontal gaze center and has neurons destined for the contralateral medial rectus subnucleus, so that a nuclear sixth lesion, most commonly from ischemia, will produce an ipsilateral gaze palsy. Fascicular lesions involving the pyramidal tract can cause an ipsilateral abduction deficit with contralateral hemiplegia (Millard-Gubler syndrome).

At Dorello's canal, the sixth nerve is vulnerable to compressive forces that are generated with increased intracranial pressure. Thus, any cause of increased intracranial pressure, including central nervous system masses and venous sinus thrombosis, can cause unilateral or bilateral sixth nerve palsies. Inflammation of the petrous portion of the temporal bone can affect the sixth nerve (Gradenigo syndrome) and inflammation of the adjacent fifth nerve ganglion can cause a painful sixth nerve palsy. Within the cavernous sinus, superior orbital fissure, and orbit, the sixth nerve is rarely affected in isolation.

As with isolated third and fourth nerve palsy, vasculopathic patients with sixth nerve palsy initially may be observed. All elderly patients should be questioned regarding signs and symptoms of GCA, as sixth nerve palsy has rarely been a presenting manifestation of this disorder.

Thyroid Eye Disease

Thyroid eye disease is the most frequent cause of acquired diplopia that is not secondary to extraocular muscle palsy (Scott and Siatkowski, 1999). It occurs more frequently in women than men and, although thyroid function testing is abnormal in most cases, patients with thyroid eye disease can be hyperthyroid, hypothyroid, or euthyroid. Furthermore, systemic treatment of thyroid dysfunction may have little or no change on the signs and symptoms of thyroid eye disease. The pathogenesis for this disorder remains unknown, but the clinical manifestations are well recognized.

Patients present with proptosis (thyroid eye disease is the most common cause of unilateral or bilateral proptosis in adults), eyelid retraction (in part because of sympathetic stimulation of Müller's muscle in the upper eyelid) causing the thyroid "stare," eyelid lag in downgaze, and disturbances in ocular motility (Fig. 12-9). Involvement of the inferior rectus muscle is most common, followed by the medial rectus, superior rectus, and lateral rectus muscles. Thus, limitation in upgaze is the most common abnormality of ocular motility, although nearly any pattern of abnormal extraocular motility can be seen. Orbital imaging with computed tomography (CT) scan or MRI shows enlargement of the extraocular muscles, with sparing of the muscle tendons, including in asymptomatic patients with thyroid eye disease (Trokel and Hilal, 1979).

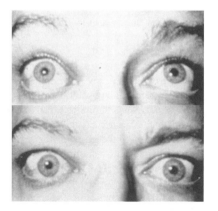

FIG. 12-9. Composite external photographs of a patient with thyroid eye disease shows restriction in upgaze (*top*), proptosis with bilateral eyelid retraction (*bottom*), and conjunctival injection over the insertion of the right lateral rectus muscle (*both*). (Courtesy of the Resident Slide Collection of the Wills Eye Hospital.)

Enlargement of the extraocular muscles can result in compression of the optic nerve at the orbital apex and subsequent visual loss with associated visual field defects. Lid and periorbital swelling may be noted, and examination of the conjunctiva may reveal chemosis (edema of the conjunctiva) and engorged vessels over the insertions of the extraocular muscles. The proptosis can lead to vision-threatening corneal exposure from inadequate eyelid closure. Corneal exposure should be managed with lubricant ointments and can, rarely, require surgical therapy.

Smoking has been associated with an increased risk of thyroid eye disease in patients with thyroid dysfunction and in a worsening of ocular symptoms in patients with preexisting thyroid eye disease (Brix et al., 2000). Recent studies suggest that treatment with radioactive iodine, without concurrent steroid treatment, has an adverse effect on thyroid eye disease (Rasmussen et al., 2000). Systemic corticosteroids can be used for patients who have acute exacerbations of thyroid eye disease. Patients who respond will typically do so within the first several weeks of therapy and, thus, prolonged courses with steroids should be avoided. Low-dose orbital radiation (20 Gy) can cause involution of active inflammation; however, acute congestion with optic neuropathy sometimes requires surgical orbital decompression to relieve crowding of the orbital apex.

The differential diagnosis of thyroid eye disease (Table 12-2) should include idiopathic orbital pseudotumor, an orbital inflammatory disorder of unknown cause, which can present with proptosis, ocular pain, and injection that mimics orbital cellulitis (Chavis et al., 1978). Orbital imaging shows inflammatory signs of the involved tissue (lacrimal gland, orbital fat, or extraocular muscles) and, in the case of extraocular muscle involvement, involvement of the tendonous insertion. Findings that help differentiate this inflammatory disorder from infection typically include the lack of fever, neutrophilia, and other systemic symptoms. Patients with orbital pseudotumor show dramatic improvement with corticosteroid therapy.

Immunosuppressed patients with ophthalmoplegia, especially diabetics, should be evaluated for fungal infections. Invasive fungal infections, such as that caused by mucormycosis, can cause progressive ophthalmoplegia with invasion of the cavernous sinus that is life-threatening, even in the absence of obvious ocular inflammatory signs (Ferry and Abedi, 1983). An otolaryngologic consultation to assess the nasal and sinus mucosa may reveal the characteristic black mucosal eschar.

TABLE 12-2. *Differential diagnosis of common orbital diseases of the elderly*

	Thyroid eye disease	Orbital pseudotumor	Orbital infection	Arteriovenous fistula
Ocular signs and symptoms	Proptosis, corneal exposure, eyelid lag, eyelid retraction, rarely visual loss, diplopia	Proptosis, pain, conjunctival injection, rarely visual loss, eyelid swelling, and erythema	Ophthalmoplegia, visual loss, eyelid swelling, and erythema	Proptosis, injection elevated intraocular pressure, pulsatile tinnitus
Orbital imaging	Enlargement of extraocular muscles sparing tendons	Enlargement of extraocular muscles, including tendons, enlargement of lacrimal gland, inflammation of orbital fat	Contiguous sinus disease, involvement of cavernous sinus	Enlargement of extraocular muscles, dilated superior ophthalmic vein
Systemic findings	History of thyroid disease, may be euthyroid	Occasional association with collagen vascular disease	Fever, immunosuppression (especially diabetes mellitus)	Hypertension

Elderly patients, especially women, are at risk for developing spontaneous low-flow dural-venous fistulas that result in proptosis, mild ocular discomfort, and conjunctival injection (Troost, 1999). These low-flow fistulae, which most commonly occur from the communication between small meningeal arteries and the cavernous sinus, can cause pulsatile tinnitus. Impaired venous return from orbital congestion can cause elevated IOP. Angiography with embolization can close these fistulas, although many will close spontaneously.

Myasthenia Gravis

Myasthenia gravis (MG) is a disorder of the voluntary muscles, commonly involving the face, limb girdle, extraocular muscles, and eyelids. Antibodies to the acetylcholine receptors found on striated muscle endplates are responsible for impaired synaptic transmission, which worsens with prolonged stimulation. Although most patients will have systemic involvement, up to 75% of them will present with only ocular involvement (Weinberg et al., 1994).

The earliest signs of MG may be ptosis and ophthalmoplegia. The ptosis is often worse at the end of the day and improves with rest. The ice test (a surgical glove filled with ice and placed over the eyelids for 2 minutes) frequently improves the ptosis caused by MG (Kubis et al., 2000). The ophthalmoplegia of MG can involve any of the extraocular muscles and produce any pattern of strabismus; however, MG does not cause clinical pupillary dysfunction. Sustained upgaze can be tested to fatigue the extraocular muscles and eyelids and elicit an ocular deviation or ptosis that may not be apparent during the initial assessment. Testing orbicularis oculi strength may reveal impairment of voluntary eyelid closure.

Although the diagnosis of MG is primarily a clinical one, several tests can aid the clinician, especially in atypical cases. Intravenous injection of edrophonium (Tensilon), a short-acting antiacetylcholinesterase agent, can improve the signs of MG within minutes after infusion (Fig. 12-10). Side effects of Tensilon include bradycardia and bronchospasm, potentially lethal in the elderly; hence, some are reluctant to perform Tensilon testing in an office setting. Antiacetylcholine receptor antibodies, found in 80% to 90% of patients with generalized MG, are seen in 50% to 60% of patients with isolated ocular myasthenia (Vincent and Newsom-Davis, 1982). Nerve conduction studies with repetitive stimulation show an abnormal decrement in approximately 70% of patients with ocular MG. Single fiber

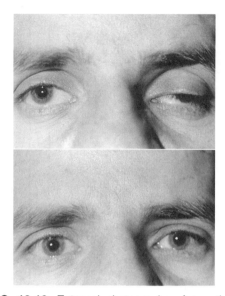

FIG. 12-10. External photographs of a patient with left upper eyelid ptosis from myasthenia gravis before edrophonium (Tensilon) (*top*) injection and improvement of ptosis after injection of Tensilon (*bottom*). (Courtesy of the Resident Slide Collection of the Wills Eye Hospital.)

electromyography of the orbicularis oculi muscle demonstrates impaired impulses, which are seen in at least 90% of ocular MG (Padua et al., 2000). Because thymomas occur in 10% of patients with MG, imaging of the mediastinum should be performed.

Although anticholinesterase agents have been the mainstay for treatment of MG, ocular myasthenia often does not respond adequately to the typical doses used for systemic MG. Corticosteroids can ease the diplopia in some patients and may reduce the risk of progression to generalized MG, but not without the risk of steroid-induced side effects (Kaminski and Daroff, 2000). Immunosuppressive agents (e.g., azathioprine and cyclosporine) can be considered, but their side effects are concerning.

DISORDERS OF GAZE

Dorsal Midbrain Syndrome

The dorsal midbrain syndrome consists of deficiency of upgaze, poorly reactive pupils that show light-near dissociation, and convergence-retraction movements with attempted upgaze. Most commonly, this occurs with mass lesions in the area of the dorsal midbrain (Leigh et al., 1999).

Progressive Supranuclear Palsy

Progressive supranuclear palsy is a progressive disorder of vertical gaze that typically begins with impaired downgaze greater than upgaze, prompting many patients to note an inability to see food at mealtime and experience difficulty walking down steps (Leigh et al., 1999). The supranuclear origin of this disorder implies that the brainstem-mediated reflexes (e.g., the oculovestibular reflex) are intact. Saccadic eye movements are affected more commonly than smooth pursuit, and patients may have a parkinsonian gait and rigidity, especially of the neck.

Vertical Ocular Deviations

Rapid downward movements of the eyes followed by a slower return is seen in ocular bobbing, most commonly from pontine lesions (Dell'Osso and Daroff, 1999). Damage within the brainstem, most commonly from ischemic insults, results in slow, pendular vertical eye movements that appear to be rhythmic with movements of the palate in oculopalatal myoclonus. A skew deviation is an acquired vertical deviation (often comitant) that cannot be ascribed to dysfunction of a single cranial nerve or extraocular muscle (Leigh et al., 1999). Skew deviation causes vertical diplopia, which often results from ischemic insults within the posterior fossa.

Internuclear Ophthalmoplegia

Internuclear ophthalmoplegia (INO) results from disruption of the medial longitudinal fasciculus (MLF), which ascends from the sixth nerve nucleus to the contralateral medial rectus subnucleus within the brainstem (Hamilton, 1999). Ischemic stroke is the most common cause of INO in the elderly. Interruption of the MLF results in an ipsilateral adduction deficit and the fellow eye will often show a jerk nystagmus that increases with abduction.

Convergence Insufficiency

The area responsible for convergence lies within the midbrain. Patients with convergence insufficiency may have diplopia or blurring at near, with the ability to fuse at distance (Siatkowski and Glaser, 1999). Examination will reveal fusion at distance but an exodeviation near, despite the presence of normal extraocular motility. Patients with this finding should have a neuroimaging study to exclude a midbrain lesion.

Divergence Insufficiency

Divergence insufficiency results in a symptomatic exodeviation at distance with fusion at near vision. It is a nonlocalizing cause of diplopia which, in the elderly, often results from pontine ischemia (Leigh et al., 1999).

NYSTAGMUS

Nystagmus is an oscillatory movement of the globes characterized by a rhythmic to-and-fro movement caused by a breakdown in fusional or gaze mechanisms (Dell'Osso and Daroff, 1999). It is categorized as "pendular" if the movements are of equal velocity in each direction and "jerk" if the movements are slow in one direction and fast in another. The direction of nystagmus is defined as the direction of the fast phase. Other descriptive features (e.g., amplitude, frequency, velocity, and axis of rotation) are used clinically to characterize the different forms of nystagmus.

Patients with acquired nystagmus often complain of oscillopsia, a visual shaking, and blurred vision; to minimize their symptoms, patients may hold their head in a position (the null point) that minimizes the nystagmus. Either pendular or jerk nystagmus can be seen in patients with poor visual acuity of longstanding duration.

Gaze-Evoked Nystagmus

Gaze-evoked nystagmus is a jerk nystagmus that occurs in the affected direction but not in primary gaze. This type of nystagmus is nonlocalizing, but often occurs from medications (ethanol, sedatives, illicit drugs) and lesions within the posterior fossa (Dell'Osso and Daroff, 1999). Poor cerebellar control is thought to contribute to impairment of the ability to hold the eyes in eccentric gaze.

Periodic Alternating Nystagmus

Periodic alternating nystagmus (PAN) is a horizontal jerk nystagmus that is intermittent, lasting 1 to 2 minutes, before spontaneously reversing (Dell'Osso and Daroff, 1999). Lesions of the cervicomedullary junction often cause this type of nystagmus. Treatment with baclofen has been successful in some of these patients.

Convergence-Retraction Nystagmus

Convergence-retraction nystagmus is characteristic of the dorsal midbrain syndrome that consists of light-near dissociation and impaired upgaze (Dell'Osso and Daroff, 1999). This eye movement, although not true nystagmus, is elicited by downward rotation of a vertical optokinetic drum, which produces fast upward reflexive movements. Instead of the normal reflexive upward movement, the globes retract and the palpebral fissures narrow.

See-Saw Nystagmus

Parachiasmal and upper midbrain lesions, rarely, result in a dissociated nystagmus in which one eye rises and intorts while the other eye falls and extorts, similar to a see-saw (Dell'Osso and Daroff, 1999).

Downbeat Nystagmus

Downbeat nystagmus is a jerk nystagmus, with the fast phase downward, which increases in downgaze (Dell'Osso and Daroff, 1999). Patients are particularly bothered when reading because of the increase in intensity on downgaze. Disorders of the cervicomedullary junction (especially the Arnold-Chiari malformation), drug intoxication, magnesium deficiency, vitamin deficiency, lithium toxicity, and ischemic stroke have all caused this form of nystagmus.

Opsoclonus

Opsoclonus is a random movement of the eyes that can be intermittent or constant. The rapid saccadic movements are in all directions and appear chaotic, without an identifiable pattern. Opsoclonus can be a marker of an underlying malignancy, most commonly a paraneoplastic syndrome, or can occur after viral encephalitis (Herishanu et al., 1985).

ANISOCORIA AND PUPILLARY DYSFUNCTION

Anisocoria is a difference in pupillary size (diameter), and a difference in pupillary diameters of 1 mm or greater is generally accepted as clinically significant (Kawasaki, 1999). To establish which eye is abnormal, measure the pupil size in light and then in dark and record the pupillary diameters. Disparity in pupil size that remains the same in light and dark is characteristic of physiologic anisocoria. To avoid the miosis that occurs with the near response, examine the pupils while the patient views a distant object.

Disparity in pupil size that increases in dark is characteristic of Horner's syndrome, with the miotic pupil failing to dilate appropriately. The presence of a Horner's syndrome can be confirmed by looking for delayed dilation of the miotic pupil with darkness (dilation lag). Pharmacologic testing with 4% to 10% cocaine in each eye will fail to dilate the pupil normally in a patient with Horner's syndrome. Hydroxyamphetamine drops can localize (preganglionic versus postganglionic see below) the Horner's syndrome.

Disparity in pupil size greater in light is generally from four causes: iris trauma, Adie's pupil, third nerve palsy, and pharmacologic dilation. Pupils that are abnormally large in light may show irregularities along the pupillary border or evidence of prior surgery, which can impair constriction to light.

An Adie's pupil (tonic pupil) is an irregularly dilated pupil that shows minimal reaction to light and is slow to constrict with convergence (Kawasaki, 1999). With slit lamp examination, sectorial constriction of the pupil may be seen, with one portion of the iris showing undulating movements. Most commonly, it occurs in women and is unilateral. Because the Adie's pupil is thought to occur from neuronal denervation, the iris demonstrates supersensitivity and constricts with 0.125% pilocarpine drops. Systemic findings can occur with decreased deep tendon reflexes (Adie's syndrome), and further evaluation rarely may be necessary as the tonic pupil has been seen in patients with syphilis and Lyme disease.

The pupillary dilation of TNP rarely occurs in the absence of other signs of third nerve dysfunction. However, in cases requiring confirmation of pupillary involvement, 1% pilocarpine instilled into the affected eye will constrict the pupil, whereas 0.125% pilocarpine generally will not (Kawasaki, 1999), although supersensitivity has been described in some cases of third nerve palsy. Pharmacologic dilation, whether knowingly self-induced or accidental, will not typically respond to 1% pilocarpine, and the pupil will remain dilated.

Light-Near Dissociation

Light-near dissociation occurs when the pupils fail to react to light but constrict with convergence. Historically, this finding was associated with tertiary syphilis (Argyll Robertson pupils), but it can be seen in diabetics, TNP with aberrant regeneration, bilateral optic nerve disease, dorsal midbrain syndrome, central nervous system lesions, and in Adie's pupils (Slamovits and Glaser, 1999).

Horner's Syndrome

Horner's syndrome results from a disturbance in the sympathetic pathway, which contains three neurons: The first neuron begins in the hypothalamus and descends to synapse in the cervical and superior thoracic spinal cord. The second neuron, with its cell body within the spinal cord, ascends to synapse in the superior cervical ganglion in the region of the angle of the mandible. The third neuron, with its body in the superior cervical ganglion, ascends with the carotid artery, through the cavernous sinus and orbital fissures, to innervate the dilator muscle of the iris via the long ciliary nerves.

Patients with Horner's syndrome may present because of ptosis, miosis, or may be diagnosed on screening examination (Fig. 12-11). Ptosis of the upper eyelid caused by Horner's syndrome is rarely greater than 2 mm and occurs because of interruption of the sympathetic pathway to Müller's muscle. The miosis and resultant pupil disparity that occur in Horner's syndrome is more apparent in dark than in light.

The causes of Horner's syndrome vary, depending on which neuron is involved (Kawasaki, 1999). The most common cause of first order Horner's syndrome in the elderly is vascular insufficiency in the brainstem, and often patients will have other neurologic signs and symptoms. Lung masses are the most common cause of second order lesions, as the apex of the lung rests adjacent to the pathway of the fibers headed to the superior cervical ganglion. Third order Horner's syndrome is frequently associated with headache syndromes (e.g., cluster headaches and migraine), cavernous sinus lesions, and internal carotid dissection.

Determining the order of the lesion in Horner's syndrome can be achieved by pharmacologic testing. Hydroxyamphetamine (1%), which stimulates the sympathetic nerve terminals to release norepinephrine, causes pupillary dilation in first and second order Horner's syndrome. Third order lesions involve the adrenergic nerve endings, which are responsible for the release of norepinephrine, hence the pupil in these lesions will not dilate with hydroxyamphetamine. It is important to note that testing with cocaine and hydroxyamphetamine should be separated by 24 hours.

An important cause of third order Horner's syndrome is internal carotid dissection. Although a history of trauma is often elicited, spontaneous dissection or exertion from the Valsalva maneuver or repetitive coughing can lead to disruption of the sympathetic chain. Patients may complain of dysgeusia, pulsatile tinnitus, and transient visual loss. These patients require immediate attention with MRI and MRA of the neck and brain to identify the intraluminal flap characteristic of carotid dissection because, within 6 days of symptom onset, 30% of patients with internal carotid dissection will have a stroke, which may be prevented by anticoagulation (Biousse et al., 1998).

NEURO-OPHTHALMIC DISORDERS OF THE EYELID AND FACE

Blepharoptosis (Ptosis)

Blepharoptosis (ptosis) is the term used when the upper eyelid margin hangs lower than its normal position. The upper eyelid normally covers the superior sclera completely, with the margin of the eyelid lying between the limbus superiorly and the superior pupillary margin. The lower lid margin rests just at the inferior limbus.

Causes of acquired ptosis are divided into the following categories: mechanical, aponeurotic, neuro-

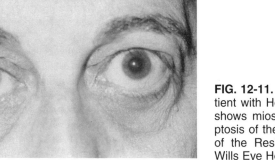

FIG. 12-11. External photograph of a patient with Horner's syndrome on the right shows miosis of the right pupil and mild ptosis of the right upper eyelid. (Courtesy of the Resident Slide Collection of the Wills Eye Hospital.)

genic, and myogenic. Mechanical ptosis arises from a compression of the upper lid, most commonly from mass lesions, scarring, and redundant skin folds. Obvious mass lesions can often be palpated through the eyelid skin. Lifting redundant eyelid skin may reveal a normal upper lid margin and eyelid function. Aponeurotic ptosis results from a dehiscence of the tendon of the levator muscle from the superior tarsus.

The most important causes of neurogenic ptosis are from third nerve palsy and Horner's syndrome. Complete TNP results in complete ptosis from involvement of the nerve to the levator; hence, levator function is impaired but position of the lid crease is normal. Thus, patients with TNP may not complain of diplopia because of occlusion of the involved visual axis. Incomplete TNP often results in incomplete ptosis, which is typically greater than 1 to 2 mm. Ptosis in Horner's syndrome occurs because of dysfunction of Müller's muscle, resulting in a mild neurogenic ptosis (1–2 mm). Myogenic ptosis most frequently occurs from myasthenia gravis. A less common cause of myogenic ptosis is chronic progressive external ophthalmoplegia (CPEO), which results from a mitochondrial abnormality. Patients present with progressive ophthalmoplegia and ptosis, which are typically bilateral. Patients with CPEO can have an associated retinal pigmentary degeneration and cardiac conduction defects (Kearns-Sayre syndrome) (Moraes et al., 1989).

Trigeminal Neuralgia

Rapid attacks of sharp, jabbing pain (lasting seconds) within the distribution of the trigeminal nerve are characteristic of trigeminal neuralgia (Troost, 1999). The onset is most common in the sixth and seventh decade, occurring more in women than men. An aberrant vessel is believed to compress the fifth nerve sensory root as it enters the pons in some cases, although multiple sclerosis (especially if bilateral) and tumors are other causes. Carbamazepine and baclofen have been used successfully in many patients, although some require surgical intervention.

Bell's Palsy

Bell's palsy is the most common cause of facial nerve dysfunction, with an increasing incidence with age. Although the pathophysiology of Bell's palsy is unknown, antecedent viral illnesses (including that from herpes zoster and simplex), diabetes mellitus, and thyroid dysfunction are predisposing factors.

Signs and symptoms develop over hours to days, with unilateral facial weakness, impaired eyelid closure, and tearing. Evaluation of patients with Bell's palsy should exclude central nervous system involvement or evidence of other cranial nerve palsies, which require neuroimaging. Other secondary causes of facial dysfunction include that caused by Lyme disease and sarcoidosis.

Ocular involvement should be assessed by testing orbicularis oculi strength, looking for lagophthalmos (inability to achieve full eyelid closure), and testing of the Bell's phenomenon (reflexive rotation of the globes superiorly with forced eyelid closure). Each of these tests will aid in determining the risk of corneal exposure.

Although 80% to 90% of patients with Bell's palsy will have spontaneous recovery, improvement of facial nerve function is most often incomplete and elderly patients have a poorer prognosis (Peitersen, 1982). Aberrant regeneration of the facial nerve can lead to abnormal facial muscle activity with movement of the mouth or excessive tearing with mastication (crocodile tears).

Corticosteroids have had a beneficial effect on the recovery of some patients with Bell's palsy. Because cases of Bell's palsy have been associated with herpes virus infections, acyclovir may be considered in these patients as well (Adour et al., 1996). Patients at risk for corneal exposure can be treated with topical lubricants, eyelid taping, and moisture chambers. Some patients may require surgical intervention with tarsorrhaphy and implanted eyelid weights to achieve eyelid closure and preserve corneal integrity.

Essential Blepharospasm

Essential blepharospasm is a repetitive, bilateral contraction of the facial musculature, most commonly affecting the orbicularis oculi and periocular muscles. Essential blepharospasm occurs more commonly in women, rarely under the age of 50. Frequently, the duration and frequency of contractions increase as the disorder progresses and complete eyelid closure can lead to a functional impairment of vision in some patients.

Examination of the ocular surface for irritants, signs of dry eye syndrome (e.g., keratopathy or poor tear film), and ocular inflammation are necessary because each of these disorders can cause a repetitive eyelid closure that mimics essential blepharospasm.

Treatment with local intramuscular injections of botulinum toxin (BTX), which interrupts release of acetylcholine from the nerve terminals, has been shown to be effective in reducing the contractions in essential blepharospasm (Jordan et al., 1989). In most patients, the effect lasts 3 to 6 months, with the need for further injections as the treatment effect wanes. Although local effects (e.g., ptosis, diplopia, and ecchymosis) can occur, reports of systemic toxicity from BTX are rare. Extensive myectomy (Anderson procedure) for patients unresponsive to BTX has been reported in some centers (Jordan et al, 1989).

Hemifacial Spasm

Repetitive, unilateral facial contractions are characteristic of hemifacial spasm. As with essential blepharospasm, the contractions, which can be localized, can progressively involve the entire side of the face (Fig. 12-12). Some patients with hemifacial spasm may have an aberrant course of a small artery that compresses the facial nerve, whereas others have rarely been associated with tumors of the parotid gland and cerebellopontine angle. Therefore, neuroimaging of the course of the facial nerve should be performed. Treatment with BTX (see above) has been effective, however some patients have undergone surgical decompression of the facial nerve at the skull base (Jannetta procedure) (Jannetta et al., 1977).

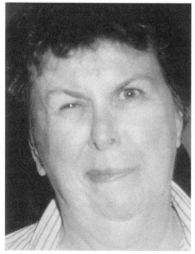

FIG. 12-12. External photograph of a patient with hemifacial spasm shows involuntary contraction of the musculature of the right side of the face. (Courtesy of the Resident Slide Collection of the Wills Eye Hospital.)

Eyelid Myokymia

Eyelid myokymia, characterized by a fine, intermittent quivering movement of the eyelids, is generally a benign condition associated with stress, fatigue, and nicotine or caffeine use; however, some pontine lesions (gliomas) can cause progressive myokymia that typically involves the platysma and other facial muscles (Waybright et al., 1979).

REFERENCES

Adour KK, Ruboyianes JM, Von Doersten PG, et al. Bell's palsy treatment with acyclovir and prednisone compared with prednisone alone: a double-blind randomized controlled trial. *Ann Otol Rhinol Laryngol* 1996;105: 371–378.

American Academy of Ophthalmology. Basic and clinical science course: Section 10. Glaucoma. San Francisco, 1998.

Beck RW, Hayreh SS, Podhajsky PA, et al. Aspirin in nonarteritic anterior ischemic optic neuropathy. *Am J Ophthalmol* 1997;123:212–217.

Beri M, Klugman MR, Kohler JA, et al. Anterior ischemic optic neuropathy. VII. Incidence of bilaterality and various influencing factors. *Ophthalmology* 1987;94: 1020–1028.

Biousse V. Carotid disease and the eye. *Curr Opin Ophthalmol* 1997;8:16–26.

Bioussie V, Touboul PJ, D'Anglejan-Chatillon J, et al. Ophthalmologic manifestations of internal carotid artery dissection. *Am J Ophthalmol* 1998;126:565–577.

Brazis PW, Lee AG. Neuro-ophthalmic problems caused by medications. *Focal points* 1998: No. 11. American Academy of Ophthalmology, San Francisco, 1998.

Brix TH, Hansen PS, Kyvik KO, et al. Cigarette smoking and risk of clinically overt thyroid disease. *Arch Intern Med* 2000;160:661–666.

Brown GC, Magargal LE. Central retinal artery obstruction and visual acuity. *Ophthalmology* 1982;89:14–19.

Brown GC, Green WR. The ocular ischemic syndrome. *Curr Opin Ophthalmol* 1994;5:14–20.

Carr RE, Siegel IM. *Visual electrodiagnostic testing: a practical guide for the clinician*, 2nd ed. Baltimore: Williams & Wilkins, 1990.

Central Vein Occlusion Study Group. Baseline and early natural history report. The central vein occlusion study. *Arch Ophthalmol* 1993;111:1087–1095.

Chavis RM, Garner A, Wright JE. Inflammatory orbital pseudotumor. A clinicopathologic study. *Arch Ophthalmol* 1978;96:1817–1822.

Dell'Osso LF, Daroff RB. Nystagmus and saccadic intrusions and oscillations. In: Glaser JS, ed. *Neuro-ophthalmology*, 3rd ed. Philadelphia: Lippincott Williams & Wilkins,1999:369–401.

Doro S, Lessell S. Cup-disc ratio and ischemic optic neuropathy. *Arch Ophthalmol* 1985;103:1143–114.

Dutton JJ. Optic nerve sheath meningiomas. *Surv Ophthalmol* 1992;37:167–183.

Ferry AP, Abedi S. Diagnosis and management of rhinoorbitocerebral mucormycosis (phycomycosis). A report of 16 personally observed cases. *Ophthalmology* 1983;90: 1096–1104.

Ghanchi FD, Dutton GN. Current concepts in giant cell (temporal) arteritis. *Surv Ophthalmol* 1997;42:99–123.

Glaser JS. Topical diagnosis: the optic chiasm. In: Glaser JS, ed. *Neuro-ophthalmology*, 3rd ed. Philadelphia: Lippincott Williams & Wilkins 1999;199–238.

Glaser JS, Siatkowski M. Infranuclear disorders of eye movement. In: Glaser JS, ed. *Neuro-ophthalmology*, 3rd ed. Philadelphia: Lippincott Williams & Wilkins, 1999: 405–460.

Hamilton SR. Neuro-ophthalmology of eye-movement disorders. *Curr Opin Ophthalmol* 1999;10:405–410.

Hayreh SS, Podhajsky PA, Zimmerman B. Ocular manifestations of giant cell arteritis. *Am J Ophthalmol* 1998;125: 509–520.

Herishanu Y, Apte R, Kuperman O. Immunological abnormalities in opsoclonus cerebellopathy. *Neuro-ophthalmology* 1985;5:271–276.

Isayama Y, Takahashi T, Inoue M, et al. Posterior ischemic optic neuropathy. Clinical diagnosis. *Ophthalmologica* 1983;187:141–147.

Jannetta PT, Abbasy M, Marion JC. Etiology and definitive microsurgical treatment of hemifacial spasm: operative techniques and results in 47 patients. *J Neurosurg* 1977; 47:321–328.

Jordan DR, Patrinely JR, Anderson RL, et al. Essential blepharospasm and related dystonias. *Surv Ophthalmol* 1989;34:123–132.

Kaminski HJ, Daroff RB. Treatment of ocular myasthenia. Steroids only when compelled. *Arch Neurol* 2000;57: 752–753.

Kawasaki A. Physiology, assessment, and disorders of the pupil. *Curr Opin Ophthalmol* 1999;10:394–400.

Keltner JL, Thirkill CE, Tyler NK, et al. Management and monitoring of cancer-associated retinopathy. *Arch Ophthalmol* 1992;110:48–53.

Klein R, Klein BEK, Jensen SC, et al. Retinal emboli and stroke: The Beaver Dam Eye Study. *Arch Ophthalmol* 1999;117:1063–1068.

Kubis KC, Danesh-Meyer HV, Savino PJ, et al. The ice test versus the rest test in myasthenia gravis. *Ophthalmology* 2000;107:1995–1998.

Lee AG, Woo Sy, Miller NR, et al. Improvement in visual function in an eye with presumed optic nerve sheath meningioma after treatment with three-dimensional conformal radiation therapy. *J Neuroophthalmol* 1996;16:247–251.

Leigh JR, Daroff RB, Troost BT. Supranuclear Disorders of Eye Movements. In: Glaser JS, ed. *Neuro-ophthalmology*, 3rd ed. Philadelphia: Lippincott Williams & Wilkins 1999;345–368.

Mantayjarvi M, Tuppurainen K, Ikaheimo K. Ocular side effects of amiodarone. *Surv Ophthalmol* 1988;42:360–366.

Mizener JB, Podhajsky P, Hayreh SS. Ocular ischemic syndrome. *Ophthalmology* 1997;104:859–864.

Moraes CT, DiMauro S, Zeviani M, et al. Mitochondrial DNA deletions in progressive external ophthalmoplegia and Kearns-Sayre syndrome. *N Engl J Med* 1989;320: 1293–1299.

North American Symptomatic Carotid Endarterectomy Trial Collaborators. Beneficial effect of carotid endarterectomy in symptomatic patients with high-grade carotid stenosis. *N Engl J Med* 1991;325:445–453.

Padua L, Stalberg E, LoMonaco M, et al. SFEMG in ocular myasthenia gravis diagnosis. *Clin Neurophysiol* 2000; 111:1203–1207.

Peitersen E. The natural history of Bell's palsy. *Am J Otol* 1982;4:107–111.

Quality of Care Committee, Glaucoma Panel. Primary open-angle glaucoma. *Preferred practice pattern*. San Francisco: American Academy of Ophthalmology, 1992.

Rasmussen AK, Nygaard B, Feldt-Rasmussen U. (131)I and thyroid-associated ophthalmopathy. *Eur J Endocrinol* 2000;143:155–160.

Regillo CD, Brown GC, Savino PJ, et al. Diabetic papillopathy: patient characteristics and fundus findings. *Arch Ophthalmol* 1995;113:889–895.

Rizzo JF, Lessell S. Tobacco amblyopia. *Am J Ophthalmol* 1993;116:84–87.

Rizzo M, Barton JJ. Retrochiasmal Visual Pathways and Higher Cortical Function. In: Glaser JS, ed. *Neuro-ophthalmology*, 3rd ed. Philadelphia: Lippincott Williams & Wilkins 1999;239–291.

Rumelt S, Dorenboim Y, Rehany U. Aggressive systematic treatment for central retinal artery occlusion. *Am J Ophthalmol* 1999;128:733–738.

Savino PJ, Glaser JS, Cassady J. Retinal stroke: is the patient at risk? *Arch Ophthalmol* 1977;95:1185–1189.

Scott IU, Siatkowski MR. Thyroid eye disease. *Semin Ophthalmol* 1999;14:52–61.

Sharma S. The systemic evaluation of acute retinal artery occlusion. *Curr Opin Ophthalmol* 1998;9:1–5.

Siatkowski MR, Glaser JB. Pediatric neuro-ophthalmology. In: Glaser JS, ed. *Neuro-ophthalmology*, 3rd ed.. Philadelphia: Lippincott Williams & Wilkins 1999; 461–487.

Slamovits TL, Glaser JS. The pupils and accommodation. In: Glaser JS, ed. *Neuro-ophthalmology*, 3rd ed. Philadelphia: Lippincott Williams & Wilkins 1999;527–552.

Teunisse RJ, Cruysberg JRM, Verbeek A, et al. The Charles Bonnet syndrome: a large prospective study in the Netherlands. *Br J Psychiatry* 1995;166:254–257.

The Central Vein Occlusion Study Group. Natural history and clinical management of central retinal vein occlusion. *Arch Ophthalmol* 1997;115:486–491.

The Ischemic Optic Neuropathy Decompression Trial Study Group. Characteristics of patients with nonarteritic anterior ischemic optic neuropathy eligible for the Ischemic Optic Neuropathy Decompression Trial. *Arch Ophthalmol* 1996;114:1366–1374.

Thompson HS, Corbett JJ, Cox TA. How to measure the relative afferent pupillary defect. *Surv Ophthalmol* 1981;26: 39–42.

Trokel SL, Hilal SK. Recognition and differential diagnosis of enlarged extraocular muscles in computed tomography. *Am J Ophthalmol* 1979;87:503–512.

Troost BT. Migraine and other headaches. In: Glaser JS, ed. *Neuro-ophthalmology*, 3rd ed. Philadelphia: Lippincott Williams & Wilkins 1999;553–587.

Troost BT, Glaser JS, Morris PP. Aneurysms, arteriovenous communications, and related vascular malformations. In: Glaser JS, ed. *Neuro-Ophthalmology*, 3rd ed. Philadelphia: Lippincott Williams & Wilkins 1999;589–628.

Vincent A, Newsom-Davis J. Acetylcholine receptor antibody characteristics in myasthenia gravis. *Clin Exp Immunol* 1982;49:266–272.

Waybright EA, Gutman L, Chou SM. Facial myokymia. Pathological features. *Arch Neurol* 1979;36:244–245.

Weinberg DA, Lesser RL, Vollmer TL. Ocular myasthenia: a protean disorder. *Surv Ophthalmol* 1994;39:169–210.

SUGGESTED READINGS

American Academy of Ophthalmology. Basic and clinical science course: Section 5. Neuro-ophthalmology, San Francisco, 1998.

Foroozan R, Bailey RS. Essentials of the ophthalmologic examination. In: Maus M, Jeffers JB, Holleran DK, eds. *The clinics atlas of office procedures: essentials of ophthalmology.* Philadelphia: WB Saunders, June 2000.

Glaser JS. *Neuro-ophthalmology*, 3rd ed. Philadelphia: Lippincott Williams & Wilkins, 1999.

Miller NR, Newman NJ. Walsh & Hoyt's clinical neuro-ophthalmology, 5th ed. Vols. 1–5. Baltimore: Williams & Wilkins, 1998.

Rhee DJ, Pyfer MF. *The Wills eye manual: office and emergency room diagnosis and treatment of eye disease*, 3rd ed. Philadelphia: Lippincott Williams & Wilkins, 1999.

13

Sleep in the Older Person

Alon Y. Avidan

By the year 2050, it is predicted that about one fifth of the population will be over 65 years of age. In 1900, only 4% were over 65. This increase will have profound medical, economic, and psychosocial consequences. Because sleep complaints increase with age, the medical community must educate itself on changes in sleep that occur with age. This chapter describes those changes, as well as the most common diagnoses and treatments of sleep disorders seen in the elderly.

Although the normal sleep architecture changes with age, with less time spent in the deeper levels of sleep, sleep disturbances in the older population are often multifactorial. The sleep disturbance can be caused by a primary sleep disorder (e.g., obstructive sleep apnea, periodic limb movements of sleep, or restless leg syndrome) or it can be secondary to circadian rhythm changes, medical problems, psychiatric conditions, polypharmacy, or psychosocial factors. Conversely, when sleep disorders become chronic, they can exacerbate medical and psychiatric illnesses. Chronic sleep disorders or associated excessive daytime sleepiness can cause disturbed intellect, impaired cognition, confusion, psychomotor retardation, or increased risk of injury, any of which can alter an individual's quality of life, or create social and economic burdens for caregivers.

SLEEP TESTS

Sleep is evaluated by recording electrical potentials from the brain (electroencephalography [EEG]); eye movements (electrooculography [EOG]); muscle activity (electromyography [EMG]); heart rhythm (electrocardiography [ECG]); body position (supine, left, right); oxymetry; and respiratory activity (airflow, thoracic and abdominal excursion). Traditionally, sleep is generally recorded in the laboratory setting for one full night. This full-night sleep recording is called a "polysomnograph" (PSG). It is a method of continuous and simultaneous recording of physio-

logic variables during sleep (Thorpy and Yager, 1991). It is indicated for the evaluation of patients suspected of having a sleep-related breathing disorder, unusual nocturnal spells, or unusual movements. A second recording, the Multiple Sleep Latency test (MSLT) can be useful in quantitating the degree of sleepiness. This test measures an individual's ability to fall asleep when given four or five nap opportunities throughout an average day. The MSLT is done during the day, following a nocturnal polysomnogram (Thory and Yager, 1991).

When patients are first recorded in the sleep laboratory, their anxiety about sleeping in a new and unfamiliar environment can lead to a recording that is not representative of their usual sleep. This is called the "first night effect" (Agnew et al., 1966). Recently, technical advances allow for these types of recordings to be done in the home. Patients are set up with instrumentation in the laboratory, sent home, and asked to come back the following day after spending the night in their own bed. These home recordings or unattended monitoring reduce the first night effect, reduce costs, increase comfort, and reduce the waiting time for a study in some cases.

SLEEP STAGING

Sleep is divided into two states: nonrapid eye movement (NREM) and REM (rapid eye movement) sleep. NREM and REM sleep alternate throughout the night in a cyclical pattern. NREM sleep is further subdivided into stages 1, 2, 3, and 4. NREM sleep progresses from stage 1 (light sleep) to slow wave sleep (SWS-stages 3 and 4). With this progression from stage 1 to 4, a relative increase occurs in the depth of sleep and the threshold for spontaneous arousals. Stage 1 sleep is a transition between wakefulness and sleep. Its characteristics include low voltage, mixed frequency EEG and slow rolling eye movements. The signatures of stage 2 sleep include sleep spindles and K-complexes. Slow wave sleep refers to stages 3 and 4 sleep. It is characterized by high amplitude (75 μV), slow frequency (delta) waves (Carskadon and Dement, 2000). REM sleep, which is very distinct from light and slow wave sleep, is characterized by increased sympathetic activity, rapid eye movements, dreaming, and an increase in the depth and rate of breathing. REM sleep manifests a low voltage, mixed frequency EEG, and reduced EMG tone (muscle atonia). This is when the most elaborate dreams emerge. A physiologic sleep paralysis manifested by low EMG tone on the polysomnogram protects the patient from acting out dreams.

AGE-RELATED CHANGES IN SLEEP

With aging, the amount of time spent in slow wave sleep decreases; thus, the time spent in a lighter level of sleep increases. The proportion of REM sleep is generally preserved. However, the latency to the first REM period decreases and the overall amount of REM sleep can decrease as a result of an overall reduction in nocturnal sleep time. Older adults also take longer to initiate sleep, having a reduced total sleep time; they have frequent awakenings and early morning awakenings, and are more likely to have diurnal naps (McGheie and Russel, 1962; Dement et al., 1996).

The prevalence of napping in older adults ranges form 25% to 80% (Prinz, 1977; Wauquier et al., 1992). Studies that have used the MSLT to evaluate sleepiness in older persons have shown that, given the opportunity, they tend to fall asleep during the day faster than younger patients (Carskadon et al., 1982). This daytime sleepiness suggests that older adults are not getting sufficient sleep at night. This is interpreted to mean that the need for sleep in older adults is not reduced, but rather that the ability to sleep is changed (Ancoli-Israel, 1997b).

Studies looking at gender differences in the sleep of healthy elderly adults have found that women sleep better than men (Benca et al., 1992) and maintain sleep better than men (Rediehs et al., 1990). Recent studies evaluating the effects of menopause on sleep have found associated subjective complaints of insomnia. Objectively, menopause was found to prolong sleep latency and reduce both REM sleep and total sleep time. Treatment with estrogen replacement therapy may alleviate these problems (Wooten, 1994).

CLINICAL HISTORY

The clinical evaluation of an elderly patient with a sleep complaint involves a multidisciplinary approach. First, the clinical approach begins with a careful history taking of the present and past sleep history, as well as detailed history of specific sleep complaints. Family history is always important as well as social history, in particular, regarding alcohol and caffeine intake. Questions regarding polypharmacy and particular use of psychiatric medications may be a key in the initial evaluation.

Important questions that need to be asked when obtaining the sleep history are provided below. This information is supplemented by having the patient keep a careful sleep diary for several weeks.

- Do you have difficulties falling asleep?
- Do you feel that you are excessively sleepy?
- What is your sleep-wake schedule during the weekdays and weekends?
- How many hours do you sleep per night?
- How long does it take you to fall asleep after deciding to go to sleep?
- How many times do you wake up during a typical night?
- How long does it take you to "get going" after you get out of bed?
- Do you snore loudly or stop breathing at night?
- Do you have crawling or aching feelings in your legs when trying to fall asleep?
- Do you kick or twitch your arms or legs during sleep?
- Do you walk in your sleep?
- Do you act out your dreams?

Questions regarding daytime behavior are also important, such as, the general quality of sleep on awakening, frequency of daytime napping, and propensity to fall asleep in unacceptable situations such as driving, during conversations, or while watching a movie. It is often crucial to interview the bed partner, as well as the patient, to obtain information regarding the patient's sleep habits, daytime functioning; alcohol, tobacco and caffeine use; snoring and recent changes in snoring intensity; apnea-like spells and nocturnal spells; morning headaches; confusion; and leg jerks. However, many older adults have no bed-partners.

ASSESSMENT OF SLEEP DISORDERS IN THE OLDER PERSON

The polysomnogram is important in the assessment of specific sleep stage abnormalities, leg movements, unusual behaviors, and the presence of underlying sleep-related breathing disorder. The MSLT serves several functions. It is useful in objective evaluation of sleepiness. It may also reveal narcolepsy, a very rare condition in the older person. The use of video PSG is especially important in the evaluation of parasomnias such as REM behavior disorder (RBD). When patients are suspected of having RBD, it is helpful to place EMG leads on all four limbs during polysomnography.

SLEEP-RELATED BREATHING DISORDER

Obstructive Sleep Apnea

Sleep-related breathing disorders are probably among the most serious of the sleep disorders. Obstructive sleep apnea (OSA) occurs because of a cessation of airflow caused by a complete or partial upper airway collapse at the level of the pharyngeal airways. Central sleep apnea is caused by cessation of both airflow and respiratory effort. Respiratory events are classified as either complete (apnea) or partial (hypopnea). The respiratory disturbance index (RDI) has been defined as the number of apneas and hypopneas per hour of sleep. At my center, an observation of at least five apneas and hypopneas per hour of sleep is thought to be consistent with a significant level of obstructive sleep apnea. However, many older persons without symptoms meet these criteria, and whether they deserve treatment has not yet been well defined.

Obstructive sleep apnea is caused by multiple factors that together can predispose an individual to develop collapse of the airways. Advanced age, neurologic and endocrine impairment, abnormal oral anatomy, obesity, and abnormal nocturnal respiratory reflexes can all contribute to the development of OSA (Shepard, 1989; Bliwise et al., 1987).

Obstructive sleep apnea is more common in the older person than in the young. In individuals over 65 years of age, 24% have five or more apneas per hour of sleep and 81% have more than 10 respiratory events per hour of sleep (Ancoli-Israel et al., 1991a). Ancoli-Israel et al. (1996) studied a population of community-dwelling geriatric men and women and found that those with severe OSA had a significant shorter survival time on follow-up when compared with those with mild to moderate OSA or minimal or no OSA. OSA, however was not a predictor of death, whereas cardiovascular and pulmonary disease was.

Obesity is a central factor contributing to OSA. Although older patients are not as overweight as clinic patients, body mass indices (BMI) is still the best predictor of whether an older individual will or will not have OSA (Ancoli-Israel et al., 1991b). Elderly patients with OSA have significantly higher BMI compared with patients with minimal or no OSA, which supports the claim that obesity is a risk factor for OSA (Ancoli-Israel et al., 1996).

Excessive Daytime Sleepiness

Excessive daytime sleepiness (EDS) is a major symptom in patients with OSA. It is unclear if the sleepiness is caused by disruption of the sleep architecture because of respiratory-related arousals, repeated episodes of hypoxemia, or factors not yet identified. The EDS may manifest itself as sleepiness during what might be considered inappropriate times. Patients with OSA with EDS report falling asleep while in conversations, reading, watching television, and even driving.

Excessive daytime sleepiness can also contribute to significant cognitive impairment. OSA is associated with difficulties with attention, memory decline, and difficulties concentrating during the day (Bliwise, 1993). Patients with OSA who experience nocturnal hypoxemia have been shown to possess reduced cognitive functioning (Ancoli-Israel and Coy, 1994). Treatment of the underlying sleep-disordered breathing may improve some of the cognitive deficiencies (Derderian et al., 1988). Elderly patients with OSA have also been reported to be at risk for disturbed vigilance, impaired ability to rapidly solve complex problems, impaired attention and concentration on formal testing of cognition when compared with subjects without OSA (Findley et al., 1991; Bliwise, 1991). Nocturnal hypoxemia can also contribute to fatal arrhythmia, hypertension, myocardial infarction, and stroke (Shepard, 1992). Other consequences of OSA include anoxia, cardiorespiratory failure, and ultimately death during sleep (Ancoli-Israel et al., 1996).

Snoring

Snoring can be a hallmark of a sleep-related breathing disorder. Snoring is often disruptive to the sleep of the bed partner who often is first to suspect that a problem exists. Snoring is caused by an incomplete upper airway obstruction and is often associated with cardiovascular disease and hypertension (Fairbanks et al., 1987). Snoring has been linked with hypertension. Research has shown that about one third of patients with hypertension have a sleep-related breathing disorder. (Ancoli-Israel et al., 1993). Repeated or chronic nocturnal hypoxemia can result in impaired cerebral function and hypersomnolence (Derderian et al., 1988).

Treatment

Continuous Positive Airway Pressure and Oral Appliances

Continuous positive airway pressure (CPAP) and, sometimes, bilevel positive airway pressure (BiPAP) are currently the main methods of treatment. Both work as a splint at the level of the upper airways to prevent their collapse (Sullivan and Grunstein, 1989; Kryger, 1989). Surgery is often an alternative for those who are unable to tolerate CPAP or BiPAP, although effective only about 50% of the time. In the elderly, surgery should be considered only in cases where no other medical problems preclude it. Various oral appliances have been recently introduced for the management of mild to moderate OSA. These act by repositioning the mandible and tongue anteriorly (mandibular-advancing device and tongue-retaining device). The net effect is an improvement in the oropharyngeal airway space. (Lowe, 2000). Oral appliances would not be appropriate for older patients with dentures or for those who are missing a significant number of teeth.

Positional Therapy

Positional therapy may be appropriate for patients with mild OSA confined to supine sleep. Teaching patients to sleep in other positions can be accomplished by sewing a pocket with a tennis ball in the back portion of the pajamas or nightgowns (Ancoli-Israel et al., 1991b).

Medications

The role of medications (e.g., tricyclic antidepressants) that can increase airway muscle tone and reduce apneas, is somewhat controversial in the elderly because of medication-related side effects and risks of polypharmacy. Strohl et al. (1981) reported that medroxyprogesterone can be effective for patients with mild OSA.

Surgery

The treatment of OSA in the elderly poses a special problem. Because their sleep is lighter and more disrupted, many patients may not tolerate CPAP very well. Major surgical interventions for OSA, such as bimaxillary advancement, genioglossus advancement, and hyoid suspension, need to be considered with caution, especially if the patient has underlying cardiovascular disease. Figure 13-1 illustrates the various therapeutic modalities used to treat OSA.

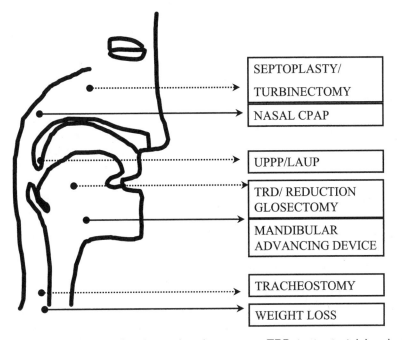

FIG. 13-1. The treatment options for obstructive sleep apnea. TRD, tongue retaining device; UPPP, uvulopalatopharyngoplasty; LAUP, laser-assisted palatoplasty. *Dotted line*, surgical intervention; *solid line*, nonsurgical intervention.

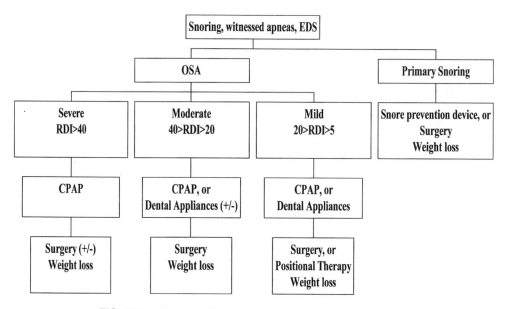

FIG. 13-2. Algorithm: Treatment of obstructive sleep apnea.

Lifestyle

Obstructive sleep apnea can be potentiated or worsened by a variety of other factors. Many older patients who suffer from insomnia may "self-medicate" themselves with alcohol, which can exacerbates OSA (Taasan et al., 1981). Sleeping in the supine position increases the respiratory disturbances (Cartwright et al., 1991). Medications such as benzodiazepines, barbiturates, and narcotics should be used with the utmost care as they can exacerbate respiratory disturbances and reduce a patient's ability to arouse when an apnea occurs (Ancoli-Israel, et al., 1993). Figure 13-2 outlines a possible algorithm for the management of OSA.

PERIODIC LIMB MOVEMENT DISORDER OF SLEEP

The hallmark of periodic limb movement disorder of sleep (PLMS), also known as "nocturnal myoclonus," is a repetitive and continuous leg jerk 0.5 to 5 seconds in duration, typically occurring usually every 20 to 40 seconds during sleep and resulting in arousals (Coleman, 1982). The polysomnographic diagnosis of PLMS is made when five or more of these movements are recorded per hour of sleep. Many patients with PLMS present to the clinician with nocturnal leg jerks associated with an uncomfortable sensation and urge to kick or move the involved limb (restless leg syndrome). Moving the limb often dissipates the uncomfortable sensation. Patients may complain of a motor restlessness, difficulties initiating sleep, and multiple nocturnal awakenings that result in hypersomnolence (Coleman et al., 1982). Bed partners of patients with PLMS are often bothered by the leg jerks that may not bother the patients themselves. The polysomnogram is often the only reliable way to document the leg movements and, thus, to make the diagnosis.

Restless leg syndrome (RLS) is often described as a "creeping" sensation in the lower extremities (Walters, 1995; Bixler et al., 1982). This sensation is improved when patients move their legs but returns when the movement ceases. Patients with RLS often complain of difficulty falling asleep. Rheumatoid arthritis, excessive caffeine intake, and iron deficiency can exacerbate RLS. Most patients with RLS have PLMS. The converse, however, is not true. Polysomnography is not indicated for making the diagnosis of RLS.

Between 5% and 6% of the population is estimated to have PLMS. This disorder increases in frequency with older age. Ancoli-Israel et al. reported that 45% of older people have this condition, with no gender predilection (1991c). The diagnosis and treatment of this disorder is extremely important as it can lead to sleep initiation insomnia in the older person.

It has been hypothesized that because dopamine agonists and opiates improve the symptoms of RLS and PLMS, related transmitter systems may be involved in the pathogenesis of these conditions.

Treatment for PLMS has included use of benzodiazepines (e.g., clonazepam or temazepam) (Mitler et al., 1986); levodopa and carbidopa (Kaplan et al., 1993); dopamine (D3) agonists (e.g., pramipexole or pergolide); or opiates (e.g., acetaminophen and codeine) (Kavey et al., 1988). Table 13-1 outlines the current treatment approaches for patients with PLMS and RLS, and possible side effects of the medications. Each pharmacologic modality has its advantages and disadvantages. Currently, the benefit-to-risk ratio is unresolved. Recently, iron has been implicated to play a central role in the physiology of RLS. Iron deficiency can produce RLS symptoms and iron replacement therapy results in an improvement.

Many patients with OSA also suffer from PLMS. It is prudent that careful analysis be made to determine if OSA and PLMS coexist in the patient because treatment of the underlying PLMS (with benzodiazepine) can worsen the OSA. Treatment of the sleep-related breathing disorder can improve or worsen the PLMS; further study of this possibility is needed.

INSOMNIA

Insomnia is the most common sleep complaint reported by older people. It is defined as the inability to either initiate or maintain sleep. Older persons are likely to experience sleep maintenance insomnia (difficulty remaining asleep) and early morning awakening (waking early in the morning with the inability to reinitiate sleep). Epidemiologic data have shown a higher prevalence of insomnia in older persons when compared to younger individuals. (Ford and Kamerow, 1989; Klink et al., 1992). For people over 60 years of age, Miles and Dement determined that up to 40% experience insomnia, frequent awakening, and light and disrupted sleep (1980).

Insomnia is a symptom, not a diagnosis. When the older person suffers from insomnia, the cause can be multifactorial. Several factors that should be considered in the differential diagnosis include medical and psychiatric illnesses as well as polypharmacy. The du-

TABLE 13-1. *Pharmacotherapy for restless leg syndrome*

Drug: Class (generic/brand)	Dose	Risks
Benzodiazepines Clonazepam (Klonopin)	0.125–0.5 mg half-hour before bedtime	Nausea, sedation, dizziness
Dopaminergic agents Levodopa/Carbidopa (Sinemet)	25/200 mg: half tablet to 3 tablets 30 minutes before bedtime	Nausea, sleepiness, augmentation of daytime symptoms, insomnia, sleepiness, gastrointestinal disturbances
Dopamine agonists Pramipexole (Mirapex)	0.125–0.5 mg, 1 hr before bedtime Start low and increase slowly	Severe sleepiness, nausea reported in some cases
Pergolide (Permax)	0.05–1.0 mg 1 hr before bedtime: divided doses; gradually increase as needed	
Ropinirole (Requip)	0.5–6 mg 1 hr before bedtime	
Anticonvulsants Gabapentin (Neurontin)	300–2,700 mg/d divided t.i.d.	Daytime sleepiness, nausea
Iron Ferrous sulfate	325 mg b.i.d./t.i.d. Recommended for ferritin <50 mg	Gastrointestinal side effects: constipation. Role in treatment under current investigation
Clonidine Catapres	0.1 mg b.i.d. May be helpful in patients with hypertension	Dry mouth, drowsiness, constipation, sedation, weakness, depression (1%), hypotension
Opioids Darvocet (Darvoset-N) Propoxyphene (Darvon) Codeine	300 mg/d 65–135 mg at bedtime 30 mg	Nausea, vomiting, restlessness, constipation Addiction, tolerance may be possible

b.i.d., twice daily; t.i.d., three times daily.

ration of insomnia—transient (<1 month), short-term (1–6 months), or chronic (>6 months) provides important diagnostic information.

In the evaluation of insomnia, a detailed medical and sleep history should be taken. Particular attention should be made to the underlying medical conditions (heart disease, diabetes), medication use or misuse (polypharmacy), and substance use or misuse (alcohol, caffeine, tobacco). Sleep history should focus on the sleep hygiene (bedtime, sleep time, wake time). Sleep diaries (sleep logs) are crucial in the evaluation. These self-reported, subjective measures allow for easy calculation of total time in bed, total sleep time, and sleep efficiency (Gillin and Byerley, 1990).

Polysomnograms are not necessary in the evaluation of most insomnia. A single PSG may not be representative of a patient's sleep at home and may not detect insomnia that is not present on a nightly basis (Hauri et al., 1983). However, in the older patient with insomnia, a PSG may be indicated if an underlying RLS, PLMS, or OSA is suspected (Edinger et al., 1989). Others have advocated a formal PSG when traditional therapy for insomnia fails and the possibility of an underlying primary sleep disorder persists (Lichstein and Reidel, 1994). Another objectively verifiable indicator of a sleep-wake schedule involves the use of an Actigraph, a device worn on the wrist to record body movements (Hauri and Wisbey, 1992; Hauri and Wisbey, 1994).

Many causes are found for insomnia in the older person. The most important to consider in this age group is insomnia caused by medical factors. These include:

Primary pulmonary problems (chronic obstructive pulmonary disease, asthma),
Neurologic disorders (cerebrovascular accidents, headaches),
Pain syndromes

Underlying psychiatric conditions are important contributors to disruption of the sleep architecture. Up to 90% of patients with depression have an abnormal sleep architecture (Reynolds, 1989). The most striking polysomnographic features of depression include a decreased REM latency and early morning awakening (Benca et al., 1992).

In addition, older patients may have sleep disruption because of the use or abuse of alcohol, nicotine, and caffeine. In the sleep practice, it is not uncommon to see alcohol being used as a sleeping aid. Although initially it does decrease the sleep latency, it produces arousals, sleep fragmentation, REM deprivation, and REM rebound later during the night. Because the me-

tabolism of alcohol is slower with advanced age, it has more powerful sedating effects (Dufour et al., 1992). Stimulants (caffeine, and medications containing stimulants) are notorious causes of insomnia (Espie, 1991). Caffeine is associated with increased sleep latency, reduced sleep efficiency, and spontaneous arousals. Caffeine withdrawal is associated with depression, irritability, and hypersomnolence. Nicotine induces insomnia and sleep fragmentation.

The role of polypharmacy is critical in assessing the older person with sleep disorders. Patients are often treated by numerous physicians and each may prescribe several medications. Patients often use over-the-counter medications, vitamins, and herbal preparations.

Treatment

Medications

Pharmacotherapy for insomnia in the older person is common, but can be complicated by age-related changes in pharmacodynamics and pharmacokinetics (Hicks et al., 1981). Some sleeping pills, particularly the longer acting ones, have multiple side effects in the older person. These range from hypersomnolence and being accident-prone (Roth et al., 1988), to having disrupted sleep architecture (reduced REM and SWS). Tolerance is a major issue when long-acting sleeping pills are taken chronically, resulting in rebound insomnia and the need of higher dosage to achieve the same clinical efficacy.

Hypnotics

Hypnotics, when used in the older person, need to be given at the lowest possible dose, for a short time. Shorter acting hypnotics are preferable and patients need to be followed closely. Potential side effects of hypnotics include anterograde amnesia and rebound insomnia. This is true for hypnotics with short to intermediate half-lives. All hypnotics, if given in appropriate doses, improve insomnia. The goal is to use the medication with the fewest side effects at the lowest dose that will be clinically effective.

Hypnotics, when prescribed to patients with underlying OSA, can produce further nocturnal hypoxemia (Gillin and Ancoli-Israel, 1992). Withdrawal from hypnotics can actually produce a worsening of insomnia and heightened anxiety. This is especially true with abrupt cessation from longer acting medications. The newer short-acting hypnotics do not have these same side effects and seem to be safer in the older patient. Examples include Zaleplon (selective for the benzodiazepine-1 receptor), and zolpidem (selective for the type-1 gamma-aminobutyric acid-A [GABAA]-benzodiazepine receptor).

Sleep Hygiene

Drug therapy alone is not appropriate if the aim is to eradicate chronic insomnia. Drug therapy, if used at all, must be combined with educational, behavioral, and cognitive interventions aimed at introducing adaptive behaviors. One of the most important educational approaches for insomnia is to modify disadvantageous sleep hygiene habits that patients may have adopted over the years (Hauri and Esther, 1990). Originally developed by Hauri, the basic elements of better sleep hygiene include limiting naps to less than 30 minutes per day, avoiding stimulants and sedatives, limiting liquids at bedtime, keeping a regular sleep schedule, and incorporating light exposure and exercise into the daily routines. Stimulus-control therapy, originally proposed by Bootzin, postulates that sleep disturbances are behaviorally conditioned and, thus, need to be reconditioned (Bootzin and Nicassio, 1978). The aim of this intervention is to recondition the bed or bedroom as cues for sleep. Patients are instructed to go to bed only when tired, to get out of bed after 20 minutes of being unable to fall asleep, and to return to bed when sleepy. They are also instructed to avoid looking at the clock, shorten daytime naps, use the bed only for sleep, and get up at a consistent time in the morning (Epsie et al., 1988; Hauri, 1998).

Among the merits of the sleep restriction therapy proposed by Spielman is the need to restrict time in bed to provide for better sleep efficiency (Spielman et al., 1987). This technique involves curtailing time in bed and total sleep time, which can initially lead to a state of sleep deprivation. It works by preventing patients from becoming frustrated by restricting the time spent in bed. Other common therapeutic modalities for insomnia include cognitive intervention, which helps patients gain insight into maladaptive beliefs and attitudes toward sleep, and relaxation technique and biofeedback, which help patients lower the degree of anxiety and arousal associated with insomnia (Bootzin and Nicassio, 1978).

CIRCADIAN RHYTHM ABNORMALITIES

The circadian modulator located in the suprachiasmatic nucleus of the anterior hypothalamus controls the sleep-wake cycle. *Zeitgebers*, external cues such as light, synchronize the circadian rhythms. Distur-bances in circadian rhythms result from a mismatch between the environmental cues and the endogenous circadian rhythms. The hypersomnolence seen in the older person may, in part, be caused by a disintegration of the normal circadian rhythm (Jacobs et al., 1989).

Advanced sleep phase syndrome (ASPS) is very common among older patients. Patients with ASPS generally get sleepy early in the evening and wake up early in the morning, and are unable to reinitiate sleep. Although older adults may get sleepier in the evening, they still try to remain awake until a "more acceptable" time (i.e., 10–11 p.m.). Then when they wake up early unable to fall back to sleep, they have not even been in bed long enough to get the sleep they need, resulting in a state of sleep deprivation (Ancoli-Israel, 1997b). ASPS can be treated with bright light therapy, as light is one of the strongest cues for synchronizing circadian rhythms. Bright light therapy involves exposure of 2,500 lux of light at 1 M eye level. Light exposure in the evening delays sleep initiation (Czeisler et al., 1989; Campbell et al., 1988; 1995).

Melatonin, a neurohormone produced by the pineal gland, can reset sleep onset by synchronization of the internal circadian clock (Dawson and Encel, 1993). With advanced age, less melatonin is produced (Reiter, 1995). Melatonin-replacement therapy may be a key for treating insomnia in the elderly. Haimov et al. (1995) showed a positive correlation between lower peak level of melatonin and poor sleep efficiency in older patients with insomnia. Melatonin treatment early in the morning may also be used for ASPS. When melatonin is given a few hours before the onset of the endogenous production, which peaks around 3 and 5 a.m., it will shift the circadian pacemaker to an earlier time and, thus, cause a phase advance (Lewy and Sacks, 1996). Currently, more data are needed to improve our understanding of the appropriate dosage, pharmacologic properties, and indications for melatonin use. More data are needed regarding the appropriate safety and efficacy of this substance. Because the US Food and Drug Administration does not regulate melatonin, care must be exercised when using it.

REM-SLEEP BEHAVIOR DISORDER

REM-sleep behavior disorder is characterized by the absence of the normal muscle atonia that usually characterizes REM sleep. Patients present with unusual intense motor activity. The range of this motor behavior can be anywhere from a simple limb movement to very complex quasi-purposeful movements

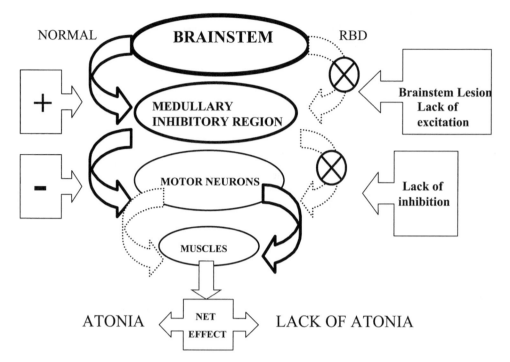

FIG. 13-3. Pathophysiology of rapid eye movement (REM)-sleep behavior disorder.

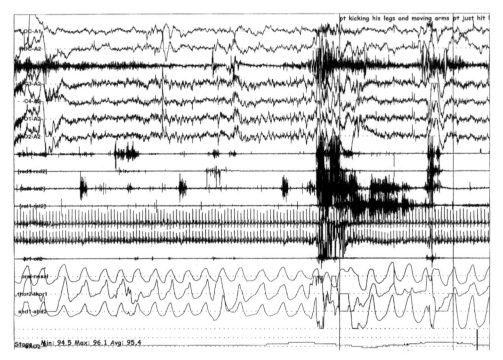

FIG. 13-4. A polysomnographic recording of rapid eye movement (REM)-sleep behavior disorder from a patient with Parkinson's disease and unusual nocturnal spells.

suggestive of dream content enactment (Chokroverty, 1996). The pontine tegmentum is the locus of the muscle tone inhibitor system that normally causes muscle atonia during REM sleep (Schenck et al., 1987). The perilocus ceruleus of the rostral tegmentum of the pons produces activation of the medullary inhibitory zone via the tegmentoreticular tract. A loss of atonia is seen during REM sleep, which facilitates the motor behaviors during dreaming (Morrison, 1998; Parkes, 1986; Schenck, 1996). Figure 13-3 summarizes the possible neuroanatomic explanation for RBD. Figure 13-4 shows a polysomnographic sample from a patient with RBD. Note the abnormally elevated limb EMG tone during REM sleep.

SLEEP AND DEGENERATIVE NEUROLOGIC DISORDERS

Alzheimer's Disease

Many neurodegenerative disorders have been shown to affect sleep (Guilleminault et al., 1992; Bliwise, 1993). Alzheimer's disease is the most common cause of irreversible dementias. Polysomnographically, patients are found to have significant sleep architecture abnormalities. The hallmarks include reduction in sleep efficiency, increase in NREM stage 1 sleep, increase in arousal and awakening frequency, decrease in total sleep time, reduction of REM sleep percentage, and reduction in sleep spindles and K complexes. A profound disruption occurs in sleep-wake rhythmicity, primarily early in disease onset. Sleep fragmentation subsequently leads to increased daytime sleepiness, nocturnal insomnia, nocturnal wandering, cognitive decline, number of daytime naps, time in bed and time spent awake in bed, frequency of nocturnal wandering, disorientation, and confusion (Ancoli-Israel, et al., 1996; Bliwise et al., 1995; Chokroverty, 1996).

Causes of Sleep Disorders in Alzheimer's Disease

Sleep-related breathing disorders in the form of obstructive sleep apnea are common in Alzheimer's disease. As a matter of fact, the severity of Alzheimer's disease is proportional to the severity of the sleep apnea (Ancoli-Israel et al., 1996). The depletion in central dopamine content and cholinergic deficits is often described as a possible cause for periodic leg movements of sleep and the sleep architectural abnormalities.

Loss of noradrenergic, serotoninergic, and cholinergic neurons in the suprachiasmatic nucleus has been linked to the inversion of sleep-wake cyclicity and circadian rhythm abnormalities seen in Alzheimer's disease. It is probably a cause for sundowning and sleep-wake schedule disturbances.

Degeneration of cholinergic neurons is probably a cause for reduced REM sleep. Degeneration of these brainstem neurons that specifically modulate REM sleep is a possible cause for REM sleep behavior disorder.

The mechanism of sleep disruption in patients with Alzheimer's disease is probably caused by two possible factors. The first, is a primary degenerative process secondary to loss of cholinergic neurons of the nucleus basalis of Meynert or the pedunculo pontine tegmentum, the lateral dorsal tegmentum nucleus, as well as depigmentation of noradrenergic brainstem nuclei. The other possibility is sleep disruptions secondary to the nature of the disease itself (i.e., immobilization, autonomic disruption, and depression).

Possible mechanism of sleep disruption in Alzheimer's disease has been linked to the progressive loss of the neuronal mechanism responsible for generating both NREM and REM sleep. Patients often are found to have EEG slowing, increased wakefulness, and reduction in REM sleep. The nucleus basalis of Meynert is found to be degenerated. It is the main source of cholinergic input, and disruption of the central cholinergic system is possibly involved in REM sleep abnormalities found in patients with Alzheimer's disease.

Sleep studies in patients with Alzheimer's disease show poor sleep quality, increase in the frequency of sleep-related breathing disorder, and sleep architectural changes, namely reductions in total sleep time, REM sleep, and NREM stage 4 sleep. Patients are found to have increased sleep fragmentation and frequent awakenings. The diagnosis of sleep disruption in patients with Alzheimer's disease is often aided by an observer (e.g., bed-partner, care provider, or family member). Sleep logs may actually underestimate the extent of the true sleep problem.

The management of sleep disorders in patients with Alzheimer's disease relies on determination of the underlying causes. First, attempt to improve hygiene by trying to regulate the patient's sleep-wake schedule abnormalities. Patients are discouraged from spending an extensive time in bed. They are also asked to reduce alcohol and caffeine intake, and limit the number of psychoactive drugs. Increasing light exposure can be useful, as patients with Alzheimer's disease may not obtain enough light secondary to underlying cataracts. Patients are also asked to reduce morning and late evening napping. The role of melatonin in the treatment of sleep problems in patients with Alzheimer's disease is still controversial and currently being investigated. Psychopharmacology use in the treatment of sleep problems in Alzheimer's disease needs to be very cautious. The use of psychotropic treatment may make the situation worse by increasing arousals and sleep disruption. Benzodiazepines often increase nocturnal confusion secondary to sedation. Tricyclic antidepressants often are found to increase cognitive deficits by virtue of their anticholinergic and sedating side effects. Antipsychotic medications can increase the risk of falls secondary to orthostatic hypertension as one of their primary side effects. Treatment of OSA in these patients is often not well tolerated.

Patients with Alzheimer's disease have a disrupted sleep-wake rhythm (Ancoli-Israel et al., 1997a). These patients have reduced slow wave and REM sleep, frequent daytime napping, and multiple nocturnal awakenings (Prinz et al., 1982). Polysomnographically, patients with dementia show increased diffuse slow wave activity, decreased sleep efficiency, and reversal of their circadian rhythmicity. This reversal in the circadian rhythmicity is the second most common cause for institutionalization after incontinence (Pollack and Perlick, 1991). Treatment of sleep problems in this special population should be multidisciplinary, including both behavioral changes, pharmacotherapy, and in some cases, light therapy. As a general rule, the time in bed should be restricted to night time hours and diurnal naps should be limited, if possible, to a short 60-minute afternoon nap. Caffeine intake should be discouraged and meals should be served in the dining room as opposed to in bed. Bright light therapy is being looked at as a possible treatment of circadian rhythm disturbances, as noted, and for the treatment of agitation in the nursing home setting (Lovell et al., 1995).

Patients with Alzheimer's disease often have nocturnal wandering and disorientation during the night. Described as the "sundowning syndrome," it is caused mostly by the loss of visual cues for orientation, and is commonly found in the nursing home setting. It is estimated that the bright light exposure in nursing home is low, averaging approximately a few minutes a day. Patients with sundowning syndrome present with loud vocalizations and disorientation, and are often found to be confused. This subsequently leads to unnecessary restraining and use of sedative medications.

Nocturnal confusional episodes, which are caused by an inversion of the sleep schedule, present as wakefulness at night and hypersomnolence during the day. Patients with Alzheimer's disease are also found to have wandering behavior during the night, increased agitation, and delirium, in advanced cases. Neuroanatomically, these patients are found to have degeneration of the suprachiasmatic nucleus, leading to nocturnal sleep fragmentation.

Several factors that can contribute to sundowning or nocturnal delirium include the following:

- Cognitive impairment
- Decrease in daytime light exposure
- Change in the living situation
- Use of psychoactive medications
- Medical illnesses, such as dehydration, malnutrition, electrolyte imbalance, and infections

Diffuse Lewy Body Dementia

Patients with diffuse Lewy body dementia (DLBD) are found to have an increased rate of REM sleep behavior disorder (Boeve et al., 1998; Turner et al., 1997). These patients often present with rapidly progressive dementia associated with attention deficit, hallucinations, and fluctuation in their cognitive abilities. RBD is often the initial manifestation of DLBD (Boeve et al., 1998).

Parkinson's Disease

Patients with Parkinson's disease can have any of several sleep disorders. On the polysomnogram, often evidence is seen of increased stage 1 sleep, reduced SWS and REM sleep, and increased nocturnal myoclonus. Almost two thirds of patients with Parkinson's disease may have sleep initiation insomnia. Close to 90% of these patients often have sleep maintenance insomnia associated with frequent awakenings (Friedman, 1980; Chokroverty, 1996).

Patients with Parkinson's disease often have difficulties and an inability to turn over during the night and get out of bed. This is most likely secondary to bradykinesia. Leg cramps and leg jerks are also common as are dystonic spasms of the limbs, face, and back. Patients may present with nocturnal vocalization and excessive nocturia (Tandberg et al., 1998).

Motor abnormalities in Parkinson's disease during sleep include the parkinsonism tremor and REM onset blepharospasm, which disappears during REM sleep. Patients have rapid blinking at sleep onset and REM intrusion into NREM sleep. REM-sleep behavior disorder is common in patients with Parkinson's disease (Chokroverty, 1996; Comella et al., 1998) and may also precede the onset of the disease (Tan et al., 1996).

One third of patients with Parkinson's disease are found to have periodic limb movement disorder of sleep based on a nocturnal polysomnogram. Patients with Parkinson's disease who have posture reflex abnormalities and autonomic impairment are at an increased risk for sleep-related breathing disorder in the form of central sleep apnea, OSA, and alveolar hypoventilation syndrome (Apps et al., 1985). Parkinson's disease can lead to a restrictive pulmonary disease. Patients with Parkinson's disease are also found to have circadian rhythm abnormalities and depression (Trenkwalder, 1998).

Cause of Sleep Disorders in Parkinson's Disease

The mechanism or biologic basis of sleep disruption in Parkinson's disease is possibly related to the alteration of dopaminergic, noradrenergic, serotonergic, and cholinergic neurons in the brainstem. Sleep-wake disturbances are often caused by mesocorticolimbic dopaminergic abnormalities and mesostriatal system abnormalities. Abnormalities of dopaminergic neurons in the ventral tegmentum area often lead to EEG desynchronization and abnormal sleep-wake schedule disorder (Eisensehr et al., 2000).

Factors often responsible for sleep disruption in Parkinson's disease are probably tremors, dystonia, rigidity, dyskinesia, RBD, periodic leg movements of sleep, REM onset blinking, and increased awakening (Partinen, 1997). These patients often have difficulty in changing position and an inability to initiate movement.

Patients with Parkinson's disease who are already on medications may have additional sleep difficulties. Low-dose dopaminergic agonists are often sedating. On the other hand, high-dose dopaminergic agonists can lead to increased hallucinations, nightmares, and increased arousals. Levodopa is often associated with increased sleep latency but an increased sleep continuity (Askenasy and Yahr, 1985; Pappert et al., 1999). Explanations for the sleep-wake disruption in Parkinson's disease have been linked to a reduction in serotonergic neurons of the dorsal raphe, noradrenergic neurons of the locus ceruleus, and cholinergic neurons of the pedunculopontine nucleus (Schneck, 1996; Stocchi et al., 1998).

The clinical suspicion of abnormal movement or parasomnias during the night is an indication for polysomnography in patients with Parkinson's disease. The polysomnographic features of patients with Parkinson's disease include reduction of sleep efficiency, increased wake after sleep onset (WASO), increased sleep fragmentation, reduction of SWS/REM sleep, disruption of NREM to REM cyclicity, loss of muscle atonia, and increased EMG activity, which is the basis for RBD (Shenck, 1996).

Possible mechanisms attributed to obstructive sleep apnea in patients with Parkinson's disease are the abnormal tone of the upper airway muscles, dystonic movements of the glottis and supraglottis, and an abnormal respiratory drive.

Treatment of sleep disorders in patients with Parkinson's disease deserves special consideration. Those who suffer from insomnia are often treated by improving their sleep hygiene abnormalities. Pharmacologic treatment with low-dose dopaminergic preparation, (i.e., 100 mg of levodopa combined with 25 mg of carbidopa; sinemet 25/100) and low doses of sedating tricyclic antidepressants (TCA) can be tried. Problems with bradykinesia and nocturia are often improved by providing patients with a portable bedside commode. For patients with RLS symptoms, an evening and nocturnal dose of dopaminergic agonist such as carbidopa/levodopa or a dopamine (D3) agonist is useful (Schenck et al., 1987). Patients with RBD are often treated with clonazepam (0.5 mg every night) (Schenck et al., 1987). Patients with OSA often have symptoms improved with nasal CPAP (nCPAP). Patients who are diagnosed with OSA in addition to autonomic dysfunction can be treated effectively with nCPAP. However, a definitive treatment (i.e., tracheostomy) for these patients is often mandatory as they may present with an increased risk for fatal cardiac arrhythmias.

Stroke

Cumulative vascular damage eventually leads to multiinfarct and vascular dementia. Patients with an underlying sleep-related breathing disorder (e.g., OSA or nocturnal hypoxemia) often present with cardiac arrhythmias, intellectual decline, and increased risk of stroke (Pressman et al., 1995). Patients with lacunar strokes in the tegmentum of the pons and periventricular white matter damage present as REM sleep without atonia, which leads to RBD (Thorpy and Glovinsky, 1987; Shimizu et al., 1990).

Patients with Binswanger's disease or subcortical leukoencephalopathy are at an increased risk for developing RBD, primarily because white matter ischemia in the vicinity of the supratentorial system is often involved in modulating REM-related atonia. Brain MRI studies in patients with RBD with underlying strokes show ischemic lesions in the pontine tegmentum, which is the locus of muscle tone inhibitor system.

Progressive Supranuclear Palsy

Many sleep problems are encountered in patients with progressive supranuclear palsy (PSP). Insomnia, which is probably the most severe sleep problem, is noted by decreased total sleep time and significant sleep disruption without a specific clinical complaint. This is probably secondary to the apathy of patients having this disease. Patients may also present with RBD.

When evaluating the eye leads of the recording polysomnographically, it is interesting to note the absence of vertical eye movement during REM sleep. Horizontal eye movements are present but are slower and reduced in amplitude. During REM sleep, polysomnography may show increased phasic twitching and increased fast activity by alpha intrusion. A few patients with PSP may have periodic leg movements of sleep and OSA. The sleep architecture profile consist of increased sleep latency, increased frequency of arousal and awakening, decreased stage 2 NREM, reduced REM sleep, and reduced REM latency (Aldrich et al., 1989; De Bruin et al., 1996).

Olivopontocerebellar Atrophy

The sleep problems encountered with olivopontocerebellar atrophy include central, obstructive and mixed sleep apnea, which is probably caused by bulbar muscle weakness. Patients may also have nocturnal stridor as well as RBD.

Shy-Drager Syndrome

Progressive autonomic failure and progressive somatic neurologic manifestations characterize patients with Shy-Drager syndrome (SDS). Patients with SDS most commonly present with sleep-related respiratory dysregulation, with frequent arousals and hypoxemia (Briskin et al., 1978). Apneas encountered in this syndrome include obstructive, mixed, and central. Cheyne-Stokes respiratory dysfunction, apneustic breathing, and inspiratory gasping are commonly seen. The hypersomnias seen in these patients are probably secondary to the dramatic sleep disruption. Patients may be at risk of dying from sudden cardiac death related to the underlying sleep-related breathing disorder. RBD disorder and insomnia are also common in this disease.

The mechanism of sleep disruption SDS is probably pathology in the brainstem structures regulating sleep-wake transition. Patients with SDS are at increased risk for developing brainstem ischemia secondary to nocturnal hypotensive episodes, which can subsequently potentiate the tendency to develop RBD.

Polysomnographically, patients are found to have reduced SWS, reduced REM sleep, reduced total sleep time, increased sleep latency, increased frequency of awakening, absence of atonia in REM sleep, and increased respiratory dysrhythmia.

Motor Neuron Disease: Amyotrophic Lateral Sclerosis

Amyotrophic lateral sclerosis (ALS) is a neurodegenerative disease of middle-aged and elderly patients. Progressive degeneration of the ventral horn of the spinal cord, motor neurons of the bulbar nuclei, and the upper motor neurons, which produces both upper and lower motor neuron deficits, cause ALS. ALS has a relentless progression, with no impairment of the mental function or sensorium. Respiratory failure in this disorder occurs late in the course of the disease, although it can also be the presenting feature of this disease. It is not uncommon for physicians to encounter patients with breathing difficulties, bulbar weakness, and stridor in the emergency room only to later diagnose ALS. The major sleep complaint of these patients is excessive daytime sleepiness likely caused by sleep-related respiratory disturbances and insomnia (Ferguson, 1996; Arnulf et al., 2000; Sivak et al., 1999).

The mechanism of respiratory disturbance in ALS disorder may be the weakness of the upper airways caused by bulbar weakness, diaphragmatic weakness from a phrenic nerve lesion, and intercostal muscle weakness caused by the degeneration of intercostal nerve nuclei. Degeneration of the central respiratory neurons also occurs, which accounts for both central and obstructive sleep apnea. Polysomnographic findings include apneas (i.e., central, obstructive, and mixed), increased awakenings, sleep fragmentation, and reduced nocturnal oxygen saturation (Culebras, 1996).

Acute Confusional State in the Elderly

Patients with acute confusional state present with reduced cognition, impaired attention, reduced alertness, and a disturbance in the sleep-wake cycle. Predisposing factors include dementia, medical illnesses, medications, sensory deprivation, and psychosocial factors, which can be transient for less than a month. During the day, patients are found to be lethargic. During the night, they are found to have fragmented sleep, hallucinations, agitation, and increased wakefulness. One likely mechanism explaining this disorder is related to cholinergic deficiency. In treating these patients, first evaluate and treat the underlying causes, and in some situations, use low-dose haloperidol.

TABLE 13-2. *Differential diagnosis of nocturnal spells in the older adult*

Variable	Nocturnal seizure	REM sleep behavior disorder	Somnambulism	Nocturnal dissociative disorder	Confusional arousals	Sleep-related panic attacks	Nightmares
Stage of sleep	NREM > REM, ictal discharges facilitated by K-complexes	REM sleep	First third of night, SWS		First third of night, during SWS	Transition from NREM stage II to SWS	Second half of night, during REM sleep, also NREM
Spell symptoms	Generalized tonic-clonic activity: Generalized epilepsy, partial epilepsy	Talking, arm movements, kicking, punching	Automatisms, getting out of bed, walking	Alteration of consciousness, identity, memory	Sudden arousal, confusion, disorientation, inappropriate behavior	Sudden awakening with subjective fear, impending doom	Sudden awakening with anxiety and dream recall
Duration	Seconds to minutes	Seconds to 20–30 minutes	1–5 minutes, 30–60 minutes rare		Seconds to 10 minutes	Several seconds to a few minutes	5–15 minutes
Postspell symptoms	Unresponsiveness—confusion, weakness, incontinence (urine/stool) tongue biting	Detailed recall of an active dream with theme of violence	Confusion, amnesia to the event; recall is rare	Amnestic to event or dreamlike mentation	No recall of event	Excessive arousal, increased sympathetic activity	Vivid recall of a frightening dream
EEG pattern during spell	Ictal EEG pattern	REM sleep	Transition from SWS to stage I, diffuse and slow high amplitude delta bursts		Slow wave activity, microsleeps, poorly reactive alpha	REM	Increased eye movement during REM
Pathophsiology	CNS vascular disease neoplasm (in the older person)	Loss of muscle atonia, pontine/CNS lesions, stress, Parkinsonian disorders	Predisposing psychopathology, sleep deprivation, alcohol, strong sleep pressure	Underlying serious psychopathology, abuse	Incomplete awakening from SWS	Predisposing anxiety disorder depression, daytime panic attacks alcohol abuse	Precipitated by daytime stress, drugs (b-blockers), psychopathology
Potential treatments	Appropriate antiepileptic drugs (i.e., valproate/phenytoin/carbamazepine)	Clonazepam Levodopa-carbidopa, diazepam	Avoid injury, protect patient, avoid precipitating factors, hypnosis, psychotherapy, benzodiazepines, tricyclic antidepressants	Psychotherapy, psychopharmacology, resistant to treatment	Relaxation techniques, avoidance of stress	Treatment of the underlying anxiety disorder, panic disorder, psychotherapy, anxiolytics	Address underlying psychiatric illness, avoid stress, psychotherapy, improve sleep hygiene, rarely REM suppressants

REM, rapid eye movement; NREM, non rapid eye movement; EEG, electroencephalogram; CNS, central nervous system; SWS, slow wave sleep

Narcolepsy

Narcolepsy is a syndrome of excessive daytime sleepiness, cataplexy, sleep paralysis, and hypnagogic hallucinations. Onset of narcolepsy is most common during the second decade of life; the onset of narcolepsy after age 50 is extremely rare. Circadian rhythm abnormalities, medication-induced REM sleep suppression, sleep-related breathing disorder, and subsequent REM sleep disruption can cause early onset of REM sleep in the older person (Bassetti and Aldrich, 1996). In the elderly, rarely is seen excessive daytime sleepiness or cataplexy that had been undiagnosed. The polysomnographic characteristics of narcolepsy include a mean sleep latency less than 5 minutes and the presence of two or more sleep-onset REM periods (Aldrich, 1998).

Fatal Familial Insomnia

A rare prion disease, fatal familial insomnia leads to premature aging and death. Seen is a loss of both neuroendocrine regulation and vegetative circadian rhythmicity. Patients develop severe progressive insomnia, loss of orthostatic stability, increased salivation, increased body temperature, and daytime stupor that alternates with wakefulness. In the final stage of the disease, patients can become very agitated, confused, and disorientated. These patients will eventually develop progressive stupor, coma, and die.

The genotypic localization of patients with fatal familial insomnia is on the short arm of the human chromosome 20. Neuropathologically, severe degeneration and gliosis of the anterior and dorsomedial nucleus of the thalamus is found (Tabernero et al., 2000; Cortelli et al., 1999).

Table 13-2 summarizes the major differential diagnosis of nocturnal spells in the older person. It outlines the common stage of sleep in which they occur, the usual symptoms, durations, after spell symptoms, EEG pattern, possible pathophysiology, and treatment (Parkes, 1986; Pedley, 1983; Thorpy and Glovinsky, 1987).

CONCLUSION

Sleep changes dramatically with old age. Both subjective and objective measures show increased sleep-wake disturbances with age. The older person has a more fragmented sleep, sleeps less deeply, and tends to have early morning awakening. The aging process itself does not cause sleep problems. The sleep requirement also does not decrease with advanced age. What remains a controversial issue is whether it is the decreased need for sleep or whether it is the ability to sleep that decreases with aging.

When encountering an older patient with daytime sleepiness, it is crucial to first review the patient's medical history, psychiatric history, medications, underlying medical illnesses, and sleep-wake schedule pattern. The prevalence of sleep-related breathing disorder, periodic limb movement disorder of sleep, and restless leg syndrome increases with aging and can lead to excessive daytime sleepiness or insomnia. Many sleep disorders are potentially reversible and a carefully thought out clinical decision-making process can greatly benefit the patient and family.

REFERENCES

Agnew HW, Webb WB, Williams RL. The first night effect: an EEG study of sleep. *Psychophysiology* 1966;2(3):263–266.

Aldrich MS. Diagnostic aspects of narcolepsy. *Neurology* 1998;50(2 Suppl 1):S2–S7.

Aldrich MS, Foster NL, White RF, et al. Sleep abnormalities in progressive supranuclear palsy. *Ann Neurol* 1989;25 (6):577–581.

Ancoli-Israel S, Klauber MR, Jones DW, et al. Variations in circadian rhythms of activity, sleep and light exposure related to severity of dementia in nursing home patients. *Sleep* 1997a;20:18–23.

Ancoli-Israel S, Kripke DF, Klauber MR, et al. Morbidity, mortality and sleep disordered breathing in community dwelling elderly. *Sleep* 1996;19(4):277–282.

Ancoli-Israel S. Sleep problems in older adults: putting myths to bed. *Geriatrics* 1997b;52(1):20–30.

Ancoli-Israel S, Bliwise DL, Mant A. Sleep and breathing in the elderly. In Saunders NA, Sullivan CE, eds. *Sleep and breathing*. New York: Marcel Dekker, 1993;673–693.

Ancoli-Israel S, Coy TV. Are breathing disturbances in elderly equivalent to sleep apnea syndrome? *Sleep* 1994;17:77–83.

Ancoli-Israel S, Jones DW, Hanger MA, et al. Sleep in the nursing home. In: Kuna ST, Suratt PM, Remmers JE, eds. *Sleep and respiration in aging adults*, New York: Elsevier, 1991a;77–84.

Ancoli-Israel S, Kripke DF, Klauber MR, et al. Sleep disordered breathing in community-dwelling elderly. *Sleep* 1991b;14(6):486–495.

Ancoli-Israel S, Kripke DF, Klauber MR, et al. Periodic limb movements in sleep in community-dwelling elderly. *Sleep* 1991c;14(6):496–500.

Apps MC, Sheaff PC, Ingram DA, et al. Respiration and sleep in Parkinson's disease. *J Neurol Neurosurg Psychiatry* 1985;48(12):1240–1245.

Arnulf I, Similowski T, Salachas F, et al. Sleep disorders and diaphragmatic function in patients with amyotrophic lateral sclerosis. *Am J Respir Crit Care Med* 2000;161(3 Pt 1):849–856.

Askenasy JJ, Yahr MD. Reversal of sleep disturbance in Parkinson's disease by antiparkinsonian therapy: a preliminary study. *Neurology* 1985;35(4):527–532.

Bassetti C, Aldrich MS. Narcolepsy. *Neurol Clin* 1996; 14(3):545–571.

Benca RM, Obermeyer WH, Thisted RA, et al. Sleep and psychiatric disorders: a meta-analysis. *Arch Gen Psychiatry* 1992;49:651–668.

Bixler EO, Kales A, Vela-Bueno A, et al. Nocturnal myoclonus and nocturnal myoclonic activity in a normal population. *Research Communications in Chemical Pathology and Pharmacology* 1982;36:129–140.

Bliwise, DL. Cognitive function and sleep disordered breathing in aging adults. In: Kuna ST, Remmers JE, Suratt PM, eds. *Sleep and respiration in aging adults.* New York: Elsevier, 1991:237–244.

Bliwise DL, Feldman DE, Bliwise N, et al. Risk factors for sleep disordered breathing in heterogeneous geriatric populations. *J Am Geriatr Soc* 1987;35:132–141.

Bliwise DL. Review: sleep in normal aging and dementia. *Sleep* 1993;16:40–81.

Bliwise DL, Hughes M, McMahon PM, et al. Observed sleep/wakefulness and severity of dementia in an Alzheimer's disease special care unit. *J Gerontol* 1995; 50A(6):M303–M306.

Boeve BF, Silber MH, Ferman TJ, et al. REM sleep behavior disorder and degenerative dementia: an association likely reflecting Lewy body disease. *Neurology* 1998; 51(2):363–370.

Bootzin RR, Engle-Friedman M. Sleep disturbances. In: Edelstein BA, Carstensen LL, eds. *Handbook of clinical gerontology.* New York: Pergamon Press, 1997.

Bootzin RR, Nicassio PM. Behavioral treatments for insomnia. In: Hersen M, Eisler RM, Miller PM, eds. *Progress in behavior modification,* Vol. 6. New York: Academic Press, 1978:1–45.

Briskin JG, Lehrman KL. Guilleminault C. Shy-Drager syndrome and sleep apnea. In: Guilleminault C, Dement WC, eds. *Sleep apnea syndromes.* New York: Liss, 1978: 317–322.

Campbell SS, Kripke DF, Gillin JC, et al. Exposure to light in healthy elderly subjects and Alzheimer's patients. *Physiol Behav* 1988;42:141–144.

Campbell SS, Terman M, Lewy A, et al. Light treatment for sleep disorders: consensus report. V. Age-related disturbances. *J Biol Rhythms* 1995;10(2):151–154.

Carskadon MA, Dement WC. Normal human sleep: an overview. In: Kryger MH, Roth T, Dement WC, eds. *Principles, and practice of sleep medicine.* Philadelphia: WB Saunders, 2000:15–25.

Carskadon MA, Brown ED, Dement WC. Sleep fragmentation in the elderly: relationship to daytime sleep tendency. *Neurobiology of Aging* 1982;3(4):321–327.

Cartwright RO, Diaz F, Lloyd S. The effects of sleep posture and sleep stage on apnea frequency. *Sleep* 1991;14(4); 351–353.

Chokroverty S. Sleep and degenerative neurologic disorders. *Neurol Clin* 1996;14(4):807–826.

Coleman RM. Periodic movements in sleep (nocturnal myoclonus) and restless legs syndrome. In: Guilleminault C, ed. *Sleeping and waking disorders: indications and techniques.* Menlo Park: Addison-Wesley Publishing, 1982; 265–296.

Coleman RM, Bliwise DL, Sajben N, et al. Daytime sleepiness in patients with periodic movements in sleep. *Sleep* 1982;5:S191–S202.

Comella CL, Nardine TM, Diederich NJ, et al. Sleep-related violence, injury, and REM sleep behavior disorder in Parkinson's disease. *Neurology* 1998;51(2): 526–529.

Cortelli P, Gambetti P, Montagna P, et al. Fatal familial insomnia: clinical features and molecular genetics. *J Sleep Res* 1999;8(Suppl 1):23–29.

Culebras A. Sleep and neuromuscular disorders. *Neurol Clin* 1996;14(4):791–805.

Czeisler CA, Kronauer RE, Allan JS, et al. Bright light induction of strong (type 0) resetting of the human circadian pacemaker. *Science* 1989;244:1328–1332.

Dawson D, Encel N. Melatonin and sleep in humans [Review]. *J Pineal Res* 1993;15:1–12.

De Bruin VS, Machado C, Howard RS, et al. Nocturnal and respiratory disturbances in Steele-Richardson-Olszewski syndrome (progressive supranuclear palsy). *Postgrad Med J* 1996;72(847):293–296.

Dement W, Richardson G, Prinz P, et al. Changes of sleep and wakefulness with age. In: Finch C, Schnieder EL, eds. *Handbook of the biology of aging,* 4th ed. New York: Van Nostrand Reinhold, 1996.

Derderian SS, Brindenbaugh RH, Rajagopal KR. Neuropsychologic symptoms in obstructive sleep apnea improve after treatment with nasal continuous airway pressure. *Chest* 1988; 94(5):1023–1027.

Dufour MC, Archer L, Gordis E. Alcohol and the elderly. *Clin Geriatr Med* 1992;8(1):127–141.

Edinger JD, Hoelscher,TJ, Webb MD, et al. Polysomnographic assessment of DIMS: empirical evaluation of its diagnostic value. *Sleep* 1989;12(4):315–322.

Eisensehr I, Linke R, Noachtar S, et al. Reduced striatal dopamine transporters in idiopathic rapid eye movement sleep behaviour disorder. Comparison with Parkinson's disease and controls. *Brain* 2000;123(Pt 6):1155–60.

Espie CA. *The psychological treatment of insomnia.* Chichester, United Kingdom: John Wiley, 1991.

Espie CA, Brooks DN, Lindsay WR. An evaluation of tailored psychological treatment of insomnia. *J Behav Ther Exp Psychiatry* 1988;19:51–56.

Fairbanks DNF, Fujita S, Ikematsu T, et al. *Snoring and obstructive sleep apnea.* New York: Raven Press, 1987.

Ferguson KA. Sleep-disorders breathing in amyotrophic lateral sclerosis. *Chest* 1996;110(3):664–669.

Findley LJ, Presty SK, Barth J, et al. Impaired cognition and vigilance in elderly subjects with sleep apnea. In: Kuna ST, Suratt JE, Remmers JE, eds. *Sleep and respiration in aging adults.* New York: Elsevier, 1991:259–265.

Ford DE, Kamerow DB. Epidemiologic study of sleep disturbances and psychiatric disorders. An opportunity for prevention? *JAMA* 1989; 262(11): 1479–1484.

Friedman A. Sleep pattern in Parkinson's disease. *Acta Med Pol* 1980;21(2):193–199.

Gillin JC, Ancoli-Israel S. The impact of age on sleep and sleep disorders. In: Salzman C, ed. *Clinical psychopharmacology.*Baltimore: Williams & Wilkins, 1992: 213–234.

Gillin JC, Byerley WF. The diagnosis and management of insomnia. *N Engl J Med* 1990;322:239–248.

Guilleminault C. Stoohs R. Quera-Salva MA. Sleep-related obstructive and nonobstructive apneas and neurologic disorders. *Neurology* 1992;42(7 Suppl 6):53–60.

Haimov I, Lavie P, Laudon M, et al. Melatonin replacement therapy of elderly insomniacs. *Sleep* 1995;18(7): 598–603.

Hauri PJ. Insomnia. *Clin Chest Med* 1998;19(1):157–168.

Hauri PJ. Esther MS. Insomnia. *Mayo Clin Proc* 1990;65 (6):869–882.

Hauri P, Roth T, Sateia M, et al. Sleep laboratory and performance evaluation of midazolam in insomniacs. *British Journal of Pharmacology* 1983; 16(Suppl1): 109S–114S.

Hauri PJ, Wisbey J. Wrist actigraphy in insomnia. *Sleep* 1992;15(4):293–301.

Hauri PJ, Wisbey J. Actigraphy and insomnia: a closer look. Part 2. *Sleep* 1994;17(5):408–410.

Hicks R, Dysken MW, Davis JM, et al. The pharmacokinetics of psychotropic medication in the elderly: a review. *J Clin Psychiatry* 1981;42:374–385.

Jacobs D, Ancoli-Israel S, Parker L, et al. Twenty-four-hour sleep-wake patterns in a nursing home population. *Psychol Aging* 1989;4(3):352–356.

Kaplan P, Allen RP, Buchholz DW, et al. A double-blind, placebo-controlled study of the treatment of periodic limb movements in sleep using carbidopa/levodopa and propoxyphene. *Sleep* 1993;16(8):717–723.

Kavey N, Walters AS, Hening W, et al. Opioid treatment of periodic movements in sleep in patients without restless legs. *Neuropeptides* 1988;11(4):181–184.

Klink ME, Quan SF, Kaltenborn WT, et al. Risk factors associated with complaints of insomnia in a general adult population. Influence of previous complaints of insomnia. *Arch Intern Med* 1992;152(8):1634–1637.

Kryger MH. Management of obstructive sleep apnea: overview. In: Kryger MH, Roth T, Dement WC, eds. *Principles and practice of sleep medicine*. Philadelphia: WB Saunders, 1989:584–590.

Lewy AJ, Sacks RL. The role of melatonin and light in the human circadian system. In: Buija RM, et al., eds. *Progress in brain research*. New York: Elsevier Science, 1996:205–216.

Lichstein KL, Reidel BW. Behavioral assessment and treatment of insomnia: a review with an emphasis on clinical application. *Behav Ther* 1994;25:659–688.

Lovell BB, Ancoli-Israel S, Gevirtz R. Effect of bright light treatment on agitated behavior in institutionalized elderly subjects. *Psychiatry Research* 1995:57(1):7–12.

Lowe AA. Dental appliances for the treatment of snoring and obstructive sleep apnea. In: Kryger MH, Roth T, Dement WC, eds. *Principles and practice of sleep medicine*. Philadelphia: WB Saunders, 2000:929–939.

McGheie A, Russel SM. The subjective assessment of normal sleep patterns. *Journal of Mental Science* 1962;108: 642–654.

Miles L, Dement WC. Sleep and aging. *Sleep* 1980;3: 119–220.

Mitler, MM, Browman CP, Menn SJ, et al. Nocturnal myoclonus: treatment efficacy of clonazepam and temazepam. *Sleep* 1986;9:385–392.

Morrison AR. The pathophysiology of REM-sleep behavior disorder. *Sleep* 1998;21(5):446–449.

Pappert EJ, Goetz CG, Niederman FG, et al. Hallucinations, sleep fragmentation, and altered dream phenomena in Parkinson's disease. *Mov Disord* 1999;14(1): 117–121.

Parkes JD. The parasomnias. *Lancet* 1986;2(8514): 1021–1025.

Partinen M. Sleep disorder related to Parkinson's disease. *J Neurol* 1997;244(4 Suppl 1):S3–S6.

Pedley TA. Differential diagnosis of episodic symptoms. *Epilepsia* 1983;24(Suppl 1)S31–S44.

Pollak CP, Perlick D. Sleep problems and institutionalization of the elderly. *J Geriatr Psychiatry Neurol* 1991;4: 204–210.

Pressman MR, Schetman WR, Figueroa WG, et al. Transient ischemic attacks and minor stroke during sleep. Relationship to obstructive sleep apnea syndrome. *Stroke* 1995; 26(12):2361–2365.

Prinz PN. Sleep patterns in the healthy aged: relationship with intellectual function. *J Gerontol* 1977;32:179–185.

Prinz PN, Vitaliano PP, Vitiello MV, et al. Sleep, EEG and mental function changes in senile dementia of the Alzheimer's type. *Neurobiol Aging* 1982: 3(4):361–370.

Rediehs MH, Reis JS, Creason NS. Sleep in old age: focus on gender differences. *Sleep* 1990;13(5):410–424.

Reimao R, Lemmi H, Bertorini T. [Excessive daytime sleepiness, central type sleep apnea and myotonic dystrophy]. [Portuguese] *Arquivos de Neuro-Psiquiatria* 1985; 43(4):391–395.

Reiter RJ. The pineal gland and melatonin in relation to aging: a summary of the theories and of the data. *Exp Gerontol* 1995:30(3–4):199–212.

Reynolds CFI. Sleep in affective disorders. In: Kryger MH, Roth T, Dement WC, eds. *Principles and practice of sleep medicine*. Philadelphia: WB Saunders, 1989:413–415.

Roth T, Roehrs T, Zorick F. Pharmacological treatment of sleep disorders. In: Williams RL, Karacan I, Moore CA, eds. *Sleep disorders: diagnosis and treatment*. New York: John Wiley & Sons, 1988:373–395.

Schenck CH. REM sleep parasomnias. *Neurol Clin* 1996; 14(4):697–720.

Schenck CH. Mahowald MW. REM sleep parasomnias. *Neurol Clin* 1996;14(4):697–720.

Schenck CH, Bundlie SR, Patterson AL, et al. Rapid eye movement sleep behavior disorder: a treatable parasomnia affecting older adults. *JAMA* 1987;257(13):1786–1789.

Shepard JWJ. Cardiorespiratory changes in obstructive sleep apnea. In: Kryger MH, Roth T, Dement WC, eds. *Principles and practice of sleep medicine*. Philadelphia: WB Saunders 1989:537–551.

Shepard JWJ. Hypertension, cardiac arrhythmias, myocardial infarction, and stroke in relation to obstructive sleep apnea. *Clin Chest Med* 1992;13(3):437–458.

Shimizu T, Inami Y, Sugita Y, et al. REM sleep without muscle atonia (stage1-REM) and its relation to delirious behavior during sleep in patients with degenerative diseases involving the brain stem. *Japanese Journal of Psychiatry & Neurology* 1990;44(4):681–692.

Sivak ED, Shefner JM., Sexton J. Neuromuscular disease and hypoventilation. *Curr Opin Pulm Med* 1999;5(6): 355–662.

Spielman AJ, Saskin P, Thorpy MJ. Treatment of chronic insomnia by restriction of time in bed. *Sleep* 1987;10: 45–56.

Stocchi F, Barbato L, Nordera G, et al. Sleep disorders in Parkinson's disease. *J Neurol* 1998;245(Suppl 1): S15–S18.

Strohl KP, Hensley MJ, Saunders NA, et al. Progesterone administration and progressive sleep apneas. *JAMA* 1981; 245:1230–1232.

Sullivan CE, Grunstein RR. Continuous positive airway pressure in sleep-disordered breathing. In: Kryger MH, Roth T, Dement WC, eds. *Principles and practice of sleep medicine*. Philadelphia: WB Saunders Company, 1989: 559–570.

Taasan VC, Block AJ, Boysen PG, et al. Alcohol increases sleep apnea and oxygen desaturation in asymptomatic men. *Am J Med* 1981;71:240–245.

Tabernero C, Polo JM, Sevillano MD, et al. Fatal familial insomnia: clinical, neuropathological, and genetic description of a Spanish family. *J Neurol Neurosurg Psychiatry* 2000;68(6):774–777.

Tan A, Salgado M, Fahn S. Rapid eye movement sleep behavior disorder preceding Parkinson's disease with therapeutic response to levodopa. *Mov Disord* 1996;11(2): 214–216.

Tandberg E, Larsen JP, Karlsen K. A community-based study of sleep disorders in patients with Parkinson's disease. *Mov Dis* 1998;13(6):895–899.

Thorpy MJ, Glovinsky PB. Parasomnias. *Psychiatr Clin North Am* 1987;10(4):623–639.

Thory MJ, Yager J. *The encyclopedia of sleep and sleep disorders.* New York: Facts on File, 1991.

Trenkwalder C. Sleep dysfunction in Parkinson's disease. *Clin Neurosci* 1998;5(2):107–114.

Turner RS, Chervin RD, Frey KA, et al. Probable diffuse Lewy body disease presenting as REM sleep behavior disorder. *Neurology* 1997;49(2):523–527.

Walters AS. Toward a better definition of the restless legs syndrome. *Mov Disord* 1995;10(5):634–642.

Wauquier A, Van Sweden B, Lagaay AM, et al. Ambulatory monitoring of sleep-wakefulness patterns in healthy elderly males and females (>88 years): The "Senieur" protocol. *J Am Geriatr Soc* 1992;40:109–114.

Wooten V. Medical causes of insomnia. In: Kryger MH, Roth T, Dement WC, eds. *Principles and practice of sleep medicine.* Philadelphia: WB Saunders, 1994:456–475.

SUGGESTED READING

Albarede JL, Morley JE, Roth T, et al., eds. Sleep disorders and insomnia in the elderly. New York: Springer Publishing, 1993.

Aldrich MS. *Sleep medicine,* vol. 53. New York: Oxford University Press, 1999.

Ancoli-Israel S. *All I want is a good night's sleep.* Chicago: Mosby-Year Book, 1996.

Chokroverty S. Sleep disorders medicine. Boston: Butterworth-Heinemann, 1998.

Dement WC, Vaughan C. The promise of sleep. New York: Delacorte Press, 1999.

Dement WC, Roth T, Kryger MH, eds. *Principles and practice of sleep medicine,* 3rd ed. New York: WB Saunders, 2000.

Morgan K. *Sleep and aging: a research-based guide to sleep in later life.* Johns Hopkins Series in Contemporary Medicine and Public Health, 1987.

WEB SITES OF NATIONAL SUPPORT GROUPS AND OTHER RELEVANT SITES

Restless Legs Syndrome Foundation: *http://www.rls.org/main.asp*, *http://www.mLists.net/judson/rls.html*

Obstructive Sleep Apnea: *http://www.apneanet.org/*

National Sleep Foundation: *http://www.sleepfoundation.org/*

Delayed Sleep Phase Syndrome: *http://www.geocities.com/HotSprings/1123/dsps.html*

REM Sleep Behavior Disorder: *http://library.thinkquest.org/25553/english/difficult/disorders/remdis.shtml*

Insomnia: *http://insomnia.zineland.net/*

14

Headaches

David W. Dodick and David J. Capobianco

Headache in the elderly, although less prevalent than in younger adults, is a common complaint that presents a special challenge to the physician. The clinician faces not only a broad differential diagnosis, but must contend with the difficulty of managing headache when comorbid illnesses can contraindicate or complicate effective treatments. Headache in the elderly can conveniently be divided into primary and secondary headaches. Primary headache disorders, such as migraine, cluster headache, and tension-type headache, are diseases unto themselves (*morbus suis generis*). Secondary headache represents a symptom of an underlying disease such as an intracranial mass lesion or a metabolic disorder. Although the overall incidence of headache declines with advancing age, the relative proportion of secondary headaches increase, thus highlighting the importance of a careful evaluation and a high level of suspicion when evaluating an elderly patient with a complaint of headache.

EPIDEMIOLOGY

Headache prevalence declines with age. Although one of the most common symptoms in the young, headache declines in old age to become the tenth most common symptom of elderly women, and the fourteenth of elderly men (Hale et al., 1986). The prevalence of headache in women and men aged 55 to 74 years is approximately 66% and 53%, respectively, compared with 92% and 74% in their younger counterparts between the ages of 21 to 34 years (Waters, 1974). The prevalence declines even further in those over the age of 75 to 55% and 22% for women and men, respectively. Despite this age-related decline, the prevalence of headache in the elderly is still high. In a community survey, the prevalence of frequent headache in the elderly was 20% for women and 10% for men, a significant public health problem by any standard (Cook et al., 1989).

CAUSES

As in the younger age groups, "benign"' primary headache disorders such as migraine and tension-type headache, account for most headaches that affect the elderly (Fig.14-1). However, an important difference is that secondary ("symptomatic") headaches are much more common in the aged, constituting up to 30% of all headache complaints (Solomon et al., 1990). The underlying causes also differ qualitatively compared with the young, in that diseases such as giant cell arteritis and subdural hematomas, are mainly disorders of the elderly. Table 14-1 outlines the various primary and secondary headaches seen in the elderly population.

PRIMARY HEADACHES

Migraine

Although migraine attenuates and often disappears with advancing age, approximately one third of individuals with migraine continue to suffer from recurrent attacks into older age. Although rare, some (2% to 3%) may experience their first migraine attack after the age of 50 years. The prevalence of migraine in the elderly has been estimated between 2.9% (Solomon et al., 1990) and 10.5% (Serratrice et al., 1985). Women continue to be affected more often than men.

The character of the migraine attack itself is generally similar to the headache in a younger individual—a unilateral or throbbing bitemporal headache, frequently associated with nausea, photophobia, and phonophobia. The headache may be accompanied by aura or, as frequently recognized in clinical practice, elderly patients may have recurrent attacks of painless aura (Waters 1974). Aura without headache, referred to as "late-life migraine accompaniments," represents reversible focal cortical dysfunction and may take the form of a recurrent hemisensory disturbance (paresthesias) or a scintillating visual scotoma.

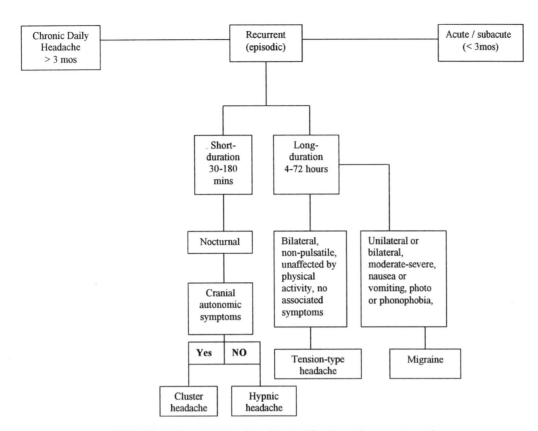

FIG. 14-1. Headache in the elderly. *(Continued on next page)*

These episodic focal neurologic disturbances can be easily confused with transient ischemic attacks. A careful evaluation is important in this setting, including a detailed history of prior migraine attacks, because the incidence and prevalence of cerebrovascular disease increase in the elderly. The key diagnostic features that differentiate late-life migraine accompaniments from transient ischemic attacks are listed in Table 14-2.

Although the effective therapeutic options for migraine are the same in the elderly, the therapeutic approach to these patients is sometimes a challenge because of coexisting medical illnesses. Managing the older patient with migraine requires a thorough familiarity with the individual's health status and a practical knowledge of pharmacology. Vascular disease, for example, precludes the use of migraine-specific medications such as ergotamine derivatives and triptans. Prophylactic medications (e.g., beta-blockers and calcium channel blockers) are difficult to use in patients with depression or congestive heart failure, whereas prostatism, glaucoma, heart failure or arrhythmias may preclude the use of tricyclic antidepressants. Moreover, even when these contraindications do not exist, the elderly are more likely to experience more side effects from certain medications such as sedation and confusion with tricyclics, or impaired renal function with nonsteroidal anti-inflammatory drugs (NSAIDS), because of diminished renal function and creatinine clearance.

In addition, medications used for certain medical disorders can exacerbate migraine in this population. For example, the use of vasodilating antihypertensive medications (e.g., nifedipine or methyldopa) can worsen migraine or lead to an increase in the frequency of attacks. Similarly, when used for ischemic heart disease, nitrates can precipitate an attack of migraine or cluster headache in those who are predisposed.

Tension-Type Headache

Tension-type headache (TTH) is a "featureless headache." It is a dull, bilateral, or diffuse headache, often described as a pressure or squeezing sensation

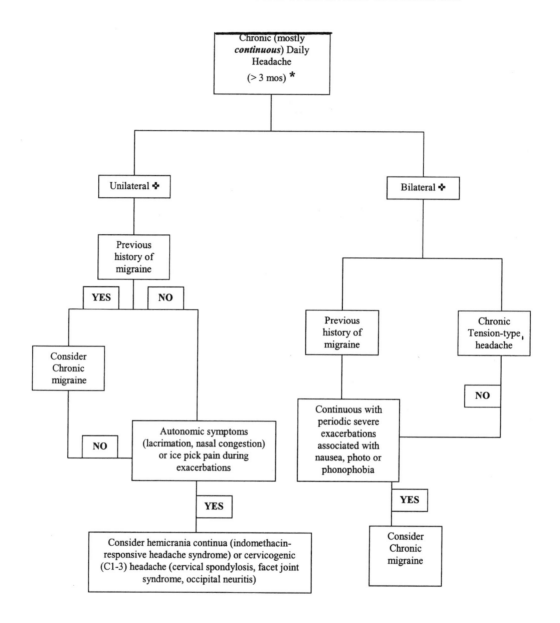

FIG. 14-1. *Continued.*

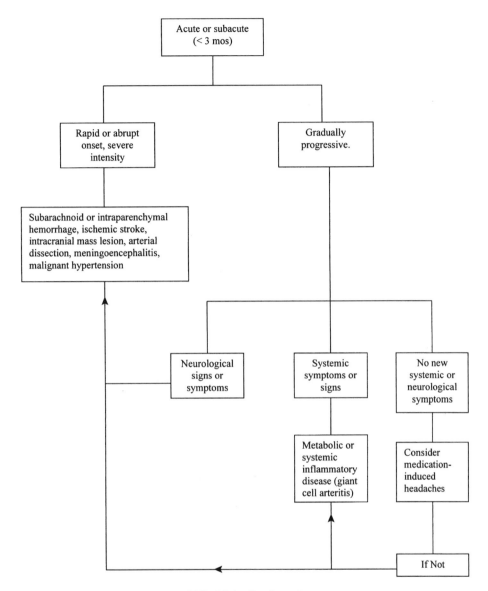

FIG. 14-1. *Continued.*

of mild to moderate intensity. It has no accompanying migraine features (nausea, emesis, photophobia, phonophobia) and the pain is not worsened with movement nor does it prohibit activity. No cranial autonomic symptoms are noted. When presenting as a new headache, especially in patients over the age of 40 years, it should be considered a diagnosis of exclusion as it is the headache phenotype most frequently mimicked by brain tumors and other organic causes of headache. The exact prevalence of TTH in the elderly is difficult to assess because of various de-

finitions used across studies and the propensity for organic disease to masquerade as TTH in this age group. However, estimates range from 18% (Strickiathachron 1991) to 52% (Serratrice et al., 1985). Although most elderly people have had TTH since youth or middle age, about 10% develop TTH after the age of 50 years. Again, a careful search for organic disease is imperative in this particular group because many underlying metabolic, systemic, and psychiatric (depression) disorders, and structural intracranial disease present with ill-defined, nonpulsatile, bi-

TABLE 14-1. *Primary and secondary headaches in the elderly*

Primary headaches
  Migraine
  Tension-type
  Cluster
  Hypnic
Secondary headaches
  Inflammatory/infectious/structural
    Giant-cell arteritis
    Cerebrovascular disease (ischemic and
      hemorrhagic stroke)
    Malignant hypertension
    Intracranial mass lesion (tumor, subdural
      hematoma)
    Intracranial injection (meningitis and encephalitis)
    Cervical spondylosis
    Fever or infection
  Metabolic/systemic
    Medications (including rebound syndromes)
    Hypoxia or hypercapnia (chronic respiratory
      diseases, sleep apnea)
    Anemia, polycythemia
    Electrolyte disturbances (hypocalcemia,
      hyponatremia)
    Depression
    Chronic renal failure

lateral headaches which could easily be mistaken for TTH.

The approach to treatment should involve nonpharmacologic treatment strategies as well as the judicious use of NSAIDS, analgesics, and tricyclic antidepressants for prophylaxis.

Cluster Headache

Cluster headache is one of the most distinctive of the primary headaches, with an unmistakable attack profile. The pain is so excruciatingly intense, it has been termed the "suicide headache." It is often maximal in the orbital region and peaks in intensity within 5 minutes. It can occur during the day or, characteristically, awaken a patient out of a sound sleep. The pain lasts between 15 minutes to 2 hours, but the average duration is 60 minutes if untreated. One or more cranial autonomic features, such as lacrimation, nasal congestion, rhinorrhea, ptosis, meiosis, and conjunctival injection, are seen in more than 97% of patients. Rarely, cluster headache can begin as late as the eighth decade, although this type of headache in elderly individuals invariably will have started at a younger age. The average age of onset is approximately 28 years, and men are affected four times more often than women (Dodick et al., 2000). Although cluster headache is uncommon in random surveys of the healthy elderly, it accounts for up to 4% of elderly patients presenting to headache clinics (Solomon et al., 1990).

As with migraine and TTH, the treatment of cluster headache in the elderly is frequently complicated by the presence of coexisting medical disorders. Subcutaneous sumatriptan, the most effective medication for the acute treatment of cluster headache, must be used with caution in those with cardiovascular risk factors, especially because cluster headache occurs more commonly in men, the majority of whom are chronic smokers. For similar reasons, the same care must be taken with methysergide, which is often used as a preventive medication. For patients with coexistent cardiovascular disease or significant risk factors, oxygen inhalation is the safest and most effective acute agent. Verapamil, usually combined with a short course of corticosteroids, is often highly effective in terminating a cluster period or reducing the frequency and intensity of attacks during this period (Dodick et al., 2000).

Hypnic Headache

Hypnic headache, a primary headache disorder that primarily affects elderly individuals, occurs exclusively during sleep (Raskin 1988; Dodick et al., 1998). The mean age of onset is approximately 60 years, and

TABLE 14-2. *Distinguishing features of late-life migraine accompaniments vs. TIA*

Migraine aura	TIA
Positive visual phenomena (scintillating scotoma)	Negative symptoms (loss of vision)
Gradual buildup	Abrupt onset
Sequential progression from one modality to another (visual–sensory–speech)	
Repetitive attacks of identical nature	Simultaneous appearance
Average duration 20–30 minutes	Variable symptomatology
Flurry of attacks in mid-life common	Average duration <15 minutes
Mild headache following attack in 50%	Flurry of attacks not common
	Headache less likely with TIA

TIA, transient ischemic attack.

women are more often affected than men. The headache typically awakens the individual from sleep, often at or near the same time each night, a feature prompting the term "alarm-clock'" headache. The headache is moderate to severe in intensity, and often bilateral and squeezing, although the pain can be unilateral in up to one third of patients. Generally, no associated "migrainous'" symptoms (nausea, emesis, photophobia, phonophobia), or cranial autonomic symptoms (lacrimation, rhinorrhea), as seen with cluster headache, occur. The pain usually lasts 30 to 60 minutes, although attacks can last several hours. Remaining in a supine position often exacerbates the pain; therefore, most individuals will report needing to rise from bed for relief. Nocturnal attacks often occur more than four nights per week, and some individuals may have several attacks through the night. In some patients, an attack can occur during a daytime nap.

Lithium carbonate is an effective treatment, but the side effects in this age group sometimes precludes its long-term use (Raskin 1988; Dodick et al., 1998). Caffeine, either by tablet or as a cup of coffee before bedtime, can be effective for some patients (Dodick et al., 1998). Other medications found to be effective include indomethacin (Dodick et al., 2000) and flunarizine (Morales-Asin et al., 1998).

SECONDARY HEADACHES

Giant Cell Arteritis

Giant cell arteritis (GCA) is a necrotizing granulomatous systemic arteritis that affects medium-sized and large arteries, especially those branching from the proximal aorta. It occurs primarily in middle-aged and elderly persons. Although it is manifest by a wide range of clinical symptoms, headache is both the most common symptom and the reason why patients with GCA are seen by neurologists. The average age of onset is approximately 70 years and the disease is rare before the age of 50. More than 90% of cases occur in those over 60 years of age. Women are affected about twice as commonly as men.

In a population-based study in Olmstead County, Minnesota, the incidence and prevalence of the disease over a 42-year period was found be 17.8 and 200 per 100,000/year, respectively, in persons aged 50 years and older (Salvarani et al., 1995). The age-specific incidence rate increases from 2.1 per 100,000 in those 50 to 59 years of age 49/100,000 in those above the age of 80, highlighting the dramatic increase in incidence with age. An autopsy series revealed arteritis in 1.6% of 899 postmortem cases, indicating that the disease may be more common than is clinically apparent (Ostberg, 1971).

Headache is not only the most frequent but also the most common initial symptom in patients with GCA. The location, quality, and severity of the headache vary from patient to patient. Although the headache is often moderate to severe, it can begin as an insidious and mild ache. The headache can be throbbing, boring, or lancinating in quality, and the pain can radiate to the neck, face, gums, jaw, or tongue. Although temporal headaches have become synonymous with this disease, the headache may be diffuse or localized to any head region, including the occiput. In one study of 24 biopsy-proved cases, headache was localized to the temporal region in only six patients, whereas seven patients had headache that did not even involve the temporal area (Solomon and Cappa,1987). Scalp tenderness is usually localized to the temporal or, less commonly, to the occipital arteries. It can be diffuse or even absent in up to one third of patients with headache. Headaches can be severe, even when the cranial arteries are normal to palpation, and may subside, even when the disease activity continues, and therefore in isolation cannot be used as a surrogate clinical marker for disease activity.

Polymyalgia rheumatica, malaise, and fatigue occur in over 50% of patients at some time during the illness. In several reports of GCA, polymyalgia rheumatica has been noted in 40% to 60% and has been the initial symptom complex in 20% to 40% of patients (Hunder, 1997).

Ocular involvement is a well-known and perhaps the most notorious complication of GCA. Visual symptoms, including amaurosis, diplopia, and permanent visual loss, are the most important early manifestations of the disease. Visual loss can be unilateral or bilateral and sequential loss of vision in one eye and then the other is not unusual. If unilateral visual loss occurs and is left untreated, involvement of the contralateral eye can occur within 1 to 2 weeks. Onset of visual loss is often sudden and irreversible, but well-documented cases of gradually progressive visual loss with recovery of vision after treatment have been described (Lipton et al., 1985). The incidence of blindness is between 8% and 20%, but can approach 40% in those patients who are not treated. Blindness is preceded by amaurosis in only about 15% of patients, which underscores the need for early diagnosis and treatment. The most common cause of visual loss is ischemic anterior optic neuropathy, although ischemic posterior optic neuropathies without disc edema can occur. Reversible ischemia can also account for other visual phenomena in this illness, including orthostatic fluctuations in vision, transient monocular visual loss, and ocular motor disturbances.

Giant cell arteritis should be considered in the diagnosis of any patient older than 50 years of age who has a new form of headache, change in a previously stable pattern of headache, jaw claudication, weight loss, abrupt loss of vision, polymyalgia rheumatica, unexplained prolonged fever or anemia, and a high erythrocyte sedimentation rate (ESR). Temporal artery biopsy is recommended for diagnosis in all patients and, when feasible and safe, the biopsy should be done before initiating treatment with steroids. The temporal artery is biopsied most frequently, but if the facial or occipital arteries are clearly involved, they can be sampled as well. If a focal abnormality can be palpated, a small biopsy of the affected segment can be performed. Skip lesions can occur pathologically, resulting in a false-positive rate of 4% to 5% (Klein et al., 1976). As such, when the arteries are normal on examination, a generous arterial specimen (3–5 cm) should be harvested and multiple histologic sections at 1-mm levels should be analyzed. In patients with a negative biopsy finding, a contralateral biopsy should be performed. Sorenson and Lorenzen (1977) found GCA-positive results in specimens from the contralateral temporal artery in 7/13 patients who initially had negative biopsy results.

Elevated sedimentation rates are characteristic of both GCA and polymyalgia rheumatica (PMR). Sedimentation rates greater than 100 mm in 1 hour (Westergren method) is common, but biopsy-proved cases with normal (0-40) sedimentation rates have been described (Wong and Kron, 1986). The prevalence of a normal ESR in patients with GCA is estimated to be between 2% and 8.7%. Other serum markers that are commonly elevated in patients with GCA include C-reactive protein, fibrinogen, alpha2 globulin, gamma globulin, complements, factor VIII or von Willebrand's factor, and interleukin-6. A mild to moderate normochromic anemia, thrombocytosis, decreased albumin, and elevated liver function tests, particularly alkaline phosphatase, are usually seen as well.

Corticosteroid therapy is the treatment of choice in all cases of GCA and is the only therapy proved to be efficacious. In general, once the diagnosis is suggested, prednisone is initiated, irrespective of the type or number of clinical manifestations. After obtaining a complete blood count and sedimentation rate, prednisone is started immediately in patients with recent or impending vascular complications (e.g., visual loss or stroke). Steroid treatment does alter the histopathologic picture and, therefore, it is preferable to obtain an arterial biopsy before or shortly after initiating treatment. However, inflammatory changes in the temporal arteries can persist for 2 to 4 weeks after steroids are begun.

Although the ideal initial prednisone dose, tapering scheme, and duration of treatment is debated, an initial starting dose of 40 to 60 mg of prednisone in single or divided daily dosages is adequate for most patients. Progression to complete bilateral blindness can occur in patients with the use of lower dosages. Alternate day steroid regimens are less effective than daily administration and cannot be relied on to control acute symptoms or disease activity. The dosage should be increased up to 120 mg/day in those who do not demonstrate a prompt clinical or laboratory response to lower dosages.

Patients with acute or impending visual loss or vascular complications should be hospitalized and administered intravenous methylprednisolone (1,000 mg/day over 3–5 days). Oral corticosteroids are then started at a dose of 1.5 to 2.0 mg/kg/day. The initial starting dosage is maintained until all reversible symptoms resolve and all aberrant laboratory parameters have normalized, which usually occurs within 2 to 4 weeks. Once resolution is maintained for 2 weeks, the dosage can be reduced by 10 mg every 2 weeks until a dose of 40 mg/day is attained. Thereafter, the dosage should not be decreased by more than 10% of the total daily dosage every 1 to 2 weeks. Once the total dosage is less than 10 mg, monthly tapering by 1 mg can be instituted. The alteration in steroid dosage should be based predominantly on clinical signs and symptoms. Most relapses appear to be related to inadequate suppression of a continuous inflammatory process rather than from spontaneous exacerbations. Although the sedimentation rate and C-reactive protein studies now are generally considered to be the most sensitive and widely available surrogate laboratory markers of disease activity, an increase in either or both does not always predict relapse; relapse can occur, despite these markers remaining within normal limits (Kyle and Hazelman, 1998). This emphasizes the importance of close clinical monitoring to determine the rate and extent to which steroids are tapered.

Treatment of GCA with long-term daily corticosteroids at high dosages can lead to frequent and potentially serious consequences. Patients must be periodically monitored for a number of potential adverse events that are commonly associated with long-standing corticosteroid administration: osteoporosis, hypertension, peptic ulcer disease, diabetes, and subcapsular cataracts. All patients on long-term corticosteroids should receive 1 to 2 g of supplemental calcium (calcium carbonate or citrate) and 400 to 800 U of vitamin D on a daily basis to prevent steroid-induced osteoporosis.

MASS LESIONS

In the elderly, the incidence of intracranial disease increases, including both metastatic and primary brain tumors. However, headache as the sole manifestation of brain tumor is uncommon in patients with a normal neurologic examination and no history of systemic cancer and occurs in only 1% of patients with brain tumors. The headache associated with intracranial mass lesions is usually intermittent and tends to develop and resolve over several hours. The most common type of brain tumor headache is a relatively bland "tension-type" headache, seen in more than two thirds of patients. Most patients describe the headache as a "dull ache" or "pressure" or "like a sinus headache." Migraine-like headaches are seen in about 10% of patients with brain tumors.

The "classic brain tumor headache"—severe headache, worse in the morning, and associated with vomiting, occurs in a minority (17%) of patients (Forsythe and Posner, 1993). In those individuals with a past history of headache, the headache associated with intracranial lesions is similar to the patient's previous headaches. This highlights the importance of carefully evaluating an elderly individual complaining of a headache that is even slightly different, more severe, more frequent, or associated with neurologic signs or symptoms, including slowed mentation. A neuroimaging study should be obtained in such a circumstance.

Headache in patients with brain tumor is more likely to be a prominent symptom when the tumor involves the leptomeninges or infratentorial compartment, which increases the likelihood of obstruction of cerebrospinal fluid pathways. Headaches are also common in those with a prior history of headache, as well as in patients with raised intracranial pressure, and in those with tumors that are associated with edema or shift of midline structures.

Some unusual headache syndromes, although uncommon, should raise the suspicion of an underlying mass lesion. These include paroxysmal headaches that are sudden in onset and peak within seconds but last only minutes to hours. This type of headache may signify a colloid cyst of the third ventricle. In addition, when this type of headache is precipitated by a Valsalva maneuver (exertion, cough, strain), it may indicate an underlying structural lesion, sometimes seen at the cervicomedullary junction. Finally, atypical facial pain in an elderly patient has been described in patients with nonmetastatic lung cancer (Capobianco, 1995). A high index of suspicion is required in patients with facial pain, especially those with a history of tobacco use or a recent history of weight loss.

Magnetic resonance imaging (MRI) with gadolinium is the imaging procedure of choice when evaluating an elderly patient with headache for an intracranial neoplasm. MRI is preferable to computed tomography (CT) because it detects smaller lesions, particularly in the brainstem or cerebellum and leptomeningeal disease, and will demonstrate involvement and enhancement of cranial nerves as well as thrombosis of venous sinuses sometimes seen in these patients. It can also assist with therapy if resection or focal radiation is contemplated.

The management of headache in a patient with a brain tumor is usually relatively straightforward. Before definitive therapy, if headache is severe and requires analgesia, simple analgesics (e.g., acetaminophen) can be used first. In cases of a significant amount of edema and central nervous system lymphoma is not in the differential diagnosis, dexamethasone (4 mg) two to four times daily is usually effective. Aspirin and other NSAIDS should generally be avoided if surgical intervention is likely because of the increased risk of bleeding. In refractory cases, opioids are effective. Codeine is usually effective, but may not be converted to morphine and lack analgesic efficacy in the presence of medications such as cimetidine and fluoxetine, which compete for enzymatic binding sites. Hydromorphone, morphine, methadone, and fentanyl can be useful, whereas meperidine and mixed opioid agonist-antagonists (e.g. pentazocine, butorphanol) should be avoided because of toxic metabolites and the potential for reverse analgesia.

CEREBROVASCULAR DISEASE

Ischemic Stroke

Headache can be an important but often neglected symptom of stroke because it is often overshadowed by other dramatic symptoms such as aphasia or hemiplegia. It is not widely recognized that ischemic strokes are associated with headache in about 25% of cases (Jensen and Gorelick, 2000). Headache occurs more often with cortical rather than subcortical infarctions and, when large, tend to be unilateral and ipsilateral to the side of the ischemia. Headache is important to recognize because it not only accompanies or follows the stroke, but it may herald the ischemic event by days or even weeks and, thus, provide an opportunity for intervention and prevention. These "'premonitory" headaches occur in up to 10% of patients with ischemic stroke (Gorelick et al., 1986). Headache is generally less common with transient ischemic attacks (TIA), but can be more common when the TIA involves the vertebrobasilar rather than the carotid circulation.

Headache associated with cerebral ischemia is sometimes unilateral and focal, but can be diffuse, nonlocalizing, and dull or throbbing in nature. The headache can last more than 24 hours. The intensity ranges from being barely noticeable, to moderately severe. Headaches associated with posterior circulation ischemia are usually more severe. When the headaches are classified according to the International Headache Society criteria, about 50% resemble tension-type headache and approximately 30% resemble migraine.

The pathophysiology is unclear, but it may be caused by vasodilation of pain-sensitive vessels by the release of vasoactive substances such as substance P, calcitonin gene-related polypeptide, and other peptides, which with cytokines, nitrous oxide, and bradykinins that are released from the vessel itself, contribute to increased nociceptive stimulation.

Hemorrhagic Stroke

Although headache is not universal in patients with hemorrhagic stroke, the frequency of headache is higher than in ischemic stroke and highest in patients with cerebellar and occipital hematomas. Overall, headache frequency appears to be in the range of 40% to 60%. When the intraparenchymal hematoma is small, headache may not be present.

Subdural Hematoma

Headache is also a frequent accompaniment of subdural hematomas in the elderly. The incidence of headache increases with the duration of the hematoma, occurring in up to 80% of those with chronic subdural hematomas (McKissock, 1960). Although a prominent complaint, few distinguishing features of the headache are reported in patients with subdural hematomas. They can be mild to moderate, but are often reported as persistent and troublesome. The headache can be paroxysmal and irregular, and occur intermittently throughout the day, sometimes with each episode lasting only minutes.

Hypertension

Although hypertension can exacerbate headache, because the two are highly prevalent conditions, the association between the two is often coincidental. Most large-scale epidemiologic studies have shown that headache in hypertensive individuals is not more prevalent than in normotensive controls. However, headache can be caused by severe hypertension, defined as a diastolic blood pressure greater than 130

mmHg (Badran et al., 1970; Bulpitt et al., 1976). Headache occurs in up to 80% of patients with paroxysmal hypertension secondary to pheochromocytoma.

The type of headache described in patients with diastolic pressure above 130 mmHg is frequently diffuse, present on awakening, and subsides over several hours. In contrast, the headache from paroxysmal hypertension is abrupt and throbbing, and subsides within several minutes.

The pathophysiology of hypertension-related headache is uncertain, but may result from hypertensive dilation and stretching of resistance vessels. In patients with malignant hypertension or paroxysmal hypertension, headache may, in part, be related to failure of autoregulation and the formation of brain edema with raised intracranial pressure.

Treatment of hypertensive headache involves aggressively treating the elevated blood pressure. Some drugs that dilate resistance vessels (e.g., calcium channel blockers and hydralazine) can exacerbate headache, and are best avoided in this patient population.

Medications-Related Headache

The illnesses that attend older age often require medications, some of which can cause headache. Table 14-3 lists some of the medications more commonly associated with headache. Alcohol and caffeine, which are often not listed on a medication list, can cause headache from either their consumption or withdrawal. Their use should be carefully determined in elderly patients complaining of headache. In addition, the elderly suffer the same analgesic, ergot, and triptan rebound headaches that afflict younger age groups. Medication-induced headaches are entirely nonspecific, but tend to be diffuse, sometimes throbbing, of mild to moderate intensity, and variable in duration. They can be persistent or episodic and temporally related to the administration of the medications (e.g., nitrates).

Treatment first and foremost involves tapering and withdrawal of the potentially offending agent(s). Withdrawal symptoms can be severe, depending on the medication being withdrawn, and therefore it is prudent, particularly in the elderly, to taper medications slowly to avoid a withdrawal syndrome. If medication is necessary, it is prudent to start low and titrate slowly to the lowest effective dose.

Cervical Spondylosis

Cervical spondylosis, which is more common with aging, is said to represent a common cause of

TABLE 14-3. *Medications causing headaches in the elderly*

Cardiovascular
    Vasodilators (nitrates, nicotinic acid, dipyridamole)
    Antihypertensives (nifedipine, methyldopa, reserpine, hydralazine)
    Antiarrythmics (quinidine, digoxin)
Nonsteroidal anti-inflammatory drugs
    Indomethacin, diclofenac, piroxicam
Antibiotics
    Tetracyclines, trimethoprim-sulfamethoxazole, isotretinoic
Gastrointestinal
    Ranitidine, cimetidine, omeprazole
Reproductive
    Estrogens
    Sildafenil
Hematologic/oncologic
    Erythropoietin
    Chemotherapeutics (tamoxifen, cyclophosphamide)
Bronchodilators
    Aminophylline, theophylline, pseudoephedrine
Central nervous system
    Sedatives (alcohol, barbiturates, benzodiazepines)
    Stimulants (caffeine, methylphenidate)
    Antiparkinsonian (amantadine, levodopa)
Antidepressant (trazodone and other selective serotonin reuptake inhibitors)

headache in the elderly. However, because radiographic evidence of cervical spondylosis is ubiquitous in the elderly and because most headache syndromes are diffuse and involve the occipitonuchal region, cervical spondylosis as a cause for headache in the elderly is likely overdiagnosed. Nevertheless, when present, the features of cervicogenic headache include occipital pain and limitation of range of motion of the neck, and spasm of cervical muscles. Associated abnormalities may be detected by physical examination of structures in the cervical root distribution, including sensory deficits, reflex changes, or muscle wasting in the arms. A local diagnostic block (short-acting local anesthetic and a corticosteroid) of the greater occipital nerve or the medial branch of C2, or a radiographically affected facet joint, may provide a diagnostic clue to the inciting structure and provide temporary pain relief. Treatment with medication may be limited, although simple analgesics or NSAIDS can be tried in conjunction with a mild muscle relaxant. Other approaches (e.g., physiotherapy and massage treatments) should be considered.

Metabolic Headaches

A number of metabolic and systemic disorders can cause headache in the elderly. According to the International Headache Society, metabolic headaches are those that occur during a metabolic disturbance and disappear within 7 days after corrective treatment.

Hypoxia-related headaches can occur in a variety of settings, including headache associated with chronic obstructive pulmonary disease, cardiac failure, and anemia. Hypoxia and hypercarbia can also occur in those with obstructive or central sleep apnea and lead to throbbing nocturnal or morning headaches that may clear after the patient rises from bed. Chronic renal failure, with or without associated anemia, can be associated with dull, diffuse, and chronic daily headaches. Dialysis can also lead to headaches, likely through an osmotic mechanism.

The Eye and Headache

A myriad of causes are found for eye pain. Ocular causes of eye pain or headache are invariably associated with a red eye, cloudy cornea (acute angle closure glaucoma), visual loss, diplopia, or an enlarged pupil. In general, "the white eye is not the cause of a painful eye." The only exceptions to this are posterior scleritis, which is best diagnosed by ultrasonography; optic neuritis where the visual loss is sometimes preceded by mild pain; and subacute angle closure glaucoma, which can only be diagnosed by gonioscopy, a procedure not routinely performed during an ophthalmologic examination. Because the incidence of glaucoma increases with advancing age, an ophthalmologic evaluation should be considered in the elderly patient with new onset ocular, frontal, or brow pain, when no other cause is evident.

Trigeminal Neuralgia

Trigeminal neuralgia is the most common neuralgic syndrome in the elderly, with an average age of onset of 50 years. A female preponderance for trigeminal neuralgia is found, with an annual incidence rate of 4.7 and 7.2 and prevalence of 108 and 200 per 1 million population in men and women, respectively.

Trigeminal neuralgia is an exquisitely severe, unilateral facial pain syndrome characterized by lancinating electric shocklike jolts of pain that are confined to the distribution of one or more divisions of the trigeminal nerve. The ophthalmic division is affected in isolation in only 4% of patients. The maxillary or mandibular divisions are more commonly affected and in more than two thirds of patients, two or more divisions of the trigeminal nerve are affected. The cardinal features of this disorder are listed in Table 14-4.

The cause of trigeminal neuralgia varies with age. Secondary trigeminal neuralgia caused by compressive mass lesions, demyelinating disease, or other structural lesions is more likely when the disorder presents before the fifth decade of life. In the elderly population, most patients have idiopathic trigeminal neuralgia, of whom approximately 80% have compression of the trigeminal root by an artery (superior cerebellar or anterior inferior cerebellar), vein, or both.

In one series of 2,972 patients with trigeminal neuralgia, 296 (10%) were found to have underlying intracranial tumors (Cheng et al., 1993). Meningiomas and posterior fossa tumors were those most commonly found, and although neurologic deficits developed on follow-up evaluation in 47% of the patients, most had no neurologic deficits and the delay in eventual tumor diagnosis was 6.3 years. These patients were younger than those with idiopathic pain, and although carbamazepine was the most effective medication used in this group, the relief was usually temporary.

The results of these studies in patients with trigeminal neuralgia underscore the need for a careful clinical evaluation of every patient, and most authorities advocate a brain MRI during the initial evaluation, even in the absence of neurologic signs or symptoms. Special attention should be given to the cerebellopontine angle and the course of the trigeminal nerve.

A diagnosis of idiopathic (primary) trigeminal neuralgia is established by its typical clinical features: a normal neurologic examination, except for the presence of trigger points, and a normal cranial imaging procedure. Impaired sensation in the distribution of any branch of the trigeminal nerve or a diminished or absent corneal reflex should raise suspicion of a structural, demyelinating, or compressive trigeminal nerve lesion.

Other diagnostic possibilities to be considered in those patients with atypical clinical features include dental pathology; tumor (intracranial, sinuses, nasopharynx, mouth, jaw, skull, chest); vascular (giant cell arteritis, aneurysm or arteriovenous malformation, carotid dissection, carotidynia); ocular (iritis, uveitis, optic neuritis, glaucoma, Tolosa Hunt syndrome, orbital pseudotumor); and idiopathic headache syndromes (cluster headache, migraine, chronic paroxysmal hemicrania, short-lasting unilateral neuralgiform pain with conjunctival injection and tearing [SUNCT]).

TABLE 14-4. *Cardinal features of the pain of trigeminal neuralgia*

Paroxysmal jabs of pain
Brief: 2–120 seconds
Sudden, intense, stabbing, superficial
Precipitated by certain activities such as brushing, chewing, talking
Associated with trigger zones: medial face (nose, lips, gums)
Paroxysms of pain separated by pain-free intervals*
Refractory phase following a paroxysm of pain, which is proportional to the length and intensity of the paroxysm, and during which pain cannot even be elicited
Spontaneous remission periods are common (50% of patients), usually last 6 months or more, and occur more commonly early in the course of the illness
No cranial nerve deficit

Medical Treatment

Medical therapy for trigeminal neuralgia is usually effective within 2 to 3 days. The most commonly used agents, the dosages, efficacy, and classes of evidence are outlined in Table 14-5. Carbamazepine has been the drug of first choice, but a related drug (oxcarbazepine) may be as effective as carbamazepine with a better tolerability profile, fewer drug interactions, and no need for hematologic and hepatic enzyme monitoring. Baclofen is also a useful agent, particularly when used in combination with carbamazepine, wherein may be a synergistic effect at lower dosages of each. More recently, some of the newer anticonvulsants (e.g., gabapentin and lamotrigine) have shown promise. The effective medications for trigeminal neuralgia, the level of evidence supporting their use, and the main side effects and dosages are listed in Table 14-5.

TABLE 14-5. *Medical treatment for trigeminal neuralgia*

Drug	Class of evidence	Standard dose (mg)	Main side effects	Special points	Efficacy: % response
Carbamazepine	Class I	Initial: 200–300	CNS (dose-dependent), rash (3%), neutropenia or pancytopenia, hyponatremia	Slow dose titration, divided dosages	60–80
L-baclofen	Class III	Initial: 600–800 Final: 600–800 Initial: 15 Final: 60–80	CNS (dose-dependent)	Synergistic effect with carbamazepine	65–75
Phenytoin	Class III	Initial: 200 Final: 300–400	CNS (dose-dependent), rash, gingival hypertrophy, acne, hirsutism, folate and vitamin D deficiency	Multiple drug influence level of serum protein binding, less effective than carbamazepine, useful as intravenous Fosphenytoin (250 mg) in acute setting	50
Gabapentin	Class III	Initial: 300 Final 600–2400	CNS (dose-dependent)	May be especially useful in TN secondary to MS	60–80**
Oxcarbazepine	Class III	Initial: 600 Final: 600–2400	Same as carbamazepine, but better tolerated	May be as if not more effective than carbamazepine, no black box warning, no monitoring of hepatic enzymes or liver function tests, fewer drug interactions; however, 2% risk of hyponatremia	75–90
Lamotrigine	Class I	Initial: 25–50 Final: 200–400	CNS (dose-dependent), rare life-threatening rash (0.3%)	Caution with co-administration with valproic acid, slow titration,	60–75
Clonazepam	Class III	Initial: 1 Final: 6–8	CNS (dose-dependent), habituation	Slow titration, gradual withdrawal	65
Valproic acid	Class III	Initial: 250–500 Final: 500–1500	CNS, tremor, alopecia, weight gain, nausea, pancreatitis and hepatotoxicity (rare)	Teratogenicity (neural tube defects), enteric coated form, SR form for once-daily dosing	50

CNS, central nervous system; MS, multiple sclerosis; SR, sustained release; TN, trigeminal neuralgia.

TABLE 14-6. *Surgical therapies for trigeminal neuralgia*

Procedure	Efficacy	Recurrence	Complications	Special points
Microvascular decompression	1 yr: 75% 10 yr: 64%	1 yr: 16% 10 yr: 33%	Persistent facial sensory loss (17%), hearing loss (2%), facial weakness (1% to 2%), cerebrospinal fluid leak (2%), major stroke/death (1%)	Recommended for patients with V1 pain, or pain involving all three divisions, who desire no sensory deficit.
Stereotactic radiosurgery	2 yr: 58% to 75% initial response for tumor-related TN	2 yr: 6%	Transient facial paresthesias (<10%), sensory loss (3%)	Non-invasive, local anasthesia, no convelescent interval, mean delay to efficacy 1 month (but up to 3–6 months)
Radiofrequency thermal rhizotomy	Initial: 96% to 100%	10–18 yr: 25% to 31%	Dysesthesias up to 50% (severe in 2%), corneal anasthesia (2% to 10%; 15% in first division procedures), keratitis (0.5% to 3%)	Stroke, diplopia, abscess, seizures (rare); death (1 patient in series of 10,000)
Glycerol rhizotomy	Initial: 80% to 95%	1.5–4 yr: 30% to 50%	Similar to RF lesions, plus oral herpes lesions, chemical aseptic meningitis.	Useful for those who wish to minimize facial sensory loss, first division pain, bilateral TN
Balloon compression	Inital: 90%	5–10 yr: 20% to 30%	Dysesthesias (4%)	Nonselective, motor division invariably transiently (<1 yr) affected
Peripheral avulsion or chemical neurolysis (phenol or absolute alcohol)	Initial: 90%	3 yr: 70%	Sensory loss (majority)—returns by 6 months	Very low risk procedure, 30% still have complete pain relief at 3 yr, may be considered in elderly or those with high operative risk

RF, radiofrequency.

A number of general caveats apply to the treatment of trigeminal neuralgia, irrespective of the agent used:

- Start *low* and titrate *slowly* to the *lowest* effective dosage.
- Clofen and clonazepam.
- Because remissions are common, withdraw medication slowly after an effective course and complete remission for 1 to 2 months.
- Combinations of medications can have additive or synergistic effect and may allow a lower dose of each with fewer side effects.
- Pain response does not exclude underlying pathology; nonresponse to a medication does not exclude diagnosis.
- In general, monitoring blood levels in patient with trigeminal neuralgia is not helpful, except to monitor compliance.
- In general, medications become less effective over time.

Surgical Treatment

Ultimately, approximately 30% of patients become resistant to or intolerant of drug therapy, and for these patients, interventional or surgical procedures are necessary. Numerous invasive approaches have been tried over the years, ranging from alcohol injection into peripheral trigeminal nerve branches to trigeminal root section. The most commonly employed procedures are outlined in Table 14-6.

Opinions differ regarding the best surgical treatment for patients with trigeminal neuralgia. When comparing different surgical approaches, consider the technical success and initial relief, long-term recurrence rate, facial numbness, facial dysesthesias, corneal anesthesia, trigeminal motor dysfunction, permanent cranial nerve deficits, intracranial hemorrhage and infarction, postoperative morbidity, and perioperative mortality.

In general, for healthy patients with idiopathic trigeminal neuralgia, a microvascular decompression is usually recommended if the first division or all three divisions are involved, or the patient desires no sensory deficit (McLaughlin et al., 1999; Barker et al., 1996). However, in some centers, stereotactic radiosurgery is becoming the treatment of first choice because it is noninvasive and associated with very low morbidity and risk for facial paresthesias (<10%) (Konzdiolka et al., 1998).

In many centers, a percutaneous technique, especially radiofrequency rhizotomy, is the procedure of choice for most patients having a first invasive surgi-

cal procedure (Taha and Tew, 1996). Compared with microvascular decompression, the results are comparable with radiofrequency rhizotomy, its side effects less morbid, and it is more cost-effective. The initial success rate is higher and recurrence rates lower compared with glycerol rhizotomy and balloon compression, but the incidence of facial dysesthesias and corneal anesthesia may be higher. Of the percutaneous procedures directed at the gasserian ganglion, balloon compression has the lowest incidence of corneal anesthesia and keratitis.

The final decision on treatment is one that weighs the patient's preference and medical risk, the rate of initial and long-term relief versus the risk of facial sensory loss and perioperative morbidity, and the comfort and expertise of the treating neurosurgeon.

REFERENCES

Badran RH, Weir RJ, McGuiness JB. Hypertension and headache. *Scand Med J* 1970;15:48–51.

Barker FG 2nd, Janetta PJ, Bissonette DJ, et al. The long-term outcome of microvascular decompression for trigeminal neuralgia. *N Engl J Med* 1996;334:1077–1083.

Bulpitt CJ, Dollery CT, Carne S. Change in symptoms of hypertension after referral to hospital clinic. *Br Heart J* 1976;38:121–128.

Capobianco DJ. Facial pain as a symptom of nonmetastatic lung cancer. *Headache* 1995;33:581–585.

Cheng TM, Cascino TL, Onofrio BM. Comprehensive study of diagnosis and treatment of trigeminal neuralgia secondary to tumors. *Neurology* 1993;43:2298–2302.

Cook NR, Evans DA, Funkelstein HH, et. al. Correlates of headache in a population-based cohort of elderly. *Arch Neurol* 1989;46:1228–1244.

Dodick DW, Jones JM, Capobianco DJ. The hypnic headache syndrome: another indomethacin responsive headache syndrome? *Headache* 2000;40(10):830–835.

Dodick DW, Mosek A, Campbell JK. The hypnic (alarm-clock) headache syndrome. *Cephalalgia* 1998;18:152–156.

Dodick DW, Rozen T, Silberstein SD, et al. Cluster headache. *Cephalalgia* 2000;20(9):787–803.

Forsythe PA, Posner JB. Headaches in patients with brain tumors: a study of 111 patients. *Neurology* 1993;43:1678–1683.

Gorelick PB, Hier DB, Caplan LR, et al. Headache in acute cerebrovascular disease. *Neurology* 1986;36:1445–1450.

Hale WE, Perkins LL, May FE, et al. Symptom prevalence in the elderly. *J Am Geriatr Soc* 1986;34:333–340.

Hunder GG. Giant cell arteritis and polymyalgia rheumatica. *Med Clin North Am* 1997;81:195–219.

Jensen TS, Gorelick PB. Headache associate with ischemic stroke and intracranial hematoma. In: Olesen J, Welch KMA, eds. *The headaches*, 2nd ed. Philadelphia: Lippincott Williams & Wilkins, 2000;781–787.

Kahn OA. Gabapentin relieves trigeminal neuralgia in multiple sclerosis patients. *Neurology* 1998;751:611–614.

Klein, RG, Campbell RJ, Hunder GG. Skip lesions in temporal arteritis. *Mayo Clin Proc* 1976;51:504–510.

Konzdiolka D, Perez B, Flickinger JC, et al. Gamma knife radiosurgery for trigeminal neuralgia. Results and expectations. *Arch Neurol* 1998;55:1524–1529.

Kyle V, Hazelman BL. Treatment of polymyalgia rheumatica and giant cell arteritis. I. Steroid regimens for the first two months. *Ann Rheum Dis* 1998;48:658–661.

Lipton RB, Soloman S, Wertenbaker C. Gradual loss and recovery of vision in temporal arteritis. *Arch Intern Med* 1985;145:2252–2253.

McKissock W. Subdural hematoma: a review of 389 cases. *Lancet* 1960;1:1365–1370.

McLaughlin MR, Janetta PJ, Clyde BL, et al. Microvascular decompression of cranial nerves: lessons learned after 4400 operations. *J Neurosurg* 90;1–8:1999.

Morales-Asin F, Mauri JA, Iniguez C, et al. The hypnic headache syndrome: report of three new cases. *Cephalalgia* 1998;18:157–158.

Ostberg G. Temporal arteritis in a large necropsy series. *Ann Rheum Dis* 1971;30:224–235.

Raskin NH. The hypnic headache syndrome. *Headache* 1988;28:534–536.

Salvarani C, Gabriel SE, O'Fallon WM, et al. The incidence of giant cell arteritis in Olmstead County, Minnesota, apparent fluctuations in cyclic pattern. *Ann Intern Med* 1995;123:192–194.

Serratrice G, Serbanesco S, Sanbuc R. Epidemiology of headache in elderly. Correlations with life conditions and socio-professional environment. *Headache* 1985;25:85–89.

Solomon GD, Kunkel RS, Frame J. Demographics of headache in elderly patients. *Headache* 1990;30:273–276.

Solomon S, Cappa K-G. The headache of temporal arteritis. *J Am Geriatr Soc* 1987;35:163–165.

Sorenson S, Lorenzen I. Giant-cell arteritis, temporal arteries and polymyalgia rheumatica: a retrospective study of 63 patients. *Acta Med Scand* 1977;201:207–213.

Strikiathachorn A. Epidemiology of headache in Thai elderly: a study in the Bangkae Home for the aged. *Headache* 1991;31:677–681.

Taha JM, Tew JM. Comparison of surgical treatments for trigeminal neuralgia: reevaluation of radiofrequency rhizotomy. *Neurosurgery* 1996;38:865–871.

Waters WE. The Pontypridd headache survey. *Headache* 1974;14:81–90.

Wong RL, Kron JH. Temporal arteritis without an elevated erythrocyte sedimentation rate. *Am J Med* 1986;80:959–964.

Young RF, Vermeulen SS, Grimm P, et al. Gamma knife radiosurgery for treatment of trigeminal neuralgia. Idiopathic and tumor related. *Neurology* 1997;48:608–614.

Zakrzewska JM, Chaudhry Z, et al. Lamotrigine in refractory trigeminal neuralgia: Results from a double-blind, placebo controlled crossover trial. *Pain* 73;223–230:1997.

SUGGESTED READING

Forsythe PA, Posner JB. Headaches in patients with brain tumors: a study of 111 patients. *Neurology* 1993;43:1678–1683.

Hunder GG. Giant cell arteritis and polymyalgia rheumatica. *Med Clin North Am* 1997;81:195–219.

Kyle V, Hazelman BL. Treatment of polymyalgia rheumatica and giant cell arteritis. I. Steroid regimens for the first two months. *Ann Rheum Dis* 1998;48:658–661.

Solomon GD, Kunkel RS, Frame J. Demographics of headache in elderly patients. *Headache* 1990;30:273–276.

15

Back and Neck Pain

H. Gordon Deen, Jr.

Acute pain in the back or neck is one of the most common symptoms experienced by older adults. Virtually every adult has experienced at least one episode of acute spinal pain. For most of these patients, extensive laboratory investigation and imaging tests are unnecessary, and rapid improvement can be expected with only simple treatment measures. It should be emphasized, however, that a few patients have significant neurologic impairment, evidence of cancer, or other serious underlying systemic illness. For these patients, an extensive differential diagnosis must be considered, and prompt workup and specialty consultation may be necessary.

DIFFERENTIAL DIAGNOSIS AND INITIAL ASSESSMENT

Primary care practitioners often do the initial evaluation and management of patients with acute back-related symptoms. Indeed, evidence shows that this is more cost-effective than similar care provided by specialists (Carey et al., 1995). The initial patient examination can be performed at the physician's office or in the hospital emergency department (Elam et al., 1995). A thorough clinical assessment is crucial to make the best decisions about diagnosis, laboratory testing, diagnostic imaging, and specialist referral. Usually, acute low back or neck pain resolves quickly, and a precise anatomic basis for the pain is never determined. These cases can be referred to as "uncomplicated" low back or neck pain. A nonspecific diagnosis (e.g., lumbar or cervical strain) is appropriate.

The clinical approach differs for patients with severe or persistent pain. In these cases, an extensive differential diagnosis must be considered (Tables 15-1 and 15-2). Several "red flags" can indicate the presence of a serious underlying disease. These include severe trauma (e.g., motor vehicle accident or sports injury), severe or progressive neurologic deficit, unrelenting nocturnal pain, unexplained weight loss, history of cancer, and fever (Table 15-3). These can be considered to be indicators of "complicated" low back or neck pain.

Severe, unremitting pain, especially at night, may indicate the presence of a spinal tumor. This is especially true in the older adult. Any patient over 65 years of age with acute, severe pain at any level of the spinal column should be considered to have a spinal metastatic

TABLE 15-1. *Differential diagnosis of low back pain with or without radiculopathy*

Discogenic or degenerative disease
  Herniated intervertebral disk
  Degenerative lumbar spondylosis
    Central lumbar canal stenosis
    Lateral recess stenosis
  Synovial cyst of facet joint
Tumor
  Primary intradural tumor of spinal cord, conus, or cauda equina
  Tumor of vertebral column or epidural space (or both)
    Metastatic tumor
    Plasmacytoma or multiple myeloma
    Primary bone tumor (e.g., chordoma)
  Extraspinal retroperitoneal malignancy
Vascular lesion
  Arteriovenous malformation of the spinal cord
  Spinal dural arteriovenous fistula
Infection
  Intervertebral diskitis or osteomyelitis
  Epidural abscess
  Urinary tract infection
  Herpes zoster or other viral radiculopathy
Intraabdominal or intrapelvic disease
  Abdominal aortic aneurysm
  Nephrolithiasis
  Posterior perforating duodenal ulcer
  Pancreatic disease
  Endometriosis
Degenerative hip disease
Neurologic complications of diabetes
  Peripheral neuropathy
  Radiculopathy
Congenital
  Tethered cord
  Intraspinal lipoma
Metabolic bone disease
  Osteoporotic compression fracture
Trauma

TABLE 15-2. *Differential diagnosis of neck pain with or without neurologic involvement*

Discogenic or degenerative disease
  Herniated intervertebral disk
  Degenerative cervical spondylosis with canal
    stenosis
  Synovial cyst of facet joint
Tumor
  Primary intradural tumor of spinal cord or adjacent
    nerve roots
  Tumor of vertebral column or epidural space (or
    both)
    Metastatic tumor
    Plasmacytoma or multiple myeloma
    Primary bone tumor (e.g., chordoma)
Vascular lesion
  Arteriovenous malformation of the spinal cord
  Spinal dural arteriovenous fistula
Infection
  Intervertebral diskitis or osteomyelitis
  Epidural abscess
  Herpes zoster or other viral radiculopathy
Degenerative shoulder disease
Neurologic complications of diabetes
Metabolic bone disease
  Osteoporotic compression fracture
Trauma

tumor until such is proved otherwise. This suspicion is heightened if the patient has a history of malignant disease or unexplained weight loss. Also be aware that low back pain can be a referred symptom and may indicate the presence of a serious disease of the abdomen or pelvis (e.g., abdominal aortic aneurysm, renal colic, pancreatitis, or retroperitoneal tumor). Low back pain can also be a manifestation of urinary tract infection, especially in women. This relatively common problem must be excluded, or treated if present, before embarking on an extensive spinal evaluation.

Patients with low back pain may also have leg pain, often referred to as "sciatica" or "radiculopathy." These terms refer to pain and paresthesias extending

TABLE 15-3. *Indicators of "complicated spinal pain"*

Severe trauma (e.g., motor vehicle accident or
  serious sports injury)
Severe or progressive neurologic deficit
  Loss of motor strength
  Numbness or loss of sensation
  Impaired bladder or bowel control
Unrelenting nocturnal pain
Unexplained weight loss (>4.5 kg in 6 months)
History of cancer
Fever

down the leg in a dermatomal pattern. The onset can be gradual or abrupt, and patients generally do not recall any trauma or unaccustomed physical activity. The most common cause of sciatica is a herniated lumbar intervertebral disk. In the general population, 95% of lumbar disk herniations occur at the L4-L5 and L5-S1 levels. In older individuals, upper lumbar disk herniations at or above the L3-L4 level are somewhat more common. Other compressive lesions that can cause sciatica include degenerative lumbar spinal stenosis, tumor, and epidural abscess. Also be aware of noncompressive causes of leg pain, including radiculopathy caused by diabetes and herpes zoster (shingles). Pain in the hip and groin occasionally indicates an upper lumbar radiculopathy, but more often indicates degenerative hip disease, especially in the older adult.

Patients with disorders of the cervical spine can also have neurologic involvement, including cervical radiculopathy, myelopathy, or a combination of the two. Cervical radiculopathy refers to pain and paresthesias radiating to the arm in a specific dermatomal pattern. Cervical myelopathy refers to symptoms caused by spinal cord compression. These symptoms are more ominous and can include weakness and clumsiness of the arms and legs, and bowel and bladder dysfunction.

CLINICAL ASSESSMENT

The importance of a detailed medical history cannot be overemphasized. The patient should be asked to describe the site, duration, and intensity of pain; extension of pain; body positions that relieve or exacerbate the pain; extremity weakness or sensory disturbance; and any bladder or bowel dysfunction. Any history of trauma, weight loss, malignant disease, or other systemic disease should be noted. Carefully review the medication history and any other treatments that have been used. It is important to take the time to obtain an accurate and thorough medication history because some patients may have obtained prescription and over-the-counter medications from multiple sources. Diet supplements and other "alternative medicine" remedies are also increasingly popular, and the patient should be asked about these as well. Inquire about previous episodes of spinal pain and what treatments had been used.

An accurate history of tobacco usage is essential. Smoking is a risk factor for osteoporosis and chronic back pain. Smoking can increase intradiskal pressure because of chronic coughing, jeopardize disk metabolism because of vascular effects of nicotine, or serve as a marker for psychosocial traits associated with frequent and prolonged pain (Deyo et al., 1990).

Secondary gain phenomena such as litigation, workers compensation issues, job dissatisfaction, psychiatric problems, and narcotic abuse should be completely explored. These psychosocial issues appear to have an important influence in magnifying symptoms of back and neck pain. If present, these are tip-offs or red flags that the patient may not respond well to treatment.

It is important to review the impact that the back pain is having on normal activities of daily living and employment. Ask whether the patient requires a cane or other ambulation aid, whether the patient has fallen, and whether the patient can function independently. It is often helpful to note how the patient arrived for examination. Ask whether the patient had to rest between the parking lot and the examination room, and whether a walker or wheelchair was needed. It is important to note whether the patient has missed work or stopped his or her usual recreational activities.

Most, but by no means all, elderly patients are retired, so employment status is not an issue for many. Ask these patients whether they have had to curtail shopping, travel, yard work, golfing, and other leisure activities.

Older adults can have preexisting medical illnesses, such as congestive heart failure; neurologic disorders (e.g., Parkinson's disease); and musculoskeletal conditions (e.g., degenerative arthritis of the hip) that magnify the impact of acute spinal symptoms. For example, the patient with an acute lumbar disk herniation, who also has Parkinson's disease, may have his or her functional status much more severely compromised than would the same patient without Parkinson's disease.

The general physical examination should include an assessment of gait, straight-leg raising (Lasegue's sign), spinal range of motion, and spinal tenderness or spasm. Straight-leg raising is the most sensitive indicator of nerve root compression. If straight-leg raising pain is absent, then another diagnosis (other than nerve root compression) should be considered. The presence of crossed straight-leg raising (exacerbation of leg pain when the contralateral leg, or "well leg" is raised) is strongly suggestive of lumbar disk herniation. Signs of malignant disease or infection should be noted. If hip and groin pain is present, the fabere maneuvers (flexion, abduction, external rotation, and extension of the hip—also known as "Patrick's test") should be performed; presence of pain during this test is suggestive of degenerative joint disease of the hip.

The trochanter should be palpated for evidence of tenderness or inflammation. Positive findings point to degenerative arthritis of the hip joint or trochanteric bursitis (or both). An inguinal hernia should be excluded.

In patients presenting with neck pain, the head and neck should be observed from all directions, looking for abnormal head posture (e.g., as seen in torticollis). Cervical range of motion should be assessed. Check for a Spurling's sign—radiating arm pain precipitated by head tilt or rotation to the symptomatic side. A positive Spurling's sign is strongly suggestive of cervical nerve root compression. The patient should be asked whether cervical flexion produces an electric shock sensation in the torso or extremities (Lhermitte's phenomenon). This finding suggests the presence of a cervical cord lesion, which could be compressive (tumor) or noncompressive (demyelinating disease). The shoulder is examined for evidence of a rotator cuff injury or degenerative joint disease.

A neurologic examination should include an assessment of strength, sensation, and deep tendon reflexes. With evidence of an acute myelopathy or cauda equina syndrome, perianal sensation and rectal tone should be assessed. A sensory level usually correlates with the anatomic level of the lesion. For example, a patient with a T-10 cord lesion will usually have a T-10 sensory level. In some cases, however, the sensory level may be several levels below the actual site of the lesion. For example, a patient harboring an intradural tumor at the T-2 vertebral level might have a T-8 dermatomal sensory level on initial evaluation.

On the basis of the initial assessment, a few patients will have a significant neurologic deficit (severe myelopathy, radiculopathy, or cauda equina syndrome) or evidence of a serious underlying disease such as cancer (Table 15-3). Patients with these findings have "complicated spinal pain" and warrant immediately radiographic investigation, usually with magnetic resonance imaging (MRI), and prompt surgical referral. Most patients, however, can be managed with simple measures, as will be described.

It should be emphasized that incomplete clinical evaluation leads to an over-reliance on diagnostic tests, notably MRI, which in turn, leads to errors in diagnosis and treatment. Patients may be given the diagnosis of lumbar disk disease or lumbar spinal stenosis on the basis of an MRI, yet ultimately prove to have a completely different diagnosis. The author has seen patients referred for neurosurgical consultation for "lumbar disk disease," who are subsequently found to have completely different diagnoses, including spinal cord tumor, spinal arteriovenous malformation, metastatic carcinoma, abdominal aortic aneurysm, spinal infection, degenerative arthritis of the hip, inguinal hernia, peripheral neuropathy, and viral radiculitis due to herpes zoster. Thus, the physician must be aware of the broad differential diagnosis of spinal column pain, and perform a thorough clinical assessment to establish the correct diagnosis and institute appropriate therapy.

INITIAL APPROACH TO DIAGNOSIS AND MANAGEMENT

The natural history of acute pain in the lower back or neck, in the absence of a tumor or other serious underlying disease process, is characterized by rapid improvement (Fig. 15-1). A substantial majority of patients will experience resolution of symptoms within 4 to 6 weeks. A nonspecific diagnosis such as lumbar or cervical strain is appropriate. Laboratory investigation and spinal imaging are usually not required.

The typical patient with "uncomplicated" acute spinal pain can be managed with short-term bed rest (2–3 days) and aspirin or nonsteroidal anti-inflammatory drugs (NSAID), such as ibuprofen. Acetaminophen is a reasonable alternative if the patient cannot tolerate NSAID because of gastrointestinal distress or other side effects. A new class of NSAID, the COX-2 inhibitors, is emerging as a useful adjunct for the treatment of spinal and musculoskeletal pain. Preliminary studies indicate that the COX-2 inhibitors have fewer gastrointestinal side effects than older NSAID, such as ibuprofen. Rofecoxib (Vioxx) is one example of a COX-2 inhibitor drug now being used clinically. Muscle relaxants (e.g., methocarbamol) may be useful on a short-term basis in selected patients with a pronounced degree of paraspinal muscle spasm. Narcotic analgesics are usually unnecessary. Narcotic medications should be used cautiously in the older patient because of cognitive side effects (e.g., confusion) that can result from their use. If narcotics are used, they should be prescribed in small quantities on a time-limited basis. A short course of oral steroids may be helpful in pa-

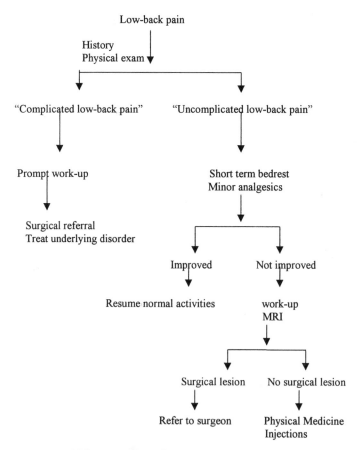

FIG. 15-1. Management of low-back pain.

tients with acute radicular pain. These medications are outlined in Table 15-4.

Patients should be cautioned about side effects and the maximum recommended doses of each medication. They should be informed when a medication has more than one active ingredient. An example of this is Darvocet-N 100, which contains propoxyphene napsylate (100 mg) and acetaminophen (650 mg). A patient who is taking Tylenol on a regular schedule and Darvocet-N 100 for breakthrough pain must avoid exceeding the maximum recommended daily dose of acetaminophen (4,000 mg), to avoid potentially serious hepatic toxicity. In older patients, the adverse effects of pharmacologic therapy must balanced against the positive effects of pain relief and functional improvement.

Diagnostic tests, physical therapy, back braces, imaging tests, and surgical referral are usually unnecessary for patients with acute spinal pain. Hospitalization is needed only in exceptional circumstances. It is important to reassure patients with nonspecific acute low back or neck pain that they most likely have a benign, self-limited condition and that symptoms should rapidly resolve without active treatment. Terms like "ruptured disk" are alarming to patients and should be avoided. Patients may resume work and normal activities of daily living as symptoms allow. Emphasize aerobic exercise, weight control, and avoidance of tobacco to them. Instruct them to avoid heavy lifting and repetitive bending and twisting of the lower back, to change positions frequently, and to use a chair with adequate lower back support. More than 90% of patients with nonspecific acute low back and neck pain will experience complete relief of symptoms by using these simple measures.

For the few patients who have not experienced improvement within 4 to 6 weeks, further assessment is warranted; attempt to establish a more precise diagnosis. Among the tests that may be done: plain radiography of the painful spinal segment, complete blood cell count, erythrocyte sedimentation rate, chemistry profile, and urinalysis. The prostate-specific antigen level should be assessed in men older than 50 years of age. The main reason for these tests is to screen for nondiskogenic causes of spinal pain.

SPINAL IMAGING

Plain radiographs can be helpful in establishing the diagnosis of spinal compression fractures in the elderly. When seen in the lower thoracic and lumbar regions, these fractures are usually the result of osteoporosis. A compression fracture at or above the T-6 level is usually not caused by osteoporosis and should raise suspicion for a tumor.

MRI should be considered for patients with 4 to 6 weeks of persistent spinal pain, especially those with neurologic symptoms or signs. This imaging test provides a wealth of anatomic information; however, be aware that the MRI is extremely sensitive, and that many "abnormalities" demonstrated by this procedure simply represent normal aging changes in the spine. Many completely asymptomatic people will have abnormal findings on lumbar and cervical MRI; thus, test results must be interpreted cautiously (Jensen et al., 1994). The phrase "gray hair of the spine" is an apt description that can be used to convey the significance of many of the positive findings seen on spinal MRI in the elderly in terms that can be understood by the lay person.

TABLE 15-4. *Medication chart: back and neck pain*

Drug	Dose	Risks	Cost/month ($)
Aspirin	325–650 mg q.i.d. p.r.n. pain; maximum 2,600 mg/d	Gastrointestinal bleeding, tinnitus, asthma	<20
Ibuprofen	600–3,200 mg/d	Gastrointestinal bleeding, hypotension	<20
Acetaminophen	1,000–4,000 mg/d	Hepatic toxicity	<20
Rofecoxib (Vioxx)	12.5–50 mg/d	Gastrointestinal symptoms, hypertension, lower extremity edema	>250
Methocarbamol	2,000–4,000 mg/d	Drowsiness, nausea, urticaria	100
Methylprednisolone (dose pack)	1-week tapering course	Gastrointestinal symptoms	<20 (1-week course)
Propoxyphene, napsylate, and acetaminophen	1–2 tablets q.i.d. p.r.n. pain; maximum 6 tablets per day	Hepatic toxicity, nausea, constipation, sedation	50

p.r.n., when needed; q.i.d., four times a day.

The so-called "open magnet" MRI is generally not helpful in the evaluation of spinal disorders. Although claustrophobic patients tolerate this type of MRI examination, image quality is suboptimal. The image quality is generally not adequate for surgical planning or even for establishing a diagnosis. As a result, patients who have open magnet MRI frequently need to have additional spinal imaging, either standard MRI with sedation or computed tomography (CT) or myelography. This adds to the time, effort, and expense of the diagnostic workup.

Although MRI plays a major role in spinal imaging, situations exist in which this examination cannot be done. Absolute contraindications include the presence of pacemakers and ferromagnetic implants, such as cochlear implants and certain intracranial aneurysm clips. Relative contraindications include claustrophobia, obesity, and the need for advanced life support in the critically ill patient. Another problem is the prolonged examination time, which can preclude technically satisfactory imaging in the patient with severe pain. These patients often are unable to hold still long enough to obtain a satisfactory MRI.

In situations where MRI would be contraindicated or technically difficult, myelography with water-soluble contrast medium, followed by CT, the so-called "myelogram-CT," remains an excellent diagnostic tool that is useful in selected patients (Miller et al., 1989). This examination allows superb visualization of the spinal canal, subarachnoid space, spinal column, and extraspinal soft tissues. Bony detail is particularly well seen. The myelogram-CT, a minimally invasive procedure, involves a spinal tap, usually in the lumbar region, for injection of contrast material, should usually be ordered only after consultation with a neurologist or neurosurgeon. The myelogram-CT should generally be reserved for those patients who are being seriously considered for surgical treatment. Similar to MRI, the myelogram-CT has a significant incidence of positive findings in asymptomatic or minimally symptomatic patients. Therefore, the examination must be interpreted cautiously and in the context of the patient's clinical findings. Unlike MRI, the myelogram-CT gives the clinician the opportunity to examine the patient's cerebrospinal fluid (CSF), a small sample of which can be removed before the contrast material is injected. Routine CSF studies include protein, glucose, and cell count. A variety of cultures and stains can be obtained if infection is a consideration. Similarly, cytologic analysis looking for malignant cells is helpful in selected cases.

The most common complication of myelography is a spinal headache caused by the lumbar puncture. This occurs in about 10% of cases. A much less common, but more serious, complication is neurologic deterioration in cases of a complete block of the spinal canal caused by tumor or other compressive lesion. It is thought that withdrawing small amounts of CSF below a complete block can cause further compression of the spinal cord, similar to the effect of a cork being pushed further into a bottle. Another uncommon, but potentially serious complication is anaphylactic reaction to the iodine-based contrast material. For this reason, any patient with a history of significant allergic reaction to iodine or shellfish should be pretreated with steroids and diphenhydramine before myelography. Oral anticoagulants (e.g., warfarin) must be discontinued for a few days before myelography to allow the international normalized ratio and prothrombin time to normalize. Fortunately, serious complications of myelography are rare and the myelogram-CT examination continues to play a major role in the evaluation of spinal disorders.

For patients with lower back and leg pain, both MRI and myelogram-CT should include the entire lumbar spine and the lower thoracic spine up to the T-10 level to rule out intradural tumors and other lesions at the thoracolumbar junction—a lumbar MRI or myelogram-CT that stops at L-3, or even at L-1, is inadequate. These examinations must image the entire spinal column from the sacrum up to T-10. Close communication between the clinician and the radiologist is necessary to avoid imaging the wrong segment of the spinal column.

The use of CT without intrathecally administered contrast enhancement (noncontrast CT) should be discouraged. This examination does not visualize the subarachnoid space and, therefore, cannot diagnose cauda equina tumors and other intradural lesions that can mimic lumbar disk herniations. A "negative" noncontrast CT does not eliminate the need for MRI or myelogram-CT in the patient with unexplained acute back or neck pain. Similarly, the patient with a "positive" noncontrast CT frequently still requires MRI or myelogram-CT for surgical decision making.

Measure bone mineral density (BMD) in individuals at increased risk for osteoporosis, in patients under 50 years of age who have atraumatic fractures, and in those with osteopenia or spinal deformities noted on plain radiographs, MRI, or CT. Bone density testing helps to establish a diagnosis of osteoporosis, to estimate future fracture risk, and to follow the response to treatment.

Dual energy x-ray absorptiometry (DEXA) is the most widely used test for measuring BMD. DEXA can measure bone density in the lumbar spine and hip, two sites that are subject to the most clinically significant fractures. The DEXA test report includes a measure of BMD in grams per centimeter^2, a calculated T-score, and a calculated Z-score. The T-score represents the number of standard deviations a bone density is above or below the mean peak bone mass of the general population. T-scores are used to define the presence of osteoporosis. For example, a T-score between +1.0 and −1.0 is normal; a T-score between −1.0 and −2.5 indicates osteopenia (low bone mass); and a T-score below −2.5 indicates osteoporosis.

Radionuclide bone scans and plain film tomography used to play a prominent role in the imaging workup of patients with back-related symptoms. Over time, MRI and CT have largely replaced these examinations. Bone scans and plain film tomography continue to play a secondary role in monitoring the progression of certain spinal diseases, notably osteomyelitis and diskitis; however, these procedures are rarely indicated in the initial diagnostic evaluation of acute back or neck pain.

In patients who have sustained neck injury, anteroposterior and lateral radiographs of the cervical spine should be obtained. It is essential for the lateral view to demonstrate the entire cervical spine, from the foramen magnum down to T-1. The most common diagnostic error in the radiographic evaluation of the cervical spine is failure to demonstrate the C-7–T-1 junction. A swimmer's view or CT may be necessary to adequately evaluate the lower cervical spine. Lateral flexion and extension views are helpful in selected cases. If neck pain persists, consider repeating imaging of the cervical spine after 3 to 6 weeks. This is important because ligamentous instability of the cervical spine may not be apparent on the initial imaging studies.

NEUROPHYSIOLOGIC TESTING

Electromyography (EMG) and nerve conduction velocity (NCV) studies can be helpful in patients with arm or leg pain. These studies can confirm a clinical impression of cervical or lumbar monoradiculopathy or indicate the presence of an unsuspected polyradiculopathy or peripheral neuropathy. In patients with upper extremity symptoms, EMG and NCV studies may indicate the presence of carpal tunnel syndrome, ulnar neuropathy, or brachial plexus lesion, which can mimic a cervical radiculopathy. In patients with atypical limb pain, normal findings on EMG can also be helpful to exclude the presence of radiculopathy as a cause for their symptoms. Somatosensory evoked potentials can be useful in patients in whom cervical myelopathy is suspected. Generally, neurophysiologic

testing is not useful in patients without evidence of radiculopathy or myelopathy, for example, the patient with midline axial spinal column pain, without neurologic involvement.

CONSERVATIVE TREATMENT

If the results of laboratory testing and imaging are unremarkable, a physical therapy program should be initiated after consultation with a physiatrist or physical therapist. Typically, a rehabilitation regimen begins with an exercise and stretching program. Physical therapy "modalities" such as traction, diathermy, application of heat or cold, ultrasound therapy, and transcutaneous electrical stimulation can be added. If physical medicine is successful, a response is generally seen within 4 to 6 weeks. Epidural steroid injections can be of benefit in selected patients (Garfin, 1995). These injections are frequently done in patients with lumbar symptoms. Cervical epidural steroid injections are less commonly done, but can safely be performed by physicians experienced in the technique. Caudal blocks, selective nerve root injections, facet blocks, and trigger point injections can benefit selected patients. A substantial majority of patients with acute and subacute spinal pain will experience relief of symptoms with these simple, minimally invasive procedures.

For most patients with back and neck pain, aerobic exercise is the best long-term conservative treatment. Aerobic exercise helps improve overall conditioning and endurance, aids with weight loss, and increases endogenous endorphins, which decreases pain and improves the sense of well-being. Most patients, even the elderly, can usually find some form of aerobic activity that they can comfortably perform.

SURGICAL CONSULTATION

Surgical referral should be considered for those patients with significant or progressing neurologic signs and symptoms and for those patients who have failed conservative treatment and whose imaging studies show a lesion that seems to explain their symptoms. Patients with pain but no structural lesion are probably best served by referral to a pain management specialist or a neurologist, rather than to a surgeon. Surgical referral of these latter cases often adds nothing but time and expense to the patient's management.

Although older patients may take longer to recover from surgery and require more rehabilitation, be aware that advanced age does not preclude consideration of elective spinal surgery in the elderly. Overall health and "physiologic age" are more important than chronologic age. Healthy individuals older than 90 years of age can be expected to have good outcomes after spinal operations, provided they meet the same criteria for operation as younger patients. One example: advanced age is not a predictor of poor outcome in patients having lumbar decompressive laminectomy for spinal stenosis.

SURGICAL MANAGEMENT

The most common indication for surgical referral of the older patient is degenerative lumbar spinal stenosis with neurogenic claudication. The optimal candidate for surgery has leg symptoms, rather than low back pain, as the primary complaint. The MRI or myelogram-CT should show significant lumbar spinal canal or lateral recess stenosis that correlates with the clinical findings. The surgical treatment is lumbar decompressive laminectomy of the stenotic spinal segments. A fusion may be needed in some cases. Lumbar decompressive laminectomy is the most common spinal operation performed on Medicare beneficiaries. Good or excellent results can be expected in 70% to 90% of cases (Atlas et al., 1996). Serious complications can occur, although uncommonly.

Lumbar disk herniation is seen more frequently in middle-aged adults, but can also occur in the elderly. The optimal candidate for a lumbar disk operation has sciatica, rather than low-back pain, as the primary symptom; an objective neurologic deficit that involves one or more spinal nerve roots; and clear-cut evidence of a herniated disk on MRI or myelogram-CT that correlates precisely with the clinical findings. Operative intervention is almost never indicated if findings on imaging studies are normal (Long, 1992).

Patients with mild to moderate neurologic deficit are considered for elective diskectomy if the aforementioned conservative treatment measures are unsuccessful. Urgent surgical treatment is usually indicated for patients with severe or rapidly progressive radiculopathy, and emergent surgical intervention should be considered for patients with an acute cauda equina syndrome. In properly selected patients, lumbar diskectomy can be expected to achieve excellent or good results in 80% to 90% of patients (Pappas et al., 1992). A fusion is usually not required. Lumbar diskectomy is a relatively safe operation. Blood loss is usually minimal. Younger patients can sometimes have this surgery on an outpatient basis, but the older adult usually requires a short hospital stay of 1 to 2 days. Serious complications (e.g., paraplegia, great vessel injury, and death) can occur, rarely.

Indications for cervical diskectomy are similar to those of lumbar diskectomy. The optimal candidate

for surgery has radicular symptoms (or myelopathy), rather than neck pain, as the primary symptom; an objective neurologic deficit; and clear-cut evidence of a herniated disk on MRI or myelogram-CT that correlates well with the clinical findings.

Patients with mild to moderate neurologic deficit are considered for elective surgery if they fail conservative treatment. Urgent surgery should be considered for those patients with severe or rapidly progressive neurologic deficit. In properly selected patients, cervical diskectomy can be expected to achieve results comparable to those seen with lumbar diskectomy, with excellent or good results in 80% to 90% of patients. The results are less favorable in patients with severe cervical myelopathy. Cervical diskectomy can be performed via anterior and posterior approaches, with or without fusion. The surgical approach will vary, depending on imaging results and surgeon preference. Serious complications (e.g., quadriplegia and death) can occur, rarely.

CONCLUSION

Acute pain in the lower back or neck is one of the most common problems encountered in clinical practice. For the few patients who have complicated spinal pain, manifested by a severe neurologic deficit or evidence of cancer or other serious underlying illness, a broad differential diagnosis must be considered. Rapid workup and surgical referral may be needed in these cases. However, most patients with uncomplicated low-back pain require no laboratory tests or imaging, and their symptoms improve with simple treatment measures. If symptoms do not improve within 4 to 6 weeks, further evaluation is required. These patients should have MRI or myelogram-CT of the symptomatic spinal segment. Physical therapy and various types of injections can be helpful in patients without clear-cut surgical lesions, or in patients who wish to defer surgery. Surgical treatment of many common degenerative spinal disorders of the elderly can be accomplished safely and result in an excellent or good result in most cases. Advanced age is not a contraindication to elective spinal surgery, provided the patient is medically fit and meets the appropriate surgical indications.

REFERENCES

Atlas SJ, Deyo RA, Keller RB, et al. The Maine lumbar spine study. Part II. 1-year outcomes of surgical and nonsurgical management of lumbar spinal stenosis. *Spine* 21;1996:1787–1795.

Carey TS, Garrett J, Jackman A, et al. The outcomes and costs of care for acute low back pain among patients seen by primary care practitioners, chiropractors, and orthopedic surgeons. *N Engl J Med* 1995;333:913–917.

Deyo RA, Loeser JD, Bigos SJ. Herniated lumber intervertebral disk. *Ann Intern Med* 1990;112:598–603.

Elam KC, Cherkin DC, Deyo RA. How emergency physicians approach low back pain: choosing costly options. *J Emerg Med* 1995;13:143–150.

Garfin SR. Clinical crossroads: a 50-year-old woman with disabling spinal stenosis. *JAMA* 1995:274:1949–1954.

Jensen MC, Brant-Zawadzki MN, Obuchowski N, et al. Magnetic resonance imaging of the lumbar spine in people without back pain. *N Engl J Med* 1994;331:69–73.

Long DM. Decision making in lumbar disc disease. *Clin Neurosurg* 1992;39:36–51.

Miller GM, Forbes GS, Onofrio BM. Magnetic resonance imaging of the spine. *Mayo Clin Proc* 1989;64:986–1004.

Pappas CTE, Harrington T, Sonntag VKH. Outcome analysis in 654 surgically treated lumbar disc herniations. *Neurosurgery* 1992;30:862–866.

SELECTED READING

Adams RD, Victor M, Ropper AH. *Principles of neurology*, 6th ed. New York: McGraw-Hill, 1997.

Deen HG. Diagnosis and management of lumbar disk disease. *Mayo Clin Proc* 1996;71:283–287.

Deyo RA, Rainville J, Kent DL. What can the history and physical examination tell us about low back pain? *JAMA* 1992;268:760–765.

Frymoyer JW. Back pain and sciatica. *N Engl J Med* 1988; 318:291–299.

Popp AJ, ed. *A guide to the primary care of neurological disorders*. Park Ridge, IL: American Association of Neurological Surgeons, 1998:101–120.

16

Incontinence and Sexual Dysfunction in the Elderly

Kathleen Hawker and Elliot M. Frohman

Bladder dysfunction, leading to incontinence, can occur in the elderly as a manifestation of a variety of diseases. When assessing these patients for incontinence, numerous factors need to be considered. Primary dysfunction of the genitourinary tract caused by estrogen deficiency in women, stress incontinence after childbearing, and prostate dysfunction in males are specific factors that predispose patients to incontinence. Furthermore, coexistent diseases (e.g., stroke, Parkinson's disease [PD], Alzheimer's disease, degenerative spine disease) and neuropathies also contribute to the risk of genitourinary dysfunction in the elderly. Loss or slowing of mobility because of joint disease, poor vision, and imbalance from a variety of disorders can contribute. Each of these problems can lead to incontinence as an independent factor. An integrated approach, including a detailed history and physical examination, urologic opinion, combined with diagnostics, can facilitate the identification of specific contributing factors and lead to the formulation of an appropriate treatment plan (Fig. 16-1).

BLADDER PHYSIOLOGY

A clear understanding of bladder physiology is crucial for the diagnosis and treatment of incontinence. The bladder wall or detrusor muscle is composed of smooth muscle and is under the control of local neural circuits consisting of cholinergic parasympathetic fibers derived from the intermediolateral cell columns of the sacral spinal cord (S2-S4). Increased activity in this pathway causes contraction of the detrusor muscle, whereas anticholinergic agents diminish or abolish the electrical activity of the bladder wall. Beta-adrenergic activity has a relaxant effect on the detrusor muscle; however, this seems to be of lesser importance for bladder control than the parasympathetic input (Blavais, 1982; De Groat and Booth, 1993).

Mechanoreceptors sense bladder filling and transmit this information along Aδ afferents from the detrusor muscle to the sacral micturition center, located in the spinal cord. Unmyelinated C-fibers respond to noxious stimuli and are usually silent in healthy individuals. These afferent inputs are transmitted rostrally in the spinal cord to a central control area, the pontine micturition center (PMC), located in the pontine tegmentum. For continence, detrusor muscle activity must be coordinated with the activity of the urethral sphincter. Uniquely composed, specialized intrinsic striated muscle cells make up the wall of the sphincter and are innervated by somatic pelvic and pudendal nerves that originate in Onuf's nucleus (S2-S3). The small anterior horn cells in Onuf's nucleus are in close proximity to the intermediolateral motor pathways of the parasympathetic system, possibly integrating the two systems. Excitatory α-adrenergic neurons originating in the hypogastric plexus from T9-L2 control the smooth muscle of the bladder neck and urethra and produce activation and muscle contraction, whereas β-adrenergic input achieves inhibition (Dasgupta and Thomas, 1999).

The PMC controls the transition between storage and voiding phases of micturition by coordinating activity between the detrusor and sphincter muscles. Barrington nucleus, located in close proximity to the locus coeruleus in the dorsal-rostral pontine tegmentum, is one anatomic component of the voiding apparatus. Lesions in these pathways could possibly disrupt the reticulospinal fibers originating in the pons, which are crucial for the integration and coordination of detrusor and urethral sphincter activity, resulting in detrusor hyperactivity and urge incontinence (Betts et al., 1992).

Descending inhibitory influences affect the ability of the PMC to regulate continence. Following a lesion in the descending pathways, unmyelinated C-fibers contribute to the establishment of new local neural circuits between the detrusor muscle to the sacral micturition center. This new circuitry is removed from descending inhibitory input. The PMC receives

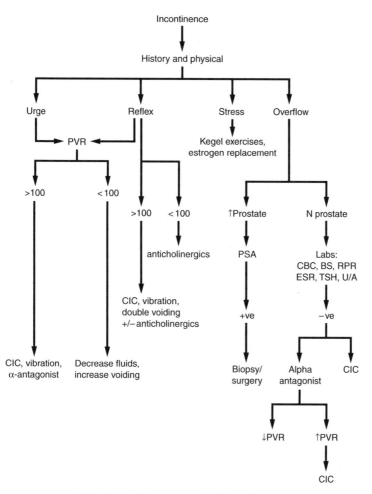

FIG. 16-1. Management of incontinence.

inhibitory input from the frontal lobe, which provides for the volitional control over micturition. Although their exact role has not yet been elucidated, the preoptic area of the hypothalamus, periaqueductal gray matter, and basal ganglia also contribute to the control of micturition (Sakakibara and Fowler, 1999).

Normal micturition consists of filling, storage, and emptying phases. With filling, intravesical pressure remains low (<10 cm H_2O), initially because of high bladder wall compliance. At larger bladder volumes (<300 mL), pressures increase and a sense of voiding urgency occurs. This evokes supraspinal, spinal, and peripheral control systems to come into play, suppressing unwanted detrusor contractions and maintaining urethral tone, and thereby continence. Volitional micturition is mediated by the frontal lobe and proceeds with complete relaxation of the sphincters

followed by contraction of the detrusor muscle (Akkus et al., 1997; Blavais, 1982). Once micturition is completed, this pattern is reversed. Complex interactions between the sacral micturition center, spinal cord, and PMC determine the coordinated control of the detrusor and sphincters during normal micturition.

BLADDER INCONTINENCE

Physiologic changes in the urinary system start in mid life, with estimates of urinary incontinence in middle age of 5% (Herzog and Fultz, 1990) among the elderly. Urinary incontinence is a more common condition among the elderly, with the prevalence being estimated at 15% in community-based studies, which rises to more than 50% in institutionalized populations (Diokno et al., 1988; Hellstrom et al.,

1990). Women have a higher predilection to incontinence than men, likely secondary to the weakening of the pelvic floor musculature following childbirth. With advancing age, detrusor contractions lessen and, therefore, postvoid residuals rise (Diokno et al., 1994). This may result from degenerative changes in both muscle and nerve cells. Prostatic enlargement, which occurs with aging in men, may contribute to urinary difficulties, including increased postvoid residuals. Most elderly, despite these changes, maintain urinary continence unless other processes come into play.

Urinary incontinence can be divided into four types, based on the patient's symptomatology and urodynamic findings: stress, urge, reflex, and overflow (Table 16-1).

Stress Incontinence

Stress incontinence tends to be more common in the elderly population, although the condition can present at any age. Studies in the frail elderly show that true, urodynamically proved stress incontinence, is a relatively rare cause of incontinence (Dubeau and Resnick, 1991). However, the incidence in the healthy elderly population does increase to levels that exceed middle age estimates. Changes in estrogen levels in postmenopausal women, as well as previous childbirths, can cause weakening of the pelvic floor, producing some laxity of the external sphincter that results in stress incontinence. The symptomatology associated with stress incontinence primarily involves the loss of small amounts of urine after coughing, sneezing, or straining. The effectiveness of pelvic floor exercises (Kegel exercises) has been well documented in numerous studies (Bump et al., 1991; Burgio et al., 1986). A trained individual can teach the exercises and the patient must be motivated to perform these on a regular basis. Estrogen replacement also improves the condition in certain cases.

Stress incontinence can coexist with other types of incontinence in elderly women and a concise history may bring out the salient features.

Urge Incontinence

Urge incontinence is defined as leakage of urine in association with urgency to void. Complaints include urgency and occasionally nocturia (Table 16-2). Contractile function of the detrusor muscle declines with age, leading to incomplete emptying and an increased postvoid residual. The residual urine can trigger unwanted detrusor contractions. These involuntary contractions of the detrusor muscle, which can be documented on urodynamics examination, may be associated with leakage of urine, in the absence of an increased abdominal pressure. The term "detrusor hyperactivity with impaired contractile function" has been coined to describe this entity (Griffiths, 1999).

Studies of normal cortical control of micturition using positron emission tomography (PET) scanning of healthy young controls demonstrate that the frontal lobe plays a prominent role in the regulation of voiding (Griffiths et al., 1996). Activity in a small area of the right inferior frontal lobe is present during volitional voiding, whereas postponement of voiding causes activation of an area in the right superior frontal region. Investigations using single photon emission computed tomography scans in elderly subjects demonstrate globally reduced perfusion in the cortex, and in the frontal lobes in particular. Based on these findings, it was postulated that superior frontal lobe and cingulate gyrus dysfunction may account for most of the detrusor hyperreflexia observed in the elderly (Griffiths, 1999).

Some studies in the elderly have suggested that cognitive abnormalities can cause urge incontinence. Cognitive testing has revealed impairment with respect to orientation and frontal lobe function. Although degenerative disorders and cerebrovascular

TABLE 16-1. *Variables between types of incontinence*

Variable	Urge	Reflex	Stress	Overflow
History	Frequency	Frequency, urgency	Incontinence with cough, sneeze	Constant dribbling
Physical	Dementia, normal	Pyramidal signs, internuclear ophthalmoplegia	Vaginal atrophy, normal	↑ Prostate, signs neuropathy
Postvoid residuals	Normal or ↑	Normal or ↑	Normal	↑
Urodynamics	↑ Contractions	↑ Contractions	Normal	↓ Contractions

TABLE 16-2. *Assessment of bladder dysfunction*

History	Physical	Tests
Frequency	Abdominal and rectal examination	Urinalysis
Urgency	Mobility	BUN/creatinine
Nocturia	Neurologic (i.e., spasticity, sensory)	PVR
Hesitancy	Mental status	Urine flow rate
Stress incontinence	Gynecologic	Urodynamics
Double voiding		Renal ultrasound
Fluid intake patterns		
Incomplete emptying		
History of obstetric or genitourinary surgery		
Medications		

BUN, blood urea nitrogen; PVR, postvoid residual.

disease have been implicated, the relationship between incontinence and cognition has not been well established. Not all cognitively impaired patients are incontinent and, correspondingly, not all patients with urge incontinence have cognitive dysfunction on formal testing (Griffiths, 1999).

The severity of incontinence can be determined by several factors. Of greatest importance are the amount of fluid intake and the pattern of voiding frequency over 24 hours. Other factors, such as urinary tract infections, mobility, underlying memory dysfunction, and impaired orientation also contribute to the severity. Medications, particularly drugs that cause sedation and cognitive changes or impair detrusor or sphincter function, can also contribute to the problem (Leach et al., 1987).

Treatment for incontinence can be challenging, as methods to lessen unwanted detrusor contractions can further impair contractility. Anticholinergic drugs can aggravate the condition by producing higher postvoid residuals, leading to the common complication of frequent urinary tract infections.

Several studies have demonstrated the effectiveness of increasing the frequency of voiding according to a specific schedule (timed voiding) (Ouslander et al., 1987). However, instituting this strategy for the institutionalized population may be impractical, given that coexistent dementia can make frequent voiding retraining difficult, if not impossible. In such a setting, an adequate and trained staff is an essential factor for successful treatment of incontinence. Along with timed voiding, decreasing fluid intake has also been shown to be effective, particularly during the evening hours. Nevertheless, concerns about adequate fluid intake have to be raised in a population of patients who may have a decline in mobility, resulting in a decreased access to fluids and a higher risk of dehydration, constipation, impaction, and renal dysfunction (Schnelle et al., 1989).

Reflex Incontinence

Reflex incontinence can occur with lesions of the spinal and supraspinal structures (e.g., PMC), which can interfere with descending impulses to the detrusor muscle and sphincters. Such lesions can disrupt the inhibitory input on detrusor contractions, leading to storage dysfunction and symptoms of urgency and frequency. Magnetic resonance imaging studies may show lesions in the midbrain and pons that correlate with the patient's urinary symptoms (Betts et al., 1992). Initial treatment is with anticholinergic drugs (Table 16-3). A more recent advance has been the development of tolterodine, which has a higher affinity for the M3 muscarinic receptor, thus decreasing side effects such as dry eyes, dry mouth, and confusion (Appell, 1997).

Desmopressin (DDAVP), an analog of antidiuretic hormone, is particularly helpful when nocturia persists despite the use of anticholinergic drugs. Periodic monitoring of the level of sodium is required and this drug should be used judiciously in the elderly. Common symptoms that are associated with DDAVP-induced hyponatremia include headache and confusion. Nevertheless, hyponatremia is extremely unusual when the use of this agent is restricted to single daily doses at night. DDAVP should be avoided in patients with concomitant renal and cardiovascular disease.

Intravesical capsaicin is another potential therapy for the hyperactive bladder. Its mechanism of action involves the blocking of C-fiber long latency responses, which results in a decrease in detrusor contractions. Capsaicin is instilled into the bladder following pretreatment with lidocaine to reduce the pain associated with capsaicin administration. The dura-

TABLE 16-3. *Pharmacologic interventions for incontinence*

Generic	Brand	Dose forms	Schedule	Drug class	Cost/month ($)
Oxybutynin	Ditropan	5 mg	b.i.d.–t.i.d.	Anticholinergics	15
	Ditropan XL	5, 10, 15 mg	q.d.	Musculotropic	75
Tolterodine	Detrol	1, 2 mg	b.i.d.	Antimuscarinic	40
Hyoscyamine	Levsin/Anaspaz	0.125, 0.15 mg	Every 4–6 hours	Anticholinergic	25
	Cystospaz				
Extended release		0.375 mg			35
	Levsinex/ Cystospaz-M		q.d.–b.i.d	.	
Propantheline	ProBanthine	7.5, 15 mg	t.i.d.	Anticholinergic	20
Flavoxate	Urispas	100 mg	1–2 b.i.d.–t.i.d.	Musculotropic	20
Imipramine	Tofranil	10, 25, 50 mg	25–50 mg q.h.s.	Tricyclic	25
Desmopressin	DDAVP	Nasal solution 10 µg/spray	1–4 puffs q.h.s.	Vasopressin analog	53
		Oral 0.2 mg	0.1–0.5 mg		10
Doxazosin	Cardura	1, 2, 4, 8 mg	1–8 mg q.h.s.	Alpha blocker	30
Terazosin	Hytrin	1, 2, 5, 10 mg	1–10 mg q.h.s.	Alpha blocker	55
Tamsulosin	Flomax	0.4 mg	0.4–0.8 mg q.h.s.	Alpha blocker	45

b.i.d., twice daily; q.d., every day; q.h.s., every night; t.i.d., three times daily.

tion of action is 3 to 4 months (Cruz et al., 1997). A newer agent, resiniferatoxin, is an ultrapotent capsaicin analog currently under investigation.

Other treatment modalities (e.g., clam ileocystoplasty, detrusor myectomy, and electrical stimulation) have been used in experienced medical centers. Outcomes are variable, with most studies reporting approximately 50% efficacy for these interventions (Burgio et al., 1986).

Emptying Dysfunction

Emptying dysfunction, in contrast to storage dysfunction, typically involves the loss of synergy between urinary sphincters and detrusor contractions, a process known as "detrusor sphincter dysynergia" (DSD). Hesitancy, interrupted stream, incomplete emptying, double voiding, nocturia, and enuresis can result, although these symptoms are not specific for DSD and can be experienced in other types of incontinence that produce emptying problems.

Neurologic and physical examination may reveal abnormalities (e.g., pyramidal signs or prostate enlargement) that often help to differentiate among causes. Although cervical spinal stenosis and pontine tegmental stroke have been cited as more common causes of reflex incontinence, compressive tumors in these regions, infections, and demyelination can also occur in the elderly (Dubeau and Resnick, 1991). Before deciding on a treatment protocol for this type of incontinence, a postvoiding residual test (PVR) must

be completed. A PVR of less than 100 mL demonstrates adequate emptying, and a variety of medications, usually with anticholinergic properties, can be used (Table 16-1). If the PVR values are greater than 100 mL, this indicates incomplete emptying and the use of anticholinergic agents may aggravate the retention of urine. If on repeat PVR and attempts at double voiding, the volume of residual urine remains high, clean intermittent catheterization (CIC) should be performed (Table 16-4). The addition of anticholinergic drugs can be used concomitantly if detrusor hyperexcitability remains a problem. Double voiding or the use of a vibrator placed over the lower abdomen during voiding may aid in emptying the bladder and avoid the need for catheterization if the urinary retention is not severe (Dasgupta et al., 1997). If DSD is suspected, the addition of α_1 antagonists (e.g., doxazosin, terazosin, or tamsulosin) may decrease sphincter tone and facilitate voiding (Griffiths et al., 1996).

TABLE 16-4. *Treatment for emptying dysfunction*

Alpha-1 antagonists
Clean intermittent catheterization (CIC)
Vibrator stimulation (Queens Square technique)
Relaxation techniques
Double voiding
Indwelling Foley catheter
Surgical procedures

PVR should be followed closely during the institution of anticholinergic therapy. Formal urologic consultation and urodynamic studies are often helpful in determining a course of action if the PVR is large or empiric drug therapy has failed.

Overflow Incontinence

Overflow incontinence is an uncommon cause of bladder dysfunction in the elderly. Lack of adequate detrusor contraction and increased urine volumes culminate in inadequate emptying. Primary dysfunction at the level of the conus medullaris, nerve roots, or peripheral nerves, leads to diminished detrusor contraction and a large PVR. When urine volumes exceed bladder capacity, urinary incontinence occurs. Patients can complain of postmicturition dribbling without the urgency and frequency that is characteristic of reflex and urge incontinence. Furthermore, inadequate bladder sensation can lead to a blunted perception of the need to void.

In the elderly, diabetes is the most common disease that produces overflow incontinence. It is present in 14% to 71% of all diabetics (Dasgupta et al., 1997). The wide variability in reporting likely stems from different criteria for the diagnosis and duration of disease. Characteristic signs include reduced sensation, increased intervals between voiding, followed by slowing of the urinary stream and difficulty in voiding. Diagnostic investigations, including bladder ultrasonography, can document the high urine residuals. An increase in bladder capacity and decreased bladder contractility is often noted on cystometrograms (Dasgupta et al., 1997).

Less frequent causes of neuropathy also reported to produce overflow incontinence include amyloidosis, Guillain-Barré syndrome; immune-mediated neuropathies; and infections (e.g., human immunodeficiency virus, Lyme disease, syphilis, and Rocky Mountain spotted fever) (Dasgupta et al., 1997). Metastatic tumors, particularly prostate cancer and lymphoma, can cause compression and, therefore, dysfunction of motor nerve roots leading to detrusor hypocontractility. Longstanding outlet obstruction can also lead to detrusor hypocontractility (Ball et al., 1981).

Incoordination of detrusor and sphincter functions can lead to high intravesical pressures, as the detrusor tries to contract against a contracted sphincter or narrowed outlet. With time, the detrusor muscle loses tone and overflow incontinence occurs. Unrecognized DSD, initially presenting as reflex incontinence, can evolve into overflow incontinence. The injudicious use of anticholinergic agents can aggravate the situation. Occasionally, α-adrenergic blockers are helpful if the cause is outlet obstruction secondary to inadequate sphincter relaxation.

Urinary Dysfunction in the Elderly with Neurologic Disease

Urinary incontinence has a high prevalence in certain neurologic diseases that present in the elderly. Recognition and treatment of the urinary dysfunction needs to be aggressive, as urinary tract infections can add to the morbidity associated with these disorders.

Parkinson's Disease

Parkinson's disease is a disorder characterized by tremor, bradykinesia, rigidity, and postural instability. Autopsy series show degeneration of pigmented dopaminergic neurons in the pars compacta of the substantia nigra, pontine cells in the locus coeruleus, and loss of neurons within the intermediolateral columns of the spinal cord. Urinary dysfunction is reported in 45% to 93% of patients and urodynamic studies typically show evidence of detrusor hyperreflexia (Anderson et al., 1976). Animal data suggest that the basal ganglia have an inhibitory effect on micturition. Intraventricular instillation of a D_1 receptor agonist inhibits contractions of the detrusor muscle induced by bladder distention, whereas no effect is seen with use of a D_2 receptor agonist. Several other animal models have confirmed the inhibitory effects of D_1 receptors (Yamamoto, 1997).

Theoretically, loss of D_1 neurons in the substantia nigra produces uninhibited detrusor contractions and occasionally urge incontinence. Despite these observations, treatment with dopaminergic agents does not necessarily correct the urinary symptoms in patients with PD. Studies using a short-acting dopaminergic agent, apomorphine, produced worsening of bladder function in some patients, while producing improvement of function in others. Alternately, small studies with pergolide, a D_1 and D_2 agonist, have shown significant improvements in voiding symptoms (Yamamoto, 1997).

A cardinal manifestation of PD is bradykinesia. Bradykinesia can impair relaxation of the urethral sphincter, producing a relative bladder outlet obstruction. In patients with this urodynamic finding, apomorphine produced improvement in voiding (Aranda and Cramer, 1993).

The significant impairment of mobility associated with PD can have a major impact on bladder dysfunction and quality of life. Patients with PD with bradykinesia and urgency and frequency often are unable to reach a bathroom in time, which can ultimately lead to incontinence. In this population, treatment should include dopaminergic agents that can improve mobility. Furthermore, it is vital to assess for detrusor contractility and possible outflow obstruction. If these dopaminergic agents do not fully improve symptoms, anticholinergic and antimuscarinic medications can be added, provided that the PVR is not elevated.

Cerebrovascular disease can be associated with incontinence; however, the incidence is variable, depending on the severity of the stroke, its location, and the resultant immobility of the patient. Following stroke, detrusor hyperreflexia is the most common abnormality identified on urodynamics, particularly when the infarct occurs in the frontal lobe, internal capsule, or putamen. Lesions within the basal ganglia or thalamus tend not to produce sphincteric abnormalities, whereas most frontal lobe and internal capsular strokes are associated with evidence of uninhibited relaxation of the sphincter during involuntary contraction of the detrusor muscle. Strokes occurring in other locations seemed to have no specific urologic correlate. Together, results of most studies seem to support the theory that the anterior medial frontal lobe and basal ganglia are important in the maintenance of normal micturition (Sakakibara and Fowler, 1999). Strokes involving Barrington's nucleus and the PMC, in the dorsal pons, produce micturition problems in about 50% of patients. The medial longitudinal fasciculus is located anatomically adjacent to the micturition center and numerous studies have documented a high correlation between internuclear ophthalmoplegia and urinary dysfunction after pontine stroke (Betts et al., 1992).

Alzheimer's Disease

Urinary incontinence is a frequent symptom seen in the later stages of Alzheimer's disease (Feldman et al., 2000). Urodynamic studies show a high incidence of detrusor hypercontractility, most likely caused by frontal lobe dysfunction. The most effective form of treatment is to increase voiding frequency and restrict fluids in the evening.

SEXUAL DYSFUNCTION

Sexuality involves the integration of emotional, intellectual, social, and moral factors, in conjunction with physiologic mechanisms that result in libido,

arousal, orgasms, and more highly complex perceptual experiences that comprise the sexual experience. Sexual dysfunction in the elderly can result from alterations in neurologic, vascular, endocrine, and psychologic functioning.

Physiology of Sexual Function

Sexual Function in Males

On a physiologic level, normal male sexual function is composed of three phases: penile erection, orgasm, and detumescence. The erectile tissue of the penis is composed of three bundles of smooth muscle: two laterally placed corpora cavernosa and a midline corpora spongiosum, which surrounds the urethra and expands distally to form the glans penis. The corpora are composed of blood-filled sinusoids and smooth muscle that are surrounded and separated by fibrous tissue, the tunica albuginea. The blood supply to the penis is principally derived from the pudendal artery, which divides into the perineal artery and two arteries to the corpus spongiosum—the bulbar and urethral arteries (Anderson et al., 1976).

Two types of erections can occur: reflexogenic and psychogenic. Each is achieved through a different neurologic pathway. Reflexogenic erections are mediated through a local neurologic loop. Direct stimulation of the genitals results in sensory information that is transmitted through the pudendal nerve to the sacral cord at S2-S4 and then back to the genitals via the S2-S4 sacral nerves. In contrast, psychogenic erections can be provoked in response to auditory, olfactory, or visual stimuli. Internally generated imagery often represents one of the most potent means by which to produce sexual arousal and erection.

The parasympathetic nervous system (derived from the sacral spinal cord at S2-S4) plays a prominent role in the development of an erection, whereas the sympathetic input is important for detumescence. In the flaccid state, the smooth muscle of the penis remains contracted because of tonic α-adrenergic activity. After parasympathetic stimulation, neurotransmitters such as nitric oxide, which mediates its effect through complimentary guanosine monophosphate (cGMP) pathways, prostaglandin E (PGE_1, PGE_2), and vasoactive intestinal peptide, are released (Kaiser, 1991). The net consequence of this neurotransmitter cascade is smooth muscle relaxation and vasodilatation of the penile artery. The sinusoids fill with blood and venous outflow is impeded by the influx of sinusoidal blood against the tunica albuginea, which results in erection.

Orgasm is divided into two phases: emission, which propagates semen into the urethra via rhythmic contractions of the bulbocavernosus, ischiocavernosus, and periurethral striated muscles, and ejaculation. Both parasympathetic and sympathetic mechanisms seem to be involved in this phase of sexual function.

Sexual Function in Females

Female sexual function is mediated through the same central and peripheral neuroanatomic pathways as described for men. Arousal from direct stimulation of the densely innervated clitoris or vaginal tissues, or through fantasy, results in increased blood flow to the vagina. These changes produce lubrication of the tissues and erection of the clitoris. Synchronous contractions of the vaginal walls, generally lasting 10 to 50 seconds, evoke orgasm in women. In contrast with men, orgasm in women can be multiple, both in number and in terms of the sites of involvement (Kaiser, 1991).

Sexual Changes with Advancing Age

A number of physiologic changes occur with advancing age that contribute to sexual dysfunction. Free testosterone or weakly bound testosterone declines with age (Nankin and Calkins, 1986; Vermeulan et al., 1972). It appears that the fall in testosterone level is caused by dysfunction of the hypothalamic-pituitary feedback loop secondary to a blunted pituitary response to gonadotropin-releasing hormone (Nankin and Calkins, 1986; Urban et al., 1982; Valenta and Elias, 1983). This results in a decrease in luteinizing hormone and testosterone.

Libido is strongly affected by testosterone and studies in the elderly have reported a reduction in libido in 30% of male patients under the age of 65, a 31% decrease between the ages of 65 to 75, and a 47% drop over the age of 75 (Tsitouras et al., 1982). Testosterone replacement can improve libido but seems to have little effect on potency (O'Carroll and Bancroft, 1986; Tsitouras et al., 1982). Penile vibration sensitivity declines with age, because of mechanoreceptor diminution (Johnson and Murray, 1992). As such, a prolonged period of tactile stimulation may be required for erection to occur. Tissue elasticity also diminishes with age, leading to a decline in erectile firmness (Johnson and Murray, 1992). Sympathetic neurotransmitter sensitivity can be upregulated, as seen by the age-dependent efficacy of phenylephrine in inducing contractions of penile smooth muscle and vascular reactivity is also increased in response to noradrenergic input (Anderson and Wagner, 1995; Christ et al., 1990; Christ et al., 1991). Animal studies have shown a defect in nitric oxide-mediated intracellular calcium fluxes resulting

in impaired erectile tissue relaxation (Haas et al., 1998). A combination of these factors can lead to greater difficulty in achieving and maintaining an erection. These factors have implications for both male and female sexual responses.

In older females, decreased vaginal blood flow and reduced thickness and elasticity of the vagina has been reported. These changes appear to be secondary to a lack of estrogen in postmenopausal women, also resulting in vaginal dryness and diminished lubrication. Such changes can be improved for many patients by hormonal replacement therapy (Campbell, 1976; Stemmons et al., 1985). Libido, however, is related to levels of circulating androgens and estrogen replacement has little effect on this aspect of sexual function (Burger et al., 1987; Dennerstein and Burrows, 1982; Morley and Kaiser, 1989; Sherwin and Gelfand, 1987). As women age, the clitoral response typically remains intact but orgasm is briefer and vaginal wall contractions are fewer and weaker.

Sexual dysfunction is reported in 25% to 55% of older men and from 28% to 90% in women. Most studies suggest that organic causes are much more likely to be responsible for these changes than are psychological reasons (Kaiser, 1991).

Contributing Factors in Sexual Dysfunction in the Aged Population

The factors that contribute to sexual dysfunction in the aged population can be divided into interpersonal and social concerns, vascular dysfunction, venous disorders, medication effects, psychological factors, endocrine function, neurologic diseases, and gynecologic and prostate disease.

In the aged society, sexual morals tend to be more conservative. Extramarital affairs are rare among widowers and divorced women, whereas they are more common among men (Greenblatt and Leng, 1972). Sexual dysfunction is noted to be higher in groups of elderly individuals who have held rigid sexual beliefs and poor sexual communication with partners when younger. People who have had frequent and full sexual experiences, tend to be more adaptable and report less sexual dysfunction with advancing age (Schreiner-Engel and Schiavi, 1986). Society fosters an image of sexuality being associated with youth, whereas aging is thought to confer a decline in sexuality. Images of sex in the elderly often are negative, which could possibly inhibit some elderly from seeking a sexually fulfilling relationship.

Social issues can have a greater impact on female sexual function than on that of men. Loss of a partner commonly leads to lack of a sexual relationship in elderly women (Christenson and Gagnon, 1965). The average current age difference between spouses is 4 years. Women have a longer life expectancy than men and these two factors combine to produce an expectation of 5 to 7 years of widowhood in western cultures. Remarriage rates for elderly women are lower because of the relative lack of elderly men and the low cultural acceptance of marriage between an older woman and younger man (Synder and Spreitzer, 1976).

Erectile Dysfunction in Men

Erectile dysfunction is defined by the inability to obtain or sustain an erection consistently for 50% of the times attempted for intercourse. It is estimated to affect 10 to 30 million men in the United States (Kaiser, 1991). Comorbid conditions that can produce dysfunction exist in 80% of people over 65 years of age, although these conditions do not always produce sexual dysfunction (Kaiser, 1999). Vascular disorders are the most common cause of erectile dysfunction in the United States (Feldman et al., 2000; Hsueh, 1988; Lochmann and Gallmetzer, 1996). Cavernosal arteries develop intimal and medial thickening and trabecular fibrosis occurs, which prevents inflow of arterial blood into the sinusoids. The noninvasive measurement of the penile-brachial indices (PBI), which is an indicator of vascular insufficiency to the penis, is diagnostic. Studies have demonstrated that the PBI also has a predictive value in determining coronary risk in men. Conversely, 64% of men with a prior myocardial infarction have complaints of erectile dysfunction (Morley et al., 1988). Cigarette smoking almost doubles the risk of dysfunction, with contributions by other risk factors such as hypertension, hyperlipidemia, diabetes, and alcohol use. In most men with erectile dysfunction, diagnostic investigations are unnecessary, as most can be empirically treated with erectile promoting agents.

Penile-occlusive disorders are common, although a poorly recognized cause of erectile dysfunction. In autopsy studies, venous outflow dysfunction was estimated to account for more than 70% of the cases producing impotence (Buvat et al., 1985). Loss in arterial compliance with aging correlates with a loss in venous compliance. This loss of compliance prevents the adequate compression of the emissary veins against the tunica albuginea by the corpora cavernosus, thereby leading to lower pressures within the penis and ultimately erectile failure.

In Peyronie's disease, a fibrous plaque develops within the tunica albuginea and the corpus cavernosus, tethering the emissary veins open, and venous outflow cannot be inhibited. In most cases, an antecedent episode of penile trauma has occurred. The resulting fibrosis can cause a curvature in the penis. The resultant fibrotic tissue can often be palpated on examination (Kaiser, 1999).

Venous leaks within the penis can occur because of weakening of venous structures from the loss of elastic tissue and the development of arteriovenous malformations. These factors can predispose to impotence in elderly men. Tests to confirm the diagnosis of venous leakage include cavernosonography and cavernosometry (Lue et al., 1986).

Although diabetes is not as common a cause of erectile dysfunction as are vascular disorders, more than 90% of diabetics develop problems and several mechanisms appear to be involved (McCullough et al., 1980). Glycosylation alters the endothelial ability to respond to neurotransmitters, whereas an autonomic neuropathy alters the cholinergic input to the erectile tissues (Lin and Bradley, 1985). Penile dorsal nerve conduction is delayed, indicating the presence of a sensory-motor neuropathy. The end products of glycosylation contribute to the accelerated atherosclerosis seen in diabetics and affect the hemodynamics of erection. Thus, a complex interplay of factors exist that may be difficult to correct (Kaiser and Korenman, 1988). Other endocrine abnormalities such as hyperprolactinemia, Cushing's disease, thyroid dysfunction, pituitary tumors, and hemachromatosis can result in decreased libido and impotence (Foster et al., 1990; Mooradian et al., 1988).

A number of drugs can produce sexual dysfunction. Several studies estimated the incidence of medication-induced sexual dysfunction to range from 9% to 25% (Buffum, 1992).

Antidepressants, including the selective serotonin reuptake inhibitors (SSRI), tricyclics, and monamine oxidase (MAO) inhibitors have been reported to cause decreased libido, erectile dysfunction, retrograde ejaculation and failure, and anorgasmia (Seagraves, 1988). Priapism has been reported with the use of trazodone, whereas lithium has produced erectile dysfunction (Lamy, 1990). The sexual dysfunction seen with neuroleptics usually is caused by higher circulating levels of prolactin; however, use of drugs with significant anticholinergics and α-adrenergic properties (e.g., chlorpromazine and thioridazine) also has a high incidence of erectile and ejaculatory dysfunction (Monterio et al., 1987). Low doses of anxiolytics are associated with sexual disinhibition, whereas higher doses are central nervous system depressants, thus producing an opposite effect on sexual function.

Compliance with antihypertensive medication can be reduced because of sexual side effects. Thiazides, sympatholytics (e.g., methyldopa and clonidine), and beta-blockers frequently produce problems, whereas angiotensin-converting enzyme inhibitors and calcium channel blockers, although implicated, have a much lower incidence of sexual dysfunction (Bauer et al., 1981). A variety of medications, including phenytoin, carbamazepine, digoxin, spirolactone, cimetidine, ranitidine, Parkinson's drugs, metoclopramide, naproxen, and morphine, have been reported to decrease libido and cause erectile dysfunction. Abused drugs, including heroin, amphetamines, marijuana, alcohol, cocaine, and nicotine can also impair sexual response by a variety of mechanisms.

Depression is coexistent in 8% to 15% of men and 31% to 50% of women with sexual dysfunction. A paucity of data exist concerning depression and sexual dysfunction and the elderly, despite the increased incidence of these two problems in this population, and a mixture of psychogenic and organic causes may be present (Derogatis et al., 1985; Matthew and Weinman, 1982).

Alcohol can affect most aspects of sexual functioning and estimates of sexual dysfunction in alcoholics range up to 95%. Causes include changes in hormone production, peripheral nerve dysfunction, and an increased incidence of vascular disease, and impaired psychosocial functioning may have an impact on personal relationships and produce depression (Schuckit, 1972). Despite the major impact that alcohol has in modern society, few studies have examined this topic and even fewer data are found on elderly alcoholics.

Anxiety disorders and schizophrenia can produce sexual dysfunction, usually by an impact on libido (Cooper, 1968; Derogatis et al., 1985; Lukoff et al., 1986). Neurologic diseases can have an impact on sexual functioning, particularly through problems with immobility and with cognitive and behavioral functioning. Patients with Alzheimer's disease have a higher prevalence of erectile dysfunction as compared with nondemented, age-matched controls; however, the disruption of sexual intimacy caused by cognitive changes probably plays a much greater role in producing sexual dysfunction (Litz et al., 1990; Zeiss et al., 1983). Cerebrovascular disease can impair multiple aspects of sexual function including cognition, erectile function, and mobility. Epilepsy, spinal cord disorders, and multiple sclerosis impair neuroanatomic pathways that are critical for proper sexual functioning. Prostate cancer is the second most common malignancy among men. Infiltration of the pelvic nerves by the carcinoma, as well as surgical treatment of the disease, can disrupt neural pathways intrinsic to normal sexual function. Treatment options, including orchiectomy and antitestosterone medications, are also likely to induce erectile failure (Schonver et al., 1984). Theoretically, transurethral prostatectomy should not affect erectile function; however, some studies have documented a 4% incidence of dysfunction, usually associated with extensive cautery of the posterolateral capsule. Gynecologic cancers and their radiation treatment can impair adjacent pelvic nerve functions. Changes in pelvic tissue can produce dyspareunia and decreased lubrication (Anderson et al., 1986; McCartney and Larson, 1987). Hysterectomy has a low impact on sexual function; however, estrogen replacement needs to be considered if a concomitant oophorectomy is performed.

Assessment of Sexual Function

A comprehensive history and physical examination are essential in the assessment of sexual dysfunction (Table 16-5). Many patients are embarrassed to voice concerns about sexual function and a nonthreatening

TABLE 16-5. *Assessment of sexual dysfunction*

History	Physical
Marital status	Urogenital examination
Presence of a sexual partner	Gynecologic examination
Sexual mores	Cardiovascular examination
Depression	Tests
Cognition	Blood glucose
Mobility	Luteinizing hormone, testosterone level
Libido	Thyroid-stimulating hormone
Lubrication	Penile brachial indices
Erection and erectile dysfunction	Cavernosonography
Ejaculation	
Orgasm	
Comorbid medical conditions	
Smoking history	
Alcohol use	
Medications	
Illicit drug use	

discussion with their physician may elicit important information. Data concerning marital status, drug history, use of alcohol and tobacco, availability of a sexual partner, comorbid medical disorders, genitourinary or gynecological problems, and a history of psychological functioning, including depressive symptomatology, can aid in diagnosis. Laboratory tests, which comprise an adjunct to the history and physical examination, can include serum estradiol, follicle-stimulating hormone, androgen levels (for women) and a testosterone and luteinizing hormone level (for males). Thyroid-stimulating hormone, prolactin level, renal function, and fasting blood sugar may be appropriate for both sexes. Depression scales and interviews with a patient's sexual partner may reveal psychological factors not initially evident. Ultimately, many patients with evidence of sexual dysfunction can benefit from consultation with a urologist experienced in the assessment and management of these disorders.

Treatment depends on the underlying problem as well as on the patient's desire to pursue therapeutic options. If primary hormonal deficiency is present, estrogen replacement therapy is indicated. If estrogen is contraindicated, local vaginal estrogen creams may alleviate vaginal atrophy and dyspareunia. Androgen supplements with methyltestosterone (2.5 mg 5 days a week) or fluoxymesterone (2 mg 5 days a week) may improve libido in women. Intramuscular testosterone can be used in males with a testosterone deficiency (Burger et al., 1987).

Erectile dysfunction can be treated initially with sildenafil, a type 5 phosphodiesterase inhibitor, which inhibits the breakdown of cGMP, thus increasing vasodilatation. The half-life of the drug is 4 hours and it has been found to be effective in 80% to 88% of patients (Anderson et al., 1976). Transurethral alprostadil (prostaglandin E), acting via a prostacyclin receptor, producing α-blockade and, thus, vasodilation, has shown efficacy in producing erections sufficient for intercourse in 65% of men (Linet and Ogrine, 1996). An intracavernosal, injectable form of alprostadil is also available, with efficacy in the 95% range (Appell, 1997). Priapism has been reported with both forms of the drug and represents a medical emergency. Patients should, therefore, be educated on the potential for an abnormally prolonged erection and the potential resultant damage that might ensue if urgent treatment is not administered. Vacuum tumescence devices are effective in 85% of patients; however, their acceptance rate is lower among patients than alternative treatments. The device consists of a negative pressure vacuum that is pumped to achieve an erection and then the erection is maintained by the application of a band or ring around

the base of the penis (Korenman et al., 1990). Finally, surgical options, with implantation of a penile prosthesis, can be considered if medical options have failed. Risks include the development of scar tissue, infection, erosion, and mechanical failure.

As the aged population grows, the diagnosis and treatment of the multiple medical and psychosocial problems will become increasingly complex. Incontinence and sexual dysfunctions are presently underdiagnosed and undertreated. An open discussion, followed by appropriate investigations can lead to an integrated, multiteam approach to improve the quality of life in this population.

REFERENCES

Akkus E, Carrier S, Baba K, et al. Structural alterations in the tunica albuginea of the penis: impact of Peyronie's disease, ageing and impotence. *Br J Urol* 1997;79:47–53.

Anderson BL, Lachenbruch PA, Anderson B, et al. Sexual dysfunction and signs of gynecological cancer. *Cancer* 1986;57:1880.

Anderson KE, Wagner, G. Physiology of penile erection. *Physiol Rev* 1995;75:191–236.

Anderson JT, Hebjorn S, Frimodt-Moller C, et al. Disturbances of micturition in Parkinson's disease. *Acta Neurol Scand* 1976;53:161–170.

Appell RA. Clinical efficacy and safety of tolterodine in the treatment of overactive bladder; a pooled analysis. *Urology* 1997;50:90–97.

Aranda B, Cramer P. Effect of apomorphine and L-dopa on parkinsonian bladder. *Neurourol Urodyn* 1993;12:203–209.

Ball AJ, Feneley RC, Abrams PH. The natural history of untreated prostatism. *Br J Urol* 1981;53:613–616.

Bauer GE, Huynor SN, Baker J, et al. Clinical side effects during antihypertensive therapy: a placebo controlled double blind study. *Postgrad Med Commun* 1981;49–59.

Betts CD, Kapoor R, Fowler CJ. Pontine pathology and micturition dysfunction. *Br J Urol* 1992;70:100–102.

Blavais JG. The neurophysiology of micturition: a clinical study of 550 patients. *J Urol* 1982;127:958.

Buffum J. Prescription drugs and sexual function. *Psychiatr Med* 1992;10:181–198.

Bump RC, Hurt WG, Fantl JA, et al. Assessment of the Kegel pelvic exercise performance after brief verbal instruction. *Am J Obstet Gynecol* 1991;165:322–329.

Burger H, Hailes J, Nelson J, et al. Effect of combined implants of oestradiol and testosterone on libido in postmenopausal women. *BMJ* 1987;294:936–937.

Burgio KL, Ives DG, Locher JL, et al. Treatment seeking for urinary incontinence in older adults. *J Am Geriatr Soc* 1994;42:208–212.

Burgio KL, Robinson JC, Engel BT. The role of biofeedback in Kegel exercise training for stress urinary incontinence. *Am J Obstet Gynecol* 1986;154:58–64.

Buvat J, Lemaire JL, Dehaene R, et al. Venous incompetence: critical study of the organic basis of high maintenance of flow rates during artificial erection test. *J Urol* 1985;135:796–798.

Campbell S. Double blind psychometric studies on the effects of natural estrogen on postmenopausal women. In:

Campbell S, ed. *Management of menopause and post-menopausal years.* Lancaster: TMP Press, 1976:149.

Christ GJ, Maayani S, Valcic M, et al. Pharmacological studies of human erectile tissue: characteristics of spontaneous contractions and alterations in alpha-adrenoceptor responsiveness with age and disease in isolated tissues. *Br J Pharmacol* 1990;101:375–381.

Christ GJ, Stone B, Melman A. Age dependent alterations in the efficacy of phenylephrine-induced contractions in vascular smooth muscle isolated from the corpus cavernosum of impotent men. *Can J Physiol Pharmacol* 1991; 69:909–913.

Christenson CV, Gagnon BA. Sexual behaviour in a group of older women. *J Gerintol* 1965;20:351.

Cooper AJ. Neurosis and disorders of sexual potency in the male. *J Psychosom Res* 1968;12:141.

Cruz F, Guimaraes M, Silva C, et al. Desensitization of bladder sensory fibers by intravesical capsaicin has long lasting clinical and urodynamic effects in patients with hyperactive or hypersensitive bladder dysfunction. *J Urol* 1997;152:285–289.

Dasgupta P, Haslam C, Goodwin R, et al. The Queens Square bladder stimulator: a device for assisting emptying of the neurogenic bladder. *Br J Urol* 1997;80:234–237.

Dasgupta P, Thomas PK. Peripheral neuropathy. In: Fowler CJ, ed. *Neurology of bladder, bowel and sexual dysfunction.* Oxford: Butterworth-Heinemann, 1999:339–352.

De Groat WC, Booth AM. Neural control of penile erection. In: Maggi CA, ed. *Nervous control of the urogenital system. Vol. 3. The autonomic nervous system.* London: Harewood Academic Publishers, 1993:465–522.

Dennerstein L, Burrows GD. Hormone replacement and sexuality in women. *Baillieres Clin Endocrinol Metab* 1982;11:661.

Derogatis LR, Meyer JK, Kourleis S. Psychiatric diagnosis and psychological symptoms in impotence. *Hillside J Clin Psychiatry* 1985;7:120–133.

Diokno AC, Brown MB, Brock BM, et al. Clinical and cystometric characteristics of continent and incontinent noninstitutionalized elderly. *J Urol* 1988;140:567–571.

Diokno AC, Brown MB, Goldstein NG, et al. Urinary flow rates and voiding pressures in elderly men living in a community. *J Urol* 1994;151:1550–1553.

Dubeau CE, Resnick NM. Evaluation of the causes and severity of geriatric incontinence: a critical appraisal. *Urol Clin North Am* 1991;18:243–256.

El-Masri WS, Fellows G. Bladder care after spinal cord injury. *Paraplegia* 1981;19:265–270.

Feldman HA, Goldstein I, Hatzichristou DG, et al. Impotence and its medical and psychosocial correlates: results of the Massachusetts Male Aging Study. *J Urol* 1994;15:54–61.

Feldman HA, Johannes CB, Derby CA, et al. Erectile dysfunction and coronary risk factors: prospective results from the Massachusetts Male Aging Study. *Prev Med*, 2000;30:328–338.

Foster RS, Mulcahy JJ, Callaghan JT, et al. Role of serum prolactin determination in the evaluation of impotent patients. *Urology* 1990;36:499–501.

Greenblatt RB, Leng JJ. Factors influencing sexual behavior. *J Am Geriatr Soc* 1972;20:49–54.

Griffiths DJ. Urinary incontinence in the elderly. In: Fowler CJ, ed. *Neurology of bladder, bowel and sexual dysfunction.* Oxford: Butterworth-Heineman, 1999:265–273.

Griffiths DJ, Mccracken PN, Harrison GM, et al. Urge incontinence in elderly people: factors predicting the severity of urine loss before and after pharmacological treatment. *Neurourol Urodyn* 1996;15:53–57.

Haas CA, Seftal AD, Razmjouel K, et al. Erectile dysfunction in aging: upregulation of endothelial nitric oxide synthase. *Urology* 1998;51(3):516–522.

Hellstrom L, Ekelund P, Milsom I, et al. The prevalence of urinary incontinence aids in 85 year old men and women. *Age Ageing* 1990;19:383–389.

Herzog AR, Fultz NH. Prevalence and incidence of urinary incontinence in community-dwelling populations. *J Am Geriatr Soc* 1990;38:273–281.

Hsueh WA. Sexual dysfunction with aging and systemic hypertension. *Am J Cardiol* 1988;61:18H–23H.

Johnson RD, Murray FT. Reduced sensitivity of penile mechanoreceptors in aging rats with sexual dysfunction. *Brain Res Bull* 1992;28:61.

Kaiser FE. Sexuality and impotence in the aging man. *Clin Geriatr Med* 1991;7:63–72.

Kaiser FE. Erectile dysfunction in the aging man. *Med Clin North Am* 1999;83:1267–1278.

Kaiser FE, Korenman SG. Impotence in diabetic men. *Am J Med* 1988;85(Suppl):147–152.

Kaiser FE, Viosca SP, Morley JE, et al. Impotence and aging: clinical and hormonal factors. *J Am Geriatr Soc* 1988;36:511–519.

Korenman SG, Viosca SP, Kaiser FE, et al. Use of a vacuum tumescence device in the management of impotence. *J Am Geriatr Soc* 1990;38:217–220.

Lamy PP. Adverse drug effects. *Clin Geriatr Med* 1990;6: 293–309.

Leach G, Yip C, Donovan B. Post-prostatectomy incontinence: the influence of bladder dysfunction. *J Urol* 1987; 138:574–578.

Lin JT, Bradley WE. Penile neuropathy in insulin dependent diabetes mellitus. *J Urol* 1985;133:213–215.

Linet OI, Ogrine FG. Efficacy and safety of intracavernosal alprostadil in men with erectile dysfunction. The Alprostadil Study Group. *N Engl J Med* 1996;334:873–877.

Litz BT, Zeiss AM, Davies HD. Sexual concerns of male spouses of female Alzheimer's disease patients. *Gerontologist* 1990;30:113.

Lochmann A, Gallmetzer J. Erectile dysfunction of arterial origin as a possible primary manifestation of atherosclerosis. *Minerva Cardioangiol* 1996;44:242–246.

Lue TF, Hricak H, Schmidt RA, et al. Functional evaluation of penile veins by cavernosography in papaverine induced erection. *J Urol* 1986;135:479–482.

Lukoff D, Gioia-Hasick D, Sullivan G. Sex education and rehabilitation with schizophrenic male outpatients. *Schizophr Bull* 1986;12:669.

Matthew RJ, Weinman ML. Sexual dysfunction in depression. *Arch Sex Behav* 1982;13:323–328.

McCartney CF, Larson DB. Quality of life in patients with gynecologic cancer. *Cancer* 1987;60:2129.

McCullough DK, Campbell IW, Wu FC, et al. The prevalence of diabetic impotence. *Diabetologia* 1980;18:279–283.

Monterio WO, Noshirvani HF, Marks IM, et al. Anorgasmia from clomipramine in obsessive-compulsive disorder: a controlled trial. *Br J Psychiatry* 1987;151:107–112.

Mooradian AD, Morley JE, Korenman SG. Endocrinology in aging. *Dis Mon* 1988;34:398–451.

Morley JE, Kaiser FE. Sexual function with advancing age. *Med Clin North Am* 1989;73:1483–1495.

Morley JE, Korenman SG, Kaiser FE, et al. Relationship of penile brachial pressure index to myocardial infarction and cerebrovascular accidents in older males. *Am J Med* 1988;84:445–448.

Nankin HR, Calkins JH. Decreased bioavailable testosterone in aging normal and impotent men. *J Clin Endocrinol Metab* 1986;63:1418–1420.

O'Carroll R, Bancroft J. Testosterone therapy for low sexual interest and erectile dysfunction in men: a controlled study. *Br J Psychiatry* 1986: 145:146–151.

Ouslander JG, Unman GC, Urman HN, et al. Incontinence among nursing home patients: clinical and functional correlates. *J Am Geriatr Soc* 1987;35:324–330.

Sakakibara R, Fowler CJ. Cerebral control of bladder, bowel and sexual function and effects of brain disease. In Fowler CJ, ed. *Neurology of bladder, bowel and sexual dysfunction*. Oxford: Butterworth-Heineman, 1999:229–243.

Schnelle JF, Traughber B, Sowell VA, et al. Prompted voiding treatment of urinary incontinence in nursing home patients: a behavior management approach for nursing home staff. *J Am Geriatr Soc* 1989;37:1051–1057.

Schonver LR, von Eschenbach AC, Smith DB, et al. Sexual rehabilitation of urologic cancer patients: a practical approach. *Cancer* 1984;34:66.

Schreiner-Engel P, Schiavi RC. Lifetime psychopathology in individuals with low sexual desire. *J Nerve Ment Dis* 1986;174:646.

Schuckit MA. Sexual disturbance in the women alcoholic. *Med Aspects Hum Sex* 1972;6:44.

Seagraves RT. Sexual side effects of psychiatric drugs. *Int J Psychiatry Med* 1988;18:242–252.

Sherwin BB, Gelfand MM. The role of androgen in the maintenance of sexual functioning in oophorectomized women. *Psychosom Med* 1987;49:397–409.

Stemmons JP, Tsai CL, Semmons EC, et al. The effects of estrogen therapy on vaginal physiology during menopause. *Obstet Gynecol* 1985;66:15–18.

Synder EE, Spreitzer ES. Attitudes of the aged toward nontraditional sexual behaviour. *Arch Sex Behav* 1976;5:249.

Tsitouras PD, Martin CE, Harman SM. Relationship of serum testosterone to sexual activity in healthy elderly men. *J Gerontol* 1982;37:288–293.

Urban RJ, Veldhais JD, Blizzard RM, et al. Attenuated release of biologically active leutinizing hormone in healthy aging men. *J Clin Endocrinol Metab* 1982;81:1020–1029.

Valenta LJ, Elias AN. Pituitary-gonadal function in the aging male: the male climacteric. *Geriatrics* 1983;38(12):67–72.

Vermeulan A, Reubens R, Verdonck L. Testosterone secretion and metabolism in male senescence. *J Clin Endocrinol Metab* 1972;34:730–735.

Yamamoto M. Pergolide improves neurogenic bladder in patients with Parkinson's disease. *Mov Disord* 1997;12 (Suppl 1):P328.

Zeiss AM, Davies HD, Wood M, et al. The incidence and correlates of problems in patients with Alzheimer's disease. *Arch Sex Behav* 1983;19:325.

SUGGESTED READING

Abelson D. Diagnostic value of the penile pulse and blood pressure: a Doppler study of impotence in diabetics. *J Urol* 1975;112:636–639.

Abrams P. Objective evaluation of bladder outlet obstruction. *Br J Urol* 1997;76:11.

Bachman GA, Leiblum SR, Sandler B, et al. Correlates of sexual desire in postmenopausal women. *Maturitas* 1985; 7:211–216.

Blackman MR, Kowatech MA, Wehmann RE, et al. Basal serum prolactin levels and prolactin responses to constant infusions of thyrotropin releasing hormone in healthy aging men. *J Gerontol* 1986;41:699–705.

Blum MD, Bahnson RR, Porter TN, et al. Effect of local alpha-adrenergic blockade on human penile tissue. *J Urol* 1985;134:479–481.

Boolell M, Gepi-Attee S, Gingell JC, et al. Sildenafil, a novel oral therapy for male erectile dysfunction. *Br J Urol* 1996;78:257–261.

Carrier S, Brock G, Kour NW. The pathophysiology of erectile dysfunction. *Urology* 1993;42:468–481.

Davidson JM, Chen JJ, Crape CL, et al. Hormonal changes and sexual function in aging men. *J Clin Endocrinol Metab* 1983;57:71–77.

Diokno AC, Brown MB, Herzog AR. Sexual function in the elderly. *Arch Intern Med* 1990;150:197.

Dow MGT, Hart DM, Forrest CS. Hormonal treatments of sexually unresponsiveness in postmenopausal women: a comparative study. *Br J Obstet Gynaecol* 1983;90:361–366.

Goldstein I. Overview of types and results of vascular surgical procedures for impotence. *Cardiovasc Intervent Radiol* 1988;11:240–244.

Gridley F, Bruskewitz R, Feyzi J. Intravenous self-injection for impotence: A long term therapeutic option: experience in 78 patients. *J Urol* 1988;140:972.

Hammerere PG, Huland H. Post prostatectomy incontinence. In: O'Donnell PD, ed. *Urinary incontinence*. St. Louis: Mosby, 1997;315–325.

Herzog AR, Dionka AC, Brown MB, et al. Urinary incontinence as a risk factor for mortality. *J Am Geriatr Soc* 1994;42:264–268.

Kent S. Impotence: the facts versus the fallacies. *Geriatrics* 1975;30:164–171.

Krane RJ, Goldstein I, Saenz de Tejada I. Impotence. *N Engl J Med* 1989;321:1648–1659.

Krant MJ. Psychosocial impact of gynecologic cancer. *Cancer* 1981;48:608.

Libman E, Fichten CS, Creti L, et al. Transurethral prostatectomy: differential effects of age category and presurgical sexual functioning on post prostatectomy sexual adjustment. *J Behav Med* 1989;12:469–485.

Lictenberg PA, Strzepek DM. Assessments of institutionalized dementia patients' competencies to participate in intimate relationships. *Gerontologist* 1990;30:117.

Madersbacher S, Pycha A, Schatzl G, et al. The aging lower urinary tract: a comparative urodynamics study of men and women. *Urology* 1998;51:206–212.

Maurice WL, Guze SB. Sexual dysfunction and associated psychiatric disorders. *Compr Psychiatry* 1970;132:172.

McCoy NC, Davidson JM. A longitudinal study of the effects of menopause on sexuality. *Maturitas* 1985;7:203–210.

Morley JE. Impotence. *Am J Med* 1986;80:897–905.

Morely JE, Korenman SG, Mooradian AD, et al. Sexual dysfunction in the elderly male. *J Am Geriatr Soc* 1987;35 (11):1014–1022.

Mulligan T, Katz PG. Why aged men become impotent. *Arch Intern Med* 1989;149:1365–1366.

Mulligan T, Retchin SM, Chinchilli VM, et al. The role of aging and chronic disease in sexual dysfunction. *J Am Geriatr Soc* 1988;36:520–524.

Munoz M, Bancroft J, Beard M. Evaluating the effects of an alpha-2-adrenoceptor antagonist on erectile function in the human male. *Psychopharmacology (Berl)* 1994;115:471–477.

O'Donnell P. Volume-interval relationship of incontinence episodes in elderly inpatient men. *Urology* 1991;41: 334–337.

O'Donnell PD, Beck C. Urinary incontinence volume patterns in elderly inpatient men. *Urology* 1991;38:128–131.

Parr D. Sexual aspects of drug abuse in narcotic addicts. *Br J Addict Alcohol Other Drugs* 1976;71:261–268.

Persson G, Nilsson LV, Svanborg A. Personality and sexuality in relation to an index of gonadal steroid hormone balance in a 70-year-old population. *Psychosom Res* 1983;27:469.

Pfeiffer E, Davis GC. Determinants of sexual behavior in middle and old age. *J Am Geriatr Soc* 1972;20:151.

Renshaw DC. Sexual problems in old age, illness and disability. *Pyschosomatics* 1981;22:975–985.

Roose SP, Glassman AH, Walsh BT, et al. Reversible loss of nocturnal penile tumescence during depression: a preliminary report. *Neuropsychobiology* 1982;8:284.

Saenz de Tejada I, Goldstein I, Azadozoi K, et al. Impaired neurogenic and endothelium mediated relaxation of penile smooth muscle from diabetic men with impotence. *N Engl J Med* 1989;320:1025–1030.

Sarrel PM. Sex problems after menopause: a study of fifty married couples. *Maturitas* 1982;4:231.

Teri L, Reifler BV. Sexual issues of patients with Alzheimers. *Med Aspects Hum Sex* 1986;2:90.

Tinetti ME, Inouye SK, Gill TM, et al. Shared risk factors for falls, incontinence, and functional dependence: unifying the approach to geriatric syndromes. *JAMA* 1995;273: 1348–1353.

Tsitouras PD, Alvarez RR. Etiology and management of sexual dysfunction in elderly men. *Psychiatric Med* 1984; 2(1):43–55.

Ware JC. Impotence and aging. *Clin Geriatr Med* 1989;5: 301–314.

Yoshimura N, Sas M, Yoshida O, et al. Dopamine D_1 receptor-mediated inhibition of micturition reflex by central dopamine from the substantia nigra. *Neurol Urodyn* 1992;11:535–545.

17

Ischemic Cerebrovascular Disease

Scott E. Kasner, Julio A. Chalela, and Susan L. Hickenbottom

DEFINITION OF TERMS

Stroke is a clinical syndrome characterized by rapidly developing symptoms or signs of focal neurologic dysfunction caused by a vascular incident. Therefore, stroke includes both ischemic and hemorrhagic cerebrovascular events.

Cerebral infarction or *ischemic stroke* is used when radiologic or pathologic confirmation of the suspected stroke is obtained.

The colloquial term *cerebrovascular accident* and the classic term *apoplexy* should be avoided as they connote a fortuitous origin, whereas stroke is usually caused by a well-defined pathogenic mechanism.

Stroke-in-evolution is sometimes used to describe stroke characterized by gradual progression of the symptoms over the first few minutes to hours.

Transient ischemic attack (TIA) is an abrupt, focal loss of neurologic function caused by temporary ischemia. Although previous thought was that TIA could persist up to 24 hours, modern imaging techniques have shown that deficits lasting more than an hour usually represent irreversible cerebral infarcts and that most true TIAs typically last less than 15 minutes (Ay et al., 1999). For the same reason, the term *reversible ischemic neurologic deficit* to refer to symptoms lasting 1 to 7 days has been abandoned (Ay et al., 1999).

Stroke in the elderly is applied in many studies to refer to strokes occurring in patients more than 60 years of age, although certain studies use the term only in patients older than 65 or 75 (Simons et al., 1998; Longstreth et al., 1998; Kaarisalo et al., 1997). *Stroke in the very old* is used in cohorts older than 80 or 85 (DiCarlo et al., 1999). Regardless of the cutoff point, stroke in the extremes of age has distinct pathophysiologic and prognostic features.

EPIDEMIOLOGY IN OLDER ADULTS

Ischemic stroke affects all age groups, but is primarily a disease of older adults. The annual incidence in the United States approaches 750,000 ischemic strokes per year (Broderick et al., 1998; Williams et al., 1999) and seems to be increasing as the population ages. Moreover, age is an independent but not modifiable risk factor for ischemic stroke. The risk of stroke approximately doubles for each successive decade of life, from about 3/1,000 people aged 55 to 64 years to about 25/1,000 people over the age of 85 years (Williams et al., 1999; Wolf and D'Agostino, 1998). The risk of stroke is greater among men up to age 75, but above age 75 it is higher among women and is the leading cause of death among women over 85 years. Blacks carry a disproportionate share of the burden of stroke at all ages, with more than double the incidence and mortality of whites. Among patients who have already survived a stroke, the only significant risk factor for recurrent stroke is age above 75 years (Hankey et al., 1998).

RISK FACTORS IN OLDER ADULTS

Many of the recognized risk factors for cerebrovascular disease are overly abundant in the elderly population and contribute to their increased stroke risk (Table 17-1). Hypertension, the leading risk factor for ischemic stroke, increases with advancing age and is found in more than half of people over 65. Furthermore, after the age of 65 years, the risk of stroke de-

TABLE 17-1. *Risk factors for ischemic stroke*

Nonmodifiable	Modifiable
Age	Hypertension
Sex	Diabetes
Race/ethnicity	Hyperlipidemia
Family history	Cardiac disease (atrial fibrillation and others)
	Elevated homocysteine
	Smoking
	Excessive alcohol use
	Physical inactivity

pends predominantly on systolic rather than diastolic pressure, and systolic pressure increases linearly with age. Primary prevention of stroke in older adults should include treatment of hypertension, including that of isolated systolic hypertension, because antihypertensive therapy reduces the risk of stroke by more than 30% (SHEP Cooperative Research Group, 1991).

Atrial fibrillation, another risk factor for ischemic stroke, also increases sharply with increasing age. Approximately 0.7% of the general US population is estimated to have atrial fibrillation; this proportion increases to 5% to 8% for persons over 65 years of age and to 10% to 15% for those above 80 (Feinberg et al., 1995). The median age for patients with atrial fibrillation in the United States is 75 years (Feinberg et al., 1995). Multiple epidemiologic studies have demonstrated that atrial fibrillation is an independent risk factor for ischemic stroke, increasing the relative risk of stroke approximately fivefold (Hart et al., 1998). In general, people with atrial fibrillation have an annual risk of stroke of about 5%, but patients stratified as "high risk" have stroke rates of up to 12% per year (Hart et al., 1998). Risk factors for stroke in atrial fibrillation include age over 75 years, congestive heart failure or reduced left ventricular fractional shortening (<25%), hypertension, or history of previous thromboembolism (Stroke Prevention in Atrial Fibrillation Investigators, 1996). The use of antiplatelet or anticoagulant therapy for stroke prophylaxis in the elderly with atrial fibrillation is somewhat controversial and will be discussed in *Treatment Options.*

Diabetes mellitus is a risk factor for ischemic stroke, and stroke is at least twice as common in patients with diabetes. The prevalence of diabetes increases steadily with age, such that approximately 18% of people aged 65 years or older in the United States have this disorder. Some of the increased risk of stroke appears to be related to concomitant hypertension, but at least some component of risk is independently related to diabetes alone (Barrett-Connor and Khaw, 1988). It remains uncertain, however, whether tight glucose control in diabetics is effective in preventing stroke.

The role of hypercholesterolemia as a stroke risk factor remains unconfirmed, although we and other authors believe that the weight of the evidence supports this association (Demchuk, et al., 1999; Futterman and Lemberg, 1999; Hess et al., 2000; Rosenson, 2000). It appears that the effect of total cholesterol seems to wane with increasing age, but high levels of low-density lipoprotein (LDL), and low levels of high-density lipoprotein (HDL) increase the risk of stroke even in elderly populations. The class of lipid-

lowering agents known either as the 3-hydroxy-3-methylglutaryl coenzyme A reductase inhibitors, or statins, appears to reduce the risk of stroke by about 30% among patients with coronary artery disease, at least in part because of mechanisms other than those that simply alter the lipid profile (Blauw et al., 1997; Bucher et al., 1998; Futterman and Lemberg, 1999; Hess, 2000; Rosenson, 2000; Warshafsky et al., 1999). It is hypothesized that statins stabilize atherosclerotic plaque, reduce platelet aggregation, and decrease inflammation, all of which in turn reduce the risk of vascular events. Relatively few data are found on the treatment of hyperlipidemia in elderly patients. It is reasonable, however, to consider primary prevention with statins if LDL levels exceed 160 mg/dL, particularly if other vascular risk factors are present (e.g., hypertension, diabetes, smoking, family history of vascular disease, or HDL levels <35 mg/dL) (Grundy et al., 1999; National Cholesterol Education Program (NCEP) Expert Panel, 1993; National Cholesterol Education Program Expert Panel, 1988). Statins are recommended for elderly patients with elevated LDL who have already suffered a TIA or minor stroke, although this approach remains to be proved in a clinical trial (Grundy et al., 1999; Shepherd et al., 1999; Weverling-Rijnsburger et al., 1997).

Elevated levels of the amino acid homocysteine have been linked to an increased risk of stroke. This association was first characterized in a relatively young population, but subsequent studies have confirmed that homocysteine is an important vascular risk factor even in elderly patients (Bots et al., 1999). The risk of stroke and myocardial infarction increases by about 7% for each 1 μmol/L increase in homocysteine. Homocysteine levels can be lowered with dietary supplementation of folic acid and vitamins B_{12} and B_6.

ETIOPATHOGENIC MECHANISMS OF ISCHEMIC STROKE

Ischemia is caused by transient or permanent occlusion of a cerebral blood vessel. The possible causes of cerebrovascular occlusion, which are myriad, are described individually below in the section *Evaluation of Causes of Stroke.* After occlusion, cerebral blood flow (CBF) is impaired, resulting in a central area (core) of severely constrained perfusion and a peripheral area of less constrained perfusion (ischemic penumbra) (Hossman, 1994). In the core, CBF is typically below 15 mL/100 g/min and will invariably succumb to infarction. In the penumbra, CBF averages 18 to 20 mL/100 g/min. The cells in the

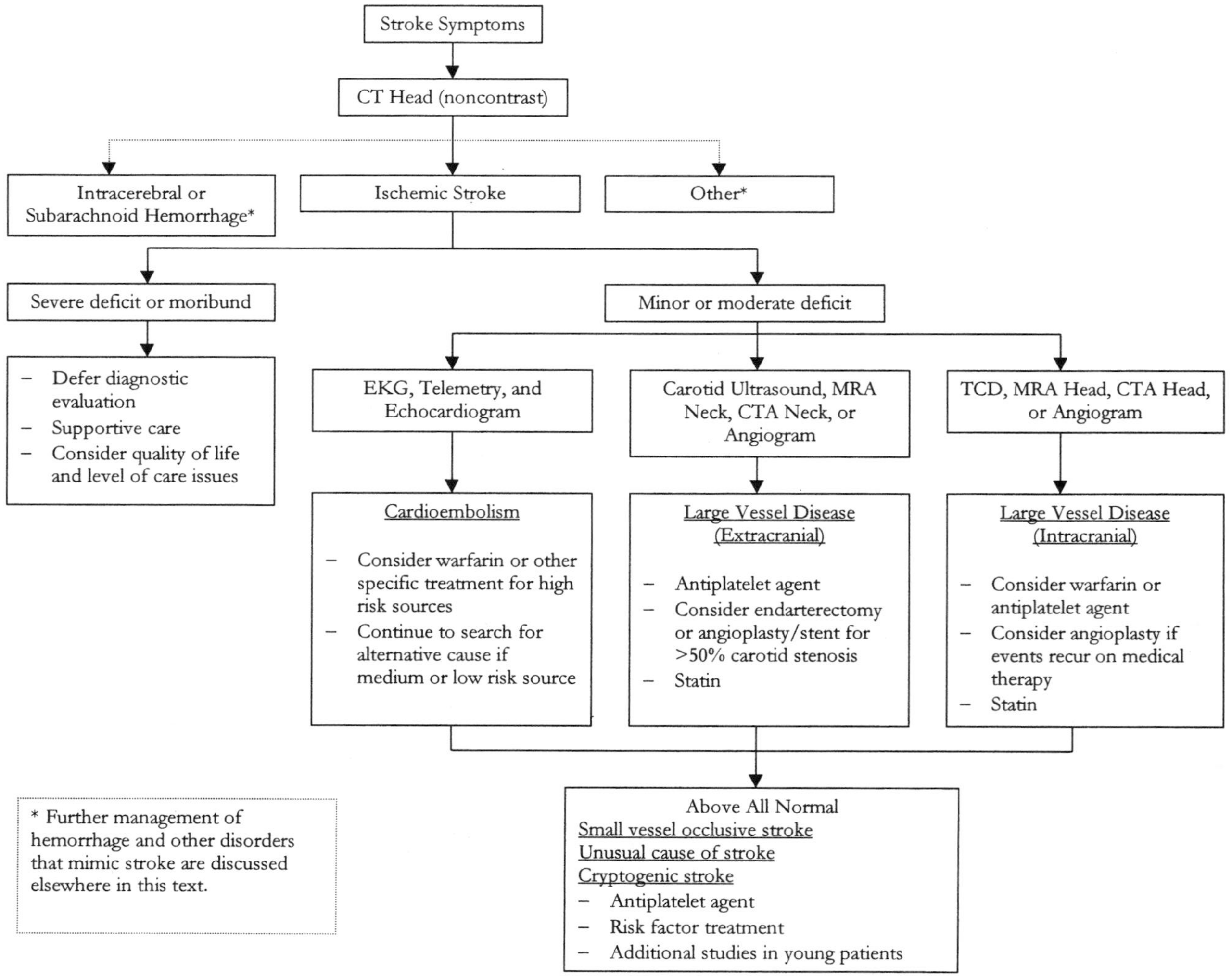

FIG. 17.1. Algorithm for the diagnosis of stroke etiology and strategies for secondary prevention.

Stroke Symptoms

CT Head (noncontrast)

Ischemic Stroke

Intracerebral or Subarachnoid Hemorrhage*

Severe deficit or moribund
- Defer diagnostic evaluation
- Supportive care
- Consider quality of life and level of care issues

Other*

Minor or moderate deficit

EKG, Telemetry, and Echocardiogram

Cardioembolism
- Consider warfarin or other specific treatment for high risk sources
- Continue to search for alternative cause if medium or low risk source

Carotid Ultrasound, MRA Neck, CTA Neck, or Angiogram

Large Vessel Disease (Extracranial)
- Antiplatelet agent
- Consider endarterectomy or angioplasty/stent for >50% carotid stenosis
- Statin

TCD, MRA Head, CTA Head, or Angiogram

Large Vessel Disease (Intracranial)
- Consider warfarin or antiplatelet agent
- Consider angioplasty if events recur on medical therapy
- Statin

Above All Normal
Small vessel occlusive stroke
Unusual cause of stroke
Cryptogenic stroke
- Antiplatelet agent
- Risk factor treatment
- Additional studies in young patients

* Further management of hemorrhage and other disorders that mimic stroke are discussed elsewhere in this text.

penumbra lose electrical function but retain structural integrity. The penumbra, thus, represents a potentially salvageable area, but the time window for intervention appears to be brief. The brain is able to tolerate low CBF only for a limited amount of time and the threshold for ischemia varies with the duration and the intensity of the ischemic insult. Thus, it is imperative to reestablish blood flow rapidly in acute stroke to minimize the cerebral injury.

Impaired cerebral perfusion sets into motion a series of events called the "ischemic cascade" (Rothman and Olney, 1986; Olney, 1994; Lipton and Rosenberg, 1994; Hickenbottom and Grotta, 1998). Neurons become unable to maintain aerobic respiration and anaerobic respiration ensues, leading to accumulation of lactic acid. With the change to a less efficient metabolic state, neurons can no longer maintain ionic balance (Kohno et al., 1995). Excitotoxicity occurs, in which glutamate and other excitatory neurotransmitters worsen the neuronal injury via excessive stimulation of neurons during their energy-depleted state. These neurotransmitters depolarize the neuronal cell membrane; an influx of sodium, chloride, and water follows, resulting in cytotoxic edema. Influx of calcium follows, which can lead to neuronal death. Several other elements amplify the ischemic cascade (Hickenbottom and Grotta, 1998). The details of this topic are beyond the scope of this chapter, but a few key elements deserve attention. Increased intracellular calcium activates several enzymatic pathways that cause proteolysis, destruction of cell wall lipids, free radical formation, further release of intracellular calcium, and increased production of nitric oxide. The enzymatic disturbances and free radical production lead to widespread disruption of neuronal and endothelial integrity. In addition, in the ischemic zone a series of cytokines are released, some of which may promote an inflammatory response and disrupt the microcirculation, thereby worsening the ischemic injury. Lastly, cell death can occur in a delayed fashion by apoptosis (Schmidt-Kastner et al., 1997), a genetically programmed form of cell death that may be induced by neuronal ischemia. It is distinct from necrosis, as it occurs in a delayed fashion, and can occur in remote areas from the core of infarction.

The sequence of events described above occurs to a different degree in all persons exposed to an ischemic injury. However, laboratory experience suggests that age has an impact on these events. Experimental evidence suggests that older animals are less resistant to ischemia than younger ones, and that the excitotoxic response can be more robust with advanced age (Glass et al., 1943; Hoffman et al., 1985; Garcia and Brown, 1992). The ability to neutralize free radicals and extrude calcium from cells is reduced in older animals than in their younger counterparts. The ability to synthesize proteins is reduced in the elderly and may lead to impaired cerebral reorganization after both trauma and stroke. The blood–brain barrier in the elderly is less efficient than in the young, and toxins normally excluded from the brain may gain access, worsening the ischemic injury (Mooradian, 1994). Although CBF is lower in older subjects, cerebral metabolism (as measured by the oxygen extraction ratio) is also lower, thus an imbalance between supply and demand does not exist. Nevertheless, the normal autoregulatory response seen in young subjects in the setting of impaired perfusion is absent in older individuals (Nagasawa et al., 1979; Choi et al., 1998). Collateral circulation may be impaired in the elderly, leading to infarcts of larger volume. The inherent elastic properties of intracranial vessels are affected by aging, thereby reducing the efficiency of the compensatory response to ischemia and acidosis. Thus, it is conceivable that in older patients comparable vascular insults may result in a more severe injury than in younger patients (Powers et al., 1984). Paradoxically, older patients with stroke may fare better when they suffer large middle cerebral artery infarcts with significant mass effect as the age-related atrophy may provide additional space for tissue displacement (Krieger et al., 1999).

NATURAL HISTORY OF ISCHEMIC STROKE

Significant advances have been made in the treatment of ischemic stroke, but most stroke survivors have some residual neurologic dysfunction. Although most patients have some improvement, it is often incomplete. In general, older patients face a worse prognosis than younger patients (Jorgensen et al., 1999). Mortality from stroke increases progressively with age, from about 10% below age 65, to 20% between ages 65 and 74, to 30% between ages 75 to 84, and 40% at age 85 and older (Nakayama et al., 1994). Functional outcome also tends to be worse in older patients, although they have similar neurologic deficits, which suggests that the ability to compensate after stroke is worse in the elderly (Jorgensen et al., 1999; Nakayama et al., 1994). Furthermore, dementia occurs in about one third of elderly stroke survivors, which further adds to the burden of disability (Zhu et al., 1998).

A major predictor of outcome after stroke is initial stroke severity, with worse outcomes in patients with more severe deficits (Reith et al., 1996). Recovery depends somewhat on the size and location of the infarction. Small infarctions, particularly subcortical lacunar strokes, can result in little permanent deficit, whereas large hemispheric infarctions can be devastating. Other diseases or medical complications after the stroke also appears to worsen outcome (Johnston et al., 1998; Pulsinelli et al., 1983) and these tend to be more common among the elderly both before and after stroke. Despite these potential prognostic indicators, the marked variability among patients makes prediction for individuals extremely difficult.

Infarcted brain tissue is irreparable, and functional improvement after stroke is believed to occur by recruitment of other neurons to serve new or additional roles. Neurons have been shown to sprout new synapses after stroke in young rodents (Stroemer et al., 1998). Electrical brain mapping in monkeys has demonstrated that the cerebral cortex can be functionally reorganized during recovery after an infarction (Nudo et al., 1996). Similarly, functional magnetic resonance imaging (MRI) in humans has shown increased activity in both hemispheres as patients improve, suggesting recruitment of neighboring cortex and corresponding areas of the contralateral cortex (Cramer et al., 1997). In general, recovery is expected to occur primarily in the first 3 months after stroke. The effect of aging on these reparative processes is unknown in humans, but it is hypothesized that they become less effective with age.

DIAGNOSIS

Emergent Evaluation

Most patients with acute stroke should initially be evaluated in the emergency department. After attention to the issues of oxygenation and hemodynamic stability, a medical history and physical examination should focus on specific stroke risk factors and causes, followed by clinical localization of the ischemic territory (Table 17-2). Other disorders that can resemble ischemic stroke must be considered and excluded, if possible, given the available information (Table 17-3). Laboratory studies, including a complete blood count, electrolytes, glucose, and coagulation parameters, should be obtained. Electrocardiography (ECG) is needed to assess for evidence of arrhythmia or cardiac ischemia. Emergent computed tomography (CT) is required to identify intracerebral hemorrhage (ICH) and early signs of cerebral ischemia. Based on these data, which can be obtained in less than 60 minutes, decisions regarding acute interventions must be reached. These basic emergent diagnostic issues are the same for young and old alike, because (as described below in *Treatment of Acute Ischemic Stroke*), age is not a major issue in the acute treatment decision (Tanne et al., 2000).

Treatment of the patient with acute stroke, ideally, should target the underlying pathophysiology. However, early determination of stroke mechanism is difficult, and many patients seen within the first 24 hours after onset are incorrectly classified (Madden et al., 1995). Because therapy for acute stroke must be initiated during this window of uncertainty, specific mechanism-directed therapy does not yet exist. Instead, treatment must have broad efficacy for all types of ischemic stroke.

Emergent imaging studies can be useful for some treatment decisions. For determination of vascular anatomy, the *gold standard* is conventional catheter arteriography that can demonstrate an acute arterial occlusion or embolus lodged at a vascular bifurcation. The vasculature can also be evaluated noninvasively with transcranial Doppler (TCD) ultrasonography, magnetic resonance angiography (MRA), or CT-angiography (CTA), but these techniques may be less accurate than conventional angiography. Furthermore, conventional angiography provides a route for interventional radiologic therapies (e.g., intraarterial thrombolysis or angioplasty), although these are currently

TABLE 17-2. *Major cerebrovascular clinical syndromes*

Artery	Clinical features
Anterior circulation	
ACA	Contralateral leg weakness
MCA	Contralateral face + arm >leg weakness, sensory loss, field cut, aphasia/neglect
Posterior circulation	
PCA	Contralateral field cut
BA	Eye movement abnormalities, ataxia, sensory/motor deficits
VA	Dysarthria, dysphagia, vertigo, ataxia, sensory/motor deficits
Small vessels	Lacunar syndrome (see text) without cortical signs[a]

ACA, anterior cerebral artery; BA, basilar artery; MCA, middle cerebral artery; PCA, posterior cerebral artery; VA, vertebral artery.

[a]Cortical signs include aphasia, apraxia, neglect, and other cognitive abnormalities.

TABLE 17-3. *Differential diagnosis of acute ischemic stroke*

Disorders that mimic stroke	Diagnostic tools
Intracerebral hemorrhage	CT/MRI
Subarachnoid hemorrhage	CT, lumbar puncture
Subdural/epidural hematoma	History of trauma, CT/MRI
Structural lesion (e.g., neoplasm, abscess)	CT/MRI
Hypo- or hyperglycemia	Finger stick glucose
Other metabolic derangements	Routine chemistry studies
Seizure	Clinical history, EEG
Migraine	Clinical history
Conversion disorder	Clinical history, psychiatric evaluation

CT, computed tomography; EEG, electroencephalogram; MRI, magnetic resonance imaging.

controversial. Physiologic imaging offers the possibility of identifying a viable "ischemic penumbra" around an infarcted core, and this viable tissue may benefit from potential treatments such as reperfusion or neuroprotection (Hossman, 1994). Discussion of these techniques is beyond the scope of this chapter, but intensive research may bring this type of neuroimaging to the clinical forefront (Baron et al., 1995).

Evaluation of Causes of Stroke

After the hyperacute period of the first few hours after stroke onset, secondary prevention therapy should be initiated for all patients with ischemic stroke. Diagnostic studies are needed to determine the risk factors and cause of the stroke, because specific treatments are available for specific stroke causes (see Fig. 17-1). No true "standard" approach exists to the evaluation of all stroke patients, and consideration must be given to each patient's medical and neurologic condition, his or her prognosis, and the possible risks and benefits of the interventions that are being considered. For example, some patients are poor candidates for carotid revascularization procedures (i.e., endarterectomy or angioplasty and stent) because of their other medical problems and, therefore, do not need carotid diagnostic studies. Testing in this situation is costly and inefficient. Similarly, some patients are comatose or moribund because of stroke and are unlikely to survive. In such patients, diagnostic studies should be deferred, at least temporarily, because information regarding cause is unlikely to alter management. These issues may be particularly important in some elderly patients, and attention should first be paid to the issues of quality of life and level of care.

Characterization of the stroke risk factors is based primarily on the medical history, but the following laboratory investigations are recommended for most patients: complete blood count, prothrombin time, partial thromboplastin time, serum glucose, fasting lipids, and serum homocysteine.

Cardioembolism

Cardioembolism should be considered as a possible cause of virtually all ischemic strokes. It is most commonly associated with atrial fibrillation, mural thrombus, focal ventricular akinesis after myocardial infarction, dilated cardiomyopathy, and valvular disease. Embolic events can be multiple and occur in the territories of any of the major vessels. Cardiac evaluation includes a clinical cardiac history and examination, an electrocardiogram (ECG), and an echocardiogram. Either transthoracic or transesophageal echocardiography (TEE) can be used as the initial screening test, but TEE is more sensitive to some abnormalities, including left atrial appendage thrombus and aortic arch atherosclerosis (McNamara et al., 1997). If cardioembolism is suspected but transthoracic echocardiography is normal, then TEE should also be performed. Treatment (described below) is aimed at preventing recurrent clot formation and cerebral embolization, often with anticoagulants.

Large Vessel Atherothromboembolism

Large vessel atherothromboembolism is usually a result of carotid artery stenosis, and less commonly caused by stenosis of the vertebral arteries or the intracranial vessels. Stenosis of the internal carotid artery can result in either a thrombotic (acute occlusive) or embolic (artery-to-artery embolic) stroke and, in either case, the treatment can include excision of the plaque by endarterectomy. Stenosis in the vertebrobasilar system or in the intracranial circulation can cause stroke by the same mechanisms, but these are not amenable to surgery. A hallmark clinical feature is recurrent similar clinical events in the same vascular territory, suggesting the involvement of a single large vessel. Examination of the large vessels should be performed, depending on the localization of the stroke. Patients with anterior circulation strokes (Table 17-2) require evaluation of the carotid arteries, whereas patients with posterior circulation strokes (Table 17-2) require evaluation of the vertebral arteries, and both may need evaluation of the intracranial vessels. The extracranial carotid arteries can be evaluated by carotid ultrasonography, whereas both the carotid and vertebral arteries can be reliably imaged with MRA or CTA. The intracranial circulation can be examined using TCD, MRA, or CTA. Conventional cerebral angiography is the definitive study, but because this invasive test carries a 1% risk of stroke and significant expense, it is often reserved for those situations in which treatment decisions require the additional information.

Small Vessel Occlusive Disease

Small vessel occlusive disease is often synonymous with "lacunar infarction." The deep small vessels in the internal capsule, corona radiata, thalamus, and pons seem most susceptible to the process of small vessel occlusive disease. Some of these infarctions can be clinically silent because they are small and can occur in a relatively less important region. However, small lesions do not necessarily cause small deficits. A microvascular infarction in the internal capsule can interrupt the entire corticospinal (motor) tract as it descends, resulting in a severe contralateral motor deficit. The most common lacunar syndromes are pure motor hemiparesis, pure sensory stroke, clumsy hand-dysarthria syndrome, and ataxic hemiparesis (Fisher, 1982). The mechanism of the small vessel occlusive process is uncertain, but it is most common in patients with longstanding diabetes or hypertension. The diagnosis of small vessel disease rests on the clinical syndrome, the finding of a small (<1.5 cm) deep infarction on CT or MRI, and the absence of an alternative cause (Adams et al, 1993).

Other Unusual Causes of Stroke

A number of uncommon causes of stroke include arterial dissection, prothrombotic disorders, genetic disorders, drug abuse (e.g., cocaine), and vasculitis (Kasner, 2000). The diagnosis of these other mechanisms may require special laboratory studies, lumbar puncture, cerebral angiography, and even brain biopsy in some circumstances. Although stroke in young patients disproportionately results from these miscellaneous causes (Bogousslavsky and Pierre, 1992), they are rare in the elderly and an extensive evaluation to identify these causes is usually not warranted. However, temporal arteritis is the one unusual cause that occurs uniquely in older adults and always requires consideration.

Consider temporal arteritis in any patient older than 50 with stroke. Clinical suspicion should be heightened by the presence of jaw or tongue claudication, transient or permanent unilateral visual impairment (amaurosis fugax or ischemic optic neuropathy, respectively), localized headache or scalp tenderness, or temporal artery abnormalities (including diminished pulse, tenderness, induration, or nodules) (Lee and Brazis, 1999). An erythrocyte sedimentation rate (ESR) is recommended, and should be considered elevated if it exceeds 50 mm/hour. If the clinical features are present, the ESR is elevated, or both, a unilateral temporal artery biopsy should be performed. If the level of suspicion is very high but the biopsy is negative, the other temporal artery should then be biopsied. Steroid therapy can be initiated before the biopsy and will not affect the results if performed within approximately 10 to 14 days (Lee and Brazis, 1999). Other methods to diagnose temporal arteritis have been proposed, including ultrasound techniques, but they remain unproved and are not widely available.

Cryptogenic Stroke

Cryptogenic (idiopathic) stroke is diagnosed when all other studies fail to identify any likely stroke mechanism. About half of strokes in young patients are diagnosed as cryptogenic, but this cause is infrequently invoked in the elderly.

TREATMENT OPTIONS

In general, treatment of the elderly patient with stroke does not differ much from that of younger patients. Following is a discussion of treatment options for both acute ischemic stroke (AIS) and for secondary stroke prevention. Special attention is given to areas of controversy in the treatment of elderly stroke patients, including acute stroke treatment with tissue plasminogen activator (tPA), anticoagulation in the setting of atrial fibrillation, and carotid endarterectomy (CEA) for symptomatic carotid artery stenosis. Treatment of temporal arteritis, an unusual cause of stroke unique to older adults, will also be addressed. A summary of medications typi-

TABLE 17-4. *Medications used in ischemic stroke*

Medication	Standard dose	Drug interactions	Adverse effects
tPA	0.9 mg/kg (maximum 90 mg); 10% as i.v. bolus over 1 minute, then remainder as i.v. infusion over 1 hour	Anticoagulants, including heparin and warfarin	Systemic and intracranial hemorrhage
Aspirin	50–325 mg q.d.	Other antiplatelet agents, NSAID, heparin, warfarin	Dyspepsia, tinnitus, gastrointestinal bleeding
Ticlopidine	250 mg b.i.d.	Aspirin and other antiplatelet agents, NSAID, heparin, warfarin, cimetidine, theophylline	Diarrhea, nausea, vomiting, rash, gastrointestinal bleeding, neutropenia, thrombotic thrombocytopenic purpura, aplastic anemia
Clopidogrel	75 mg q.d.	Aspirin and other antiplatelet agents, NSAID, heparin, warfarin. At high concentrations, can inhibit certain hepatic enzymes and decrease metabolism of various medications	Rash, diarrhea, dyspepsia, gastrointestinal bleeding
Dipyridamole	75–100 mg t.i.d. to q.i.d. Modified-release formulation (200 mg) given in combination with 25 mg aspirin b.i.d.	None	Headache, dizziness, flushing, abdominal distress, diarrhea, vomiting
Warfarin	Individualized according to patient response as measured by international normalized ratio (INR) Usual dosages vary from 1–10 mg q.d. and titrated to keep INR between 2.0 and 3.0.	Aspirin and other antiplatelet agents, NSAID, ticlopidine, clopidogrel, heparin. Interacts with multiple other medications through pharmacokinetic mechanisms. Consult literature (Wells, 1994) before initiating therapy	Gastrointestinal and other systemic bleeding, warfarin necrosis syndrome, systemic atheromatous embolization ("purple toe" syndrome)

b.i.d., twice daily; i.v., intravenous; NSAID, nonsteriodal anti-inflammatory drugs; q.d., every day; q.i.d., four times daily; t.i.d., three times daily; tPA, tissue plasminogen activator.

cally used in stroke treatment and prevention can be found in Table 17-4.

Treatment of Acute Ischemic Stroke

Intravenous tPA, at a dose of 0.9 mg/kg used within 3 hours of symptom onset, is the only US Food and Drug Administration-approved treatment for AIS. Its approval arose largely as a result of the National Institute of Neurological Disorders and Stroke (NINDS) t-PA stroke study (The National Institute of Neurological Disorders and Stroke t-PA Stroke Study Group, 1995). This study documented an 11% to 13% absolute and 30% to 50% relative increase in favorable outcomes on four different outcome scales at 3 months following stroke. Although a statistically significant increase was seen in the rate of symptomatic

ICH in the tPA-treated group (6.4% vs 0.6% in the placebo group, $P < 0.0001$), no significant difference was found in mortality at 3 months. The European Cooperative Acute Stroke Study (ECASS I) found no significant benefit for tPA therapy in AIS and high rates of treatment-associated ICH. However, a longer time window (6 hours) and higher dose (1.1 mg/kg) were used in this study than in the NINDS tPA trial. It was also complicated by a very high rate of protocol violations (109 of 620 patients enrolled) (Hacke et al., 1995). A second European trial, ECASS II, again used a 6-hour time window, but used the NINDS dosing regimen (0.9 mg/kg) and required rigorous CT training for its investigators (Hacke et al., 1998). Again, no significant difference in outcome was seen between placebo- and tPA-treated patients, but few patients were enrolled with the 0- to 3-hour time window. Symptomatic ICH occurred more frequently in the tPA-treated group (8.8% vs 3.4% in the placebo group), but no difference in mortality was seen at 3 months. In summary, the trials for intravenous (i.v.) tPA for AIS demonstrated improved outcome following treatment in selected patients within 3 hours of stroke onset. Although treatment with i.v. tPA appears to be safe when given up to 6 hours after symptom onset, efficacy has not been proved beyond the 3-hour time window.

It should be noted that the ECASS trial excluded patients over 80 years of age. Nevertheless, the initial results from ECASS I did suggest that age was a risk factor for parenchymatous hematoma; this finding was not supported in the subsequent ECASS II trial (Hacke et al., 1995; Hacke et al., 1998). Moreover, subgroup analysis of the NINDS t-PA Stroke Study results did not find age to be predictive of ICH (The NINDS t-PA Stroke Study Group, 1997). These studies, therefore, demonstrated no age-associated increased risk of ICH in the setting of a carefully monitored clinical trial. A recent postmarketing trial in 189 patients treated with i.v. tPA within 3 hours of stroke onset found no difference in the rates of fatal, symptomatic, or total ICH in patients (80 years of age as compared with those younger than 80) (Tanne et al., 2000). In addition, older and younger patients had equal likelihood of favorable outcome following treatment with tPA (Tanne et al., 2000). In another postmarketing study, the Standard Treatment with Alteplase to Reverse Stroke (STARS), the incidence of symptomatic ICH (3.3%) was too low to perform analysis for predictors of ICH; however, age less than 85 years was a predictor of favorable clinical outcome (Albers et al., 2000).

Together, the results of these trials indicate that the elderly are not at increased risk for ICH with the use of i.v. tPA for AIS, and indicate that they may be as likely as younger patients to benefit from such treatment. Other acute therapies for AIS (e.g., intraarterial thrombolysis, mechanical reperfusion strategies, defibrinogenating agents) have been evaluated more recently, but thus far few data are available evaluating the specific risks and benefits of these therapies for elderly stroke patients. A general discussion of newer acute stroke therapies can be found elsewhere (Hickenbottom and Barsan, 2000).

Prevention of Ischemic Stroke

Strategies for secondary prevention of stroke include risk factor modification, pharmacologic treatment with antiplatelet or anticoagulant therapies, and surgical management of carotid artery disease. The American Academy of Neurology (AAN) has issued practice parameters for stroke prevention in atrial fibrillation (Report of the Quality Standards Subcommittee of the American Academy of Neurology, 1998). In the general population with atrial fibrillation, warfarin with dosing adjusted to yield an international normalized ratio (INR) of 2 to 3 reduces the risk of stroke by about 70% and is recommended for stroke prophylaxis in patients who can be appropriately monitored. Despite this recommendation, warfarin is generally underutilized, with perhaps only one third to one half of eligible patients with atrial fibrillation being managed appropriately (Albers et al., 1997). In elderly populations, underutilization of warfarin may be even more problematic. Several studies designed to assess practice patterns and attitudes about anticoagulation in the elderly with atrial fibrillation have demonstrated decreased willingness on the part of physicians to use warfarin in their older patients (McCrory et al., 1995; Mendelson and Aronow, 1999). Some of this hesitance may result from concerns about increased risk for ICH in elderly patients on chronic anticoagulation. The Stroke Prevention in Atrial Fibrillation II (SPAF II) found that patients with atrial fibrillation above 75 years of age who were treated with adjusted dose warfarin were at significantly higher risk for ICH than younger patients (Stroke Prevention in Atrial Fibrillation Investigators, 1994). Unfortunately, a regimen of fixed, low-dose warfarin (INR 1.2–1.5) and aspirin was found to be significantly less effective in preventing stroke than adjusted dose warfarin (INR 2–3) and cannot be recommended as an alternative (Stroke Prevention in Atrial Fibrillation Investigators, 1996). Therefore, the AAN included an additional practice option that states that patients over 75 years of age may be treated with a lower INR target range (1.6–2.5). The efficacy of this option, however, has not been established, so that even for elderly patients the higher target INR of 2 to 3 is still recommended.

Antiplatelet therapy is also used in secondary prevention of ischemic stroke. To date, clinical trials involving antiplatelet agents for stroke prevention have not focused specifically on treatment of elderly patients. Thus, this section briefly outlines antiplatelet treatment options that are available for all stroke patients; more detailed discussion of antiplatelet therapy selection can be found elsewhere (Albers et al., 1998). Aspirin currently remains the standard initial medical treatment for secondary stroke prevention, and numerous trials and metaanalyses have documented an approximate 25% reduction in the odds of stroke recurrence or vascular death in aspirin recipients compared with placebo (Antiplatelet Trialists' Collaboration, 1988; Antiplatelet Trialists' Collaboration, 1994). The best dose of aspirin for stroke prevention has been controversial in the past, but most authors now agree that a low to moderate dose of aspirin (50–325 mg) is as effective as high dose and has fewer side effects (Albers et al., 1998). Several newer antiplatelet agents have been introduced that have marginal to modest benefit for secondary stroke prevention over aspirin: ticlopidine (Hass et al., 1989; Gent et al., 1989); clopidogrel (CAPRIE Steering Committee, 1998); and an extended-release dipyridamole–low-dose aspirin combination (Diener et al., 1996). Ticlopidine use has been curtailed because of its adverse safety profile, including the risk of severe neutropenia and thrombotic thrombocytopenic purpura (Bennett et al., 1998).

In addition to pharmacologic agents, surgical intervention with CEA can also be appropriate preventive therapy for selected stroke patients. The North American Symptomatic Carotid Endarterectomy Trial (NASCET) and the European Carotid Surgery Trial (ECST) demonstrated marked benefit for CEA over best medical management in symptomatic patients with high-grade carotid stenosis (defined as >70% in NASCET and >80% in ECST) (North American Symptomatic Carotid Endarterectomy Trial Collaborators, 1991; European Carotid Surgery Trialists' Collaborative Group, 1998). More recently, NASCET results for symptomatic patients with moderately severe stenosis (50% to 69%) have been published and demonstrate a less robust, but still significant, benefit for CEA in this population (Barnett et al., 1998).

Patients over 80 years of age were excluded from the first phase of NASCET (the study of both moderate and severe stenosis through early 1991), but were included in the second phase involving the continuing study of moderate stenosis. Analysis of the complete NASCET data set did not reveal age to be a predictor of perioperative stroke or death (Barnett et al., 1998). However, a study using community hospital discharge data from the Healthcare Cost and Utilization Project (HCUP-3) nationwide inpatient sample demonstrated that age was a predictor of in-hospital mortality following CEA, although not as strong a predictor as surgical complications or performing CEA simultaneously with coronary artery bypass grafting (Lanska, 1998). The difference may be related to practice variability among the institutions at which the surgery was performed. In NASCET, enrolling centers were required to meet stringent criteria regarding perioperative morbidity and mortality simply to participate in the trial, whereas the HCUP-3 data represent results from community practice. Thus, these data emphasize the importance of knowing the CEA perioperative complication rates of particular surgeons to whom patients may be referred. Elderly patients can definitely have CEA safely in the hands of well-trained surgeons who perform the procedure often.

In some elderly patients with ischemic stroke, treatment of temporal arteritis must be considered (Flynn and Hellmann, 1997). Long-term daily administration of corticosteroids is the mainstay of therapy. For patients presenting with acute visual loss, treatment with high-dose intravenous methylprednisolone (1,000 mg daily) should begin immediately and be continued for 3 to 5 days. Maintenance therapy with daily oral prednisone (starting at 60–80 mg daily) should then be initiated with a gradual taper over 12 months. The taper should be adjusted according to the patient's clinical response and ESR can also be monitored. The prednisone dose should be increased by 20 to 40 mg/day for symptom recurrence or increase in ESR; after 2 to 3 weeks on the higher dose, the taper can then be re-instituted. Experience with other immunosuppressive agents for temporal arteritis is limited.

PSYCHOSOCIAL IMPACT

Stroke is far more often disabling than lethal. It is estimated that stroke currently disables more than 4 million Americans. The financial, social, and familial impact of stroke is staggering. The decline in stroke mortality seen in recent years may result in a longer period of disability before death, with significant costs for individuals and society. In 1997 the US Bureau of the Census and the National Center for Health Statistics estimated the economic cost of stroke was $40.9 billion. Some $26.2 billion was the direct cost of hospital care, medical care, and drugs, and $14.7 billion represented subsequent lifelong expenses and lost income. In Scotland, the cost of each stroke to the National Health Service in 1988 was £6,000 (approximately $9,000), including only hospital costs (Warlow, 1998). When community, social service, and family costs were computed, the average cost was £70,000 (approximately $100,000). It is obvious that the financial burden imposed by stroke is mainly caused by long-term care and, to a lesser extent, lost income. Older patients are more likely to be discharged to a nursing home and to be handicapped at 3 months, accounting for a significant part of the financial burden of stroke (DiCarlo et al., 1999). Older patients also tend to be institutionalized more often before the stroke and that, in itself, is a predictor of poststroke institutionalization and increased cost. Even after treatment with intravenous tPA, patients above 80 are more likely to be discharged to a nursing home than younger patients. (Tanne et al., 2000).

Stroke has a significant impact on the ability to return to work. Of all stroke survivors, only 53% are able to return to work (Wozniak et al., 1999). Of those who return to work, 20% do so only on a parttime basis. Advanced age is inversely related to the chance of returning to work. On the other hand, many older stroke survivors are retired or unemployed before the stroke, thus confounding the interpretation of poststroke employment status. Stroke severity and cortical involvement also predict inability to return to work. Older patients appear to have more difficulty with instrumental activities of daily living (ambulation outdoors, shopping, public transportation), which hampers their ability to return to work (Grimby et al., 1998).

Depression and anxiety are extremely common after stroke, occurring in approximately 40% of survivors (Pohjasvara et al., 1998). Major depression occurs in about 25% and minor depression in 15%. Depression after stroke is not directly caused by the functional deficit, as patients with similar deficits from nonvascular causes do not develop depression with the same frequency. Stroke severity correlates weakly with the risk of development of depression, whereas a prior history of depression and marked dependency on caregivers correlate strongly. Depression is more frequent in elderly stroke victims than in younger ones. Lack of social support seems to exacerbate poststroke functional and cognitive impairment, and may increase the risk of depression in older subjects (Kauhanen et al., 1999). The prevalence of depression after stroke decreases after 3 months, but remains elevated up to 1 year. Language impairment appears to be correlated with the risk of developing depression. Poststroke cognitive impairment can be aggravated by depression, and may manifest as "pseudodementia." Treatment of poststroke depression may improve cognitive performance.

Sexual functioning is affected by stroke, which can have a significant psychosocial impact on the patient. Up to 50% of survivors of stroke and their spouses recommend that sexual counseling should be a part of stroke rehabilitation (Korpelainen et al., 1999). Of stroke patients, 57% and of spouses 65% note diminished libido after stroke. Penile erection decreases in 75% of men and decreased vaginal lubrication occurs in 46% of women, whereas anorgasmia occurs in 55%. Sexual dysfunction does not appear to be related to stroke location, stroke cause, or marital status. Sexual dysfunction is more common among diabetic men and among women taking cardiovascular medicines. A strong correlation exists between impaired sexual performance and depression, as determined by the Geriatric Depression Scale (Weatherall, 2000).

Finally, stroke takes an enormous toll on the caregivers and family members of the stroke victim. Emotional support, personal hygiene, feeding, ambulation, and nursing care are often under the direct responsibility of the loved ones. Of stroke survivors, 43% depend entirely on family members for assistance with activities of daily living (Dennis et al., 1998). The most common causes for dependency are sphincter incontinence; inability to walk, transfer, and eat; and difficulty dressing. Caring for a stroke patient poses constraints on the social life of the caregiver as well, and is particularly burdensome if the caregiver is also elderly or functionally impaired. A retrospective European study found that a significant proportion of stroke victims' family members felt lonely and that their social performance had declined; they experienced emotional distress and felt that their role as spouse was impaired (Scholte op Reimer et al., 1998). Furthermore, caregiver anxiety and depression are directly related to stroke severity and functional dependence, which tends to be worse in elderly patients (Dennis et al., 1998). Anxiety and depression also appear to be more common in female caregivers.

REFERENCES

Adams HP, Bendixen BH, Kappelle LJ, et al. Classification of subtype of acute ischemic stroke. Definitions for use in a multicenter clinical trial. *Stroke* 1993;24:35–41.

Albers GW, Bates VE, Clark WM, et al. Intravenous tissue-type plasminogen activator for treatment of acute stroke. The Standard Treatment with Alteplase to Reverse Stroke (STARS) Study. *JAMA* 2000;283:1145–1150.

Albers GW, Bittar N, Young L, et al. Clinical characteristics and management of acute stroke in patients with atrial fibrillation admitted to US university hospitals. *Neurology* 1997;48:1598–1604.

Albers GW, Easton JD, Sacco RL, et al. Antithrombotic and thrombolytic therapy for ischemic stroke. *Chest* 1998; 114:683S–698S.

Antiplatelet Trialists' Collaboration. Secondary prevention of vascular disease by prolonged antiplatelet treatment. *BMJ* 1988;296:320–331.

Antiplatelet Trialists' Collaboration. Collaborative overview of randomised trials of antiplatelet therapy. I. Prevention of death, myocardial infarction, and stroke by prolonged antiplatelet therapy in various categories of patients. *BMJ* 1994;308:81–106.

Ay H, Buonanno FS, Rordorf G, et al. Normal diffusion-weighted MRI during stroke-like deficits. *Neurology* 1999;52:1784–1792.

Baron JC, von Kummer R, del Zoppo GJ. Treatment of acute ischemic stroke. Challenging the concept of a rigid and universal time window. *Stroke* 1995;26:2219–2221.

Barnett HJM, Taylor DW, Eliasziw MA, et al., for the North American Symptomatic Carotid Endarterectomy Trial Collaborators. Benefit of carotid endarterectomy in patients with symptomatic moderate or severe stenosis. *N Engl J Med* 1998;339:1415–1425.

Barrett-Connor E, Khaw KT. Diabetes mellitus: an independent risk factor for stroke? *Am J Epidemiol* 1988;128:116–123.

Bennett CL, Weinberg PD, Brozenberg-ben-Dror K, et al. Thrombotic thrombocytopenic purpura associated with ticlopidine. A review of 60 cases. *Ann Intern Med* 1998;128:541–544.

Blauw GJ, Lagaay AM, Smelt AH, et al. Stroke, statins, and cholesterol. A meta-analysis of randomized, placebo-controlled, double-blind trials with HMG-CoA reductase inhibitors. *Stroke* 1997;28:946–950.

Bogousslavsky J, Pierre P. Ischemic stroke in patients under age 45. *Neurol Clin* 1992;10:113–124.

Bots ML, Launer LJ, Lindemans J, et al. Homocysteine and short-term risk of myocardial infarction and stroke in the elderly: the Rotterdam Study. *Arch Intern Med* 1999;159:38–44.

Broderick J, Brott T, Kothari R, et al. The Greater Cincinnati/Northern Kentucky Stroke Study: preliminary first-ever and total incidence rates of stroke among blacks. *Stroke* 1998;29:415–421.

Bucher HC, Griffith LE, Guyatt GH. Effect of HMG-CoA reductase inhibitors on stroke: a meta-analysis of randomized, controlled trials. *Ann Intern Med* 1998;128:89.

CAPRIE Steering Committee. A randomized, blinded trial of clopidogrel versus aspirin in patients at risk of ischemic events (CAPRIE). *Lancet* 1998;348:1329–1339.

Choi JY, Morris JC, Hsu CY. Aging and cerebrovascular disease. *Neurol Clin* 1998; 16: 687–711.

Cramer SC, Nelles G, Benson RR, et al. A functional MRI study of subjects recovered from hemiparetic stroke. *Stroke* 1997;28:2518–2527.

Demchuk AM, Hess DC, Brass LM, et al. Is cholesterol a risk factor for stroke? Yes. *Arch Neurol* 1999;56:1518–1520; discussion 1524.

Dennis M, O'Rourke S, Lewis S, et al. A quantitative study of the emotional outcome of people caring for stroke survivors. *Stroke* 1998;29:1867–1872.

DiCarlo A, Lamassa M, Pracucci G, et al. Stroke in the very old. *Stroke* 1999;30:2313–2319.

Diener HC, Cuhna L, Forbes C, et al. European Stroke Prevention Study 2. Dipyridamole and acetylsalicylic acid in the secondary prevention of stroke. *J Neurol Sci* 1996;143:1–13.

European Carotid Surgery Trialists' Collaborative Group. Randomised trial of endarterectomy for recently symptomatic carotid stenosis: final results of the MRC European Carotid Surgery Trial (ECST). *Lancet* 1998;351:1379–1387.

Feinberg WM, Blackshear JL, Laupacis A, et al. Prevalence, age distribution, and gender of patients with atrial fibrillation. *Arch Intern Med* 1995;155:469–473.

Fisher CM. Lacunar strokes and infarcts: a review. *Neurology* 1982;32:871–876.

Flynn JA, Hellmann DB. Giant cell arteritis and cerebral vasculitis. In: Johnson RT, Griffith JW, eds. *Current therapy in neurologic disease.* St. Louis: Mosby, 1997:214–219.

Futterman LG, Lemberg L. Stroke risk, cholesterol and statins. *Am J Crit Care* 1999;8:416–419.

Garcia JH, Brown GG. Vascular dementia: neuropathologic alterations and metabolic brain changes. *J Neurol Sci* 1992;109:121–131.

Gent M, Blakely JA, Easton JD, et al., and the CATS Group. The Canadian American Ticlopidine Study (CATS) in thromboembolic stroke. *Lancet* 1989;1:1215–1220.

Glass HG, Snyder FF, Webster E. The rate of decline in resistance to anoxia of rabbits, dogs, and guinea pigs from the onset of viability to adult life. *Brain* 1943;140:609–614.

Grimby G, Andren E, Daving Y, et al. Dependence and perceived difficulty in daily activities in community living stroke survivors 2 years after stroke. *Stroke* 1998:1843–1849.

Grundy SM, Cleeman JI, Rifkind BM, et al. Cholesterol lowering in the elderly population. Coordinating Committee of the National Cholesterol Education Program. *Arch Intern Med* 1999;159:1670–1678.

Hacke W, Kaste M, Fieschi C, et al., for the ECASS Study Group. Intravenous thrombolysis with recombinant tissue plasminogen activator for acute ischemic stroke: the European Cooperative Acute Stroke Study (ECASS). *JAMA* 1995;274:1017–1025.

Hacke W, Kaste M, Fieschi C, et al., for the Second European-Australian Acute Stroke Study Investigators. Randomised double-blind placebo-controlled trial of thrombolytic therapy with intravenous alteplase in acute ischaemic stroke (ECASS II). *Lancet* 1998;352:1245–1251.

Hankey GJ, Jamrozik K, Broadhurst RJ, et al. Long-term risk of first recurrent stroke in the Perth Community Stroke Study. *Stroke* 1998;29:2491–2500.

Hart RG, Sherman DG, Easton JD, et al. Prevention of stroke in patients with nonvalvular atrial fibrillation. *Neurology* 1998;51:674–681.

Hass WK, Easton JD, Adams HP, et al., for the Ticlopidine Aspirin Stroke Study Group. A randomized trial comparing ticlopidine hydrochloride with aspirin for the prevention of stroke in high-risk patients. Ticlopidine Aspirin Stroke Study Group. *N Engl J Med* 1989;321:501–507.

Hess DC, Demchuk AM, Brass LM, et al. HMG-CoA reductase inhibitors (statins): a promising approach to stroke prevention. *Neurology* 2000;54:790–796.

Hickenbottom SL, Barson WG. Acute ischemic stroke therapy. *Neurologic Clinics* 2000;18:379–397.

Hickenbottom SL, Grotta J. Neuroprotective therapy. *Semin Neurol* 1998;18: 485–492.

Hoffman WE, Pelligrino DJ, Miletich DJ, et al. Brain metabolism changes in young vs. aged rats during hypoxia. *Stroke* 1985;16:860–863.

Hossman K-A. Viability thresholds and the penumbra of focal ischemia. *Ann Neurol* 1994;36:557–565.

Johnston KC, Li JY, Lyden PD, et al. Medical and neurological complications of ischemic stroke: experience from the RANTTAS trial. RANTTAS Investigators. *Stroke* 1998;29:447–453.

Jorgensen HS, Reith J, Nakayama H, et al. What determines good recovery in patients with the most severe strokes? The Copenhagen Stroke Study. *Stroke* 1999;30:2008–2012.

Kaarisalo MM, Immonen-Raiha P, Marttila RJ, et al. Atrial fibrillation in older stroke patients: association with recurrence and mortality after first ischemic stroke. *J Am Geriatr Soc* 1997; 45:1297–1301.

Kasner SE. Stroke treatment—specific considerations. *Neurol Clin* 2000;19:399–417.

Kauhanen ML, Korpelainen JT, Hiltunen P, et al. Poststroke depression correlates with cognitive impairment and neurological deficits. *Stroke* 1999;30:1875–1880.

Kohno K, Hoehn-Berlage M, Mies G, et al. Relationship between diffusion-weighted MR images, cerebral blood flow, and energy state in experimental brain infarction. *Magn Reson Imaging* 1995;13:73–80.

Korpelainen JT, Nieminen P, Myllyla VV. Sexual functioning among stroke patients and their spouses. *Stroke* 1999; 30: 715–719.

Krieger DW, Demchuk AM, Kasner SE, et al. Early clinical and radiological predictors of fatal brain swelling in ischemic stroke. *Stroke* 1999; 30:287–292.

Lanska DJ, Kryscio RJ. In-hospital mortality following carotid endorterectomy. *Neurology* 1998;51:440–447.

Lee AG, Brazis PW. Temporal arteritis: a clinical approach. *J Am Geriatr Soc* 1999;47:1364–1370.

Lipton SA, Rosenberg PA. Excitatory amino acids as a final common pathway for neurological disorders. *N Engl J Med* 1994;330:613–622.

Longstreth WT, Shemanski L, Leftowitz D, et al. Asymptomatic internal carotid artery stenosis defined by ultrasound and the risk of subsequent stroke in the elderly. *Stroke* 1998;29:2371–2376.

Madden KP, Karanjia PN, Adams HP, et al. Accuracy of initial stroke subtype diagnosis in the TOAST study. *Neurology* 1995;45:1975–1979.

McCrory DC, Matchar DB, Samsa G, et al. Physician attitudes about anticoagulation for nonvalvular atrial fibrillation in the elderly. *Arch Intern Med* 1995;155:277–281.

McNamara RL, Lima JA, Whelton PK, et al. Echocardiographic identification of cardiovascular sources of emboli to guide clinical management of stroke: a cost-effectiveness analysis. *Ann Intern Med* 1997;127:775–787.

Mendelson G, Aronow WS. Underutilization of warfarin in older persons with chronic nonvalvular atrial fibrillation at high risk for developing stroke. *J Am Geriatr Soc* 1999; 46:1423–1424.

Mooradian AD. Potential mechanisms of the age-related changes in the blood-brain barrier. *Neurobiol Aging* 1994; 15:751–755.

Nagasawa S, Handa H, Okumura A, et al. Mechanical properties of human cerebral arteries. Part 1: Effects of age and vascular smooth muscle activation. *Surg Neurol* 1979;12:297–304.

Nakayama H, Jorgensen HS, Raaschou HO, et al. The influence of age on stroke outcome. The Copenhagen Stroke Study. *Stroke* 1994;25:808–813.

National Cholesterol Education Program Expert Panel. Report of the National Cholesterol Education Program Expert Panel on Detection, Evaluation, and Treatment of High Blood Cholesterol in Adults. *Arch Intern Med* 1988; 148:36–69.

National Cholesterol Education Program (NCEP) Expert Panel. Summary of the second report of the National Cholesterol Education Program (NCEP) Expert Panel on Detection, Evaluation, and Treatment of High Blood Cholesterol in Adults (Adult Treatment Panel II). *JAMA* 1993;269:3015–3023.

The National Institute of Neurological Disorders and Stroke t-PA Stroke Study Group. Tissue plasminogen activator for acute ischemic stroke. *N Engl J Med* 1995;333:1581–1587.

The NINDS t-PA Stroke Study Group. Intracerebral hemorrhage after intravenous t-PA therapy for ischemic stroke. *Stroke* 1997;28:2109–2118.

North American Symptomatic Carotid Endarterectomy Trial Collaborators. Beneficial effects of carotid endarterectomy in symptomatic patients with high-grade carotid stenosis. *N Engl J Med* 1991;325:445–453.

Nudo RJ, Wise BM, SiFuentes F, et al. Neural substrates for the effects of rehabilitative training on motor recovery after ischemic infarct. *Science*, 1996;272:1791–1794.

Olney JW. Excitatory transmitter neurotoxicity. *Neurobiol Aging* 1994;15:259–260.

Pohjasvaara T, Leppavuori A, Siira I, et al. Frequency and clinical determinants of poststroke depression. *Stroke* 1998;29:2311–2317.

Powers WJ, Grubb RL, Raichle ME. Physiological responses to focal cerebral ischemia in humans. *Ann Neurol* 1984; 16:546–552.

Pulsinelli WA, Levy DE, Sigsbee B, et al. Increased damage after ischemic stroke in patients with hyperglycemia with or without established diabetes mellitus. *Am J Med* 1983; 74:540–544.

Reith J, Jorgensen HS, Pedersen PM, et al. Body temperature in acute stroke: relation to stroke severity, infarct size, mortality, and outcome. *Lancet* 1996;347: 422–425.

Report of the Quality Standards Subcommittee of the American Academy of Neurology. Practice parameter: stroke prevention in patients with nonvalvular atrial fibrillation. *Neurology* 1998;51:671–673.

Rosenson RS. Biological basis for statin therapy in stroke prevention. *Curr Opin Neurol* 2000;13:57–62.

Rothman SM, Olney JW. Glutamate and the pathophysiology of hypoxic-ischemic brain damage. *Ann Neurol* 1986; 19:105–111.

Schmidt-Kastner R, Fliss H, Hakim AM. Subtle neuronal death in striatum after short forebrain ischemia in rats detected by in situ end-labeling for DNA damage. *Stroke* 1997;28:163–170.

Scholte op Reimer WJM, de Haan RJ, Rijnders PT, et al. The burden of caregiving in partners of long-term stroke survivors. *Stroke* 1998;29:1605–1611.

SHEP Cooperative Research Group. Prevention of stroke by antihypertensive drug treatment in older persons with isolated systolic hypertension. Final results of the Systolic Hypertension in the Elderly Program (SHEP). *JAMA* 1991;265:3255–3264.

Shepherd J, Blauw GJ, Murphy MB, et al. The design of a prospective study of Pravastatin in the Elderly at Risk (PROSPER). PROSPER Study Group. Prospective Study of Pravastatin in the Elderly at Risk. *Am J Cardiol* 1999; 84:1192–1197.

Simons LA, McCallum J, Friedlandler Y, et al. Risk factors for ischemic stroke: Dubbo study of the elderly. *Stroke* 1998;29:1341–1313.

Stroemer RP, Kent TA, Hulsebosch CE. Enhanced neocortical neural sprouting, synaptogenesis, and behavioral recovery with D-amphetamine therapy after neocortical infarction in rats. *Stroke* 1998;29:2381–2393.

Stroke Prevention in Atrial Fibrillation Investigators. Warfarin versus aspirin for prevention of thromboembolism in atrial fibrillation: Stroke Prevention in Atrial Fibrillation II Study. *Lancet* 1994;343:687–691.

Stroke Prevention in Atrial Fibrillation Investigators. Adjusted-dose warfarin versus low-intensity, fixed-dose warfarin plus aspirin for high-risk patients with atrial fibrillation: Stroke Prevention in Atrial Fibrillation III randomized clinical trial. *Lancet* 1996;348:633–638.

Tanne D, Gorman MJ, Bates VE, et al., and the tPA Stroke Survey Group. Intravenous tissue plasminogen activator for acute ischemic stroke in patients aged 80 years and older. The tPA Stroke Survey experience. *Stroke* 2000; 31:370–375.

Warlow CP. Epidemiology of stroke. *Lancet* 1998;352 (Suppl):1–4.

Warshafsky S, Packard D, Marks SJ, et al. Efficacy of 3-hydroxy-3-methylglutaryl coenzyme A reductase inhibitors for prevention of stroke. *J Gen Intern Med* 1999;14: 763–774.

Weatherall M. A randomized trial of the Geriatric Depression Scale in an inpatient ward for older adults. *Clin Rehabil* 2000;14:186–191.

Weverling-Rijnsburger AW, Blauw GJ, Lagaay AM, et al. Total cholesterol and risk of mortality in the oldest old. *Lancet* 1997;350:1119–1123.

Williams GR, Jiang JG, Matchar DB, et al. Incidence and occurrence of total (first-ever and recurrent) stroke. *Stroke* 1999;30:2523–2528.

Wolf PA, D'Agostino RB. Epidemiology of stroke. In: Barnett HJM, Mohr JP, Stein BM, Yatsu FM, eds. *Stroke: pathophysiology, diagnosis, and management*, 3rd ed. New York: Churchill Livingstone, 1998:3–28.

Wozniak MA, Kittner SJ, Price TR, et al. Stroke location is not associated with return to work after first ischemic stroke. *Stroke* 1999;30:2568–2573.

Zhu L, Fratiglioni L, Guo Z, et al. Association of stroke with dementia, cognitive impairment, and functional disability in the very old. A population based study. *Stroke* 1998;29: 2094–2099.

SUGGESTED READINGS

Alberts MJ, Hademenos G, Latchaw RE, et al. Recommendations for the establishment of primary stroke centers. Brain Attack Coalition. *JAMA* 2000; 283: 3102–3109.

Hart RG, Halperin JL. Atrial fibrillation and thromboembolism: a decade of progress in stroke prevention. *Ann Intern Med* 1999;131:688–695.

Hickenbottom SL, Barsan WG. Acute ischemic stroke therapy. *Neurol Clin* 2000;18:379–397.

Kasner SE, Grotta JC. Emergency identification and treatment of acute ischemic stroke. *Ann Emerg Med* 1997;30: 642–653.

Sacco RL, Elkind MS. Update on antiplatelet therapy for stroke prevention. *Arch Intern Med* 2000;160:1579–1582.

WEB SITES OF NATIONAL SUPPORT GROUPS

National Stroke Association: *http://www.stroke.org/*
American Stroke Association (a division of American Heart Association): *http://www.strokeassociation.org/*
The Stroke Network: *http://www.strokenetwork.org/*

18

Cognitive Effects of Stroke and Hemorrhage

Henry J. Riordan and Laura A. Flashman

RELATIONSHIP BETWEEN STROKE AND COGNITION

As the incidence of stroke risk increases sharply with age, doubling every decade after the age of 55 years, the cognitive and behavioral sequelae of stroke will undoubtedly become the most challenging illnesses that our society must face. Efforts to describe the relationship between stroke and cognition have driven neuropsychological thought with mounting evidence on various neurobehavioral disorders following stroke. This is helping us to revise our current understanding of brain-behavior relationships. In general, cerebrovascular lesions, including damage caused by stroke and hemorrhage, can have three distinct effects on cognition and behavior: a loss of function, a release of function, and a disorganization of function. The most obvious and direct effect of cerebral lesions is a loss of function in which the patient can no longer perform a specific cognitive or behavioral task. A release of function is said to occur when a new behavior appears or the frequency of a behavior is drastically increased after a brain lesion occurs. When bits or pieces of behavior still occur, but not in the correct order, or if behaviors occur at the wrong time and place, a disorganization of function is said to have occurred.

Often, a number of behavioral changes are transient following brain damage from stroke or hemorrhage. This recovery of function may take place over the course of days, weeks, or even years. To date, the processes involved in this recovery are poorly understood and are complicated by the variability of recovery across individuals. It should also be noted that some of the cognitive decline *recognized* following a stroke may have been the result of preexisting cognitive deficits. For example, Pohjasvaara et al. (1999) reported that the frequency of prestroke cognitive decline, including dementia, was approximately 9%. Older age, poorer education, and history of prior stroke were the most frequent factors associated with prestroke cognitive decline. Therefore, the possibility of two or more underlying disease processes should be considered in the diagnosis and treatment of cognitive dysfunction caused by stroke and hemorrhage.

NEUROBEHAVIORAL CONSEQUENCES OF CEREBRAL VASCULAR LESIONS

Below is a summary of some of the more common neurobehavioral disorders associated with cerebral vascular damage. In this chapter, specific cognitive deficits are viewed as being the direct result of an isolated lesion. However, in clinical practice rarely do patients present with a cognitive deficit that is caused by a lesion confined to a single functional region. Damage to any number of cerebral regions can result in similar and related patterns of cognitive deficits or constellations of behavioral deficits. To complicate matters, very few neuropsychological tasks are specifically designed to assess unitary cognitive areas, as almost all cognitive tasks rely on a complex networking among various functional areas. For example, many neuropsychological tests, even tests that require only a verbal response, involve the visual modality and assume some minimal levels of arousal, attention, organizational abilities, and the ability to make a behavioral response. Thus, few (arguably if any) neuropsychological tests have been devised to elicit a specific functional deficit in a cognitive domain such as memory, attention, or executive functioning. Therefore, this chapter is meant to serve as a general guide to some of the more common, if not more interesting, deficits in cognitive and behavioral functioning following stroke and hemorrhage. Although the extent of lesion is certainly important in the assessment of cognitive dysfunction following stroke, some appreciation of the basic tenants of the localization theory of brain function is also essential. For a much more comprehensive review of the behavioral geography of the human brain, as well as the neurobehavioral consequences of stroke, see Lezak (1995) or Robinson (1998).

CORTICAL LESIONS

Occlusion of the carotid arteries can result in infarction of the border zones between the anterior and middle, or middle and posterior, cerebral arteries. Clinical presentation in these instances includes primarily cortical deficits, including transcortical aphasia with preserved repetition, visuospatial deficits, and sensorimotor changes involving the proximal arm and leg (Stuss and Cummings, 1990). Occlusion of the anterior, middle, or posterior cerebral artery produces hemisphere-specific deficits related to the role of the affected tissue in the irrigated territory of the artery. Characteristic left hemisphere deficits include aphasia, apraxia, alexia, agraphia, and acalculia, whereas more representative right hemisphere deficits include visuospatial deficits, amusia, and impaired prosody.

Frontal Cortex

Comprising nearly one third of the mass of the cerebral hemispheres, the frontal lobes are the largest of the lobes of the brain and the most recently developed portion of the cerebrum. The frontal lobe has been called the "executor," maintaining control over all other cognitive processes. Although not directly responsible for many overt behaviors, the frontal lobes play an executive role in the planning, purpose, and performance of many behaviors. Additionally, damage to the prefrontal cortex can result in deficits in self-awareness that, in turn, can affect almost all areas of cognitive function. Damage to selective areas in the frontal lobe can interfere with motor or language functioning as well as relatively higher order cognitive processes such as abstract reasoning, planning, selective attention, complex problem-solving, concept formation, and cognitive flexibility (Walsh, 1987).

The frontal lobes are organized in an asymmetric manner. Together, they play an important role in nearly all cognitive processes. Language-mediated tasks tend to be under control of the dominant, usually left, hemisphere and nonverbal tasks are usually associated with the nondominant hemisphere. Thus, damage to the left frontal lobe can produce deficits in verbal behavior, including naming and fluency, whereas damage to the right frontal lobe can result in deficits in figural or design fluency (Cummings, 1993; Jones-Gottman and Milner, 1977). However, verbal fluency deficits, albeit less severe, have also been noted following right frontal lobe lesions, suggesting that the degree of laterality is relative. Some of the more commonly seen neurobehavioral disorders following damage to the prefrontal cortex, which

are described below, include Broca's aphasia, memory difficulties, difficulties in abstract thought, difficulties in initiation and stopping an action, and difficulties in attention and making mental shifts to changing task demands (Lezak,1995; Kolb and Wishaw, 1985).

Broca's Aphasia

Damage to the opercular and triangular portions of the inferior frontal gyrus (also known as Brodmann area 44) causes a constellation of deficits in expressive language commonly referred to as Broca's aphasia (Goodglass, 1975). Broca's aphasia is also known as expressive, nonfluent, or motor aphasia, suggesting that most of the deficits are in expressive rather than receptive language processing. In fact, patients with Broca's aphasia tend to have relatively good language comprehension skills. Patients who have a lesion of this area tend to produce very few words orally or in written form, exhibit extreme difficulty in word production, have impaired repetition and naming abilities, tend to leave out articles and qualifiers, and speak and write in a manner best described as "telegraphic."

Memory Deficits

Patients with prefrontal lobe lesions tend to have difficulty with the initial acquisition of new information because of their poor attention and organizational skills. They also tend to make numerous errors of perseveration and commission (e.g., false-positive errors, on cued memory recall tasks), as they have difficulty inhibiting inappropriate responses. Working memory, which refers to holding a limited amount of information in mind for a few seconds while manipulating it, depends on intact frontal lobe functioning (Goldman-Rakic, 1993). Impairments in working memory can result in diminished declarative memory performance by limiting the amount of material that is acquired initially. Although the frontal cortex plays a role in various memory processes, deficits in retention of new information are more likely to be seen following a lesion of the temporal lobes (see below for more detail).

Attentional Deficits

The prefrontal cortex is intrinsically involved in the capacity to focus or shift attention as required by changing task demands (Milner, 1963; Mirsky, 1989). Damage to the prefrontal cortex can result in numerous types of attentional deficits. For example, patients may be slow to react to stimuli and have attentional difficulties that are characterized by an inability to maintain or sustain focus, an inability to shift mental sets, and poor cognitive flexibility. Patients with prefrontal lesions can be described as having a "rigid" approach to problem-solving in general and are often unable to benefit from contextual cues or even direct instructional sets that direct them to the correct solution. Once again, their cognitive style can be characterized by numerous errors of perseveration, a deficit that may be seen across a variety of mental tasks and settings. An extreme example of this is when a patient is unable to stop making the same erroneous perseverative responses even though he or she can accurately state a correct answer.

Related to this "rigid" cognitive style is an inability to overcome literal associations. These patients tend to view events and interactions at face value and are unable to detect more subtle nuances and, therefore, the genuine meaning of events. This concrete approach also results in an inability to generate or appropriately use abstract notions, such as symbols, proverbs, and metaphors.

Volitional Deficits

Finally, as alluded to, many patients with prefrontal lesions tend to have difficulties in both initiating and stopping behavior, a deficit that can dramatically affect cognitive functioning. Difficulties in initiation can be related to apathy, poor spontaneity, and productivity, whereas difficulties in stopping and disinhibition may be more related to poor impulse control or an inability to benefit from feedback, suggesting the cessation of a behavior is warranted. As seen before, difficulties in stopping behavior can be caused by an inability to overcome perseverative responses. This type of disinhibition is often seen following lesions of the orbitofrontal circuitry, whereas symptoms such as spontaneity and apathy are more likely to follow injury to the anterior cingulate circuitry (Cummings, 1993).

Temporal Cortex

Because of the complex organization and the numerous and diverse tasks mediated by the temporal cortex, both the anatomic boundaries and the functional specialization of the temporal lobes are relatively less well defined than other lobes of the brain (Walsh, 1987). The temporal cortex serves various functions related to the primary perception of audition, olfaction, and visual information, and serves to integrate all aspects of our senses into a unified and meaningful experience. The temporal cortex also plays a critical role in memory and is intrinsically tied to the limbic system. Thus, the temporal lobe plays a role in associating emotional and motivational aspects of information to various sensory experiences and helps form impressions and knowledge of the world. Although numerous cognitive deficits can arise from stroke or hemorrhage of the temporal neocortex and adjacent medial temporal lobe structures, some of the more commonly observed and interesting neurobehavioral disorders include those of auditory perception, visual perception, and memory.

Wernicke's Aphasia

One of the most notable, if not the most disabling, disorders of auditory perception is referred to as "Wernicke's aphasia" (also known as sensory, fluent, or jargon aphasia), which can result from a lesion of the left temporal association cortex (Brodmann area 22). In this disorder, patients typically have very poor language comprehension but relatively intact speech production abilities (Goodglass, 1975). This pattern of preserved language production but impaired comprehension is at direct odds with Broca's aphasia in that patients with Wernicke's type aphasia can be characterized as being hyperverbal, despite the fact that their speech itself is nonsensical. In fact, these patients may even show signs of an anosognosia or inability to recognize their impaired speech and, therefore, can have difficulties benefiting from feedback in speech therapy. Interestingly, patients with similar lesions of the right temporal cortex may experience similar problems with nonverbal sound recognition and discrimination (McGlone and Young, 1986). In some cases, right temporal lesions can result in a deficit in music perception (i.e., amusia, where patients are unable to differentiate various musical tones or rhythms) (Shuppert et al., 2000).

Visual Perceptual Deficits

Lesions of the temporal cortex can cause deficits in visual discrimination, visual word recognition, pattern recognition, and even object recognition. These visual perceptual deficits can occur despite relatively normal performance on standard visual spatial tasks. For example, patients with right temporal lobe lesions may have difficulty recognizing objects from incomplete or partially drawn figures, may fail to recognize salient aspects of pictures, and may have relatively poor spatial reasoning abilities (Walsh, 1987).

Material-Specific Memory Deficits

Damage to the temporal cortex and medial temporal structures have long been known to result in material-specific memory deficits (De Renzi et al., 1982; Pillon et al.,1999). Lesions of the left temporal lobe can result in impairment in the ability to encode and recall a list of words, numbers, and letters presented aurally; semantic memory; and verbal paired-associate learning (Walsh, 1987). Patients with left temporal lobe lesions can have difficulty recalling words, which can also adversely affect fluent speech production. When severe, this inability is referred to as "anomia." Patients with this disorder can have impaired comprehension of complex information and, therefore, find it difficult to learn new verbal material.

Patients with right temporal lobe lesions are more likely to have memory difficulties involving visual spatial stimuli such as faces, nonverbalizable designs and figures. They can also have difficulty with maze learning as well as difficulties with any stimuli or task that does not readily lend itself to verbal tagging or labeling. Deficits in material-specific memory caused by unilateral temporal lobe lesions tend to produce relatively mild cognitive dysfunction that may only be notable on neuropsychological testing. However, bilateral temporal lobe lesions can result in a global amnesia (i.e., a severe and pervasive deficit in forming new conscious memories for all types of material). Although amnesia has been noted after unilateral temporal lobe lesions (typically of the dominant hemisphere), the most likely cause of an amnestic stroke is bilateral infarction of the posterior cerebral arteries affecting inferomedial structures of the temporal lobe, including the hippocampus and amygdala. This type of bilateral infarction is not exceptional, as both posterior cerebral arteries arise from a single basilar artery (Walsh, 1987).

Parietal Cortex

Situated between the frontal, temporal, and occipital lobes, the parietal lobe shares many of the functional features of the other lobes. In fact, it could be argued that lesions of the parietal lobes are associated with a greater variety of cognitive and behavioral disorders than any other lobe of the brain. However, unlike other cerebral regions, the cognitive deficits associated with parietal lesions often require specialized neuropsychological and behavioral techniques to bring forth. Some of the more commonly seen neurobehavioral disorders following a stroke or hemorrhage of the parietal lobe include agraphia or

acalculia, disorders of spatial orientation, alexia, constructional apraxia, and anosognosia. When lesions are located within the angular gyrus, which is the inferior lobule of the dominant parietal lobe (Brodmann area 39), a constellation of deficits known as "Gerstmann syndrome" (right-left disorientation, dysgraphia, acalculia, and finger agnosia) often occurs.

Agraphia

Agraphia, an inability to write, has been associated with lesions in the angular gyrus itself or connections to this region within the left parietal lobe. Although not as common, these deficits can also be seen following right hemisphere lesions as well. Several types of agraphia are seen, and the particular type of agraphia seen following posterior dominant hemisphere lesions tends to be characterized by well-formed letters joined together but with incorrect spellings, abnormal word order, and frequent omissions (Benson and Geschwind, 1985). This is in contrast to the more anterior type of agraphia characterized by large, crude, scrawling output that is poorly constructed and agrammatic. Isolated agraphia (not in the context of aphasia), which can also be seen following lesions of the angular gyrus, can co-occur with acalculia.

Acalculia

Acalculia refers to the inability to perform certain mathematical operations. It can be seen following damage of the left parietal lobe and often co-occurs with agraphia. Several types of agraphia and acalculia reflect a disruption of more complicated higher order cognitive processes. One form of acalculia in which patients cannot comprehend or write numbers correctly, or even substitute one number for another, can be seen after damage to the dominant hemisphere language areas. Damage to the nondominant parietal-occipital junction can result in a visual-spatial discrimination problem that causes an acalculia. This is characterized by poor placement of numbers in space such that the numbers are not aligned properly to allow for complex calculations. In this case, patients can understand numbers, symbols, and computation signs and may even be able to successfully complete most mathematical operations.

Spatial Neglect and Disorders of Spatial Orientation

Disorders of spatial orientation, including contralateral neglect, are seen after right parietal lesions.

In contralateral neglect there is often a neglect of visual, tactile, and auditory stimulation confined to one side of the body that is contralateral to the site of the lesion. Allegri (2000) reported that left-sided neglect after right hemisphere lesions is more common (31% to 46%) than right-sided neglect following lesions in the left hemisphere (2% to 12%). Thus, although unilateral neglect can be seen following left parietal infarcts, this is relatively rare compared with most patients who present with a left-neglect corresponding to right parietal damage. Unilateral neglect has also been observed following frontal and subcortical vascular damage as well. Patients with parietal lesions can also experience route-finding problems and an inability to recognize objects that might ordinarily serve as landmarks (i.e., topographical agnosia). Additionally, patients with left parietal lesions can also present with significant right-left spatial disorientation problems.

Apraxia

Apraxia can be simply defined as an inability to carry out purposeful movement in the absence of some type of motor disturbance such as a paralysis. Many different types of apraxia occur, one of the most notable forms being constructional apraxia or the inability to perform familiar sequences of movements when making or preparing something (Walsh, 1987). Interestingly, this deficit is seen when patients can still perform all of the individual actions or steps involved in a particular sequence. For example, a patient may be able to perform all of the individual steps needed to mail a letter (e.g., licking the stamp and sealing the envelope), but is unable to make the proper sequence of movements to actually complete the task of mailing the letter. Constructional disorders characterized by an inability to draw or construct objects or shapes have also been observed following lesions to either hemisphere, with qualitative differences in the process and product of the construction providing valuable clues as to lesion laterality. For example, the drawings of patients with right hemisphere lesions are frequently seen as fragmented and characterized by poor spatial relations. These drawings can also be characterized by poor or faulty orientation. Conversely, patients with left hemisphere lesions may produce better spatial orientation and relations but their drawing can be overly simple, lack detail, and be especially labored to produce. Not surprisingly, constructional apraxia caused by right hemisphere damage appears to be more chronic and resistant to recovery (Sunderland et al., 1994).

Anosognosias

Anosognosia can be defined generally as the failure to perceive illness. Numerous types of anosognosias exist. Asomatognosia or loss of knowledge about the body or about a bodily condition is a disorder that can be seen following damage to the parietal cortex of either hemisphere, of which many varieties exist. Anosodiaphoria refers to an unawareness or denial of a disorder. It also refers to a general indifference to a disorder. An inability to name and localize body parts is known as autotopagnosia. These agnosias all stem from lesions to the left parietal cortex. Patients with right parietal or frontal infarcts have been shown to have significantly fewer introspective capacities and less concern over their illness than patients with infarcts in other regions, despite similar degrees of cognitive impairment (Hutter and Gilsbach, 1995).

Occipital Cortex

Although small lesions of the visual cortex can often produce defects or "blind spots" in the visual field, these types of lesions are unlikely to affect higher cognitive functioning as related to visual perception and comprehension. However, when other subcortical and associative cortices are involved, several neurobehavioral deficits can result. These neurobehavioral disorders include cerebral blindness, Anton's syndrome, and the visual agnosias.

Cerebral Blindness and Anton's Syndrome

Occlusion of the posterior cerebral artery resulting in bilateral visual cortex damage can lead to a condition known as cerebral or cortical blindness, a condition characterized by an inability to distinguish forms or patterns, despite intact responsiveness to light changes (Luria, 1966). Cerebral blindness may be accompanied by a period of confusion or even unconsciousness and is often accompanied by an amnestic syndrome such as that described above. Astonishingly, patients who are cerebrally blind (or more commonly referred to as "cortically blind") can exhibit visually responsive behaviors and be able to detect visual stimuli in the blind field without the experience of vision (Poppel et al., 1973), a phenomenon called "blindsight." Hartmann et al. (1991) described a patient with cerebral blindness resulting from bioccipital and left parietal lesions who, although denying visual perception, correctly named objects, colors, and famous faces; recognized facial emotions; and read various types of single words with greater than 50% accuracy when they were presented in the upper right visual field. On confrontation regarding his apparent visual abilities, the patient continued to deny visual perceptual awareness, typically stating "I feel it." The authors suggest that this type of denial of visual perception is best explained as a disconnection of the parietal lobe attention system from regions controlling visual perception. In direct opposition to "blindsight," patients with Anton's syndrome fail to appreciate the fact that they are blind and make elaborate confabulations and rationalizations as to their impaired performance. Anton's syndrome typically stems from lesions of the bilateral occipital lobe and most likely is caused by the disruption of corticothalamic connections (Damasio, 1985a).

Visual Agnosia

Visual agnosias characterized by defective visual perception or distortion of visual stimuli, despite normal visual input, can be seen following infarction of the visual association areas (Benson, 1989). For example, visual object agnosia is characterized by intact visual perception of the visual stimulus but an inability to recognize the object. Patients with this neurobehavioral disorder can often draw the object or copy a picture of it, confirming intact visual perceptual abilities. This type of agnosia can be seen after lesions of the dominant occipital lobe (Walsh, 1987). One particular example of a visual agnosia is known as "simultag-

nosia" or "Balint's syndrome." This syndrome is characterized by an inability to perceive more than one aspect of a stimulus at one time, despite the ability to identify and remember single aspects of features of an object. This neurobehavioral deficit may be partially caused by an inability to shift attentional focus and direct gaze (Benson, 1989). Another more rare type of visual agnosia is characterized by an inability to recognize familiar faces. This disorder is referred to as "prosopagnosia" and in severe cases some patients do not even recognize their own reflection in the mirror. The neuroanatomic underpinnings of this disorder are still in question; however, prosopagnosia has been associated with bilateral, left, and right hemisphere lesions of both the parietal and occipital lobe (Lopera, 2000). Some suggestion exists for a relatively greater frequency of bilateral and nondominant lesions to a greater degree (De Romanis and Benfatto, 1973), as well as for a relatively greater degree of dysfunction seen following right versus left hemisphere lesions (Lezak, 1995). Finally, another type of visual agnosia for colors has also been known to follow occipital lobe lesions. This type of neurobehavioral disorder can take on various manifestations, including an inability to distinguish color hues (i.e., achromatopsia); an inability to name colors (i.e., color anomia); and an inability to associate particular colors with objects and vice versa (i.e., color agnosia) (Kolb and Wishaw, 1985). Table 18-1 summarizes some of the more common neurobehavioral disorders following cortical stroke and hemorrhage that have been described in more detail above. The anatomic localization of some of these disorders is somewhat equivocal and deficits assigned solely to left hemisphere lesions assume left hemisphere language dominance.

TABLE 18-1. *Common neurobehavioral disorders associated with cortical vascular lesions*

	Right hemisphere	Left hemisphere[a]	Bilateral hemisphere
Frontal lobe	Figural fluency	Broca's aphasia (area 44) Verbal fluency	Working memory Cognitive flexibility
Temporal lobe	Visual discrimination Visual reasoning and memory Amusia	Wernicke' aphasia (area 22) Verbal reasoning and memory Dysnomia	Amnesia
Parietal lobe	Unilateral (left) neglect Constructional apraxia Anosognosia Anosodiaphoria	Agraphia/acalculia Right-left confusion Topographic agnosia Autotopagnosia	
Occipital lobe	Visual object agnosia Prosopagnosia Color agnosia Achromatopsia	Simultagnosia Color anomia	Cerebral blindness Anton's syndrome Prosopagnosia

[a]Assumes left hemisphere dominance.

COGNITIVE EFFECTS OF SUBCORTICAL LESIONS

Multiinfarct Dementia

Vascular dementia can be caused by both white-matter ischemia and multiple occlusions of blood vessels (a series of small strokes) that result in focal areas of dead tissue. Hachinski et al. (1975) introduced the term "multiinfarct dementia" (MID), and concluded that most infarctions were secondary to disease of the heart and of extracranial blood vessels. Clinical dementia can be caused by a multiinfarct state, but the neuropathology is often complicated by the presence of more than one disease process. Histopathologic studies have variously concluded that vascular factors are involved in 10% to 40% of cases (Semple, 1998). The prevalence of vascular dementia is difficult to establish as the criteria for diagnosis are inexact and, when diagnosing vascular dementia, it is essential to rule out the presence of Alzheimer's disease.

Lacunar Strokes

Small infarcts deep in the cerebral hemispheres and in the brainstem caused by occlusion of perforating end arteries originating in the circle of Willis, and of the proximal middle, posterior cerebral, and basilar arteries, are often described as "lacunar" (Fisher, 1982). The most commonly encountered lacunar syndrome is pure motor hemiplegia, affecting the face, arm, and leg as a result of infarction in the internal capsule or in the basis pontis (Semple, 1998). By definition, aphasia, visuospatial neglect, agnosia, apraxia, and visual field defects do not occur in lacunar syndromes, but can be present as a result of larger striatocapsular infarcts, which probably have a different cause.

A lacunar state refers to the occurrence of multiple lacunes, which usually results in both motoric and intellectual dysfunction. Most patients who present with a lacunar state describe a series of discrete cognitive or behavioral episodes, each representing a new vascular event that involves the appearance of new symptoms. However, it has been noted, in up to one third of patients with demonstrable lacunar infarctions, that the deterioration appears gradual and the syndrome is often mistaken for a degenerative process (Weisberg, 1982). The clinical presentation of multiple lacunar infarctions typically involves prominent motor dysfunction with more limited somatosensory and visual impairment. Pyramidal signs are common, and include spasticity, gait abnormali-

ties, hyperreflexia, and extensor plantar response. Pseudobulbar palsy with dysarthria, dysphagia, facial paresis, hyperreflexive gag response, and emotional incontinence can also occur (Ishii et al., 1986). Extrapyramidal symptoms are often intermixed with the upper motor neuron signs.

Single Infarctions

Small subcortical infarctions can result in disruption of multiple cognitive domains, depending on their location. Circumscribed damage to the thalamus, caudate nucleus, or globus pallidus can produce multifaceted cognitive deficits because of disruption of specific subcortical cortical circuits. The caudate nucleus, globus pallidus, and thalamus are neuroanatomically connected to the dorsolateral prefrontal cortex. Damage to any part of this circuit results in deficits, primarily in executive functions and motor programming. The exact nature of the behavioral changes depends on which structure in the circuit is damaged. Single infarctions to the caudate or pallidal nuclei are rare in humans and, therefore, little is known about them. In contrast, many studies have examined the effects of thalamic lesions on neuropsychological functioning.

Thalamic Stroke

Neuropsychological syndromes resulting from thalamic infarctions vary widely and are largely determined by the specific thalamic nuclei involved. The thalamus contains at least three principal types of cortical projection nuclei (specific sensory, nonspecific, association), as well as nuclei that project to the limbic system and frontal lobes (Aggleton and Mishkin, 1983; Martin, 1968; Mishkin, 1982). Despite the wide range of neurobehavioral features associated with thalamic infarct, three cardinal clinical features of thalamic hemorrhage have been generally reported (Fisher, 1959). In the dominant hemisphere, these include greater sensory than motor loss; oculomotor impairments (particularly abnormalities of vertical gaze with the eyes deviated downward and inward); and moderate dysphasia. Transcortical sensory aphasias and memory impairment can also occur.

Numerous other neurobehavioral consequences of thalamic stroke are seen. Given the degree of thalamic-cortical interconnectivity (with almost the entire neocortex and striatum receiving fibers from the thalamus), it is not surprising that many of the neurobehavioral disorders following thalamic lesions are qualitatively similar in nature to some of the neurobehavioral deficits following cortical lesions. Some of the more common of these disorders, including disorders of arousal and attention, executive functioning, language, and memory, are described below.

Disorders of Arousal and Attention

Disorders of arousal, including loss of consciousness, are commonly observed following thalamic hemorrhage. Although this is seen most commonly after bilateral paramedian thalamic infarction, coma and extreme disturbances of consciousness have been known to occur with unilateral lesions as well (Friedman, 1985; Graff-Radford et al., 1985; Stuss et al., 1988). In patients who display an initial disturbance of consciousness, generally, a gradual improvement is seen over time marked by considerable fluctuations in arousal level (Archer et al., 1981; Guberman and Stuss, 1983; Katz et al., 1987). As recovery proceeds, patients with thalamic hemorrhage may be fully alert, but slow to respond; apathetic; and susceptible to hypersomnolence if not stimulated (Katz et al., 1987; Van Der Werf et al., 1999). It is believed that the hypersomnolence noted in these patients results from local pressure on the reticular activating system of the rostral brainstem (Castaigne et al., 1981; Katz et al., 1987; Graff-Radford et al., 1985). Individuals with thalamic lesions can have other attentional problems that can be easily seen when they are trying to complete less structured tasks (e.g., digit span may be intact, but maze learning is impaired [Stuss et al., 1988]).

Disorders of Executive Functioning

Patients with lesions of the thalamus often demonstrate behavioral changes consistent with those previously described following lesions to the frontal lobes or to the frontal-limbic circuitry (Bogousslavsky et al., 1988; Damasio, 1985b; Stuss and Benson, 1984; Stuss and Benson, 1986). For example, confabulation and reduplicative paramnesia can be present (Brion et al., 1983; Swanson and Schmidley, 1985; Stuss et al., 1988). Various alterations in mood have been described, including apathy, akinesia, lack of concern, and euphoria (Katz et al., 1987; Mills and Swanson, 1978; Speedie and Heilman, 1982). Other executive characteristics that have been reported include perseveration, increased susceptibility to interference, problems sequencing information, and inability to maintain sustained interest in a topic or task.

Disorders of Language

Language disorders occur almost universally after damage to the left thalamus (Barraguer-Bordas et al., 1981; Karussis et al., 2000), although controversy exists about the necessary lesion within the thalamus. Most studies suggest that involvement of the pulvinar (see Crosson, 1984 for a review) or the ventrolateral nucleus (Davous et al., 1984; Graff-Radford et al., 1985) is necessary. The type of language disturbance following thalamic damage can be best described as multifarious and resulting from a disruption of cortical-subcortical integration (Crosson, 1985); the language disturbances following thalamic infarct can be attributable to multiple dysfunctions, including alterations in alerting, arousal, and monitoring.

However, in general, mutism may occur initially, followed by poor initiation of speech, with limited output and many pauses. Word list generation can be moderately to severely impaired and speech characterized by diminished volume, impaired prosody, and variable dysarthria. Perseverations, perceptual errors, intrusions, and nonaphasic misnaming have been observed.

Disorders of Memory

Significant memory dysfunction secondary to thalamic insult, which has been frequently reported, is characterized primarily by anterograde memory disturbance (Markowitsch, 1982; Winocur et al., 1984). As with cortical lesions, this memory disturbance appears to be hemisphere specific. Bilateral lesions result in a severe and persistent memory disturbance, whereas unilateral left and right lesions produce verbal and nonverbal memory disturbances, respectively (Speedie and Heilman, 1982; Stuss et al., 1988). In patients with bilateral thalamic damage, a subcortical dementia syndrome has also been reported, with impairment noted in memory, attention, language, and visuospatial ability as well as changes in personality. This syndrome appears to be more consistent with the impairment noted in other "subcortical" dementias rather than Alzheimer's disease due to the absence of apraxia, agnosia, or definite aphasia and the presence of slowed information processing speed, inertia, and apathy (Cummings and Benson, 1983). Unlike other subcortical dementias, however, the dementia syndrome associated with bilateral thalamic insult combines frontal-subcortical dysfunction with a severe memory disorder (Stuss et al., 1988).

Cerebellar Stroke

Although it is well established that the cerebellum is essential for the coordination of movement, more recent evidence suggests that the cerebellum is also involved in higher order cognitive functioning (Heath et al., 1979; Schmahmann and Sherman, 1998). Studies evaluating patients with damage limited to the cerebellum as a result of cerebellar degeneration or cerebellar stroke indicate neurobehavioral impairment that appears related to the cerebellum itself (Appollonio et al., 1993; Grafman et al., 1992; Levisohn et al., 1997). Furthermore, recent functional neuroimaging studies have demonstrated cerebellar activation during nonmotor tasks (Allen et al., 1997; Andreasen et al., 1995; Feiz and Raichle, 1997), suggesting that it plays a role in other cognitive functions such as learning and memory, attention, and language.

Cerebellar Cognitive Affective Syndrome

Schmahmann and colleagues (Schmahmann, 1997; Schmahmann and Sherman, 1998) have described a pattern of behavioral and cognitive abnormalities resulting from cerebellar insult, referred to as the "cerebellar cognitive affective syndrome." The syndrome includes impairment in executive functions that is characterized by perseveration, distractibility or inattention, visual-spatial disturbances, difficulties with language production, and personality changes. Remote episodic and semantic memory is preserved, and new learning is only mildly affected. The net effect of these neurobehavioral disturbances is a general lowering of intellectual functioning, despite the fact that arousal and alertness levels are not affected (Schmahmann and Sherman, 1998). These core features set this syndrome apart from nonspecific confusional states as well as other currently accepted notions of dementia. For example, features of a more typical cortical dementia (e.g., aphasia, apraxia, and agnosia) are largely absent (Schmahmann and Scherman, 1998). Dementia is also more often noted in patients with evidence of more widespread central nervous system involvement (i.e., cerebellar signs as well as extrapyramidal and pyramidal tract disorders) than in patients manifesting spinal and cerebellar syndromes exclusively (Hier and Cummings, 1990).

Behavioral changes related to cerebellar damage have been characterized by personality change, with blunting of affect or disinhibition or inappropriate behavior, as well as impairment of a number of executive functions, including planning, impaired ability to shift set, and difficulties with abstract reasoning. Cognitive disturbances associated with lesions of the posterior lobe of the cerebellum and the vermis include other executive abilities (e.g., decreased verbal fluency and impaired working memory, problems with spatial cognition, including visual-spatial organization and memory) (Botez-Marquard et al., 1994; Schmahmann and Sherman, 1998), and language deficits including agrammatism, dysprosody, and mild anomia (Schmahmann and Sherman, 1998; Silveri et al., 1994).

PROGNOSIS AND REHABILITATION

Improved treatment regimens, coupled with educational efforts designed to reduce the amount of time elapsed between initial stroke symptoms and treatment, have significantly reduced the mortality associated with stroke and hemorrhage. However, this increased survival rate also means that increasingly more patients need a rehabilitation program (Sisson, 1995). In response to this, the last decade has seen an increase in research focusing on functional outcomes following stroke and hemorrhage. However, relatively little research has investigated the relationship between cognitive functioning and stroke outcome. This is surprising, as cognition and affective functioning are well known to be important contributors to quality of life.

Numerous studies support the utility of clearly defining stroke subtypes on admission that are based on cognitive test performance and lesion laterality, and suggest that rehabilitation programs can be specifically tailored to meet various stroke subtypes in an effort to maximize functional outcome. In fact, Hajek et al. (1997) suggest that rehabilitation outcome could be better predicted if the results of functional assessment were coupled with in-depth cognitive assessment. Therefore, a comprehensive and standardized neuropsychological evaluation of all stroke patients at admission and intermittently during the recovery process is warranted.

Although some other researchers (Kwa et al., 1996) failed to find a significant impact of cognitive impairment on the quality of life of stroke survivors, larger studies (Tatemici, 1994) suggest that cognitive impairment is a significant independent predictor of functional outcome, after adjusting for age and physical impairment. Specifically, they reported that the degree of cognitive impairment was related to increased functional impairment, and a lack of cognitive impairment was associated with frequency of independent living after discharge. In another study of 59 patients (aged 75 years and older) Kong et al. (1998) reported that admissions scores on cognitive tests, as well as the Modified Barthel Index (MBI), could predict discharge MBI scores. Feigenson et al. (1977) reported that the presence of severe cognitive and perceptual dysfunction or a homonymous hemianopsia, in addition to a motor deficit, have been shown to be related to an unfavorable outcome and longer length of hospital stay in a retrospective analysis of 248 patients with stroke. In another study involving 199 elderly stroke victims who had rehabilitation treatment, Kanemarau et al. (1998) examined the effect of various factors on discharge in a multiple regression analysis with discharge place as the dependent variable. They reported that higher scores on the Wechsler Adult Intelligence Scale (Performance IQ measures), along with older age and higher levels of activities of daily living, were significantly related to the likelihood of home discharge.

Given the importance of laterality on cognitive functioning, it is also unexpected that only modest research to date supports the effects of lateralized stroke on functional outcome. Although some researchers have reported that laterality is not an important factor in stroke outcome, others have suggested that, in fact, it is. One such study by Sisson (1995) reported that patients with right parietal and temporal lobe stroke had greatest difficulties with memory, concentration, and mental fatigue at four time periods after stroke (10 days, 1 month, 3 months, and 6 months). Sisson also reported a positive association between cognitive functioning and physical abilities that remained over the study period. Chae and Zorowitz (1998) examined the effects of cortical and subcortical nonhemorrhagic infarct and lesion laterality on functional outcome of stroke victims and reported that both level of lesion (subcortical versus cortical) and laterality are important determinants of outcome during inpatient rehabilitation. Specifically, subcortical stroke survivors were reported to have higher self-care, better mobility function, and higher communication and social cognition than cortical stroke survivors. Importantly, this effect was seen only for patients with left hemisphere lesions. Additionally, left hemisphere stroke survivors tended to have relatively poorer communication and social cognitive functioning than right hemisphere stroke survivors.

In sum, it may be beneficial to define stroke subtypes based on age, cognitive test performance, and lesion laterality on admission, as rehabilitation programs are likely to be more effective in terms of functional outcome when they are specifically tailored to these prognostic indicators.

REFERENCES

Aggleton JP, Mishkin M. Visual recognition impairment following medial thalamic lesions in monkeys. *Neuropsychologia* 1983;21:189–197.

Allegri RF. Attention and neglect: neurological basis, assessment and disorders. *Rev Neurology* 2000;30:491–494.

Allen G, Buxton RB, Wong EC, et al. Attentional activation of the cerebellum independent of motor involvement. *Science* 1997;275:1940–1943.

Andreasen NC, O'Leary DS, Arndt S, et al. Neural substrates of facial recognition. *J Neuropsychiatry Clin Neurosci* 1995; 8:139–146.

Appollonio IM, Grafman J, Schwartz V, et al. Memory in patients with cerebellar degeneration. *Neurology* 1993;43:1536–1544.

Archer CR, Ilinsky IA, Goldfader PR, et al. Aphasia in thalamic stroke: CT stereotactic localization. *J Comput Assist Tomogr* 1981;5:427–432.

Barraguer-Bordas L, Illa I, Escartin A, et al. Thalamic hemorrhage. A study of 23 patients with diagnosis by computed tomography. *Stroke* 1981;12:524–527.

Benson DF. Disorders of visual gnosis. In: Brown JW, ed. *Neuropsychology of visual perception* New York: The IRBN Press, 1989.

Benson DF, Geschwind N. Aphasia and related disorders: a clinical approach. In: Mesulam M, ed. *Principles of behavioral neurology.* Philadelphia: FA Davis, 1985: 193–238.

Bogousslavsky J, Regli F, Uske A. Thalamic infarcts: clinical syndromes, etiology and prognosis. *Neurology* 1988; 38:837–848.

Botez-Marquard T, Leveille J, Botez MI. Neuropsychological functioning in unilateral cerebellar damage. *Can J Neurol Sci* 1994;21:353–357.

Brion S, Mikol J, Plas J. Memoire et specialization fonctionnelle hemispherique. Rapport anatomo-clinique. *Revue Neurologique (Paris)* 1983;139:39–43.

Castaigne P, Lhermitte F, Buge A, et al. Paramedian thalamic and midbrain infarcts: clinical and neuropathological study. *Ann Neurol* 1981;10:127–148.

Chae J, Zorowitz R. Functional status of cortical and subcortical nonhemorrhagic stroke survivors and the effect of lesion laterality. *Am J Phys Med Rehabil* 1998;77:415–420.

Crosson B. Role of the dominant thalamus in language: a review. *Psychol Bull* 1984;96:491–517.

Crosson B. Subcortical functions in language: a working model. *Brain Lang* 1985;25:257–292.

Cummings JL, Benson DF. *Dementia: a clinical approach.* Boston: Butterworth-Heineman, 1983.

Cummings JL. Frontal-subcortical circuits and human behavior. *Arch Neurol* 1993;50:873–880.

Damasio AR. Disorders of complex visual processing: agnosias, achromatopsia, Balint's syndrome, and related difficulties of orientation and construction. In: Mesulam M, ed. *Principles of behavioral neurology.* Philadelphia: FA Davis, 1985a:259–288.

Damasio AR. The frontal lobes. In: Heilman KM, Valenstein E, eds. *Clinical neuropsychology.* New York: Oxford University Press, 1985b:339–375.

Davous P, Bianco C, Duval-Lota AM, et al. Aphasie par infarctus thalamique paramedian gauche. Observation anatomo-clinique. *Revue Neurologique (Paris)* 1984;140:711–719.

DeRenzi E. Memory disorders following focal neocortical damage. *Philos Trans R Soc Lond B Biol Sci* 1982;298:73–83.

De Romanis F, Benfatto B. Presentazione e discussione di quattro casi di prosopagosia. *Rivista di Neurologia* 1973;43:111–132.

Feigenson JS, McDowell FH, Meese P, et al. Factors influencing outcome and length of stay in a stroke rehabilitation unit. Part 1. Analysis of 248 unscreened patients—medical and functional prognostic indicators. *Stroke* 1977;8:651–656.

Fiez JA. Raichle ME. Linguistic processing. *Int Rev Neurobiol* 1997;41:233–254.

Fisher CM. The pathologic and clinical aspects of thalamic hemorrhage. *Transactions of the American Neurological Association* 1959;84:56–59.

Fisher CM. Lacunar strokes and infarct: a review. *Neurology* 1982;32:871–876.

Friedman JH. Syndrome of diffuse encephalopathy due to nondominant thalamic infarction. *Neurology* 1985;35:1524–1526.

Goldman-Rakic PS. Specification of higher cortical functions. *J Head Trauma Rehabil* 1993;8:13–23.

Goodglass H. Phonological factors in aphasia. In: Brookshire RH, ed. *Clinical aphasiology.* Minneapolis: BRK Publishers, 1975:28–44.

Graff-Radford NR, Damasio H, Yamada T, et al. Nonhemorrhagic thalamic infarction. Clinical, neuropsychological, and electrophysiological findings in four anatomical groups defined by computed tomography. *Brain* 1985;108:485–516.

Grafman J, Litvan I, Massaquoi S, et al. Cognitive planning deficit in patients with cerebellar atrophy. *Neurology* 1992;42:1493–1496.

Guberman A, Stuss D. The syndrome of bilateral paramedian thalamic infarction. *Neurology* 1983;33:540–546.

Hachinski VC, Iliff LD, Zilhka E, et al. Cerebral blood flow in dementia. *Arch Neurol* 1975;32:632–637.

Hajek VE, Gagnon S, Ruderman JE. Cognitive and functional assessments of stroke patients: an analysis of their relation. *Arch Phys Med Rehabil* 1997;78:1331–1337.

Hartmann JA, Wolz WA, Roeltgen DP, et al. Denial of visual perception. *Brain Cogn* 1991;16:29–40.

Heath RG, Franklin DE, Shraberg D. Gross pathology of the cerebellum in patients diagnosed and treated as functional psychiatric disorders. *J Nerv Ment Dis* 1979;167:585–592.

Hier DB, Cummings JL. Rare acquired and degenerative subcortical dementias. In: Cummings JL, ed. *Subcortical dementia.* New York: Oxford University Press, 1990:199–217.

Hutter BO, Gilsbach JM. Introspective capacities in patients with cognitive deficits after subarachnoid hemorrhage. *J Clin Exp Neuropsychol* 1995;17:499–517.

Ishii N, Nishahara Y, Imamura T. Why do frontal lobe symptoms predominate in vascular dementia with lacunes? *Neurology* 1986;36:340–345.

Jones-Gotman M, Milner B. Design fluency: the invention of nonsense drawings after focal cortical lesions. *Neuropsychologia* 1977;15:653–674.

Kanemaru A, Takahashi R, Yamanaka T, et al. Relationship between cognitive function and discharge place among stroke patients after rehabilitation. *Nippon Ronen Igakkai Zasshi* 1998;35:307–312.

Karussis D, Leker RR, Abramsky O. Cognitive dysfunction following thalamic stroke: a study of 16 cases and review of the literature. *J Neurol Sci* 2000;172:25–29.

Katz DI, Alexander MP, Mandell AM. Dementia following strokes in the mesencephalon and diencephalon. *Arch Neurol* 1987;44:1127–1133.

Kolb B, Whishaw IQ. *Fundamentals of human neuropsychology.* New York: WH Freeman and Company, 1985.

Kong KH, Chua KS, Tow AP. Clinical characteristics and functional outcome of stroke patients 75 years old and older. *Arch Phys Med Rehabil* 1998;79:1535–1539.

Kwa VI, Linburg M, de Haan RJ. The role of cognitive impairment in the quality of life after ischaemic stroke. *J Neurol* 1996;243:599–604.

Levisohn L, Cronin-Golomb A, Schmahmann JD. Neuropsychological sequelae of cerebellar tumors in children. *Society for Neurosciences Abstracts* 1997;23:496.

Lezak MD. *Neuropsychological assessment.* New York: Oxford University Press, 1995.

Lopera F. Processing of faces: neurological bases, disorders and evaluation. *Rev Neurol* 2000;30:486–490.

Luria AR. *Higher cortical functions in man.* New York: Basic Books, 1966.

Markowitsch HJ. Thalamic mediodorsal nucleus and memory: a critical evaluation of studies in animals and man. *Neurosci Biobehav Rev* 1982;6:351–380.

Martin JJ. Thalamic syndromes. In: Vincken PJ, Bruyn GW, eds. *Handbook of clinical neurology,* Vol. 2. Amsterdam: North Holland Press, 1968:469–496.

McGlone J, Young B. Cerebral localization. In: Baker AB, ed. *Clinical neurology.* Philadelphia: Harper & Row, 1986.

Mills RP, Swanson PD. Vertical oculomotor apraxia and memory loss. *Ann Neurol* 1978;4:149–153.

Milner B. Effects of different brain lesions on card sorting. *Arch Neurol* 1963;9:90–100.

Mirsky AF. The neuropsychology of attention: elements of a complex behavior. In: Perecman E, ed. *Integrating theory and practice in clinical neuropsychology.* Hillsdale, NJ: Laurence Erlbaum, 1989.

Mishkin M. A memory system in the monkey. In: Broadbent DE, Weiskrantz L, eds. *The neuropsychiatry of cognitive function.* London: The Royal Society, 1982:85–95.

National Stroke Association. *Be stroke smart* [Newsletter]. Englewood, CO: NSA, 1995.

Pillon B, Bazin B, Deweer B, et al. Specificity of memory deficits after right or left temporal lobectomy. *Cortex* 1999;34:561–571.

Pohjasvaara T, Mantyla R, Aronen HJ, et al. Clinical and radiological determinants of prestroke cognitive decline in a stroke cohort. *J Neurol Neurosurg Psychiatry* 1999;67:742–748.

Poppel E, Held R, Front D. Residual visual function after brain wounds involving the central visual pathways. *Nature*1973;243:295–296.

Robinson RG. *The clinical neuropsychiatry of stroke: cognitive, behavioral, and emotional disorders following vascular brain injury.* Cambridge, UK: Cambridge University Press, 1998.

Schmahmann JD. Rediscovery of an early concept. *Int Rev Neurobiol* 1997;41:3–27.

Schmahmann JD, Sherman JC. The cerebellar cognitive affective syndrome. *Brain* 1998;121:561–579.

Schuppert M, Munte TF, Wieringa BM, et al. Receptive amusia: evidence for cross-hemispheric neural networks underlying music processing strategies. *Brain* 2000;123:546–549.

Semple PF. *An atlas of stroke.* New York: The Parthenon Publishing Group, 1998.

Silveri MC, Leggio MG, Molinari M. The cerebellum contributes to linguistic production: a case of agrammatic speech following a right cerebellar lesion. *Neurology* 1994;44:2047–2050.

Sisson RA. Cognitive status as a predictor of right hemisphere stroke outcomes. *J Neurosci Nurs* 1995;27: 152–156.

Speedie LJ, Heilman KM. Amnestic disturbance following infarction of the left dorsomedial nucleus of the thalamus. *Neuropsychologia* 1982;20:597–604.

Stuss DT, Benson DF. Neuropsychological studies of the frontal lobes. *Psychol Bull* 1984;95:3–28.

Stuss DT, Benson DF. *The frontal lobes*. New York: Raven Press, 1986.

Stuss DT, Cummings JL. Subcortical vascular dementias. In: Cummings JL, ed. *Subcortical dementia*. New York: Oxford University Press, 1990:145–163.

Stuss DT, Guberman A, Nelson R, et al. The neuropsychology of paramedian thalamic infarcts. *Brain Cogn* 1988;8: 348–378.

Sunderland A, Tinson D, Bradley L. Differences in recovery from constructional apraxia after right and left hemisphere stroke? *J Clin Exp Neuropsychol* 1994;16:916–920.

Swanson RA, Schmidley JW. Amnestic syndrome and vertical gaze palsy: early detection of bilateral thalamic infarction by CT and NMR. *Stroke* 1985;16:823–827.

Tatemichi TK, Desmond DW, Stern Y, et al. Cognitive impairment after stroke: frequency, patterns, and relationship to functional abilities. *J Neurol Neurosurg Psychiatry* 1994;57:202–207.

Van Der Werf YD, Weerts JG, Jolles J, et al. Neuropsychological correlates of a right unilateral lacunar thalamic infarction. *J Neurol Neurosurg Psychiatry* 1999;66:36–42.

Walsh K. *Neuropsychology: a clinical approach*, 2nd ed. New York: Churchill Livingstone, 1987.

Weisberg LA. Lacunar infarcts. Clinical and computed tomographic correlations. *Arch Neurol* 1982;39:37–40.

Winocur G, Oxbury S, Roberts R, et al. Amnesia in a patient with bilateral lesions to the thalamus. *Neuropsychologia* 1984;22:123–143.

SUGGESTED READINGS

Lezak MD. *Neuropsychological assessment.* New York: Oxford University Press, 1995.

McCrum R. *My year off: rediscovering life after a stroke.* New York: WW Norton, 1998.

Robinson RG. *The clinical neuropsychiatry of stroke: cognitive, behavioral, and emotional disorders following vascular brain injury.* Cambridge, UK: Cambridge University Press, 1998.

WEB SITES OF NATIONAL SUPPORT GROUPS

National Stroke Association: *http://www.stroke.org/NS804.0 Recov&Rehab.html*

American Heart Organization: *http://www.americanheart. org/*

The Stroke Network: *http://www.strokenetwork.org/*

National Stroke & Quality Of Life Medical Education Institute: *http://www.lifethreat.org/NS&Qmedu.htm*

American Society of NeuroRehabilitation: *http://www.asnr. com/*

A general resource for clinicians, survivors and family members of stroke victims: http://www.strokehelp.com/ resourceinformation.htm

19

Spontaneous and Traumatic Cerebral Hemorrhage in the Elderly

Ricardo F. Izurieta and Eelco F.M. Wijdicks

Cerebral hemorrhage, which is common in the vulnerable elderly population, commonly refers to hypertensive cerebral hemorrhage, traumatic lobar contusions, or subdural hematoma. Intracerebral hemorrhage is more frequent in the elderly for several reasons: falls, amyloid deposition producing brittle cortical arteries, and the long-term effects of hypertension. Its management is complicated because of both associated morbidity and unexpected responses to pharmacy, nosocomial infections, and in-hospital complications. Age is an important independent and also overpowering risk factor for poor outcome in all types of cerebral hemorrhage. Clinical findings, complications, diagnosis, therapeutic modalities, and prognosis of hemorrhagic stroke in the older adult are reviewed in this chapter.

EPIDEMIOLOGY

The elderly population, which has been growing over the last 30 years, specifically those aged 85 years and older, has been accompanied by an increased incidence of cerebrovascular disease. This older aged group has a two- to threefold greater frequency of both ischemic and hemorrhagic stroke than the group composed of those aged 65 to 74 years (Kurtzke, 1985).

In a study of acute stroke in very old people (≥85 years) by Arboix et al. (2000), data were collected on 2,000 patients of all ages between 1986 to 1995. The incidence of stroke was 13% in those 85 years or older, 37% in patients aged 75 to 84 years, and 28% in those 65 to 74 years of age. Stroke was more prevalent in women than in men. The main cardiovascular risk factors were hypertension, atrial fibrillation, and diabetes. As expected, hemorrhagic stroke was less frequently present in 14% and ischemic stroke occurred in 86%, but the ratio of hemorrhagic versus ischemic stroke remained similar over the years. The elderly population had the worst outcome, with longer hospitalizations and the greatest in-hospital mortality rate. Altered consciousness, limb weakness, sensory deficit, parietal and temporal lobe involvement, internal capsule involvement, intraventricular hemorrhage, and respiratory and cardiac events were considered predictive factors of in-hospital morbidity and mortality.

ETIOLOGY

Cerebral hemorrhages can involve the subcortical (ganglionic) or lobar structures. These localizations are equally prevalent, but the causes are different. Hemorrhage from a ruptured arteriovenous malformation is uncommon. Although the cumulative risk of rupture increases, most patients who experience hemorrhage are between 10 and 35 years of age. Hemorrhage into a metastasis or anticoagulation-associated hemorrhages should be considered as well. In the elderly population, important consideration should be given to hypertension, in particular isolated systolic hypertension, and cerebral amyloid angiopathy as common causes of intracerebral hemorrhage.

Longstanding hypertension is probably a common cause of intracerebral hemorrhage in the elderly. Its presentation can be biphasic, at the onset of the hypertension or later when a significant injury occurring to the penetrating arteries has resulted in formation of fibrinoid degeneration and, possibly, microaneurysms. The predilection sites in the basal ganglia, pons, and cerebellum attest to that.

Cerebral amyloid angiopathy is a common cause of hemorrhage in the old-oldest. It is usually diagnosed at autopsies, suggested by magnetic resonance imaging (MRI), or found in surgical specimens. In many instances, amyloid deposits involve leptomeningeal or cortical vessels and can completely and continuously involve the blood vessel wall. Severe angiopathy can cause lobar cerebral hemorrhage from rupture of a cortical or meningeal vessel and dementia, which is noted by family members. Schutz et al. (1990) found that the incidence is 30 to 40/00,000 in patients 70 years of age and older, which would make cerebral amyloid angiopathy responsible for 30% to 50% of cerebral hemorrhage in this age group. Autopsies have also revealed that the prevalence is 2.3% for those between 65 and 74 years; 8% for ages 75 to 84 years; and 12% for those older than 85 years (Greenberg et al., 1998).

As alluded to, a coagulopathy is an important cause of hemorrhage in this age group, particularly because warfarin is commonly initiated to prevent ischemic stroke in conditions such as atrial fibrillation, prosthetic heart valves, and rheumatic mitral stenosis. When stroke occurs, it has a high morbidity and mortality rate. To complicate matters even further, the Massachusetts General Hospital group documented a clear link between cerebral amyloid angiopathy and warfarin-associated lobar hemorrhage.

Trauma can also lead to cerebral hemorrhage, and is probably the predominant cause in elderly patients. Hemorrhage caused by trauma is often characterized by frontal and temporal lobe contusions or a blood collection located between the dura and the underlying brain. According to the time interval between the trauma and the onset of symptoms, such hemorrhages are divided into acute (≤24 hours), subacute (1–10 days), and chronic (>10 days). They are typically located over the convexity and in some occasions can be bilateral.

CLINICAL COURSE

The clinical findings are manifestations of initial tissue destruction and subsequent mass effect. A tendency is seen for progression of the focal neurologic deficits over a few hours.

Patients with intracerebral hemorrhage complain of headaches, vomiting, and a decreased level of consciousness. The headaches are more common with lobar or cerebellar hematomas. Because the location is near to the meningeal surface, meningeal signs may appear.

A decreased level of consciousness is present in large hematomas and when the lesion is located primary in the posterior fossa. Although the decreased level of alertness is considered an adverse prognostic sign, it may simply reflect a larger volume, more tissue shift, or the development of hydrocephalus. Vomiting is also present as a consequence of the increased pressure or pressure on the vomiting center in the floor of the fourth ventricle. Seizures can be present in cases of a lobar hemorrhage, but are rare in putaminal and thalamic hemorrhage. Most often, seizures occur at the time of the bleeding. One recent large study by Bladin et al. (2000) found early onset seizures (within 2 weeks) in 8%, late onset seizures in 2.6%, with recurrent seizures only in patients with late onset seizures.

Fever has been significantly associated with intracerebral hemorrhage and with the presence of mass effect, transtentorial herniation and intraventricular blood on computed tomography (CT) scan. Patients who developed fever were older, but also had larger volume hemorrhages.

The physical findings depend on the location of the hemorrhage. Level of consciousness involves arousal and content. Content disturbances can be more prevalent as a premorbid condition in the elderly, and diminished attention and lack of integration should not be interpreted as altered state of consciousness. Acute confusional state commonly affects the elderly patient who also may be susceptible because of underlying dementia. Sleep becomes quickly disturbed and additional sedative drugs can cause a more profound state. In putaminal hemorrhage, patients present with hemiplegia, homonymous hemianopia, and eye deviation to the side of the hemorrhage. Mild and transient contralateral hemiparesis and a clinical picture similar to subarachnoid hemorrhage characterize a caudate hemorrhage. Hydrocephalus is a common feature because of the early extension of the bleeding to the ventricles. Hemiplegia, hemisensory syndrome, upward gaze paralysis, and small nonreactive pupils are seen in thalamic hemorrhage. Also is seen frequent communication with the ventricular system, and prognosis is related to the size of the hematoma. A poor prognosis is seen in cases of hydrocephalus caused by aqueductal obstruction.

Lobar hemorrhages are characterized by hemiparesis of upper limb in frontal hematomas, sensory motor deficit and hemianopia in parietal location, fluent aphasia in dominant temporal hematomas and homonymous hemianopia in occipital hemorrhages. Because of their superficial location, a better prognosis is seen for lobar hemorrhages than for other types of hematomas because they are easily approached surgically.

In cerebellar hemorrhage, patients complain of sudden vertigo, vomiting, headache, and an inability to stand and walk. Ipsilateral limb ataxia, horizontal gaze palsy, and peripheral facial palsy are present. Pontine hemorrhage is typically massive, bilateral, and characterized by quadriplegia, decerebrate posturing, horizontal ophthalmoplegia, pinpoint reactive pupils, respiratory rhythm abnormalities, coma, and hyperthermia. The clinical features are summarized in Table 19-1.

Acute subdural hematomas are usually associated with severe brain damage. Additional contusions not only are found in direct proximity to the subdural hematoma but can be scattered throughout both hemispheres. The mortality rate for acute subdural hematomas in elderly is extremely high. Age older than 65 years, no motor response or eye opening to pain, in combination with no verbal response and

TABLE 19-1. *Clinical features of cerebral hemorrhage*

Primary site	Extension	Telltale signs
Caudate nucleus	Localized intraventricular hemorrhage	Headache, confusion, drowsiness-stupor, abulia
	Capsule, putamen, diencephalon	Hemiparesis, eye deviation, Horner's syndrome
Putamen	Localized	Hemiparesis, eye deviation, global aphasia
	Posterior extension	Fluent aphasia
Thalamus	Localized	Paresthesia, hemineglect, nonfluent aphasia (often preserved repetition), disorientation to place
	Mesencephalon	Marked bradykinesia
Cerebellum	Localized	Dysarthria, appendicular ataxia, headache
	Vermis	Deterioration in consciousness, marked gait ataxia
Pons	Localized	Ataxic hemiparesis ophthalmoplegia, ocular bobbing
	Mesencephalon	Hyperthermia, coma, pinpoint pupils

Adapted from Intracerebral hematoma. In: Wijdicks EFM, ed. *Neurologic catastrophies.* Boston: Butterworth-Heineman, 2000:127.

postoperative intracranial pressure greater than 45 mmHg are poor predictors of outcome. Chronic subdural hematomas are characterized by persistent headaches for several days, followed by decreased consciousness. They can develop after unrecognized trauma and their clinical picture is similar to subacute processes. Importantly, in the elderly, brain atrophy provokes stretching of cortical veins, making this age group more susceptible to ruptures.

However, age has at least one advantage: shrinkage of the brain allows for accommodation of large clots. Thus, brain shift is less common and large volume hemorrhages are more easily tolerated in the posterior fossa. Therefore, the volume needs to be large or the hematoma located in a strategic location (e.g., pons) to cause immediate permanent damage.

NEUROIMAGING

Although MRI has much better resolution, a CT scan of the brain remains the first mode of imaging in cerebral hemorrhage. Imaging time has been reduced to a matter of minutes and information about potential life-threatening lesions is quickly available.

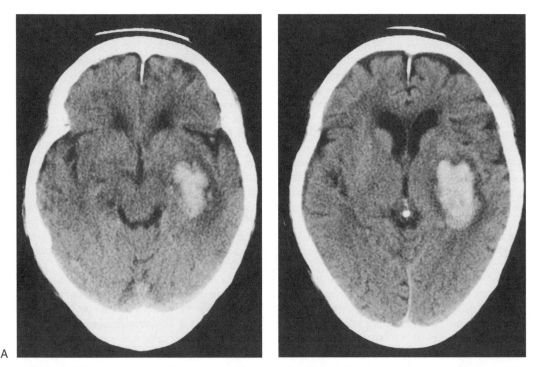

A   B

FIG. 19-1. CT scan in a 92-year-old man with a putaminal (hypertensive) hemorrhage. Note marked sulci and fissures. Despite large volume of hemorrhage, no shift is seen and the additional volume is well-tolerated.

Several specific features are evident in the elderly. These are profound sulci, large ventricles, and less common brain shift (Fig. 19-1). Commonly, prior lacunar strokes and white matter hypodensity are seen with ganglionic hemorrhages, a reflection of long-standing effects of hypertension. Subdural hematomas can be difficult to detect when they become isodense. A typical CT scan feature is the "supernormal CT" in which the CT scan image looks like it was that of a much younger person (the isodense subdural hematoma effaces the sulci).

Acute subdural hematoma in the elderly is often accompanied by additional contusions, which may determine outcome rather than subdural hematoma itself. These contusions may not be apparent on admission CT scan. The number of contusions, as well as localization, can have a dramatic impact on long-term outcome. An example of a patient with massive subdural hematoma with comparatively little mass effect but multiple contusions resulting in poor outcome in this particular case is shown in Figure 19-2.

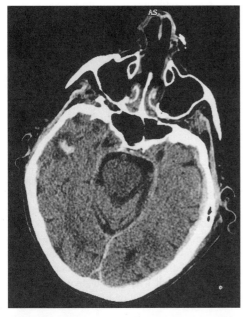

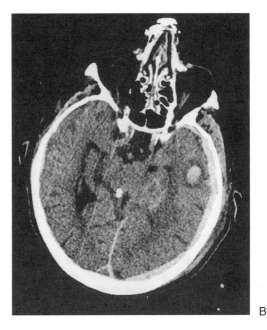

A B

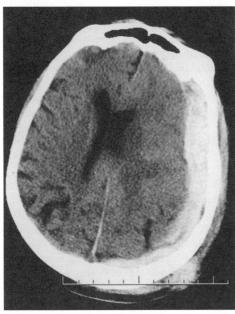

FIG. 19-2. CT scan in a 95-year-old woman who fell on the ice showing large subdural hematoma with mass effect and bilateral temporal lobe contusions.

C

TABLE 19-2. *Neuroimaging findings in elderly patients with cerebral hemorrhage*

Leukoaraiosis, silent strokes, and lacunes
Enlarged ventricles
Less brain shift with large volume hematoma
Isodense subdural hematoma
Hemosiderin associated with prior hemorrhages

The combination of MRI and magnetic resonance angiography is important in documenting vascular lesions and underlying primary tumors or metastasis, but more commonly demonstrates earlier small size hemorrhages suggestive of amyloid angiopathy. Common neuroimaging features of cerebral hemorrhage seen in the elderly are summarized in Table 19-2.

MANAGEMENT

Few data exist about specific management of brain hemorrhage in the elderly. Nonetheless, well-recognized aspects in management include the need of mechanical ventilation, management of increased intracranial pressure (ICP), blood pressure control, a surgical approach, and management of complications.

Mechanical Ventilation

Decreased intracranial pressure and airway protection are the main goals of mechanical ventilation. For those patients with midline shift, hyperventilation aiming at a Paco$_2$ between 30 and 35 mmHg will decrease cerebral blood flow and intracranial pressure. This can be better controlled with sedation and the assist control mode. The beneficial effect is transient and usually decreases after 3 to 4 days. Hyperventilation to levels less than 25 mmHg has not proved to be beneficial.

A retrospective study by Gujjar et al. (1998) reviewed indications, timing, and outcome of mechanical ventilation in hemorrhagic and ischemic stroke, in 230 patients. The rates of intubation were higher with hemorrhagic strokes and 75% of patients required intubation at arrival. Older age, intubation on arrival, intubation because of neurologic deterioration rather than primary pulmonary causes, and absence of corneal, pupillary, and oculocephalic reflexes were considered predictors of high mortality.

It is important to emphasize that aging is associated with changes in pulmonary function such as decrease in elastic recoil, expiratory flow rates, and oxygen diffusing capacity; increased pulmonary compliance, and ventilation-perfusion mismatch. Furthermore, cardiopulmonary comorbidity such as chronic obstructive pulmonary disease, congestive heart failure, and coronary artery disease are much more common in the elderly, which contributes to a high mortality rate.

The incidence of hospital-acquired pneumonia (HAP) increases with age. Risk factors for HAP in the elderly are underlying diseases that decrease immune function (e.g., diabetes, cirrhosis, malnutrition, and malignancy); oropharyngeal colonization with gram-negative organisms; presence of nasogastric tubes; recent antibiotic use; neutralization of gastric pH; and aspiration caused by a neurologic deficit. A study using age-matched elderly control subjects found that endotracheal intubation is also an important risk factor for HAP in elderly. Several studies have identified prognostic factors of mortality. Some found that age could be an independent risk factor for death from pneumonia, but others found that the presence of concomitant cardiopulmonary illnesses contributed to the higher mortality rate.

A prospective cohort study was conducted attempting to determine if age had an independent effect on the outcome of patients treated with mechanical ventilation. Enrolled were 63 patients 75 years of age or older and 237 patients younger than 75 years of age. In-hospital mortality rate, duration of mechanical ventilation, length of stay (intensive care unit and hospital), and cost of care were measured. After adjusting for the severity of illness, elderly patients were found to have a similar length of stay and time with mechanical ventilation.

Management of Intracranial Pressure

Patients with cerebral hemorrhage may have an ICP causing decreased responsiveness. Monitoring of ICP could provide important information and is required in those patients with multiple contusions. The normal ICP is between 5 and 20 mmHg and patients with values above 20 mmHg need emergent intervention. The increased ICP compromises cerebral perfusion pressure (CPP), which is obtained after subtracting ICP from mean arterial pressure. Ideal values of CPP above 70 mmHg should be pursued.

All attempts are directed at decreasing the ICP. Different approaches can be used, such as hyperventilation, osmotic diuretics, and barbiturate coma. Once the patients are mechanically ventilated, they need to be adequately sedated to decrease the ICP.

Mannitol and glycerol are the most common agents used to decrease ICP. They have a transient beneficial effect and sometimes can cause a rebound increase of ICP when they are discontinued. A study by Node and Nakazawa (1990), using different modes of infusion of mannitol and glycerol, found that when an urgent reduction of ICP is required, a dose of 1 g/kg mannitol should be given in 30 minutes. Mannitol has side effects such as hyperosmolarity and renal failure. In addition, theoretical concerns exist that these hypertonic agents could increase the size of the hematoma.

Other approaches used to decrease ICP are elevating the head of the bed to 30 degrees and avoiding endotracheal suctioning and intermittent drainage of cerebrospinal fluid (CSF) with a ventricular catheter. Continuous CSF drainage is not recommended because of inability to measure ICP. No study has documented the benefit of ventriculostomy in patients with cerebral hemorrhage.

Surgical options for increased ICP are subtemporal decompression, subfrontal decompressive craniectomy, internal decompression, or removal of existing bone flaps. In our experiences and that of others, these aggressive measures are of no use and in virtually all instances family members object. Corticosteroids do not improve outcome and can increase the risk of nonketotic hyperosmolar coma in an elderly patient.

Blood Pressure Control

Blood pressure management in the elderly after a cerebral hemorrhage is very complicated. Dandapani et al. (1995) found that a significantly high blood pressure on admission and inadequate control negatively affected the prognosis of hypertensive cerebral hemorrhage. Marked blood pressure reduction may not be tolerated (particularly with use of propofol) and persistent blood pressure elevation can trigger congestive heart failure. Obviously, the goal is to decrease the blood pressure while avoiding hypoperfusion, but target levels are not known. It is recommended to use short-acting agents (e.g., labetalol or esmolol). It is prudent to gradually lower the blood pressure, probably not more than 10% to 20%. Nitroprusside should be avoided in patients with increased ICP because of its possible deleterious effects in the CPP.

Much more is known about long-term control of blood pressure. Arakawa et al. (1998) conducted a prospective study about blood pressure control and recurrence of brain hemorrhage in 74 patients with hypertensive brain hemorrhage who were followed for 2.8 years. They compared different clinical parameters, including blood pressure, between patients with and without rebleeding and found a higher diastolic blood pressure was associated with increase rate of rebleeding.

A recent multicenter study was published in JAMA about the effects of treating isolated systolic hypertension in elderly patients. Patients were randomized to receive chlorthalidone as a first-line drug, atenolol or reserpine as a second-line drug, or placebo. A significant reduction was seen in the incidence of hypertension when treatment was provided to patients with isolated systolic hypertension.

Seizure Control

The incidence of seizures with intracerebral hemorrhage is between 5% and 15%. It is the initial manifestation in 30% of patients with hemorrhage, and in the remaining 70% seizure usually occurs within 72 hours. The seizures are commonly isolated and self-limited events. The higher incidence of seizures is seen with lobar hematomas, as was alluded to. Predisposition to develop epilepsy is greater if the seizures present weeks after the ictus. Prophylaxis with anticonvulsants is not recommended in most patients with intracerebral hemorrhage. The concerns with pharmacodynamics in the elderly are outlined elsewhere in this text.

Surgical Approach

Clear indications for a surgical approach have been developed, but only for superficially located hematoma. Thus, cerebellar and lobar hemorrhages are mostly considered.

In cerebellar hemorrhage, ventriculostomy followed by suboccipital craniotomy is recommended. In a retrospective study by Dunne et al. (1987), both conscious and comatose patients benefited from immediate surgery because of risk of brainstem compression. In comatose patients on arrival, morbidity is greater but a chance for recovery still exists. Bulbar dysfunction, bilateral gaze paresis, limb weakness, severe hypertension, and moderate to severe hydrocephalus are considered to be predictors of clinical deterioration in conscious patients.

In lobar hemorrhage, according to a study by Kase (1991), a hematoma less than 20 mL in diameter could be approached conservatively, but those between 20 and 44 mL had better outcomes with surgery. In addition, their superficial location has a reduced risk of additional neurologic trauma than the already established deficit.

Cerebral amyloid angiopathy severity fluctuates from asymptomatic amyloid deposition to complete replacement and breakdown of vessel wall. Presump-

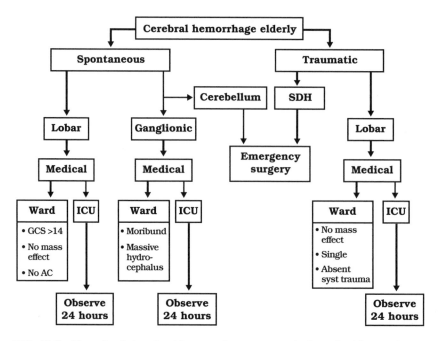

FIG. 19-3. Flow chart showing triage and management of cerebral hemorrhage.

tive diagnosis is made in elderly patients with multiple lobar hemorrhages without apparent cause. The treatment in amyloid angiopathy is not different than any other type of cerebral hemorrhage. Anticoagulant or antiplatelets withdrawal is important for preventing cerebral amyloid angiopathy-related hemorrhage.

A surgical approach is typically needed for acute subdural hematoma. Management of chronic subdural hematoma depends on the size and the patient's reliability. If the hematoma is small and the patient is without neurologic deficits, surgery can be postponed.

The triage and initial management is shown in the flow chart seen in Figure 19-3.

PROGNOSIS

Prognosis is poor when the initial level of consciousness is reduced or the volume of hematoma exceeds 50 mL. Other important prognostic factors are severe hypertension on admission and failure to control blood pressure. The presence and duration of fever in patients who survive more than 72 hours is also associated with poor prognosis. Diringer et al. (1998) recognized that hydrocephalus is an independent predictor of mortality after intracerebral hemorrhage.

A retrospective study was conducted at the Mayo Clinic to identify predictive features for poor neuro-

logic outcome with cerebellar hematomas. In the study, 72 patients were enrolled for clinical and neuroimaging analysis. The presence of systolic pressure greater than 200 mmHg, pinpoint pupils, abnormal corneal or oculocephalic reflexes, hematoma size more than 3 cm in diameter, hemorrhage extending in the vermis, brainstem distortion, intraventricular hemorrhage, upward herniation, and acute hydrocephalus were considered predictors of neurologic deterioration.

Another study recently analyzed patients with deep cerebral hemorrhage (putaminal hemorrhage and thalamic-caudate hemorrhage). Hydrocephalus was present in 40% of these patients, with a 30-day mortality rate of 29%. This trial concluded that a Glasgow Coma Scale score equal to or less than 8 and hydrocephalus were predictors of 30-day mortality. When to withdraw support or defer surgical intervention is determined by a reasonable period of observation (5–7 days in coma), expected disability (aphasia or ataxia), intervening systemic medical complication (aspiration pneumonitis or sepsis), and prior expressed wishes.

CONCLUSION

The best care and management of intracerebral hematoma in the elderly is not well defined. Only generalizations apply. Prognosis is decisively worse in the elderly because an aggressive approach may not be permitted because of existing living wills. The harsh reality is that prolonged rehabilitation and care may not be adequately provided or funded in these patients who have lived to an old age.

REFERENCES

Arakawa S, Saku Y, Ibayashi S, et al. Blood pressure control and recurrence of hypertensive brain hemorrhage. *Stroke* 1998;29:1806–1809.

Arboix A, Garcia-Eroles L, Massons J, et al. Acute stroke in very older people: clinical features and predictors of in-hospital mortality. *J Am Geriatr Soc* 2000;48:36–41.

Bladin CF, Alexander AV, Bellevance A, et al. Seizures after stroke: a prospective multicenter study. *Arch Neurol* 2000; 57:1617–1622.

Dandapani B, Suzuki S, Kelley R, et al. Relation between blood pressure and outcome in intra-cerebral hemorrhage. *Stroke* 1995;26:21–24.

Diringer M, Edwards D, Zazulia A. Hydrocephalus: a previously unrecognized predictor of poor outcome from supratentorial intra-cerebral hemorrhage. *Stroke* 1998;29: 1352–1357.

Dunne J, Chakera T, Kermode S. Cerebellar hemorrhage. Diagnosis and treatment: a study of 75 consecutive cases. *Q J Med* 1987;245:739–754.

Greenberg, Steven M. Cerebral amyloid angiopathy: prospects for clinical diagnosis and treatment. *Neurology* 1998;51(3):690–694.

Gujjar A, Deibert E, Manno E, et al. Mechanical ventilation for ischemic stroke and intra-cerebral hemorrhage: indications, timing and outcome. *Neurology* 1998;51:447–451.

Kase C. Diagnosis and management of intra-cerebral hemorrhage in elderly patients. *Clin Geriatr Med* 1991;7: 549–567.

Kurtzke JF. Epidemiology of cerebrovascular disease. Cerebrovascular Report. Bethesda, MD: National Institute of Neurological and Communicative Disorders and Stroke, 1985.

Node Y, Nakazawa S. Clinical study of mannitol and glycerol on raised intracranial pressure and on their rebound phenomenon. *Neurology* 1990;52:359–363.

SUGGESTED READING

Adams R, Diringer M. Response to external ventricular drainage in spontaneous intra-cerebral hemorrhage with hydrocephalous. *Neurology* 1998;50:519–523.

Akdemir H, Selcuklu A, Pasaoglu A, et al. Treatment of severe intra-ventricular hemorrhage by intra-ventricular infusion of urokinase. *Neurosurg Rev* 1995;18:95–100.

Allen CMC. Predicting the outcome of acute stroke: a prognostic score. *J Neurol Neurosurg Psychiatry* 1984;47: 475–480.

Berger A, Lipton R, Lesser M, et al. Early seizures following intra-cerebral hemorrhage: implications for therapy. *Neurology* 1988;38:1363–1365.

Broderick JP, Brott TG, Tomsick T, et al. Ultra-early evaluation of intra-cerebral hemorrhage. *J Neurosurg* 1990;72: 195.

Broderick JP, Brott TG, Tomsick T, et al. Lobar hemorrhage in the elderly. The undiminishing importance of hypertension. *Stroke* 1993;24:49–51.

Broderick JP, Brott TG, Duldner JE, et al. Initial and recurrent bleeding are the major causes of death following subarachnoid hemorrhage. *Stroke* 1994;25:1342–1347.

Caplan LR. Intra-cerebral hemorrhage revisited. *Neurology* 1988; 38:624–627.

Caplan LR. *Hypertensive intracerebral hemorrhage.* 1994: 99–116.

Chambers BR, Norris JW, Shurvell BL, et al. Prognosis of acute stroke. *Neurology* 1997;37:221–225.

Chan E, Welsh C. Geriatric respiratory medicine. *Chest* 1998;114:1704–1733.

Chung-Yang S, Nai-Shin C. Epileptic seizures in intra-cerebral hemorrhage. *J Neurol Neurosurg Psychiatry* 1989; 52:1273–1276.

Cole F, Yates P. Intra-cerebral microaneurysms and small cerebrovascular lesions. *Brain* 1967;90:759–768.

Davis SM, Andrews JT, Lichtenstein M, et al. Correlations between cerebral arterial velocities, blood flow and delayed ischemia after subarachnoid hemorrhage. *Stroke* 1992;23:492–497.

Ely W, Evans G, Haponik E. Mechanical ventilation in a cohort of elderly patients admitted to an intensive care unit. *Ann Intern Med* 1999;131:96–104.

Faught E, Peters D, Bartolucci A, et al. Seizures after primary intra-cerebral hemorrhage. *Neurology* 1989;39: 1089–1093.

Georgilis K, Plomaritoglou A, Dafni U, et al. Etiology of fever in patients with acute stroke. *J Intern Med* 1999; 246:203–209.

Graff-Radford N, Torner J, Adams HP. Factors associated with hydrocephalus after subarachnoid hemorrhage. *Arch Neurol* 1989;46:744–752.

Grotta J, Pasteur W, Khwaja G, et al. Elective intubation for neurologic deterioration after stroke. *Neurology* 1995;45: 640–644.

Hijdra A, Van Gijn J, Stefanko S, et al. Delayed cerebral ischemia after aneurysmal subarachnoid hemorrhage: clinico-anatomic correlations. *Neurology* 1986;36:329–333.

Howard MA III, Gross AS, Dacey RG Jr., et al. Acute subdural hematomas: an age-dependent clinical entity. *J Neurosurg* 1989;71:858–863.

Kazama T, Ikeda K, Morita K, et al. Comparison of the effect-site keOs of propofol for blood pressure in elderly and young patients. *Anesthesiology* 1999;90:1517–1527.

Ludwig UG, Baechrendtz S, Wanecek M, et al. Mechanical ventilation in medical and neurological diseases: 11 years of experience. *J Intern Med* 1991;229:798–802.

Mello T, Pinto AN, Ferro JM. Headache in intra-cerebral hematomas. *Neurology* 1996;47:494–500.

Morfis L, Schwartz R, Poulos R, et al. Blood pressure changes in acute cerebral infarction and hemorrhage. *Stroke* 1997;28:1401–1405.

Phan TJ, Koh M, Vierkant RA, et al. Hydrocephalus is a determinant of early mortality in putaminal hemorrhage. *Stroke* 2000;31:2157–2162.

Poungvarin N, Bhoopat W, Viriyavejakul A, et al. Effects of dexamethasone in primary supratentorial intra-cerebral hemorrhage. *N Engl J Med* 1987;316:1229–1233.

Radberg J, Olsson J, Radberg C. Prognostic parameters in spontaneous intra-cerebral hematomas with special reference to anticoagulant treatment. *Stroke* 1991;22:571–576.

Schutz H, Bodeker R, Damian M, et al. Age-related spontaneous intra-cerebral hematoma in a German community. *Stroke* 1990;21:1412.

Stephan F, Cheffi A, Bonnet F. Nosocomial infection and outcome of critically ill elderly patients after surgery. *Anesthesiology* 2001;94:407–417.

St. Louis EK, Wijdicks EF, Li H. Predicting neurologic deterioration in patients with cerebellar hematomas. *Neurology* 1998;51:1364–1369.

Stober T, Sen S, Anstatt T, et al. Correlation of cardiac arrhythmias with brainstem compression in patients with intra-cerebral hemorrhage. *Stroke* 1988;19:688–692.

Thurim S, Dambrosia JM, Price TR, et al. Predilection of intra-cerebral hemorrhage survival. *Ann Neurol* 1988;24:258–263.

Tone O, Ito U, Tomita H, et al. High colloid oncotic therapy for brain edema with cerebral hemorrhage. *Acta Neurochir* 1994;60:568–570.

Touho H, Karasawa J, Shishido H, et al. Neurogenic pulmonary edema in the acute stage of hemorrhagic cerebrovascular disease. *Neurosurgery* 1989;25:762–768.

Wilberger JE, Harris M, Diamond DL. Acute subdural hematoma: morbidity, mortality and operative timing. *J Neurosurg* 1991;74:212–218.

Wood JH, Kee DB. Hemorheology of the cerebral circulation in stroke. *Stroke* 1985;16:765–772.

Yu Y, Kumana C, Lauder I, et al. Treatment of acute cerebral hemorrhage with intravenous glycerol. *Stroke* 1992;23:967–971.

20

Cognitive Effects of Head Trauma
in the Older Adult

Laurie M. Ryan and Judith R. O'Jile

Head injury, a frequent occurrence in the United States and other industrialized nations, is the leading cause of brain injury. Centers for Disease Control estimates suggest that annually about 100 of every 100,000 people in the United States sustain head injuries that result in brain damage. Severity of head injury varies, but most (70% to 90%) are mild (Frankowski, 1986; Rimel et al., 1981), and most are closed or nonpenetrating (i.e., intact skull with no exposure of brain tissue) (Lezak, 1995). Given the much less frequent occurrence of open head injury, this chapter focuses exclusively on the diffuse damage associated with closed head trauma. The terms head trauma, traumatic brain injury, and head injury are used interchangeably.

Research in the area of geriatric head trauma has been limited. This chapter delineates the known information about geriatric head trauma, provides information regarding possible pharmaceutical interventions, and elaborates on areas for future study. The incidence of head injury is related to age and gender as well as other sociodemographic variables. Three age-related peaks of head injury occurrence seem to exist: ages 1 to 5, 15 to 24, and above 65 years, and, of these, the highest incidence rates are seen among people in the 15 to 24 age range (Frankowski, 1986; Naugle, 1990). Persons most at risk of sustaining head injuries are those just entering young adulthood. In terms of gender, males have consistently outnumbered females in rates of head injury among the younger age groups but, no gender differences are seen among older adults (Fields, 1997). In younger adults, motor vehicle accidents account for most head injuries, whereas in older adults, falls predominate. It has been estimated that 73% of all head injuries in those over 65 years of age are the result of falls (Fife et al., 1986). The second most common cause of geriatric head injury appears to be motor vehicle acci-

dents, with a larger proportion involving pedestrian injuries (Naugle, 1990).

INJURY SEVERITY

Head injury is usually characterized as mild, moderate, or severe and should be measured by a number of methods, including loss of consciousness (LOC), posttraumatic amnesia (PTA), and magnetic resonance imaging or computerized tomography (CT). The length of LOC at the time of injury is often related to severity; however, it is now well established that brain injury can occur without complete LOC (Bigler, 1990). Alteration of consciousness or mental status (i.e., being dazed, disoriented, or confused) following head trauma is considered the minimal grade of concussion or cerebral injury (Ommaya and Gennarelli, 1974). The Glasgow Coma Scale (Teasdale and Jennett, 1974) quantifies level of consciousness, ranging from alert to comatose, with scores of 13 to 15 (of a maximum score of 15) considered mild; scores of 9 to 12 indicate moderate injury; and scores of 8 or less suggest severe injury. Posttraumatic amnesia presupposes that the patient is alert and functioning and has recovered from the comatose state, but has persistent, severe deficits in retaining new information and processing new memories (Bigler, 1990). It is generally accepted that the greater the length of PTA, the greater the severity of the head injury (Smith, 1961).

Magnetic resonance imaging or CT can provide additional information to help in the estimation of injury severity. Neuroradiographic evidence of abnormality (i.e., edema, hemorrhage, and any other structural lesion) can suggest a greater level of severity of injury than indicated by PTA or LOC alone (Bigler, 1990). Because of the complexity of head injury, all of the measures listed should be considered in determining severity level, when available.

PATHOLOGY

A large body of evidence indicates that neuropathologic changes occur with even mild head injury. Mild head injury represents the low end of a spectrum in that pathologic changes increase as the severity of injury increases (Dixon et al., 1993). In all head injuries, mechanical force to the head, either through direct impact or acceleration-deceleration motion, leads to a rapid displacement of the skull, which if sufficiently severe can cause differential motion between the brain and skull. The path of head motion, the anatomic surfaces surrounding the brain, and the violence of the motion determine the severity of displacement. Deformation of brain tissue is a result of such displacement and is thought to be the primary factor in traumatic brain damage. Cerebral deformation can result in structural alterations of neurons such as axonal and cytoskeletal injury, vascular changes (e.g., contusions and hemorrhage), generation of oxygen radicals, and excessive neural depolarization causing abnormal neurochemical agonist-receptor interactions related to excitotoxic processes (Dixon et al., 1993). Evidence suggests that activation of muscarinic cholinergic or N-methyl-D-aspartatic acid (NMDA) glutamate receptors is involved (Hayes et al., 1992). Such neurochemical alterations may play a role in the behavioral changes associated with head injury.

Diffuse axonal injury has been demonstrated in clinical and laboratory studies of head injury and seems to be a consistent feature of all injuries, regardless of severity, with the distribution and number of axons involved increasing with injury severity (Povlishock et al., 1992). Axonal injury can come from physical shearing or tearing at the time of injury or be a delayed pathophysiologic reaction that occurs over several hours. Povlishock et al. (1983) found that axonal changes occurred without the presence of focal parenchymal or vascular damage even in mild head injuries. In addition, axonal injury can contribute to neurotransmitter changes by tissue destruction and deafferentation (Dixon et al., 1993).

Orbitofrontal and anterior temporal regions are particularly vulnerable to contusions, lacerations, abrasions, hematomas, and intercerebral hemorrhages caused by forceful contact with the rough bony surface of the skull in these areas during head injury (Mattson and Levin, 1987; Varney and Menefee, 1993). In addition, diffuse axonal damage can disrupt frontal pathways to other cortical and subcortical regions, including the limbic system. Damage to these regions has been linked to deficits in complex neurocognitive functioning, including attention, memory, and emotional changes (Mattson and Levin, 1987).

With aging, a greater risk exists for postinjury neurologic changes, including subdural hematomas, intracranial hemorrhage, and post-traumatic infections. The elderly are at increased risk because brain atrophy increases the distance between the brain surface and the venous sinuses. Bridging veins are more vulnerable to rupture, increasing the risk of subdural bleeds, even with less severe injuries (Cummings and Benson, 1992). In addition, subdural hematomas are common consequences of falls (Fields, 1997). The elderly, however, are not at greater risk than younger adults for skull fracture, edema, or seizures following head injury (Richardson, 1990). In addition to these increased risks, the course of the geriatric patient can be complicated by comorbid medical or neurologic disease (e.g., cardiovascular disease, dementia, diabetes, or chronic obstructive pulmonary disease).

DIFFERENTIAL CLINICAL PRESENTATION IN THE OLDER ADULT

The clinical presentation of older individuals with head trauma can differ from that of younger adults because of differences in demography (e.g., live alone, no close family or friends), cause, and prevalence of comorbidity (Fogel and Duffy, 1994). Older adults with head injuries may have a delayed presentation for medical care, even hours to days after a traumatic brain injury. For example, an older person may fall, lose consciousness, and not be brought for medical treatment until they are found unconscious or confused or they recover enough to call for help themselves. Alternatively, an older patient may gradually develop a subdural hematoma after a relatively minor injury. Such a patient may present as much as 3 months after the onset of mental status changes and even longer after the injury (Jennett, 1982; Velasco et al., 1995). Moreover, urgent orthopedic or medical problems may supersede or even prevent recognition of the traumatic brain injury. Common situations include hip fractures with head trauma or head trauma from a fall, precipitated by a medical problem such as syncope. Even when head trauma is recognized, severity can be difficult to assess because the medical problems may contribute to the altered mental status. Finally, older individuals may present with a chronic progressive cognitive impairment and disability; for example, patients may be brought to medical attention by family or neighbors because of a change in their ability to perform day-to-day activities. Although evidence of physical trauma may be seen, the patient may be unable to provide details. In such case, head trauma should be suspected as contributing to or exacerbating the patient's preexisting cognitive difficulties (e.g., dementia) (Fogel and Duffy, 1994).

OVERALL COGNITIVE OUTCOME

In general, both injury severity and the patient's age at the time of injury, influence the neuropsychological outcome following head injury. With increasing age, is seen increasing risk of negative outcome as well as greater risk for mortality (Rakier et al., 1995; Pentland et al., 1986). The cognitive effects of a diffuse head injury emerge after resolution of PTA and have been well documented in younger patients (Lezak, 1995; McAllister, 1992). Although deficits vary with injury severity, these generally include problems with executive or attention functions, speed of information processing, mental flexibility, memory, and naming. Each of these cognitive functions is discussed below.

Executive and Attention Functioning

Executive function refers to those higher level cognitive abilities that enable an individual to successfully engage in independent goal-directed behavior. Initiation of action, planning and organization, problem-solving, information-processing, and self-monitoring are all part of executive functioning. Diffuse injury is often manifested by diminished mental speed, concentration, cognitive efficiency, and higher level reasoning abilities. Related to these decreased abilities, patients' complaints include distractibility, difficulty performing more than one task at a time, confusion and perplexity in thinking, irritability, fatigue, and increased effort to perform even simple tasks (Gentilini et al., 1989). Such problems are easily identified on a neuropsychological examination, but otherwise may be misinterpreted as the onset of dementia. For example, slowed speed of mental processing can result in significantly lowered scores on timed tests, despite the capacity to perform the required task accurately (Lezak, 1995). In general, patients with diffuse damage perform relatively poorly on measures requiring concentration and working memory (i.e., limited capacity memory system where material is held temporarily while it is manipulated for complex cognitive tasks such as learning and reasoning). Tasks involving these abilities include mental arithmetic, serial calculations,

and reasoning problems (Gronwall and Wrightson, 1981). In addition, mental inflexibility is problematic, as evidenced by disturbed behavioral or conceptual shifting in response to changing circumstances (Levin et al., 1991).

It should be noted that patients with mental efficiency problems frequently interpret their slowed processing and attentional deficits as memory problems, even when recall is intact. Although they report memory loss, analysis of their neuropsychological performance often indicates reduced auditory attention span and difficulty with divided attention and verbal retrieval problems. Many patients are acutely aware of these cognitive difficulties and try to use various strategies to compensate. One such strategy is a continual rechecking of their actions (Lezak, 1995).

With the most severe injuries, additional executive deficits often include impaired capacity for self-determination, self-direction, and self-control and regulation, all of which depend on intact awareness of one's self and the environment. Such impairments are often the most crippling as well as the most intractable disorders to remediate. Compromised self-awareness is reflected in diminished insight, which can lead to dysfunctional social interactions, but more importantly increased safety risks when unsupervised. For example, geriatric head-injured patients with poor insight and other cognitive dysfunction may leave food cooking unattended on the stove, or wander away from familiar places when taking a walk. Perseveration in thoughts and behavioral responses is typical and can compromise both cognitive and social functioning. Often, patients have the ability to perform tasks, but their ability to initiate actions or to plan and choose alternatives is impaired. It is these types of deficits that often account for the poor outcome and lack of independence seen in severely injured patients (Lezak, 1995). However, it is important to note that in the elderly, even less severe injuries can result in such disability.

Memory

Following traumatic head injury, complaints of learning and memory dysfunction are common, with problems usually found in the acquisition and retrieval of information. Patients may have difficulty learning information, but once encoded, the information is generally retained. However, patients may have problems retrieving material from memory once it has been stored (Gronwall and Wrightson, 1981). Thus, patients tend to perform better on recognition or with cueing than from free recall. In addition, because of cerebral lateralization of functions, verbal and visual memory can be affected differentially, depending on the location of focal injury. Left-sided injuries often result in problems with verbal memory and right-sided lesions are often associated with nonverbal memory deficits. In very severe injuries, memory can be affected to such an extent that new learning is almost completely disrupted. However, even in these cases, procedural memory (e.g., skill learning) is typically preserved (Lezak, 1995).

Language

Classic aphasia syndromes are atypical after closed head injury, except when associated with focal lesions (Lezak, 1995). However, a decline can be seen in certain language abilities, typically including defective or slowed naming and word-finding problems that lead to circumlocution and semantic word substitutions. Circumlocution involves using an unnecessarily large number of words to express an idea. Semantic word substitution refers to the use of a word that is within the category that one wants to convey but is not the exact word (e.g., using the word toy instead of ball). Even with more mild injuries, a breakdown in the ability to effectively communicate and understand thoughts and ideas (i.e., linguistic competence) can also occur and affects the pragmatic aspects of language. Pragmatic language skills include conversational turn taking, gestures, loudness of speech, verbal appropriateness, making inferences, and understanding humor.

COGNITIVE SEQUELAE OF HEAD TRAUMA IN THE OLDER ADULT

Despite the comprehensive literature on the cognitive sequelae of head injury in younger adults, the data are limited and relatively recent for older adults. Research suggests that deficits experienced by elderly individuals after head injury are similar to those of younger adults (Goldstein et al., 1999). Initial studies of geriatric patients generally focused on global outcome measures such as the Mini-Mental State Examination (Folstein et al., 1975), whereas only recently have data on specific cognitive functions been generated. Goldstein et al. (1994) examined the neurocognitive effects of mild to moderate closed head injury in adults aged 50 years and older who were relatively early in the recovery process (<7 months). These subjects were found to have sig-

nificantly worse performance than matched elderly controls on measures of memory, attention, information processing speed, and executive functioning, with particular difficulties for naming, verbal fluency, and memory. Moreover, the pattern of deficits observed in the older subjects was similar to that typically seen in younger traumatic brain injury survivors. Findings of several other recent studies (Fields, 1997; Johnstone et al., 1998; Ginsberg and Long, 1996) have also demonstrated that older head-injured individuals' performance did not differ significantly from that of younger head-injured subjects when they were compared with people of the same age. Improvement at 6 months and 1 year after mild to moderate head injury was noted on some measures of memory and verbal fluency in a group of elderly people (Goldstein et al., 1997). Moreover, in a group of high functioning older individuals without additional risk factors such as previous head injury, substance abuse, or psychiatric or neurologic condition, a single uncomplicated mild head injury did not result in clinically significant cognitive deficits at 2 months after injury (Goldstein et al., 2000). No studies have yet investigated long-term cognitive recovery from head injury in the elderly.

PSYCHOSOCIAL OUTCOME IN THE OLDER ADULT

On the whole, a negative relationship appears to exist between age and psychosocial outcome. Advancing age at the time of head injury is associated with increased long-term functional disability (Pentland et al., 1986). For example, in one sample of head-injured elderly, 72% of survivors had experienced a change in functional status that necessitated increased family involvement and use of community support services (Wilson et al., 1987). Similarly, studies (Fields, 1997; Fife et al., 1986) have shown that older adults who have sustained a head injury are less likely to be discharged from the hospital to their home and are more likely to be placed in a nursing home. Moreover, a significantly greater proportion of older individuals is rated as disabled compared with younger adults 1 year after injury (Rothweiler et al., 1998). Persons 60 years and older were more disabled than those under 50, and those from 30 to 49 were more disabled than those under 30. Significantly fewer older adults returned to their former living status 1 year after injury compared with younger adults, with most requiring a more supervised living environment. For those employed before the injury, a smaller percentage of those individuals over 50 returned to work. It is noteworthy that, although increasing dependence is associated with increasing age, variability in psychosocial outcome was marked in the older sample. Older individuals showed a greater range of outcomes, from good outcome in 20% of the sample to death in 32%.

HEAD TRAUMA AND ALZHEIMER'S DISEASE

Differential Cognitive Effects of Head Trauma and Alzheimer's Disease

Cognitive deficits observed in the head-injured elderly could reflect premorbid dementia, a magnification of such a preexisting condition, or the sequelae of head trauma. Without a good history, it is often difficult to differentiate the cause of a cognitive disturbance in the elderly because, although falling in the elderly is the primary cause of head injury, cognitive dysfunction (e.g., dementia) can be a predisposing factor for falls (Luukinen et al., 1999). Differential diagnosis is further complicated by overlap in cognitive symptoms in head injury and dementing disorders, including difficulties with memory, verbal fluency, and naming (Ginsberg and Long, 1996; Goldstein et al., 1996). Research comparing the neuropsychological performance of subjects with dementia and head injury is sparse but available data suggest that the cognitive effects of head injury in the elderly can be differentiated from those of dementia.

Evidence so far, suggests that elderly head-injured subjects perform better than a group of subjects with mild dementia on measures of verbal memory and executive functioning (Young et al., 1995). Furthermore, qualitative differences emerged between groups such that (Goldstein et al., 1996) memory deficits appear to be caused by retrieval deficits in head injury and encoding problems in Alzheimer's disease.

Head Trauma as a Risk Factor for Alzheimer's Disease

A relationship between head injury and increased risk for Alzheimer's disease has been postulated, but results have been inconclusive. Some investigators found that head injury is a risk factor for Alzheimer's disease (Rasmusson et al., 1995). On the other hand, others (Gedye et al., 1989; Nemetz et al., 1999) reported that head trauma does not increase the risk for the disease but does reduce the time to onset in those patients with Alzheimer's disease. Moreover, it has been suggested (Mayeux et al., 1995) that head injury alone does not increase the risk of Alzheimer's disease, but head injury in persons with the ApoE e4 allele increases the risk tenfold compared with those who lack both factors. Yet, a different study (Salib and Hillier, 1997) found that head injury was a risk factor for Alzheimer's disease as well as other types of dementia, but only in male patients.

Severity of head injury may also play a role in increasing the risk of Alzheimer's disease. A recent large case-controlled study (Guo et al., 2000) that was part of the Multi-Institutional Research in Alzheimer's Genetic Epidemiology Project (MIRAGE) found that the risk of Alzheimer's disease for those with head injury with LOC was double that of those with head injury without LOC. This suggests that the magnitude of risk was proportional to head injury severity. Moreover, even head injury without LOC significantly increased the risk of Alzheimer's disease in first-degree relatives of patients with the disease, suggesting a link between head injury without LOC and family history. However, in contrast to findings from other investigations (Katzman et al., 1996; Mayeux et al., 1995), this study did not find an increased risk of Alzheimer's disease for those with both a history of head injury and apolipoprotein e4 (ApoE e4).

TREATMENT

Cognitive Rehabilitation

Only a paucity of research has investigated cognitive rehabilitation of the older head-injured patient. The few rehabilitation studies to date suggest that older persons do demonstrate functional improvement, albeit at a slower rate and subsequently greater cost (Cifu et al., 1996; Gershkoff et al., 1993). Even patients with head injury and progressive neurodegenerative disorders such as Alzheimer's disease have been found to benefit from cognitive remediation strategies using standard mnemonic techniques (Gouvier et al., 1997). Although the data are limited, given the apparent efficacy for even these more impaired individuals, cognitive rehabilitation should be considered for older head-injured persons (Fig. 20-1). For a comprehensive review of the cognitive rehabilitation literature, see the chapter by Gouvier et al. (1997).

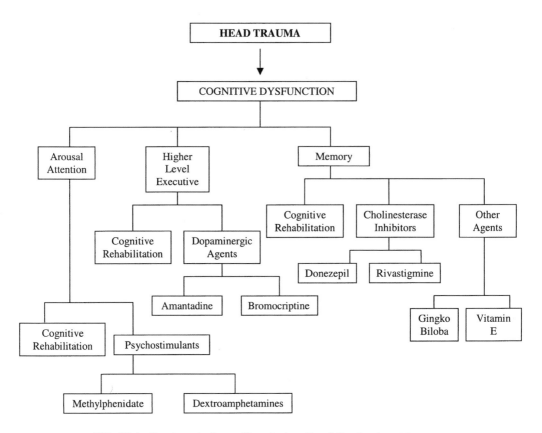

FIG. 20.1. Treatment of cognitive dysfunction following head trauma.

Pharmacologic Interventions

Psychostimulants

Psychostimulants are probably the most commonly used medication in the treatment of attentional problems following head injury, although no studies have been conducted solely on elderly head-injured subjects (Table 20-1; Fig. 20-1). Psychostimulant medications (e.g., methylphenidate) increase activity in the catecholamine system, which is one of the neurotransmitter systems disturbed in traumatic brain injury (Malone et al., 1994; Wroblewski and Glenn, 1994). Recent placebo-controlled studies suggest good efficacy of methylphenidate in head injury (Glenn, 1998), and other studies have shown that its use results in significant improvement in attention over that expected from natural recovery and was well tolerated by patients (Kaelin et al., 1996). Another study (Whyte et al., 1997) found improvements in speed of information processing but not for sustained attention in postacute head injury patients. None of these studies, however, included elderly head-injured patients.

Dopaminergic Agents

Dopaminergic agents have also been used to improve cognitive functioning in patients with head injury, although no studies have been performed with older head-injured subjects (Table 20-1; Fig. 20-1). Of the studies done, most have been small case series. The rationale for the use of dopaminergic medications is based on the finding of lowered levels of dopamine metabolites following traumatic brain injury. Moreover, dopamine is important for frontal system functioning, which is often affected in traumatic brain injury (Brown et al., 1979; Pearlson and Robinson, 1981). Investigations of dopaminergic medications have included amantadine and bromocriptine. In addition to the dopaminergic ef-

TABLE 20-1. *Cognitive enhancing medications*

Drug type	Medication	Cognitive indications	Medical contraindications
Psychostimulants	Methylphenidate	Arousal/attention deficits	Motor tics, Tourette's syndrome, family history of Tourette's Significant anxiety, tension, agitation, glaucoma, hypersensitivity to methylphenidate
	Dextroamphetamines	Same as above	Advanced arterosclerosis, symptomatic cardiovascular disease, moderate to severe hypertension, hyperthyroidism, hypersensitivity to sympathomimetic amines, glaucoma, agitation, history of drug abuse, MAO inhibitor use *Cautions:* Mild hypertension, Tourette's syndrome
Dopaminergic agents	Amantadine	Frontal-executive dysfunction	Renal dysfunction, hypersensitivity to amantadine *Cautions:* Seizures, CHF, peripheral edema, liver disease, orthostatic hypertension, psychosis, CNS stimulant use
	Bromocriptine	Same as above	Uncontrolled hypertension, hypersensitivity to ergot alkaloids, pregnancy *Cautions:* Renal disease, liver disease
Cholinesterase inhibitors	Donepezil	Memory	Hypersensitivity to donepezil or piperidine derivatives *Cautions:* Supraventricular cardiac conduction conditions, ulcers, asthma, COPD, seizures
	Rivastigmine	Same as above	Hypersensitivity to rivastigmine or carbamate derivatives *Cautions:* Same as above
Other cognitive agents	Gingko Biloba	Same as above	Not known *Cautions:* Anticoagulant or NSAID use
	Vitamin E	Same as above	Not known

CHF, congestive heart failure; CNS, central nervous system; COPD, chronic obstructive pulmonary disease; MAO, monoamine oxidase; NSAID, nonsteroidal anti-inflammatory drug.

fects of amantadine, it is an NMDA glutamate receptor antagonist, and, as such, might provide a protective effect against excitotoxic release following head trauma (Weller and Kornhuber, 1992). In a recent study (Kraus and Maki, 1997) examining the efficacy of amantadine in the treatment of cognitive and behavioral sequelae of brain injury patients at least 1 year after injury, all patients showed some degree of positive response in executive functions to amantadine, based on improved neuropsychological test performance. Similarly, bromocriptine was found to be effective in improving executive functioning in head-injured patients evaluated in a double-blind, placebo-controlled, crossover study (McDowell et al., 1998).

Cholinesterase Inhibitors

Similar to Alzheimer's disease, cholinergic dysfunction has also been found in traumatic brain injury, raising the question of possible usefulness of cholinesterase inhibitors such as physostigmine, tacrine, and donepezil as a treatment for cognitive dysfunction associated with head injury (Table 20-1; Fig. 20-1). Donepezil appears especially well suited because it has a longer duration of inhibitory action, greater specificity for brain tissue, and is well tolerated by most patients, even at high doses (Vandewoude, 1999). In a recent study (Taverni et al., 1998), donepezil was reported to be effective in the treatment of memory problems in two severely head-injured patients during postacute rehabilitation. Another selective cholinesterase inhibitor, rivastigmine, has just been approved for clinical use and, in preliminary studies, has shown positive results in the treatment of cognitive dysfunction in Alzheimer's disease (Birks et al., 2000; Jann, 2000; Vandewoude, 1999). Studies are needed to determine whether this medication will also be useful in the treatment of cognitive effects of head injury.

Other Cognitive Enhancers

Gingko biloba, a botanical supplement, has been found in a number of studies to show multiple pharmacologic effects on neuronal functioning, including improved glucose metabolism, antioxidant effects, increased acetylcholine synthesis and release, as well as an increase in cholinergic receptors (Vandewoude, 1999; Wettstein, 2000). Results of initial studies of cognitive symptom progression suggest similar efficacy in patients with Alzheimer's disease between gingko biloba extract (EGb 761) and several cholinesterase inhibitors (Wettstein, 2000). Although these results are intriguing, well-designed clinical trials are needed in patients both with Alzheimer's disease and with head injury (Table 20-1; Fig. 20-1).

Vitamin E has also provided some interesting results in the treatment of cognitive dysfunction in patients with dementia, but further study is necessary to determine if it will be effective in remediating cognitive deficits resulting from head injury in the elderly (Table 20-1; Fig. 20-1).

REFERENCES

Bigler ED. Neuropathology of traumatic brain injury. In: Bigler ED, ed. *Traumatic brain injury: mechanisms of damage, assessment, intervention, and outcome.* Austin: Pro-Ed Inc., 1990:13–49.

Birks J, Iakovidou V, Tsolaki M. Rivastigmine for Alzheimer's disease. *Cochrane Database System Review* 2000: 2:CD001191.

Brown RM, Crane AM, Goldman PS. Regional distribution of monoamines in the cerebral cortex and subcortical structures of the rhesus monkey: concentrations and in vivo synthesis rates. *Brain Res* 1979;168:133–150.

Cifu DX, Kreutzer JS, Marwitz JH, et al. Functional outcomes of older adults with traumatic brain injury: a prospective, multicenter analysis. *Arch Phys Med Rehabil* 1996;77:883–888.

Cummings JL, Benson DF. *Dementia: a clinical approach*, 2nd ed. Stoneham, MA: Butterworth-Heinemann, 1992.

Dixon CE, Taft WC, Hayes RL. Mechanisms of mild traumatic brain injury. *J Head Trauma Rehabil* 1993;8:1–12.

Fields RB. Geriatric head injury. In: Nussbaum PD, ed. *Handbook of neuropsychology and aging.* New York: Plenum Press, 1997;281–297.

Fife D, Faich G, Hollinshead W, et al. Incidence and outcome of hospital-treated head injury in Rhode Island. *Am J Public Health* 1986;76:773–778.

Fogel BS, Duffy J. Elderly patients. In: Silver J, Udosfky SC, Hales RE, eds. *Neuropsychiatry of traumatic brain injury.* Washington, DC: American Psychiatric Press, 1994:412–441.

Folstein MF, Folstein SE, McHugh PR. "Mini-mental state." *J Psychiatr Res* 1975;12;189–198.

Frankowski RF. Descriptive epidemiologic studies of head injury in the United States: 1974-1983. *Adv Psychosom Med* 1986;16:153–172.

Gedye A, Beattie BL, Tuokko H, et al. Severe head injury hastens age of onset of Alzheimer's disease. *J Am Geriatr Soc* 1989;37:970–973.

Gentilini N, Nichelli P, Schoenhuber R. Assessment of attention in mild head injury. In: Levin HS, Eisenberg HM, Benton AL, eds. *Mild head injury.* New York: Oxford University Press, 1989:163–175.

Gershkoff AM, Cifu DX, Means KM. Geriatric rehabilitation: social, attitudinal, and economic factors. *Arch Phys Med Rehabil* 1993;74 (Suppl):S402–S405.

Ginsberg JP, Long CJ. Acceleration of age-related decline in neuropsychological performance after recovery from severe traumatic brain injury. *Arch Clin Neuropsychol* 1996; 11(5):394.

Glenn MB. Methylphenidate for cognitive and behavioral dysfunction after traumatic brain injury. *J Head Trauma Rehabil* 1998;13:87–90.

Goldstein FC, Clark A, McGuire C, et al. Detection of dementia: comparison of informant reports versus objective patient screening. *J Neuropsychiatry Clin Neurosci* 1997; 9:173.

Goldstein FC, Levin HS, Goldman WP, et al. Cognitive and behavioral sequelae of closed head injury in older adults according to their significant others. *J Neuropsychiatry Clin Neurosci* 1999;11:38–44.

Goldstein FC, Levin HS, Presley RM, et al. Neurobehavioral consequences of closed head injury in older adults. *J Neurol Neurosurg Psychiatry* 1994;57 (8):961–966.

Goldstein FC, Levin HS, Roberts VJ, et al. Neurocognitive recovery in older adults with closed head injury. *J Int Neuropsychol Soc* 2000;6:183.

Goldstein FC, Levin HS, Roberts VJ, et al. Neuropsychological effects of closed head injury in older adults: a comparison with Alzheimer's disease. *Neuropsychology* 1996;10(2):147–154.

Gouvier WD, Ryan LM, O'Jile JR, et al. Cognitive retraining with brain-damaged patients. In: Wedding D, Horton A, Webster J, eds. *The neuropsychology handbook: clinical and behavioral perspectives,* 2nd ed., Vol. 2. New York: Springer Publishing, 1997:3–46.

Gronwall D, Wrightson P. Memory and information processing capacity after closed head injury. *J Neurol Neurosurg Psychiatry* 1981;44:889–895.

Guo Z, Cupples LA, Kurz A, et al. Head injury and the risk of AD in the MIRAGE study. *Neurology* 2000;54:1316–1323.

Hayes RL, Jenkins LW, Lyeth BG. Neurotransmitter-mediated mechanisms of traumatic brain injury: acetylcholine and excitatory amino acids. *J Neurotrauma* 1992;9 (Suppl 1):173–187.

Jann MW. Rivastigmine, a new-generation cholinesterase inhibitor for the treatment of Alzheimer's disease. *Pharmacotherapy* 2000;20:1–12.

Jennett B. Head injuries. In: *Neurological disorders in the elderly*. Littleton, MA: John Wright & Sons, 1982: 202–211.

Johnstone B, Childers MK, Hoerner J. The effects of normal ageing on neuropsychological functioning following traumatic brain injury. *Brain Inj* 1998;12:569–576.

Kaelin DL, Cifu DX, Matthies B. Methylphenidate effect on attention deficit in the acutely brain-injured adult. *Arch Phys Med Rehabil* 1996;77:6–9.

Katzman R, Galasko DR, Saitoh T, et al. Apolipoprotein epsilon4 and head trauma: synergistic or additive quirks? *Neurology* 1996;46:889–891.

Kraus MF, Maki PM. Effect of amantadine hydrochloride on symptoms of frontal lobe dysfunction in brain injury: case studies and review. *J Neuropsychiatr Clin Neurosci* 1997; 9:222–230.

Levin HS, Goldstein FC, Williams DH, et al. The contribution of frontal lobe lesions to the neurobehavioral outcome of closed head injury. In: Levin HS, Eisenberg HM, Benton AL, eds. *Frontal lobe function and dysfunction*. New York: Oxford University Press, 1991:318–337.

Lezak MD. *Neuropsychological assessment*, 3rd ed. New York: Oxford University Press, 1995.

Luukinen H, Viramo P, Koski K, et al. Head injuries and cognitive decline among older adults: a population-based study. *Neurology* 1999;52:557–562.

Malone MA, Kerschner JR, Swanson JM. Hemispheric processing and methylphenidate effects in attention-deficit hyperactivity disorder. *J Child Neurol* 1994;9:181–189.

Mattson AG, Levin HS. Frontal lobe dysfunction following closed head injury: a review of the literature. *J Nerv Ment Dis* 1987;178:282–291.

Mayeux R, Ottman R, Maestre G, et al. Synergistic effects of traumatic head injury and apolipoprotein-epsilon 4 in patients with Alzheimer's disease. *Neurology* 1995;45: 555–557.

McAllister, TW. Neuropsychiatric sequelae of head injuries. *Psychiatr Clin North Am* 1992;15:395–413.

McDowell S, Whyte J, D'Esposito M. Differential effect of a dopaminergic agonist on prefrontal function in traumatic brain injury patients. *Brain* 1998;121:1155–1164.

Naugle RI. Epidemiology of traumatic brain injury in adults. In: Bigler ED, ed. *Traumatic brain injury: mechanisms of damage, assessment, intervention, and outcome*. Austin: Pro-Ed Inc., 1990:69–103.

Nemetz PN, Leibson C, Naessens JM, et al. Traumatic brain injury and time to onset of Alzheimer's disease: a population-based study. *Am J Epidemiol* 1999;149:32–40.

Ommaya, AK, Gennarelli TA. Cerebral concussion and traumatic unconsciousness. *Brain* 1974;97:633–654.

Pearlson GD, Robinson RG. Suction lesions of the frontal cerebral cortex in the rat induced asymmetrical behavioral and catecholaminergic responses. *Brain Res* 1981; 218:233–242.

Pentland B, Jones PA, Roy CW, et al. Head injury in the elderly. *Age Aging* 1986;15:193–202.

Povlishock JT, Becker DP, Cheng CLY, et al. Axonal change in minor head injury. *J Neuropathol Exp Neurol* 1983; 42:225–242.

Povlishock JT, Erb DE, Astrug J. Axonal response to traumatic brain injury: reactive axonal change, deafferentation, and neuroplasticity. *J Neurotrauma* 1992;9(Suppl 1): 189–200.

Rakier A, Guilburd JN, Soustiel JF, et al. Head injuries in the elderly. *Brain Inj* 1995;9:187–193.

Rasmusson DX, Brant J, Martin DB, et al. Head injury as a risk factor in Alzheimer's disease. *Brain Inj* 1995;9(3): 213–219.

Richardson JTE. *Clinical and neuropsychological aspects of closed head injury*. London: Taylor & Francis, 1990.

Rimel RW, Giordani B, Barth JT, et al. Disability caused by minor head injury. *Neurosurgery* 1981; 9:221–228.

Rothweiler B, Temkin NR, Dikmen SS. Aging effect on psychosocial outcome in traumatic brain injury. *Arch Phys Med Rehabil* 1998;79:881–887.

Salib E, Hillier V. Head injury and the risk of Alzheimer's disease: a case control study. *Int J Geriatr Psychiatry* 1997;2 (3):363–368.

Schneider LS. New therapeutic approaches to cognitive impairment. *J Clin Psychiatry* 1998;59(Suppl 11):8–13.

Shue KL, Douglas VI. Attention deficit hyperactivity disorder and the frontal lobe syndrome. *Brain Cogn* 1992; 20:104–142.

Smith A. Duration of impaired consciousness as an index of severity in closed head injuries. *Diseases of the Nervous System* 1961;22:1–6.

Sohlberg MM, Mateer CA. *Introduction to cognitive rehabilitation: theory and practice*. New York: Guilford Press, 1989.

Taverni JP, Seliger G, Lichtman SW. Donepezil medicated memory improvement in traumatic brain injury during post acute rehabilitation. *Brain Inj* 1998;12:77–80.

Teasdale G, Jennett B. Assessment of coma in impaired consciousness: a practical scale. *Lancet* 1974;2:81–84.

Vandewoude MF. The pharmacological management of cognitive dysfunction in Alzheimer's disease. *Acta Clinica Belgica* 1999;54:306–311.

Varney NR, Menefee L. Psychosocial and executive deficits following closed head injury: implications for orbitofrontal cortex. *J Head Trauma Rehabil* 1993;8:32–44.

Velasco J, Head M, Farlin E, et al. Unsuspected subdural hematoma as a differential diagnosis in elderly patients. *South Med J* 1995; 88:977–979.

Weller M, Kornhuber J. A rationale for NMDA receptor antagonist therapy for neuroleptic malignant syndrome. *Med Hypotheses* 1992;38:329–333.

Wettstein A. Cholinesterase inhibitors and gingko extracts— are they comparable in the treatment of dementia? Comparison of published placebo-controlled efficacy studies of at least six months' duration. *Phytomedicine* 2000;6: 393–401.

Whyte J, Hart T, Schuster K, et al. Effects of methylphenidate on attentional function after traumatic brain injury. A randomized, placebo-controlled trial. *Am J Phys Med Rehabil* 1997;76:440–450.

Wilson JA, Pentland B, Currie CT, et al. Outcome after severe head injury in the elderly. *Brain Inj* 1987;1:183–188.

Wroblewski BA, Glenn MB. Pharmacological treatment of arousal and cognitive deficits. *J Head Trauma Rehabil* 1994;9:19–42.

Young L, Fields RB, Lovell M. Neuropsychological differentiation of geriatric head injury from dementia. *J Neuropsychiatr Clin Neurosci* 1995;7:414.

SUGGESTED READINGS

Fields RB. Geriatric head injury. In: Nussbaum PD, ed. *Handbook of neuropsychology and aging.* New York: Plenum Press, 1997:281–297.

Guo Z, Cupples LA, Kurz A, et al. Head injury and the risk of AD in the MIRAGE study. *Neurology* 2000;54:1316–1323.

Goldstein FC, Levin HS, Presley RM, et al. Neurobehavioral consequences of closed head injury in older adults. *J Neurol Neurosurg Psychiatry* 1994;57 (8):961–966.

WEB SITES

Brain Injury Association: *www.biausa.org*
Alzheimer's Association: *www.alz.org*

21.1

Diagnostic Evaluation and Treatment of Dementia

David S. Knopman

DEFINITION

Dementia is a syndrome defined by a subacute or insidious decline in cognition from a previously higher level (American Psychiatric Association, 1994). The specificity of the diagnosis of dementia is enhanced by also requiring that the patient's cognitive and behavioral deficits interfere "significantly" with daily function and independence. Dementia, in contrast to disorders defined by deficits in only one cognitive or behavioral domain, is diagnosed when deficits are seen in multiple domains. Besides memory dysfunction, the other cognitive and behavioral manifestations of the dementia syndrome include abnormalities in speech and language, visuospatial function, abstract reasoning and executive function, and mood and personality. Alzheimer's disease, the dementia associated with cerebrovascular disease, vascular dementia, the dementias associated with Parkinson's disease, and Lewy body dementia are the most common causes of dementia in the elderly.

DIAGNOSIS

Distinguishing Dementia from Aging

The most difficult aspect of the diagnosis of dementia is in first recognizing that the patient is experiencing lapses in mental function or behavior that are outside the normal variability of everyday life. Cognitive and functional decline from a previously higher level is not compatible with a diagnosis of "normal aging." Patients themselves rarely seek medical attention for the symptoms of dementia. Family members are usually the ones who seek out medical attention, not the patient. However, family members are often tardy in recognizing that the changes in the affected individuals represent early dementia. Denial on the part of family members of the early symptoms of dementia is pervasive. Several studies have shown that

dementia is under-recognized in clinical practice (Callahan et al., 1995; Eefsting et al., 1996; Ross et al., 1997).

Depression

Depression, a common disorder in the elderly, is often associated with impaired memory and concentration. Depression must certainly be considered in the differential diagnosis of dementia, but several key points help to clarify the relationship between depression and dementia. In depressed elderly without dementia, cognitive function is usually close to the normal range. Depression is often an early symptom of dementia (Levy et al., 1996; Forsell and Winblad, 1998). As a consequence, the two syndromes often coexist. Depressed patients who have clear-cut cognitive deficits should be treated for their depression, but the diagnosis of dementia should also be shared with the patient's family. Families are generally better in identifying depressive symptomatology than the patient with dementia (Mackenzie et al., 1989; Teri and Wagner, 1991). Treating depression on the strength of the caregiver's observations, without necessarily obtaining affirmation of feelings of depression from the patient, is the preferred approach in such a situation.

Systemic Metabolic Disorders

Many metabolic disorders have been associated with dementia, but in the past 20 years, surveys of demented patients contain few such examples (White et al., 1996). A practice parameter published by the American Academy of Neurology (AAN) (1994), recently updated, recommends routine laboratory screening with a complete blood count, calcium, electrolytes, blood urea nitrogen, creatinine, transaminases, vitamin B_{12} levels, and thyroid-stimulating hormone levels. These measures are unlikely to yield diagnoses that will substantially change the cognitive disorder. However, elderly patients with dementia may not have regular preventive health check-ups. Screening for common co-morbidities in the elderly patient with dementia is simply a part of good general care.

Structural Brain Lesions

Brain tumors, subdural hematomas, and normal pressure hydrocephalus can cause cognitive deficits indistinguishable from the dementia of Alzheimer's disease. Usually, however, these disorders produce gait abnormalities, other motor findings, seizures, and headaches of subacute (rather than longer duration) onset. These associated abnormalities can help to distinguish them from those of Alzheimer's disease, but analyses (Martin et al., 1987; Corey-Bloom et al., 1995) have shown that no clinical decision rule will detect all structural lesions in patients being evaluated for dementia. Hence, the revised AAN practice parameter recommends that a neuroimaging study be performed routinely at the time of initial diagnosis in a patient with dementia.

Mild Cognitive Impairment

Between the state of normal cognitive and functional abilities and that of mild but definite dementia is a diagnostic gray zone referred to as "mild cognitive impairment" (MCI) (Petersen et al., 1995). Others have referred to this state as possible dementia prodrome, or very mild Alzheimer's disease (Rubin et al., 1989). The term "age-associated memory impairment" appears to describe a similar group of patients, but the memory impairment that is of concern is not *age-associated*, but rather is *disease-associated*. MCI is often a precursor of Alzheimer's disease, but not always (Hanninen et al., 1995; Petersen et al., 1995). Proposed diagnostic criteria (Petersen et al., 1995) for MCI include a memory complaint, objective evidence of impaired recent memory, intact daily function, and intact non-memory cognitive functions. Intact function in daily affairs is perhaps the major distinction between MCI and mild Alzheimer's disease. Approximately 15% of MCI patients deteriorate and qualify for a diagnosis of Alzheimer's disease each year (Petersen et al., 1995). Patients with mild cognitive impairment are sometimes identified because they are discovered coincidentally to have poor performance on mental status testing. Sometimes, patients with MCI refer themselves to physicians because of concerns about their own memory.

ALZHEIMER'S DISEASE

Diagnostic Considerations

Alzheimer's disease is the most common of the dementias in the elderly. It can be diagnosed clinically with confidence in a patient with the gradual and progressive impairment of recent memory and dysfunction in at least one other cognitive or behavioral domain. In routine clinical practice, the diagnostic criteria of the NINCDS-ADRDA workgroup (McKhann et al., 1984) yield an accurate view of the diagnosis of Alzheimer's disease in most instances.

Presentation

Disturbances in recent memory function are the typical symptoms that lead to the suspicion and eventual diagnosis of Alzheimer's disease. Patients repeat themselves in conversation, repeat the same question, or forget recent conversations (Rubin et al., 1989; Koss et al., 1993; Oppenheim, 1994; Petersen et al., 1994). The symptoms can be so insidious in onset that they can be overlooked by family caregivers or physicians. Patients with Alzheimer's disease usually ignore their own shortcomings and deny or minimize their deficits (Grut et al., 1993; Lopez et al., 1994; Starkstein et al., 1996; Seltzer et al., 1997). Symptoms are typically present for 1 to 3 years before family members bring the patient to medical attention. Loss of the ability to carry out key daily tasks such as shopping, handling money, or doing chores around the house may be more powerful triggers than forgetfulness for seeking medical attention. Neuropsychiatric symptoms also are more likely to prompt an evaluation than forgetfulness itself.

On occasion, Alzheimer's disease presents in ways other than as a disorder of recent memory. Sometimes, impaired judgment, social misbehavior, and other manifestations of a frontotemporal dementia are as prominent as the memory disorder (Neary et al., 1988; Brun, 1993; Miller et al., 1997). Another rare alternative presentation of Alzheimer's disease is that of a visual disturbance, visual agnosia. The visual agnosia manifests as impaired figure-ground perceptions, impaired reading, impaired face recognition, and impaired object recognition (Crystal et al., 1982; Mendez et al., 1990; Graff-Radford et al., 1993; Levine et al., 1993). Rarely, will a patient with Alzheimer's disease present exclusively with anomia or expressive language deficits (Green et al., 1990), although name- and word-finding complaints are common.

Natural History

The natural history of Alzheimer's disease is variable. The average length of time from onset of symptoms until diagnosis is about 2 to 3 years (Morris et al., 1989; Galasko et al., 1990; Walsh et al., 1990). The average duration of time from diagnosis to nursing home placement (a marker of severe dementia) is approximately 3 to 6 years (Severson et al., 1994; Knopman et al., 1996; Heyman et al., 1997; Scott et al., 1997; Stern et al., 1997). Patients with Alzheimer's disease spend 3 years in nursing homes prior to death (Welch et al., 1992). Thus, the total duration of the disease is approximately 9 to 12 years.

Across patients whose initial Mini-Mental State Examination (MMSE) (Folstein et al., 1975) scores ranged from 10 to 26, the average rate of change per year is about 3 ± 4 points (Salmon et al., 1990; van Belle et al., 1990; Galasko et al., 1991). The rate of decline follows a curvilinear relationship to the cognitive test scores (Morris et al., 1993; Stern, Mohs, and Davidson, 1994). Faster rates of decline occur in the mid-portions of the scales, and slower rates occur among patients with milder and more severe diseases. Parkinsonian signs, hallucinations, and delusions have been shown to be associated with more rapid decline (Chui et al., 1994; Stern, Albert, and Brandt, 1994; Lopez et al., 1997).

Mortality in Alzheimer's disease averages under 10% per year (Katzman et al., 1994; Kukull et al., 1994; Bowen et al., 1996; Heyman et al., 1996). Causes of death from the disease include pneumonia, sepsis, and other common causes of mortality in the elderly, such as cardiovascular disease and stroke (Kukull et al., 1994; Beard et al., 1996).

Laboratory Aids for the Diagnosis

At the present time, no accepted laboratory procedures or tests are routinely of value in supporting the diagnosis of Alzheimer's disease. Some that are under investigation include apolipoprotein E genotyping, cerebrospinal fluid markers, structural neuroimaging, and functional neuroimaging. None of these appear to provide sufficient improvement in diagnostic accuracy beyond that accomplished by competent clinical diagnoses. Neuropsychological testing, on the other hand, is a valuable extension of the mental status examination; it can yield important clues about the diagnosis of dementia versus other syndromes and about the precise nature of the dementia.

Diagnostic Composition of Alzheimer's Disease in Population Samples

At least 50% to 80% of patients with dementia in clinical epidemiologic surveys have Alzheimer's disease (Evans et al., 1989; Kokmen et al., 1989; Bachman et al., 1992; Canadian Study of Health and Aging, 1994; Hendrie et al., 1995; Graves et al., 1996; White et al., 1996; Hofman et al., 1997; Fillenbaum et al., 1998). In clinicopathologic studies, Alzheimer's disease comprises 70% to 80% of dementias (Wade et al., 1987; Galasko et al., 1994; Victoroff et al., 1995; Berg et al., 1998; Jobst et al., 1998; Mayeux et al., 1998; Holmes et al., 1999; Lim et al., 1999; Massoud et al., 1999).

Prevalence

The prevalence of dementia and Alzheimer's disease increases with advancing age (Pfeffer et al., 1987; Evans et al., 1989; Kokmen et al., 1989; Bachman et al., 1992; 1994; Hendrie et al., 1995; Ott et al., 1995; Graves et al., 1996; White et al., 1996; Hofman et al., 1997; Fillenbaum et al., 1998). In those 65 to 70 years of age, the prevalence of dementia is approximately 1/100 individuals. With each subsequent 5-year increment, the prevalence of dementia and Alzheimer's disease doubles. Over age 85 years, estimates of the prevalence of dementia vary between 20% to nearly 50%. Beyond age 85, it appears that dementia prevalence continues to rise.

Incidence

The incidence of AD also rises dramatically with advancing age (Bachman et al., 1993; Stern et al., 1994; Hebert et al., 1995; Fillenbaum et al., 1998; Gao et al., 1998; Jorm and Jolley, 1998; Ott, Breteler, et al., 1998; Rocca et al., 1998). Because patients with dementia tend to live for several years to as long as a decade or more, incidence rates are considerably lower than prevalence rates.

Conditions Associated with Increased Risk

The two most prominent risk factors for Alzheimer's disease are advancing age and a family history of dementia. Genetic factors will be covered in the next section. The remainder of this section will be devoted to several characteristics that might potentially be risk factors.

Very low educational achievement (<8th grade education) has been a consistently observed, but modestly potent, risk factor that increases a person's odds of developing Alzheimer's disease by two- to three-fold (Cobb et al., 1995; Ott et al., 1995; Stern et al., 1995; Callahan et al., 1996). A threshold effect for education may exist, whereby the effect is only operative in those with less than an 8th grade education. Even when diagnostic methods are specifically modified to reduce educational or cultural biases, the education effect remains (Stern et al., 1995).

Cardiovascular disease confers a small to moderate increased risk for Alzheimer's disease (Elias et al., 1993; Launer et al., 1995; Hofman et al., 1997; Carmelli et al., 1998). The cardiovascular risk factors associated with the disease include atherosclerosis (broadly defined), history of stroke, history of midlife hypertension, and carotid artery disease.

Occupational exposure to industrial solvents and agricultural chemicals have not been consistently shown to increase the risk for Alzheimer's disease (Kukull et al., 1995). The evidence against aluminum (Graves et al., 1990; Bjertness et al., 1996; Salib and Hillier, 1996; Hachinski, 1998) as a risk factor for Alzheimer's disease outweighs suggestions (Crapper et al., 1975; Good et al., 1992) of its possible role.

Two protective factors that have been observed prospectively include estrogen replacement therapy (ERT) (Paganini-Hill and Henderson, 1996; Tang et al., 1996; Kawas et al., 1997) and the use of nonsteroidal anti-inflammatory drugs (NSAID) (Breitner et al., 1994; Andersen et al., 1995; McGeer et al., 1996; Stewart et al., 1997). However, epidemiologic associations do not prove causality. ERT or NSAID use could have been associated with some other factor that actually mediated the risk of Alzheimer's disease. Cigarette smoking has appeared in most studies as a protective factor against Alzheimer's disease (Graves et al., 1991; Hebert et al., 1992; Brenner et al., 1993; Ford et al., 1996), although in some studies it has been a risk factor (Prince et al., 1996; Galanis et al., 1997; Ott, Slooter, et al., 1998).

Genetics

The lifetime risk to first-degree relatives of patients clinically diagnosed as having Alzheimer's disease is approximately 15% by 80 years of age and 39% by 96 years of age (Lautenschlager et al., 1996). Two patterns of genetic risk for Alzheimer's disease are seen: One is through autosomal dominant transmission of mutations in one of three genes; the other is mediated by susceptibility genes, of which only one, the APOE gene, has been identified with certainty.

About 30% to 40% of early onset Alzheimer's disease has been shown to be caused by mutations in either the Alzheimer precursor protein (APP) located on chromosome 21, the presenilin 1 (PS1) gene located on chromosome 14 (Sherrington et al., 1995; Hutton et al., 1996; Hardy, 1997), and its homolog presenilin 2 (PS2) located on chromosome 1 (Rogaev et al., 1995). Approximately 150 families have been identified worldwide with mutations in one of these three genes (Blacker and Tanzi, 1998). Other genes are suspected of contributing to the cause of Alzheimer's disease, but have not been proved as of early 2001 (St George-Hyslop, 2000).

Late onset familial Alzheimer's disease is mediated through susceptibility genes such as apolipoprotein E (ApoE). In humans, ApoE is found in three allelic variations that differ from one another by two amino acid substitutions at positions 112 and 158. The ApoE e4 allele had been known for some time to be associated with cardiovascular disease, before it was shown that the e4 allele was substantially over-represented among patients with Alzheimer's disease (Corder et al., 1993; Poirier et al., 1993). The homozygous state carries the most risk, mainly between the ages of 60 and 80 (Farrer et al., 1997). The heterozygous state is associated with a lower risk. Homozygosity for the e4 allele confers an approximately 50% lifetime risk for Alzheimer's disease (Henderson et al., 1995; Hyman et al., 1996; Myers et al., 1996).

Pathogenesis

The hippocampal formation is the region first affected by neuronal pathology. As the disease progresses, other limbic and cortical association areas become involved. Microscopically, prominent cell loss and synapse loss in the hippocampus and neocortex are seen in patients with Alzheimer's disease. A strong correlation is seen between these features and cognitive status (DeKosky and Scheff, 1990; Terry et al., 1991; Gomez-Isla et al., 1997). A variety of mechanisms might be the proximate causes of reduction in synaptic density and eventually neuronal loss (e.g., inflammation-induced cell injury, oxidative cellular injury, apoptotic cell death) or alteration in cellular respiratory function. Convergent evidence from the autosomal-dominant genetic defects associated with familial Alzheimer's disease, from *in vitro* molecular studies and from transgenic animal models of Alzheimer's disease, imply that the overproduction of the 42-43 amino-acid amyloid beta peptide (Abeta) is the primary mechanism that drives the pathologic process. The Abeta peptide is derived from a larger protein, the amyloid precursor protein (APP). APP and its processing are discussed further in the therapy section of this chapter.

VASCULAR DEMENTIA: DEMENTIAS ASSOCIATED WITH STROKE

Cerebrovascular disease occurs commonly in the elderly (Wolf et al., 1992). Dementia associated with stroke was previously referred to as "multiinfarct dementia," but more recently, the term "vascular dementia" has been adopted. Studies in dementia clinics yield very low numbers of patients with vascular dementia, wherein pure vascular dementia occurred in only 2.4% of cases, whereas another 7.1% of patients had both Alzheimer's disease and "significant" vascular pathology (Larson et al., 1985). In contrast, population-based prevalence studies have found rates of 15% to 20% (Evans et al., 1989; Bachman et al., 1992; Canadian Study of Health and Aging, 1994; Hendrie et al., 1995; White et al., 1996). Incidence studies found about the same rate relative to Alzheimer's disease (Fratiglioni et al., 2000).

Dementia caused by a series of large cortical infarctions will have different clinical manifestations than dementia caused by arteriolar infarctions (lacunar infarctions) in the striatum and thalamus. Multiple lacunar infarctions can produce a pattern of cognitive impairment that is similar to frontotemporal dementia, caused by the deafferentation and de-efferentation of the prefrontal regions by subcortical infarctions (Wolfe et al., 1990).

Diagnostic criteria for vascular dementia (Chui et al., 1992; Roman et al., 1993) require cognitive impairment in several domains, a temporal profile of the illness compatible with a vascular cause, imaging evidence of infarctions, and neurologic examination evidence of residual deficits typical of stroke. A temporal link between stroke and dementia onset is an important feature. These criteria (Chui et al., 1992; Roman et al., 1993) have been shown to be highly specific, but somewhat insensitive. The Hachinski Ischemic Scale (Hachinski et al., 1974), which also embodies these features, excepting the imaging criteria, has been validated neuropathologically (Rosen et al., 1980; Moroney et al., 1997).

Cerebrovascular pathology in a patient with slowly evolving dementia plays an important supporting role behind Alzheimer's disease pathology (Snowdon et al., 1997; Heyman et al., 1998). Vascular risk factors—hypertension, in particular—and not just stroke specifically increase the probability of dementia (Launer et al., 1995; Prince et al., 1996; Hofman et

al., 1997). Stroke is associated with a greatly increased risk for the subsequent development of dementia (5.5 to 9 greater risk compared with nonstroke) (Tatemichi et al., 1992; Tatemichi et al., 1994; Kokmen et al., 1996). For most patients being assessed for dementia, the clinical diagnosis of vascular dementia as the exclusive and highly certain diagnosis rarely applies. Instead, clinicians will be confronted with patients having some vascular features together with Alzheimer's disease.

Recognition of vascular disease in the setting of dementia has therapeutic implications. Because individuals are occasionally found to have cerebral infarctions without antecedent clinical history (Bryan et al., 1997; Longstreth et al., 1998), detection of "silent" infarctions in a demented patient might prompt treatment with antiplatelet drugs. It might also induce a more careful look at other stroke risk factors (e.g., hypertension, smoking, or possible embolic sources).

DEMENTIAS ASSOCIATED WITH EXTRAPYRAMIDAL FEATURES

The most common disorder causing dementia associated with extrapyramidal features is one with a newly minted name, "dementia with Lewy bodies" (DLB) (McKeith et al., 1996). Other entities in the differential diagnosis of dementia with extrapyramidal features include progressive supranuclear palsy, corticobasal degeneration, striatonigral degeneration, Huntington's disease, and Wilson's disease.

Clinical Syndrome of Dementia with Lewy Bodies

The diagnostic criteria for DLB (McKeith et al., 1996) include gait and balance disturbances, dementia, prominent visual hallucinations and delusions, fluctuations in cognitive status or arousal, sleep disturbances, sensitivity to dopaminergic blocking drugs (e.g., first generation antipsychotics), and other less consistently seen symptoms and signs.

In the Framingham study (Bachman et al., 1992), for example, dementia with extrapyramidal features was diagnosed in 7.7% of cases in an epidemiologic sample. In autopsy series, DLB accounted for 25.5% of cases, and ranked behind Alzheimer's disease as the second most common dementing disorder (Galasko et al., 1994). The threefold discrepancy between epidemiologic and the neuropathologic estimates of DLB suggests that the distinct clinical manifestations of Lewy body pathology are under-recognized.

The treatment implications of a clinical diagnosis of DLB are considerable. Antipsychotic agents with dopaminergic blocking properties should not be used in these patients. Quetiapine and clozapine are the preferred antipsychotics for patients with DLB. Levodopa should be used if needed, but be alert to the possibility of worsening of delusions, hallucinations, or agitation.

FRONTOTEMPORAL DEMENTIAS

The frontotemporal dementias (FTD) are much less common than either AD, vascular dementia, or dementia associated with Parkinsonism (Stevens et al., 1998). FTD is the preferred label for this clinicopathologic entity because the FTD encompass a broader neuropathologic spectrum than just Pick's disease. Primary progressive aphasia (PPA) is a disorder with prominent expressive language disturbance relative to anterograde amnesia, and shares the same neuropathologic differential diagnosis as FTD.

Clinical Syndrome

The term "dysexecutive syndrome" has been applied to the cognitive syndrome of patients with FTD who have grossly disturbed abstract reasoning, poor judgment, and reduced mental flexibility (Neary et al., 1988; Gustafson, 1993; The Lund and Manchester Groups, 1994). Psychometric testing plays an essential role in the diagnosis of FTD because the bedside mental status examination lacks sensitivity for early signs of executive dysfunction. Behavioral disturbances, which are particularly prominent, can erroneously be attributed to primary psychiatric diseases. Patients may become very withdrawn, and may be treated for depression to no avail. Alternatively, patients may become socially inappropriate, excessively ebullient, inappropriately aggressive, or get themselves into trouble because of grossly impaired judgment. Diagnostic criteria for FTD that come from a recent consensus conference (Neary et al., 1998) reflect the cognitive and behavioral characteristics of FTD observed in pathologically verified cases.

Neuroimaging may show evidence of frontal or anterior temporal atrophy, although not in all cases, especially early in the disease (Knopman et al., 1990). Functional imaging with single photon emission computed tomography (SPECT) or positron emission tomography (PET) may be more sensitive for the early diagnosis of FTD (Kamo et al., 1987; Miller et al., 1991; Friedland et al., 1993; Read et al., 1995; Talbot et al., 1998). Data are still limited on the actual clinical utility of functional imaging in the differential diagnosis of dementia and FTD.

Some cases of FTD have been associated with amyotrophic lateral sclerosis (Neary et al., 1990). In these cases, the bulbar dysfunction that occurs is associated with a much reduced life expectancy.

Primary Progressive Aphasia

The distinctive features of PPA are the excess dysfunction of expressive language and the relative absence of anterograde amnesia (Kirshner et al., 1987; Snowden and Neary, 1993; Kertesz et al., 1994; Snowdon et al., 1996). Conversational speech is nonfluent, hesitant, and filled with stammering and pauses for word finding. Comprehension is affected but sometimes only to a minor degree. Other cognitive functions may be spared. The mental status examination scores and a history of deficits are pivotal in the diagnosis of PPA. Variability is seen in the extent to which progressive aphasia progresses to global dementia. As with FTD, patients with PPA may show focal atrophy on structural imaging, especially of the dominant hemisphere's peri-Sylvian region. Similarly, functional imaging may detect hypometabolism in that region. Neither feature is necessary for the diagnosis, however.

Genetics

Many patients with FTD have a positive family history for similar dementias. Mutations in the *tau* gene located on chromosome 17 are associated with the FTD (Hutton et al., 1998; Poorkaj et al., 1998; Spillantini et al., 1998). These mutations lead to altered proportions of the various forms of *tau* that, in turn, lead to deposition of hyperphosphorylated *tau*. A number of other families with FTD but no linkage to the *tau* gene have also been recognized (Foster et al., 1997), but not yet linked to a specific gene.

Treatment and Management

Correct diagnosis of the FTD spares the patient from futile attempts to treat depression or mania. If patients with PPA are incorrectly diagnosed with stroke, they may be unnecessarily subjected to carotid angiography or surgery. Patients with PPA will be managed differently from those with Alzheimer's disease. Because their recent memory is not severely impaired, they may be given more independence than the typical patient with Alzheimer's disease. Although a diagnosis of FTD or PPA carries the prognosis of inexorable decline, families appreciate the more accurate prognostication that comes with the proper diagnosis. The agitation that occurs in patients with

FTC can be treated in the same manner as that in Alzheimer's disease. Nonpharmacologic behavior management is often sufficient to control the disruptive behaviors in patients with FTD once the caregivers understand the nature of the disease.

PRIMARY PHARMACOTHERAPY FOR ALZHEIMER'S DISEASE

Cholinesterase Inhibitor Drugs

Drugs used to treat patients with Alzheimer's disease are found in Table 21-1.

Autopsy-based neurochemical studies have demonstrated deficits in the enzymes responsible for synthesis of acetylcholine (Davies and Maloney, 1976; Perry et al., 1978). Based on these findings, clinical trials with various approaches have led to the commercial availability of two cholinesterase inhibitors (ChEI), donepezil and rivastigmine, by prescription in the United States.

Although tacrine (Knapp et al., 1994) was the first of the ChEI to be marketed, its short half-life and hepatotoxicity foiled its chances for success. This opened the door for several other agents. Pivotal trials for donepezil (Rogers, Farlow, et al., 1998; Burns et al., 1999), rivastigmine (Corey-Bloom et al., 1998; Rosler et al., 1999), and galantamine (Raskind et al., 2000; Tariot et al., 2000) have appeared.

Without doubt, the ChEI drugs have effects on the symptoms of Alzheimer's disease, although their effect beyond 1 year of therapy is still poorly understood. Several lines of evidence—the clinical trials cited above, open-label long-term extension studies with donepezil (Rogers and Friedhoff, 1998), and a recently completed 1-year study (Mohs et al., 2001)—put the effect size of these drugs in the range of about 6 to 9 months in delay of symptoms.

In a dose-related fashion, gastrointestinal side effects (e.g., nausea, diarrhea, vomiting, or anorexia) occur in a subset of patients. These side effects are more likely with more rapid dose escalation regimens. Differences between donepezil, galantamine, and rivastigmine in rates of nausea, diarrhea, and vomiting are somewhat difficult to interpret when taken from clinical trials that employed different dose escalation strategies. Taking the adverse event profiles of the drugs at their face values, rivastigmine appears to have the highest rate of gastrointestinal side effects, whereas donepezil had the lowest, and galantamine intermediate.

Strategies Aimed at Beta-Amyloid Processing

The Abeta molecule in its soluble form is considered to be the pathogenic molecule in Alzheimer's disease (McLean et al., 1999); hence, it has become the focus for therapeutic interventions. The fate of APP and the subsequent production of the Abeta peptide are determined by the actions of three secretases that cleave APP into different fragments. Overactivity of the beta or gamma secretases or an underactivity of the alpha secretase could lead to overproduction of the Abeta peptide. The gamma secretase has been found to be closely linked to presenilin (Xia et al., 1998; Wolfe et al., 1999; Li et al., 2000). Mutations in the presenilin gene are assumed to produce a gain in function of gamma secretase, thereby generating the higher loads of Abeta observed in models of presenilin mutants (Duff et al., 1996). The beta secretase has also been identified (Hussain et al., 1999; Sinha et al., 1999; Vassar et al., 1999; Yan et al., 1999). Armed with the knowledge about the secretases as a prime target for preventing Alzheimer's disease at the molecular level, initial human studies of such agents were in phase I testing at the end of 2000. Important questions about safety must, of course, first be answered. Ultimately, if these agents prove to be safe, trials meant to prove efficacy have to be designed and executed.

The Immunization Hypothesis

Schenk et al. (1999) reported protective effects of monthly intraperitoneal injections of the Abeta peptide itself into transgenic mice that carried the APP

TABLE 21-1. *Drugs for the treatment of Alzheimer's disease*

Drug	Dosage	Side effects
Donepezil	Dose escalation from 5 mg q.d. to 10 mg	Nausea, diarrhea
Rivastigmine	Dose escalation from 1.5 mg b.i.d. to 6 mg b.i.d.	Nausea, diarrhea, vomiting
Galantamine	Dose escalation from 4 mg b.i.d. to 12 mg b.i.d.	Nausea, diarrhea
Vitamin E	800–1,000 IU b.i.d.	None

b.i.d., twice daily; q.d., every day.

717 mutation (Games et al., 1995) and that developed Abeta-centered neuritic plaques by 1 year of age. With immunizations near birth, Abeta pathology was virtually prevented when the mice were killed at 18 months of age. Immunizations at 11 months of age produced nearly as dramatic results. Others (Weiner et al., 2000) reported replication of the findings, but in this latter study, Abeta peptide was delivered to the mice via intranasal administration. The immunization model is now being assessed in phase I safety trials. It is not clear when efficacy trials will begin, assuming that safety is demonstrated in phase I trials.

Estrogen Studies

Despite a sound basis in epidemiologic studies and basic neuroscience, expectations for estrogen as a treatment for symptomatic Alzheimer's disease suffered a serious blow with the publication of two negative studies (Henderson et al., 2000; Mulnard et al., 2000). The larger of the two involved more than 120 women with mild Alzheimer's disease. Orally administered equine estrogens had no effect on cognitive function or any other measure of the disease. Other studies with estrogen are ongoing. In a study with a prevention design, the Women's Health Initiative Memory study (Shumaker and Rapp, 1996) 8,000 women treated with estrogen-progesterone or placebo are being followed for many years to establish definitively whether estrogen-progesterone has any protective effects against the development of Alzheimer's disease.

Antiinflammatory Drugs

A 1-year trial of low dose prednisone (1 month of 20 mg/d followed by 11 months of 10 mg/d) versus placebo in 138 patients with symptomatic mild to moderate Alzheimer's disease (Aisen et al., 2000) failed to show benefits. A small study with the NSAID diclofenac failed to demonstrate any differences between placebo-treated and diclofenac-treated patients, except in dropout rates (Scharf et al., 1999). Half of those treated with NSAID withdrew before the end of the 25-week trial. Other studies of NSAID are underway.

Memantine

Memantine antagonizes glutamate-gated NMDA receptor channels. Studies a decade ago suggested that it was effective in treating patients with Alzheimer's disease, but findings from two new studies focusing on moderately to severely demented patients (Winblad and Poritis, 1999; Reisberg et al., 2000) might be propelling it to approval as an anti-dementia agent.

Gingko Biloba

A study of gingko biloba that appeared in 1997 (Le Bars et al., 1997) generated interest in this alternative medicine. However, a second multicenter study with gingko biloba that involved 214 subjects with dementia, either from Alzheimer's disease or vascular disease, failed to show any benefits (van Dongen et al., 2000).

TREATMENT OF AGITATION

Disruptive, troublesome behaviors, generically referred to as "agitation," occur commonly in severe dementia, and may occur at earlier stages as well (Levy et al., 1996; Mega et al., 1996; Devanand et al., 1997; Marin et al., 1997). Managing agitation can require both pharmacologic and nonpharmacologic techniques. Education and training of family and professional caregivers can reduce agitation. When any form of agitation occurs in a patient with dementia, it is possible that the disruptive behavior is being caused by some underlying physical ailment, such as an unrecognized urinary tract function. Physical aggressiveness often, but not always, requires pharmacologic treatment. Hallucinations and delusions may not require active treatment if they are not disruptive, anxiety-provoking, or frightening. Caregivers can become intensely uncomfortable or embarrassed when the patient reports strangers in the home or other bizarre occurrences, but reassurance can be sufficient in some cases. Once the nature of the delusions or hallucinations is explained to the caregivers, they tend to become much more tolerant of the patient's behavior.

No consensus exists regarding a choice of medication to use as a first-line treatment of agitation. Medications that are sometimes used include benzodiazepines, trazodone, buspirone, valproic acid, or carbamazepine (1998; Tariot et al., 1998). If these fail, antipsychotics might be the next choice. Most physicians who treat patients with dementia regard the antipsychotics as the most effective agents (1998). Clozapine, risperidone, olanzapine, and quetiapine are the currently available second-generation antipsychotics. Low dose risperidone is well tolerated, although not free of extrapyramidal side effects in the treatment of agitation in institutionalized patients with dementia (Goldberg and Goldberg, 1997). Two recent clinical trials showed that risperidone was superior to placebo in treating agitation (De Deyn et al., 1999; Katz et al.,

1999). Quetiapine, on the other hand, may be a preferred agent, in that it does not produce as much extrapyramidal dysfunction as risperidone.

TREATMENT OF SLEEP DISTURBANCES

Disturbances of nocturnal sleep, which are also common in dementia, are a source of considerable caregiver burden and stress. Disruptive nighttime sleep in a patient with dementia is often caused by daytime sleeping or allowing the patient to retire for the evening too early. When sleep disturbances result from either of these causes, sedative use is likely to be ineffective. Management of sleep disorders, therefore, often involves service interventions to manage the daytime and early evening behavior, which in turn may require the use of such social services as daycare or home health aides. Involving a patient in daycare may keep the patient occupied and more active during the daytime and, hence, more likely to sleep at night. If the sleep disorder proves to be caused by disordered sleep patterns independent of daytime sleeping, trazodone was the first choice in the expert consensus survey, with zolpidem and the short-acting benzodiazepines being remote second-line choices (Anonymous, 1998).

TREATMENT OF ANXIETY

Anxiety is a common symptom in patients with Alzheimer's disease (Mega et al., 1996). It is often accompanied by symptoms of depression (e.g., tearfulness, claims of feeling worthless) or symptoms of paranoia (e.g., delusions and hallucinations). In the former context, patients appear primarily depressed but become very anxious and agitated if, for example, their caregivers leave them at a daycare facility or if they simply leave the patient's sight. Treatment with trazodone or buspirone was the first-line choice in the consensus survey (Anonymous, 1998). Sometimes patients with dementia experience considerable anxiety in the context of disturbing hallucinations or delusions. The anxiety, rather than the delusion, may become the major management focus. Use of antipsychotic agents might be more appropriate when anxiety occurs in the context of delusional thinking. (Treatment of depression in dementia is covered in depth in Chapter 31.)

ACKNOWLEDGMENTS

This work was supported in part by grants AG 08031 (Mayo Alzheimer's Disease Center) and AG 06786 (Mayo Alzheimer's Disease Patient Registry) from the National Institute on Aging.

Disclosure: Dr. Knopman has served as a paid consultant to Janssen, Takeda, Parke-Davis, Bayer, Eisai/Pfizer, and Novartis in the past 5 years.

REFERENCES

Anonymous. Treatment of agitation in older persons with dementia. *Postgrad Med* 1998;Spec No:1–88.

Canadian study of health and aging: study methods and prevalence of dementia. CMAJ. 1994;150:899–913.

Practice parameter for diagnosis and evaluation of dementia [summary statement]. Report of the Quality Standards Subcommittee of the American Academy of Neurology. *Neurology* 44: 2203–2206.

Treatment of special populations with the atypical antipsychotics. Collaborative Working Group on Clinical Trial Evaluations. *J Clin Psychiatry* 1998;59(Suppl 12): 46–52.

Aisen PS, Davis KL, Berg JD, et al. A randomized controlled trial of prednisone in Alzheimer's disease. Alzheimer's Disease Cooperative Study. *Neurology* 2000; 54:588–593.

American Psychiatric Association. *Diagnostic and statistical manual of mental disorders*, 4th ed. Washington, DC: American Psychiatric Association, 1994.

Andersen K, Launer LJ, Ott A, et al. Do nonsteroidal anti-inflammatory drugs decrease the risk for Alzheimer's disease? The Rotterdam Study. *Neurology* 1995;45:1441–1445.

Bachman DL, Wolf PA, Linn R, et al. Prevalence of dementia and probable senile dementia of the Alzheimer type in the Framingham Study. *Neurology* 1992; 42:115–119.

Bachman DL, Wolf PA, Linn RT, et al. Incidence of dementia and probable Alzheimer's disease in a general population: the Framingham Study. *Neurology* 1993;43:515–519.

Beard CM, Kokmen E, Sigler C, et al. Cause of death in Alzheimer's disease. *Ann Epidemiol* 1996;6:195–200.

Berg L, McKeel DW Jr, Miller JP, et al. Clinicopathologic studies in cognitively healthy aging and Alzheimer's disease: relation of histologic markers to dementia severity, age, sex, and apolipoprotein E genotype. *Arch Neurol* 1998;55:326–335.

Bjertness E, Candy JM, Torvik A, et al. Content of brain aluminum is not elevated in Alzheimer disease. *Alzheimer Dis Assoc Disord* 1996;10:171–174.

Blacker D, Tanzi RE. The genetics of Alzheimer disease: current status and future prospects. *Arch Neurol* 1998;55: 294–296.

Bowen JD, Malter AD, Sheppard L, et al. Predictors of mortality in patients diagnosed with probable Alzheimer's disease. *Neurology* 1996;47:433–439.

Breitner JC, Gau BA, Welsh KA, et al. Inverse association of anti-inflammatory treatments and Alzheimer's disease: initial results of a co-twin control study. *Neurology* 1994; 44:227–232.

Brenner DE, Kukull WA, van Belle G, et al. Relationship between cigarette smoking and Alzheimer's disease in a population-based case-control study. *Neurology* 1993;43: 293–300.

Brun A. Frontal lobe degeneration of non-Alzheimer type revisited. *Dementia* 1993;4:126–131.

Bryan RN, Wells SW, Miller TJ, et al. Infarctlike lesions in the brain: prevalence and anatomic characteristics at MR imaging of the elderly—data from the Cardiovascular Health Study. *Radiology* 1997;202:47–54.

Burns A, Rossor M, Hecker J, et al. The Effects of donepezil in Alzheimer's disease. Results from a multinational trial. *Dement Geriatr Cogn Disord* 1999;10:237–244.

Callahan CM, Hall KS, Hui SL, et al. Relationship of age, education, and occupation with dementia among a community-based sample of African Americans. *Arch Neurol* 1996;53:134–140.

Callahan CM, Hendrie HC, Tierney WM. Documentation and evaluation of cognitive impairment in elderly primary care patients. *Ann Intern Med* 1995;122:422–429.

Carmelli D, Swan GE, Reed T, et al. Midlife cardiovascular risk factors, ApoE, and cognitive decline in elderly male twins. *Neurology* 1998;50:1580–1585.

Chui HC, Lyness SA, Sobel E, et al. Extrapyramidal signs and psychiatric symptoms predict faster cognitive decline in Alzheimer's disease. *Arch Neurol* 1994;51:676–681.

Chui HC, Victoroff JI, Margolin D, et al. Criteria for the diagnosis of ischemic vascular dementia proposed by the State of California Alzheimer's Disease Diagnostic and Treatment Centers. *Neurology* 1992;42:473–480.

Cobb JL, Wolf PA, Au R, et al. The effect of education on the incidence of dementia and Alzheimer's disease in the Framingham Study. *Neurology* 1995;45:1707–1712.

Corder EH, Saunders AM, Strittmatter WJ, et al. Gene dose of apolipoprotein E type 4 allele and the risk of Alzheimer's disease in late onset families. *Science* 1993;261:921–923.

Corey-Bloom J, Anand R, Veach J, for the ENA 713 B352 Study Group. A randomized trial evaluating the efficacy and safety of ENA 713 (rivastigmine tartrate), a new acetylcholinesterase inhibitor, in patients with mild to moderately severe Alzheimer's disease. *International Journal of Geriatric Psychopharmacology* 1998;1:55–65.

Corey-Bloom J, Thal LJ, Galasko D, et al. Diagnosis and evaluation of dementia. *Neurology* 1995;45:211–218.

Crapper DR, Krishnan SS, De Boni U, et al. Aluminum: a possible neurotoxic agent in Alzheimer's disease. *Transactions of the American Neurological Association* 1975;100:154–156.

Crystal HA, Horoupian DS, Katzman R, et al. Biopsy-proved Alzheimer disease presenting as a right parietal lobe syndrome. *Ann Neurol* 1982;12:186–188.

Davies P, Maloney AJ. Selective loss of central cholinergic neurons in Alzheimer's disease. *Lancet* 1976;2:1403.

De Deyn PP, Rabheru K, Rasmussen A, et al. A randomized trial of risperidone, placebo, and haloperidol for behavioral symptoms of dementia. *Neurology* 1999;53:946–955.

DeKosky ST, Scheff SW. Synapse loss in frontal cortex biopsies in Alzheimer's disease: correlation with cognitive severity. *Ann Neurol* 1990;27:457–464.

Devanand DP, Jacobs DM, Tang MX, et al. The course of psychopathologic features in mild to moderate Alzheimer disease. *Arch Gen Psychiatry* 1997;54:257–263.

Duff K, Eckman C, Zehr C, et al. Increased amyloid-beta42 (43) in brains of mice expressing mutant presenilin 1. *Nature* 1996;383:710–713.

Eefsting JA, Boersma F, Van den Brink W, et al. Differences in prevalence of dementia based on community survey and general practitioner recognition. *Psychol Med* 1996;26:1223–1230.

Elias MF, Wolf PA, D'Agostino RB, et al. Untreated blood pressure level is inversely related to cognitive functioning: the Framingham Study. *Am J Epidemiol* 1993;138:353–364.

Evans DA, Funkenstein HH, Albert MS, et al. Prevalence of Alzheimer's disease in a community population of older persons. Higher than previously reported. *JAMA* 1989;262:2551–2556.

Farrer LA, Cupples LA, Haines JL, et al. Effects of age, sex, and ethnicity on the association between apolipoprotein E genotype and Alzheimer disease. A meta-analysis. APOE and Alzheimer Disease Meta Analysis Consortium. *JAMA* 1997;278:1349–1356.

Fillenbaum GG, Heyman A, Huber MS, et al. The prevalence and 3-year incidence of dementia in older black and white community residents. *J Clin Epidemiol* 1998;51:587–595.

Folstein MF, Folstein SE, McHugh PR. "Mini-mental state." A practical method for grading the cognitive state of patients for the clinician. *J Psychiatr Res* 1975;12:189–198.

Ford AB, Mefrouche Z, Friedland RP, et al. Smoking and cognitive impairment: a population-based study. *J Am Geriatr Soc* 1996;44:905–909.

Forsell Y, Winblad B. Major depression in a population of demented and nondemented older people: prevalence and correlates. *J Am Geriatr Soc* 1998;46:27–30.

Foster NL, Wilhelmsen K, Sima AA, et al. Frontotemporal dementia and parkinsonism linked to chromosome 17: a consensus conference. Conference participants. *Ann Neurol* 1997;41:706–715.

Fratiglioni L, Launer LJ, Andersen K, et al. Incidence of dementia and major subtypes in Europe: a collaborative study of population-based cohorts. Neurologic Diseases in the Elderly Research Group. *Neurology* 2000;54:S10–S15.

Friedland RP, Koss E, Lerner A, et al. Functional imaging, the frontal lobes, and dementia. *Dementia* 1993;4:192–203.

Galanis DJ, Petrovitch H, Launer LJ, et al. Smoking history in middle age and subsequent cognitive performance in elderly Japanese-American men. The Honolulu-Asia Aging Study. *Am J Epidemiol* 1997;145:507–515.

Galasko D, Corey-Bloom J, Thal LJ. Monitoring progression in Alzheimer's disease. *J Am Geriatr Soc* 1991;39:932–941.

Galasko D, Hansen LA, Katzman R, et al. Clinical-neuropathological correlations in Alzheimer's disease and related dementias. *Arch Neurol* 1994;51:888–895.

Galasko D, Klauber MR, Hofstetter CR, et al. The Mini-Mental State Examination in the early diagnosis of Alzheimer's disease. *Arch Neurol* 1990;47:49–52.

Games D, Adams D, Alessandrini R, et al. Alzheimer-type neuropathology in transgenic mice overexpressing V717F beta-amyloid precursor protein. *Nature* 1995;373:523–527.

Gao S, Hendrie HC, Hall KS, et al. The relationships between age, sex, and the incidence of dementia and Alzheimer disease: a meta-analysis. *Arch Gen Psychiatry* 1998;55:809–815.

Goldberg RJ, Goldberg J. Risperidone for dementia-related disturbed behavior in nursing home residents: a clinical experience. *Int Psychogeriatr* 1997;9:65–68.

Gomez-Isla T, Hollister R, West H, et al. Neuronal loss correlates with but exceeds neurofibrillary tangles in Alzheimer's disease. *Ann Neurol* 1997;41:17–24.

Good PF, Perl DP, Bierer LM, et al. Selective accumulation of aluminum and iron in the neurofibrillary tangles of Alzheimer's disease: a laser microprobe (LAMMA) study. *Ann Neurol* 1992;31:286–292.

Graff-Radford NR, Bolling JP, Earnest FT, et al. Simultanagnosia as the initial sign of degenerative dementia. *Mayo Clin Proc* 1993;68:955–964.

Graves AB, Larson EB, Edland SD, et al. Prevalence of dementia and its subtypes in the Japanese American population of King County, Washington state. The Kame Project. *Am J Epidemiol* 1996;144:760–771.

Graves AB, van Duijn CM, Chandra V, et al. Alcohol and tobacco consumption as risk factors for Alzheimer's disease: a collaborative re-analysis of case-control studies. EURODEM Risk Factors Research Group. *Int J Epidemiol* 1991;20(Suppl 2):S48–S57.

Graves AB, White E, Koepsell TD, et al. The association between aluminum-containing products and Alzheimer's disease. *J Clin Epidemiol* 1990;43:35–44.

Green J, Morris JC, Sandson J, et al. Progressive aphasia: a precursor of global dementia? *Neurology* 1990;40: 423–429.

Grut M, Jorm AF, Fratiglioni L, et al. Memory complaints of elderly people in a population survey: variation according to dementia stage and depression. *J Am Geriatr Soc* 1993; 41:1295–300.

Gustafson L. Clinical picture of frontal lobe degeneration of non-Alzheimer type. *Dementia* 1993;4:143–148.

Hachinski V. Aluminum exposure and risk of Alzheimer disease. *Arch Neurol* 1998;55:742.

Hachinski VC, Lassen NA, Marshall J. Multi-infarct dementia. A cause of mental deterioration in the elderly. *Lancet* 1974;2:207–210.

Hanninen T, Hallikainen M, Koivisto K, et al. A follow-up study of age-associated memory impairment: neuropsychological predictors of dementia. *J Am Geriatr Soc* 1995;43:1007–1015.

Hardy J. Amyloid, the presenilins and Alzheimer's disease. *Trends Neurosci* 1997;20:154–159.

Hebert LE, Scherr PA, Beckett LA, et al. Age-specific incidence of Alzheimer's disease in a community population. *JAMA* 1995;273:1354–1359.

Hebert LE, Scherr PA, Beckett LA, et al. Relation of smoking and alcohol consumption to incident Alzheimer's disease. *Am J Epidemiol* 1992;135:347–355.

Henderson AS, Easteal S, Jorm AF, et al. Apolipoprotein E allele epsilon 4, dementia, and cognitive decline in a population sample. *Lancet* 1995;346:1387–1390.

Henderson VW, Paganini-Hill A, Miller BL, et al. Estrogen for Alzheimer's disease in women: randomized, double-blind, placebo-controlled trial. *Neurology* 2000;54: 295–301.

Hendrie HC, Osuntokun BO, Hall KS, et al. Prevalence of Alzheimer's disease and dementia in two communities: Nigerian Africans and African Americans. *Am J Psychiatry* 1995;152:1485–1492.

Heyman A, Fillenbaum GG, Welsh-Bohmer KA, et al. Cerebral infarcts in patients with autopsy-proven Alzheimer's disease: CERAD, part XVIII. Consortium to Establish a Registry for Alzheimer's Disease. *Neurology* 1998;51: 159–62.

Heyman A, Peterson B, Fillenbaum G, et al. The consortium to establish a registry for Alzheimer's disease (CERAD). Part XIV: Demographic and clinical predictors of survival in patients with Alzheimer's disease. *Neurology* 1996;46: 656–660.

Heyman A, Peterson B, Fillenbaum G, et al. Predictors of time to institutionalization of patients with Alzheimer's disease: the CERAD experience, part XVII. *Neurology* 1997;48:1304–1309.

Hofman A, Ott A, Breteler MM, et al. Atherosclerosis, apolipoprotein E, and prevalence of dementia and Alzheimer's disease in the Rotterdam Study. *Lancet* 1997; 349:151–154.

Holmes C, Cairns N, Lantos P, et al. Validity of current clinical criteria for Alzheimer's disease, vascular dementia and dementia with Lewy bodies. *Br J Psychiatry* 1999; 174:45–50.

Hussain I, Powell D, Howlett DR, et al. Identification of a novel aspartic protease (Asp 2) as beta-secretase. *Mol Cell Neurosci* 1999;14:419–427.

Hutton M, Busfield F, Wragg M, et al. Complete analysis of the presenilin 1 gene in early onset Alzheimer's disease. *Neuroreport* 1996;7:801–805.

Hutton M, Lendon CL, Rizzu P, et al. Association of missense and 58-splice-site mutations in tau with the inherited dementia FTDP-17. *Nature* 1998;393:702–705.

Hyman BT, Gomez-Isla T, Briggs M, et al. Apolipoprotein E and cognitive change in an elderly population. *Ann Neurol* 1996;40:55–66.

Jobst KA, Barnetson LP, Shepstone BJ. Accurate prediction of histologically confirmed Alzheimer's disease and the differential diagnosis of dementia: the use of NINCDS-ADRDA and DSM- III-R criteria, SPECT, X-ray CT, and apo E4 in medial temporal lobe dementias. Oxford Project to Investigate Memory and Aging. *Int Psychogeriatr* 1998;10:271–302.

Jorm AF, Jolley D. The incidence of dementia: a meta-analysis. *Neurology* 1998;51:728–733.

Kamo H, McGeer PL, Harrop R, et al. Positron emission tomography and histopathology in Pick's disease. *Neurology* 1987;37:439–445.

Katz IR, Jeste DV, Mintzer JE, et al. Comparison of risperidone and placebo for psychosis and behavioral disturbances associated with dementia: a randomized, double-blind trial. Risperidone Study Group. *J Clin Psychiatry* 1999;60:107–115.

Katzman R, Hill LR, Yu ES, et al. The malignancy of dementia. Predictors of mortality in clinically diagnosed dementia in a population survey of Shanghai, China. *Arch Neurol* 1994;51:1220–1225.

Kawas C, Resnick S, Morrison A, et al. A prospective study of estrogen replacement therapy and the risk of developing Alzheimer's disease: the Baltimore Longitudinal Study of Aging. *Neurology* 1997;48: 1517–1521.

Kertesz A, Hudson L, Mackenzie IR, et al. The pathology and nosology of primary progressive aphasia. *Neurology* 1994;44:2065–2072.

Kirshner HS, Tanridag O, Thurman L, et al. Progressive aphasia without dementia: two cases with focal spongiform degeneration. *Ann Neurol* 1987;22:527–532.

Knapp MJ, Knopman DS, Solomon PR, et al. A 30-week randomized controlled trial of high-dose tacrine in patients with Alzheimer's disease. The Tacrine Study Group. *JAMA* 1994;271:985–991.

Knopman D, Schneider L, Davis K, et al. Long-term tacrine (Cognex) treatment: effects on nursing home placement and mortality, Tacrine Study Group. *Neurology* 1996;47: 166–177.

Knopman DS, Mastri AR, Frey et al. Dementia lacking distinctive histologic features: a common non-Alzheimer degenerative dementia. *Neurology* 1990;40:251–256.

Kokmen E, Beard CM, Offord KP, et al. Prevalence of medically diagnosed dementia in a defined United States population: Rochester, Minnesota, January 1, 1975. *Neurology* 1989;39:773–776.

Kokmen E, Whisnant JP, O'Fallon WM, et al. Dementia after ischemic stroke: a population-based study in Rochester, Minnesota (1960-1984). *Neurology* 1996;46: 154–159.

Koss E, Patterson MB, Ownby R, et al. Memory evaluation in Alzheimer's disease. Caregivers' appraisals and objective testing. *Arch Neurol* 1993;50:92–97.

Kukull WA, Brenner DE, Speck CE, et al. Causes of death associated with Alzheimer disease: variation by level of cognitive impairment before death. *J Am Geriatr Soc* 1994;42:723–726.

Kukull WA, Larson EB, Bowen JD, et al. Solvent exposure as a risk factor for Alzheimer's disease: a case- control study. *Am J Epidemiol* 1995;141:1059–1071.

Larson EB, Reifler BV, Sumi SM, et al. Diagnostic evaluation of 200 elderly outpatients with suspected dementia. *J Gerontol* 1985;40:536–543.

Launer LJ, Masaki K, Petrovitch H, et al. The association between midlife blood pressure levels and late-life cognitive function. The Honolulu-Asia Aging Study. *JAMA* 1995; 274:1846–1851.

Lautenschlager NT, Cupples LA, Rao VS, et al. Risk of dementia among relatives of Alzheimer's disease patients in the MIRAGE study: what is in store for the oldest old? *Neurology* 1996;46:641–650.

Le Bars PL, Katz MM, Berman N, et al. A placebo-controlled, double-blind, randomized trial of an extract of ginkgo biloba for dementia. North American EGb Study Group. *JAMA* 1997;278:1327–1332.

Levine DN, Lee JM, Fisher CM. The visual variant of Alzheimer's disease: a clinicopathologic case study. *Neurology* 1993;43:305–313.

Levy ML, Cummings JL, Fairbanks LA, et al. Longitudinal assessment of symptoms of depression, agitation, and psychosis in 181 patients with Alzheimer's disease. *Am J Psychiatry* 1996;153:1438–1443.

Li YM, Lai MT, Xu M, et al. Presenilin 1 is linked with gamma-secretase activity in the detergent solubilized state. *Proc Natl Acad Sci USA* 2000;97:6138–6143.

Lim A, Tsuang D, Kukull W, et al. Clinico-neuropathological correlation of Alzheimer's disease in a community-based case series. *J Am Geriatr Soc* 1999;47:564–569.

Longstreth WT Jr, Bernick C, Manolio TA, et al. Lacunar infarcts defined by magnetic resonance imaging of 3660 elderly people: the Cardiovascular Health Study. *Arch Neurol* 1998;55:1217–1225.

Lopez OL, Becker JT, Somsak D, et al. Awareness of cognitive deficits and anosognosia in probable Alzheimer's disease. *Eur Neurol* 1994;34:277–282.

Lopez OL, Wisnieski SR, Becker JT, et al. Extrapyramidal signs in patients with probable Alzheimer disease. *Arch Neurol* 1997;54:969–975.

The Lund and Manchester Groups. Clinical and neuropathological criteria for frontotemporal dementia. *J Neurol Neurosurg Psychiatry* 1994;57:416–418.

Mackenzie TB, Robiner WN, Knopman DS. Differences between patient and family assessments of depression in Alzheimer's disease. *Am J Psychiatry* 1989;146: 1174–1178.

Marin DB, Green CR, Schmeidler J, et al. Noncognitive disturbances in Alzheimer's disease: frequency, longitudinal course, and relationship to cognitive symptoms. *J Am Geriatr Soc* 1997;45:1331–1338.

Martin DC, Miller J, Kapoor W, et al. Clinical prediction rules for computed tomographic scanning in senile dementia. *Arch Intern Med* 1987;147:77–80.

Massoud F, Devi G, Stern Y, et al. A clinicopathological comparison of community-based and clinic-based cohorts of patients with dementia. *Arch Neurol* 1999;56: 1368–1373.

Mayeux R, Saunders AM, Shea S, et al. Utility of the apolipoprotein E genotype in the diagnosis of Alzheimer's disease. Alzheimer's Disease Centers Consortium on Apolipoprotein E and Alzheimer's Disease. *N Engl J Med* 1998;338:506–511.

McGeer PL, Schulzer M, McGeer EG. Arthritis and anti-inflammatory agents as possible protective factors for Alzheimer's disease: a review of 17 epidemiologic studies. *Neurology* 1996;47:425–432.

McKeith IG, Galasko D, Kosaka K, et al. Consensus guidelines for the clinical and pathologic diagnosis of dementia with Lewy bodies (DLB): report of the consortium on DLB international workshop. *Neurology*. 1996;47: 1113–1124.

McKhann G, Drachman D, Folstein M, et al. Clinical diagnosis of Alzheimer's disease: report of the NINCDS-ADRDA Work Group under the auspices of Department of Health and Human Services Task Force on Alzheimer's Disease. *Neurology* 1984;34:939–944.

McLean CA, Cherny RA, Fraser FW, et al. Soluble pool of Abeta amyloid as a determinant of severity of neurodegeneration in Alzheimer's disease. *Ann Neurol* 1999;46: 860–866.

Mega MS, Cummings JL, Fiorello T, et al. The spectrum of behavioral changes in Alzheimer's disease. *Neurology* 1996;46:130–135.

Mendez MF, Mendez MA, Martin R, et al. Complex visual disturbances in Alzheimer's disease. *Neurology* 1990;40: 439–443.

Miller BL, Cummings JL, Villanueva-Meyer J, et al. Frontal lobe degeneration: clinical, neuropsychological, and SPECT characteristics. *Neurology* 1991;41:1374–1382.

Miller BL, Ikonte C, Ponton M, et al. A study of the Lund-Manchester research criteria for frontotemporal dementia: clinical and single-photon emission CT correlations. *Neurology* 1997;48:937–942.

Mohs RC, Doody RS, Morris JC , et al. A 1-year placebo-controlled preservation of function survival study of donepezil in AD patients. *Neurology* 2001;57:481–488..

Moroney JT, Bagiella E, Desmond DW, et al. Meta-analysis of the Hachinski Ischemic Score in pathologically verified dementias. *Neurology* 1997;49:1096–1105.

Morris JC, Edland S, Clark C, et al. The consortium to establish a registry for Alzheimer's disease (CERAD). Part IV. Rates of cognitive change in the longitudinal assessment of probable Alzheimer's disease. *Neurology* 1993; 43:2457–2465.

Morris JC, Heyman A, Mohs RC, et al. The Consortium to Establish a Registry for Alzheimer's Disease (CERAD).

Part I. Clinical and neuropsychological assessment of Alzheimer's disease. *Neurology* 1989;39:1159–1165.

Mulnard RA, Cotman CW, Kawas C, et al. Estrogen replacement therapy for treatment of mild to moderate Alzheimer disease: a randomized controlled trial. Alzheimer's Disease Cooperative Study. *JAMA* 2000;283:1007–1015.

Myers RH, Schaefer EJ, Wilson PW, et al. Apolipoprotein E epsilon4 association with dementia in a population- based study: The Framingham study. *Neurology* 1996;46: 673–677.

Neary D, Snowden JS, Gustafson L, et al. Frontotemporal lobar degeneration: a consensus on clinical diagnostic criteria. *Neurology* 1998;51:1546–1554.

Neary D, Snowden JS, Mann DM, et al. Frontal lobe dementia and motor neuron disease. *J Neurol Neurosurg Psychiatry* 1990;53:23–32.

Neary D, Snowden JS, Northen B, et al. Dementia of frontal lobe type. *J Neurol Neurosurg Psychiatry* 1988;51: 353–361.

Oppenheim G. The earliest signs of Alzheimer's disease. *J Geriatr Psychiatry Neurol* 1994;7:116–120.

Ott A, Breteler MM, van Harskamp F, et al. Prevalence of Alzheimer's disease and vascular dementia: association with education. The Rotterdam study. *BMJ* 1995;310: 970–973.

Ott A, Breteler MM, van Harskamp F, et al. Incidence and risk of dementia. The Rotterdam Study. *Am J Epidemiol* 1998;147:574–580.

Ott A, Slooter AJ, Hofman A, et al. Smoking and risk of dementia and Alzheimer's disease in a population- based cohort study: the Rotterdam Study. *Lancet* 1998;351: 1840–1843.

Paganini-Hill A, Henderson VW. Estrogen replacement therapy and risk of Alzheimer disease. *Arch Intern Med* 1996; 156:2213–2217.

Perry EK, Tomlinson BE, Blessed G, et al. Correlation of cholinergic abnormalities with senile plaques and mental test scores in senile dementia. *BMJ* 1978;2:1457–1459.

Petersen RC, Smith GE, Ivnik RJ, et al. Memory function in very early Alzheimer's disease. *Neurology* 1994;44: 867–872.

Petersen RC, Smith GE, Ivnik RJ, et al. Apolipoprotein E status as a predictor of the development of Alzheimer's disease in memory-impaired individuals. *JAMA* 1995; 273:1274–1278.

Pfeffer RI, Afifi AA, Chance JM. Prevalence of Alzheimer's disease in a retirement community. *Am J Epidemiol* 1987;125:420–436.

Poirier J, Davignon J, Bouthillier D, et al. Apolipoprotein E polymorphism and Alzheimer's disease. *Lancet* 1993; 342:697–699.

Poorkaj P, Bird TD, Wijsman E, et al. Tau is a candidate gene for chromosome 17 frontotemporal dementia. *Ann Neurol* 1998;43:815–825.

Prince M, Lewis G, Bird A, Blizard R, et al. A longitudinal study of factors predicting change in cognitive test scores over time, in an older hypertensive population. *Psychol Med* 1996;26:555–568.

Raskind MA, Peskind ER, Wessel T, et al. Galantamine in AD: a 6-month randomized, placebo-controlled trial with a 6-month extension. *Neurology* 2000;54:2261–2268.

Read SL, Miller BL, Mena I, et al. SPECT in dementia: clinical and pathological correlation. *J Am Geriatr Soc* 1995;43:1243–1247.

Reisberg B, Windscheif U, Ferris S, et al. Memantine in moderately severe to severe Alzheimer's disease: Results of a placebo controlled 6-month trial. *Neurobiol Aging* 2000;21(Suppl 1):S275.

Rocca WA, Cha RH, Waring SC, et al. Incidence of dementia and Alzheimer's disease: a reanalysis of data from Rochester, Minnesota, 1975-1984. *Am J Epidemiol* 1998; 148:51–62.

Rogaev EI, Sherrington R, Rogaeva EA, et al. Familial Alzheimer's disease in kindreds with missense mutations in a gene on chromosome 1 related to the Alzheimer's disease type 3 gene. *Nature* 1995;376:775–7778.

Rogers SL, Farlow MR, Doody RS, et al. A 24-week, double-blind, placebo-controlled trial of donepezil in patients with Alzheimer's disease. *Neurology* 1998;50:136–145.

Rogers SL, Friedhoff LT. Long-term efficacy and safety of donepezil in the treatment of Alzheimer's disease: an interim analysis of the results of a US multicentre open label extension study. *Eur Neuropsychopharmacol* 1998;8:67–75.

Roman GC, Tatemichi TK, Erkinjuntti T, et al. Vascular dementia: diagnostic criteria for research studies. Report of the NINDS-AIREN International Workshop. *Neurology* 1993;43:250–260.

Rosen WG, Terry RD, Fuld PA, et al. Pathological verification of ischemic score in differentiation of dementias. *Ann Neurol* 1980;7:486–488.

Rosler M, Anand R, Cicin-Sain A, et al. Efficacy and safety of rivastigmine in patients with Alzheimer's disease: international randomised controlled trial. *BMJ* 1999;318:633–640.

Ross GW, Abbott RD, Petrovitch H, et al. Frequency and characteristics of silent dementia among elderly Japanese-American men. The Honolulu-Asia Aging Study. *JAMA* 1997;277:800–805.

Rubin EH, Morris JC, Grant EA, et al. Very mild senile dementia of the Alzheimer type. I. Clinical assessment. *Arch Neurol* 1989;46:379–382.

Salib E, Hillier V. A case-control study of Alzheimer's disease and aluminium occupation. *Br J Psychiatry* 1996; 168:244–249.

Salmon DP, Thal LJ, Butters N, et al. Longitudinal evaluation of dementia of the Alzheimer type: a comparison of 3 standardized mental status examinations. *Neurology* 1990;40:1225–1230.

Scharf S, Mander A, Ugoni A, et al. A double-blind, placebo-controlled trial of diclofenac/misoprostol in Alzheimer's disease. *Neurology* 1999;53:197–201.

Schenk D, Barbour R, Dunn W, et al. Immunization with amyloid-beta attenuates Alzheimer-disease-like pathology in the PDAPP mouse. *Nature* 1999;400:173–177.

Scott WK, Edwards KB, Davis DR, et al. Risk of institutionalization among community long-term care clients with dementia. *Gerontologist* 1997;37:46–51.

Seltzer B, Vasterling JJ, Yoder JA, et al. Awareness of deficit in Alzheimer's disease: relation to caregiver burden. *Gerontologist* 1997;37:20–24.

Severson MA, Smith GE, Tangalos EG, et al. Patterns and predictors of institutionalization in community-based dementia patients. *J Am Geriatr Soc* 1994;42:181–185.

Sherrington R, Rogaev EI, Liang Y, et al. Cloning of a gene bearing missense mutations in early-onset familial Alzheimer's disease. *Nature* 1995;375:754–760.

Shumaker S, Rapp S. Hormone therapy in dementia prevention: the Women's Health Initiative memory study. *Neurobiol Aging* 1996;17:S9.

Sinha S, Anderson JP, Barbour R, et al. Purification and cloning of amyloid precursor protein beta-secretase from human brain. *Nature* 1999;402:537–540.

Snowden JS, Neary D. Progressive language dysfunction and lobar atrophy. *Dementia* 1993;4:226–231.

Snowdon DA, Greiner LH, Mortimer JA, et al. Brain infarction and the clinical expression of Alzheimer disease. The Nun Study. *JAMA* 1997;277:813–817.

Snowdon DA, Kemper SJ, Mortimer JA, et al. Linguistic ability in early life and cognitive function and Alzheimer's disease in late life. Findings from the Nun Study. *JAMA* 1996;275:528–532.

Spillantini MG, Bird TD, Ghetti B. Frontotemporal dementia and parkinsonism linked to chromosome 17: a new group of tauopathies. *Brain Pathol* 1998;8:387–402.

St. George-Hyslop PH. Genetic factors in the genesis of Alzheimer's disease. *Ann N Y Acad Sci* 2000;924:1–7.

Starkstein SE, Sabe L, Chemerinski E, et al. Two domains of anosognosia in Alzheimer's disease. *J Neurol Neurosurg Psychiatry* 1996;61:485–490.

Stern RG, Mohs RC, Davidson M, et al. A longitudinal study of Alzheimer's disease: measurement, rate, and predictors of cognitive deterioration. *Am J Psychiatry* 1994; 151:390–396.

Stern Y, Albert M, Brandt J, et al. Utility of extrapyramidal signs and psychosis as predictors of cognitive and functional decline, nursing home admission, and death in Alzheimer's disease: prospective analyses from the Predictors Study. *Neurology* 1994;44:2300–2307.

Stern Y, Gurland B, Tatemichi TK, et al. Influence of education and occupation on the incidence of Alzheimer's disease. *JAMA* 1994;271:1004–1010.

Stern Y, Tang MX, Albert MS, et al. Predicting time to nursing home care and death in individuals with Alzheimer disease. *JAMA* 1997;277:806–812.

Stern Y, Tang MX, Denaro J, et al. Increased risk of mortality in Alzheimer's disease patients with more advanced educational and occupational attainment. *Ann Neurol* 1995;37:590–595.

Stevens M, van Duijn CM, Kamphorst W, et al. Familial aggregation in frontotemporal dementia. *Neurology* 1998; 50:1541–1545.

Stewart WF, Kawas C, Corrada M, et al. Risk of Alzheimer's disease and duration of NSAID use. *Neurology* 1997;48: 626–632.

Talbot PR, Lloyd JJ, Snowden JS, et al. A clinical role for 99mTc-HMPAO SPECT in the investigation of dementia? *J Neurol Neurosurg Psychiatry* 1998;64:306–313.

Tang MX, Jacobs D, Stern Y, et al. Effect of oestrogen during menopause on risk and age at onset of Alzheimer's disease. *Lancet* 1996;348:429–432.

Tariot PN, Erb R, Podgorski CA, et al. Efficacy and tolerability of carbamazepine for agitation and aggression in dementia. *Am J Psychiatry* 1998;155:54–61.

Tariot PN, Solomon PR, Morris JC, et al. A 5-month, randomized, placebo-controlled trial of galantamine in AD. *Neurology* 2000;54:2269–2276.

Tatemichi TK, Desmond DW, Mayeux R, et al. Dementia after stroke: baseline frequency, risks, and clinical features in a hospitalized cohort. *Neurology* 1992;42: 1185–1193.

Tatemichi TK, Paik M, Bagiella E, et al. Risk of dementia after stroke in a hospitalized cohort: results of a longitudinal study. *Neurology* 1994;44:1885–1891.

Teri L, Wagner AW. Assessment of depression in patients with Alzheimer's disease: concordance among informants. *Psychol Aging* 1991;6:280–285.

Terry RD, Masliah E, Salmon DP, et al. Physical basis of cognitive alterations in Alzheimer's disease: synapse loss is the major correlate of cognitive impairment. *Ann Neurol* 1991;30:572–580.

van Belle G, Uhlmann RF, Hughes JP, et al. Reliability of estimates of changes in mental status test performance in senile dementia of the Alzheimer type. *J Clin Epidemiol* 1990;43:589–595.

van Dongen MC, van Rossum E, Kessels AG, et al. The efficacy of ginkgo for elderly people with dementia and age-associated memory impairment: new results of a randomized clinical trial. *J Am Geriatr Soc* 2000;48:1183–1194.

Vassar R, Bennett BD, Babu-Khan S, et al. Beta-Secretase cleavage of Alzheimer's amyloid precursor protein by the transmembrane aspartic protease BACE. *Science* 1999; 286:735–741.

Victoroff J, Mack WJ, Lyness SA, et al. Multicenter clinicopathological correlation in dementia. *Am J Psychiatry* 1995;152:1476–1484.

Wade JP, Mirsen TR, Hachinski VC, et al. The clinical diagnosis of Alzheimer's disease. *Arch Neurol* 1987;44:24–29.

Walsh JS, Welch HG, Larson EB. Survival of outpatients with Alzheimer-type dementia. *Ann Intern Med* 1990; 113:429–434.

Weiner HL, Lemere CA, Maron R, et al. Nasal administration of amyloid-beta peptide decreases cerebral amyloid burden in a mouse model of Alzheimer's disease. *Ann Neurol* 2000;48:567–579.

Welch HG, Walsh JS, Larson EB. The cost of institutional care in Alzheimer's disease: nursing home and hospital use in a prospective cohort. *J Am Geriatr Soc* 1992;40:221–224.

White L, Petrovitch H, Ross GW, et al. Prevalence of dementia in older Japanese-American men in Hawaii: the Honolulu-Asia Aging Study. *JAMA* 1996;276:955–960.

Winblad B, Poritis N. Memantine in severe dementia: results of the 9M-Best Study (Benefit and efficacy in severely demented patients during treatment with memantine). *Int J Geriatr Psychiatry* 1999;14:135–146.

Wolf PA, Cobb JL, D'Agostino RB. Epidemiology of stroke. In: Barnett HJM, Mohr JP, Stein, BP, et al. *Stroke. Pathophysiology, diagnosis and management*. New York: Churchill Livingstone, 1992:3–27.

Wolfe MS, Xia W, Ostaszewski BL, et al. Two transmembrane aspartates in presenilin-1 required for presenilin endoproteolysis and gamma-secretase activity. *Nature* 1999;398:513–517.

Wolfe N, Linn R, Babikian VL, et al. Frontal systems impairment following multiple lacunar infarcts. *Arch Neurol* 1990;47:129–132.

Xia W, Zhang J, Ostaszewski BL, et al. Presenilin 1 regulates the processing of beta-amyloid precursor protein C-terminal fragments and the generation of amyloid beta-protein in endoplasmic reticulum and Golgi. *Biochemistry* 1998;37:16465–16471.

Yan R, Bienkowski MJ, Shuck ME, et al. Membrane-anchored aspartyl protease with Alzheimer's disease beta-secretase activity. *Nature* 1999;402:533–537.

21.2

Dementia Disorders: Behavioral and Cognitive Aspects

Barbara L. Malamut

Recognition that a patient is experiencing a decline in mental status can often be obvious, especially to the physician who is well acquainted with the person over a period of many years. Determining the cause of the mental decline, however, can be more challenging. Depression, anxiety, metabolic disorders, drug interactions, or alcohol use can often result in behavioral and cognitive difficulties that resemble those of dementia and, therefore, often lead to a misdiagnosis. Furthermore, many different forms of dementia are seen, each with its own cognitive and behavioral manifestation. As new medications are developed, diagnostic accuracy will become essential to form different treatment decisions.

In this chapter, the neuropsychological and psychosocial aspects of the most common neurodegenerative dementing illnesses are discussed. Particular emphasis is placed on Alzheimer's disease because of the prevalence of this disorder.

According to the American Psychiatric Association's *Diagnostic and Statistical Manual of Mental Disorders*, 4th edition (DSM-IV, 1994), the cognitive manifestations of dementia must include impairment in at least two or more of the following domains: short and long-term memory, abstract thinking, impaired judgment, language or other disturbances of higher cortical functioning, or personality change. Dementia affects an individual's social and occupational skills as well as the ability for self-care. The cognitive and behavioral disturbances must not be caused by psychiatric mental disorders. Once the physician suspects mental status changes, performs a screening test of mental status, and runs the appropriate battery of medical tests to rule out a reversible process, the patient should be referred for a neuropsychological assessment.

THE ROLE OF THE NEUROPSYCHOLOGIST

Neuropsychology contributes greatly to the diagnosis of dementia. Distinguishing between age-related decline, mild cognitive impairment, and dementia such as Alzheimer's disease can be difficult, requiring careful evaluation across many cognitive functions as well as a person's day-to-day functional status. For example, an impairment in memory is not specific to any one dementing disorder and should be viewed as a symptom of cognitive dysfunction rather than a diagnostic certainty. Problems in free recall, which is characteristic of confusional states, depression, or attentional disorders, can reflect a deficit in activating encoding processes. Memory problems, which are observed in depression, frontal lobe dementias, subcortical dementias, or a frontal lobe-related deficit, can also be caused by impairment in retrieval of information. Alternatively, poor performance on a free recall measure could be a symptom of a pure amnestic disorder caused by hippocampal or temporal lobe damage. It is the role of the neuropsychologist to measure the pattern and level of cognitive impairment.

The neuropsychologist also contributes to the diagnostic process by addressing issues related to a person's ability to safely carry out instrumental activities of daily living (IADL), such as driving, medication management, handling finances, and so on, and activities of daily living (ADL), such as bathing, toileting, and so forth. By definition, dementia interferes with a person's ability to function normally in everyday life. Skills needed for self-care, social and occupational functioning, and financial management are greatly affected, but the degree and pattern of functional impairment vary widely. In the early and middle stages of a dementing process, evaluation of cognitive status is critical to help assure the individual's day-to-day safety and to determine a diagnosis. In the later stages, a neuropsychological evaluation is usually requested to help with problematic behaviors such as wandering, screaming or verbal abuse. If behavioral or environmental interventions are appropriate to individual abilities, problematic behaviors can be minimized and use of psychotropic medication to control these behaviors can be reduced.

DIAGNOSIS

A first step in determining a diagnosis is to understand the nature of the cognitive disturbance and to narrow the causes for the change in mental status. Other than medical and psychiatric history, four key features are important when forming a diagnosis: information regarding when the problems began (i.e., time of onset of initial symptoms); the course of the symptomatology (i.e., insidious, acute presentation with little change, or step-wise); rate of progression of the disorder (i.e., slow or rapidly progressing); and presenting symptoms. Demographic information (e.g., education, occupation) and social history (e.g., living situation, hobbies, alcohol and drug consumption) are also pertinent variables. Tables 21-2 and 21-3 illustrate differences between the pattern of presentation and rate of progression among the various dementing syndromes.

When obtaining the history, even in the early stages of a dementing process, it is important to interview the patient and another person who knows the patient well. Informant reports of memory loss have been shown to distinguish individuals who are demented from those who are not and also to predict future diagnosis of Alzheimer's disease, whereas patient reports are usually not related to cognitive performance (Carr et al., 2000). With regard to functional capacity, however, informant reports were not always reliable. Loewenstein et al. (2001) found that caregivers were accurate in predicting the functional performance of patients with Alzheimer's disease who were not impaired on objective tests of functional status. In contrast, caregivers overestimated the functional abilities of patients with Alzheimer's disease who were impaired on objective testing. Caregivers tended to overestimate the patient's ability to tell time, identify currency, make change for a purchase, and use eating utensils. In this study, higher Mini-Mental Status Examination (MMSE) scores were associated with caregivers' overestimation of functional capacity.

SCREENING MEASURES

The most commonly used clinical screening tool for the presence of dementia is the Mini Mental State Examination, which is easily administered in about 5 to 10 minutes (Folstein et al., 1975). Although it has proved to be highly sensitive to changes in mental status, the MMSE does not distinguish between different forms of dementia (i.e., specificity). One reason for its lack of specificity is that the MMSE does not measure long-term memory, recognition memory, or executive functions (Malloy et al., 1997). Another drawback is that the MMSE is not informative about the level of care needed for patients with mild to moderate levels of dementia.

The MMSE has a total score of 30 points, with a score of 23 or lower usually considered indicative of organic dysfunction. However, age and education must be taken into account when interpreting the to-

TABLE 21-2. *Patterns of progression and onset of dementing disorders*

| Onset | Disease progression | | |
	Slow	Rapid	Step-wise
Insidious	Alzheimer's disease Vascular dementia CSH Alcoholism Parkinson's disease NPH HD PSP	Pick's disease Jakob-Creutzfeld disease Lewy body disease	AD + VaD
Acute	Vitamin B deficiency	Herpes encephalitis Meningitis	MID, stroke Head trauma Encephalitis Abscess Anoxia

AD, Alzheimer's disease; CSH, chronic subdural hematoma; HD, Huntington's chorea; MID, multiinfarct dementia; NPH, normal pressure hydrocephalus; PSP progressive supranuclear palsy; VaD, vascular dementia.
Reprinted from Tuokko H, Hadjistavropoulos T. Screening instruments for cognitive impairment. In: An assessment guide to geriatric neuropsychology. Mahwah, NJ: Lawrence Erlbaum, 1998:28–43, with permission.

TABLE 21-3. *Most common presenting signs for various dementia syndromes and depression*

AD	DLB	PD	FTD	DFT	Vascular	Depression
Memory loss	Visual hallucinations Fluctuating cognition	EPS	Language impaired	Executive dysfunction	Executive dysfunction	Complaints of memory loss Apathy

AD, Alzheimer's disease; DFT, dementia frontal type; DLB, dementia with Lewy bodies; EPS, extrapyramidal signs; FTD, frontotemporal degeneration; PD, Parkinson's disease.

tal score. As individuals grow older (age ≤80 years) or education level is low (<9 years), the cutoff score suggestive of dementia decreases. It has been suggested that for people with fewer than 9 years of education, a score of 17 should be considered as the cutoff (Tuokko and Hadjistavropoulos, 1998). Likewise, a cutoff score of 26 or less has been suggested as optimum to detect mild to moderate dementia in people with higher education (Van Gorp et al., 1999). Cultural background has also been shown to affect MMSE scores. For example, Hispanics performed worse than non-Hispanics on the serial subtraction subtest when both groups were matched on education, age, and overall level of dementia. Similar results were found when spelling a word in reverse was substituted for serial subtraction (Hohl et al., 1999).

Another screening test that is often administered along with the MMSE is the Clock Drawing Test. In this test, the person is asked to draw the face of a clock, put all the numbers in the correct location, and set the clock to a specific time. To correctly execute the multiple steps needed for a clock drawing, several diverse skills are required, including planning, visual attention, spatial conceptualization, and graphomotor control. The time to which the hands are set is important and two times (i.e., 10 after 11 or 20 after 8) have been shown to be most sensitive to dementia because they are sensitive to hemi-inattention as well as problems in spatial conceptualization (Freedman et al., 1994). Several different scoring systems of the clock have been devised to objectively quantify the presence and level of impairment (Libon et al., 1996; Freedman et al., 1994). In general, the clocks are evaluated for accuracy, general planning and organization, spatial planning, visuoperceptual, visuomotor, and spatial conceptualization skills. Together with MMSE scores, Clock Drawing Test performance has been shown to be sensitive to the presence of dementia, especially in those with very mild disease. However, on its own, it is not useful in discriminating between different causes of dementia.

The Alzheimer's Disease Assessment Scale (ADAS) is used mostly in research settings, but it is mentioned here because of its wide use in drug trials

(Rosen et al., 1984). It is designed to evaluate the severity of both cognitive and noncognitive functions that are characteristic of Alzheimer's disease. The scale is composed of 21 items tapping memory, language and praxis, mood, and behavioral changes (e.g., depression, agitation, psychosis, and vegetative symptoms). It is administered in an interview format and takes about 45 minutes.

NEUROPSYCHOLOGICAL PROFILES OF DEMENTING DISORDERS

Alzheimer's Disease

Alzheimer's disease is the most common form of dementia, affecting an estimated 6% to 8% of people over 65 years of age, and 30% to 40% of people above the age of 85 (Small et al., 1997). The initial presentation for most patients with Alzheimer's disease often involves memory lapses with an insidious onset. Families often report that a holiday meal was burned or a parent became lost while driving a familiar route. Often, relatives of the effected individual will only realize in hindsight that certain episodes that had occurred several years earlier were actually the beginning signs of the dementia. The rate of disease progression is slow, and estimate is that typically 10 years pass from the initial diagnosis until death. However, Alzheimer's disease is frequently superimposed on other disorders (e.g., Parkinson's disease or Lewy Body dementia) and, in these cases, the rate of progression and neuropsychological profiles vary.

Three diagnostic categories for Alzheimer's disease are definite, probable, and possible. The National Institute of Neurological and Communicative Disorders and Stroke and the Alzheimer's Disease and Related Disorders Association Workgroup have set forth the criteria listed in Table 21-4 for diagnosing *probable* and *possible* Alzheimer's disease (McKhann, 1984). A diagnosis of *definite* Alzheimer's disease can be made only postmortem . The individual must have met criteria for *probable* and the histopathologic findings indicating the disease are also required.

TABLE 21-4. *NINCDS-ADRDA criteria for diagnoses of probable and possible AD*

Probable AD
1. Dementia is established by clinical examination and documented by performance on a mental status examination, and
2. Confirmed by neuropsychological testing, documenting deficits in two or more areas of cognition, and
3. Characterized by a history of progressive worsening of memory and other cognitive deficits, with
4. No disturbance in level of consciousness, and
5. Symptom onset between the ages of 40 and 90 years, most typically after age 65, and
6. An absence of systemic disorders or other brain diseases that of themselves could account for the progressive deficits.

The diagnosis of probable AD is further supported by evidence (i.e., from neuropsychological reexamination) of progressive deterioration of specific cognitive functions, impairment in activities of daily living, a family history of similar disorders, and results of particular laboratory tests (e.g., lumbar puncture, normal pattern or nonspecific changes in the electroencephalogram, evidence of cerebral atrophy on computerized topographic scanning).

The clinical diagnosis of possible AD is made when:
1. The syndrome of dementia is present, and
2. There is an absence of other neurologic, psychiatric, or systemic disorders that are sufficient to cause the dementia, but
3. There are present variations from criteria for probable AD in the onset, presentation, or clinical course.

Possible AD may also be diagnosed when there is a systemic or brain disease that is sufficient to produce a dementia, but which (for various reasons) is not considered to be the cause of the patient's dementia.

AD, Alzheimer's disease; NINCDS-ADRDA, National Institute of Neurological and Communicative Disorders and Stroke and the Alzheimer's Disease and Related Disorders Association.
From McKhann G, Drachman D, Folstein M, et al. Clinical diagnosis of Alzheimer's disease: Report of the NINCDS-ADRDA work group under the auspices of department of health and human services on Alzheimer's disease. *Neurology* 1984;34:939–944, with permission.

Neuropsychological Profile of Presymptomatic Alzheimer's Disease Patients

Although patients with Alzheimer's disease most often present to their physicians in the mild to moderate stages of the disease, some individuals complain of memory loss before any other signs of disease are evident, including normal performance on the MMSE. It is now understood that Alzheimer's disease has a long preclinical period during which memory deficits are detectable on neuropsychological testing.

Problems in delayed recall memory of a word list and executive functioning as measured by the Trail Making Test B (Reitan, 1958) in individuals who were clinically presymptomatic at the time of neuropsychological testing, could discriminate those who would manifest Alzheimer's disease 18 months later from those who would remain normal (Chen et al., 2000).

In another population-based prospective study, recall memory distinguished those individuals who would develop Alzheimer's disease from those who would remain healthy from *three to six years* in advance of a diagnosis (Backman et al., 2001). No differences were noted in digit span forward and reverse between those who remained healthy and those who developed the disease.

Changes in the identification of smells can also be a way of detecting those individuals with mild cognitive impairment who will develop Alzheimer's disease. Because the hippocampus and entorhinal cortex are affected very early in the disease and the lateral portions of the entorhinal cortex are directly innervated by the lateral olfactory tract, researchers began examining the olfactory system in Alzheimer's disease. In their study using patients with suspected Alzheimer's disease, Nordin and Murphy (1996; 1998) concluded that tests of odor detection could be useful in the early detection of the disease. In a more recent study, patients with normal MMSE scores who had impairment in olfactory identification and were *unaware* of their deficit were more likely to develop Alzheimer's disease than those with olfactory deficits but who were *aware* of their poor performance on the test (Devanand, et al. 2000). Further research is needed to determine whether impairment in olfactory identification is a reliable indicator of early Alzheimer's disease.

Presenting Neuropsychological Signs

The core features of individuals who were shown to have only Alzheimer's disease pathology determined at autopsy are a progressive decline in explicit memory, anomia, executive function difficulties, visuospatial deficits, as well as a variety of other behavioral features discussed below. The rate and order in which these functions decline is variable among patients and reflects the differential competencies premorbidly as well as differences in the progressive accumulation of neuritic plaques and neurofibrillary tangles within the various association cortices (Stern et al., 1999).

Most patients with Alzheimer's disease present initially with the greatest problems in episodic memory, but great variability is seen in the pattern of decline among the other neuropsychological domains such that some skills remain preserved longer than others. Results from several studies have demonstrated three qualitatively distinct patterns of performance on neuropsychological testing and on functional imaging (Martin et al., 1986, Fisher et al., 1999). All three groups had severe episodic memory impairment. One group of patients with Alzheimer's disease demonstrated severe impairment on semantic variables with more favorable visual spatial skills (i.e., severe naming impairment in relation to drawing skills); another group demonstrated the opposite pattern (i.e., severe impairment in drawing skills and average naming ability), whereas the third group demonstrated global decline across most measures (i.e., profound anomia and drawing skills). Further support for clinical heterogeneity among patients with early Alzheimer's disease comes from a study of monozygotic twins concordant for the disease (Resnick et al., 1988). One twin presented with greater involvement of the right hemisphere, whereas the other demonstrated greater involvement of the left hemisphere as measured by CT scan atrophy, electroencephalogram (EEG), positron emission tomography (PET), and neuropsychological profiles. In all cases of AD, however, patients eventually become globally impaired with further progression of the disease.

Memory

Verbal and visual episodic memory loss is the hallmark of Alzheimer's disease. On tests of episodic memory (e.g., story recall or list learning), patients with the disease demonstrate a rapid rate of forgetting and often do not recall the new information after 10 to 20 minutes (i.e., savings score) (Becker et al., 1987; Larrabee et al., 1993; Troster et al., 1993). Furthermore, the normal pattern of learning a list of words—the *serial position effect* (i.e., better immediate recall of items from the beginning and end of a word list, with poorest recall of words in the middle

of the list)—is also disrupted early in the disease process (Bayley et al., 2000; Simon et al., 1994). Patients demonstrate a *recency effect* (i.e., they tend to recall the last few words of a supraspan word list immediately after it is read aloud). In contrast, normal elderly people demonstrate primacy and recency (i.e., recall most words from the beginning and end of the list immediately after it is presented). Patients with Alzheimer's disease also tend to make more intrusion and perseverative errors on memory tests when compared with normal elderly controls (Cahn et al., 1997). In addition to new learning, the disease also effects memories from the remote past (i.e., remote memory). In the early stages of the disease, patients perform worse than normal control subjects in their ability to recall and recognize famous faces, public events, and autobiographical information, but some memories from the past remain preserved. Controversy exists to whether a pattern of remote memory loss is such that earlier autobiographical memories remain intact longer than more recent memories (i.e., temporal gradient). In any case, their impairment appears to worsen with disease progression (Dorrego et al., 1999).

Executive Functioning

Deficits in executive functioning are evident in the early stages of Alzheimer's disease, although they are usually not as prominent as episodic memory loss. The term "executive functioning" refers to the capacity to plan and carry out complex goal-oriented behaviors and is most often evaluated with tests of problem solving (i.e., Wisconsin Card Sorting; Heaton et al., 1993), working memory (i.e., Digit Span backward), and mental flexibility (i.e., Trail Making Test B; Reitan, 1958). Executive functioning allows a person to independently adapt his or her behavior to changing contingencies, which is necessary for the performance of all independent goal-directed activities including IADL. Deficits in executive functioning have been shown to be related to a decline in IADL in patients with mild or moderate Alzheimer's disease and, therefore, have important implications for safety issues regarding medication management and driving (Ryan et al., in submission).

Language and Semantic Memory

Early in the course of Alzheimer's disease, patients demonstrate impairments in the linguistic aspects of speech. Their conversations are often vague and their discourse is filled with circumlocutions and overlearned phrases. On formal testing, these patients have deficits on tests of word list generation and naming and they tend to make more lexical and semantic naming errors on fluency and naming tests compared with normal elderly controls (Cahn et al., 1997; Bayles and Tomaeda, 1983; Suhr and Jones., 1998; Cummings et al., 1985). With disease progression, paraphasic errors and impairment in written and oral comprehension develops. In the late stages, dysarthria and mutism may occur.

Typically, the linguistic aspects of speech are examined through category fluency tests (i.e., rapidly name items within a specific category) and letter fluency tests (i.e., rapidly name words beginning with specific letters). At one time, having better category than letter fluency, was thought to be evidence of cortical dementias, such as Alzheimer's disease, whereas the reverse pattern was thought to indicate a subcortical dementia such as in Parkinson's disease, Huntington's disease, or vascular dementia (Rosen, 1980; Butters et al., 1987). More recently, however, several studies have disputed these findings and found no difference in performance on category and fluency tests between patients with dementia due to different causes (Suhr and Jones, 1998; Sherman and Massman, 1999). Given the discrepancy in the literature, differences in performance between these two tests should not be used to distinguish different types of dementia.

Semantic memory refers to knowledge of words (vocabulary) and factual information and is affected in the beginning stages of Alzheimer's disease as noted by consistent impairments in naming and fluency tasks. The level of the semantic memory impairment is related to the level of dementia. Semantic memory for generic knowledge (e.g., how many days are there in a week?) has also been shown to be impaired relatively early in the course of the disease and declines further as the disease progresses (Norton, 1997). Although no disagreement is seen about the presence of a semantic memory impairment in Alzheimer's disease, much controversy exists regarding the underlying cause of the impairment. One explanation is that degradation of the organization and content of semantic knowledge causes the impairment. The alternative is based on an information processing deficit such that the person has problems in accessing information from an intact semantic store (Salmon et al., 1999; Thompson-Schill et al., 1999; Bayles et al., 1999; Ford et al., 2001). Although this debate has not been resolved, studies have shown that task difficulty (i.e., requiring active searches of semantic memory or greater attentional resources) is one of the intervening variables.

Praxis

Ideomotor apraxia is a disorder of skilled movement or gestural behavior to verbal command or imitation, and it is thought to be caused by disruption in the access to stored memories of familiar action patterns. It usually emerges in Alzheimer's disease after memory and language disturbances, but it can be seen in the early stages of the disease (Crowe and Hoogenraad, 2000). Ideomotor praxis can be evaluated in many ways. When the four types of movements listed in Table 21-5 were evaluated in a group of patients with moderate to severe disease, transitive limb movements to command were found to decline before intransitive limb, buccofacial, and axial actions (Rapcsak et al., 1989). The most common errors on transitive limb praxis testing occurred because patients used their body part as the object. Deficits are also found in ideational praxis where a person is asked to perform a series of actions using objects to accomplish a goal such as "fold a paper, put it in the envelope, seal, and address it." In ideational praxis, the deficits are usually a result of sequencing errors (e.g., sealing the envelope before putting the paper in). Evaluation of praxis is an important part of a dementia evaluation in patients suspected of having Alzheimer's disease, as it has been shown to differentiate depressed elderly patients with cognitive impair-

TABLE 21-5. *Apraxia battery*

Buccofacial
  Show me how you. . . .
  1. Cough
  2. Stick out your tongue
  3. Suck through a straw
  4. Blow out a match
  5. Sniff a flower
Limb intransitive
  Show me how you . . .
  1. Wave goodbye
  2. Beckon "come here"
  3. Hitchhike
  4. Salute
  5. Signal "Stop"
Limb transitive
  Show me how you . . .
  1. Brush your teeth
  2. Stir coffee with a spoon
  3. Comb your hair
  4. Saw a board
  5. Use a screwdriver
Ideational
  1. Fold paper, place it in envelope, seal and address it
  2. Prepare a cup of instant coffee with sugar
  3. Put candle in holder, light it, and blow it out

ment from those with probable disease (Crowe and Hoogenraad, 2000).

Visuospatial

Visuospatial functioning is often impaired early in Alzheimer's disease and declines further as the disease progresses. Visual agnosia usually does not appear until the middle to late stages of the disorder. Visual spatial constructional apraxia can be seen early in the disease process. This is usually tested with tasks involving graphomotor skills such as drawing a clock, copying simple and complex drawings, as well as tasks involving manipulation of materials (i.e., constructing a design with blocks to look like a model). When drawing a clock to command, patients with the disease often fail to include the numbers or clock hands, or they have problems in spatial conceptualization. In the moderate to severe stages of the disease, patients often will write the time rather than draw clock hands (Fig. 21-1). Their performance often reflects a loss of the knowledge or a deficit in accessing the attributes of a clock. Usually, their copy of a clock is much better than their spontaneous drawing. In drawing tasks, the patient is usually asked to copy geometric forms that increase in complexity (e.g., circle, Red Cross sign, diamond, cube). In Alzheimer's disease, as the disease progresses, pa-

tients' performance will often decline in the reverse order of the developmental sequence (Rosen, 1984). Thus, in the mild stages of the disease, patients may demonstrate problems copying a cube but have no difficulty copying a diamond or circle. As the disease progresses, problems develop when copying the diamond. In the moderate to severe stages, patients often draw over the shape or use part of the form in their drawing (i.e., closing in) rather than draw in the space provided.

Motor

Extrapyramidal signs (EPS) (e.g., bradykinesia, rigidity, gait disturbance, tremor, postural instability) are common in Alzheimer's disease. They appear more frequently as the disease progresses, and are important predictors of decline in patients with the disease. Patients who have at least one EPS at baseline evaluation are reported to demonstrate a more rapid cognitive and functional decline than those with Alzheimer's disease who do not show EPS (Richards et al., 1993).

Atypical Neuropsychological Presentations

Although the three subtypes discussed above are the most common patterns of presentation of Alzheimer's disease, atypical presentations involving circumscribed

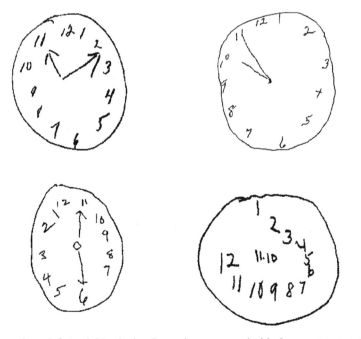

FIG 21.1. Top row from left to right, clocks drawn by: a normal elderly woman, a patient with Mild AD. Second row from left to right, clocks drawn by a patient with moderate AD, and a patient with moderate to severe AD.

deficits related to other cognitive functions have also been reported. The neurobiological basis for this clinical heterogeneity appears related to variations in the distribution of the pathogenic changes occurring with the disease. Functional imaging (i.e., PET and single photon emission computerized tomography [SPECT]), has been helpful in illustrating the relationship between specific neuropsychological deficits and various locations of abnormal metabolic activity. Similarly, neuropathologic studies have shown that differences in the distribution of pathogenic changes associated with Alzheimer's disease account for some of the variability in cognitive profiles. In one study, a group of patients who presented with disproportionate frontal lobe impairments on neuropsychological testing while in the mild stages of dementia were followed to autopsy (Hodges et al., 1999). The results indicated as much as a tenfold increase in neurofibrillary tangles (NFT), but not plaques, in the frontal lobes when compared with individuals with typical Alzheimer's disease neuropsychological presentations. Both groups had the expected NFT hippocampal pathology but, of the five regions sampled, the patients with neuropsychologically frontal impairment had the greatest proportion of NFT in the frontal region. The patients with initial frontal presentations eventually demonstrated memory and visuospatial deficits characteristic of Alzheimer's disease, but their performance was worse on tests sensitive to frontal lobe functioning. Similarly, subgroups of patients have presented with isolated visual disturbances early in the disease without memory impairments (Furey-Kurkjian et al., 1996). In another subgroup of patients demonstrating a selective impairment of episodic and semantic memory, SPECT showed focal temporal lobe dysfunction (FTLD). In contrast, the group with typical disease demonstrated the bilateral mesial temporal hypoperfusion but also the posterior parietal and temporal parietal hypoperfusion. The authors suggested that FTLD is a rare but a distinct anatomoclinical form of Alzheimer's disease with a slower rate of cognitive decline (Cappa, 2001). Thus, although memory loss is the most common initial symptom of Alzheimer's disease, circumscribed impairments in other cognitive domains can also be seen. It has been suggested that these subcategories of the disease may represent different gene combinations with different rates of progression and prognosis, and patients falling into these subcategories may possibly respond to different treatment regimens (Furey-Kurkjian et al., 1996).

Behavioral Manifestations

Many patients with Alzheimer's disease have concomitant psychiatric symptoms at some point in their illness (Cummings and Benson, 1986). Early in the disease process, decreased spontaneity and increased passivity are the most common behavioral changes, although not noted in all individuals. Other patients demonstrate restlessness, hyperactivity, and disinhibited behavior. Agitation is also seen, which increases with disease severity. Estimates of the incidence of psychosis in AD (i.e., hallucinations and delusions) range from 10% to 75%, with delusions occurring more often than hallucinations (Paulsen et al., 2000). Psychotic symptoms in earlier stages of Alzheimer's disease have been associated with increased rates of aggression, cognitive impairment, and functional decline (Rapoport et al., 2001; Paulsen et al., 2000; Stern et al., 1987; Mayeux et al., 1985; Lopez et al., 1991). Hallucinations are most common toward the end stages of the disease.

Lewy Body

Dementia with Lewy bodies (DLB) is thought to be the second most frequent type of dementia in the elderly, affecting as many as 20% to 30% of people with dementia (Jellinger, 2000). Lewy bodies are intraneuronal inclusions in the neocortex and subcortical regions of the brain that can be found in individuals with Parkinson's disease and, less often, Alzheimer's disease. Until recently, it was not understood whether DLB was a subtype of Parkinson's disease, Alzheimer's disease, or an illness unto itself. The current consensus is that DLB is a distinct dementing illness with specific clinical and pathologic features rather than a part of the spectrum of either Alzheimer's or Parkinson's disease (Brown, 1999; McKeith et al., 1999; Gomez-Isla et al., 1999; Gomez-Tortosa et al., 2000). As in Alzheimer's disease where the severity of dementia is related to the density of cortical neuritic plaques and neurofibrillary tangles, in DLB the density of Lewy bodies appears to be strongly related to dementia severity (Haroutunian et al., 2000).

According to the criteria established by the Consortium on Dementia with Lewy bodies (Table 21-6), the clinical presentation usually has an insidious onset, with progressive and disabling mental impairment that develops into a dementia within months to several years (McKeith et al., 1996; 1999). To make a diagnosis of possible DLB, one of the following three core features must by present: fluctuation in the level of cognitive functioning, prominent visual hallucinations, and extrapyramidal motor features of parkinsonism. Fluctuation in cognition, as measured by choice reaction time tests and vigilance reaction time

TABLE 21-6. *Consensus criteria for the clinical diagnosis of dementia with Lewy bodies (DLB)*

Progressive cognitive decline of sufficient magnitude to interfere with normal social or occupational function.
Two of the following are essential for the diagnosis of probable DLB; one for a diagnosis of possible DLB:
   Fluctuating cognition
   Recurrent visual hallucinations
   Spontaneous parkinsonism
Features supportive of the diagnosis
   Repeated falls
   Syncope
   Transient losses of consciousness
   Neuroleptic sensitivity
   Systematized delusions
   Hallucinations in other modalities
Diagnosis less likely in the presence of:
   Stroke confirmed by clinical local findings and/or brain imaging
   Evidence of other physical illness or brain disorder that may account for the clinical findings

From McKeith IG, Galasko D, Kosaka K, et al. Consensus guidelines for the clinical and pathologic diagnosis of dementia with Lewy bodies (DLB): report of the consortium on DLB international workshop. *Neurology* 1996;47:1113–1124, with permission.

tests, has been shown to be more common and severe in DLB than in Alzheimer's disease or vascular dementia (VaD) (Walker et al., 2000).

Neuropsychological Profile

Very few autopsy-confirmed neuropsychological studies have been done of individuals who had DLB without some Alzheimer's, vascular, or parkinsonians pathology. The reports of pure DLB indicate that the core neuropsychological features evident early in the disease involve attention and visuospatial difficulties. Vision-related cognitive and behavioral symptoms were most frequently observed in a recent study of 24 patients with DLB (Shimomura et al., 2000). Problem-solving and executive functioning deficits have also been reported, but do not appear as prominent as attentional and visuospatial difficulties. Memory impairment is also reported in DLB, but it is not as severe as in Alzheimer's disease (Ballard et al., 1999b). The memory dysfunction may be caused by problems in retrieval of information rather than memory acquisition and consolidation that is characteristic of Alzheimer's disease. Conversely, visuoconstructive and psychomotor impairments are more severe in DLB than in Alzheimer's disease (Salmon DP et al., 1996). Although language problems are generally not reported in the early stages, one case study of autopsy-confirmed pure DLB reported that the patient presented with distinctive verbal fluency deficits in the context of mild language impairment, intact recognition memory, and impaired paragraph recall (Gurd et al., 2000). As the disease progresses, people

with DLB demonstrate global impairment across all neuropsychological domains.

Behavioral Manifestations

In the early stages, DLB is associated with psychiatric morbidity such as visual and auditory hallucinations, depression, delusions, and delusional misidentification (Ballard et al., 1999a). A number of psychiatric symptoms were found in common when DLB was compared with Alzheimer's disease, but visual hallucinations were found to be more persistent in DLB (Ballard et al., 2001). Hirono et al. (1999) found that most of their DLB subjects had visual hallucinations but the frequency and severity of visual hallucinations did not differ between DLB and Alzheimer's disease. Instead, they reported that the type of delusion distinguished the two groups such that misidentification delusions were more common in DLB than in Alzheimer's disease. Shimomura et al. (2000) suggested that defective visual perception plays a role in the development of visual hallucinations, delusional misidentifications, visual agnosias, and visuoconstructive disability.

In individuals who have both Lewy body and Alzheimer's disease pathology, the clinical presentation is different than is characteristic of either condition alone. This is especially true at the beginning stages of the disease process. When patients with mixed disease pathologies were compared with individuals with Alzheimer's disease pathology only, delusions and hallucinations were more frequent; greater impairment was noted on visuospatial and executive tasks and lesser impairment on memory and praxis tasks (Galasko et al., 1996; Connor et al., 1998; Del Ser, 2001).

Vascular Dementia

It is estimated that dementia caused solely by cerebral vascular disease varies between 2% and 18% of all dementias (Larson et al., 1985; White et al., 1996). In contrast with Alzheimer's disease, dementia from cerebral vascular disease has not been as well defined, and criteria for a diagnosis of VaD are not yet uniform. Estimates of the incidence of VaD vary because the term "vascular dementia" incorporates different vascular mechanisms and changes in the brain that result in different clinical manifestations. VaD can result from cerebral ischemic episodes, multiple infarction, cerebral hemorrhages, or ischemia and hypoxia secondary to cardiac arrest. The neuropsychological results can vary greatly, depending on the criteria used to make a diagnosis. Hachinski et al.

(1974) first introduced the term "multiinfarct dementia" (MID) and developed a scale that rates 13 clinical features (e.g., fluctuating course or nocturnal confusion) and yields an ischemic score (Hachinski et al., 1974). Rosen (1980) modified the Hachinski scale to 8 of the 13 features and found good differentiation between patients with vascular dementia and Alzheimer's disease. However, it is clear that pathogenic mechanisms different than those of MID (i.e., small vessel disease in the periventricular and deep white matter of the brain) can also result in a dementia (Pohjasvaara et al., 2000; Desmond et al., 1999). Therefore, new research criteria (Table 21-7) for the diagnoses of *probable* and *possible* vascular disease were proposed (Roman et al., 1993). These criteria emphasize the heterogeneity of vascular syndromes and leukoencephalopathic lesions (i.e., ischemic and hemorrhagic strokes, ischemic-hypoxic lesions, and senile leukoencephalopathic lesions). The definitions of the cognitive syndrome can vary significantly, depending on the cause of the vascular disease being

TABLE 21-7. *NINDS-AIREN International Workgroup criteria for probable and possible vascular dementia (VaD)*

The diagnosis of probable VaD is made when:
1. Dementia is present, defined by (a) cognitive decline from a previously higher level of functioning; (b) impairment of memory and two or more cognitive domains (preferably established by clinical examination and documented by neuropsychological testing); (c) sufficient severity as to interfere with activities of daily living; and (d) is not caused by the physical (i.e., sensorimotor) effects of stroke alone, and
2. The patient does not show disturbance of consciousness, delirium, psychosis, severe aphasia, sensorimotor impairment sufficient to preclude neuropsychological testing, system disorders, or other brain diseases (e.g., Alzheimer's disease) that could account for the cognitive deficits, and
3. Cerebrovascular disease is present, defined by (a) the presence of focal neurologic signs (e.g., hemiparesis, sensory deficit, hemianopia, dysarthria, lower facial weakness, Babinski sign); (b) evidence of relevant features consistent with cerebrovascular disease on brain imaging (i.e., computed tomography, magnetic resonance imaging) including: multiinfarctions involving cortical and/or subcortical regions, single infarct, small-vessel disease, hypoperfusion, hemorrhagic lesion, or combinations of the above lesions, and
4. A relationship is established between the dementia and the cerebrovascular disease, inferred from one or more of the following: (a) onset of dementia within 3 months of a recognized stroke; (b) abrupt deterioration in cognitive functioning; or (c) fluctuating, stepwise progression of cognitive deficits.

The diagnosis of probable VaD is further supported by (a) the early presence of a gait disturbance (small-step gait, or magnetic, apraxic-ataxic, or parkinsonian gait); (b) a history of unsteadiness and frequent falls; (c) early urinary urgency, frequency, and other urinary symptoms not explained by urologic disease; (d) pseudobulbar palsy; and (e) mood and personality changes, abulia, depression, emotional incontinence, or other subcortical deficits including psychomotor retardation and abnormal executive function.

The clinical diagnosis of possible VaD is made when:
1. The patient meets criteria for the presence of dementia, with focal neurologic signs, but
2. In whom brain imaging studies to confirm cerebrovascular disease are missing, or
3. When there is an absence of clear temporal relationship between dementia and stroke, or
4. In patients with subtle onset and variable course (improvement or plateau) of cognitive deficits and evidence of relevant cerebrovascular disease.

NINDS-AIREN, Neuroepidemiology Branch of the National Institute of Neurological Disorders and Stroke and the Association internationale pour la recherche et l'Enseignment en Neurosciences.
From Roman GC, Tatemichi TK, Erkinjuntti T, et al. Vascular dementia: diagnostic criteria for research studies. Report of the NINDS-AIREN International Workshop. *Neurology* 1993;43:250–260, with permission.

studied. Erkinjuntti et al. (2000), therefore, proposed a modification of the criteria listed in Table 21-7 that would emphasize *small vessel disease* (i.e., ischemic white matter lesions and lacunar infarcts) as the type of brain lesion and *subcortical location* as the primary location of lesion. *The Diagnostic and Statistical Manual of Mental Disorders*, 4th edition (DSM-IV, 1994) no longer uses the term MID and has adopted vascular dementia as the new terminology. Table 21-8 lists the DSM-IV criteria for a diagnosis of vascular dementia. Chapter 18 discusses the cognitive manifestations of stroke, MID, and cerebral hemorrhages, including thalamic and caudate strokes that can be thought of as acute VaD. For the purpose of this chapter, VaD refers to dementia caused by subcortical small vessel disease resulting in ischemic injury (i.e., Binswanger's type) or small lacunar infarct(s) in the basal ganglia, pons, and white matter of the centrum ovale (i.e., lacunar state). These types of brain lesions usually present subacutely, with an insidious onset and negative neurologic examination (Erkinjuntt et al., 2000). On magnetic resonance imaging (MRI), subcortical lacunar infarctions,

periventricular white matter hyperintensity (WMH), and deep white matter alterations are noted. This clinical entity represents the most frequent type of subcortical dementia, particularly among people older than 75 years of age.

Neuropsychological Profile

Although WMH are commonly found on MRI in the elderly, the clinical significance of these alterations is not fully understood because some individuals demonstrate cognitive decline or a dementia, whereas others appear cognitively intact. When MRI first became available, early reports suggested little to no relationship between neuropsychological functioning and the presence of white matter changes. It is now generally accepted, however, that it is the extent of the disease rather than its cause that determines the development of dementia (Rao et al., 1989; O'Brien, 1994; Gunning-Dixon and Raz, 2000). A recent meta-analysis of 23 studies examining the relationship between WMH and cognitive functioning in nondemented elderly, found processing speed, executive functioning, and immediate and delayed explicit memory were sensitive to WMH. On the other hand, they found intelligence and fine motor functioning did not appear related to the presence or extent of WMH (Gunning-Dixon and Raz, 2000). In other recent studies, it was suggested that the neuropsychological profile of patients with significant white matter ischemic disease is similar to that of other subcortical dementias such as Parkinson's or Huntington's disease (Doody et al., 1998; Libon et al., 2001). Thus, studies have suggested that the neuropsychological profile of VaD is characterized by impairment in executive functions, greater perseverative errors, and slowed mental processing speed (Roman and Royal, 1999; Doody et al., 1998; Libon et al., 1997; Lamar et al., 1997). In their study, Boon et al. (1992) reported that functions associated with frontal functioning (e.g., executive function) occurred before the onset of memory problems in VaD. Similarly, in a recent meta-analysis that was performed on 27 published studies of VaD and Alzheimer's disease, patients with VaD had more impairment in frontal executive functioning compared with patients with Alzheimer's disease when they were matched for age, education, and severity of dementia (Looi and Sachdev, 1999).

In contrast to Alzheimer's disease, patients with VaD show less forgetting and demonstrate better recall and recognition memory (i.e., superior long-term memory) (Libon et al., 1997; 2001; Looi and Sachdev, 1999). Pa-

---

TABLE 21-8. *DSM-IV diagnostic criteria for vascular dementia*

The development of multiple cognitive deficits manifested by both
1. Memory impairment (impaired ability to learn new information or to recall previously learned information)
2. One (or more) of the following cognitive disturbances:
   a. aphasia
   b. apraxia
   c. agnosia
   d. disturbance in executive functioning

The cognitive deficits in criteria 1 and 2 above each cause significant impairment in social or occupational functioning and represent a significant decline from a previous level of functioning.

Focal neurologic signs and symptoms (e.g., exaggeration of deep tendon reflexes, extensor plantar response, pseudobulbar palsy, gait abnormalities, weakness of an extremity) or laboratory evidence indicative of cerebrovascular disease (e.g., multiple infarctions involving cortex and underlying white matter) that are judged to be etiologically related to the disturbance.

The deficits do not occur exclusively during the course of a delirium.

From American Psychiatric Association. *The diagnostic and statistical manual of mental disorders,* 4th ed. Washington, DC: American Psychiatric Association, 1994, with permission.

tients with extensive subcortical cerebrovascular disease often demonstrate memory deficits but the nature of the memory impairment usually differs from Alzheimer's disease or other disease states affecting the temporal lobe. In mild to moderate VaD, patients usually demonstrate problems in initiating strategies to more efficiently acquire the new material (i.e., deficit in working memory). Once information is acquired, however, retention of the learned information is intact when measured by recognition tests. In mild to moderate Alzheimer's disease, the patients have the most difficulty retaining the new material over long delays on recall and recognition tests (i.e., deficit in declarative memory), but they also demonstrate problems in initiating strategies (Libon et al., 1998). Thus, the pattern of memory deficits in VaD is consistent with the interruption of frontal-subcortical circuits rather than temporal lobe dysfunction. Functional imaging has supported these distinctions in memory functioning. In one [18F]-fluorodeoxyglucose PET study, during a continuous verbal memory task, performance in VaD patients correlated with prefrontal hypometabolism, whereas in Alzheimer's disease, memory correlated with left hippocampal and temporal lobe metabolism (Reed et al., 2000).

Behavior

Behavioral changes such as depression, apathy, delusions, hallucinations, and aggression have frequently been reported in patients with VaD, regardless of the severity of cognitive decline. In patients with small infarct volumes (<15 mL), the combination of microinfarction, diffuse white matter disease, and perivascular changes were found to be associated with depression (Ballard et al., 2001). Frontal white matter lesions have been associated with high depression scores in nondemented elderly and in patients with all types of dementia (VaD, Alzheimer's disease, DLB), suggesting that it is caused by a common pathophysiology such as a disturbance in the frontostriatal pathways (O'Brien et al., 2000; Boland, 2000). Although similar types of changes are also noted in Alzheimer's disease without vascular changes, they were usually related to the level of dementia and were most prevalent during the later stages of the disease. In VaD, behavioral changes are thought to be more common than in Alzheimer's disease and independent of level of severity of dementia (Aharon-Peretz, 2000; Groves et al., 2000; Hargrave et al., 2000). In cases where Alzheimer's disease and microvascular changes were present, patients were particularly vulnerable to depression (Ballard et al., 2001).

Frontotemporal Degeneration

Compared with neuropsychological studies in Alzheimer's disease, relatively few studies have been conducted on patients with frontotemporal degeneration (FTD) and these studies have resulted in conflicting findings. In a review of past studies, Hodges et al. (1999) found support of the belief raised by others that FTD may not be a uniform disorder (Pachana et al., 1996; Neary and Snowden, 1998). Furthermore, they suggested that two distinct forms of FTD exist, one with the initial presentation of predominantly frontal impairment and frontal atrophy on imaging (DFT), and one that initially presents with predominantly temporal lobe impairment and temporal lobe atrophy on imaging (FTD). In either case, the neuropathology can involve Pick's cells and Pick's bodies or nonspecific neuronal loss with spongiosis. These patients present with different clinical syndromes, depending on the lobe initially affected. With progression of the disease, both types of impairments usually emerge. Part of the difficulty in previous neuropsychological studies may be that the FTD group was composed of pathologically heterogeneous individuals. It has also been suggested that Pick's disease, semantic dementia, and primary progressive aphasia are subtypes of FTD (1999). For a comprehensive review of the pattern of language disorder in these dementias, the reader is referred to Chapter 10.

Differentiating the Dementias

At times, it is difficult initially to differentiate FTD from Alzheimer's disease or other progressive dementias in a clinical setting early in the disease process because family members of individuals with FTD usually voice similar complaints about cognition as do those having a family member with Alzheimer's disease (i.e., change in memory and language skills). However, rapidly progressive language deterioration distinguishes the two disease entities as does a change in personality (Binetti et al., 2000; Mendez et al., 1993). Often, patients with FTD present with aphasic syndromes where their speech remains fluent but becomes devoid of content words. Reported changes in language from various case studies indicate anomia, surface dyslexia, neologisms, echolalia, phonemic paraphasias, and verbal stereotypy can be present (Graff-Radford et al., 1990; Hodges et al., 1999), but it appears that the *rapid* deterioration in expressive language is of greatest diagnostic importance. These language deficits appear to be caused by a progressive breakdown in semantic memory, including loss of general knowledge that results in impairment on tests of both nonverbal and verbal semantic knowledge. The phonological and syntactical aspects of language are preserved. Other areas of preserved neuropsychological functioning include visuospatial and perceptual abilities (Judgment of Line Orientation and Rey Figure Copy), nonverbal problem solving (Wisconsin Card Sorting Test), working memory, and good day-to-day episodic memory (Hodges et al., 1999). In contrast to patients with FTD, those with DFT in the same study presented with prominent deficits in executive functioning that was reflected in impairment on tests that involved organization and planning (i.e., Rey copy, category fluency). Mild deficits in episodic memory and verbal fluency have been reported. Semantic memory was usually intact. Changes in personality, which are early signs of the DFT, include disengagement or apathy, social impropriety, decreased personal hygiene, and possibly hyperorality and disinhibited behavior (Mendez et al., 1993). Emotional changes in DFT are also present and often include lability, depression, and delusional thinking.

With regard to the cognitive profile over time, studies reported that results of initial testing of the FTD group was worse than normal controls on all neuropsychological tests, except on a measure of visuospatial function (Pachana et al., 1996). On the other hand, the Alzheimer's disease group performed worse than controls on all measures. Patients with FTD were superior on visuospatial functioning. During the course of the disease, measures of explicit memory and visuospatial and reasoning skills worsened equally. Demented Parkinson's disease patients have been shown to decline faster than those with dementia due to Alzheimer's disease on language tests (i.e., category fluency, naming), global measures of dementia severity, and ADLs (Huber et al., 1989; Stern et al., 1998).

Dementias Associated with Extrapyramidal Signs

For a full description of the specific neuropsychologic consequences associated with various movement disorders, see Chapter 23. For comparative purposes, however, Table 21-9 includes the typical neuropsychological profile of Parkinson's disease.

Dementia Syndrome of Depression

Depression in the elderly can cause cognitive changes that are often misinterpreted as early signs of a dementia; however, in depression cognitive functioning improves once a person is effectively treated. Although depressed patients demonstrate improvement with treatment, not all of these individuals return to

their baseline level of cognitive functioning. This has led some researchers to conclude that in a subset of elderly in whom depression is associated with residual cognitive dysfunction, their depression may actually be a prodromal phase of irreversible dementia (Alexopoulos et al., 1993; Kral et al., 1989). Others have argued that with longer follow-up (i.e., 8–10 years) depressed patients with residual cognitive decline have a poorer prognosis in terms of global psychiatric morbidity (Ron et al., 1979). This remains an area of ambiguity and further prospective neuropsychological and neuropsychiatric longitudinal studies are ongoing.

The reversible decline accompanying depression is often known as pseudodementia or dementia syndrome of depression (DSD). More recently, the term "pseudodementia" has fallen out of favor because it refers to several clinical conditions, including hysterical dementias, and the use of the term "dementia syndrome of depression" is in favor. Reports of the neuropsychological profile in DSD vary widely, with no clear consensus regarding whether depression affects all cognitive domains equally or separate functions (e.g., memory or attention). Neuropsychological studies have reported that, in depression, elderly patients often demonstrate intact speech but limited spontaneous elaboration as well as impairment in psychomotor speed, speed of information processing, attention, and memory efficiency (secondary to attentional problems). Conversely, deficits in language, visuospatial abilities, and mathematical skills are often observed in dementia (Stoudemire et al., 1989; Abas et al., 1990). Furthermore, depressed patients often have heightened awareness of their memory problems in contrast with patients with Alzheimer's disease who are usually unaware of their memory decline (Bolla et al., 1991). When patients demonstrate depression, and impairment in language, recognition memory, and visual constructional praxis, consider diagnoses of depression and dementia.

PSYCHOSOCIAL ASPECTS OF DEMENTIA

Medication Management

Overall level of cognitive dysfunction in dementia, as assessed by global screening measures, is associated with impairment in the ability to carry out IADL, with an increase in functional problems typically seen in individuals with greater cognitive impairment (Agüero-Torres et al., 1998; McCue, 1996). Determining whether a person is able to self-manage medication is an important consideration in deciding if a person can live safely alone. To date, no specific neuropsychological test has been shown to be associated with medica-

TABLE 21-9. *Comparison of neuropsychological findings in the early stages of different dementing disorders and depression*

Domain	AD	DLB	PD	FTD (temporal)	DFT (frontal)	VaD	Depression
Attention	Distractible	Impaired	Normal	Normal	Distractible	Distractible	Poor
Digit span	Normal	Unknown	Normal	Normal	Impaired	Variable	Variable
Executive	Impaired	Variable	Impaired	Intact	Impaired	Impaired	Slowed
Language							
Naming	Impaired	Intact	Intact	Impaired	Intact	Intact	Intact
Fluency	Impaired	Intact	Slow	Impaired	Mild $\downarrow$	Intact	Slow
Comprehension	Normal	Intact	Intact	Impaired	Intact	Intact	Intact
Praxis	Impaired	Intact	Intact	Impaired	Unknown	Intact	Intact
Memory							
Acquisition	Impaired	Intact	Mild $\downarrow$	Impaired	Mild $\downarrow$	Impaired	Poor
Storage	Impaired	Intact	Mild $\downarrow$	Impaired	Intact	Intact	Intact
Recall	Impaired	Intact	Impaired	Impaired	Variable	Mild $\downarrow$	Impaired
Recognition	Impaired	Preserved	Intact	Impaired	Intact	Mild $\downarrow$	Intact
Remote	Impaired	Unknown	Intact	Unknown	Intact	Intact	Intact
Motor	Intact	Impaired, EPS	Impaired	Intact	Intact	Impaired	Slow
Handwriting	Intact	Impaired	Small	Intact	Intact	Intact	Intact
Visuoperception	Agnosia	Agnosia	Intact	Intact	Intact	Variable	Intact
Constructional	Impaired	Severely impaired	Impaired	Intact	Impaired	Impaired	Intact
Reasoning	Impaired	Impaired	Impaired	Intact	Impaired	Variable	Slowed
Personality change	Variable, apathetic, agitated	Visual hallucinations, delusions	Blunted affect	Apathetic	Hyperoral and/or disinhibited	Variable, but depression is common	Apathetic, $\downarrow$ motivation, irritable
Emotional	Paranoid, depression	Depression	Depression, anxiety	Apathy	Labile, depression	Depression	Hopelessness, helplessness

AD, Alzheimer's disease; DFT, dementia frontal type; DLB, dementia with Lewy bodies; EPS, extrapyramidal signs; FTD, frontotemporal degeneration; PD, Parkinson's disease; VaD, vascular dementia; $\downarrow$, decline.

tion compliance. This is probably because taking medication involves diverse skills such as telling time, memory, sequencing, and motor skills and an impairment in any one can result in problems with taking medication. A recent study (Edelberg, et al., 1999) reported a relationship between medication management and Mini-Mental State Examination (MMSE) scores in a group of geriatric medical outpatients such that level of global cognitive dysfunction strongly correlated with the inability to take medications independently. However, these results are skewed because of the inclusion of severely demented patients who perform poorly on the MMSE and have problems taking medications on their own. It is generally accepted that multiple neuropsychological measures are needed to maximize the prediction of functional skills. The most common situation where medication management is discussed occurs in patients who are in the early stages of a disease and are likely to be living on their own. In a personal study where a large battery of neuropsychological tests were administered, praxis was found to be predictive of medication management for individuals with mild dementia (Ryan et al., in submission). If individuals have difficulty carrying out simple, overlearned gestures, then it is reasonable to assume that they would have difficulty performing higher order motor sequences such as taking medications, preparing meals, and dialing the telephone. Although patients are less likely to demonstrate impairment in praxis early on in the dementia process, when they do, it is likely to have a significant negative effect in their ability to perform most IADL, as they all involve sequences of behavior.

Driving

With the increasing numbers of people developing dementing disorders, determining a person's fitness to drive has become an increasingly important issue. A decline in response time, sensory and perceptual changes, and a decline in some cognitive functions that are associated with aging are just a few reasons why some normal healthy elderly individuals become unfit to drive. In people with a dementia, normal age-related changes can increase their vulnerability to problems when driving because they may no longer be able to compensate for their weaknesses. Furthermore, they may not even be aware of these normal changes. In one study, individuals with dementia had 2.5 times the crash rate of other age-matched nondemented residents randomly selected from their community (Tuokko et al., 1995). Another group who were not demented but had medical problems had a crash rate that was 2.2 times that of healthy elderly community residents.

Since the late 1980s, an increasing number of studies have tried to determine what factors distinguish safe from unsafe drivers. Early studies were inconclusive in finding specific cognitive variables that predict a person's driving fitness; some later studies have reported that visual perceptual and attentional aspects are likely to correlate with unsafe driving. Trails B test from the Trail Making Test (Reitan 1958), a test requiring the conceptual shifting between two alternating sequences of numbers and letters, was the only neuropsychological test that was repeatedly related to traffic violations or crashes (Withaar et al., 2000). These results lead to the conclusion, however, that people with mild dementia who have intact visual perceptual skills and normal performance on the Trails B test may still be safe drivers. Therefore, a diagnosis of dementia alone may not justify terminating a person's driving privileges.

To develop a practice parameter regarding driving and Alzheimer's disease, the Quality Standards Subcommittee of the American Academy of Neurology recently completed a review of the literature regarding automobile accident frequency among drivers with the disease. It concluded that *level* of dementia was an important factor (Dubinsky et al. 2000). Specifically, driving was found to be mildly impaired in those drivers with *probable* Alzheimer's disease and a clinical dementia rating (CDR) of 0.5, but drivers with the disease and a severity of CDR 1 were found to pose a significant traffic safety problem, both from crashes and from driving performance measurements. The Committee recommended that patients and their families be told that those with Alzheimer's disease whose CDR is 1 should not drive because of a substantially increased risk of crashing, and that patients with *possible* disease and a CDR of 0.5 pose a significant traffic problem compared with other elderly drivers. It was also recommended that driving performance of the milder group be evaluated by a qualified examiner with a reevaluation of dementia severity and driving privileges every 6 months. In the future, it is imperative to develop a better understanding of the variables that make a person unfit to drive so that a person's independence can be maximized while minimizing the risk of accidents. Important ethical and legal considerations related to decisions about driving competency are discussed in Chapter 35.

CONCLUSION

Although researchers have made great progress in identifying and defining the various dementing syndromes over the past 30 years, problems with diagnostic criteria continue to exist. More prospective, longitudinal neuropsychological studies are needed to better elucidate similarities and differences among various dementing disorders. In particular, further work must be done to refine these criteria and develop diagnostic tools that are more sensitive early in the disease process so that the effects of potential therapies can be accurately measured.

REFERENCES

Abas MA, Sahakian BJ, Levy R. Neuropsychological deficits and CT scan changes in elderly depressives. *Psychol Med* 1990;20:507–520.

Agüero-Torres H, Fratiglioni L, Guo Z, Viitanen M, et al. Dementia is the major cause of functional dependence in the elderly: 3-year follow-up data from a population-based study. *Am J Public Health* 1998;88:1452–1456.

Aharon-Peretz J, Kliot D, Tomer R. Behavioral differences between white matter lacunar dementia and Alzheimer's disease: a comparison of the neuropsychiatric inventory. *Dement Geriatr Cogn Disord* 2000;11:294–298.

Alexopoulos GS, Meyers BS, Young RC, et al. The course of geriatric depression with "reversible dementia": a controlled study. *Am J Psychiatry* 1993;150:1693–1699.

American Psychiatric Association. *The diagnostic and statistical manual of mental disorders*, 4th ed. Washington, DC: American Psychiatric Association, 1994.

Backman L, Small BJ, Fratiglioni. Stability of the preclinical episodic memory deficit in Alzheimer's disease. *Brain* 2001; 124:96–102.

Ballard CG, Ayre G, O'Brien J, et al. Simple standardized neuropsychological assessments aid in the differential diagnosis of dementia with Lewy bodies from Alzheimer's disease and vascular dementia. *Dement Geriatr Cogn Disord* 1999b;10:104–108.

Ballard C, Holmes C, McKeith I, et al. Psychiatric morbidity in dementia with Lewy bodies: a prospective clinical and neuropathological comparative study with Alzheimer's disease. *Am J Psychiatry* 1999a;156:1039–1045.

Ballard CG, O'Brien J, Swann AG, et al. The natural history of psychosis and depression in dementia with Lewy bodies and Alzheimer's disease: persistence and new cases over 1 year of follow-up. *J Clin Psychiatry* 2001;62: 46–49.

Bayles KA, Tomoeda CK. Confrontation naming impairment in dementia. *Brain Lang* 1983;19:98–114.

Bayles KA, Tomoeda CK, Cruz RF. Performance of Alzheimer's disease patients in judging word relatedness. *J Int Neuropsychol Soc* 1999;5:668–675.

Bayley PJ, Salmon DP, Bondi MW, et al. Comparison of the serial position effect in very mild Alzheimer's disease, mild Alzheimer's disease, and amnesia associated with electroconvulsive therapy. *J Int Neuropsychol Soc* 2000;6: 290–298.

Becker JT, Boller F, Saxton J, et al. Normal rate of forgetting of verbal and non-verbal material in Alzheimer's disease. *Cortex* 1987;23:59–72.

Binetti G, Locascio JJ, Corkin S, et al. Differences between Pick disease and Alzheimer disease in clinical appearance and rate of cognitive decline. *Arch Neurol* 2000;57: 225–232.

Boland RJ. Depression in Alzheimer's disease and other dementias. *Curr Psychiatry Rep* 2000;2:427–433.

Bolla KI, Lindgren KN, Bonaccorsy C, et al. Memory complaints in older adults. Fact or fiction? *Arch Neurol* 1991; 48:61–64.

Boone K, Miller BL, Lesser IM, et al. Neuropsychological correlates of white-matter lesions in healthy elderly subjects. *Arch Neurol* 1992;49:549–554.

Brown DF. Lewy body dementia. *Ann Med* 1999;31:188–196.

Butters N, Granholm E, Salmon DP, et al. Episodic and semantic memory: a comparison of amnestic and demented patients. *J Clin Exp Neuropsychol* 1987;9:585–589.

Cahn DA, Salmon DP, Bondi MW, et al. A population-based analysis of qualitative features of the neuropsychological test performance of individuals with dementia of the Alzheimer type: implications for individuals with questionable dementia. *J Int Neuropsychol Soc* 1997;3:387–393.

Cappa A, Calcagni ML, Villa G, et al. Brain perfusion abnormalities in Alzheimer's disease: comparison between patients with focal temporal lobe dysfunction and patients with diffuse cognitive impairment. *J Neurol Neurosurg Psychiatry* 2001;70:22–27.

Carr DB, Gray S, Baty J, et al. The value of informant versus individual's complaints of memory impairment in early dementia. *Neurology* 2000;55:1724–1727.

Chen P, Ratcliff G, Belle SH, et al. Cognitive tests that best discriminate between presymptomatic AD and those who remain nondemented. *Neurology* 2000;55:1847–1853.

Connor DJ, Salmon DP, Sandy TJ, et al. Cognitive profiles of autopsy-confirmed Lewy body variant vs. pure Alzheimer disease. *Arch Neurol* 1998;55:994–1000.

Crowe SF, Hoogenraad K. Differentiation of dementia of the Alzheimer's type from depression with cognitive impairment on the basis of a cortical versus subcortical pattern of cognitive deficit. *Arch Clin Neuropsychol* 2000;15:9–19.

Cummings JL, Benson DF. Dementia of the Alzheimer's type: an inventory of diagnostic clinical features. *J Am Geriatr Soc* 1986;34:12–19.

Cummings JL, Benson DF, Hill MA, et al. Aphasia in dementia of the Alzheimer's type. *Neurology* 1985;29: 394–397.

Del Ser T, Hachinski V, Merskey H, et al. Clinical and pathological features of two groups of patients with dementia with Lewy bodies: effect of coexisting Alzheimer-type lesion load. *Alzheimer Dis Assoc Disord* 2001;15:31–44.

Desmond DW, Erkinjuntti T, Sano M, et al. The cognitive syndrome of vascular dementia: implications for clinical trials. *Alzheimer Dis Assoc Disord* 1999;13(Suppl 3):S21–S29.

Devanand DP, Michaels-Martson KS, Liu X, et al. Olfactory deficits in patients with mild cognitive impairment predict Alzheimer's disease at follow-up. *Am J Psychiatry* 2000;157:1399–1405.

Doody RS, Massman PJ, Mawad M, et al. Cognitive consequences of subcortical magnetic resonance imaging changes in Alzheimer's disease: comparison to small vessel ischemic vascular dementia. *Neuropsychiatry Neuropsychol Behav Neurol* 1998;11:191–199.

Dorrego MF, Sabe L, Cuerva AG, et al. Remote memory in Alzheimer's disease. *J Neuropsychiatry Clin Neurosci* 1999;11:490–497.

Dubinsky RM, Stein AC, Lyons K. Practice parameter: risk of driving and Alzheimer's disease (an evidence-based review). Report of the Quality Standards Subcommittee of the American Academy of Neurology. *Neurology* 2000; 54:2205–2211.

Edelberg HK, Shallenberger E, Wei JY. Medication management capacity in high functioning community-living older adults: detection of early deficits. *J Am Geriat Soc* 1999;47:592–596.

Erkinjuntti T, Inzitari D, Pantoni L, et al. Research criteria for subcortical vascular dementia in clinical trials. *J Neural Transm* 2000;59(Suppl):23–30.

Fisher NJ, Rourke BP, Bieliauskas LA. Neuropsychological subgroups of patients with Alzheimer's disease: an examination of the first 10 years of CERAD data. *J Clin Exp Neuropsychol* 1999 21:488–518.

Folstein MF, Folstein SE, McHugh PR. "Mini-mental state." A practical method for grading the cognitive state of patients for the clinician. *J Psychiatr Res* 1975;12:189–198.

Ford JM, Askari N, Gabrieli JD, et al. Event-related brain potential evidence of spared knowledge in Alzheimer's disease. *Psychol Aging* 2001;16:161–176.

Freedman M, Leach L, Kaplan E, et al. *Clock drawing: a neuropsychological analysis*. New York: Oxford University Press, 1994.

Furey-Kurkjian ML, Pietrini P, Graff-Radford NR, et al. Visual variant of Alzheimer disease: distinctive neuropsychological features. *Neuropsychology* 1996;10:294–300.

Galasko D, Katzman R, Salmon DP, et al. Clinical and neuropathological findings in Lewy body dementias. *Brain Cogn* 1996;31:166–175.

Gomez-Isla T, Growdon WB, McNamara M, et al. Clinicopathologic correlates in temporal cortex in dementia with Lewy bodies. *Neurology* 1999;53:2003–2009.

Gomez-Tortosa E, Irizarry MC, Gomez-Isla T, et al. Clinical and neuropathological correlates of dementia with Lewy bodies. *Ann NY Acad Sci* 2000;920:9–15.

Graff-Radford NR, Damasio AR, Hyman BT, et al. Progressive aphasia in patients with Pick's disease: a neuropsychological, radiological, and anatomic study. *Neurology* 1990;40:620–626.

Groves WC, Brandt J, Steinberg M, et al. Vascular dementia and Alzheimer's disease: is there a difference? A comparison of symptoms by disease duration. *J Neuropsychiatry Clin Neurosci* 2000;12:305–315.

Gunning-Dixon FM, Raz N. The cognitive correlates of white matter abnormalities in normal aging: a quantitative review. *Neuropsychology* 2000;14:224–232.

Gurd JM, Herzberg L, Joachim C, et al. Dementia with Lewy bodies: a pure case. *Brain Cogn* 2000;44:307–323.

Hachinski VC, Lassen NA, Marshall J. Multi-infarct dementia. A cause of mental deterioration in the elderly. *Lancet* 1974;2:207–210.

Hargrave R, Reed B, Mungas D. Depressive syndromes and functional disability in dementia. *J Geriatr Psychiatry Neurol* 2000;13:72–77.

Haroutunian V, Serby M, Purohit DP, et al. Contribution of Lewy body inclusions to dementia in patients with and without Alzheimer disease neuropathological conditions. *Arch Neurol* 2000;57:1145–1150.

Heaton RK, Chelune GJ, Talley JL, et al. *Wisconsin card sorting test manual*, revised and expanded. Odessa, FL: Psychological Assessment Resources, 1993.

Hirono N, Mori E, Tanimukai S, et al. Distinctive neurobehavioral features among neurodegenerative dementias. *J Neuropsychiatry Clin Neurosci* 1999;11:498–503.

Hodges JR, Patterson K, Ward R, et al. The differentiation of semantic dementia and frontal lobe dementia (temporal and frontal variants of frontotemporal dementia) from early Alzheimer's disease: a comparative neuropsychological study. *Neuropsychology* 1999;13:31–40.

Hohl U, Grundman M, Salmon DP, et al. Mini-mental examination and Mattis dementia rating scale performance differs in Hispanic and non-Hispanic Alzheimer's disease patients. *J Int Neuropsychol Soc* 1999;5:301–307.

Huber SJ, Shuttleworth EC, Freidenberg DL. Neuropsychological differences between the dementias of Alzheimer's and Parkinson's diseases. *Arch Neurol* 1989;46:1287–1291.

Jellinger KA. Morphological substrates of mental dysfunction in Lewy body disease: an update. *J Neural Transm* 2000;59(Suppl):185–212.

Kral VA, Emery OB. Long-term follow-up of depressive pseudodementia of the aged. *Can J Psychiatry* 1989;34:445–446.

Lamar M, Podell K, Carew TG, et al. Perseverative behavior in Alzheimer's disease and subcortical ischemic vascular dementia. *Neuropsychology* 1997;11:523–534.

Larrabee GJ, Youngjohn JR, Sudilovsky A, et al. Accelerated forgetting in Alzheimer-type dementia. *J Clin Exp Neuropsychol* 1993;15:701–712.

Larson EB, Reifler BV, Sumi SM, et al. Diagnostic evaluation of 200 elderly outpatients with suspected dementia. *J Gerontol* 1985;40:536–543.

Libon DJ, Malamut BL, Swenson R, et al. Further analyses of clock drawings among demented and nondemented older subjects. *Archives of Clinical Neuropsychology* 1996;11:193–205.

Libon DJ, Bogdanoff B, Leopold N, et al. Neuropsychological profile associated with subcortical white matter alterations and Parkinson's disease—implications for the diagnosis of dementia. *Archives of Clinical Neuropsychology* 2001;16:19–32.

Libon DJ, Bogdanoff B, Bonavita J, et al. Neuropsychological deficits associated with ischemic vascular dementia caused by periventricular and deep white matter alterations. *Archives of Clinical Neuropsychology* 1997;12:239–250.

Libon DJ, Bogdanoff B, Cloud BS, et al. Declarative and procedural learning, quantitative measures of the hippocampus and subcortical white alterations in Alzheimer's disease and ischemic vascular dementia. *J Clin Exp Neuropsychol* 1998;20:30–41.

Loewenstein DA, Arguelles S, Bravo M, et al. Caregivers' judgments of the functional abilities of the Alzheimer's disease patient: a comparison of proxy reports and objective measures. *J Gerontol B Psychol Sci Soc Sci* 2001;56:78–84.

Looi JC, Sachdev PS. Differentiation of vascular dementia from AD on neuropsychological tests. *Neurology* 1999;53:670–678.

Lopez OL, Becker JT, Brenner RP, et al. Alzheimer's disease with delusions and hallucinations: neuropsychological and electroencephalographic correlates. *Neurology* 1991;41:906–912.

Malloy PF, Cummings JL, Coffey CE, et al. Cognitive screening instruments in neuropsychiatry: a report of the committee on research of the American Neuropsychiatric Association. *J Neuropsychiatry Clin Sci* 1997;9:189–197.

Martin A, Brouwers P, Lalonde F, et al. Towards a behavioral topology of Alzheimer's patients. *J Clin Exp Neuropsychol* 1986;8:594–610.

Mayeux R, Stern Y, Spanton S. Heterogeneity in dementia of the Alzheimer type: evidence of subgroups. *Neurology* 1985;35:453–461.

McCue M. The relationship between neuropsychology and functional assessment in the elderly. In Nussbaum P, ed. *The handbook of neuropsychology and aging*. New York: Plenum Press, 1996:394–408.

McKeith IG, Galasko D, Kosaka K, et al. Consensus guidelines for the clinical and pathologic diagnosis of dementia with Lewy bodies (DLB): report of the consortium on DLB international workshop. *Neurology* 1996;47:1113–1124.

McKeith IG, Perry EK, Perry RH. Report of the second dementia with Lewy body international workshop: diagnosis and treatment. Consortium on Dementia with Lewy bodies. *Neurology* 1999;53:902–905.

McKhann G, Drachman D, Folstein M, et al. Clinical diagnosis of Alzheimer's disease: report of the NINCDS-ADRDA work group under the auspices of department of health and human services on Alzheimer's disease. *Neurology* 1984;34:939–944.

Mendez MF, Selwood A, Mastri AR, et al. Pick's disease versus Alzheimer's disease: a comparison of clinical characteristics. *Neurology* 1993;43:289–292.

Neary D, Snowden J. Fronto-temporal dementia: nosology, neuropsychology, and neuropathology. *Brain Cogn* 1996; 31:176–187.

Nordin S, Murphy C. Impaired sensory and cognitive olfactory function in questionable Alzheimer's disease. *Neuropsychology* 1996;10:113–119.

Nordin S, Murphy C. Odor memory in normal aging and Alzheimer's disease. *Ann NY Acad Sci* 1998;885:686–693.

Norton LE, Bondi MW, Salmon DP, et al. Deterioration of generic knowledge in patients with Alzheimer's disease: evidence from the Number Information Test. *J Clin Exp Neuropsychol* 19:857–866.

O'Brien JT, Metcalfe S, Swann A, et al. Medial temporal lobe width on CT scanning in Alzheimer's disease: comparison with vascular dementia, depression and dementia with Lewy bodies. *Dement Geriatr Cogn Disord* 2000;11: 114–118.

O'Brien MD. How does cerebrovascular disease cause dementia? *Dementia* 1994;5:133–136.

Pachana NA, Boone KB, Miller BL, et al. Comparison of neuropsychological functioning in Alzheimer's disease and frontotemporal dementia. *J Clin Exp Neuropsychol Soc* 1996;2:505–510.

Paulson JS, Salmon DP, Thal LJ, et al. Incidence of and risk factors for hallucinations and delusions in patients with probable AD. *Neurology* 2000;54:1965–1971.

Pohjasvaara T, Mantyla R, Ylikoski R, et al. Comparison of different clinical criteria (S\DMS-III, ADDTC, IDC-10, NINDS-AIREN, DSM-IV) for the diagnosis of vascular dementia. National Institute of Neurological Disorders and Stroke-Association Internationale pour la Recherche et l'Enseignment Neurosciences. *Stroke* 2000;31:2952–2957.

Rao SM, Mittenberg W, Bernardin L, et al. Neuropsychological test findings on subjects with leukoariosis. *Arch Neurol* 1989;46:40–47.

Rapcsak SZ, Croswell SC, Rubens AB. Apraxia in Alzheimer's disease. *Neurology* 1989;39:664–668.

Rapoport MJ, van Reekum R, Freedman M, et al. Relationship of psychosis to aggression, apathy and function in dementia. *Int J Geriatr Psychiatry* 2001;16:123–130.

Reed BR, Eberling JL, Mungas D, et al. Memory failure has different mechanisms in subcortical stroke and Alzheimer's disease. *Ann Neurol* 2000;48:275–284.

Reitan RM. Validity of the Trailmaking test as an indicator of organic brain damage. *Percept Mot Skills* 1958;8:271–276.

Resnick SM, Gottlieb GL, Gur RE, et al. Identical twins with probable Alzheimer's disease: behavior, anatomy, and physiology. *Neuropsychiat Neuropsychol Behav Neurol* 1988;1:62–72.

Richards M, Bell K, Dooneief F, et al. Patterns of neuropsychological performance in Alzheimer's disease patients with and without extrapyramidal signs. *Neurology* 1993; 43:1708–1711.

Roman GC, Royall DR. Executive control function: a rational basis for the diagnosis of vascular dementia. *Alzheimer Dis Assoc Disord* 1999;13(Suppl 3): S69–S80.

Roman GC, Tatemichi TK, Erkinjuntti T, et all. Vascular dementia: diagnostic criteria for research studies. Report of the NINDS-AIREN International Workshop. *Neurology* 1993;43:250–260.

Ron MA, Toone BK, Garralda ME, et al. Diagnostic accuracy in presenile dementia. *Br J Psychiatry* 1979;34:1;61–168.

Rosen WG. Verbal fluency in aging and dementia. *J Clin Neuropsychol* 1980;2:135–146.

Rosen WG. Neuropsychological patterns with focus on constructional apraxia. In: Symposium, longitudinal studies of dementia of the Alzheimer type: neuropsychological and neurophysiological patterns. INS meetings, Houston, 1984.

Rosen WG, Mohs RC, Davis KL. A new rating scale for Alzheimer disease. *Am J Psychiatry* 1984;141:1356–1364.

Ryan LM, Malamut BL, Hill SK, et al. Neuropsychological tests predict instrumental activities of daily living in patients with dementia (*submitted for publication*).

Salmon DP, Galasko D, Hansen LA, et al. Neuropsychological deficits associated with diffuse Lewy body disease. *Brain Cogn* 1996;31:148–165.

Salmon DP, Heindel WC, Lange KL. Differential decline in word generation from phonemic and semantic categories during the course of Alzheimer's disease: implications for the integrity of semantic memory. *J Int Neuropsychol Soc* 1999;5:692–703.

Sherman AM, Massman PJ. Prevalence and correlates of category versus letter fluency discrepancies in Alzheimer's disease. *Arch Clin Neuropsychol* 1999;14:411–418.

Shimomura ME, Fujimora M, Hirono N, et al. Visuoperceptual impairment in dementia with Lewy bodies. *Arch Neurol* 2000;57:489–493.

Simon E, Leach L, Winocur G, et al. Intact primary memory in mild to moderate Alzheimer disease: indices from the California Verbal Learning Test. *J Clin Exp Neuropsychol* 1994;16:414–422.

Small GW, Rabins PV, Barry PP, et al. Diagnosis and treatment of Alzheimer disease and related disorders. Consensus statement of the American Association, and American Geriatrics Society. *JAMA* 1997 1997;278:1363–1371.

Stern Y, Albert M, Tang MX, et al. Rate of memory decline in AD is related to education and occupation: cognitive reserve? *Neurology* 1999;53:1942–1947.

Stern Y, Mayeux R, Sano M, et al. Predictors of disease course in patients with probable Alzheimer's disease. *Neurology* 1987;37:1649–1653.

Stern Y, Ming-Xin T, Jacobs DM, et al. Prospective comparative study of the evolution of probable Alzheimer's disease and Parkinson's disease dementia. *J Int Neuropsychol Soc* 1998;4:279–284.

Stoudimire A, Hill C, Gulley L, et al. Neuropsychological and biomedical assessment of depression-dementia syndromes. *J Neuropsychiatry Clin Neurosci* 1989;1:347–361.

Suhr JA, Jones RD. Letter and semantic fluency in Alzheimer's, Huntington's, and Parkinson's dementias. *Arch Clin Neuropsychol* 1998;13:447–454.

Thompson-Schill SL, Gabrieli JD, Fleischman DA. Effects of structural similarity and name frequency of picture naming in Alzheimer's disease. *J Int Neuropsychol Soc* 1999;5:659–667.

Troster AI, Butters N, Salmon DP, et al. The diagnostic utility of savings scores: differentiating Alzheimer's and Huntington's diseases with the logical memory and visual reproduction tests. *J Clin Exp Neuropsychol* 1993;15:773–788.

Tuokko H, Hadjistavropoulos T. Screening instruments for cognitive impairment. In: *An assessment guide to geriatric neuropsychology*. Mahwah, NJ: Lawrence Erlbaum, 1998:28–43.

Tuokko H, Tallman K, Beattie BL, et al. An examination of driving records in a dementia clinic. *J Gerontol B Psychol Sci Soc Sci* 1995;50:S173–S181.

Van Gorp WG, Marcotte TD, Sultzer D, et al. Screening for dementia: comparison of three commonly used instruments. *J Clin Exp Neuropsychol* 1999;21:29–38.

Walker MP, Ayre GA, Cummings JL, et al. Quantifying fluctuation in dementia with Lewy bodies, Alzheimer's disease, and vascular dementia. *Neurology* 2000;25: 1616–1625.

White L, Petrovitch H, Ross GW, et al. Prevalence of dementia in older Japanese-American men in Hawaii: the Honolulu-Asia Aging Study. *JAMA* 1996;276:955–960.

Withaar FK, Brouwer WH, Van Zomeren AH. Fitness to drive in older drivers with cognitive impairment. *J Int Neuropsychol Soc* 2000;6:480–490.

WEB SITES

4 Anything Network *www.4alzheimers.4anthing.com*

Alzheimer's Disease Education & Referral Service *www.alzheimers.org*

Internet Mental Health *www.mentalhealth.com*

U.S. Public Health Service *www.surgeongeneral.gov/library/mentalhealth*

American Psychiatric Association *www.psych.org*

22

Movement Disorders in the Older Adult

Bernard Ravina and Howard Hurtig

INTRODUCTION

Several movement disorders increase in incidence and prevalence with old age. However, normal aging is associated with changes (e.g., slowed motor speed) that can resemble common findings of movement disorders. Also, older adults are more likely to take multiple prescription medications, and to experience drug-induced side effects and movement disorders (Rajput, 1997). Thus, the clinician caring for the older adult must distinguish between age-related findings and true movement disorders as well as target therapeutic interventions to the specific needs of the elderly patient.

HYPOKINETIC MOVEMENT DISORDERS: PARKINSONISM

For clinical purposes, movement disorders can be divided into *hypokinetic* and *hyperkinetic* disorders. Parkinsonism, the most common of the hypokinetic disorders, is a "syndrome" of slowed movements, rigidity, postural instability, and tremor. Idiopathic parkinsonism or Parkinson's disease (PD) is the most common parkinsonian syndrome, accounting for approximately 75% of the total number of patients with a parkinsonian diagnosis (Paulson and Stern, 1997). It is a progressive, degenerative disease with distinctive clinical features, a specific histopathology characterized by degeneration of pigmented neurons in the substantia nigra of the midbrain, and a strongly positive response to levodopa replacement therapy by most patients. Parkinsonism caused by other degenerative disorders such as progressive supranuclear palsy, multiple system atrophy, stroke, brain tumor, infections, and intoxications comprise the other 25% of cases.

Parkinsonism is a disorder of aging. Parkinson's disease is rare before the age of 50, and incidence and prevalence increase steadily until the 9th or 10th decades (Tanner et al., 1997). Although PD can begin in childhood or early adulthood (juvenile PD), the median time of onset is likely in the sixth decade (Hoehn and Yahr, 1967).

Pathogenesis

Although the cause of PD is unknown, the disease pathology is well described. On gross inspection of the brain sliced through the midbrain, can be seen pallor of the normally pigmented substantia nigra and a histologic depletion of dopaminergic cells that project from the substantia nigra to the caudate and putamen (referred to together as the "striatum"). The severity of the clinical disability in PD is proportional to the loss of dopaminergic neurons in the substantia nigra. The neuropathologic hallmark of the disease is the eosinophilic, intraneuronal, intracytoplasmic inclusion known as the "Lewy body," which can be found in the substantia nigra, locus ceruleus, dorsal motor nucleus of the vagus nerve, thalamus, hypothalamus, and substantia innominata (nucleus basalis of Meynert) (Lowe et al., 1997).

Clinical Manifestations

Parkinson's disease remains a clinical diagnosis, despite recent advances in computerized isotopic brain imaging (positron emission and single photon emission computed tomography) that make it possible to visualize the abnormalities in the basal ganglia caused by the disease. The cardinal features—rest tremor, rigidity, and bradykinesia—usually appear asymmetrically, often only affecting one side of the body in the early stages of the disease. Most movement disorders specialists believe that a patient must have two of the three cardinal features and a strongly positive response to levodopa before a diagnosis of PD can be seriously considered (Hughes et al., 1992). Patients with other parkinsonian syndromes (e.g., progressive supranuclear palsy and multisystems atrophy) rarely respond as well to levodopa as do patients with PD. Postural instability (tendency to fall) is a relatively late feature of the disease, in contrast to the other parkinsonian syndromes, in which it appears relatively early in the course.

Tremor, often the initial symptom, is eventually present in 75% of patients with PD. It has a frequency of 5 to 7 Hz and usually starts on one side in a hand or foot (Findley et al., 1981). Tremor is typically most prominent when the affected part is at rest, but it can also be evident with sustention and action. As the disease progresses, the tremor may involve both sides as well as the lips and chin. *Rigidity* (increased tone) is resistance to passive movement in a relaxed limb that occurs throughout the whole range of movement. During the examination of a patient with PD, the physician may detect increased tone that starts and stops as the limb is moved passively back and forth. The term "cogwheeling" has been used to describe this finding on neurologic examination. Rigidity is an inconstant finding, but can occur in all stages of disease. *Bradykinesia* refers to slowness of movement and initiation of movements. Bradykinesia and tremor are the most noticeable physical sign of parkinsonism. Bradykinesia underlies many of the symptoms of PD, including difficulty with dexterity, fine motor movements, and gait.

Gait dysfunction in PD reflects a composite of bradykinesia, rigidity, and impairment of postural righting reflexes. Stride length is shortened and the feet shuffle. Arm swing is decreased, usually on the more affected side. Posture is stooped and the arms assume a flexed and adducted position. Turning in the act of walking is done *en bloc*, without pivoting or twisting the torso and with multiple small steps that describe a wide arc. As the disease progresses, gait is interrupted by transient freezing of the feet, as though they were glued to the ground, especially on initiating the first step or when entering a narrow space such as a doorway.

Loss of balance and falling tend to occur later in the course of the disease. Patients who present with postural instability or frequent falls early in the course of illness should be evaluated for other causes of parkinsonism such as *progressive supranuclear palsy* (PSP) or *multiple systems atrophy* (MSA). A modest backward pull on the patient's shoulders can be used to test postural instability. The patient should be instructed to take only one step back if necessary to prevent going backward. If more than two steps are required to regain balance, postural reflexes are impaired. More severely affected patients may fall like solid objects (Sudarsky, 1990) and the examiner must be prepared to catch the patient. Stooped posture, combined with a loss of postural reflexes, leads to uncontrolled running as the patient's torso leans forward and moves his or her feet faster to catch up with the upper body. This type of forward locomotion is referred to as a "festinating gait."

Many manifestations of PD are seen (Table 22-1), which are considered secondary features, not sufficient by themselves to confirm a diagnosis of the disease. However, some secondary symptoms may be the presenting complaint and may be more debilitating than the primary features of PD.

Diagnosing Parkinson's Disease in the Elderly

Some signs of parkinsonism can be a part of normal aging. In one study, bradykinesia was present in 37% of normal elderly community residents (Rajput, 1997). No increase was noted in tone in normal elderly subjects, but joint stiffness caused by arthritis can limit mobility and be confused with increased tone. Similarly, posture tends to become flexed at the neck and trunk as part of normal aging. Dizziness can lead to gait instability and stride length is shorter in the elderly (Parker, 1994). The descriptive terms "senile gait" and "old person's gait" are two of the many default labels used to define the nonspecific, but sometimes incapacitating, abnormality of walking by the elderly when no obvious other cause can be found. Rest tremor does not occur as a manifestation of normal aging and is one of the more specific indicators of PD in the elderly. If bradykinesia and postural instability alone were used in the diagnosis of

TABLE 22-1. *Secondary symptoms of Parkinson's disease*

Cognitive and behavioral	Craniofacial	Autonomic	Other
Dementia	Masked facies	Orthostatic hypotension	Cramps
Anxiety	Decreased blinking	Impaired gastric motility	Paresthesias
Depression	Decreased sense of smell	Urinary bladder dysfunction	Seborrhea
Sleep disturbance	Dysphagia	Abnormal thermoregulation	Micrographia
	Dysarthria	Sexual dysfunction	
	Sialorrhea		

the disease, many normal elderly patients might be misdiagnosed. Therefore, to make a diagnosis of PD, older patients (and younger ones) should meet the standard criteria of two of the three cardinal features and a good response to levodopa.

Other Causes of Parkinsonism in the Elderly

Most cases of parkinsonism are ultimately classified as PD, although the differential diagnosis of secondary parkinsonism is broad (Fig. 22-1). Structural lesions of the basal ganglia (stroke, hydrocephalus, tumor), drugs, infections, or metabolic disorders can rarely mimic those typical of PD. In general, these patients do not have a rest tremor and do not respond to levodopa (Murrow et al., 1990).

Vascular Parkinsonism

Parkinsonism caused by strokes can occur after a single stroke in the basal ganglia or brainstem, or as the cumulative result of several strokes. Patients with vascular parkinsonism tend to have a long history of hypertension and a step-wise progression of symptoms. Evidence for stroke may be noted on examination. Gait may be shuffling or *apraxic*, a term used synonymously with transient freezing. Patients

should have evidence of cerebrovascular disease on computed tomography (CT) scan or magnetic resonance imaging (MRI), although asymptomatic ischemic changes are common in older patients and do not independently make the diagnosis of vascular parkinsonism (Hurtig, 1993).

Hydrocephalus

Hydrocephalus can cause parkinsonian signs and symptoms. Normal pressure hydrocephalus (NPH) is a syndrome, characterized by the triad of gait instability, incontinence, and cognitive dysfunction (Krauss et al., 1997; Shannon, 1993). As with vascular parkinsonism, gait in NPH is classically apraxic, but any gait disturbances, especially "gait ignition failure" and "frontal gait" (Nutt, 1995), have been described in NPH. Brain imaging (CT or MRI) shows communicating hydrocephalus with ventricles enlarged out of proportion to atrophy of the cerebral cortical sulci.

Drug-Induced Parkinsonism

Drug-induced parkinsonism is a critically important entity because it is one of the few reversible causes of parkinsonism. The most common offenders

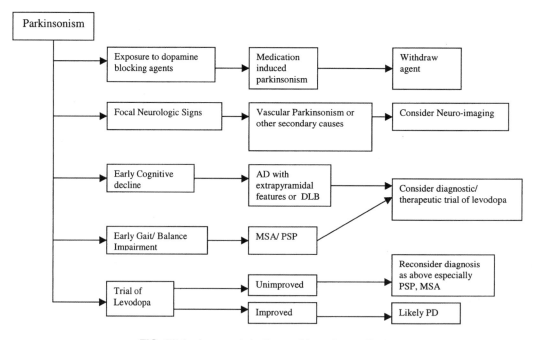

FIG. 22-1. Approach to the parkinsonian patient.

are members of the class of drugs known as neuroleptics, which are dopamine receptor antagonists, usually used as antipsychotics. These include phenothiazines, butyrophenones, and thioxanthenes (Jankovic, 1995). The antiemetic prochlorperazine (Compazine) and the gastrointestinal promotility agent metoclopramide (Reglan) are also dopamine receptor blockers that have the potential to induce parkinsonism and other "extrapyramidal" involuntary movements, such as dystonia and tardive dyskinesia (Indo and Ando, 1982). Clozapine (Clozaril), the first "atypical" neuroleptic, was introduced to the American market in 1990 as a major breakthrough for treating schizophrenia without causing parkinsonism or other extrapyramidal side effects. Several other atypical neuroleptics have followed in the last decade, including quetiapine (Seroquel), olanzapine (Zyprexa), and risperidone (Risperdal), although they produce varying degrees of extrapyramidal side effects. Other problematic drugs include the antihypertensives methyldopa (Aldomet), verapamil (Hubble, 1993), and reserpine (Serapsil). Reserpine can induce signs of parkinsonism by depleting dopamine storage vesicles presynaptically instead of blocking postsynaptic dopamine receptors. Lovastatin (Mevacor) has also been reported as a potential cause of parkinsonism (Muller, 1995). Treatment of parkinsonism in this setting consists of a combination of a high index of suspicion and prudent withdrawal of the offending drug.

Alzheimer's Disease and Dementia with Lewy Bodies

Neurodegenerative diseases other than Parkinson's often have clinical parkinsonian features. Alzheimer's disease, the most common cause of dementia, may be accompanied by varying degrees of parkinsonism in up to 50% of patients (Chen et al., 1991). In Alzheimer's disease, the dementia precedes the parkinsonian signs and is disproportionately more severe. Dementia and parkinsonism also co-occur in the pathologic entity diffuse Lewy body disease, also known clinically as "dementia with Lewy bodies" (DLB). The clinical presentation in DLB consists of prominent and early cognitive decline, fluctuations in cognitive function, spontaneous visual hallucinations that are not drug-induced, and parkinsonism (Consortium on DLB, 1996). The parkinsonian signs consist of bradykinesia, rigidity, and a prominent gait disorder; rest tremor is seen less frequently than in PD (Galasko et al., 1996; Mega et al., 1996). A diagnosis of DLB may be difficult to differentiate from

Alzheimer's disease or from typical PD and dementia. However, in PD the interval between the onset of parkinsonism and onset of the cognitive disturbance is usually more than 2 years.

Progressive Supranuclear Palsy and Multiple System Atrophy

Progressive supranuclear palsy (PSP) and multiple system atrophy (MSA) closely resemble PD and may be clinically indistinguishable in the early stages of progression, but they are distinct pathologic and clinical entities. PSP presents as an akinetic-rigid syndrome with a prominent gait disorder early in the disease course. In contrast, walking is usually not a major issue in PD until late in the course. Truncal posture tends to be upright instead of stooped, and axial and asymmetric limb dystonia may be present (Golbe, 1997). Tremor is much less common in PSP than in PD (Globe 1997). Cognitive impairment occurs earlier than in PD, but the dementia of PSP is usually not as severe as that in PD and the other parkinsonian syndromes. Many patients demonstrate a pseudobulbar affect, marked by uncontrollable laughing or crying. Several characteristic eye movement abnormalities are seen, the most important of which is a supranuclear paresis of conjugate gaze, beginning with symptomatic slowing of gaze in the vertical plane. Patients often complain of having trouble looking at their food during meals or hitting a golf ball. Examination may reveal impaired voluntary gaze, spontaneous mini-myoclonic jerks of the eyes (square wave jerks), and loss of optokinetic nystagmus, which can be elicited in the normal subject by passing a sequence of stripes or other repetitively occurring graphic objects horizontally or vertically across the field of vision (Globe 1997). Reflex eye movements are preserved, hence, the application of the term "supranuclear" in PSP. These reflexive eye movements may be demonstrated using the doll's head maneuver, in which the patient is asked to visually fixate a target while the examiner gradually moves the patient's head in the horizontal or vertical plane. Preserved reflexive eye movements allow patients to hold their eyes on target despite the head movements. In the late stages of PSP, voluntary and reflexive eye movements in all directions, including the horizontal plane, are severely impaired. MRI may show atrophy of the dorsal midbrain (Savoiardo et al., 1989).

Multiple system atrophy is a diagnostic grouping of three disorders that are distinguished by a combination of parkinsonism, cerebellar ataxia, autonomic insufficiency, and pyramidal tract deficits. By convention, the most prominent neurologic finding determines the subclassification under the MSA umbrella, although any assortment of the four types of signs can occur in the same patient. Thus, a mix of parkinsonism and severe autonomic dysfunction (orthostatic hypotension, atonic bladder and impotence) would be called autonomic MSA or the Shy-Drager syndrome. Pure parkinsonism is called "striatonigral MSA"; and cerebellar ataxia without a family history is called "cerebellar MSA," or olivopontocerebellar atrophy in the old terminology (Litvan et al., 1997). Autonomic failure and postural instability are early findings. As in PSP, tremor is rare. The MRI scan, which is normal in PD, and in most cases of MSA, may sometimes show a combination of shrinkage of the brainstem and cerebellum and an abnormally large area of low signal in the striatum (Gillman, 1998). The course of MSA is generally faster than that of PD. In most patients with MSA, especially striatonigral, cognitive function is preserved.

Both PSP and MSA have limited responses to levodopa and other agents used for the treatment of PD. However, a trial of levodopa may be useful as a diagnostic test, particularly in striatonigral degeneration. A strongly positive response would suggest PD and cast doubt on the diagnosis of MSA or PSP. Doses of up to 1,000 mg/day of levodopa or more may be needed to achieve any symptomatic benefit. The therapeutic response in patients with PSP or MSA is usually disappointing and the drugs may aggravate orthostatic hypotension, particularly in MSA. If patients fail to respond to levodopa, other dopaminergic agents generally should not be tried. Botulinum toxin (BTX) injections may be useful for dystonia associated with PSP and MSA. Autonomic insufficiency can be treated with specific drugs (see below). Nonpharmacologic therapies such as speech therapy, swallowing therapy for dysphagia, and physical therapy are also an important part of patient care.

Treatment of Parkinson's Disease

The objective of treating PD is to suppress symptoms and improve neurologic function. No treatment has yet been proved to alter the underlying progression of the disease. Some therapeutic strategies, however, may avert or delay the complications that are associated with long-term dopaminergic therapy. The first decision for doctor and patient after the diagnosis is

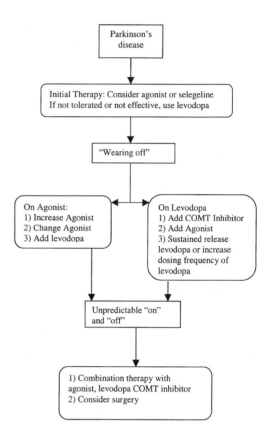

FIG. 22-2. Approach to the pharmacological management of Parkinson's disease.

whether the symptoms require treatment. As a general rule, pharmacotherapy should be considered when symptoms begin to interfere with a patient's ability to function at home or work. Once initiated, treatment should be individualized, taking the patient's age, stage of disease, mental state, and tolerance of side effects into account. The algorithm shown in Figure 22-2 outlines a common approach to treatment.

Nonpharmacologic Therapies

The care of patients with PD is best accomplished through a multidisciplinary approach, which should include access to psychological counseling; occupational, physical, and speech therapy; and support groups. Nonpharmacologic intervention can be as important as medications and should be started early in the course of PD. Exercise is especially important in a program of general health maintenance for almost every patient.

Pharmacotherapy

Levodopa

Levodopa was introduced to the marketplace over 30 years ago as the first truly effective drug for treating parkinsonism, and today it is still the most potent (Table 22-2). Levodopa works most efficiently and with fewest side effects when administered in combination with carbidopa, an inhibitor of the peripheral catabolic enzyme dopa decarboxylase. Carbidopa is joined with levodopa in different ratios (10/100, 25/100, 25/250) as well as regular and controlled release preparations. A typical starting dose of carbidopa/levodopa (Sinemet) is one half of a 25/100 mg tablet three times a day (with meals to prevent nausea). Once tolerance is established at a low dose, the amount of carbidopa/levodopa per dose can be slowly increased to an optimal therapeutic level compatible with realistic expectations for the individual patient. Average daily consumption ranges between 300 and 600 mg/day in three divided doses; few patients require more than 1,000 mg/day (Calne, 1993). Most patients with typical PD will have a gratifying and smooth initial response to levodopa. Many symptoms improve, but most patients will observe that bradykinesia improves the most. Tremor suppression often lags behind but it, too, can be well controlled by levodopa.

One of the major drawbacks of levodopa is its short half-life of 90 minutes, which has an impact on long-term therapy. When patients with relatively mild disability first use levodopa, the overall response is positive and smooth throughout the day. Few doses per 24 hours are required because of the brain's ability to store the drug in the axon terminals of the intact nigrostriatal neurons. As more neurons degenerate, the brain's storage capacity declines and at some point, which varies with the individual inherent rate of progression, the long, smooth duration response (LDR) gives way to the short duration response (SDR). Clinical expression of the SDR occurs in the form of motor fluctuations, which are characterized by a "wearing off" of the benefit of a dose of carbidopa/levodopa, usually 3 to 4 hours after a dose is taken. The patient will notice a gradual reemergence of parkinsonian symptoms during this interlude, which at its nadir is called the "off" period. The reciprocal "on" response is gradually reestablished (usually within 30 minutes) after the next dose of levodopa is swallowed. Levodopa-induced choreiform or dystonic involuntary movements, called "dyskinesias," commonly begin to occur at the stage of the disease when motor fluctuations start to appear, usually at

peak effect 1 to 2 hours after a dose (Fahn et al., 1984). In most patients, dyskinesias are dose-related and can be so severe and disabling to greatly interfere with all activities of daily living.

Fluctuations of one sort or another occur as a matter of course in over half of all patients with typical PD who use levodopa for more than 5 years. Initially, this can be remedied by shortening the interval between doses. In extreme cases, however, the SDR will contract so much that it will conform to the actual 90 minute half-life of levodopa and patients will be forced to use levodopa as frequently as every 2 hours. Controlled-release carbidopa/levodopa was developed in the 1980s as a practical approach to combat the problems of the SDR, namely the hyperkinetic dyskinesias of the "on" period and the bradykinesia of the "off" period. Controlled-release drug is more slowly released into the small intestine by the stomach than is regular carbidopa/levodopa, and its peak blood level following absorption is lower. Unfortunately, the benefit attributable to controlled release has been modest at best, although some patients can reduce the frequency of dosing and experience a partial restoration of the LDR as well as a lessening of the intensity of peak dose dyskinesias. Many find its effect disappointing because of its slow onset of action and the tendency for it to cause an increase in the intensity of dyskinesias at the end of the day.

Active debate occurs in the neurological literature over when to start using levodopa in a patient with advancing symptoms because of its alleged potential for accelerating the progression of PD. Although no clear clinical evidence exists, some investigators and authors claim that levodopa is toxic to nigral neurons because of its *in vitro* ability to induce oxidant stress, a process that can destroy the lipid membrane of the cell wall (Olanow and Koller, 1998). According to this hypothesis, early use of levodopa not only increases the rate of nigral cell death but also hastens the onset of motor fluctuations and the associated disabilities. There is no definitive resolution of this debate, but neurologists who believe that levodopa is toxic will postpone the use of levodopa until late in the course of the illness, substituting the less potent dopamine agonists as a temporizing therapeutic measure. Other neurologists who are unconvinced that levodopa is toxic, will use it early on. Most with expertise in PD initiate levodopa therapy when the doctor, patient, and family determine sufficient compromise in social and occupational functioning warrants such treatment, especially if other medications to control symptoms have been inadequate.

TABLE 22-2. Selected medications for Parkinson's disease

Medication	Action	Usual dose range	Common side effects	Warnings and contraindications
Carbidopa/Levodopa (Sinemet)	Dopamine replacement	Carbidopa ≥75 mg Levodopa: 300–1,000 mg divided t.i.d.	Orthostasis Nausea Vomiting Confusion/hallucinations Dyskinesias	Do not use with nonselective MAO inhibitor
Pramipexole (Mirapex)	Dopamine agonist	0.375–4.5 mg divided t.i.d.	Similar to levodopa + somnolence?	Known sensitivity to drug or its ingredients Use with caution in patients who drive
Pergolide (Permax)	Dopamine agonist	0.05–5 mg/d divided t.i.d.	Similar to levodopa + somnolence?	Ergot sensitivity
Ropinirole (Requip)	Dopamine agonist	0.75–24 mg/d divided t.i.d.	Similar to levodopa + somnolence?	Known sensitivity to drug or its ingredients Use with caution in patients who drive
Entacapone (Comtan)	Inhibits dopamine metabolism	200 mg with each carbidopa/levodopa dose to maximum of 1,600 mg/d	Similar to levodopa + diarrhea	Known sensitivity to drug or its ingredients
Selegiline (Eldepryl)	Selective MAO-B inhibitor in doses up to 10 mg/d	10 mg/d or less, divided b.i.d.	Similar to levodopa	Risk of hypertensive crisis caused by MAO-A inhibition at doses >10 mg/d Do not use with meperidine and other opioids

b.i.d., twice daily; MAO, monoamine oxidase; t.i.d., three times daily.

Dopamine Agonists

Dopamine agonists are a class of drugs that directly stimulate dopamine receptors and require no metabolism to the active form. Bromocriptine, the first agent of this class, was developed and introduced in the early 1970s to complement and enhance the effect of levodopa. Although not as clinically effective as levodopa, dopamine agonists have the advantages of a longer pharmacologic half-life and no need for conversion from precursor to active agent. Four agonists are available in the United States. Two are ergot derivatives (pergolide or Permax and bromocriptine or Parlodel) have been available for more than 20 years. Two are non-ergots (pramipexole or Mirapex and ropinirole or Requip) were marketed in the United States in 1997. Agonists initially were used as an adjunct to levodopa for patients with motor complications (Calne 1993), but more recently, they have been studied in early stages of PD as monotherapy in an effort to postpone the initiation of levodopa. For example, a recent randomized, controlled trial comparing ropinirole with levodopa as initial monotherapy showed a significantly lower incidence of motor complications in the group of patients taking ropinirole, although levodopa supplements were required by many in this group (Rascol et al., 2000). For this reason, many patients and doctors have chosen to use dopamine agonists as the first line of treatment, particularly in young people, and to save levodopa for later when agonist monotherapy is no longer sufficient. Although the side effects of levodopa and agonists are similar, many patients, especially the elderly and cognitively impaired, do not tolerate agonists because of drug-induced confusion, hallucinations, orthostasis, and excessive daytime somnolence (Ferreira and Galitzky, 2000; Schapira, 2000). It cannot be overstated that drug treatment of patients with PD must be individualized.

Anticholinergics and Selegiline

Drugs with a primary dopaminergic effect are the mainstay of treatment for PD, but other, secondary drugs can complement and augment the primary impact of the dopaminergics. *Anticholinergics*, such as trihexyphenidyl (Artane) and benztropine (Cogentin), may be useful in treating tremor. They are less effective in alleviating rigidity and bradykinesia. These agents are often poorly tolerated by older patients because of the high potential for causing short-term memory dysfunction, confusion, prostatism, and blurred vision. *Amantadine*, a drug with anticholinergic, dopaminergic, and putative glutamate-blocking properties, is inconsistently effective in relieving mild

symptoms of PD. It has recently been shown to suppress levodopa-induced dyskinesias in some patients (Metman et al., 1998). *Selegiline (*Deprenyl, Eldepryl) is a selective monoamine oxidase (MAO)–inhibitor. It has well-documented symptomatic benefits in treating PD (Parkinson's Study Group [PSG], 1996). Selegiline has been studied as a potential neuroprotective agent (PSG, 1989; Olanow et al., 1995), although its ability to delay disease progression remains unproved. Some experts use selegiline as initial therapy; others prefer dopamine agonists, which have more potent symptomatic benefits.

Catechol-O-Methyltransferase Inhibition

Catechol-O-methyltransferase (COMT) inhibitors work by reducing metabolism and increasing the availability of levodopa. These agents, tolcapone (Tasmar) and entacapone (Comtan), augment and prolong the response to levodopa. They are used in patients who are experiencing "wearing-off." COMT inhibitors decrease "off" time by approximately an hour per day (Adler et al., 1998). Tolcapone has been removed from the pharmaceutical market in Europe and Canada because of potential hepatotoxicity, but is still available in the United States under the condition of mandatory biweekly monitoring of liver function tests. Mild, transient elevations of transaminase were reported in clinical trials before tolcapone received unrestricted US Food and Drug Administration (FDA) approval. Three European patients with PD who were taking tolcapone, among other drugs, died of liver failure, although the exact role of tolcapone was not established (Assal et al., 1998).

Natural substances, vitamins, and other "alternative" therapies for PD are popular but largely unproved. A single controlled trial of high dosage vitamin E (2,000 U/day) showed no effect on symptom relief or the natural history of disease progression when compared with placebo (PSG, 1996).

Surgical Therapies

The neurosurgical treatment of PD has a long and uneven history. The first effort to ablate the basal ganglia was made in the late 1930s and became popular in the 1950s and early 1960s because of the void of pharmacotherapy. The motor region of the thalamus became a favored target for lesioning, particularly in patients with severe tremor, and although serious complications were frequent, many patients who survived the procedure experienced satisfactory tremor suppression. With the introduction of levodopa in the late 1960s, neurosurgical treatment of patients with PD all but disappeared. However, the development of computerized imaging and improved neurosurgical techniques brought about a revival of lesioning of the internal globus pallidus (pallidotomy), thalamus (thalamotomy), and, more recently, deep brain stimulation (DBS) of the subthalamic nucleus and other sites. Many PD centers can perform both ablative and DBS procedures in various brain nuclei in appropriate patients with PD who meet strict criteria for operative treatment. Thalamic DBS is useful for treating parkinsonian and essential tremor and is the only FDA approved DBS procedure. DBS of the internal globus pallidus and subthalamic nucleus appears to alleviate more features of parkinsonism than thalamic DBS, but target selection remains controversial (Hallett and Litvan, 1999). Currently under investigation are cell implantation in humans and gene therapy in experimental animals.

Particular Problems of Parkinson's Disease in the Elderly

Cognitive impairment and psychiatric symptoms (e.g., depression and psychosis) may be prominent features of PD, especially in the elderly. The neuropsychiatric complications of this disease are discussed in Chapter 23.

Prominent autonomic dysfunction is usually a hallmark of MSA, but mild autonomic insufficiency is common in PD. Findings can include abnormal thermoregulatory responses, with hyperhidrosis, orthostatic hypotension, constipation, urinary frequency and urge incontinence, and impotence. In the elderly, urinary symptoms and syncope caused by orthostatic hypotension are the most clinically troublesome. Urinary tract infection and outflow obstruction caused by prostatic hypertrophy must be considered as causes of disturbed bladder function. Urodynamic studies of the bladder in PD have shown that detrusor hyperreflexia is the most common finding (Pavlakis et al., 1983). Peripheral anticholinergic drugs (e.g., oxybutynin) may effectively relax the detrusor, but central side effects, especially confusion, are a potential risk. Consultation with a urologist is essential (and usually helpful) in this setting.

Orthostatic hypotension occurs in PD both because of degenerative changes in the neurons of the autonomic nervous system and antiparkinson drugs tend to aggravate this already compromised state of blood pressure control. Even without symptoms of orthostatic hypotension, blood pressure in these patients is low, often in the range of 90 to 100 systolic. It is important, therefore, to monitor brachial blood pressure sitting and standing when adjusting medications for patients with PD. Mild orthostasis (e.g., light headedness) can often be controlled by increasing fluid and salt intake or by using simple compression stockings. Severe symptoms (e.g., recurrent syncope) may require the use of the mineralocorticoid fludrocortisone (Florinef) in a single daily dose of 0.1 mg with salt supplements or the α_{1a} agonist midodrine (ProAmatine) (McTavish and Goa, 1989).

HYPERKINETIC MOVEMENT DISORDERS: TREMOR, CHOREA, TARDIVE SYNDROMES, AND DYSTONIA

Tremor

Tremor is the most common hyperkinetic involuntary movement in adults (Rautakorpi I 1982). This topic is discussed in Chapter 11.

Chorea

Chorea consists of involuntary, continuous, rapid movements that flow randomly from one body part to another. In contrast to tremor, choreiform movements are not predictable. Numerous causes of chorea can manifest during childhood or early adulthood; this chapter focuses on those that predominate among the elderly.

Huntington's disease, the most common hereditary cause of chorea, is transmitted in an autosomal dominant pattern with complete penetrance. In general, Huntington's chorea afflicts young and middle-aged adults (fourth to sixth decade), but it can appear for the first time in the elderly. The gene for Huntington's chorea is located on the short arm of chromosome 4; the abnormality is an excessively long repetition of the trinucleotide sequence CAG. Age of onset is inversely related to the length of the trinucleotide repeat; paternal transmission is often associated with onset in the late teens or early twenties (Huntington's Disease Collaborative Group, 1993). The main manifestation of the disease are choreiform and athetoid movements, accompanied by cognitive and behavioral changes, eventually evolving to severe dementia. Chorea and athetosis gradually are accompanied by numerous other features such as dysarthria, dysphagia, ataxia, rigidity, dystonia (Jankovic, 1995), and abnormal supranuclear gaze problems (Penny et al., 1990). Behavioral symptoms typically consist of agitation, anxiety, depression, mania, and psychosis (Litvan et al., 1998).

Senile or idiopathic chorea is an uncommon, insidious, generalized disorder that occurs among patients above 60 years of age. Patients have no family history and lack the cognitive and behavioral changes seen in Huntington's chorea. The pathogenesis and pathophysiology are poorly understood; no specific pathology is seen, based on findings in the few cases that have come to autopsy. Choreiform or dyskinetic movements restricted to the mouth and tongue can be seen in the elderly and are more common among edentulous patients. The movements improve with proper dental appliances (Mark, 1997).

Generalized chorea, hemichorea, and hemiballism can be caused by vascular disease. Strokes, hemorrhage, and vascular malformations have all been associated with chorea (Mark 1997). Lesions in many areas of the basal ganglia, but particularly the subthalamic nucleus and globus pallidus, have been noted to cause ballism and choreiform movements (Vidakovic et al., 1994; Fukui et al., 1993). The onset of vascular chorea is usually abrupt, but it can follow the acute insult by weeks or months. The symptoms can resolve spontaneously or persist. When treatment is required, drugs that deplete dopamine from the presynaptic terminals (reserpine or tetrabenazine) or block postsynaptic receptors (typical neuroleptics) can be effective.

Tardive Dyskinesia

The syndrome of tardive dyskinesia results from treatment with dopamine receptor blocking agents (DRBA), especially when high doses of typical neuroleptics are required to treat severe mental illness. However, chronic exposure to any dose of a neuroleptic, including prochlorperazine (Compazine) for nausea and metoclopramide (Reglan) for gastrointestinal dysmotility, imposes a risk of tardive dyskinesia. In contrast to acute dystonia or subacute parkinsonism associated with the use of these agents, tardive syndromes occur later in the course of treatment or in the setting of drug withdrawal (Faurbye et al., 1964). Tardive syndromes have various manifestations, including akathisia, dystonia, parkinsonism, mycoclonus, and tics (Fahn, 1984). The most common manifestation is a pattern of repetitive, stereotyped movements of the mouth and tongue that are suppressed by action. Typically, classic tardive dyskinesia consists of repetitive chewing movements, tongue thrusting, or writhing movements of the mouth and tongue. Similar movements can occur in the limbs, trunk, and respiratory muscles. Tardive movements can resemble chorea but

tend to be more repetitive and stereotyped than chorea.

A diagnosis of a tardive syndrome requires exposure to one or more DRBA, with onset of symptoms within 6 months of use of a DRBA, and persistence of symptoms for 1 month after withdrawal of the agent (Stacy and Jankovic, 1991). Additionally, patients should have no other clear cause for a movement disorder (Baldessarini et al., 1980). In exceptional cases, a diagnosis of tardive dyskinesia should be seriously considered if all other criteria are in place and exposure to an offending drug is less than 3 months.

Among the atypical neuroleptics, clozapine and quetiapine appear to be least likely to induce tardive syndromes. Olanzapine is more likely to induce tardive dyskinesia and drug-induced parkinsonism, but less readily than risperidone and typical neuroleptics (Wood, 1998). Risperidone has a significantly greater propensity to induce extrapyramidal syndromes than the other atypical neuroleptics (Gutierrez-Esteinou, et al., 1997).

Epidemiologic studies of tardive dyskinesia have been hampered by discrepancies in diagnostic criteria and biased study samples. Data in one study suggest an incidence rate of approximately 5% per year for the 4 years studied (Chakos et al., 1996). Older age and female gender have been consistent risk factors (Kane et al., 1988). Prevalence rates in a study of patients above 54 years of age using neuroleptics were 25%, 34%, and 53% at 1, 2, and 3 years, respectively (Woerner et al., 1998). Longer duration of exposure and higher total cumulative dose also appear to increase the risk of tardive dyskinesia (Kane et al., 1988).

The treatment of patients with tardive dyskinesia is always challenging and often unsatisfactory. Once the involuntary movements appear, the offending agent should be slowly withdrawn or substituted with a safer drug, such as clozapine or quetiapine. Increasing the dose of the DRBA may suppress the movements but at the expense of perpetuating or even aggravating the underlying process. This approach should be avoided. If the offending agent is withdrawn reasonably soon after onset of the tardive movements, remission can occur, but can take several years. Remissions are more likely in younger patients (Smith and Baldessarini, 1980).

Dopamine depleting agents (e.g., reserpine and tetrabenazine) have shown the most consistent results in the treatment of patients with tardive dyskinesia and do not cause the disease. Tetrabenazine is not readily available in the United States. Reserpine has been shown to be beneficial in a randomized clinical trial at doses of 0.75 mg to 1.5 mg/day (Huang et al., 1980). Side effects include hypotension, parkinsonism, and depression. Atypical neuroleptics, particularly clozapine (Clozaril), have also been reported to improve the symptoms of tardive dyskinesia (Bassit and Neto, 1998). The mechanism of action is unclear, because the atypical neuroleptics have a low affinity for dopamine receptors.

Dystonia

Dystonia is a syndrome of sustained muscle contractions, causing twisting, repetitive movements, and abnormal postures. Dystonic movements are distinguished from chorea by the sustained nature of the movement. Dystonia is classified etiologically as *primary* or *secondary* and anatomically by affected body region—generalized or focal. *Generalized* dystonia typically starts in the leg with onset before age 20 and is often hereditary. *Focal* dystonias, in contrast, usually involve the upper extremities or neck and head, start after the age of 20, and are sporadic (Greene et al., 1995). Several secondary causes of dystonia are seen in the adult, including focal lesions of the central and peripheral nervous system, degenerative disorders such as PD and PSP, and drugs. The same drugs that cause classic tardive dyskinesia can also cause tardive dystonia. Patients with primary dystonia should have no findings on neurologic examination except for dystonia and, possibly, essential tremor, which frequently coexist. Dystonic tremor tends to be less regular than essential tremor (Jednyak et al., 1991). The workup for primary dystonia is negative, by definition, including a normal CT or MRI scan. Dystonia is considered *focal* if one body area is affected (a hand or the neck), *segmental* if two contiguous areas are affected (neck and arm), and *generalized* if both legs and another body area are affected or if both legs and the trunk are involved. The "sensory trick" is a characteristic feature of dystonia. Patients may be able to alleviate the dystonic movement, by tactile or proprioceptive input, such as touching or supporting the affected body part against gravity.

Primary Segmental Dystonia

The head and neck are the most common sites for primary segmental dystonia (Tolosa and Marti, 1997). Examples include cervical dystonia (also known as spasmodic torticollis), blepharospasm, oromandibular dystonia (OMD), and spasmodic dysphonia. *Cervical dystonia* can present with rotation, flexion, extension, tilting of the head, or a combination of these. Sudden spasms of head jerking or head tremor are frequently associated. *Blepharospasm* can manifest as increased blinking or forced episodic eye closure. Blepharospasm is often exacerbated by reading, driving, or other visual triggers. *Meige syndrome* is the combination of blepharospasm and OMD. OMD involves the muscles of facial expression causing grimacing, puckering, lip smacking, and several other movements, including jaw opening, jaw closing, or bruxism (Tolosa et al., 1988). OMD must be distinguished from tardive dyskinesia, which tends to have more regular movements, but the overlap can be considerable. Spasmodic dysphonia is a form of dystonia causing muscles in and around the larynx to assume excessively adducted or abducted positions. Patients with adduction dysphonia tend to have choked or staccato speech, whereas those with abduction dysphonia tend to have breathy, whispered speech (Hartman and Aronson, 1991).

Focal Limb Dystonia

Focal limb dystonias can affect the leg or, more commonly in adults, the arm. Primary limb dystonias are frequently task specific, such as writer's dystonia or writer's cramp. In writer's cramp, the force of the grip may be exaggerated and the wrist and forearm can assume a flexed or extended posture. Writing becomes shaky and laborious. Several other task-specific dystonias have been described, including dystonias in string musicians and sportsmen (e.g., golfer's dystonia) (Tolosa and Marti, 1997). Dystonias that are initially task specific rarely generalize to other activities at a later time or spread to the homologous opposite limb.

Pathogenesis

The pathogenesis of dystonia is unknown. The physiologic hallmark of dystonia is sustained contraction of agonist and antagonist muscle pairs (Rothwell and Obeso,1987). In primary dystonia, the cortex and basal ganglia may be involved, according to one study using PET, which showed a relative metabolic overactivity of the lentiform nucleus and premotor cortices (Eidelberg et al., 1995). This suggests that a relative imbalance or metabolic dissociation within the basal ganglia may be responsible for the hyperkinetic movements. Primary dystonia is not associated with any known histopathologic or biochemical lesion, although the volume of the putamen is increased by about 10% in one report (Black et al., 1998).

Treatment

Nonpharmacologic treatments (e.g., physical therapy) may be useful in preventing contractures and increasing range of motion, particularly in cervical dystonia. In some cases, braces can be fitted to provide moderating sensory input similar to a sensory trick. The pharmacologic treatment of dystonia is largely based on empiric and anecdotal evidence. However, several randomized clinical trials have reported that anticholinergic agents (e.g., trihexyphenidyl and benztropine) are effective in young onset generalized dystonia (Greene et al., 1988). Most older adults are unable to tolerate the relatively high doses required to relieve symptoms and signs. Benzodiazepines (e.g., clonazepam and lorazepam) and γ-aminobutyric acid (GABA)ergic agents such as baclofen (Lioresal) can also be helpful and these agents can be used in combination.

The introduction of BTX, subtype A, in the 1980s revolutionized the treatment of dystonia and is now the first line of treatment in most cases. The primary effect of BTX is to induce a transient paralysis of skeletal muscles by inhibiting presynaptic release of acetylcholine across the neuromuscular junction (Jankovic and Brin, 1991). BTX has been well studied and has been proved effective and safe in numerous types of focal dystonia, especially cervical dystonia and blepharospasm. Approximately 85% to 90% of patients will achieve satisfactory and sustained improvement, lasting 3 to 4 months in most cases (Jankovic et al., 1990; Jankovic, 1997). Repeat injections are needed as symptoms return. Adverse effects are uncommon and mild, depending on the site injected and dose delivered. For patients who are unresponsive to BTX, a variety of surgical procedures, including rhizotomy, intradural sectioning of the nerve root, or ramisectomy, extradural sectioning of a nerve division, have been attempted with mixed results (Bertrand and Molina-Negro. 1987). DBS has been shown to be effective in selected cases of generalized and focal dystonia (Coubes, 2000).

SUMMARY

The diagnosis of movement disorders in the elderly is particularly challenging, as clinicians must distinguish between features of normal aging and true disease states. Movement disorders encompass a wide array of clinical phenomenology, which remains the basis for the most accurate diagnosis, despite advances in the technology of neuroimaging. Effective treatment of movement disorders in the elderly depends entirely on the accuracy of the diagnosis and can be gratifying for both patient and clinician. Recent therapeutic advances (e.g., BTX) have dramatically brightened the horizons of patients with chronic neurologic disabilities. Treatment strategies must, however, be tailored to the individual patient, with particular attention to medication side effects.

REFERENCES

Adler CH, Singer C, O'Brien C, et al. Randomized, placebo-controlled study of tolcapone in patients with fluctuating Parkinson's disease treated with levodopa-carbidopa. *Arch Neurol* 1998;55:1089–1095.

Assal F, Spahr L, Hadengue A, et al. Tolcapone and fulminant hepatitis. *Lancet* 1998;352:958.

Baldessarini RJ, Cole JO, Davis JM, et al. Tardive dyskinesia. Summary of a task force report of the American Psychiatric Association. *Am J Psychiatry* 1980;137:1163–1172.

Bassitt DP, Neto MRL. Clozapine efficacy in tardive dyskinesia in schizophrenia patients. *Eur Arch Psychiat Clin Neurosi* 1998;248:209–211.

Bertrand CM, Molina-Negro P. Selective peripheral denervation in 111 cases of spasmodic torticollis: rationale and results. *Adv Neurol* 1987;50:637–643.

Black K, Ongur D, Perlmutter JS. Putamen volume in idiopathic focal dystonia. *Neurology* 1998;51:819–824.

Calne DB. Treatment of Parkinson's disease. *N Engl J Med* 1993;329:1021–1027.

Chakos MH, Alvir JMJ, Woerner MG, et al. Incidence and correlates of tardive dyskinesia in first episode schizophrenia. *Arch Gen Psychiatry* 1996;53:313–319.

Chen JY, Stern Y, Sano M, et al. Cumulative risks of developing extrapyramidal signs, psychosis, or myoclonus in the course of Alzheimer's disease. *Arch Neurol* 1991;48:1141–1143.

Consortium on Dementia with Lewy Bodies. Consensus guidelines for the clinical and pathological diagnosis of dementia with Lewy Bodies. *Neurology* 1996;47:113–1124.

Coubes P, Roubertie A, Vayssiere N, et al. Treatment of DYT-1—generalized dystonia by bilateral stimulation of the internal globus pallidus. *Lancet* 2000;355(9222):2220–2221.

Eidelberg D, Moeller JR, Ishikawa T, et al. The metabolic topography of idiopathic torsion dystonia. *Brain* 1995;118:1473–1484.

Fahn S. The varied clinical expressions of dystonia. *Neurol Clin* 1984;2:541–554.

Fahn S, Bressman SB. Should levodopa therapy for Parkinsonism be started early or late? Evidence against early treatment. *Can J Neurol Sci* 1984;11:200–205.

Faurbye A, Rasch PJ, Peterson PB, et al. Neurological symptoms in pharmacotherapy of psychosis. *Acta Psychiatr Scand* 1964;40:10–27.

Ferreira JJ, Galitzky M, Montrastruc JL, et al. Sleep attacks and Parkinson's disease treatment. *Lancet* 2000;355:1333–1334.

Findley LJ, Gresty MA, Halmagyi GM. Tremor, the cogwheel phenomenon and clonus in Parkinson's disease. *J Neurol Neurosurg Psychiatry* 1981;44:534–546.

Fukui T, Hasegawa Y, Seriyama S, et al. Hemiballism-hemichorea induced by subcortical ischemia. *Can J Neurol Sci* 1993;20:324–328.

Galasko D, Katzman R, Salmon DP, et al. Clinical and neuropathological findings in Lewy body dementias. *Brain Cogn* 1996;31:166–175.

Gillman S. Multiple system atrophy. In: Jankovic J, Tolosa E, eds. *Parkinson's disease and movement disorders*, 3rd ed. Baltimore: Williams & Wilkins, 1998:245–262.

Golbe LI. Progressive supranuclear palsy. In: Watts RL, Koller WC, eds. *Movement disorders, neurologic principles and practice*. New York: McGraw-Hill, 1997: 279–296.

Golbe LI. Young-onset Parkinson's disease: a clinical review. *Neurology* 1991;41:168–173.

Greene P, Kang UJ, Fahn S. Spread of symptoms in idiopathic torsion dystonia. *Mov Disord* 1995;10:143–152.

Greene P, Shale H, Fahn S. Analysis of open label trials in torsion dystonia using high dosage anticholinergics and other drugs. *Mov Disord* 1988;3:46–60.

Gutierrez-Esteinou R, Grebb JA. Risperdone: an analysis of the first three years in general use. *Int Clin Psychopharmacol* 1997;12;S3–S10.

Hallett M. Litvan I. Evaluation of surgery for Parkinson's disease: a report of the Therapeutics and Technology Assessment Subcommittee of the American Academy of Neurology. The Task Force on Surgery for Parkinson's Disease. *Neurology* 1999;53(9):1910–1921.

Hartman DE, Aronson AE. Clinical investigations of intermittent breathy dysphonia. *J Speech Hear Disord* 1991; 46:428–432.

Hoehn MM, Yahr MD. Parkinsonism: onset, progression and mortality. *Neurology* 1967;17:427–442.

Huang CC, Wang RIH, Hasegawa A, et al. Evaluation of reserpine and alpha-methyldopa in the treatment of tardive dyskinesia. *Psychopharmacol Bull* 1980;16:41–43.

Hubble J. Drug-induced parkinsonism. In: Stern MB, Koeller WC, eds. *Parkinsonian syndromes*. New York: Marcel Dekker, 1993:111–122.

Hughes AJ, Daniel SE, Kilford L, et al. Accuracy of the clinical diagnosis of idiopathic Parkinson's disease: a clinicopathological study of 100 cases. *J Neurol Neurosurg Psychiatry* 1992;55:181–184.

Huntington's Disease Collaborative Research Group. A novel gene containing a trinucleotide repeat that is expanded and unstable on Huntington's disease chromosomes. *Cell* 1993;72:971–982.

Hurtig HI. Vascular parkinsonism. In: Stern MB, Koeller WC, eds. *Parkinsonian Syndromes*. New York: Marcel Dekker, 1993:81–93.

Indo T, Ando K. Metoclopramide-induced parkinsonism. *Arch Neurol* 1982;39:494–496.

Jankovic J. Treatment of dystonia. In: Watts RL, Koller WC, eds. *Movement disorders, neurologic principles and practice*. New York. McGraw-Hill, 1997:443–454.

Jankovic J. Tardive syndromes and other drug induced movement disorders. *Clin Neuropaharmacol* 1995;18: 197–214.

Jankovic J, Brin MF. Therapeutic uses of botulism toxin. *N Engl J Med* 1991;324:1186–1194.

Jankovic J, Schwartz K, Donovan DT. Botulism toxin treatment of cranial-cervical dystonia, spasmodic dysphonia, other focal dystonias, and hemifacial spasm. *J Neurol Neurosurg Psychiatry* 1990;53:633–639.

Jankovic J, Ashizawa T. Huntington's disease. In: Appel SH, eds. *Current neurology*. Chicago: Mosby-Year Book, 1995;5:29–60.

Jednyak CP, Bonnet AM, Agid Y. Tremor and idiopathic dystonia. *Mov Disord* 1991;6:230–236.

Kane JM, Woerner MW, Lieberman J. Tardive dyskinesia: prevalence, incidence and risk factors. *J Clin Psychopharmacol* 1988;8:S52–S56.

Kessler II. Epidemiologic studies of Parkinsons's disease. III. A community-based survey. *Am J Epidemiol* 1972;96: 242–254.

Krauss JK, Regel JP, Droste DW, et al. Movement disorders in adult hydrocephalus. *Mov Disord* 1997;12:53–60.

Litvan I, Goetz CG, Jankovic J, et al. What is the accuracy of the clinical diagnosis of multiple system atrophy? *Arch Neurol* 1997;54:937–944.

Litvan I, Paulsen JS, Mega MS, et al. Neuropsychiatric assessment of patients with hyperkinetic and hypokinetic movement disorders. *Arch Neurol* 1998;55:1313–1319.

Lowe J, Lennox G, Leigh PN. Disorders of movement and system degenerations. In: Graham DI, Lantos PL, eds. *Greenfield's neuropathology*, 6th ed., Vol 2. London: Arnold 1997:281–366.

Mark HM. Other choreatic disorders. In: Watts RL, Koller WC, eds. *Movement disorders, neurologic principles and practice*. New York: McGraw-Hill, 1997:527–539.

Mayeux R, Stern Y, Rosenstein R. An estimate of the prevalence of dementia in idiopathic Parkinson's disease. *Arch Neurol* 1988;45:260–262.

McTavish D, Goa KL. Mididrine: a review of the pharmacological properties and therapeutic use in orthostatic hypotension and secondary hypotensive disorders. *Drugs* 1989;38:757–777.

Mega MS, Masterman DL, Benson DF, et al. Dementia with Lewy bodies: reliability and validity of clinical and pathologic criteria. *Neurology* 1996;47:1403–1409.

Metman LV, Del Dotto P, van den Munckhof P, et al. Amantadine as treatment for dyskinesias and motor fluctuations in Parkinson's disease. *Neurology* 1998;50: 1323–1326.

Muller T, Kuhn W, Pohlau D, et al. Parkinsonism unmasked by lovastatin. *Ann Neurol* 1995;37(5):685–686.

Murrow RW, Schweiger GD, Kepes JJ, et al. Parkinsonism due to basal ganglia lacunar state: clinicopathological correlation. *Neurology* 1990;40:897–900.

Nutt JG. Classification of gait and balance disorders. *Adv Neurol* 2001;87:135–141.

Olanow CW, Hauser RA, Gauger L, et al. The effect of deprenyl and levadopa on the progression of Parkinson's disease. *Ann Neurol* 1995;38:771–777.

Olanow CW, Koller WC. An Algorithm (decision tree) for the management of Parkinson's disease: treatment guidelines. *Neurology* 1998;50(3 Suppl 3):S5–S7.

Parker SW. Dizziness in the elderly. In: Albert ML Knoefel JE, eds. *Clinical neurology of aging*, 2d ed. New York: Oxford University Press, 1994:569–579.

Parkinson Study Group. Effect of deprenyl on the progression of disability in early Parkinson's disease. *N Engl J Med* 1989;321:1364–1371.

Parkinson Study Group. Impact of deprenyl and tocopherol treatment on Parkinson's disease in DATATOP patients requiring levodopa. *Ann Neurol* 1996;39:37–45.

Paulson H, Stern MB. Clinical manifestations of Parkinson's disease. In: Watts RL, Koller WC, eds. *Movement disor-*

ders, neurologic principles and practice. New York: Mc-Graw-Hill, 1997:181–199.

Pavlakis AJ, Siroky MB Goldstein I, et al. Neurourologic findings in Parkinson's disease. *J Urol* 1983;129:80–83.

Penny JB, Young AB, Snodgrass SR, et al. Huntington's disease in Venezuela: 7 years of follow-up on symptomatic and asymptomatic individuals. *Mov Disord* 1990;5:93–99.

Rascol O, Brooks DJ, Korczyn AD, et al. A five-year study of the incidence of dyskinesia in patients with early Parkinson's disease who were treated with ropinirole or levodopa. *N Engl J Med* 2000;342:1484–1491.

Rajput AH. Movement disorders and aging. In: Watts RL, Koller WC, eds. *Movement disorders, neurologic principles and practice.* New York: McGraw-Hill, 1997:674–686.

Rautakorpi I, Marttila RJ, Takal J, et al. Occurrences and causes of tremors. *Neuroepidemiology* 1982;1:209–215.

Rajput AH, Offord KP, Beard CM, et al. Epidemiology of Parkinsonism: incidence, classification, and mortality. *Ann Neurol* 1984;16:278–282.

Rothwell JC, Obeso JA. The anatomical and physiological basis of torsion dystonia. In: Marsden CD, Fahn S, eds: Movement Disorders. London: Butterworths, 1987:313–331.

Savoiardo M, Strada L, Girotti F, et al. MR imaging in progressive supranuclear palsy and Shy-Drager syndrome. *J Comput Assist Tomogr* 1989;13:555–560.

Schapira AHV. Sleep attacks (sleep episodes) with pergolide. *Lancet* 2000;355:1332–1333.

Shannon KM. Hydrocephalus and parkinsonism. In: Stern MB, Koeller WC, eds. *Parkinsonian syndromes.* New York: Marcel Dekker, 1993:123–136.

Shulman LM, Weiner WJ. Multiple-system atrophy. In: Watts RL, Koller WC, eds. *Movement disorders, neurologic principles and practice.* New York: McGraw-Hill, 1997:297–306.

Smith JM, Baldessarini RJ. Changes in prevalence, severity, and recovery in tardive dyskinesia with age. *Arch Gen Psychiatry* 1980;37:1368–1373.

Stacy M, Jankovic J. Tardive dyskinesia. *Curr Opin Neuro Neurosurg* 1991;4:343–349.

Sudarsky L. Geriatrics: gait disorders in the elderly. *N Engl J Med* 1990;322:1441–1446.

Tanner C, Hubble JP, Chan P. Epidemiology and genetics of Parkinson's disease. In: Watts RL, Koller WC, eds. *Movement disorders, neurologic principles and practice.* New York: McGraw-Hill, 1997:137–152.

Tolosa E, Kulisevsky J, Fahn S. Meige syndrome: primary and secondary forms. *Adv Neuol* 1988;50:509–515.

Tolosa E, Marti JFM. Adult-onset idiopathic torsion dystonia. In: Watts RL, Koller WC, eds. *Movement disorders, neurologic principles and practice.* New York: McGraw-Hill, 1997:429–442.

Vidakovic A, Dragasevic N, Kostic VS. Hemiballism: report of 25 cases. *J Neurol Neurosurg Psychiatry* 1994;57: 945–949.

Woerner MG, Alvir JMJ Saltz BL, et al. Prospective study of tardive dyskinesia in the elderly: rates and risk factors. *Am J Psychiatry* 1998;155:1521–1528.

Wood A. Clinical experience with olanzapine, a new atypical antipsychotic. *Int Clin Psychopharmacol* 1998;13: S59–S62.

23

Cognitive Effects of Movement Disorders

Enrique Noé and Yaakov Stern

INTRODUCTION

Although Parkinson's disease, progressive supranuclear palsy (PSP), corticobasal ganglionic degeneration (CBGD), multiple system atrophy (MSA), and Huntington's disease have traditionally been described as neurodegenerative processes preserving mental functions, cognitive impairment is now accepted as an integral part of the clinical presentation of these diseases (Table 23-1). Disturbed cognitive function and neurobehavioral abnormalities, which are also a common source of disability for patients and of distress to caregivers and families, are powerful predictors of institutionalization. Because of the high prevalence and great impact of these disturbances, they must be clearly recognized and treated. This chapter reviews the main clinical characteristics, pathophysiological mechanisms, and pharmacologic treatment of these features of movement disorders.

PARKINSON'S DISEASE

Parkinson's disease represents between 70% to 75% of all the parkinsonisms. It is the most common movement disorder in the elderly and one of the most common causes of disability in this population. The prevalence of Parkinson's disease is up to 1% of the population over 65 years of age, and this percentage increases with age. In fact, aging is the most consistent recognized risk factor for the disease. The age of onset varies between 40 and 70 years, with an incidence peak above 60 years of age. Less than 20% of the cases have onset before 50 years of age. The progression and evolution of Parkinson's disease varies from one patient to another, with a mean survival time around 10 to 15 years. The impact of the disease is clear if we consider that the risk for death or developing dementia in this disease is more than twofold greater than in an age-adjusted population (Louis et al., 1997).

Psychosocial Aspects and Healthcare

Since the advent of levodopa therapy, the mortality rate for patients with Parkinson's disease is not different than for age and sex-matched controls. Today, approximately 60% of patients are over 75 years at death and the prevalence of the disease is as high as 3% among individuals older than 85 years of age. The decrease in elderly mortality and the improvement in treatment for early Parkinson's disease is generating an increasing number of families living with affected relatives, and a greater percentage of patients living to experience the advanced stages of this disease.

The combination of the progressive course of the disease, the prolonged survival, and the broad range of impairment, suggests that a high proportion of patients with Parkinson's disease may eventually need long-term care. However, general healthcare is important from the very first moment the disease was diagnosed. At early stages, advice is necessary for understanding the information related to the disease and reducing stress. A second stage would be to focus on maintenance of good health and to reduce complications. Third, in the late stages of Parkinson's disease, palliative care begins to be required and some patients need to be institutionalized (MacMahon, 1999). European and American studies have estimated the prevalence of patients with Parkinson's disease in nursing homes is about 5% to 10% and that up to 20% of older patients with the disease will eventually be institutionalized. Risk factors for nursing home placement are old age, living alone, motor disability, impairment of activities of daily living, dementia, and psychosis (Aarsland et al., 1999; Mitchell et al., 1996).

Parkinson's disease markedly reduces patient's health-related quality of life, generates an important dysfunction on family roles and activities, and places a major socioeconomic impact on society. The economic costs of Parkinson's disease, including both direct healthcare costs (for drugs, physician services, and

TABLE 23-1. *Neuropsychological pattern in patients with movement disorders*

	PD	PD-D	CBGD	PSP	MSA	HD	AD
Orientation	−	++	−	−	−	−/+	+++
Language							
Naming	−/+	+	−/+	−/+	−/+	−/+	++
Fluency	++	+++	++	++	++	+++	+
Aphasia/paraphasia	−	−/+	++	−	−	−/+	+
Visuospatial function							
Visual memory	−/+	++	−/+	−/+	−/+	+	+++
Spatial reasoning	+	+++	+	++	+	++	++
Visuoconstructive	+	++	++	+	+	++	++
Memory							
Immediate recall	+	++	−/+	−/+	+	+	++
Delayed recall	−/+	++	−/+	−/+	−/+	+	+++
Recognition	−	+	−	−	−	−/+	+++
Praxis	−	++	+++	−/+	−	−/+	++
Executive function	++	+++	++	+++	++	++	+
Attention	+	+++	+	++	+++	++	++

(−) Normal function; (+) mild impairment; (++) moderate impairment; (+++) severe impairment.
AD, Alzheimer's disease; CBGD, corticobasal ganglionic degeneration; HD, Huntington's disease; MSA, multiple system atrophy; PD, Parkinson's disease; PD-D, Parkinson's disease-dementia; PSP, progressive supranuclear palsy.
Shading underlines the principal symptoms of each disease.

hospitalization) and indirect costs (for lost worker productivity) have been estimated to be around $25 billion per year (Scheife et al., 2000). The total mean societal burden per individual with Parkinson's disease in the United States is more than $6,000/year ($4,000 for drugs, physician services, and hospitalization, and $2,000 for earnings loss) (Whetten-Goldstein et al., 1997). The largest per capita compensated healthcare costs are physician visits and hospital expenses component of care (39% of costs), followed by ancillary care (30%), and drug therapy (22%) (LePen et al., 1999). Physician visits cost society an average of $1,324/year/patient with Parkinson's disease in the United States (Whetten-Goldstein et al., 1997). Obviously, medical costs are strongly correlated with most clinical indicators and the cost generally progresses in line with the severity of the disease.

The largest components of family burden are not direct healthcare costs, but providing informal caregiving and earnings loss. The caregiver, usually the spouse, provides an average of 22 hours of care per week. After income loss ($12,000/patient/year), informal caregiving is the single most expensive element of burden attributable to Parkinson's disease ($5,000/patient/year) (Whetten-Goldstein et al., 1997).

Circumscribed Cognitive Deficits

Typical cognitive alterations present in Parkinson's disease include circumscribed deficits in memory, vi-

suospatial, attention, and executive functions. Although mild cognitive deficits can be present in nearly all patients with the disease, they usually remain stable. A clear progression to dementia can be shown in up to 20% of patients with this disease (Marder et al., 1995).

Executive Function

The broad set of abilities that comprise executive function include initiating and planning activities, attentional shifts, concept formation, problem-solving, implementing behavior, self-control, and maintenance of socially appropriate behavior. All these processes are known to be disturbed after damage to the frontal lobes. Numerous authors have reported executive deficits in patients with Parkinson's disease assessed with different tests. Set-shifting deficits have been reported in these patients who have been tested using the Wisconsin Card Sorting Test (WCST), a conditional associative learning task based on three categorical sorting rules (number-color-shape). Patients with Parkinson's disease show a diminished number of categories and an increased number of perseverative errors. These deficits are present even in *de novo* patients, regardless the age of onset, and especially if they are depressed (Kuzis et al., 1997; Levin et al., 1989; Tsai et al., 1994). Similarly, set-shifting and set-maintenance difficulties (Odd-Man-Out Test, Stroop Test) have been reported in patients with parkinsonian symptoms, even at the beginning of the disease (Heniket al., 1993; Richards et al., 1993). Many other attentional and executive tasks are also altered in patients with Parkinson's disease (Cooper et al., 1992; Tsai et al., 1994), including the following:

- Working-memory: Digit Span, the Arithmetic subtest of the Wechsler Adult Intelligence Scale (WAIS)
- Problem-solving (Tower of London/Hanoi)
- Verbal or visuospatial abstract reasoning (Raven Progressive Matrices, Similarities and Comprehension subtests of the WAIS)
- Switching or planning: Trail-making Test

Results of these tests taken by patients with Parkinson's disease suggest that these patients initially have difficulties in focusing attention and mental flexibility, which are necessary to shift and maintain mental sets. Deficits in initiation and in planning strategies needed to solve problems can occur later in the evolution of the disease.

Visuospatial Function

Visuospatial impairments are among the most common deficits described in Parkinson's disease for tasks including visual recognition, visual analysis and synthesis, spatial planning and attention, visual orientation, and visuoconstructive praxis. Deficits in facial recognition, which can appear 2 to 3 years after the diagnosis of the disease, may be the earliest affected visuospatial function in patients with Parkinson's disease (Levin et al., 1991). This impairment might not be noted in juvenile forms, suggesting that age might influence performance on this test (Tsai et al., 1994). Deficits in perception, construction and mental management of objects and figures, and alterations in judgment of direction, orientation, and distance, can appear later in the evolution of the disease, whatever the age of onset (Pillon et al., 1997; Tsai et al., 1994). Patients show deficits in almost all the performance subtests of the WAIS, including Picture Completion, Block Design, and Object Assembly. These deficits usually appear some years after the diagnosis of the disease, even in the juvenile onset, and are not related to motor dysfunction (Levin et al., 1991). Other studies have reported deficits in visuoconstructive graphomotor tasks, including difficulties copying complex figures (Rey-Osterrieth Figure) and impairments in copying simple designs (e.g., house or a clock) with the evolution of the disease (Cooper et al., 1991; Jagust et al., 1992).

Most of the visuospatial tests studied in patients with Parkinson's disease demand manual dexterity or require active planning and strategy formation. However visuoperceptual impairments have been reported even when motoric task demands are minimized. These impairments were not correlated with the duration of the disease or the severity of motor dysfunction (Boller et al., 1984; Hovestadt et al., 1987). A significant correlation between executive and visuospatial tasks have been described, as have beneficial effects of problem-solving clues in visuospatial tasks in patients with Parkinson's disease (Bondi et al., 1993). Qualitative analysis of visuoconstructive test performance shows figures reduced in size, distortions, poor organization, and significant omissions. These data suggest that impoverished performance on visuospatial function in patients with this disease is more related to difficulties in executive tasks and shifting attention than to pure visuospatial difficulties (Brown and Marsden, 1986).

Memory

Explicit (declarative) memory deficits and implicit (procedural) memory impairments have consistently been reported in nondemented patients with Parkinson's disease. *Explicit* memory refers to the conscious recollection (free recall and cued recall) or recognition of a previous event or experience, whereas *implicit* memory includes perceptual or motor skills learned during life and not readily accessible to conscious recollection. Semantic explicit material (memory for conceptual knowledge and relations that are context-free) is usually preserved compared with episodic explicit memory (memory for personally experienced events or episodes). However, some aspects of episodic memory, especially immediate memory, are more affected than long-term memory, cued retrieval, and recognition tasks. Verbal learning and working-memory are also commonly affected.

Verbal memory is usually affected later than visuospatial memory because visuospatial material is not semantically related and the recall process requires a greater cognitive effort. As less external supports (fewer cues) are offered and more cognitive demand or self-initiated activities are required, more difficulties appear. For example, conditional associative learning would be more impaired than cue-dependent, paired associative learning because the former requires learning by trial and error. Also, recall of a text or a paragraph that has a semantic structure sufficient to guide memory is less affected than word-list learning tasks in which organization must be self-elaborated (Pillon et al., 1996; Cooper et al., 1992). This factor could also explain the superior performance of patients with Parkinson's disease on recognition (which relies on external cues) as opposed to free recall tasks (relying on own internal cues), and their ability to benefit from cueing (Appollonio et al., 1994). Long-term memory is generally less (and later) impaired than immediate memory, reflecting a problem in acquisition of information (immediate organization) more than a genuine storage, retention, and retrieval deficit (long-term recall) (Brown and Marsden, 1990). Remote memory is generally preserved.

Although some controversial results have been seen, performance on implicit memory tasks can be affected in patients with Parkinson's disease (Bondi and Kaszniak, 1991). Because implicit memory refers to a form of remembering that can be expressed only through the performance of tasks operations, these deficits represent a slowness in the acquisition of new motor, perceptual, and cognitive skills. Some authors have also reported patients having difficulty maintaining these skills against competing stimulus, suggesting again an attentional deficit (Dubois and Pillon, 1998).

Language

Typically, Parkinson's disease affects mechanical aspects of speech, especially articulatory components (e.g., speed, tone, and volume). These alterations generate monotonous, hypophonic, and dysarthric speech that can compromise communication with these patients. Handwriting is limited by motor impairments. It can start with normal size script but usually becomes smaller and cramped.

Regarding nonmotor components, patients with Parkinson's disease without dementia have been shown to be only slightly impaired in syntax and grammar tests and in lexical and semantic tasks. Lack of spontaneous speech, delayed responses, single word answers, and reduction in the length of the phrases can reflect difficulty planning linguistic sentences and an effort to generate as much information as possible in single sentences (Cummings et al., 1988; Illes et al., 1988). Vocabulary and naming tasks are usually preserved in nondemented patients with Parkinson's disease at the beginning of the disease and they become affected with the evolution of the disease (Globus et al., 1985). Verbal fluency can be affected, even at early stages of the disease, especially if loosely defined categories (e.g., objects) or alternating categories (e.g., birds/colors) are included. Letter verbal fluency tasks are usually affected later than category tasks, suggesting that a "letter" rather than a "category" might act as a cueing device to facilitate semantic retrieval (Cools et al., 1984; Cooper et al., 1991). Perseverative intrusions in fluency tasks suggest a difficulty shifting between letter categories under a time constraint. Similarly to visuospatial and memory dysfunction, it is not clear whether verbal fluency deficits represent a specific language dysfunction or are the expression of an impairment in planning and initiating a systematic search in semantic memory (executive dysfunction).

Dementia in Parkinson's Disease

It is generally accepted that the prevalence of dementia in Parkinson's disease is approximately 20%, with an estimated incidence of 3% new cases per year in patients under 60 years of age, and up to 14% new cases per year in those older than 80 years of age (Marder et al., 1995; Mayeux et al., 1990). Incidence is a better estimate than prevalence of the frequency of dementia in Parkinson's disease because dementia significantly reduces survival in this disease (Louis et al., 1997). Risk factors for dementia in the disease include increased age, a lower educational background, older age at onset, depression, and longer duration or more severe disease (Table 23-2). Demented patients respond poorly to levodopa, and are more likely to present adverse psychiatric effects (depression and psychosis) related to dopaminergic therapy. Their parkinsonism is more likely to consist of rigidity, bradykinesia, and postural instability instead of tremor (Marder et al., 1995; Stern et al., 1993). Neuropsychological data suggest that for nondemented patients with Parkinson's disease, greater early impairment on letter and category fluency tests or attentional and visuoperceptual tasks increases the likelihood of later incident dementia (Jacobs et al., 1995; Mahieuxet al., 1998).

Dementia in Parkinson's disease has often been termed "subcortical dementia," which involves slowness of thought processes, altered personality, impaired arousal and motivation, and difficulty manipulating acquired knowledge, but with a relative sparing of memory, perceptual, language, and praxis functions. Although the concept of subcortical dementia was useful in prodding the investigation of different dementia syndromes, it may not be useful to delineate the features associated with each type of dementia.

The Mattis Dementia Rating Scale (MDRS) is more appropriate than the Mini-Mental State Examination (MMSE) or the *Diagnostic and Statistical*

TABLE 23-2. *Risk factors for dementia in Parkinson's disease*

Risk factors	Risk ratio
Demographic factors	
Age	1.06
Education	1.01
Gender (female)	0.73
Clinical factors	
Age of onset of Parkinson's disease (>60 years)	4.1
Duration of Parkinson's disease (years)	1.01
Unified Parkinson's Disease Rating Scale-Motor Scale (>25)	1.04–3.56
Hamilton Depression Scale (>10)	1.11–3.55
Neuropsychological factors	
Picture Completion of the Wechsler Adult Intelligent Scale (<10)	4.9
Stroop Test (interference <21)	3.8
Letter fluency (CFL <27, M <9)	3.3–2.7
Category fluency (animal, food, clothing <42)	6.01

Data from Jacobs DM, Marder K, Cote LJ, et al. Neuropsychological characteristics of preclinical dementia in Parkinson's disease. *Neurology* 1995;45:1691–1696; Marder K, Tang MX, Cote L, et al. The frequency and associated risk factors for dementia in patients with Parkinson's disease. *Arch Neurol* 1995;52:695–701; and Mahieux F, Fenelon G, Flahault A, et al. Neuropsychological prediction of dementia in Parkinson's disease. *J Neurol Neurosurg Psychiatry* 1998;64:178–183, with permission.

Manual of Mental Disorders (DSM-IV) to evaluate cognitive function in Parkinson's disease because it includes attentional and executive measures. The presence of depression, the motor stage during neuropsychological evaluation, and the confusional side effects of any concomitant medication should be addressed as confounding factors before establishing the diagnosis of dementia.

As in nondemented patients, almost all patients with Parkinson's disease and dementia show an early prominent executive dysfunction that includes difficulties with planning, problem-solving, concept formation, and abstract reasoning, when evaluated with frontal-executive tests previously described (Litvan et al., 1991). Visuospatial, visuoperceptual, and visuoconstructive problems are common, even when patients are evaluated performing tasks requiring minimal motor demands. Demented patients with Parkinson's disease demonstrate difficulties recognizing faces, assembling objects, drawing figures, mentally assembling puzzles, formulating line and angular judgments, and identifying embedded figures. Most of these deficits are similar to those found in Alzheimer's disease, however, patients with Parkinson's disease performed significantly better on visuospatial memory tasks and worse visual abstract reasoning when compared with patients with Alzheimer's disease. Both declarative and procedural memory may be affected in a similar pattern described previously in nondemented patients with Parkinson's disease.

Cross-sectional studies comparing demented patients with Parkinson's with those with Alzheimer's disease have shown that the former performs worse on verbal fluency tasks, shows better recognition memory (despite equally impaired recall), and a slower rate of forgetting from immediate to delayed recall. Longitudinal studies have confirmed these results and have reported a more rapid decline in naming, delayed recall, and category verbal fluency in demented patients with Parkinson's disease. They also described how patients with Alzheimer's disease had a poorer performance on delayed recognition (Heindel et al., 1989; Huber et al., 1989; Stern et al., 1993; Stern et al., 1998).

Although aphasia is rare, language deficits are present in Parkinson's disease dementia and include naming and word-finding difficulties, perseverations, decreased phrase length, diminished verbal fluency, and impaired strategies in sentence comprehension (Cummings et al., 1988; Huber et al., 1989). Compared with those with Alzheimer's disease, patients with Parkinson's disease are less likely to have poorer semantic than phonemic fluency. Parkinson's disease dementia becomes less distinguishable from other dementias (e.g., Alzheimer's disease or dementia with Lewy bodies) as it becomes more severe.

Psychiatric Complications

Up to 60% of patients with Parkinson's disease experience psychiatric complications. The most frequent are mood disorders, anxiety syndromes, and drug-induced psychosis (Table 23-3) (Aarsland et al., 1999).

TABLE 23-3. *Neuropsychiatric disturbances in movement disorders*

	PD %	CBGD %	PSP %	MSA %	HD %	AD %
Depression	5–90	38–75	18	30–50	9–44	20–50
Apathy	41	40	91	90	34–50	70–90
Anxiety	20–66	13	18	8	34	40–60
Delusions	10–20	7	0	15	6–25	20–50
Hallucinations	4–40	0	0	15	10	5–40
Irritability	30	20	9	?	38–50	42
Euphoria	2–33	0	0	?	10–17	3–17
Disinhibition	12–30	20	36	?	24	36
Agitation	30	20	5	?	50	48–70
Sleep disorders	67–88	?	? (Most)	? (Most)	20	45

AD, Alzheimer's disease; CBGD, corticobasal ganglionic degeneration; HD, Huntington's disease; MSA, multiple system atrophy; PD, Parkinson's disease; PSP, progressive supranuclear palsy.
Shading underlines the principal symptoms of each disease. (?) means that no epidemiologic studies are published yet.
Data are from: Cummings et al., 1992a, 1992b; Aarsland et al., 1999; Burns et al., 1990; Celesia et al., 1970; Chokroverty et al., 1996; Dubois et al., 1998; Esmonde et al., 1996; Fentoni et al., 1999; Folstein et al., 1983; Inzelberg et al., 1998; Litvan et al., 1996b, 1998a, 1998b; Pilo et al., 1996; Sanchez-Ramos et al., 1996; Stein et al., 1990.

Depression

The prevalence rate of depression in Parkinson's disease is unclear, ranging from 5% to 90%, a percentage significantly higher than in age-matched control groups. Depression in Parkinson's disease may be difficult to recognize because many of the traditional symptoms associated with the diagnosis of depression may be present because of motor disability. Major depression is present in 20% of the cases, whereas others experience adjustment disorders, dysthymia, or bipolar disorders (Cummings, 1992). Depression in Parkinson's disease shares symptoms of primary affective depressive disorders, including feelings of poor self-esteem and loss of social, family, and interpersonal relationships. Other atypical features include comorbid anxiety and panic attacks (40% of the cases), irritability and disinhibition (30%), and psychosis (10%) (Schiffer et al., 1988).

Depressive symptoms in Parkinson's disease are a combination of endogenous and exogenous factors. Depression can antedate any recognizable motor symptoms and occur independently of disease duration and motor impairment. These data suggest that the depressive syndrome may be caused by endogenous deficiency in monoamines, especially serotonin, more than a reaction to physical impairment. On the other hand, some studies have shown that successful treatment of depression can be associated with better motor function, and a motor improvement may be associated with improved mood. So, reactive depression in response to having an inexorably progressive and debilitating disease can predominate at some point in the evolution of the disease (Starkstein et al., 1992).

Apathy can be present in Parkinson's disease as a symptom of major depression, delirium, and dementia, or as an independent syndrome. Emotional lability is present in 40% of patients from the onset of the disease.

Anxiety

Generalized anxiety disorders occur in 20% to 40% of patients with Parkinson's disease; social phobia or panic disorder is seen in up to 25% of the patients; and mania or euphoria can appear in 10%. These symptoms may precede the onset of motor features, accompany major depressive syndrome, and persist after the depressive illness is treated (Stein et al., 1990; Celesia and Barr, 1970). Commonly, anxiety appears in fluctuating patients ("on-off" motor fluctuations) during "off" periods, when the patient experiences worsening of parkinsonian symptoms. Anxiety syndromes have to be differentiated from the understandable psychological response to motor impairment, the somatic complaints related to autonomic symptoms, and from akathisia (the necessity to be in constant motion), a frequent feature of Parkinson's disease.

Sleep Disorders

Sleep disturbances occur in more than 75% of patients with Parkinson's disease, especially in those with advanced disease and older onset. These patients may experience difficulty falling asleep because of anxiety, but most commonly they complain of fragmentation of nocturnal sleep, with frequent awakenings, and sleepiness in the morning (Chokroverty, 1996). These disturbances are generally related to difficulty in turning over in bed, vivid dreams or nightmares, painful limb dystonia or cramps, and nocturia (Nausieda et al., 1982).

Psychosis

Psychosis, which occurs in up to 40% of patients with Parkinson's disease, is generally drug-related, and a major precipitant of nursing home placement. Psychosis can occur in up to 80% of demented patients with Parkinson's disease, but also in up to 20% of cognitively intact patients (Sanchez-Ramos et al., 1996; Inzelberg et al., 1998). Although psychoses are often considered a levodopa effect, they occur with all dopaminergic drugs. Prevalence rates of psychosis increase with the presence of cognitive impairment, depressive symptoms, sleep-wake disturbances, older age, and longer duration of the disease (Cummings, 1991).

Hallucinations usually occur as a late complication of antiparkinsonian medication in the context of a clear sensorium, but can also be present as features of major depressive episodes, mania syndromes, or as a part of a drug-induced toxic delirium. Polymodal, disturbing, and vague in content hallucinations are more common during delirium. Visual, well-formed, not frightening, and nocturnal hallucinations are more common in the context of a clear mental sensorium (Saint Cyr et al., 1993). In these cases, the most frequent types of hallucinations are the vivid sensation of the presence of somebody, brief visions of a person or an animal passing sideways, and elaborate visual hallucinations (Masterman et al., 1998).

Illusions (10% to 20%) and auditory hallucinations (10%) are less common, and usually accompany visual hallucinations. Delusions are present in approximately 10% of the patients after some years of dopaminergic treatment. They are usually accompanied or preceded by vivid dreams, nightmares, or visual hallucinations. Delusions are complex in content and well structured. Paranoid, grandiosity, erotomanic, and auto-referential contents are common (Cummings, 1991). Although a decrease in sexual activity with loss of libido is present in the early stages of Parkinson's disease, hypersexuality and altered sexual behavior (e.g., paraphilia, exhibitionistic thoughts, voyeurism, pedophilia) have also been reported in 1% to 13% of the patients after initiating dopaminergic treatment (Uitti et al., 1989).

Pathology

The pathologic hallmark of Parkinson's disease is the progressive loss of dopaminergic cells in the substantia nigra and other aminergic nuclei of the basal forebrain. The prominent impairment on executive tasks described in the disease, and most of the psychiatric complications associated with it, has been attributed to degeneration of frontosubcortical circuits. These systems link specific areas of frontal cortex involved in executive function (dorsolateral cortex), motivation (orbitofrontal cortex), and social behavior (anterior cingular cortex), with the striatum, globus pallidus, and thalamus (Alexander et al., 1986). It has been suggested that the decreased dopaminergic nigrostriatal stimulation induces cognitive and behavior abnormalities, reflecting interruption of these circuits.

Degeneration of the medial substantia nigra, with associated loss of dopaminergic nigral projections to the limbic cortex (mesolimbic pathway) and frontal areas (mesocortical pathway), has also been implicated in cognitive dysfunction. In addition to the predominant dopaminergic deficiency, degeneration of subcortical ascending systems with neuronal losses in serotonergic, cholinergic, and noradrenergic nuclei have also been reported in Parkinson's disease. Involvement of these neurotransmitter systems has been related to depression and cognitive dysfunction in some patients with the disease. Finally, coincident Alzheimer or Lewy body cortical changes, with loss of synapses and neuronal death, have been proposed as some of the possible neuropathologic basis for dementia in Parkinson's disease (Dubois and Pillon, 1998).

Treatment

Cognitive Impairment

The management of cognitive impairment in patients with Parkinson's disease involves nonspecific symptomatic treatment and counseling of the patient and the family. Consensus is lacking regarding the effect of drug therapy on cognition in Parkinson's disease. It has been shown that neither deprenyl, tocopherol, nor piracetam improve cognitive testing in patients with Parkinson's disease. Studies of levodopa have reported improvement, worsening, or no change in attentional, executive, or memory tasks. Similarly, it is accepted that levodopa cannot improve the cognitive deficits of demented patients with this disease.

Longitudinal studies have shown a transient and limited improvement in overall cognitive functioning—especially in executive tasks—in patients with parkinsonian under levodopa therapy compared with drug-naive patients (Downes et al., 1989). Similarly, an initial cognitive improvement that gradually reverses to baseline performance has been described in patients with *de novo* Parkinson's disease after several months of dopaminergic treatment (Growdon et al., 1998). Cross-sectional studies have reported a greater impairment in executive, memory, and visuospatial tasks in patients treated long term compared with drug-naive *de novo* patients. However, the effect of disease progression in the former group should be considered (Owen et al., 1992; 1993).

The most efficient way to study the effect of drug therapy on cognition in patients with Parkinson's disease is probably by comparing "on" versus "off" conditions. Most such studies have reported no change in memory and visuospatial tests when comparing *on* and *off* stages (Pillon et al., 1989). Differences arise when comparing executive or attentional tasks. Improvement on these tasks during *on* stage has been related to a secondary effect of improved attention or vigilance, whereas worsening has been related to a toxic effect of levodopa on speed of processing information (Malapani et al., 1994; Poewe et al., 1991).

Anticholinergic drugs have a recognized negative effect on memory (Wechsler Memory Scale), executive (WCST), and attentional (Digit Span) tasks in the context of confusional states in Parkinson's disease (Cooper et al., 1992; Dubois et al., 1990). Cognitive side effects of anticholinergic drugs are more likely to occur in older and demented patients, so this kind of treatment should be reserved for younger nondemented patients at earlier stages of the disease. Short-term memory may recover, at least partly, after withdrawal of long-term anticholinergic medication.

Surgical procedures (e.g., thalamotomy, pallidotomy, fetal tissue transplantation) do not seem to have a negative effect on cognition in nondemented patients with parkinsonian (frequently limited to verbal fluency decrements), but long-term follow-up studies are needed (Masterman et al., 1998).

Psychiatric Symptoms

The most important consideration when prescribing a medication for patients with parkinsonian symptoms is that the underlying brain disease and older age renders them especially vulnerable to adverse effects. Often, patients respond to low doses of medicine. Increasing the dose runs the risk of aggravating motor and cognitive symptoms. Before adding any new treatment, a careful review of antiparkinsonian and other medications should be done in an effort

to reduce polypharmacy and drug interactions. Systemic and other causes of cognitive or behavioral symptoms should be ruled out (e.g., infections, metabolic alterations, and endocrine imbalances). Finally, when prescribing any new drug, increase dosage slowly, and taper over a long period when discontinuing (Valldeoriola et al., 1997).

Antidepressants

Depression treatment should not be delayed, because early treatment of depressed patients can result in a less severe cognitive decline. Most patients should be treated with antidepressants because levodopa has only short beneficial effect on depression in Parkinson's disease. The use of the classic nonselective monoamine oxidase inhibitors, and the combination of these drugs with other antidepressants, should be avoided because of the high prevalence of side effects. The overall efficacy of most antidepressants is similar, but the selective serotonin reuptake inhibitors (SSRI) have advantages over tricyclics (TCA) because of the absence of anticholinergic features. The doses of SSRI for depression in patients with Parkinson's disease are the same as for depression in general population. Some reported cases have suggested that SSRI worsen the motor condition for patients with this disease. Electroconvulsive therapy is another effective treatment for depression in patients with Parkinson's disease (Cummings, 1992a).

Anxiolytics and Hypnotics

Anxiety associated with *off* periods should be managed by strategies designed to lessen the severity of the motor symptoms and to increase *on* time. If this does not control the anxiety, benzodiazepines, buspirone, and antidepressants can be used in the management of these symptoms. Short-acting benzodiazepines—alprazolam and lorazepam—are better tolerated (less confusion) in older populations but have the disadvantage of their repeated administration. Diphenhydramine, hydroxyzine and beta-blockers can also be used in patients with symptoms of autonomic dysfunction or anxiety-related palpitations, respectively. Buspirone does not have the sedative side effects of benzodiazepines and seems to be effective in reducing aggressivity and anxiety symptoms. Sedative TCA can be used as anxiolytics, whereas stimulating SSRI may be useful in apathy. However, because of the anticholinergic and orthostatic hypotensive properties of the TCA, the SSRI are preferred for the treatment of anxiety associated with agitated depression.

Levodopa can cause sleep disruption in patients with mild to moderate disease, but has a beneficial effect on those nocturnal disabilities that cause sleep disruption in more severely affected patients. Hypnotic sedative agents, as well as diphenhydramine, TCA, trazodone, or atypical antipsychotics, can help with insomnia (Cummings, 1991; Saint Cyr et al., 1993).

Antipsychotics

Traditional antipsychotic agents (e.g., haloperidol) block dopamine type II receptors and have long been associated with parkinsonian symptoms and, thus, should be avoided in the patient with Parkinson's disease. Novel antipsychotic agents that selectively block cortical dopamine III, IV, and V receptors (e.g. clozapine, olanzapine, quetiapine, and risperidone) have been recommended to treat these behavioral symptoms at low doses without this adverse effect. Sedation is the most frequent side effect of clozapine (20%), whereas granulocytopenia (1% to 3%) is the most serious. Hematologic complications are more common in older patients at the beginning of the treatment, initially requiring weekly white cell monitoring. This drug should be avoided in patients with history of blood dyscrasia and should never be combined with other bone marrow depression drugs. Risperidone is better tolerated than clozapine, but seems to have lower antipsychotic efficacy and produces more extrapyramidal side effects. Olanzapine and quetiapine do not need hematologic control. The main adverse side effects of this drug are dose-related drowsiness and sedation. Odansetron, a 5-HT3 antagonist, has also been used with success in parkinsonian patients with drug-induced psychosis with no remarkable side effects, but its expense often precludes continuing treatment. Cholinergic agents may also reduce psychosis in patients with Parkinson's disease (Factor et al., 1995).

CORTICOBASAL GANGLIONIC DEGENERATION

Corticobasal ganglionic degeneration (CBGD) represents approximately 5% of all the parkinsonisms. The age of onset is between 60 and 70 years, but earlier onset has been reported. The mean evolution is around 7 years. The major features of the disease are cortical (e.g., aphasia, apraxia, and agnosia) and subcortical (e.g., parkinsonism, limb dystonia, and bulbar abnormalities). The parkinsonism responds poorly to levodopa; it is usually asymmetric with rigidity and bradykinesia more common than tremor, and is frequently associated with atypical signs (e.g., myoclonus or a Babinski sign) (Riley et al., 1990; Gibb et al., 1989).

Circumscribed Cognitive Deficits

Aphasia occurs in up to 53% of patients with CBGD. Aphasia is typically nonfluent and associated with dysnomia, perseverations, and paraphasias. Speech is almost always abnormal, especially as the disease progresses, and has been described as slow, slurred, dysphonic, mute, echolalic (involuntary repetition of words and phrases spoken by others), or palilalic (repetition of a phrase involuntarily with increasing rapidity) (Frattali et al., 2000).

Apraxia, defined as the inability to carry out purposeful movements despite intact comprehension, muscular power, sensibility, and coordination, can occur in more than 70% of patients with CBGD. *Ideomotor* apraxia is when the implementation of a gesture in a motor program is disrupted such that the patient uses an incorrect gesture but can imitate a movement. *Ideational* apraxia is when the gesture is lacking so the patient does not know how to do or imitate a movement. *Constructive* apraxia is an inability to represent graphically geometric patterns. Dressing apraxia, apraxia of gaze, apraxia of eyelids, buccofacial apraxia, apraxia of speech, and apraxia of gait have all been reported as well. Limb apraxia, the most common form, can be asymmetric, frequently affecting the right upper extremity; it is sometimes difficult to evaluate because of other coexisting motor disturbances (Pillon et al., 1995b; Leiguarda et al., 1994). Both aphasia and apraxia can be the symptoms of the disease, but nearly all cases presenting with progressive aphasia eventually evolve to show impairment in other cognitive spheres (Table 23-1).

Although neglect syndromes have been noted in a few patients, "alien limb phenomenon" (limb movements without patient awareness) are reported to occur in 50% of patients with CBGD. Alien limb phenomena include levitation and posturing of the arm when attention is diverted or the eyes are closed, mechanical movement against patient's wishes, and a tendency to "forget" the limb while walking. Cortical sensory loss (impaired stereognosis, graphesthesia, two-point discrimination, and double simultaneous stimulation) has also been reported (Riley et al., 1990).

Dementia

Approximately 25% to 45% of the patients with CBGD become demented as the disease evolves (Riley et al., 1990). The clinical characteristics of dementia accompanying CBGD are similar to those found in other parkinsonisms, with the exception of an increased number of cortical symptoms (aphasia, apraxia, agnosia) and a high prevalence of visuospatial and constructional deficits accompanying the executive difficulties. Immediate and delayed recall of verbal material is generally preserved compared with patients with Alzheimer's disease, whereas praxis, motor programming, sustained attention, and mental control tasks are moderately impaired (Massman et al., 1996). Frontotemporal dementia is the principal clinical differential diagnosis, which can be difficult to differentiate in the absence of typical motor features (Kertesz et al., 1999). Impaired attention, acalculia, difficulties in recall and learning, abstract reasoning deficits, and left-right confusion have been noted in a number of patients.

Psychiatric Complications

More than 75% of the patients with CBGD manifest neuropsychiatric features, mostly depressive symptoms (73%), personality changes including irritability (20%), increased aggression (20%), apathy (40%) and, less commonly, anxiety, disinhibition, or drug-induced psychoses (Table 23-3) (Litvan et al., 1998a).

Pathology

The characteristic combination of both cortical and subcortical cognitive changes in CBGD is mirrored by similar mixed neuropathologic changes. Subcortical pathology includes neuronal loss and gliosis in the substantia nigra, locus ceruleus, thalamus, subthalamic nucleus, red nucleus, and midbrain tegmentum (Gibb et al., 1989). Similar to Parkinson's disease, degeneration of multiple subcortical ascending systems may be responsible for some of the cognitive dysfunction found in these patients, especially the executive deficits.

On the other hand, cortical changes include cell loss, gliosis, and the presence of *tau*-positive astrocytic plaques, especially in frontoparietal regions contralateral to the side of the body with pronounced motor symptoms. The hippocampus is typically spared. Involvement of these cortical areas has been related to the presence of ideomotor apraxia, ideational apraxia, visuospatial and constructional disorders, and neglect syndromes (Okuda et al., 1992). Both cortical and subcortical changes contribute to aphasic syndromes.

PROGRESSIVE SUPRANUCLEAR PALSY

Progressive supranuclear palsy is a rare neurodegenerative disorder accounting for approximately 5% of all the parkinsonisms. The age of onset (50–75 years) and the clinical symptoms resemble Parkinson's disease, although the presence of early gait disturbances with falls, pseudobulbar palsy, nuchal dystonia, and supranuclear gaze palsy may help in the differential diagnosis. The prevalence is around 1×10^5 and increases with age. The mean interval from onset of symptoms to diagnosis is approximately 3 to 4 years and the median survival time from onset to death 6 years (Litvan et al., 1996a). The presence of cognitive and behavioral abnormalities in PSP was first described by Steele, Richardson and Olszewski in 1964. The prominent features they reported included emotional and personality disturbances associated with mild cognitive deficits early in the clinical course of the disease.

Circumscribed Cognitive Deficits

More than half of patients with newly diagnosed disease and almost all long-term patients, show some kind of cognitive impairment on neuropsychological assessment (Table 23-1).

Visuospatial Function

The performance subtests of the WAIS and other visuoconstructive tests are impaired in patients with PSP (Milberg and Albert, 1989). These deficits should be interpreted cautiously because most patients present with oculomotor abnormalities and motor disabilities, which may interfere with their task performance. This is especially true in cases where the evaluation includes tasks relying heavily on visual search and scanning ability (digit symbol), timed tests (block design, picture completion and picture arrangement), or graphomotor abilities (drawing tests) (Esmonde et al., 1996).

Memory

Although complaints of forgetfulness are common, the memory disorder of PSP is generally mild and affects semantic more than episodic memory (van der Hurk and Hodges, 1995). Most of the recall difficulties are relayed in the executive component of memory tasks, which generates abnormally rapid forgetting, increased sensitivity to interference, and difficulty using strategic mechanisms searching information. This can also explain why most of these abnormalities are considerably alleviated or even normalized by controlled encoding associated with cued recall.

Language

Semantic and syntactic components of language are often preserved, but motor components are severely affected. Dysarthria associated with a severe reduction of spontaneous speech often impairs communicative ability. Letter and semantic verbal fluency tasks are equally affected (Rosser and Hodges, 1994). Reading difficulties, visual dyslexia, constructional dysgraphia, an increased rate of self-corrections, misnaming, and disturbances of handwriting have also been reported (Podoll et al., 1991).

Executive Function

Comparative studies of patients with Parkinson's disease, SND, and progressive supranuclear palsy have shown that the latter presents the earliest and most severe deficits on tasks sensitive to frontal lobe function (Pillon et al., 1995a; Pillon et al., 1995b) Neuropsychologically, this represents problems in response initiation (verbal fluency tasks are impoverished), planning (decrease motor speed and information process in Trail Making Tests), shifting of attention (increase interference effect on Stroop test), or problem-solving (failure to develop logical strategies to solve the WCST). This produces an abnormal regulation of behavior, associated with a loss of interest in the environment, inertia, lack of initiative, and a marked reduction in spontaneous activity.

Dementia

Estimates of the prevalence of dementia in PSP range from 20% to 70%. The term "subcortical dementia" was originally used to describe this condition, although the overlap with frontal executive deficits led to the term "frontosubcortical dementia" being proposed (Mayeux et al., 1983). This pattern can be useful in distinguishing patients with PSP who are demented from other cortical dementias (e.g., Alzheimer's disease). On the other hand, dementia in PSP is more frequent, more severe—especially in frontal tasks—and appears earlier than dementia in other parkinsonisms.

Psychiatric Complications

Apathy is the dominant behavior change found in PSP (91%) and is only occasionally accompanied by depression (18%). Disinhibition, obsessive disorders, inappropriate sexual behavior, aggressiveness, and impulsive behavior occur in one third of patients with this disease. Lability of mood, emotional incontinence, perseverative responses and grasping, imitation and utilization behaviors have also been reported. Sleep disorders are present in almost all cases of PSP (Table 23-3) (Chokroverty, 1996; Litvan et al., 1996b).

Pathology

Pathologic changes in PSP occur in diffuse regions of the basal ganglia (caudate, globus pallidus, and subthalamic nucleus), thalamus, and brainstem (substantia nigra, red nucleus, reticular formation, locus ceruleus, superior colliculus, third and fourth cranial nerve nuclei, and vestibular and dentate nuclei), with minimal changes in the frontal cerebral cortex (Daniel et al., 1995). Involvement of the dopaminergic nigrostriatal pathway, associated with damage in several output nuclei (striatum, thalamus) and afferent areas (frontal cortex), has been related to the greater dysexecutive syndrome found in PSP. Dementia has been attributed to a disruption of the subcorticofrontal connections needed to activate frontal lobe function as well as a dysfunction of cholinergic substantia innominata cortical and septohippocampal systems involved in memory processes. Uncontrolled behaviors are considered to result from the lack of inhibitory frontal lobe control.

MULTIPLE SYSTEM ATROPHY

The term "multiple system atrophy" (MSA) includes three different entities considered to be different manifestations of a single disease process: olivopontocerebellar atrophy (OPCA), striatonigral degeneration (SND), and Shy-Drager syndrome (SDS). Autopsy studies show that 7% to 20% of patients diagnosed with Parkinson's disease have pathologic evidence of MSA. The median age of onset is 60 years and the median survival from onset of motor symptoms is 7.5 years. Although motor symptoms are the prominent and distinguishing features of MSA, cognitive changes are commonly associated symptoms (Table 23-1) (Berciano, 1982).

Circumscribed Cognitive Deficits and Dementia

Olivopontocerebellar Atrophy

Dementia has been reported in up to 60% of the familial and 40% of the sporadic forms of olivopontocerebellar atrophy (OPCA), respectively. Dementia tends to occur both in the mild to late and also in the early course of the disease (3%) (Berciano, 1982). Although WAIS and Wechsler Memory Scale (WMS) quotients may be normal, mild but definite cognitive abnormalities affecting memory (Logical Memory of the WMS), visuospatial (Block Design of the WAIS, Rey Complex Figure, Visual Hooper Organization Test), and predominantly executive tasks (WCST, Verbal Fluency, Tower Tests, Similarities and Comprehension of the WAIS) have been described consistently in patients with OPCA (Arroyo-Anllo and Botez-Marquard, 1998; Botez-Marquard, Botez, 1993; 1997; Berent et al., 1990). Almost all patients show mixed dysarthria, with combinations of hypokinetic, ataxic, and spastic components (Kluin et al., 1996).

Striatonigral Degeneration and Shy-Drager Syndrome

Patients with MSA (SND-SDS) rarely develop dementia. The cognitive profile of these patients is similar to that found in other forms of parkinsonisms. Specifically, there is a recall memory deficit solved with cues or recognition, a reduced speed of processing information, and increasing difficulty depending on the "effort-demanding" gradient of the tasks. A recent comparative study showed no disturbance of apraxic functions in patients with MSA compared with those with PSP and Parkinson's disease (Leiguarda et al., 1997).

Executive impairment (Verbal Fluency, Trail Making Test), even in the absence of intellectual deterioration, is the most consistent finding described in patients with striatonigral degeneration and Shy-Drager syndrome. The dysexecutive syndrome found in SND is far less dramatic than in PSP and more selective than in Parkinson's disease because performance in the WCST seems to be preserved in patients with SND compared with those with Parkinson's disease. However, consistent greater impairment is seen in attentional resources (Stroop test) in patients with SND than in patients with Parkinson's disease (Meco et al., 1996). Other language, memory, or perceptual tasks are relatively preserved. Mild visuospatial organizational abnormalities and memory deficits (Buschke Selective Reminding Test) have also been reported in SND and interpreted as resulting from an inefficient planning of visuospatial or memory processes.

Psychiatric Complications

Patients with MSA were reported to exhibit depression similar to that seen in patients with Parkin-

son's disease (Table 23-3). Few descriptive studies have reported a high prevalence of apathy (90%), a low percentage of anxiety (8%), and dopaminergic-induced psychotic features (15%) (Fetoni et al., 1999; Pilo et al., 1996).

Pathology

Pathologic features of MSA vary among patients. In patients with prominent cerebellar symptoms (OPCA), prominent atrophy of the cerebellum and brainstem nuclei is seen, whereas striatal degeneration predominates in patients with prominent parkinsonism symptoms (SND and SDS). As described, corticosubcortical deafferentation processes may explain some cognitive deficits found in patients with MSA. Besides, cerebellar pathology can interfere with visuospatial and executive tasks because of defective cerebellocortical (cerebelloparietal and cerebellofrontal) and cerebello-brainstem-cortical loops (Arroyo-Anllo and Botez-Marquard, 1998).

HUNTINGTON'S DISEASE

Huntington's disease is a progressive neurodegenerative disease determined by an excessive number of CAG repeats in the short arm of chromosome 4, transmitted with complete penetrance. Although Huntington's disease typically begins in midlife (30–55 years), late-onset forms (>50 years) occur in up to 25% of the cases. The prevalence of Huntington's disease is about 5 to $10/10^5$. The average life span is 15 to 20 years from onset, with the worst course in early-onset cases. The presentation of Huntington's disease can be variable. The onset is generally insidious and can be manifested by different combinations of hyperkinetic (choreic) movements (although a small percentage of patients may have parkinsonian features), cognitive impairment, and neuropsychiatric disturbances.

Circumscribed Cognitive Deficits

Cognitive abnormalities, which usually begin with psychomotor skills, are among the earliest indicators of functional decline (Table 23-1) (Mayeux et al., 1986). In fact, neuropsychological impairment can be even more disabling than motor symptoms, especially when the disease progresses and dementia appears (Bamford et al., 1995). Cognitive disturbances have been described in gene carriers with motor symptoms and also in self-reported asymptomatic gene carriers. Psychomotor retardation has also been recognized in medically reported unaffected gene carriers (De Boo et al., 1997; Foroud et al., 1995; Kirkwood et al., 1999).

Intelligence

Patients with Huntington's disease present with a decrement in full-scale intelligence quotient and in both verbal, and predominantly, performance subtests of the WAIS (Caine et al., 1978). Impairment is seen in motor, problem-solving, memory, and concentration skills of the Halstead-Reitan battery as are difficulties in the initiation/perseveration and construction subscales of the MDRS (Paulsen et al., 1995). The gradual decline in global measures of cognitive function has been associated with longer disease duration, greater severity of motor impairment (akinesia), more trinucleotide repeats, and later onset of motor symptoms (>51 years) (Brandt et al., 1984; Girotti et al., 1988; Gomez-Tortosa et al., 1998; Jason et al., 1997).

Memory

Memory problems may be the initial symptom of the disease and tend to worsen as the disease progresses. Registration of information is usually normal, but verbal or visual acquisition is slowed and vulnerable to interference effects. Most memory scores are well correlated with performance on tests of executive functions, suggesting that memory impairment in patients with Huntington's disease results primarily from an inability to initiate systematic retrieval strategies. In accordance with this hypothesis, recent memory is impaired particularly in those tasks that require the ability to spontaneously generate efficient strategies and to use internally guided behavior (Pillon et al., 1993). This failure of retrieval with normal encoding and storing mechanisms also account for the deficits in remote memory found in patients with Huntington's disease.

Language

Motor, syntactical (grammar and syntax), and semantic (vocabulary and naming) components of language are affected. Dysarthria may be present even in the early stages and can make the speech unintelligible as the disease evolves. Verbal fluency is reduced, and the grammatical form, the length of the phrases, and the syntactical complexity of speech are reduced (Rich et al., 1999). Paraphasic errors and naming difficulties have been described, especially late in the disease course, but at lesser frequency and intensity than in other cortical dementias (Hodges et al., 1991).

Comprehension is remarkably well preserved. Motor disturbances can make patient's writing slow, difficult, or even impossible, but dysgraphic errors and perseverations have also been described (Podoll et al., 1988).

Visuospatial Function

Graphomotor visuospatial deficits (Rey-Osterrieth Complex Figure, Clock Drawing), visual memory impairments (Benton Visual Retention Tests), visuoconstructional disturbances (Block Design and Object Assembly of the WAIS), and spatial disorientation (Road-map Test of Direction) have been identified in Huntington's disease (Mohr et al., 1991) A deficit in visual tracking tasks (Trail Making Test, Digit Symbol) should be interpreted cautiously because eye movements are frequently disturbed in these patients.

Executive Function

Even at early stages of the disease, patients with Huntington's disease present with deficits in planning and organizing activities (Tower of London/Hanoi), perseverative tendencies (WCST), and an inability to shift mental sets (WCST, Trail Making Test, Stroop Test) (Lawrence et al., 1996; Watkins et al., 2000). Abstract reasoning and concept formation can be preserved at early stages but decline as the disease progresses (Similarities, Comprehension and Calculation subtests of the WAIS). In general, patients with Huntington's disease present with more difficulties when the task includes novel material, timed tasks, manipulation, or reasoning. As mentioned, slowed mental processing and set-shifting or set-maintenance difficulties can also contribute to performance failures in visuospatial, language and memory tasks.

Dementia

The prevalence rate of dementia varies from 15% to 95% among studies (Pillon et al., 1991). Sample differences as well as the method for assessing dementia may be partially responsible for these discrepancies. Cognitive decline seems to be related to the number of years affected more than with age at onset. Dementia is consistently present at final stages of the disease if survival is long enough, although the time of its onset is difficult to determine precisely.

The dementia of Huntington's disease is classified as subcortical, so apraxia, agnosia, and aphasia are not common symptoms. Attentional disorders, retrieval deficits, and executive impairments are present at early stages of the dementing process. As described, free recall of information from both episodic and semantic memory is impaired at this stage. Although cued recall and recognition are generally normal, these mechanisms can also be affected with disease progression (Huber and Paulson, 1987).

Huntington's Disease Versus Alzheimer's Disease

Neuropsychological evaluation of patients with Huntington's disease shows an inability to shift mental sets; concept formation, initiation, and problem-solving deficits; and perseverative errors. This pattern can be useful in differentiating cognitive impairment between patients with Huntington's disease and Alzheimer's disease (Lange et al., 1995; Hodges et al., 1990). Patients with Huntington's disease demonstrate greater impairment on serial sevens of the MMSE and performed worse on the initiation subscale of the MDRS, whereas patients with Alzheimer's disease are more impaired on memory tasks of both scales. Moreover, differences between groups exist at mid and severe stages of the disease, with an additional impairment in constructional praxis seen in patients with Huntington's disease (Brandt et al., 1988; Paulsen et al., 1995). Demented patients with Alzheimer's disease commonly present graphic difficulties in visuoconstructive tests such as the Clock Drawing Test, whereas conceptual errors are almost exclusively seen in patients with Huntington's disease. In the copy condition, only those patients with Alzheimer's disease showed a marked improvement in performance (Rouleau et al., 1992). They were more impaired in semantic than in letter verbal fluency tasks and produced a larger proportion of responses earlier in the recall period. By contrast, patients with Huntington's disease had similar difficulties in both tasks and produced a larger proportion of their responses late in the recall period (Rohrer et al., 1999; Rosser and Hodges, 1994). Deficits in verbal recognition tasks may be similar in both disease entities, but patients with Alzheimer's disease tend to have lower discrimination indexes (Brandt et al., 1992). Finally, patients with Huntington's disease tend to have more difficulties in egocentric (right-left) than extrapersonal (constructional skills) spatial perception, just the opposite to what described in those with Alzheimer's disease (Bylsma et al., 1992). So far as implicit memory is concerned, patients with Huntington's disease are impaired on motor learning but not lexical priming tasks, whereas those with Alzheimer's disease evidence the opposite relationship on these tasks (Heindel et al., 1989).

Psychiatric Features

The prevalence of psychiatric symptoms in Huntington's disease varies between 35% and 75% (Table 23-3). Psychiatric symptoms may be the presenting manifestation of the disease in up to 50% of the cases and may precede the onset of motor or cognitive symptoms by as much as 10 years, so they cannot readily be ascribed to declining cognitive or motor abilities (Zappacosta et al., 1996).

Globally, irritability (50%), agitation (50%), apathy (50%), depression (30%), psychosis (20%), and mania (10%) are the most common symptoms (Folstein and Folstein, 1983; Burns et al., 1990). A gradient is seen, with anxiety, impulsivity, lability, irritability, and aggressiveness more commonly associated with suicidal and homicidal behavior in the early stages of the illness. Depression, dysthymia, mania, dysphoria, and psychosis (persecutory delusions and auditory hallucinations) are seen in the middle phases, with apathy, abulia, and dementia appearing in the late stages. Depression may antedate the onset of neurologic symptoms in up to 75% of the cases, suggesting that it is not simply a reaction to motor disabilities. The risk of suicide is 8 to 20 times higher than in the general population, especially in the middle-aged group. Obsessions and compulsions are present in most of patients (Cummings and Cunningham, 1992b). Sleep disturbances have been reported in about 20% of patients with late-onset Huntington's disease (Chokroverty, 1996). Paraphilias and altered sexual behavior have also been reported, especially in the early phases of the disease, and have also been associated with mania or hypomania (Fedoroff et al., 1994).

Pathology

The core pathologic feature of Huntington's disease is the selective loss of inhibitory gamma-aminobutyric acidergic striatal neurons projecting to the globus pallidus and substantia nigra pars reticulata. This process generates an increase in the activity of the excitatory neurotransmitters, which can have neurotoxic effects. The degenerative process may also involve the cerebellum, thalamic nuclei, subthalamic nucleus, and frontal and prefrontal cortex. Most of the early cognitive and psychiatric deficits reported in Huntington's disease have been related to an increased excitatory subcortical output flow to the dorsolateral (executive impairment), orbitofrontal (mania, obsessive-compulsive disorder), and anterior cingular cortex (abulia, and apathy). At later stages, depression, apathy, and other cognitive impairment may be secondary to more widespread frontal or caudate degeneration (Litvan et al., 1998b).

Treatment

No specific treatment exists for cognitive disturbances in Huntington's disease. An irregular improvement in cognitive function has been described after bilateral transplantation of human fetal striatal tissue, but follow-up studies are needed (Philpott et al., 1997). Neuroleptics can be used to treat psychosis, although some patients may be resistant to treatment with conventional antipsychotic agents. These drugs may decrease chorea but usually worsen cognitive function. Propanolol and buspirone have also been reported to relieve aggression. Depression and suicidal behavior are treated with conventional antidepressant agents and reportedly also responds to treatment with electroconvulsive therapy. Mania has been found to respond to treatment with carbamazepine, lithium, clonazepam, and valproic acid. Obsessive-compulsive disorder can be ameliorated by treatment with serotonergic agents.

REFERENCES

Aarsland D, Larsen JP, Lim NG, et al. Range of neuropsychiatric disturbances in patients with Parkinson's disease. *J Neurol Neurosurg Psychiatry* 1999;67:492–496.

Aarsland D, Larsen IP, Tandberg E, et al. Predictors of nursing home placement in Parkinson's disease: a population-based, prospective study. *J Am Geriatr Soc* 2000;48: 938–942.

Alexander GE, DeLong MR, Strick PL. Parallel organization of functionally segregated circuits linking basal ganglia and cortex. *Annu Rev Neurosci* 1986;9:357–381.

Appollonio I, Grafman J, Clark K, et al. Implicit and explicit memory in patients with Parkinson's disease with and without dementia. *Arch Neurol* 1994;51:359–367.

Arroyo-Anllo EM, Botez-Marquard T. Neurobehavioral dimensions of olivopontocerebellar atrophy. *J Clin Exp Neuropsychol* 1998;20:52–59.

Bamford KA, Caine ED, Kido DK, et al. A prospective evaluation of cognitive decline in early Huntington's disease: functional and radiographic correlates. *Neurology* 1995; 45:1867–1873..

Berciano J. Olivopontocerebellar atrophy. A review of 117 cases. *J Neurol Sci* 1982;53:253–272.

Berent S, Giordani B, Gilman S, et al. Neuropsychological changes in olivopontocerebellar atrophy. *Arch Neurol* 1990;47:997–1001.

Boller F, Passafiume D, Keefe NC, et al. Visuospatial impairment in Parkinson's disease. Role of perceptual and motor factors. *Arch Neurol* 1984;41:485–490.

Bondi MW, Kaszniak AW. Implicit and explicit memory in Alzheimer's disease and Parkinson's disease. *J Clin Exp Neuropsychol* 1991;13:339–358.

Bondi MW, Kaszniak AW, Bayles KA, et al. Contribution of frontal system dysfunction to memory and perceptual abilities in Parkinson's disease. *Neuropsychology* 1993;7: 89–102.

Botez-Marquard T, et al. Cognitive behavior in heredodegenerative ataxias. *Eur Neurol* 1992;33:351–357.

Botez-Marquard T, et al. Olivopontocerebellar atrophy and Friedreich's ataxia: neuropsychological consequences of bilateral versus unilateral cerebellar lesions. *Int Rev Neurobiol* 1997;41:387–410.

Brandt J, Strauss ME, Larus J, et al. Clinical correlates of dementia and disability in Huntington's disease. *J Clin Neuropsychol* 1984;6:401–412.

Brandt J, Folstein SE, Folstein MF. Differential cognitive impairment in Alzheimer's disease and Huntington's disease. *Ann Neurol* 1988;23:555–561.

Brandt J, Corwin J, Krafft L. Is verbal recognition memory really different in Huntington's and Alzheimer's disease. *J Clin Exp Neuropsychol* 1992;14:773–784.

Brown RG, Marsden CD. Visuospatial function in Parkinson's disease. *Brain* 1986;109:987–1002.

Brown RG, Marsden CD. Cognitive function in Parkinson's disease: from description to theory. *Trends Neurosci* 1990;13:21–29.

Burns A, Folstein S, Brandt J, et al. Clinical assessment of irritability, aggression, and apathy in Huntington and Alzheimer disease. *J Nerv Ment Dis* 1990;178:20–26.

Bylsma FW, Brandt J, Strauss ME. Personal and extrapersonal orientation in Huntington's disease patients and those at risk. *Cortex* 1992;28:113–122.

Caine ED, Hunt RD, Weingartner H, et al. Huntington's dementia. Clinical and neuropsychological features. *Arch Gen Psychiatry* 1978;35:377–384.

Celesia GG, Barr AN. Psychosis and other psychiatric manifestations of levodopa therapy. *Arch Neurol* 1970;23: 193–200. 1970.

Chokroverty S. Sleep and degenerative neurologic disorders. *Neurol Clin* 1996;4:807–826.

Cools AR, van den Bercken JH, Horstink MW, et al. Cognitive and motor shifting aptitude disorder in Parkinson's disease. *J Neurol Neurosurg Psychiatry* 1984;47:443–453.

Cooper JA, Sagar HJ, Jordan N, et al. Cognitive impairment in early, untreated Parkinson's disease and its relationship to motor disability. *Brain* 1991;114:2095–2122.

Cooper JA, Sagar HJ, Doherty SM, et al. Different effects of dopaminergic and anticholinergic therapies on cognitive and motor function in Parkinson's disease. A follow-up study of untreated patients. *Brain* 1992;115:1701–1725.

Cummings JL. Behavioral complications of drug treatment of Parkinson's disease. *J Am Geriatr Soc* 1991;39:708–716.

Cummings JL. Depression and Parkinson's disease: a review. *Am J Psychiatry* 1992a;149:443–454.

Cummings JL, Cunningham K. Obsessive-compulsive disorder in Huntington's disease. *Biol Psychiatry* 1992b;31: 263–270.

Cummings JL, Darkins A, Mendez M, et al. Alzheimer's disease and Parkinson's disease: comparison of speech and language alterations. *Neurology* 1988;38:680–684.

Daniel SE, de Bruin V, Lees AJ. The clinical and pathological spectrum of Steele-Richardson-Olszewski syndrome (progressive supranuclear palsy): a reappraisal. *Brain* 1995;118:759–770.

De Boo GM, Tibben A, Lanser JB, et al. Early cognitive and motor symptoms in identified carriers of the gene for Huntington disease. *Arch Neurol* 1997;54:1353–1357.

Downes JJ, Roberts AC, Sahakian BJ, et al. Impaired extra-dimensional shift performance in medicated and unmedicated Parkinson's disease: evidence for a specific attentional dysfunction. *Neuropsychologia* 1989;27:1329–1343.

Dubois B, Pillon B, Lhermitte F, et al. Cholinergic deficiency and frontal dysfunction in Parkinson's disease. *Ann Neurol* 1990;28:117–121.

Dubois B, Pillon B. Cognitive and behavioral aspects of movement disorders. In: Jankovic J, Tolosa E, eds. *Parkinson's disease and movement disorders*, 3rd ed. Baltimore: Williams & Wilkins, 1998:837–859.

Esmonde T, Giles E, Gibson M, et al. Neuropsychological performance, disease severity, and depression in progressive supranuclear palsy. *J Neurol* 1996;243:638–643.

Factor SA, Molho ES, Podskalny GD, et al. Parkinson's disease: drug-induced psychiatric states. *Adv Neurol* 1995; 65:115–138.

Fedoroff JP, Peyser C, Franz ML, et al. Sexual disorders in Huntington's disease. *J Neuropsychiatry Clin Neurosci* 1994;6:147–153.

Fetoni V, Soliveri P, Monza D, et al. Affective symptoms in multiple system atrophy and Parkinson's disease: response to levodopa therapy. *J Neurol Neurosurg Psychiatry* 1999;66:541–544.

Folstein SE, Folstein MF. Psychiatric features of Huntington's disease: recent approaches and findings. *Psychiatr Dev* 1983;1:193–205.

Foroud T, Siemers E, Kleindorfer D, et al. Cognitive scores in carriers of Huntington's disease gene compared to noncarriers. *Ann Neurol* 1995;37:657–664.

Frattali CM, Grafman J, Patronas N, et al. Language disturbances in corticobasal degeneration. *Neurology* 2000;54: 990–992.

Gibb WR, Luthert PJ, Marsden CD. Corticobasal degeneration. *Brain* 1989;112:1171–1192.

Girotti F, Marano R, Soliveri P, et al. Relationship between motor and cognitive disorders in Huntington's disease. *J Neurol* 1988;235:454–457.

Globus M, Mildworf B, Melamed E. Cerebral blood flow and cognitive impairment in Parkinson's disease. *Neurology* 1985;35:1135–1139.

Gomez-Tortosa E, del Barrio A, Garcia Ruiz PJ, et al. Severity of cognitive impairment in juvenile and late-onset Huntington disease. *Arch Neurol* 1998;55:835–843.

Growdon JH, Kieburtz K, McDermott MP, et al. Levodopa improves motor function without impairing cognition in mild non-demented Parkinson's disease patients. Parkinson Study Group. *Neurology* 1998;50:1327-1331.

Heindel WC, Salmon DP, Shults CW, et al. Neuropsychological evidence for multiple implicit memory systems: a comparison of Alzheimer's, Huntington's, and Parkinson's disease patients. *J Neurosci* 1989;9:582–587.

Henik A, Singh J, Beckley DJ, et al. Disinhibition of automatic word reading in Parkinson's disease. *Cortex* 1993; 29:589–599.

Hodges JR, Salmon DP, Butters N. Differential impairment of semantic and episodic memory in Alzheimer's and Huntington's diseases: a controlled prospective study. *J Neurol Neurosurg Psychiatry* 1990;53:1089–1095.

Hodges JR, Salmon DP, Butters N. The nature of the naming deficit in Alzheimer's and Huntington's disease. *Brain* 1991;114:1547–1558.

Hovestadt A, de Jong GJ, Meerwaldt, J. D. Spatial disorientation as an early symptom of Parkinson's disease. *Neurology* 1987;37:485–487.

Huber SJ, Paulson GW. Memory impairment associated with progression of Huntington's disease. *Cortex* 1987; 23:275–283.

Huber SJ, Shuttleworth EC, Freidenberg DL. Neuropsychological differences between the dementias of Alzheimer's and Parkinson's diseases. *Arch Neurol* 1989;46:1287–1291.

Illes J, Metter EJ, Hanson WR, et al. Language production in Parkinson's disease: acoustic and linguistic considerations. *Brain Lang* 1988;33:146–160.

Inzelberg R, Kipervasser S, Korczyn AD. Auditory hallucinations in Parkinson's disease. *J Neurol Neurosurg Psychiatry* 1998;64:533–535.

Jacobs DM, Marder K, Cote LJ, et al. Neuropsychological characteristics of preclinical dementia in Parkinson's disease. *Neurology* 1995;45:1691–1696.

Jagust WJ, Reed BR, Martin EM, et al. Cognitive function and regional cerebral blood flow in Parkinson's disease. *Brain* 1992;115:521–537.

Jason GW, Suchowersky O, Pajurkova EM, et al. Cognitive manifestations of Huntington disease in relation to genetic structure and clinical onset. *Arch Neurol* 1997;54: 1081–1088.

Kertesz A, Davidson W, Munoz DG. Clinical and pathological overlap between frontotemporal dementia, primary progressive aphasia and corticobasal degeneration: the Pick complex. *Dement Geriatr Cogn Disord* 1999;10 (Suppl 1):46–49.

Kirkwood SC, Siemers E, Stout JC, et al. Longitudinal cognitive and motor changes among presymptomatic Huntington disease gene carriers. *Arch Neurol* 1999;56: 563–568.

Kluin KJ, Gilman S, Lohman M, et al. Characteristics of the dysarthria of multiple system atrophy. *Arch Neurol* 19996;53:545–548.

Kuzis G, Sabe L, Tiberti C, et al. Cognitive functions in major depression and Parkinson disease. *Arch Neurol* 1997; 54:982–986.

Lange KW, Sahakian BJ, Quinn NP, et al. Comparison of executive and visuospatial memory function in Huntington's disease and dementia of Alzheimer type matched for degree of dementia. *J Neurol Neurosurg Psychiatry* 1995; 58:598–606.

Lawrence AD, Sahakian BJ, Hodges JR, et al. Executive and mnemonic functions in early Huntington's disease. *Brain* 1996;119:1633–1645.

Leiguarda R, Lees AJ, Merello M, et al. The nature of apraxia in corticobasal degeneration. *J Neurol Neurosurg Psychiatry* 1994;57:455–459.

Leiguarda RC, Pramstaller PP, Merello M, et al. Apraxia in Parkinson's disease, progressive supranuclear palsy, multiple system atrophy and neuroleptic-induced parkinsonism. *Brain* 1997;120:75–90.

Lepen C, Wait S, Moutard-Martin F, et al. Cost of illness and disease severity in a cohort of French patients with Parkinson's disease. *Pharmacoeconomics* 1999;16:59–69.

Levin BE, Llabre MM, Weiner WJ. Cognitive impairments associated with early Parkinson's disease. *Neurology* 1989;39:557–561.

Levin BE, Llabre MM, Reisman S, et al. Visuospatial impairment in Parkinson's disease. *Neurology* 1991;41: 365–369.

Litvan I, Mohr E, Williams J, et al. Differential memory and executive functions in demented patients with Parkinson's and Alzheimer's disease. *J Neurol Neurosurg Psychiatry* 1991;54:25–29.

Litvan I, Mangone CA, McKee A, et al. Natural history of progressive supranuclear palsy (Steele-Richardson-Olszewski syndrome) and clinical predictors of survival: a clinicopathological study. *J Neurol Neurosurg Psychiatry* 1996a;60:615–620.

Litvan I, Mega MS, Cummings JL, et al. Neuropsychiatric aspects of progressive supranuclear palsy. *Neurology* 1996b;47:1184–1189.

Litvan I, Cummings JL, Mega M. Neuropsychiatric features of corticobasal degeneration. *J Neurol Neurosurg Psychiatry* 1998a;65:717–721.

Litvan I, Paulsen JS, Mega MS, et al. Neuropsychiatric assessment of patients with hyperkinetic and hypokinetic movement disorders. *Arch Neurol* 1998b;55:1313–1319.

Louis ED, Marder K, Cote L, et al. Mortality from Parkinson disease. *Arch Neurol* 1997;54:260–264.

Macmahon DG. Parkinson's disease nurse specialists: an important role in disease management. *Neurology* 1999; 52(Suppl 3):21–25.

Mahieux F, Fenelon G, Flahault A, et al. Neuropsychological prediction of dementia in Parkinson's disease. *J Neurol Neurosurg Psychiatry* 1998;64:178–183.

Malapani C, Pillon B, Dubois B, et al. Impaired simultaneous cognitive task performance in Parkinson's disease: a dopamine-related dysfunction. *Neurology* 1994;44:319–326.

Marder K, Tang MX, Cote L, et al. The frequency and associated risk factors for dementia in patients with Parkinson's disease. *Arch Neurol* 1995;52:695–701.

Massman PJ, Kreiter KT, Jankovic J, et al. Neuropsychological functioning in cortical-basal ganglionic degeneration: differentiation from Alzheimer's disease. *Neurology* 1996;46:720–726.

Masterman D, DeSalles A, Baloh RW, et al. Motor, cognitive, and behavioral performance following unilateral ventroposterior pallidotomy for Parkinson disease. *Arch Neurol* 1998;55:1201–1208.

Mayeux R, Stern Y, Rosen J, et al. Is "subcortical dementia" a recognizable clinical entity? *Ann Neurol* 1983;14:278–283.

Mayeux R, Stern Y, Herman A, et al. Correlates of early disability in Huntington's disease. *Ann Neurol* 1986;20:727–731.

Mayeux R, Chen J, Mirabello E, et al. An estimate of the incidence of dementia in idiopathic Parkinson's disease. *Neurology* 1990;40:1513–1517.

Meco G, Gasparini M, Doricchi F. Attentional functions in multiple system atrophy and Parkinson's disease. *J Neurol Neurosurg Psychiatry* 1996;60:393–398.

Milberg W, Albert M. Cognitive differences between patients with progressive supranuclear palsy and Alzheimer's disease. *J Clin Exp Neuropsychol* 1989;11:605–614.

Mitchell SL, Kiely DK, Kiel DP, et al. The epidemiology, clinical characteristics, and natural history of older nursing home residents with a diagnosis of Parkinson's disease. *J Am Geriatr Soc* 1996;44:394–399.

Mohr E, Brouwers P, Claus JJ, et al. Visuospatial cognition in Huntington's disease. *Mov Disord* 1991;6:127–132.

Nausieda PA, Weiner WJ, Kaplan LR, et al. Sleep disruption in the course of chronic levodopa therapy: an early feature of the levodopa psychosis. *Clin Neuropharmacol* 1982;5:183–194.

Okuda B, Tachibana H, Kawabata K, et al. Slowly progressive limb-kinetic apraxia with a decrease in unilateral cerebral blood flow. *Acta Neurol Scand* 1992;86:76–81.

Owen AM, James M, Leigh PN, et al. Fronto-striatal cognitive deficits at different stages of Parkinson's disease. *Brain* 1992;115:1727–1751.

Owen AM, Beksinska M, James M, et al. Visuospatial memory deficits at different stages of Parkinson's disease. *Neuropsychologia* 1993;31:627–644.

Paulsen JS, Butters N, Sadek JR, et al. Distinct cognitive profiles of cortical and subcortical dementia in advanced illness. *Neurology* 1995;45:951–956.

Philpott LM, Kopyov OV, Lee AJ, et al. Neuropsychological functioning following fetal striatal transplantation in Huntington's chorea: three case presentations. *Cell Transplant* 1997;6:203–212.

Pillon B, Dubois B, Lhermitte F, et al. Heterogeneity of cognitive impairment in progressive supranuclear palsy, Parkinson's disease, and Alzheimer's disease. *Neurology* 1986;36:1179–1185.

Pillon B, Dubois B, Bonnet AM, et al. Cognitive slowing in Parkinson's disease fails to respond to levodopa treatment: the 15-objects test. *Neurology* 1989;39:762–768.

Pillon B, Dubois B, Agid Y. Severity and specificity of cognitive impairment in Alzheimer's, Huntington's, and Parkinson's diseases and progressive supranuclear palsy. *Ann N Y Acad Sci* 1991;640:224–227.

Pillon B, Deweer B, Agid Y, et al. Explicit memory in Alzheimer's, Huntington's, and Parkinson's diseases. *Arch Neurol* 1993;50:374–379.

Pillon B, Blin J, Vidailhet M, et al. The neuropsychological pattern of corticobasal degeneration: comparison with progressive supranuclear palsy and Alzheimer's disease. *Neurology* 1995a;45:1477–1483.

Pillon B, Gouider Khouja N, Deweer B, et al. Neuropsychological pattern of striatonigral degeneration: comparison with Parkinson's disease and progressive supranuclear palsy. *J Neurol Neurosurg Psychiatry* 1995b;58:174–179.

Pillon B, Ertle S, Deweer B, et al. Memory for spatial location is affected in Parkinson's disease. *Neuropsychologia* 1996;34:77–85.

Pillon B, Ertle S, Deweer B, et al. Memory for spatial location in 'de novo' parkinsonian patients. *Neuropsychologia* 1997;35:221–228.

Pilo L, Ring H, Quinn N, et al. Depression in multiple system atrophy and in idiopathic Parkinson's disease: a pilot comparative study. *Biol Psychiatry* 1996;39:803–807.

Podoll K, Caspary P, Lange HW, et al. Language functions in Huntington's disease. *Brain* 1988;111:1475–1503.

Podoll K, Schwarz M, Noth J. Language functions in progressive supranuclear palsy. *Brain* 1991;114:1457–1472.

Poewe W, Berger W, Benke T, et al. High-speed memory scanning in Parkinson's disease: adverse effects of levodopa. *Ann Neurol* 1991;29:670–673.

Rich JB, Troyer AK, Bylsma FW, et al. Longitudinal analysis of phonemic clustering and switching during word-list generation in Huntington's disease. *Neuropsychology* 1999;13:525–531.

Richards M, Cote LJ, Stern Y. Executive function in Parkinson's disease: set-shifting or set-maintenance? *J Clin Exp Neuropsychol* 1993;15:266–279.

Riley DE, Lang AE, Lewis A, et al. Cortical-basal ganglionic degeneration. *Neurology* 1990;40:1203–1212.

Rohrer D, Salmon DP, Wixted JT, et al. The disparate effects of Alzheimer's disease and Huntington's disease on semantic memory. *Neuropsychology* 1999;13:381–388.

Rosser A, Hodges JR. Initial letter and semantic category fluency in Alzheimer's disease, Huntington's disease, and progressive supranuclear palsy. *J Neurol Neurosurg Psychiatry* 1994;57:1389–1394.

Rouleau I, Salmon DP, Butters N, et al. Quantitative and qualitative analyses of clock drawings in Alzheimer's and Huntington's disease. *Brain Cogn* 1992;18:70–87.

Saint Cyr JA, Taylor AE, Lang AE. Neuropsychological and psychiatric side effects in the treatment of Parkinson's disease. *Neurology* 1993;43(Suppl 6):47–52.

Sanchez-Ramos JR, Ortoll R, Paulson GW. Visual hallucinations associated with Parkinson disease. *Arch Neurol* 1996;53:1265–1268.

Scheife RT, Schumock GT, Burstein A, et al. Impact of Parkinson's disease and its pharmacologic treatment on quality of life and economic outcomes. *Am J Health Syst Pharm* 2000;57:953–962.

Schiffer RB, Kurlan R, Rubin A, et al. Evidence for atypical depression in Parkinson's disease. *Am J Psychiatry* 1988; 145:1020–1022.

Starkstein SE, Mayberg HS, Leiguarda R, et al. A prospective longitudinal study of depression, cognitive decline, and physical impairments in patients with Parkinson's disease. *J Neurol Neurosurg Psychiatry* 1992;55:377–382.

Steele JC, Richardson JC, Olzewski J. Progressive supranuclear palsy: a heterogeneous degeneration involving the brain stem, basal ganglia, and cerebellum with vertical gaze and pseudobulbar palsy, nuchal dystonia and dementia. *Arch Neurol* 1964;10:333–359.

Stein MB, Heuser IJ, Juncos JL, et al. Anxiety disorders in patients with Parkinson's disease. *Am J Psychiatry* 1990; 147:217–220.

Stern Y, Marder K, Tang MX, et al. Antecedent clinical features associated with dementia in Parkinson's disease. *Neurology* 1993;43:1690–1692.

Stern Y, Richards M, Sano M, et al. Comparison of cognitive changes in patients with Alzheimer's and Parkinson's disease. *Arch Neurol* 1993;50:1040–1045.

Stern Y, Tang MX, Jacobs DM, et al. Prospective comparative study of the evolution of probable Alzheimer's disease and Parkinson's disease dementia. *J Int Neuropsychol Soc* 1998;4:279–284.

Tsai CH, Lu CS, Hua MS, et al. Cognitive dysfunction in early onset parkinsonism. *Acta Neurol Scand* 1994;89: 9–14.

Uitti RJ, Tanner CM, Rajput AH, et al. Hypersexuality with antiparkinsonian therapy. *Clin Neuropharmacol* 1989;12: 375–383.

Valldeoriola F, Nobbe FA, Tolosa E. Treatment of behavioural disturbances in Parkinson's disease. *J Neural Transm* 1997;(Suppl 51):175–204.

Van der Hurk PR, Hodges JR. Episodic and semantic memory in Alzheimer's disease and progressive supranuclear palsy: a comparative study. *J Clin Exp Neuropsychol* 1995;17:459–471.

Watkins LH, Rogers RD, Lawrence AD, et al. Impaired planning but intact decision making in early Huntington's disease: implications for specific fronto-striatal pathology. *Neuropsychologia* 2000;38:1112–1125.

Whetten-Goldstein K, Sloan F, Kulas E, et al. The burden of Parkinson's disease on society, family, and the individual. *J Am Geriatr Soc* 1997;45:844–849.

Zappacosta B, Monza D, Meoni C, et al. Psychiatric symptoms do not correlate with cognitive decline, motor symptoms, or CAG repeat length in Huntington's disease. *Arch Neurol* 1996;53:493–497.

SUGGESTED READINGS

Behavioral neurology of movement disorders. Weiner WJ, Lang AE, eds. *Advances in Neurology* Vol. 65. New York: Raven Press, 1995.

Dubois B, Pillon B. Cognitive and behavioral aspects of movement disorders. In: Jankovic J, Tolosa E, eds. *Parkinson's disease and movement disorders*, 3rd ed. Baltimore: Williams & Wilkins, 1998;37:837–859.

Jacobs DM, Stern Y, Mayeux R. Dementia in Parkinson disease, Huntington disease, and other degenerative conditions. In: Feinberg TE, Farah MJ, eds. *Behavioral neurology and Neuropsychology*. New York: McGraw-Hill, 1997;579–603.

Lezak MD. Neuropathology for neuropsychologist. In: Lezak MD, eds. *Neuropsychological assessment*, 3rd ed. New York: Oxford University Press, 1995;7:223–238.

WEB SITES

Information regarding local support organizations and educational materials can be obtained by contacting:

American Parkinson Disease Association, Inc.: *www.apdaparkinson.com*

National Parkinson Foundation, Inc.: *www.parkinson.org*

The Parkinson's Disease Foundation: *www.pdf.org*

The Parkinson Action Network: *www.parkinsonaction.org*

The Parkinson Foundation of Canada: *www.parkinson.ca*

World Parkinson Disease Association: *www.wpda.org*

Society for Progressive Supranuclear Palsy, Inc.: *www.psp.org*

Huntington's Disease Society of America: *www.hdsa.org*

The Shy-Drager/Multiple System Atrophy Support Group: *www.shy-drager.com*

National Ataxia Foundation: *www.ataxia.org*

Worldwide Education and Awareness for Movement Disorders: *www.wemove.org*

24

Diseases of the Spinal Cord and Vertebrae

H. Gordon Deen, Jr.

A wide range of disease processes can affect the vertebral column of the older adult. The spinal cord, cauda equina, and spinal nerve roots may also be involved. This chapter provides an overview of these diseases, with an emphasis on the more common disorders, which the primary care practitioner or neurologist will be more likely to encounter in clinical practice.

OSTEOPOROSIS

Osteoporosis is a common problem in the elderly. Despite increased attention in medical publications and in the lay press, this disorder often remains unrecognized and untreated. Osteoporosis is seen more frequently in women, but can also occur in men. From a conceptual standpoint, osteoporosis can be defined as a systemic skeletal disease characterized by low bone mass and microarchitectural deterioration, with a consequent increase in bone fragility and susceptibility to fracture (Eastell, 1998). From an operational standpoint, osteoporosis is defined as a bone mineral density (T-score) score that is 2.5 SD below the mean peak value in young adults. Patients with osteoporosis can sustain fractures with minimal trauma. The vertebral column, proximal femur, and distal forearm are most commonly involved, but fracture of any bone can occur. Vertebral compression fractures are the most common manifestation of osteoporosis of the spine. The lower thoracic and upper lumbar vertebrae are the most common sites of involvement. A compression fracture above the T-7 level is rarely caused by osteoporosis, and the diagnosis of tumor or infection should be considered in such cases.

Osteoporotic spinal compression fractures cause back pain, with or without radiculopathy. Symptoms often respond poorly to treatment. Multiple vertebral fractures occurring over time can lead to secondary spinal disorders such as spinal stenosis, scoliosis, or kyphotic deformity.

"Benign" osteoporotic compression fracture should be a diagnosis of exclusion (Fig. 24-1). Always consider the possibility that an acute spinal compression fracture can be caused by neoplasm or infection. Magnetic resonance imaging (MRI) usually provides some clues in this regard. In osteoporotic spinal compression fractures, the adjacent epidural and paraspinal soft tissues are normal, and the pedicle is not involved. Usually only one acute fracture is seen; however, old, healed compression fractures may have occurred in other vertebral bodies. In cases where the fracture is caused by metastatic tumor, abnormalities are often seen in the adjacent epidural and paraspinal soft tissues and in the pedicle. Often, acute lesions occur at other levels of the spinal column. In cases where the fracture is caused by infection, the abnormalities are centered in the intervertebral disk space. Abnormal T1 signal is seen in the vertebral bodies, adjacent to the disk. The epidural and paraspinal soft tissues are often involved. In most cases, the MRI, coupled with clinical findings, enables the physician to determine whether the patient has a benign osteoporotic compression fracture, or whether a more ominous diagnosis is present. A few patients, initially felt to have benign spinal compression fractures, have persistent or worsening pain or indeterminate MRI findings. These individuals should have a follow-up MRI examination in 6 weeks to 3 months.

When a diagnosis of osteoporosis is suspected, inquire about risk factors, including family history, cigarette smoking, alcohol abuse, sedentary lifestyle, low body weight, inadequate dietary calcium, low exposure to sunlight, early menopause, and chronic medication therapy with steroids, certain anticonvulsants (phenytoin), and anticoagulants. Also be aware that a variety of endocrine diseases (e.g., Cushing's syndrome), hematologic diseases (e.g., multiple myeloma), rheumatologic diseases (e.g., rheumatoid arthritis), and gastrointestinal diseases (e.g., malabsorption syndromes) can be associated with osteoporosis. Radiotherapy that includes the spinal column

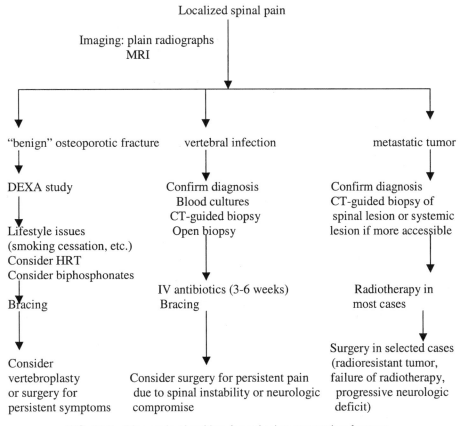

FIG. 24.1. Diagnosis algorithm for spinal compression fracture.

in the treatment fields can also predispose to loss of skeletal bone mass.

Management of osteoporosis involves both prevention and treatment. First focus on the patient's lifestyle issues, emphasizing the importance of smoking cessation and avoidance of excessive alcohol, while encouraging an adequate level of physical exercise and dietary calcium. Patients should be counseled to avoid heavy lifting and to take care to avoid falls. The risk of falling can be decreased by eliminating sedating medications. Some patients benefit from using a cane or walker. Estrogen replacement therapy is the treatment of choice for women with postmenopausal osteoporosis. Other pharmacologic options include biphosphonates, raloxifene, and calcitonin nasal spray.

An acute osteoporotic spinal compression fracture is managed with short-term activity reduction, analgesics, and bracing. A lightweight corset is better tolerated and less expensive, and appears to be

as effective as more rigid, custom-made orthoses. Narcotics may be necessary for short-term pain control.

Percutaneous vertebroplasty is emerging as a useful treatment for spinal compression fractures that fail to respond to 4 to 6 weeks of conservative treatment. This procedure involves the percutaneous injection of methylmethacrylate bone cement, under fluoroscopic guidance, into the symptomatic, compressed vertebral body. The goal of this treatment is to restore or improve the structural integrity of the vertebral body and anterior spinal column. This is an outpatient procedure done under local anesthesia and intravenous sedation. Vertebroplasty is a new procedure; therefore, long-term results are unknown. Early experience indicates that the procedure can be done safely, with encouraging short-term pain relief. Vertebroplasty is contraindicated in cases of significant compromise of the spinal canal from compressed bone fragment retropulsion.

Open surgery is usually not needed for osteoporotic spinal compression fractures. An occasional patient with significant spinal canal compromise and myelopathy or cauda equina syndrome will need to be considered for spinal canal decompression and stabilization via anterior or posterior surgical approaches. Unfortunately, these surgical procedures are often lengthy and complex, with the potential for significant blood loss and other complications. Prolonged hospital care and rehabilitation may be required. Furthermore, the patients who harbor osteoporotic compression fractures are often elderly and debilitated. Therefore, a decision to intervene surgically should not be taken lightly by the physician or the patient.

SPINAL METASTATIC TUMOR

The diagnosis of spinal metastatic tumor should be strongly considered in the older adult who presents with acute, severe spinal pain. The patient typically reports intense, localized, persistent pain at the level of the lesion. The pain is often worse at night. A wide range of neurologic involvement may exist. The patient may have a monoradiculopathy, myelopathy, or cauda equina syndrome from neural compression. Some patients have no neurologic symptoms or signs, whereas others present with a rapidly progressive, severe neurologic deficit. Some patients have an established diagnosis of systemic cancer, whereas many others do not. Be aware that the metastatic component of a tumor can cause symptoms before the primary lesion. For example, a patient with carcinoma of the lung may present with spinal metastasis, with the primary lesion being discovered only during subsequent evaluation. Occasionally is encountered the patient with spinal metastatic cancer, in whom a primary tumor is never identified, despite aggressive workup. Metastases account for 70% of all tumors of the spine. The most common primary tumor types are carcinoma of the breast, carcinoma of the lung, lymphoma, and carcinoma of the prostate. Carcinoma of the kidney and colon and a wide range of less common tumors can also have metastatic involvement of the spinal column.

Plain radiographs of the spine still play a useful role in the evaluation of spinal metastatic disease. The first radiographic evidence of spinal metastasis is the "winking owl" sign, which is caused by obliteration of the pedicle (Connolly and Hamilton, 1996). Spinal compression fractures may be seen. These lesions can be osteolytic, osteoblastic, or mixed. Carcinoma of the prostate and Hodgkin's disease can cause osteoblastic bony changes with the so-called "ivory vertebrae." MRI is more sensitive than plain radiographs and should be performed whenever spinal metastasis is a diagnostic possibility. MRI shows bony lesions before they become apparent on plain radiographs, and also reveals their soft tissue components, epidural spread, and neural compromise. Patients with spinal metastatic disease often have involvement of multiple spinal segments. Therefore, if one lesion is identified, the clinician must diligently search for lesions at other levels.

Spinal metastatic tumors are almost always extradural in location. Intradural metastases from primary brain tumors such as glioblastoma multiforme and medulloblastoma are uncommon. These so-called "drop metastases" have a characteristic MRI appearance of multiple nodules on the spinal cord and cauda equina. Intramedullary metastasis of non-central nervous system tumors into the substance of the spinal cord is rare. The lesion is usually well seen on MRI. These cases are characterized by rapid neurological deterioration. Prognosis is poor.

The mainstay of treatment is radiotherapy of the involved spinal segments. Surgery is reserved for patients harboring tumors known to be radioresistant, patients with a rapidly progressive neurologic deficit or severe pain, and those who have failed radiation therapy. A surgical approach may also be necessary to obtain diagnostic tissue in the occasional patient in whom the diagnosis is uncertain. Laminectomy as a stand-alone procedure is seldom indicated. Surgical treatment usually involves both decompression and stabilization from anterior or posterior (or combined) surgical approaches.

Prognosis depends on the biological activity of the underlying neoplasm. For example, spinal metastasis from carcinoma of the prostate often pursues an indolent course with little morbidity. In contrast, spinal metastasis from carcinoma of the lung carries a poorer prognosis. Outcome is variable with multiple myeloma. Some patients with this disease have a rapidly progressive downhill course, whereas others have prolonged survival for 5 years or more. Prognosis also depends on whether the spinal lesions are single or multiple, and on whether any neurologic involvement is present. An isolated spinal metastatic lesion without neurologic compromise can generally be controlled with radiotherapy and surgery, provided the malignancy is not progressing elsewhere in the body. In contrast, the prognosis is much worse in patients with multiple spinal metastases and significant cord compression, and in patients with rapidly progressive extraspinal disease.

PRIMARY BONE TUMORS AFFECTING THE SPINE

A number of primary bone tumors can be found in the spinal column. In contrast to metastatic tumors, primary bone tumors of the spine are uncommon, and are seen infrequently, even by spinal surgeons. These lesions can be benign or malignant. Benign tumors include osteochondroma, osteoid osteoma, aneurysmal bone cyst, hemangioma, giant cell tumor, and eosinophilic granuloma. Malignant tumors include chordoma, sarcoma, and chondrosarcoma (Boriani and Weinstein, 1997).

Similar to spinal metastases, the hallmark of primary bone tumors of the spine is intractable pain. Neurologic deficits caused by neural compression may also be present.

Treatment usually involves radical surgery using anterior or posterior or combination approaches. Postoperative radiotherapy is needed in selected cases.

SPINAL INTRADURAL TUMORS

A wide variety of tumors and other mass lesions can occur within the spinal dura. Most are uncommon in the elderly and will rarely be encountered by the primary care physician. Even a neurologist or neurosurgeon will see only a handful of these cases each year.

Lesions arising within the substance of the spinal cord are referred to as "intramedullary" tumors. All other intradural tumors are considered to be intradural, extramedullary in location. This includes tumors of the spinal nerve roots, cauda equina, and meninges. The most common intramedullary tumors are ependymoma and astrocytoma. Less common lesions include hemangioblastoma, lipoma, and metastasis. Nonneoplastic mass lesions are occasionally seen in the spinal cord, including cavernoma, epidermoid cyst, neuroglial cyst, and sarcoid granuloma (Fischer and Brotchi, 1996). The most common intradural, extramedullary tumors are meningioma and Schwannoma. Both are benign lesions.

Although a wide range of pathologic processes can occur within the spinal dura, the clinical presentation, evaluation, and treatment are similar for each type of lesion.

Intradural tumors usually present with localized pain and progressive neurologic deficit, which can include radiculopathy, myelopathy, or cauda equina syndrome. Symptoms usually develop insidiously, but lesions that hemorrhage can cause acute, even catastrophic, neurologic deterioration. Examples of spinal cord lesions that can be associated with hemorrhage include cavernoma and true arteriovenous malformations.

The imaging modality of choice for patients with intradural tumors is MRI, which accurately demonstrates the level of the lesion and whether the lesion is intramedullary or extramedullary. Spinal cord expansion, cystic and solid components of the tumor, and presence of an associated syrinx can be identified.

Surgical excision, usually via a posterior (laminectomy) approach, is the treatment of choice. Prognosis depends on the histology of the lesion and the extent of the preoperative neurologic deficit. Postoperative radiotherapy is recommended in selected cases.

SPINAL INFECTIONS

Spinal infections are uncommon, but must be considered in the older adult with back pain. These infections can be pyogenic, tuberculous, or fungal. The term "spinal infection" encompasses a spectrum of specific entities, including intervertebral diskitis, osteomyelitis of the vertebral bodies, epidural abscess, infection of the paravertebral structures (e.g., psoas abscess), or some combination of these. Early symptoms may be vague and not worrisome to the patient or the physician. Thus, the diagnosis is sometimes delayed. As time goes on, the patient often develops intense, localized pain, similar to spinal metastatic disease. Neurologic involvement is variable. Patients often have no neurologic symptoms or signs, but may have radiculopathy, myelopathy, or cauda equina syndrome.

Spinal infections can be divided into two groups. The first group includes spinal infections that occur as a complication of spinal surgery. These typically present within 2 to 3 weeks of surgery, although more indolent infections may not manifest for 6 to 8 weeks.

The second group includes patients who have not had recent spinal surgery. In these patients, spinal infection presumably is caused by hematogenous spread of bacteria from some distant site. A wide range of infections can lead to secondary involvement of the spinal column. Urinary tract infection, subacute bacterial endocarditis, septic arthritis, and sinusitis are frequent antecedent sources of infection. Also, be aware that infections of the skin, respiratory system, and gastrointestinal tract can also lead to spinal infection. Ask about recent invasive procedures that can cause bacteremia (e.g., cytoscopy and dental work). Diabetes mellitus, advancing age, and intravenous drug abuse are risk factors associated with spinal infection. Other factors that can play a contributing role include alcoholism, long-term steroid therapy, rheumatoid arthritis, immunosuppression, coexisting malignancy, and osteoporosis.

Strongly consider the possibility of spinal infection in the patient with fever and back pain; however, most patients harboring spinal infections are afebrile. Thus, the presence of a fever can help establish the diagnosis of spinal infection, but the absence of fever in no way excludes this diagnosis. Surprisingly, the white blood cell count and differential are often normal, even in the face of active spinal infection, and provide little guidance in establishing this diagnosis. In contrast, the erythrocyte sedimentation rate (ESR) is very helpful. An elevated ESR suggests the presence of infection, whereas a normal ESR strongly suggests that a spinal infection is not present. The ESR is also a good way to follow the disease and the response to antibiotic treatment. The C-reactive protein is also sensitive for spinal infection, but may not be widely available in some centers. Blood cultures should be obtained in all cases where spinal infection is suspected.

Early in the course of the illness, plain radiographs and even MRI may show no abnormality. The radiographic hallmark of infection is that the epicenter of involvement of the spinal column is the disk space, with secondary spread to the adjacent vertebral bodies. In contrast, metastatic tumor usually starts in the vertebral body and spares the disk space, at least initially. The MRI can help define whether the patient has diskitis, osteomyelitis, epidural abscess, paraspinal infection (e.g., psoas abscess), or some combination of these processes. MRI is also useful in assessing the response to antibiotic treatment.

It is important to obtain an accurate microbiologic diagnosis before proceeding with treatment. If blood cultures are positive, and the clinical and imaging findings support the diagnosis of vertebral osteomyelitis or diskitis, antibiotic treatment can be initiated. If blood cultures are negative, a computed tomography (CT)-guided percutaneous biopsy of the involved spinal segment should be performed. If the CT-guided biopsy is negative, an open surgical biopsy should be performed. With each biopsy procedure, a full range of aerobic, anaerobic, fungal, and mycobacterial cultures and stains should be obtained.

The most common organisms found in spinal infections are coagulase-positive and coagulase-negative staphylococci. *Escherichia coli* and other gram-negative organisms, tuberculosis, and fungi can be seen in intravenous drug abusers and in immunocompromised individuals.

Antibiotics represent the primary treatment for spinal infection. Spinal infections are typically treated with 3 to 6 weeks of intravenous antibiotics, often followed by a course of oral therapy.

Early surgery is sometimes needed for patients with spinal cord or cauda equina compression, and late surgery is occasionally needed for patients who develop spinal instability or deformity as a result of the infectious process. It is uncommon to find a localized collection of purulent fluid that is amenable to drainage. Dural enhancement usually just represents a secondary inflammatory response, but is often over-diagnosed as representing an epidural abscess. Thus, the MRI diagnosis of epidural abscess must be interpreted cautiously and in the context of the clinical findings.

Bracing, usually with a lightweight corset, is helpful for symptomatic relief. Patients may continue with their usual physical activities as tolerated. Much of the treatment of these patients can be conducted in the outpatient setting. Hospitalization is needed only for surgical procedures, and occasionally for pain control.

LUMBAR SPINAL STENOSIS

Degenerative lumbar spinal stenosis is a common spinal disorder in older adults. In its more advanced forms, lumbar spinal stenosis causes neurogenic claudication, which refers to leg pain and paresthesias, precipitated by standing and walking, and relieved by sitting down. This diagnosis is being made with increasing frequency, partly as a result of the widespread availability of MRI, and partly as a result of increased recognition of the clinical syndrome of neurogenic claudication. Patients present with varying degrees of low back pain, but intervention usually depends on whether leg symptoms are present.

A careful history is essential to establish the diagnosis. Patients with neurogenic claudication give varying descriptions of their lower extremity symptoms. Some patients report true leg pain, whereas others describe tingling, heaviness, or a sensation that their legs are going to "give out." The leg symptoms can be unilateral or bilateral.

Be aware that lumbar spinal stenosis, vascular occlusive disease, degenerative joint disease of the hip, and peripheral neuropathy are all common in the elderly, and can cause similar symptoms. Patients with vascular claudication develop leg pain with walking, but gain relief by standing still. In contrast, patients with neurogenic claudication must sit down to gain relief. Patients with degenerative joint disease of the hip describe hip and groin pain, without distal radiation. Patients with peripheral neuropathy typically describe painless numbness affecting both legs symmetrically in a stocking distribution.

In patients with lumbar spinal stenosis, the neurologic examination is usually normal, or reveals only mild abnormalities. If the patient has a moderate or severe neurologic deficit, a second diagnosis may be present. For example, the patient might have lumbar spinal stenosis with a superimposed acute disk herniation. It is important to check distal pulses to assess vascular status and also to do the Fabere maneuvers to assess for degenerative joint disease of the hip.

MRI or myelogram-CT should be used to establish the diagnosis of lumbar spinal stenosis. These studies may reveal stenosis of the central canal, lateral recess, or neural foramina. A degenerative spondylolisthesis or scoliosis may be present. Plain radiographs with flexion and extension views should also be obtained.

Symptoms may wax and wane early in the course of the disease process; however, the natural history of lumbar spinal stenosis is one of gradual progression of discomfort and functional limitation over time.

Conservative treatment, including physical therapy with or without modalities, and lumbar epidural steroid injections, helps in selected cases. Patients with disabling neurogenic claudication, coupled with severe spinal stenosis, usually require surgical treatment.

Before making a surgical referral, it is important to ask how much the patient is limited in his or her usual activities of daily living. For example, the patient who develops mild leg aching after walking 5 kilometers in 30 minutes probably does not need any active treatment, even with radiographic evidence of lumbar spinal stenosis. In contrast, the patient who consistently develops severe leg pain after walking 50 meters in 2 minutes should be considered for surgery.

Surgical treatment involves a lumbar decompressive laminectomy of the stenotic spinal segments. A fusion may be required for some patients with spondylolisthesis or scoliosis. A good or excellent result can be expected in 70% to 90% of cases at 1-year follow-up. With longer follow-up, a few patients who had good or excellent outcomes at 1-year, will develop recurrent symptoms and require further investigation and treatment. Despite this, surgical results are superior to those in patients treated nonoperatively at 4-year follow-up (Atlas et al., 2000).

Risk factors for poor outcome after decompressive laminectomy include coexisting illness (severe arthritis at sites other than the spine, rheumatoid arthritis, cardiac disease), single-interspace laminectomy, female gender, and presence of a preoperative neurologic deficit (Katz et al., 1991). Advanced age does not appear to be a risk factor for poor outcome.

SPINAL SYNOVIAL CYST

Synovial cysts can occur in the spine, causing neurologic symptoms as they enlarge. These cysts arise from the lining of the facet joint and can be viewed as a subset of degenerative spinal stenosis. They are most common in the lumbar region, but can occur in the cervical spine. Synovial cysts are typically solitary, but can be multiple. Conservative treatment is usually not helpful. MRI is the imaging procedure of choice, although the myelogram-CT can also be used.

Synovial cysts usually cause radicular pain and paresthesias because of compression of the underlying spinal nerve root(s). Symptoms usually develop gradually; however, patients occasionally present with the sudden onset of severe pain if an acute hemorrhage into a synovial cyst has occurred.

Clinical indications for surgery are similar to those for other lumbar spinal operations. The ideal candidate for surgery has intractable leg pain (rather than back pain) as the primary symptom. The imaging studies should demonstrate a synovial cyst in a location that correlates well with the clinical findings.

The surgical procedure consists of a lumbar laminectomy and cyst removal. A concomitant fusion is occasionally needed if spondylolisthesis has occurred at the level of the cyst. Surgical results are excellent, and the cyst recurrence rate is low.

HERNIATED INTERVERTEBRAL DISK

Intervertebral disk herniations are most common in middle-aged adults, but are also frequently seen in the elderly. Disk herniations occur most commonly in the lumbar region, somewhat less frequently in the cervical spine, and occasionally in the thoracic spine. MRI is the imaging procedure of choice; however, the myelogram-CT remains a superb diagnostic tool for those patients in whom MRI is contraindicated. The natural history of disk herniation at any level of the vertebral column is one of spontaneous improvement. Most patients will improve without any active treatment. Conservative treatment, including physical therapy (exercises or modalities) and epidural steroid injections can be of benefit in selected patients. Surgery is needed in only a small percentage of cases. The management of intervertebral disk disease is discussed in more detail in Chapter 15.

INFLAMMATORY SPINAL DISORDERS

The most common inflammatory spinal disorders are ankylosing spondylitis and rheumatoid arthritis. The spine can also be affected by other rheumatologic processes, including gout, pseudogout, acromegaly, amyloidosis, lupus, and diffuse idiopathic skeletal hyperostosis.

Ankylosing spondylitis is a chronic inflammatory disease that chiefly affects the spine. This disease is characterized by involvement of the sacroiliac joint and spinal column and has an association with the histocompatibility antigen HLA-B27. The disease typically has its onset between puberty and age 45. Men are affected more often than women. The pathologic picture includes inflammation, bony erosion, and ankylosis. Over time, complete ossification of the anterior longitudinal ligament occurs and bridging osteophytes develop. The radiographic appearance is described as a "bamboo" spine.

Patients with ankylosing spondylitis usually present with the insidious onset of low back pain and stiffness. Symptoms are usually worse in the morning and improve with exercise. Buttock pain that spreads diffusely to the posterior thighs may be present. Leg pain with ankylosing spondylitis usually does not radiate below the knee and does not represent sciatica caused by nerve root compression.

Ankylosing spondylitis is a chronic disease with a variable course, most often characterized by spontaneous remissions and exacerbations. Symptoms typically begin in the lumbosacral region and progress rostrally over time to involve the thoracic and cervical regions. Patients can have extraspinal involvement as well. Constitutional symptoms, peripheral arthritis, ocular disease, cardiovascular disease, and pulmonary complications can occur.

The primary goals of management are to optimize functional status and minimize pain and stiffness. Physical therapy and exercise are important for maintaining good functional status and joint mobility. Standard pharmacologic treatment includes nonsteroidal anti-inflammatory drugs (NSAID), analgesics, and muscle relaxants for symptomatic relief. Recent interest has focused on using disease-modifying antirheumatic drugs such as sulfasalazine, methotrexate, or corticosteroids. These agents can be helpful in selected patients with an active inflammatory component, manifested by acute pain and an elevated ESR. Unfortunately, none of these antirheumatic drugs have been shown to prevent disease progression.

Spinal fracture represents a frequent complication of ankylosing spondylitis. These fractures can occur after minor trauma, and often remain undiagnosed. Some of these cases can be managed nonoperatively with bracing, whereas others require surgical treatment. Surgery is also needed in a limited number of cases to correct severe spinal deformity, for example, the "chin-on-chest" deformity, or for management of progressive myelopathy.

Rheumatoid arthritis is another inflammatory disorder that often affects the spine. In contrast to ankylosing spondylitis, rheumatoid arthritis has a female preponderance and more significant polyarticular joint involvement. Patients typically present with pain and stiffness of multiple joints, fatigue, and low-grade fever. Extraarticular manifestations include ocular involvement, pericarditis, myocarditis, pleural effusions, and pulmonary nodules, which can be difficult to distinguish from malignancies. Neurologic involvement includes peripheral neuropathy, mononeuritis multiplex, and compression neuropathies, such as carpal tunnel syndrome. Patients may also develop cervical myelopathy from cord compression.

Many different spinal abnormalities are seen in patients with rheumatoid arthritis, including cervical spine instability with subluxation. Atlantoaxial subluxation is the most common spinal deformity seen in rheumatoid arthritis; however, subluxations can occur at any level of the cervical spine.

The overall management of rheumatoid arthritis involves a team approach, including internists, rheumatologists, neurologists, physiatrists, and orthopedic specialists. Social and psychological support is essential. The overall goals of therapy include pain relief and maintaining or improving functional capacity. These patients often have neck pain caused by rheumatoid involvement of the cervical spine. Conservative management with physical therapy, exercises, NSAID, and various types of cervical collars is usually helpful. Surgery may be required if the cervical spine is unstable or in cases of a significant neurologic deficit.

SPINAL TRAUMA

Spinal injury should be suspected in patients with severe systemic trauma, patients with minor trauma who report spinal pain or have sensory or motor symptoms, and patients with an impaired level of consciousness after trauma (Chiles and Cooper, 1996). Patients with acute spinal injury usually present to a hospital emergency department, but may also be seen at urgent care centers or other outpatient facilities. The cervical spine is the most mobile segment of the spinal column, and is the most common site of spinal cord injury. The thoracic spine from T-1 to T-10 has intrinsic stability because of the rib cage and is relatively immobile. Injuries to this region are uncommon. The thoracolumbar junction (T-11 to L-2), a transition zone between the rigid thoracic spine and the more mobile lumbar spine, is the second most common site of spinal fractures and dislocations. Fractures of the lower lumbar spine are less common.

Patients with acute spinal trauma report pain at the site of injury. The unconscious patient should be considered to have a cervical spine injury until proved otherwise with appropriate imaging studies. General physical examination may reveal bruising, tenderness, and muscle spasm at the site of injury. A detailed neurologic examination should include motor testing, sensory testing (light touch, pinprick, joint position sense) of the entire body including the perianal region, deep tendon reflexes, rectal tone, and bulbocavernosus reflex.

The neurologic assessment can reveal a wide spectrum of findings from a completely normal examination to a severe spinal cord injury. It is important to distinguish between complete and incomplete spinal cord injury. Patients with complete cord injuries rarely improve, whereas patients with incomplete spinal cord injuries can have substantial neurologic recovery.

Incomplete spinal cord injury syndromes can occur and should be carefully documented. The central cord syndrome is characterized by weakness that is more profound in the upper extremities than the lower extremities. Elderly patients are at particular risk for this syndrome, which typically occurs with acute hyperextension of the neck in patients with cervical spinal canal stenosis on a congenital or acquired basis. Brown-Sequard syndrome is a unilateral spinal cord injury, usually caused by penetrating trauma. These patients have loss of motor function and joint position sense ipsilateral to the injury, and loss of pain and temperature sensation contralateral to the injury.

Be aware that patients with acute spinal injury can have other severe injuries, including head injury that require rapid diagnosis and treatment.

The imaging assessment begins with plain radiographs of the symptomatic spinal segment. In the cervical region, the lateral radiograph is the most important view. The film must demonstrate the entire cervical spine, from the occipitocervical junction down to the top of T-1. If the lower cervical spine cannot be adequately seen, a Swimmer's view or CT scan should be obtained. A CT scan should also be obtained to further evaluate all positive findings seen on plain radiographs. Lateral radiographs of the cervical spine in flexion and extension should be considered if the stability of the spine is uncertain after plain films and CT have been obtained. Be in attendance while these views are obtained. The patient should be asked to move his or her neck without force or assistance from medical personnel. Flexion and extension views are contraindicated if the patient has a neurologic deficit or a subluxation seen on standard radiographs. MRI can demonstrate compression, edema, or hemorrhage of the spinal cord and traumatic disk herniations. The disadvantage of MRI is prolonged scanning times and the difficulty in imaging patients on advanced life support. These factors may preclude MRI in the unstable, multiple trauma patient.

The basic principles of management of acute spinal injury include immobilization, airway management, and cardiovascular resuscitation. Pharmacologic treatment is indicated for acute spinal cord injury. For patients seen within 3 hours of injury, high-dose methylprednisolone is administered intravenously, with an initial bolus of 30 mg/kg, followed by a continuous infusion of 5.4 mg/kg for 23 hours. For patients seen between 3 and 8 hours following injury, the methylprednisolone infusion is continued for 48 hours. For patients seen more than 8 hours following injury, methylprednisolone should not be given (Bracken et al., 1997).

Patients with acute, unstable fractures of the cervical spine should be placed in traction to immobilize the spine. Some spinal injuries can be managed nonoperatively with bracing, whereas others require surgery to decompress neural elements and to realign and stabilize the spinal column. An active rehabilitation program is needed for patients with spinal cord injury. The acute management of the injury should be carried out as expeditiously as possible, so that the patient can be mobilized and into rehabilitation as soon as possible. This is especially important in the elderly. Rapid mobilization will help minimize the complications of bedrest, including deep venous thrombophlebitis, skin breakdown, and pneumonia.

Steady progress has been made in the management of spinal cord injury, and the mortality rate has been significantly reduced. Despite these improvements, traumatic spinal cord injury remains a devastating condition that alters every aspect of the victim's life.

CONCLUSIONS

Many spinal disorders may be encountered in the older adult. Some affect the bony structures of the spinal column primarily. Examples include osteoporosis, metastatic cancer, and vertebral infection. Neurologic symptoms or signs can occur in cases of compression of the spinal cord, cauda equina, or spinal nerve roots caused by pathologic fracture of the vertebral body or extension of the disease process into the spinal canal itself. Degenerative spinal disorders, including spinal canal stenosis and disk herniations, are very common in the elderly. Inflammatory arthropathies, which are chronic illnesses that develop in young and middle-aged adults, present in more advanced forms in the elderly. Acute spinal injury is most common in young adult men, but can be seen at any age. A wide range of primary intradural tumors can occur in the elderly. Most are uncommon, and will be encountered rarely by the primary care physician. Prompt, accurate diagnosis of each of these disorders is essential. Treatment is individualized, based on the underlying disease process.

REFERENCES

Atlas SJ, Keller RB, Robson D, et al. Surgical and nonsurgical management of lumbar spinal stenosis: four-year outcomes from the Maine lumbar spine study. *Spine* 2000;25:556–562.

Boriani S, Weinstein JN. Differential diagnosis and surgical treatment of primary benign and malignant neoplasms. In: Frymoyer JW, ed. *The adult spine: principles and practice, 2nd ed. Philadelphia: Lippincott-Raven, 1997:951–987.*

Bracken MB, Shepard MJ, Holford TR, et al. Administration of methylprednisolone for 24 or 48 hours or tirilazad mesylate for 48 hours in the treatment of acute spinal cord injury. *JAMA* 1997;277:1597–1604.

Chiles BW, Cooper PR. Acute spinal injury. *N Engl J Med* 1996;334:514–520.

Connolly ES, Hamilton HB. Metabolic and other nondegenerative causes of low back pain. In Youmans JR, ed. *Neurological surgery, 4th ed. Philadelphia: WB Saunders, 1996:2354.*

Eastell R. *Treatment of postmenopausal osteoporosis.* N Engl J Med 1998;338:736–746.

Fischer G, Brotchi J. *Intramedullary spinal cord tumors.* New York: Thieme Medical Publishers, 1996:21–23.

Katz JN, Lipson SJ, Larson MG, et al. The outcome of decompressive laminectomy for degenerative lumbar stenosis. *J Bone Joint Surg (Am)* 1991;73:809–816.

SELECTED READINGS

Adams RA, Victor M, Ropper AH. *Principles of neurology*, 6th ed. New York, McGraw-Hill, 1997:194–223.

Hazzard WR, Blass JP, Ettinger WH, et al. *Principles of geriatric medicine and gerontology*, 4th ed. New York: McGraw-Hill, 1999:1174–1190.

Popp AJ, ed. *A guide to the primary care of neurological disorders.* Park Ridge, IL: American Association of Neurological Surgeons, 1998:101–120.

Wilkins RH, Rengachary SS. *Neurosurgery*, 2nd ed. New York: McGraw-Hill, 1996:3749–3892.

WEB SITES OF NATIONAL SUPPORT GROUPS AND OTHER RESOURCES

Arthritis Foundation: *www.arthritis.org*

National Osteoporosis Foundation: *www.nof.org*

National Spinal Cord Injury Association: *www.spinalcord. org*

National Scoliosis Foundation (*scoliosis@aol.com*)

NIH/National Institute of Arthritis and Musculoskeletal and Skin Diseases: *www.nih.gov/niams*

25

Peripheral Nervous System Disorders: Neuropathies, Myopathies, Motor Neuron and Neuromuscular Junction Disorders

Enrica Arnaudo and Jay D. Varrato

Peripheral nervous system disorders frequently encountered in the older adult include diseases that affect the anterior horn cells, peripheral nerves, neuromuscular junctions, and muscles. A careful history and physical examination are crucial in evaluating patients with neuromuscular disorders, keeping in mind that the boundaries of "normal findings" in the elderly can be different than in younger people. For instance, it is not unusual to detect mild vibratory sensory loss in the feet of a patient 70 years of age. Loss of ankle reflexes or mild distal muscular wasting in people above 60 is not pathologic *per se*, but can be caused by chronic spondylotic disc disease or multifactorial (e.g., related to arthritis, peripheral vascular, or skin disease). Normal aging is associated with some loss of large myelinated fibers, nerve demyelination and remyelination, and mild neurogenic changes in the distal limb muscles. Because of this, it can be challenging to distinguish what is old and what is new, such as recognizing the impact of a new muscle disease superimposed on a chronic neuropathy or polyradiculopathy.

EVALUATION OF THE PATIENT

Based on the patient's history and complaints, the physician can usually discern among the disorders affecting the motor, the sensory, or the autonomic nervous system. However, most commonly, these systems are affected in combination, which makes recognizing how and where symptoms began crucial for proper diagnosis and treatment.

Disorders of the motor system can affect motor neurons, motor axons, neuromuscular junctions, or muscles, causing weakness in all cases. Initial evaluation begins by asking the patient to describe how the weakness impairs him or her and what tasks the patient has difficulty performing. This allows the physician to predict which muscle groups are weak. Weakness can be generalized, with fatigue or fluctuation of severity, or it can be localized to certain muscle groups: shoulders, hands and forearms, hips and thighs, and distal leg muscles. Proximal weakness, with difficulty combing hair, getting up from a low chair, and climbing stairs is typically found in myopathic disorders. Weakness of distal muscles, leading to ankle sprains or foot or wrist drop, is commonly seen among patients with neuropathy. Chronically weak muscles usually show wasting, because of either a neurogenic or myopathic disorder. If spontaneous muscle twitching is seen, indicating lower motor neuron dysfunction, the process may be localized to the peripheral nerves, spinal roots, or the anterior horn cells. The presence or absence of sensory symptoms allows such distinctions: if present, think of radiculopathies or neuropathies; if absent, suspect a motor neuron disease (Figs. 25-1 and 25-2).

Fluctuation of weakness, including eyelid droopiness and double vision caused by extraocular muscle involvement, suggests a neuromuscular junction disorder, such as myasthenia gravis.

Pure sensory syndromes can affect the sensory nerves or ganglions. The type of sensory complaint helps distinguishing small-fiber and large-fiber neuropathies, whereas the distribution of symptoms helps localize a lesion to certain peripheral nerves or roots (Table 25-1).

If both sensory and motor symptoms are present in one, chronologically unified disease, the peripheral nerves are affected. Symptom onset and distribution help to distinguish among diffuse, symmetric, segmental, focal or multifocal nerve lesions that can be acute or chronic. This kind of information restricts the differential diagnosis to a small list of peripheral nerve system disorders, as indicated in Table 25-1 and Figures 25-1 and 25-2.

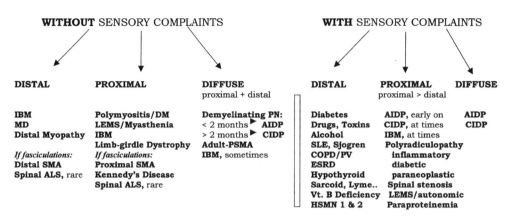

FIG. 25-1. Symmetric weakness. IBM, inclusion body myopathy; MD, myotonic dystrophy; SMA, spinal muscular atrophy; PSMA, progressive adult-SMA; AIDP/CIDP, acute or chronic inflammatory demyelinating polyradiculoneuropathy; PM/DM, polymyositis or dermatomyositis; LEMS, Lambert-Eaton myasthenic syndrome; PN, polyneuropathies; ALS, amyotrophic lateral sclerosis.

MOTOR NEURON DISEASES

Degenerative disorders of the motor neurons typically manifest with insidious, progressive muscle weakness, atrophy, and fasciculations. If only the lower motor neurons (LMN) are affected, the differential diagnosis includes:

1. *Adult-onset progressive spinal muscular atrophy* (PSMA), with symmetric weakness, wasting, and areflexia in a segmental distribution
2. *Monomelic amyotrophy*, with similar findings in a focal distribution (one arm or leg)
3. Spinal onset of *amyotrophic lateral sclerosis* (ALS), which can begin in a segmental or monomelic distribution

4. LMN degeneration caused by irradiation, electrocution, viral infection (e.g., poliomyelitis), toxic, or heavy-metal exposure
5. Paraneoplastic motor neuron disease (MND)

The most common of all of these disorders is ALS, a rapidly progressive fatal disorder. Patients with ALS display a peculiar combination of signs indicating concurrent lower and upper motor neuron dysfunction, typically spreading to all body muscles in a few months.

These patients show spasticity, and brisk and pathologic reflexes in the distribution of weak and wasted muscles, where reduced or absent reflexes would be expected to be found. Because of this, the clinical diagnosis of ALS is not a difficult one in ad-

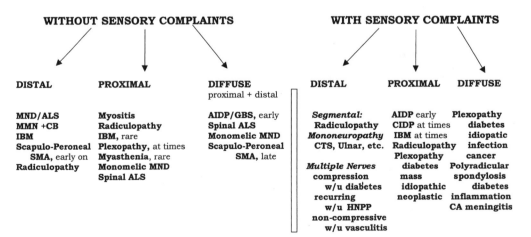

FIG. 25-2. Asymmetric weakness.

TABLE 25-1. *Sensory loss/complaints without weakness*

Symmetric	Asymmetric	Painful/autonomic	Sensory ataxia
Diabetes/metabolic/ vitamin B_{12} deficiency Drugs/toxins: Cis-platinum, megadose pyridoxine Cryptogenic sensory polyneuropathy (CSPN)	Inflammatory sensory polyganglionopathy Paraneoplastic sensory neuronopathy	Diabetes mellitus Tabes dorsalis (and ataxia) Amyloidosis Paraneoplastic neuropathy (and ataxia) Acute pandysautonomia Hereditary sensory and autonomic neuropathy	Vitamin B_{12} deficiency MAG-associated neuropathy Megadose pyridoxine/ Cis-platinum toxicity Inflammatory sensory polyganglionopathy Herpes zoster Friedreich and other spinocerebellar ataxias

MAG, myelin-associated glycoprotein.

vanced cases, but it remains a delicate and frustrating experience for the clinician, because no specific diagnostic test or cure is available.

Amyotrophic lateral sclerosis is a sporadic disorder 90% of the times, with a uniform worldwide incidence of 1/100,000 general population, more common in the sixth to seventh decade and slightly more frequent in men. Prognosis is grim in all cases, but worse in the older individuals: the older the age of onset, the poorer the prognosis. Initially, patients complain of painless, patchy weakness in a distal arm or leg, neck extensor weakness, and nocturnal cramps. They can present with hand clumsiness, and "dissociated wasting" is seen of the medial versus lateral hand muscles. Early bulbar symptoms such as dysarthria, difficulty swallowing, choking, weight loss, dyspnea on exertion, and shortness of breath at rest are bad prognostic signs. Slightly better prognosis is associated with younger age of onset, a long interval from onset to diagnosis, spinal onset, predominant upper motor neuron (UMN) or LMN involvement, absent or slowly progressive pulmonary impairment, fewer fasciculations, milder muscle involvement at diagnosis, and a psychological sense of well-being.

In older patients, cervical or lumbar stenosis and polyradiculopathy is initially suspected, unless the tongue or bulbar muscles are affected early. Cervical and lumbar magnetic resonance imaging (MRI) are obtained to rule out chronic spondylotic myelopathy, syringomyelia, or syringobulbia. Brain MRI is obtained to look for unusual compressive lesions (e.g., a meningioma of the foramen magnus) or prominent white matter disease.

The patient in whom ALS is suspected must have a thorough electrophysiologic evaluation with nerve conduction (NCV) and electromyography (EMG), because these modalities are the gold standard of diagnosis. Nerve conduction testing is necessary to assure that sensory fibers are spared and no demyelinating

features are in the motor potentials (e.g., partial motor conduction block), which may steer the diagnosis to a treatable condition (i.e., multifocal motor neuropathy). EMG is necessary to look for subclinical evidence of acute and chronic denervation in muscles of different nerves and roots. If at least two muscles of different nerves and roots in three of the four body regions (i.e., cervical, lumbar, thoracic and bulbar) are affected, no single anatomic location can account for such widespread motor neuron degeneration, leaving motor neuron disease the only possible diagnosis.

With the development of research treatment protocols, it became important to have guidelines for the early diagnosis of ALS. In 1990, the World Federation of Neurology generated a consensus document on clinical, electrophysiologic, neuroimaging, and neuropathologic features of ALS. These features are subdivided into those that are *required, supportive, compatible with,* or *rule out* the diagnosis of ALS (Table 25-2). Rarely, treatable conditions can cause or mimic a motor neuronopa-

TABLE 25-2. *World Federation of Neurology El Escorial criterial for the diagnosis of ALS*

Required
1. Lower motor neuron signs in one or more of four regions: *bulbar, cervical, thoracic, and lumbosacral*
2. Upper motor neuron signs in one or more of these four regions
   and
3. Progression of signs within a region, and involving other regions

Inconsistent with diagnosis of ALS
1. Sensory and/or autonomic dysfunction
2. Sphincter abnormalities
3. Anterior visual pathway abnormalities
4. Movement abnormalities seen in Parkinson's disease
5. Cognitive abnormalities seen in Alzheimer's disease

ALS, amyotropic lateral sclerosis.
Adapted from World Federation of Neurology (320).

thy, including hyper- or hypothyroidism, autoimmune or paraneoplastic diseases, paraproteinemia, and heavy-metal intoxication with lead or mercury.

The workup for ALS should include blood testing and cerebrospinal fluid analysis (Fig. 25-3), but it can extend to a muscle and nerve biopsy, paraneoplastic screening with chest and abdomen computer tomography scans, or an extensive search for rare deficiencies, such as hexosaminidase A. This costly workup is appropriate in cases with predominant-LMN signs and a prolonged clinical course, or in cases of a positive family history, occupational history, or unusual associated symptoms. However, ALS cases with clear upper and lower motor neuron dysfunction fully confirmed by EMG do not typically require such an extensive and low-yield evaluation.

Effective treatment for ALS is still lacking. Riluzole is the only US Food and Drug Administration-approved drug shown to prolong the time to tracheostomy by 2 to 3 months. The management of patients with ALS requires a competent multidisciplinary team providing medical interventions to treat weakness, fatigue, spasticity, pain, depression, and respiratory failure aggressively, and psychological counseling for the patient and family.

PERIPHERAL NEUROPATHIES

Neuropathy in adults is relatively common in the United States, with an annual incidence of 40/100,000. Diagnosing neuropathy is not difficult, but identifying the underlying pathophysiology and

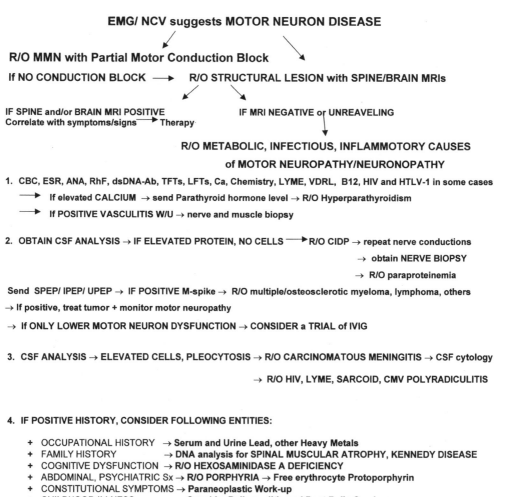

EMG/ NCV suggests MOTOR NEURON DISEASE

R/O MMN with Partial Motor Conduction Block

If NO CONDUCTION BLOCK ⟶ **R/O STRUCTURAL LESION with SPINE/BRAIN MRIs**

IF SPINE and/or BRAIN MRI POSITIVE
Correlate with symptoms/signs ⟶ Therapy

IF MRI NEGATIVE or UNREAVELING

**R/O METABOLIC, INFECTIOUS, INFLAMMOTORY CAUSES
of MOTOR NEUROPATHY/NEURONOPATHY**

1. CBC, ESR, ANA, RhF, dsDNA-Ab, TFTs, LFTs, Ca, Chemistry, LYME, VDRL, B12, HIV and HTLV-1 in some cases
    ⟶ If elevated CALCIUM → send Parathyroid hormone level → R/O Hyperparathyroidism
    ⟶ If POSITIVE VASCULITIS W/U → nerve and muscle biopsy

2. OBTAIN CSF ANALYSIS → IF ELEVATED PROTEIN, NO CELLS ⟶ R/O CIDP → repeat nerve conductions
    → obtain NERVE BIOPSY
    → R/O paraproteinemia

    Send SPEP/ IPEP/ UPEP → IF POSITIVE M-spike → R/O multiple/osteosclerotic myeloma, lymphoma, others
    → If positive, treat tumor + monitor motor neuropathy

    → If ONLY LOWER MOTOR NEURON DYSFUNCTION → CONSIDER a TRIAL of IVIG

3. CSF ANALYSIS → ELEVATED CELLS, PLEOCYTOSIS → R/O CARCINOMATOUS MENINGITIS → CSF cytology
    → R/O HIV, LYME, SARCOID, CMV POLYRADICULITIS

4. IF POSITIVE HISTORY, CONSIDER FOLLOWING ENTITIES:

    + OCCUPATIONAL HISTORY → **Serum and Urine Lead, other Heavy Metals**
    + FAMILY HISTORY   → **DNA analysis for SPINAL MUSCULAR ATROPHY, KENNEDY DISEASE**
    + COGNITIVE DYSFUNCTION → **R/O HEXOSAMINIDASE A DEFICIENCY**
    + ABDOMINAL, PSYCHIATRIC Sx → **R/O PORPHYRIA → Free erythrocyte Protoporphyrin**
    + CONSTITUTIONAL SYMPTOMS → **Paraneoplastic Work-up**
    + CHILDHOOD ILLNESS   → **Consider Poliomyelitis and Post-Polio Syndrome**
    + HISTORY of Radiation Therapy → **Post-XRT MOTOR NEURONOPATHY, myokymia**

FIG. 25-3. Workup for suspected amyotrophic lateral sclerosis.

TABLE 25-3. *Diseases associated with neuropathy*

Diabetes mellitus	Chronic liver disease
Chronic renal insufficiency	Herpes zoster
Carcinoma	Leprosy
Plasma cell dyscrasias	Diphtheria
Multiple myeloma	Vitamin deficiency:
Waldenström macroglobulinemia	Thiamine (B_1) deficiency
Other monoclonal gammopathies	Riboflavin (B_2) deficiency
Primary nonfamilial amyloidosis	Pyridoxine (B_6) deficiency
Osteosclerotic myeloma	Pernicious anemia (B_{12} deficiency)
Rheumatoid arthritis	Malnutrition
Sjögren syndrome	Postgastrectomy state
Scleroderma	Tropical (nutritional) ataxia
Systemic lupus erythematosus	Chronic obstructive pulmonary disease
Cranial arteritis	Polycythemia vera
Hypothyroidism	Gout
Polyarteritis nodosa	Lymphoma
Cryoglobulinemia	Sarcoidosis

cause is challenging. Peripheral neuropathies result from a large number of conditions, including systemic metabolic derangements, endocrine and inflammatory disorders, failure of organs such as liver and kidney, toxin or drug exposure, and direct or remote effects of cancer (Table 25-3). Because of this, physicians usually engage in an extensive blood screening of possible causes of neuropathy. Indeed, it is unlikely for the neuropathy to be the presenting manifestation of an unrecognized metabolic disorder. Diabetes occasionally presents with a lumbosacral radiculoplexopathy (diabetic amyotrophy or Bruns-Garland syndrome). Some disorders such as vasculitis can cause a neuropathy concurrently with other organ involvement, and recognizing the real sequence of events and cause has obvious and profound treatment implications.

Clinicians use the electrodiagnostic (EDX) testing with NCV and EMG as an extension of the neurologic examination to confirm the diagnosis, localize the abnormalities, focus the differential diagnosis, and, most importantly, distinguish primary axonal from primary demyelinating lesions. Demyelination can have a *uniform* pattern of involvement, as in hereditary neuropathies (e.g., Charcot-Marie-Tooth disease type-Ia) or a *multifocal* pattern as in acquired demyelinating polyneuropathies, which are more common in the elderly.

The identification of acquired demyelinating polyneuropathies is important because they are treatable conditions and frequently associated with an underlying systemic illness. These neuropathies include the acute Guillain-Barré syndrome (GBS) and chronic inflammatory demyelinating polyneuropathy (CIDP). They both present with progressive weakness, areflexia, decreased sensation, and ele-

vated cerebrospinal fluid protein. They differ in the timing of symptom onset, which is rapid: less than 6 weeks in GBS and more than 2 months in CIDP. The disease course is also different, usually monophasic and self-limited in GBS and progressive or relapsing in CIDP.

GUILLAIN-BARRÉ SYNDROME

Guillain-Barré syndrome is probably the most common acute paralytic disease in the Western countries, with a uniform annual incidence of 1–2/100,000 cases in the general populations. It occurs at all ages, although it is more common in the young adult and the elderly, with a mean age of presentation approximately 40 years, and a slight male preponderance. Two thirds of patients report a preceding viral illness, usually upper respiratory infection or gastroenteritis.

Guillain-Barré syndrome is a dynamic disease with a variable rate of progression and inconsistent involvement of the peripheral nervous system (i.e., proximal vs distal involvement) from one patient to the next, particularly during the first several weeks (Table 25-4). Most patients follow a "typical" GBS pattern, with initial sensory complaints of tingling paresthesias in the hands and feet, often associated with back pain or burning dysesthesias, followed by leg weakness that rapidly ascends to the arms. In about 10% of cases, weakness begins in the arms. Cranial nerve involvement is seen in 45% to 75% of patients, affecting mainly facial and extraocular muscles. More than 50% of patients reach the nadir of their symptoms by 2 weeks, 80% by 3 weeks, and 90% by 4 weeks. It is extremely unusual for symptoms to worsen after 1 month. Respiratory failure

TABLE 25-4. *Variants of Guillain-Barré syndrome*

Miller Fisher Syndrome
  Ophthalmoplegia, ataxia, areflexia
Areflexic paraparesis with back pain
  May resemble a cord lesion
Pharyngeal-cervical-brachial weakness
  May resemble botulism
Ptosis without ophthalmoplegia
Facial diplegia with paresthesias
Sixth nerve palsies with paresthesias
Axonal
  Rapidly progressive weakness
  Prolonged paralysis and respiratory failure
  Associated with *Campylobacter jejuni*
  Usually predominantly motor symptoms

TABLE 25-5. *Differential diagnosis in Guillain-Barré syndrome*

Spinal cord compression, infarction
Brainstem (pontine) infarction
Acute myelopathy, skull base lesions
Polymyositis
Defects of neuromuscular junction
Myasthenia gravis, LEMS, botulism
Tick paralysis
Acute intermittent porphyria
Diphtheria
Hypokalemic periodic paralysis
Hypophosphatemia and hypermagnesemia
Critical illness polyneuropathy
Paraneoplastic acute polyneuropathy
Meningoradiculitis of:
  Lyme disease
  Epstein-Barr virus
  Hepatitis
  Human immunodeficiency virus disease
  Carcinomatous meningitis
  Sarcoidosis

LEMS, Lambert-Eaton myasthenic syndrome.

occurs in 30% of patients, usually because of diaphragmatic and respiratory muscle weakness, bulbar weakness, and aspiration of secretions. Autonomic dysfunction occurs in two thirds of patients, causing unpredictable episodes of hypertension or hypotension, and sudden potentially fatal cardiac arrhythmia

Several conditions present with GBS-like features and need to be differentiated using a thorough history, physical examination, and appropriate investigations (Table 25-5).

In the first week of disease, nerve conduction studies may show only minimal changes, such as low-amplitude motor potentials and prolonged motor latencies and F waves, which indicate a predilection for nerve roots and terminals. After the first week, 90% of GBS cases show increased spinal fluid protein without concomitant pleocytosis, called "albuminocytologic dissociation." Antibodies to various gangliosides (GM1, GM1b, GD1b, and others) have been documented in several series of patients with GBS. A number of these patients have evidence of *Campylobacter jejuni* infection, a bacterium with GM1-like oligosaccharides on the surface that may cross-react with GM1, explaining why an antibody directed against bacteria can also produce a neuropathy. Some antibodies appear to be specific for certain syndrome. For instance, the Miller-Fisher syndrome is a well-recognized variant of GBS, consisting of ophthalmoplegia, ataxia, and areflexia and associated with GQ1b antibodies in 95% of cases.

The outcome for patients with GBS is generally good, with virtually full recovery in most cases. However, the older the patient and the more preexisting medical conditions, the greater the risk of death or severe sequelae. Mortality rates are less than 5% in the modern intensive care units. Plasma exchange is the treatment of choice for patients with GBS, but high-dose intravenous immunoglobulins (IVIG) can be used as an alternative or adjunct therapy, if plasma exchange is not available. Most authorities use 2 g/kg IVIG infusion over 4 or 5 days, monitoring for improvement in the following 2 weeks.

CHRONIC INFLAMMATORY DEMYELINATING POLYNEUROPATHY

The most common form of treatable neuropathy encountered by the physician is CIDP, although no population-based incidence study has been performed and, therefore, no clear estimate is known of its frequency. In tertiary care centers, it can represent up to 30% of previously undiagnosed cases of neuropathy. Diagnostic criteria for this condition have been established (Table 25-6), but not all cases fulfill these criteria and the condition is often misdiagnosed.

Although CIDP can occur at any age, it is more common in the adult population, with a peak incidence in those 50 to 60 years of age. It is often associated with an underlying systemic illness, including plasma-cell dyscrasia, lymphoma, Waldenström's macroglobulinemia, gamma heavy-chain disease, cryoglobulinemia, systemic lupus erythematous, Castleman's disease, an occult malignancy, and human immunodeficiency virus (HIV) infection. Recognition of CIDP is important for therapy and for treatment of possible

TABLE 25-6. *Diagnostic criteria for CIDP*

Mandatory clinical features
    Progression of muscle weakness in proximal and distal muscles of upper and lower extremities for 2 months
    Areflexia or hyporeflexia
Major laboratory features
    Electrophysiologic studies (three of four required):
        Reduction of nerve conduction velocity in two or more motor nerves
        Partial conduction block or temporal dispersion in one or more motor nerves
        Prolonged distal latencies in two or more nerves
        Absent or prolonged F wave latencies in at least two motor nerves
    CSF studies:
        CSF protein >45 mg/dL
        Cell count <10/mm
    Nerve biopsy features:
        Segmental demyelination, remyelination (onion-bulbs) and inflammation
Mandatory exclusion criteria (patients must be devoid of these features)
    Clinical features, including pure sensory neuropathy, mutilation of hands or feet, retinitis pigmentosa,
        ichthyosis, orange tonsils, exposure to drugs or toxins causing peripheral neuropathy
    Laboratory findings of low cholesterol, abnormal porphyrins, CSF white blood cell >50, low vitamin B_{12},
        hypothyroidism, high fasting glucose, heavy metal intoxication
    Nerve biopsy specimen with vasculitis, neurofilamentous swollen axons, intramyelinic blebs, amyloid
        deposits, Schwann cells with storage material as in Fabry's disease, adrenal leukodystrophy,
        metachromatic leukodystrophy, globoid cell leukodystrophy, or Refsum disease
    Electrodiagnostic features of neuromuscular transmission defect, myopathy, or anterior horn cell disease

CIDP, chronic inflammatory demyelinating polyneuropathy; CSF, cerebrospinal fluid.

concurrent illnesses. CIDP characteristically presents with slowly progressive weakness and sensory loss. Weakness must be progressive for at least 2 months, a feature that distinguishes CIDP from GBS, and it is commonly symmetric, involving proximal and distal muscles of the upper and lower extremities. Facial and neck flexor muscle weakness can occur. Deep tendon reflexes are usually absent or depressed. Sensory complaints of numbness, tingling, loss of balance, and even painful paresthesias are not uncommon, but can also be absent or undetected, making it difficult at times to differentiate CIDP from motor neuron disease. Table 25-7 summarizes the major differences between the two diseases.

TABLE 25-7. *Differences between CIDP and ALS*

	CIDP	ALS
Anatomy	Sensory-motor myelinopathy	Motor neuronopathy
Age of onset	All ages 40–60	50–60
Sex	M > F = 1.5:1	M > F = 2:1
Weakness	Symmetric	Asymmetric
Distribution	Sensory and motor nerves	Myotomes
	Onset proximal > distal	Onset distal > proximal
	Lower > upper limbs	Including bulbar, respiratory
Progression	Insidious	Rapid, fatal 3–5 years
Fasciculations	Some	Many
Muscle cramps	Uncommon	Very common
Reflexes	Reduced	Pathologically brisk
Stiffness, spasticity	No	Yes
Facial weakness	Yes	Late, asymmetric
Pseudobulbar affect	No	Yes
Prognosis	Relapses, may remit	Invariably fatal
CSF protein	Increased	Normal
Nerve conductions	Abnormal	Normal
	Motor and sensory	Late low amplitude
Needle EMG	Symmetric Fib/PSW	Widespread Fib/PSW
Effective treatment	Yes	No

ALS, amyotrophic lateral sclerosis; CIDP, chronic inflammatory demyelinating polyneuropathy; CSF, cerebrospinal fluid; EMG, electromyograph; Fib/PSW, fibrillations/positive sharp waves.

Rarely, patients with CIDP persistently show focal or markedly asymmetric sensorimotor deficits, mimicking a mononeuritis multiplex. In such cases, a sural nerve biopsy may be needed to confirm that the neuropathy is indeed a multifocal *demyelinating* neuropathy. Nerve biopsy specimens of CIDP demonstrate segmental demyelination or remyelination and inflammation.

Cerebrospinal fluid analysis of patients with CIDP shows albuminocytologic dissociation in 90% of cases. Nerve conduction testing shows slow conduction velocities, prolonged motor latencies and F-waves, partial motor conduction block, or temporal dispersion of the motor potentials. However, only 70% of patients ever meet the strict EDX demyelinating criteria. In the other cases, a sural nerve biopsy can help to exclude processes as amyloidosis or vasculitis. Although no need is seen to obtain a spine MRI in most cases, gadolinium-enhanced MRI of the lumbosacral spine may show root enhancement in both acute and chronic inflammatory demyelinating neuropathy.

All patients suspected of having CIDP should be checked for serum paraproteinemia. If an IgM paraprotein is found, search for malignancy such as lymphoma and osteosclerotic myeloma. In addition, antibody against myelin-associated glycoprotein should be sent, because patients with CIDP with anti-myelin-associated glycoprotein antibodies are usually more refractory to treatment.

Neuropathies associated with osteosclerotic myeloma are usually motor neuropathies, and could be mistaken for the progressive muscular atrophy form of ALS. Skeletal bone survey reveals a small number of bony abnormalities, either sclerotic or mixed with lytic lesions. Some patients develop one or more of other manifestations, such as organomegaly, endocrinopathy, hypertrichosis, digital clubbing and gynecomastia, as part of the POEMS syndrome (i.e., polyneuropathy, organomegaly, endocrinopahty, monoclonal gammopathy, and skin changes). In such cases, radiotherapy or the surgical excision of a solitary bony lesion may lead to substantial improvement.

Chronic inflammatory demyelinating polyneuropathy can be difficult to diagnose in the setting of diabetes mellitus, because even asymptomatic patients with diabetes can demonstrate nerve conduction slowing. However, patients with diabetes complain more commonly of distal sensory loss and dysesthesias, which predominate symmetrically in the distal lower extremities. Later, they may develop distal leg weakness, in contrast with the early proximal weakness seen in patients with CIDP.

Treatment options for patients with CIDP include steroids, plasma exchange, and IVIG. Prednisone can be initiated at a high dose (100 mg/d). Once improvement begins, usually within 2 to 4 weeks, it can be switched to alternate day therapy. When strength has returned to normal or reached a plateau, prednisone is slowly tapered by 5 mg every 2 to 3 weeks. Plasma exchange was shown to be more effective than "sham" pheresis for CIDP in two important studies, and is typically used in patients who are severely weak or relapse on prednisone. IVIG has been shown to be as effective as plasma exchange at the dose of 2 g/kg over 5 days, with monthly maintenance doses of 0.4 or 1 g/kg. IgA-deficiency must be excluded before initiating IVIG therapy, and caution should be used in giving IVIG to elderly patients with borderline renal dysfunction or cardiac dysfunction. Cyclosporin and cyclophosphamide are used as a third-line oral therapy in difficult cases.

MULTIFOCAL MOTOR NEUROPATHY

Multifocal motor neuropathy (MMN) is an acquired demyelinating neuropathy with clinical and electrophysiologic manifestations similar but distinct from CIDP. The disorder is also more prevalent in men, with a male-to-female ratio of 3:1, mean age of onset in the fifth decade, and disease duration from several months up to 30 years (average, 7.5 years). It typically presents with progressive, asymmetric, predominantly distal weakness, causing wrist drop, foot drop, and grip weakness over several years. Most patients retain useful function and continue working for a long time. Muscle weakness is located in the distribution of peripheral nerves without sensory involvement of those nerves. Cramps and fasciculations are common, sensory symptoms are absent or minimal, and the sensory examination is normal. Weakness is often more pronounced than the degree of atrophy would suggest, so that marked weakness is frequently detected in muscles where the bulk is preserved. Tendon reflexes are asymmetrically reduced in the affected limbs and at times also in the asymptomatic limbs.

The diagnosis of MMN relies on detecting demyelination outside the usual sites of nerve entrapment in a well-localized short nerve segment showing persistent reproducible motor conduction block.

In the absence of careful electrodiagnostic studies, this disorder is often misdiagnosed as progressive muscular atrophy. Difficulty can arise in those cases where the patient has a pure lower motor neuron syndrome, but no obvious demyelinating physiology. In such cases, careful follow-up at 3- to 6-month intervals will show the disorder either evolving into ALS with diffuse widespread denervation and pyramidal signs, or not changing significantly over months, as in MMN. High titers of GM1-antibodies are reported in 22% to 84% of patients with MMN.

Treatment consists of high-dose IVIG (2 g/kg over 2–5 days) and is effective in 90% of patients, so much so that a lack of response to the first IVIG course should make the clinician question the diagnosis. Beneficial effects begin within days, sometimes hours, after the infusion and last for several weeks to months. Most patients require periodic maintenance doses of IVIG.

NEUROMUSCULAR JUNCTION DISORDERS

Neuromuscular junction disorders can be presynaptic, as in Lambert-Eaton myasthenic syndrome (LEMS), or postsynaptic, as in myasthenia gravis (MG). Table 25-8 summarizes the differences and similarities between myasthenia gravis and ALS.

Lambert-Eaton Myasthenic Syndrome

Lambert-Eaton myasthenic syndrome is a neuromuscular junction disorder of mid to late life, slightly more frequent in men, and associated with small cell lung carcinoma (SCLC) in approximately 60% of patients. The underlying defect is a reduction in the release of the neurotransmitter acetylcholine (Ach)

TABLE 25-8. *Differences between myasthenia gravis and ALS*

Characteristic	Myasthenia	ALS
"Elderly men" 6th–7th decade	Yes	Yes
Bulbar symptoms (dysarthria, dysphagia, dyspnea)	Yes	Yes
Neck extensor weakness	Yes	Yes
Double vision, ptosis	Yes	No
Facial weakness	Yes	
Late, asymmetric		
Early proximal weakness	Yes	No
Early distal weakness	No	Yes
Fluctuating course	Yes	No
Muscle cramps	No	Yes
Muscle ache	Yes	No
Stiffness, spasticity	No	Yes
Sensory loss	No	No
Brisk reflexes, Babinski	No	Yes
Cognitive dysfunction	No	No
Pseudobulbar affect	No	Yes
Effective treatment	Yes	No

ALS, amyotrophic lateral sclerosis.

from the presynaptic nerve terminal at the neuromuscular junction. Autoantibodies directed against voltage-gated calcium channels in the nerve terminals are found in up to 75% of patients with LEMS and lung cancer, less than 50% of LEMS with no cancer, and up to 25% of LEMS with cancer other than lung. The voltage-gated calcium channel antibody titer does not correlate with disease severity. Usually, LEMS precedes the identification of lung cancer. In most patients, the cancer is discovered in 2 years and in all patients after 4 years.

Lambert-Eaton myasthenic syndrome is characterized by insidious proximal muscle weakness, affecting mainly thighs and hips. The weak muscle may be sore and tender. Ptosis and diplopia are seen in 25% of patients, and respiratory muscle weakness is detected by spirometry in most patients with LEMS. Muscle stretch reflexes are reduced or absent, but can be brought out by a brief contraction. Strength facilitation is seen in half the patients with LEMS. Autonomic dysfunction is common, and most patients have dry mouth, postural hypotension, or impotence.

Most patients with LEMS are either undiagnosed or misdiagnosed with myopathy, neuropathy, or myasthenia. EDX evaluation is crucial to make the correct diagnosis. It shows low motor amplitudes, often less than 10% of normal, which fall further with repetitive nerve stimulation (RNS) at frequencies between 1 and 5 Hz. With RNS frequencies at 20 to 50 Hz, the motor amplitude increases and becomes at least twice the size of the initial response. Similar increase immediately after brief maximal muscle contraction is also diagnostic. Treatment of LEMS is described in Table 25-9.

Autoimmune Myasthenia Gravis

Myasthenia gravis one of the best-characterized immunopathologically mediated disorders of humans. A total prevalence of the disease is 50 to 125 cases per million, an annual incidence of 1/300,000 general population, and a bimodal pattern of onset. In the second and third decade, myasthenia gravis most often affects women, but after the sixth decade the incidence increases in both sexes with a slight male predominance. Autoimmune MG is rarely a familial disorder. Characteristic of the disease is fluctuating, fatigable weakness of striated muscles, varying according to the involvement of specific muscle groups. Initially, patients may have symptoms only late in the day or after exertion.

Presenting symptoms are ocular in 50% of cases: fluctuating eyelid droopiness and binocular double vision occur typically toward the end of the day or af-

TABLE 25-9. *Treatment of LEMS*

Cancer therapy, if associated with a tumor
Mestinon 30–60 mg every 4–6 h
Guanidine hydrochloride 5–10 mg/kg/d (maximum 30 mg/kg/d)
    It inhibits uptake of calcium by subcellular organisms, increasing acetylcholine (Ach) release. Pyridostigmine enhances response to guanidine
3,4 Diaminopyridine 5–25 mg p.o. t.i.d. or q.i.d.
    It facilitates Ach-release from the motor nerve terminals, improving strength and autonomic function in most patients with LEMS
    The therapeutic effects are augmented by concurrent pyridostigmine.
Prednisone 60–80 mg/d until improvement, then change to 100–120 mg every other day, then taper over months to the smallest dose that maintains improvement.
Azathioprine 50 mg/d, then increase by 50 mg every week to a total of 150–200 mg/d.
    Follow CBC, LFT once a week the first month, then once a month for 6 months.
Cyclosporine, if patient did not respond or cannot take azathioprine.
    The dose is 5–6 mg/kg/d, divided in two doses every 12 h.
    Follow cyclosporine level, BUN/creatinine.
Plasma exchange or *IVIG* for temporary improvement of severe weakness

BUN, blood urea nitrogen; CBC, complete blood count; IVIG, intravenous immunoglobulin; LEMS, Lambert-Eaton myasthenic syndrome; LFT, liver function tests; p.o., by mouth; q.i.d., four times daily; t.i.d., three times daily.

ter extensive reading, driving, or working at the computer. Initial symptoms or exacerbations can occur during a systemic illness (i.e., hypo- or hyperthyroid dysfunction), a viral upper respiratory infection, or after a surgical intervention. Factors that can aggravate myasthenia gravis weakness are emotional stress, excessive heat, pregnancy, and certain medications. About 65% of patients with ocular MG develop generalized weakness with involvement of limb or bulbar muscles within the first year after diagnosis. Once the diagnosis of myasthenia gravis is confirmed, patients with ocular signs should be watched closely during the first 3 years for evidence of generalized weakness. Some degree of facial weakness is present in 95% of patients. Neck flexor muscle involvement is common and, in general, upper extremity muscles are weaker than leg muscles. Deltoid and wrist or finger extensor muscles are most commonly involved, and the triceps is more likely to be weaker than the biceps. Dysarthria, weak mastication, dysphagia associated with poor gag reflex and palate elevation, and tongue weakness can result in aspiration

pneumonia. Pneumonia with respiratory failure, usually caused by diaphragmatic and intercostal muscle weakness, can be life threatening, and is an indication for a rapidly acting therapeutic intervention, such as plasma-exchange. Respiratory distress can occur precipitously in a patient with myasthenia gravis with recent worsening of symptoms, especially if oropharyngeal muscles are involved, and respiratory support may be required. In elderly patients with predominant bulbar involvement, motor neuron disease may be suspected at first.

Autoantibodies directed against the Ach-receptors (AchR), which are responsible for the muscle weakness in myasthenia gravis, are specific for the diagnosis of the disease. Approximately 90% of patients with generalized acquired disease have detectable antibodies to AchR (AchR-Ab) in their serum. Among the patients with ocular myasthenia gravis, the incidence of detectable AchR-Ab is about 50%.

In a patient with suspected myasthenia but negative AchR-Ab, the diagnostic workup should include other studies, such as the Tensilon test, ice and sleep test, repetitive nerve stimulation test, and EMG, as described in the diagnostic algorithm of Figure 25-4.

Specifically, the Tensilon test consists of an intravenous injection of the short-acting cholinesterase-inhibitor edrophonium (Tensilon). This helps diagnose myasthenia gravis in patients with ptosis and ophthalmoplegia, because it causes improvement of the ocular weakness within 10 seconds from the injection, reaching its maximum in about 5 minutes and then declining. The prompt improvement of muscle function with this test differentiates myasthenia gravis from a myopathy, Lambert-Eaton myasthenic syndrome, neurosis, and cranial nerve palsy. The Tensilon test has a reported diagnostic sensitivity of 86% in ocular MG, and 95% in systemic MG. The best results are obtained in the patients with clearly weak muscles in which improvement can be easily identified (e.g., eyelid ptosis). Side effects including bradycardia, hypotension, and cardiac arrest, occur rarely. False-positive results have been observed in a variety of conditions, including tumors, multiple sclerosis, and diabetic third nerve palsy.

A frozen ice pack applied to a closed ptotic lid for 2 minutes is also reported to show improvement of 2 mm or greater ptosis in 80% of patients with myasthenia gravis and in none of the patients without MG, yielding a sensitivity of 80% and a specificity of 100% for this test. The sleep test is based on the fatigable nature of myasthenia gravis and the patient is evaluated before and after 30 minutes of rest with

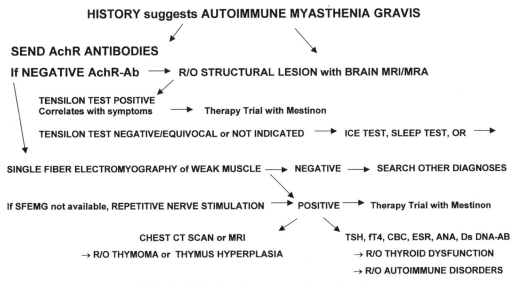

FIG. 25-4. Workup for suspected myasthenia.

eyes closed. The repetitive nerve stimulation test and single-fiber electromyography are the most useful electrophysiologic tests for the diagnosis of myasthenia gravis. RNS shows a higher sensitivity in generalized MG (60% to 85%) than in ocular MG (18% to 35%); however, false-positive responses to RNS are encountered in a variety of other conditions. The single-fiber is positive in up to 90% to 100% of patients with generalized MG and 80% to 88% of patients with ocular MG. Performing the single-fiber EMG on the orbicularis oculi or frontalis muscle can increase the test sensitivity. False-positive single-fiber EMG results are observed in several other neuromuscular diseases, such as ocular myopathies, ALS, and nerve injuries. Chronic progressive external ophthalmoplegia is a syndrome consisting of ptosis, symmetric progressive ophthalmoplegia, and mild proximal limb weakness, caused by a deletion in the mitochondrial DNA. Single-fiber EMG may be positive in chronic progressive external ophthalmoplegia, but a good clinical history and physical examination will differentiate this syndrome, usually without diplopia, from myasthenia gravis.

Once the diagnosis of myasthenia gravis is made, it is necessary to exclude the presence of a thymoma or thymus hyperplasia, commonly associated with MG. The relationship between the thymus and the pathogenesis of myasthenia gravis is not precisely understood. However, more than 50% of patients having a thymectomy have sustained improvement of muscle weakness.

No reliable relationship exists between any of the laboratory tests and response to therapy, and consensus is found among the experts in the field on which therapeutic approach is best. The clinical course is to choose the appropriate treatment plan, as described in Table 25-10.

TABLE 25-10. *Therapeutic options in myasthenia gravis (MG)*

Cholinesterase inhibitors (pyridostigmine [Mestinon]) provide symptomatic improvement for most patients with MG for a period of time. These drugs impede the hydrolysis of acetylcholine at the neuromuscular junction.

Thymectomy is indicated in selected patients <60 years of age with generalized weakness and for all patients with thymoma.

Immunosuppressant drugs, such as *azathioprine*, are indicated in older adult patients with no cancer, and are avoided in reproductive young women. They may take months to show effect, and need initial white blood cell count monitoring to rule out neutropenia.

Prednisone 1 mg/kg up until sustained improvement is demonstrated, then slowly taper over months. Therapy of choice in ocular MG without contraindications for steroids.

Plasma exchange is useful in case of exacerbation, in preparation for surgery; it usually provides rapid improvement of weakness.

Intravenous immunoglobulins (IVIG) can also provide rapid improvement. They are not indicated in the patients with IgA deficiency, renal disease, cardiac failure or important stroke risk factors.

In the patients with myasthenia gravis onset after 60 years of age, the treatment mainly relies on medical therapy. Thymectomy is generally not performed unless a thymoma is present. Azathioprine is the treatment of choice in older people, because steroid-related side effects are more frequent than those related to azathioprine. Combination therapy with prednisone and azathioprine is more effective than prednisone alone, and may be the only choice if the patient has congestive heart failure or renal insufficiency, and cannot receive plasma exchange and IVIG. The prognosis of myasthenia gravis in older people seems to be favorable, although full remission is rare and MG weakness, treatment side-effects, and associated thymoma can contribute to a higher mortality rate.

INFLAMMATORY MYOPATHIES

The inflammatory myopathies represent a rare but severe group of disorders causing progressive muscle weakness in the elderly patient. The three most common myopathies are polymyositis, dermatomyositis, and inclusion body myositis (IBM). They are clinically, pathologically, and systemically distinct entities that frequently overlap with other connective tissue disorders and manifest with systemic symptoms.

The annual incidence of inflammatory myopathies is approximately 1/100,000. Polymyositis is more common in women than in men, with a ratio of 2:1. Dermatomyositis is also more common in women over the age of 20. Inclusion body myositis typically presents over the age of 50, and has a male preponderance. The clinical cardinal features of these myopathies are summarized in Table 25-11.

Polymyositis

Polymyositis typically presents in adults over 20 years of age with proximal arm and leg weakness and pain, gradually worsening over weeks or months. Patients complain of difficulty lifting their arms over the head, an inability to get out of chairs or climb stairs, mild facial weakness, muscle pain, cramping, and dysphagia in one third of cases. Cardiac and respiratory muscles can also be involved, manifesting as dysrhythmia, pericarditis, and respiratory failure. Reflexes and sensation are normal.

Dermatomyositis

Dermatomyositis presents in a similar fashion, with the addition of skin involvement, including a red-purple heliotrope rash on the face and upper eyelids, Gottron's sign, red-purple keratotic rash, erythematous macules or papules on the extensor surfaces of the metacarpophalangeal, proximal interphalangeal, and distal interphalangeal joints, and also a pruritic rash. Nailfold lesions (e.g., petechiae), erythema, uveitis, and conjunctivitis can also be seen in patients with dermatomyositis.

Both dermatomyositis and polymyositis cause systemic involvement, and are associated with connec-

TABLE 25-11. *Clinical features of the inflammatory myopathies*

Myopathy	PM	DM	IBM
Age of onset	Adults >20	Adults >20 Children 5–14	Adults >50
Gender preference	Females 2:1	Females	Males
Skin rash	Rare	Yes	No
Sensory symptoms	Myalgias/cramps	Myalgias/cramps	Numbness
Dysphagia	30% of cases	30% of cases	40% of cases
Pattern of muscle weakness	Symmetric proximal > distal	Symmetric proximal > distal	Asymmetric distal proximal
Muscle enzymes CK	Elevated	Elevated	Normal-to-mild, increase
Interstitial lung disease (ILD)	10% of cases	10% of cases 50% of Jo-1 Ab	Rare
Associated malignancy	±	Yes	No
Associated connective tissue disease	Common	Common	No
Poor prognostic factors	Older age AntiJo-1, SRP, ILD, cardiac disease, treatment delay	Older age, ILD, cardiac disease, malignancy, treatment delay	None
Treatment response	Adequate	Good	Poor

DM, dermatomyositis; IBM, inclusion body myositis; Jo-1, anti-histidyl-tRNA synthetase antibodies; PM, polymyositis; SRP, signal recognition particle antibodies.

tive tissue disorders, including scleroderma, Sjö-gren's syndrome, mixed connective tissue disease, systemic lupus erythematosus, and rheumatoid arthritis. The presence of such disorders should be evaluated clinically and with appropriate serologic tests. Evaluation for associated malignancy is somewhat controversial, but indicated in selected cases. Interstitial lung disease is seen in both polymyositis and dermatomyositis.

Inclusion Body Myopathy

Onset of weakness in inclusion body myopathy can involve both proximal and distal musculature, with distal involvement predominating in up to 20% of cases. It is commonly misdiagnosed as motor neuron disease early on. Marked asymmetry can present with focal weakness of finger and wrist flexors with quadriceps involvement and relative sparing of deltoid, pectoralis, and hand intrinsics muscles. Progression of symptoms is typically slower than in dermatomyositis and polymyositis and dysphagia is present in 30% to 40% of patients. Reflexes can be reduced especially with disease progression. Unlike dermatomyositis and polymyositis, systemic involvement is rare.

Laboratory Evaluation of Myopathies

Laboratory evaluation is crucial in the assessment and treatment of an inflammatory myopathy (Fig. 25-5). Given the large number of overlap syndromes and associated connective tissue disorders, the serologic workup can be revealing. The creatine kinase is elevated in more than 90% of patients with polymyositis and dermatomyositis, and as much as 50 times the normal value, whereas creatine kinase is normal or only mildly elevated in IBM. Other muscle enzymes such as lactate dehydrogenase, aldolase, aspartate aminotransferase, and alanine aminotransferase may also be increased. Erythrocyte sedimentation rate is normal in half of the patients with inflammatory myopathy, and positive antinuclear antibodies are seen in 24% to 60% of dermatomyositis, 16% to 40% of polymyositis, and 19% to 23% of IBM cases. In addition, myositis-specific antibodies can be detected in a minority of patients with inflammatory myopathy, and have been used as a predictor for prognosis and response to therapy. In particular, anti-Jo1 antibodies are found in up to 20% of patients with dermatomyositis and polymyositis. They are present in 50% of patients with myositis with associated interstitial lung disease, more commonly those with polymyosi-

tis, and associated with poor response to treatment and long-term prognosis. The anti-skeletal recognition protein (anti-SRP) is seen in 5% of patients with polymyositis and is associated with treatment resistance and a 5-year survival of 25%. After a confirmatory diagnosis of inflammatory myopathy is made one should check for the presence and type of myositis-specific antibodies.

Nerve conduction studies are typically normal in the setting of an inflammatory myopathy, although motor amplitudes can be reduced in the patients with severe weakness. In contrast with the other myopathies, IBM has been associated peripheral neuropathy, although sometimes without obvious clinical manifestation.

Characteristic EMG findings of polymyositis and dermatomyositis include marked spontaneous activity with fibrillation potentials and positive sharp waves in limb and paraspinal muscles, and small-duration, low-amplitude polyphasic "myopathic" motor units with early recruitment pattern. Spontaneous activity helps in differentiating a polymyositis or dermatomyositis "flare" from a myopathy induced by steroid therapy. IBM demonstrates a more heterogeneous EMG profile, with a mixed pattern of large and small motor units in about one third of cases, and occasionally only "neurogenic" motor units.

Muscle biopsy remains the gold standard in the diagnosis of myopathy, even though the pathologic process can be patchy and multifocal within the biopsy specimen. Special attention should be made to biopsy a clinically weak muscle or a contralateral muscle. Generally, proximal muscles (e.g., the quadriceps and deltoids) have higher yields. The muscle biopsy confirms the presence of a myopathy, distinguishing the various inflammatory myopathies, which are pathologically distinct disorders. Polymyositis shows scattered necrotic and regenerating fibers, marked endomysial inflammation, and invasion of non-necrotic fibers. Dermatomyositis specimens show perifascicular atrophy, scattered necrotic fibers, and less invasion of non-necrotic fibers. Rimmed vacuoles with granular material and amyloid deposits on the Congo-red staining are seen in biopsy of patients with IBM.

Although somewhat controversial, an increased incidence is seen of underlying malignancy among patients with inflammatory myopathy, especially dermatomyositis. The malignancies most often associated with myopathy include ovarian, lung, breast, pancreatic, gastrointestinal, and prostate cancer. Screening for malignancy is appropriate in selected cases, and treatment of it occasionally results in improved muscle strength.

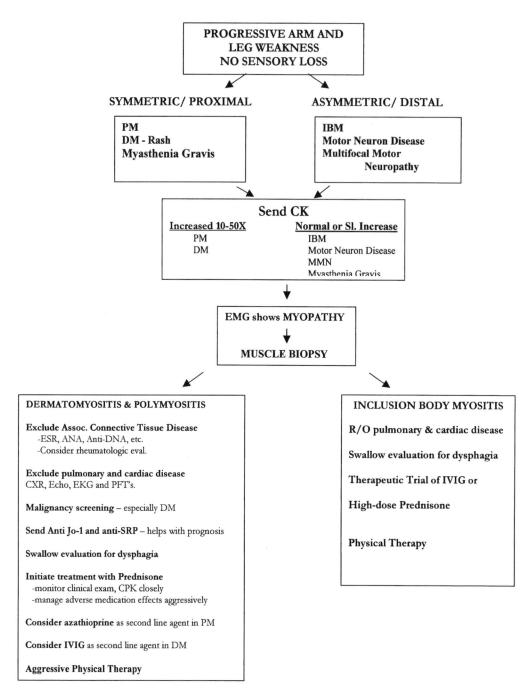

FIG. 25-5. Workup for myopathy.

TABLE 25-12. *Treatment of inflammatory myopathy*

Therapy	Dose	Things to monitor	Adverse effects
Prednisone	1 mg/kg/d for 4–6 weeks, then alternate day dosing for 4–6 months	Blood pressure, weight, glucose, bone density	HTN, weight gain, increase glucose, GI upset, osteoporosis
Azathioprine	50 mg daily, with gradual increase to 2 mg/kg/d over several months	Bimonthly CBC, LFT, GGT for 6 months, then monthly	Bone marrow toxicity, hepatotoxicity, leukopenia, flulike symptoms, neoplasia, teratogenicity
Methotrexate	7.5 mg weekly, with gradual increase by 2.5 mg weekly to 20 mg/wk	Monthly CBC, LFT Routine chest x-ray Consider liver biopsy at 2 g cumulative dose	Alopecia, interstitial lung disease, renal toxicity, hepatotoxicity, leukopenia, neoplasia, teratogenicity
Intravenous immunoglobulin	Start 0.5 g/kg × 4 doses, then maintenance every month as needed. First dose in monitored setting.	Electrolytes, BUN, creatine, blood pressure, fluid status	Flulike symptoms, fluid overload, renal failure, flushing, headache, aseptic meningitis, rare anaphylaxis
Cyclophosphamide	1–2 mg/kg/d	Monthly CBC, urinalysis	GI upset, alopecia, hemorrhagic cystitis, bone marrow suppression, teratogenicity, neoplasia

BUN, blood urea nitrogen; CBC, complete blood count; GGT, γ-glutamyl transpeptidase; GI, gastrointestinal; HTN, hypertension; LFT, liver function test.

Table 25-12 summarizes the various treatment options, according to our practice and literature review. Immunosuppressant treatments usually improve muscle strength and function in patients with polymyositis and dermatomyositis, but not those with IBM. Corticosteroids are recommended as first-line therapy for polymyositis and dermatomyositis, at an initial dose of 1 mg/kg/day prednisone until sustained improvement is achieved, usually requiring 4 to 6 weeks. We use concurrent H2-blockers, calcium, and vitamin D. Steroid dose is then tapered to alternate-day dosing, and later a very slow steroid taper is instituted, according to clinical improvement or relapse. Physical therapy, diet counseling, and blood pressure and glucose monitoring are always required. If the patient improves on steroids after 4 to 6 months, the dose is tapered by 5 mg weekly to the lowest effective dose. If improvement does not occur after 4 to 6 months of steroid treatment, then a second-line agent is added.

Because of the side effects of steroids in older adults, a second-line steroid-sparing agent (e.g., azathioprine) can be instituted early on, particularly in severely affected patients or those at risk for steroid complications. An initial 50-mg dose of azathioprine daily is gradually increased over several months to 2 mg/kg/day. Maximal effect is reached only 6 to 9 months after drug initiation, and the possible adverse effects of bone marrow suppression, hepatotoxicity, leukopenia, and flulike symptoms are monitored by a monthly screen of complete blood count, liver function tests, and g-glutamyltranspeptidase. Methotrexate and cyclophosphamide are options in patients refractory to steroids. Methotrexate is initiated at 7.5 mg weekly with a gradual increase by 2.5 mg/week to 20 mg weekly, depending on the patient response. Major adverse effects include alopecia, interstitial lung disease, and renal- and hepatotoxicity. Methotrexate should not be used in patients with myositis associated with interstitial lung disease. Cyclophosphamide is reserved for the patient refractory to steroids, azathioprine, and methotrexate. The recommended dose is 1 to 2 mg/kg/day and side effects include gastrointestinal upset, alopecia, teratogenicity, malignancy, and hemorrhagic cystitis.

For refractory myositis, IVIG can be used. Recent trials have shown a benefit, particularly in dermatomyositis, and some authorities recommend it as a second-line treatment of choice for patients with this disorder. IVIG can be of mild benefit in IBM. Initial dose is 2 g/kg given over 4 or 5 days, with monthly maintenance doses of 0.5 g/kg. Possible side effects include renal failure, fluid overload, flulike symptoms, and aseptic meningitis.

Monitoring inflammatory myopathy in elderly patients can be challenging, especially in view of the numerous adverse effects of treatment, such as deciding if new recurrent weakness is steroid induced or caused by disease relapse. Relapsing myositis typically produces acute denervation changes on EMG and elevated creatine kinase, and can occur during the steroid taper, whereby in steroid myopathy, creatine kinase levels and EMG are usually normal.

SUMMARY

The spectrum of neuromuscular disorders includes diseases affecting anterior horn cells, peripheral nerves, neuromuscular junctions, and muscles. In evaluating the patient with a neuromuscular disorder, it is crucial to understand the basic anatomy and pathophysiology of the various peripheral nervous system diseases, and appreciate valuable diagnostic clues in the patient's history and clinical examination. After addressing key questions from the patient history and neurologic examination, neuropathic disorders can be classified into several patterns, each with a limited differential diagnosis. This lead to a preliminary diagnosis and the formulation of a plan, which includes radiologic, laboratory, and electrodiagnostic tests. Specifically, the EDX evaluation is used to confirm the presence of a peripheral nervous system disorder, quantitate its severity, and look for sensory or motor abnormalities that are not apparent by clinical examination. If the EDX results suggest new diagnostic considerations, other tests may be required to reach a final diagnosis.

Neuromuscular clinicians appreciate the value of tests when the initial question is clear and grounded on solid anatomic and pathophysiologic knowledge. We teach our students that only good questions have potential for useful answers. Even when the EDX results cannot fully address how a peripheral neuropathy will progress, they are often useful in reassuring the patient's fear of a rapidly incapacitating disease, as most undiagnosed neuropathies are usually very slowly progressive.

SUGGESTED READING

Academy of Neurology. Assessment of plasmapheresis. *Neurology* 1996;47:840–843.

Ad Hoc Subcommittee of the AAN AIDS Task Force. Research criteria for diagnosis of chronic inflammatory demyelinating polyneuropathy (CIDP). *Neurology* 1991;41: 617–618.

Albers JW, Kelly JJ. Acquired inflammatory demyelinating polyneuropathies: clinical and electrodiagnostic features. *Muscle Nerve* 1989;12:435–451.

Amato AA, Barohn RJ. Idiopathic inflammatory myopathies. *Neurol Clin* 1997;15:615–648.

Asbury AK, Cornblath DR. Assessment of current diagnostic criteria for Guillain-Barré syndrome. *Ann Neurol* 1990;27:S21–S24.

Barohn RJ. Approach to peripheral neuropathy and neuronopathy. *Semin Neurol* 1998;18 (1):7–18.

Belsh JM, Schiffman PL, eds. *Amyotrophic lateral sclerosis: diagnosis and management for the clinician.* Armonk, NY: Futura, 1996.

Engel AG, Franzini-Armstrong C, eds. *Myology.* New York: McGraw-Hill 1994:1335–1383.

Fisher CM. An unusual variant of acute idiopathic polyneuritis (syndrome of ophthalmoplegia, ataxia, and areflexia). *N Engl J Med* 1956;255:57–65.

Kelly JJ Jr. Peripheral neuropathies associated with monoclonal proteins: a clinical review. *Muscle Nerve* 1985;8: 138–150.

Kornberg AJ, Pestronk A. The clinical and diagnostic role of anti-GM1 antibody testing. *Muscle Nerve* 1994;17: 100–104.

Mastaglia FL, Phillips BA, Zilko P. Treatment of inflammatory myopathies. *Muscle Nerve* 1997;20:651–664.

Mendell JR, Kissel JT, Cornblath DR. *Diagnosis and management of peripheral nerve disorders,* Contemporary Neurology Series #59. New York: Oxford University Press, 2001.

Mitsumoto H, Chad DA, Pioro EP, eds. *Amyotrophic lateral sclerosis.* Philadelphia: CNS FA Davis, 1998.

Parry GJ. Motor neuropathy with multifocal conduction block. *Semin Neurol* 1993;13:266–275.

Schaumburg HH, Berger AR, Thomas PK. Disorders of peripheral nerves. In: *Disorders of peripheral nerves.* Philadelphia: FA Davis, 1992.

Therapeutics and Technology Assessment Subcommittee of the American Academy of Neurology: assessment of plasmapheresis. *Neurology* 1996;47:840–843.

Van Doorn PA, Brand Q, Strengers PFW, et al. High-dose intravenous immunoglobulin treatment in chronic inflammatory demyelinating polyneuropathy: a double blind, placebo-controlled, crossover study. *Neurology* 1990;40: 209–212.

Walter MC, Lochmuller H, Toepfer M, et al. High dose immunoglobulin therapy in sporadic inclusion body myositis: a double-blind, placebo-controlled study. *J Neurol* 2000;247:22–28.

World Federation of Neurology Research Group on Neuromuscular Diseases and Subcommittee on Motor Neuron Diseases/Amyotrophic Lateral Sclerosis. El Escorial World Federation of Neurology criteria for the diagnosis of amyotrophic lateral sclerosis. *J Neurol Sci* 1994; 24 (Suppl.):96–107.

WEB SITES

Guillain-Barré Syndrome Foundation International: *http://www.webmast.com/gbs/*

Neuromuscular home page: *www.neuro.wustl.edu*

26

Nonviral Infectious Diseases of the Nervous System

Karen L. Roos

INTRODUCTION

An acquired immunodeficiency occurs with aging, which increases an individual's susceptibility to infection. The older adult is at risk for disseminated disease, which in a younger person may remain localized to the primary site of infection. The older adult is at risk for reactivation of latent infection in the central nervous system (CNS) that has remained latent for years because of intact cell-mediated immunity. The increased risk for tuberculous meningitis with aging is a classic example of this. The older adult may also have chronic illness (diabetes mellitus, cardiopulmonary disease, chronic renal insufficiency) or cancer or be treated with immunosuppressive therapy or corticosteroid therapy, all of which contribute to impaired cell-mediated immunity. For these reasons, the older adult is at risk for CNS infections that are classically considered opportunistic infections.

This chapter reviews the nonviral infectious diseases of the nervous system, which include bacterial, fungal and tuberculous meningitis, and brain abscess. A concise discussion of the infectious causes of stroke and of dementia is provided. An understanding of the acquired immunodeficiency that occurs with aging is needed to prevent the reactivation of latent CNS infections (viruses and tuberculosis) and the acquisition of opportunistic CNS infections in the older adult. Until then, a high degree of suspicion for the possibility of these infectious diseases in the older adult should be maintained.

MENINGITIS

Bacterial Meningitis

Bacterial meningitis is an acute purulent infection in the subarachnoid space that is associated with an inflammatory reaction in the brain parenchyma and cerebral blood vessels that causes decreased consciousness, seizure activity, raised intracranial pressure (ICP), and stroke.

Epidemiology in Older Adults

The most common causative organisms of bacterial meningitis in older adults are *Streptococcus pneumoniae* and gram-negative bacilli (*Acinetobacter calcoaceticus, Escherichia coli, Klebsiella* species, *Pseudomonas aeruginosa*, and *Enterobacter* species). *Listeria monocytogenes* is a causative organism of meningitis in older adults with impaired cell-mediated immunity from chronic illness, malignancy, organ transplantation, acquired immunodeficiency syndrome or immunosuppressive therapy. *Streptococcus agalactiae*, a leading cause of bacterial meningitis and sepsis in neonates, is increasingly seen in older adults with underlying diseases. *Haemophilus influenzae* type b, once the most common causative organism of bacterial meningitis in children, is now rarely seen in children but remains a causative organism of bacterial meningitis in older adults, especially those with chronic lung disease, those that have had a splenectomy, and patients who are immunocompromised. The most common causative organisms of bacterial meningitis in patients who have had a neurosurgical procedure are gram-negative bacilli and staphylococci.

Clinical Presentation

The classic triad of symptoms of meningitis is composed of fever, headache, and stiff neck. An altered level of consciousness, ranging from lethargy to stupor or coma, and seizure activity can accompany or follow the initial symptoms. The combination of fever, headache, stiff neck, and an altered level of consciousness is highly suggestive of bacterial meningitis. Nuchal rigidity, the pathognomonic sign of meningeal irritation, is present when the neck resists passive flexion. Neck stiffness is sometimes difficult to interpret in the older adult. In this age group, resistance to passive movement of the neck may be caused by meningeal infection or inflammation, cervical spondylosis, parkinsonism, or paratonic rigidity. When neck stiffness is caused by meningitis, the neck resists flexion but can usually be passively rotated from side to side. When neck stiffness is caused by cervical spondylosis, parkinsonism, or paratonic rigidity, any passive movement of the neck (lateral rotation, extension or flexion) meets with resistance. The possibility that nuchal rigidity is caused by meningeal infection or inflammation is supported by a positive Brudzinski's or Kernig's sign. Brudzinski's sign, which is elicited with the patient in the supine position, is positive when passive flexion of the neck results in spontaneous flexion of the hips and knees. Kernig's sign is elicited with the patient in the supine position and the thigh is flexed on the abdomen with the knee flexed. Passive extension of the leg is limited by pain when meningeal irritation is present.

Seizures occur as part of the initial presentation of bacterial meningitis or during the course of the illness in up to 40% of patients. Most seizures have a focal onset, suggesting that focal arterial ischemia or infarction is a major cause of seizure activity in bacterial meningitis. Focal seizures can also be caused by cortical venous thrombosis with hemorrhage or focal edema. Generalized seizure activity and status epilepticus are caused by fever, anoxia from decreased cerebral perfusion, spread from a focal onset to a generalized tonic clonic convulsion, or less commonly as a result of toxicity from antimicrobial agents.

Raised ICP, an expected complication of bacterial meningitis, is the major cause of obtundation and coma in this disease. Signs of increased ICP include an altered or deteriorating level of consciousness, papilledema, dilated poorly reactive pupils, sixth nerve palsies, decerebrate posturing, and the Cushing reflex (bradycardia, hypertension, and irregular respirations).

Diagnosis

When the clinical presentation is suggestive of bacterial meningitis, blood cultures should be immediately obtained and empiric antimicrobial therapy initiated without delay (Fig. 26-1). The diagnosis of bacterial meningitis is made by examination of the cerebrospinal fluid (CSF) (Table 26-1). As stated, raised ICP is an expected complication of bacterial meningitis, and is the major cause of obtundation and

coma in this disease. The role of lumbar puncture as a causative factor for cerebral herniation in patients with acute bacterial meningitis has been debated for years, and remains unresolved. The risk of cerebral herniation from acute bacterial meningitis independent of lumbar puncture is approximately 6% to 8%. When the possibility of increased ICP exists because of a decreased level of consciousness, either delay lumbar puncture (but initiate empiric antimicrobial therapy) until the increased ICP can be treated, or perform lumbar puncture with a 22-gauge needle, 30 to 60 minutes after 1 g/kg mannitol has been administered intravenously. The patient can also be intubated and hyperventilated, in addition to being treated with mannitol, to decrease ICP before lumbar puncture. CSF should be obtained for cell count (1.0 mL), glucose and protein concentrations (1.0 mL), Gram's stain and bacterial culture (1.0 mL), and latex agglutination test (0.5 mL). The last tube of CSF should be sent to the polymerase chain reaction (PCR) laboratory for viral DNA, as herpes simplex virus encephalitis is the leading disease in the differential diagnosis of bacterial meningitis. It is recommended that the fourth tube of CSF be sent to the PCR laboratory, as this is the tube that is least likely to contain red blood cells. PCR should not be done on bloody CSF, as porphyrin compounds from the degradation of heme in erythrocytes can give a false-negative PCR result.

The classic CSF abnormalities in bacterial meningitis are (a) increased opening pressure; (b) a pleocytosis of polymorphonuclear leukocytes (10–10,000 cells/mm^3); (c) decreased glucose concentration (<45 mg/dL or a CSF-to-serum glucose ratio of <0.31); and (d) an increased protein concentration. CSF bacterial cultures are positive in more than 80% of patients, and CSF Gram's stain demonstrates organisms in more than 60%.

Opening pressure should be measured with the patient in the lateral recumbent position. The normal opening pressure for adults is less than 180 mm H$_2$O. In obese adults, however, the normal opening pressure is less than 250 mm H$_2$O. In adults, in uninfected CSF, the normal white blood cell (WBC) count ranges from 0 to 5 mononuclear cells (lymphocytes and monocytes) per mm^3. In normal uninfected CSF in the adult, no polymorphonuclear leukocytes should be seen; however, a rare polymorphonuclear leukocyte can be found in concentrated CSF specimens. If the total WBC count is less than 5 cells per mm^3, the presence of a single polymorphonuclear leukocyte can be considered normal. The latex particle agglutination test for the detection of bacterial antigens of *Streptococcus pneumoniae*, *Neisseria*

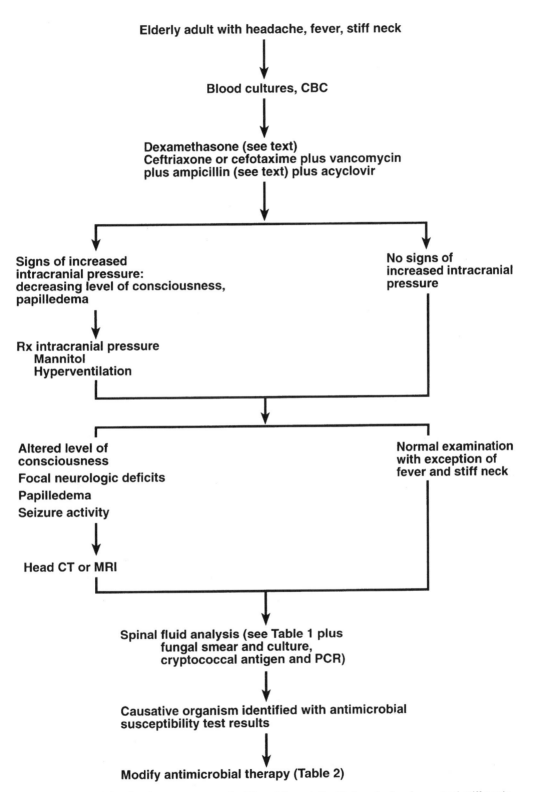

FIG. 26-1. Algorithm for the management of the older adult with headache, fever, and stiff neck.

TABLE 26-1. *Cerebrospinal fluid analysis in bacterial meningitis*

Opening pressure	>180 mm H_2O
White blood cells	>10 to <10,000/mm³—neutrophils predominate
Red blood cells	Absent unless traumatic tap
Glucose	<40 mg/dL
Cerebrospinal fluid: serum glucose ratio	<0.40
Protein	>50 mg/dL
Gram's stain	Positive in 70%–90% of untreated cases
Culture	Positive in 80% of cases
Latex agglutination	Specific for antigens of *Streptococcus pneumoniae, Neisseria meningitidis, Escherichia coli,* Hib, and group B streptococcus
Limulus amebocyte lysate assay	Positive in gram-negative meningitis
Polymerase chain reaction	Sensitivity and specificity unknown

meningitidis, H. influenzae type b, *S. agalactiae,* and *E. coli* K1 strains in the CSF is useful for making a rapid diagnosis of bacterial meningitis, and in making a diagnosis of bacterial meningitis in those patients who have been pretreated with antibiotics, in whom Gram's stain and CSF culture are negative. This test has a rapid turnaround time, usually less than a few hours, but negative findings on the test do not rule out bacterial meningitis. PCR is not as useful in the diagnosis of the causative organism of bacterial meningitis as it is in identifying the virus causing encephalitis. Commercial assays are available. The turnaround time for PCR is, however, several days. Gram's stain and the latex agglutination technique can be completed in a matter of minutes, making these the superior tests to identify the causative organism of bacterial meningitis. The Limulus amebocyte lysate assay is a rapid diagnostic test for the detection of gram-negative endotoxin in CSF and, thus, for making a diagnosis of gram-negative meningitis.

All patients with bacterial meningitis should have neuroimaging performed, either before or after lumbar puncture. Indications for neuroimaging before lumbar puncture are an altered level of consciousness, papilledema, focal neurologic deficits, and focal or generalized seizure activity. Magnetic resonance imaging (MRI) is preferred over computed tomography (CT) because of its superiority in demonstrating areas of cerebral edema and ischemia.

Treatment

Antimicrobial therapy should be initiated immediately in every older adult with fever, headache, and stiff neck. There is a heightened sense of urgency in initiating antimicrobial therapy when an altered level of consciousness is seen with these symptoms. The choice of antimicrobial therapy should be based on the predisposing conditions for bacterial meningitis. There are a number of predisposing conditions that increase the risk of pneumococcal meningitis in the older adult, the most important of which is pneumococcal pneumonia. Because of the emergence of penicillin- and cephalosporin-resistant *S. pneumoniae,* empiric therapy of community-acquired bacterial meningitis in the older adult should include a third generation cephalosporin, vancomycin, and acyclovir. Acyclovir is added to the initial empiric regimen, as herpes simplex virus encephalitis is the leading disease in the differential diagnosis. A third generation cephalosporin, either ceftriaxone or cefotaxime, provides good coverage for *S. pneumoniae* and *H. influenzae.* Ampicillin should be added to the empiric regimen for coverage of *L. monocytogenes* in individuals over 55 years of age with suspected impaired cell-mediated immunity caused by chronic illness, organ transplantation, malignancy, or immunosuppressive therapy. In hospital-acquired meningitis, and particularly meningitis following neurosurgical procedures, staphylococci and gram-negative organisms, including *Pseudomonas aeruginosa,* are the most common causative organisms. In these patients, empiric therapy should include a combination of vancomycin and ceftazidime. Ceftazidime should be substituted for ceftriaxone or cefotaxime in neurosurgical patients and in neutropenic patients, as *P. aeruginosa* may be the meningeal pathogen, and ceftazidime is the only cephalosporin with sufficient activity against *P. aeruginosa* in the CNS. Once the organism has been identified by Gram's stain or by bacterial culture of CSF, and the results of antimicrobial susceptibility tests are known, antimicrobial therapy can be modified accordingly (Table 26-2). Some strains of pneumococci are sensitive to penicillin, but in clinical practice few physicians use penicillin to treat pneumococcal meningitis. A CSF isolate of *S. pneumoniae* is considered to be susceptible to penicillin with a minimal inhibitory concentration (MIC) less than 0.06 µg/mL, to have intermediate resistance when the MIC is 0.1 to 1.0 µg/mL, and to be highly resistant when the MIC is greater than 1.0 µg/mL. Isolates of *S. pneumoniae* that have cephalosporin MIC of 0.5 µg/mL or

TABLE 26-2. *Antimicrobial therapy of bacterial meningitis*

Organism	Antibiotic	Total daily adult dose (dosing interval)
Streptococcus pneumoniae		
Sensitive to penicillin	Penicillin G	20–24 million U/d (every 4 h)
Relatively resistant to penicillin	Ceftriaxone	4 g/d (every 12 h)
	OR	
	Cefotaxime	12 g/d (every 4 h)
Resistant to penicillin	Vancomycin	2–3 g/d (every 8–12 h)
	PLUS	
	Ceftriaxone	4 g/d (every 12 h)
	OR	
	Cefotaxime	12 g/d (every 4 h)
	±Intraventricular vancomycin	20 mg/d
Gram-negative bacilli (except	Ceftriaxone	4 g/d (every 12 h)
Pseudomonas aeruginosa)	OR	
	Cefotaxime	12 g/d (every 4 h)
Pseudomonas aeruginosa	Ceftazidime	6 g/d (every 8 h)
Staphylococci		
Methicillin-sensitive	Nafcillin	9–12 g/d (every 4 h)
Methicillin-resistant	Vancomycin	2 g/d (every 6 h)
Listeria monocytogenes	Ampicillin	12 g/d (every 4 h)
	PLUS	
	Gentamicin	6 mg/kg/d (every 8 h)
Haemophilus influenzae	Ceftriaxone	4 g/d (every 12 h)
	OR	
	Cefotaxime	12 g/d (every 4 h)
Streptococcus agalactiae	Ampicillin	12 g/d (every 4 h)
	OR	
	Penicillin G	20–24 million U/d (every 4 h)

All antibiotics are administered intravenously. Doses indicated are for patients with normal renal function.

greater are considered sensitive to the cephalosporins (cefotaxime, ceftriaxone, cefepime). Those with MIC equal to 1 µg/mL are considered to have intermediate resistance, and those with MIC of 2 µg/mL or greater are considered resistant (National Committee for Clinical Laboratory Standards, 1994). For meningitis caused by pneumococci with cefotaxime or ceftriaxone MIC of 0.5 µg/mL or less, treatment with cefotaxime or ceftriaxone is usually adequate. If the MIC are 1 µg/mL or greater, vancomycin is the antibiotic of choice. Patients with *S. pneumoniae* meningitis should have a repeat lumbar puncture performed 24 to 36 hours after the initiation of antimicrobial therapy to document sterilization of the CSF. Use of intraventricular vancomycin should be considered when intravenous vancomycin fails to sterilize the CSF after 24 to 36 hours of therapy. The intraventricular route of administration is preferred over the intrathecal route because adequate concentrations of vancomycin in the cerebral ventricles are not always achieved with intrathecal administration. Intrathecal administration of vancomycin is safe, and is not associated with a risk of seizure activity. Cefepime is a broad-spectrum, fourth generation cephalosporin that is increasingly seen on the medication charts of hospitalized patients. Cefepime has *in vitro* activity similar to that of cefotaxime or ceftriaxone against *S. pneumoniae*, and greater activity against *Enterobacter* species and *P. aeruginosa*. The dose of cefepime (2 g) is given intravenously every 12 hours in adults. In clinical trials, cefepime has been demonstrated to be equivalent to cefotaxime in the treatment of pneumococcal meningitis, but its efficacy in bacterial meningitis caused by penicillin- and cephalosporin-resistant pneumococcal organisms, *Enterobacter* species, and *P. aeruginosa* has not been established. A 2-week course of intravenous antimicrobial therapy is recommended for pneumococcal meningitis.

The third generation cephalosporins, cefotaxime, ceftriaxone, and ceftazidime, are equally efficacious for the treatment of gram-negative bacillary meningitis, with the exception of meningitis caused by *P. aeruginosa*, for which ceftazidime is the drug of choice. A 3-week course of intravenous antimicrobial therapy is recommended for meningitis caused by gram-negative bacilli. Meningitis caused by *S. aureus* or by coagulase-negative staphylococci is treated with nafcillin or oxacillin. Vancomycin is the drug of choice for methicillin-resistant staphylococci. The CSF should be monitored during therapy, and if the spinal fluid continues to yield viable organisms after 48 hours of intravenous therapy, then intraventricular vancomycin (20 mg once daily) can be added.

A 3- to 4-week course of ampicillin is recommended for *L. monocytogenes* meningitis. Gentamicin should be added to ampicillin in critically ill patients, as the combination of ampicillin and gentamicin has greater bactericidal activity than ampicillin alone in experimental models of meningitis (Quagliarello and Scheld, 1997).

Adjunctive Therapy

Neurologic complications of bacterial meningitis (raised ICP, seizure activity, stroke) continue long after the CSF has been sterilized by antimicrobial therapy (Tauber and Moser, 1999). The pathophysiology of the neurologic complications of bacterial meningitis are shown in Figure 26-2. The release of bacterial cell wall components by the multiplication of bacteria and the lysis of bacteria by bactericidal antibiotics

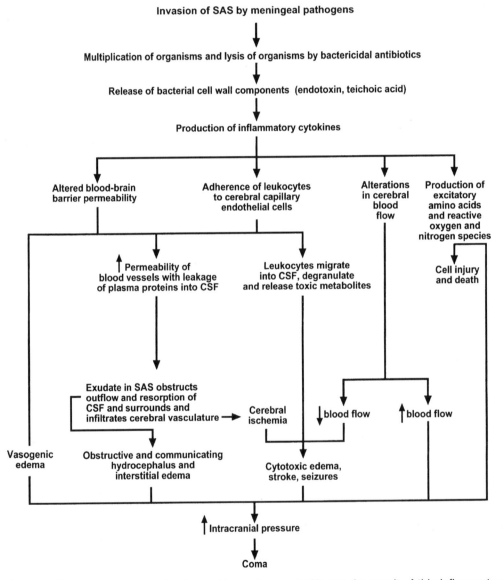

FIG. 26-2. The neurologic complications of bacterial meningitis are the result of this inflammatory cascade. © Roos.

leads to the production of the inflammatory cytokines, interleukin-1 (IL-1) and tumor necrosis factor (TNF), in the subarachnoid space, which initiates a cascade of events that ultimately leads to increased ICP, coma, stroke, seizures, and obstructive and communicating hydrocephalus. Dexamethasone has a beneficial effect by inhibiting the synthesis of IL-1 and TNF at the level of mRNA, and by decreasing CSF outflow resistance and stabilizing the blood—brain barrier. Microglia, astrocytes, monocytes, and macrophages produce IL-1 and TNF. The rationale for giving dexamethasone before antibiotic therapy is that dexamethasone inhibits the production of TNF if administered to macrophages and microglia before they are activated by bacterial cell wall components. There are ongoing clinical trials to evaluate the efficacy of dexamethasone in adults with bacterial meningitis. A metaanalysis of randomized, concurrently controlled trials of dexamethasone therapy in childhood bacterial meningitis published from 1988 to 1996 confirmed its benefit for *H. influenzae* type b meningitis, if begun with or before intravenous antibiotics, and suggested benefit for pneumococcal meningitis in children (McIntyre et al., 1997). At a May 1999 meeting of physician-scientists working in the area of the molecular basis of neurologic injury in bacterial meningitis, universal support was given for the use of dexamethasone in adults with bacterial meningitis because of its beneficial effect on inhibiting the synthesis of the inflammatory cytokines. The recommended dose of dexamethasone is 0.15 mg given intravenously every 6 hours for 4 days.

Fungal Meningitis

Aging is associated with immune dysfunction, especially cell-mediated immunity (Yoshikawa, 2000). This places older adults at risk for fungal meningitis. A number of fungi can cause meningitis, the most common of which are *Cryptococcus neoformans*, *Histoplasma capsulatum*, and *Coccidioides immitis*. *Blastomyces dermatitidis*, *Candida* species, and *Sporothrix schenckii* can also be the causative organisms of meningitis as can the rare fungi, *Paracoccidioides brasiliensis*, *Chaetomium atrobrunneum*, *Cladophialophora bantiana*, *Pseudallescheria boydii*, and *Schizophyllum commune*.

Epidemiology in Older Adults

Cryptococcus neoformans is an encapsulated yeast that is found worldwide in soil and in bird feces, particularly in pigeon droppings. Infection is acquired by inhaling cryptococcal organisms. Host resistance depends primarily on cell-mediated immunity. The loss of an efficient cell-mediated response by CD4 cells, cytotoxic lymphocytes, natural killer cells, and activated macrophages is the most important risk factor for cryptococcal meningitis. Humoral immunity also has an important role in the prevention of invasive disease by this fungus (Gottfredsson and Perfect, 2000). Corticosteroid use is a risk factor for cryptococcal meningitis, and many older adults are treated with prednisone for a variety of illnesses.

Histoplasma capsulatum, endemic in the midwestern United States and in Central and South America, causes a common, usually benign and self-limited fungal disease. Disseminated disease and CNS infection occurs primarily in individuals with impaired cell-mediated immunity. CNS infection is usually a subacute or chronic meningitis. Chronic steroid therapy is a risk factor for disseminated histoplasmosis.

Coccidioides immitis is endemic to the southwestern United States principally California, Arizona, and Texas, and also to Mexico and Central and South America. The fungus lives in the soil. Infection is acquired by inhaling airborne arthroconidia. Of people who are infected with *C. immitis*, 70% have no symptoms or have an illness indistinguishable from an upper respiratory infection. Signs and symptoms of a lower respiratory infection may also be seen with fever, sweating, anorexia, weakness, arthralgias, cough, sputum production, and chest pain. The acute infection almost always resolves without specific therapy. If the acute pulmonary infection does not resolve, a progressive pneumonia or chronic lung infection develops. Symptomatic extrapulmonary disease is more common in immunocompromised individuals, including those who are immunocompromised by aging (Stevens, 1995). When *C. immitis* infects the CNS, it is usually in the form of a subacute meningitis.

Clinical Presentation

Most patients with fungal meningitis have fever and headache for 2 weeks or longer, a subacute meningitis syndrome. They may also have stiff neck, lethargy, and weight loss. As the disease progresses, patients develop cranial nerve palsies, cognitive difficulty, and eventually signs of increased ICP. Fungal meningitis can be associated with a history or signs of pulmonary infection, and patients with coccidioidomycosis and cryptococcosis may also have skin lesions.

Diagnosis

The diagnosis of fungal meningitis is made by examination of the CSF (Table 26-3). The characteristic CSF abnormalities are a mononuclear or lymphocytic pleocytosis, increased protein concentration, and decreased glucose concentration. *C. immitis* is unique among the common fungal pathogens in that it may have a CSF eosinophilia. It is difficult to grow fungi in culture of CSF with the exception of *C. neoformans*. Because microscopy and culture of CSF are often negative, large volumes (>10 mL) of CSF should be cultured on at least three occasions to increase the yield of fungi isolation. If fungi fail to grow in cultures obtained from CSF by lumbar puncture, cisternal puncture should be performed. The cryptococcal polysaccharide antigen test is a highly sensitive and specific test for cryptococcal meningitis. A reactive CSF cryptococcal antigen test establishes the diagnosis of cryptococcal meningitis. The typical neuroimaging abnormalities in cryptococcal meningitis are enhancement of the basilar meninges after the administration of gadolinium, and progressive hydrocephalus (Fig. 26-3). The finding of progressive hydrocephalus in an older adult with fever and headache is highly suggestive of either fungal or tuberculous meningitis. The histoplasma polysaccharide antigen can be sent on CSF to make a diagnosis of histoplasma meningitis. Histoplasma polysaccharide antigen is reported to be positive in 40% of patients with histoplasma meningitis, but it can be falsely positive in coccidioidal meningitis (Wheat et al., 1989). Complement fixation antibody titers should be sent on CSF to make a diagnosis of coccidioidal meningitis. The complement fixation antibody test on CSF is reported to have a specificity of 100% and a sensitivity of 75% in the setting of active disease. Measurement of antibodies against a 33-kDa antigen from spherules of *C. immitis* in CSF is also a sensitive indicator of coccidioidal meningitis (Gottfredsson and Perfect, 2000).

Treatment

Amphotericin B is the mainstay of therapy of fungal meningitis. The treatment of cryptococcal meningitis is divided into three stages. Therapy is initiated with a combination of amphotericin B (0.7 mg/kg/day) plus flucytosine (100 mg/kg/day in four divided doses) for 2 weeks. Flucytosine blood levels should be monitored and kept at 50 to 100 μg/mL. In patients with renal dysfunction, the liposomal form of amphotericin B (AmBisome) (4 mg/kg/day) or amphotericin B lipid complex (5 mg/kg/day) can be substituted for amphotericin B. After 2 weeks of induction therapy, patients who are responding to treatment can be switched to fluconazole (400 to 800 mg/day) for 8 weeks. CSF should be recultured at the end of 10 weeks. If CSF fungal cultures are negative, the dose of fluconazole can be decreased to 200 mg/day. Fluconazole therapy is continued for 1 year (Gottfredsson and Perfect, 2000). Meningitis caused by *H. capsulatum* is treated with amphotericin B (0.7–1.0 mg/kg/day) for at least 4 weeks, and often as long as 12 weeks (until CSF fungal cultures are sterile). The addition of intrathecal amphotericin B (0.25–1.0 mg/dose) every other day or twice weekly may be required to eradicate the infection. After completing a course of amphotericin B, maintenance therapy with itraconazole (400 mg/day) is initiated and continued for at least 6 months to 1 year. During that time, the CSF should be periodically reexamined for fungal smear and culture and histoplasma polysaccharide antigen. Initial therapy of *C. immitis* meningitis is intravenous amphotericin B (0.5–0.7 mg/kg/day). When meningeal loculi and hydrocephalus from arachnoiditis or vasculitis complicate *C. immitis* meningitis, intrathecal amphotericin B (0.25-1.5 mg/dose) three times a week is often added (Davis, 1999). Intrathecal amphotericin B use can be associated with headache, fever, nausea, and vomiting. The addition of 15 mg of hydrocortisone to the intrathecal mixture may lessen these symptoms. Life-long therapy with fluconazole (400 mg) every day is recommended to prevent relapse of *C. im-*

TABLE 26-3. *Cerebrospinal fluid analysis in fungal meningitis*

White blood cells	Mononuclear or lymphocytic pleocytosis
Glucose	<40 mg/dL
Cerebrospinal fluid: serum glucose ratio	<0.40
Protein	>50 mg/dL
India ink and fungal culture	Positive in 10% to 30% of cases
Cryptococcus neoformans	Cryptococcal polysaccharide antigen
Histoplasma capsulatum	Histoplasma polysaccharide antigen
Coccidioides immitis	Complement fixation antibodies
	Anti-33–kDa antibodies

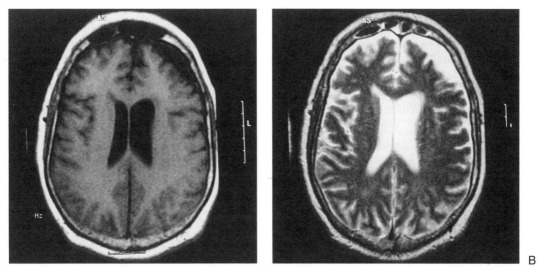

A   B

FIG. 26-3. T_1-weighted magnetic resonance (MR) scan (**A**) and T_2-weighted MR scan (**B**) in patient with cryptococcal meningitis demonstrating hydrocephalus, meningeal enhancement, and a subdural effusion.

mitis meningitis. Patients who develop hydrocephalus during the course of fungal meningitis need a CSF diversion device. Shunts can be placed in patients receiving antifungal therapy. Shunting procedures are a safe and effective therapy for hydrocephalus. Shunt placement in patients with acute infection will not disseminate cryptococcal infection into the peritoneum or bloodstream, nor does shunting provide a nidus from which cryptococcal organisms are difficult to eradicate (Park et al., 1999). A ventriculostomy can be used until CSF fungal cultures are sterile, and then the ventriculostomy is replaced by a ventriculoperitoneal shunt. The treatment of fungal meningitis is summarized in Table 26-4.

Tuberculous Meningitis

Tuberculous meningitis is the result of endogenous reactivation of infection in caseous tuberculous foci adjacent to the subarachnoid space that developed

TABLE 26-4. *Antimicrobial therapy of fungal meningitis*

Fungus	Therapy
Cryptococcus neoformans	Induction therapy (for 2 wk):
	Amphotericin B 0.7 mg/kg/d
	PLUS
	Flucytosine 100 mg/kg/d (in 4 divided doses)
	FOLLOWED BY
	Fluconazole 400–800 mg/d for 8–10 wk
	OR
	Itraconazole 400 mg/d for 8–10 wk
	If cerebrospinal fluid sterile: fluconazole 200 mg/d 6–12 mo
Histoplasma capsulatum	Amphotericin B 0.7–1.0 mg/kg/d for 4 wk
	FOLLOWED BY
	Itraconazole 400 mg/d
Coccidioides immitis	Amphotericin B 0.5–0.7 mg/kg/d
	May need intrathecal amphotericin B (0.25–1.5 mg/dose)
	Fluconazole 400 mg/d for life
Treatment failure	Ambisome 4 mg/kg/d or amphotericin B lipid complex 5 mg/kg/d
	OR
	Intraventricular amphotericin B

during hematogenous spread of tubercle bacilli in the course of an earlier primary infection, usually pulmonary tuberculosis. Meningitis is the result of the discharge of bacilli and tuberculous antigens into the subarachnoid space.

Epidemiology in Older Adults

As stated, tuberculous meningitis is the result of reactivation of infection in tuberculous foci that seeded the CNS during the course of an earlier primary infection. Most adults become infected with *Mycobacterium tuberculosis* when they inhale aerosolized droplet nuclei containing tubercle bacilli. Not all infected persons have the same risk of developing pulmonary disease. An immunocompetent adult with untreated *M. tuberculosis* has a 5% to 10% lifetime risk of disease. The risk is greatest in the first 2 to 3 years after infection. Approximately 10% of persons with tuberculosis who are immunocompetent develop CNS disease (Udani et al., 1971). Risk factors for tuberculous meningitis include age, malnutrition, alcoholism, diabetes mellitus, chronic corticosteroid therapy, and the human immunodeficiency virus infection.

Clinical Presentation

In the older adult, in developed countries, tuberculous meningitis typically presents as a subacute or chronic meningitis characterized by fever, headache, night sweats, and malaise. As the disease progresses, seizure activity, stroke, progressive hydrocephalus, raised ICP, and eventually coma complicate the clinical course. The possibility of tuberculous meningitis should be strongly considered in the older adult with unrelenting headache, night sweats, and progressive hydrocephalus by neuroimaging.

Diagnosis

The diagnosis of tuberculous meningitis is made by examination of CSF. The characteristic CSF abnormalities are an elevated opening pressure, a lymphocytic pleocytosis (10–500 cells/mm^3), a mildly decreased glucose concentration (20–40 mg/dL), and an elevated protein concentration. Spinal fluid should be examined by acid-fast stains and cultures, and molecular diagnostic techniques for *M. tuberculosis* DNA. The last tube of fluid collected at lumbar puncture is the best tube to send for acid-fast bacilli smear. A pellicle can form in the CSF in tuberculous meningitis or a cobweb-like clot on the surface of the fluid. Tubercle bacilli are best demonstrated in a smear of

the clot or sediment. Positive smears are reported in 10% to 40% of cases. The growth of the organism is slow, so cultures take weeks to be positive. Cultures are reported to be positive in 25% to 75% of cases of tuberculous meningitis, requiring 3 to 6 weeks for growth to be detectable (Traub et al., 1984; Leonard and Des Prez, 1990). The PCR technique has yet to be perfected for the detection of *M. tuberculosis* DNA in CSF, but it is available in most laboratories. False-negative results are caused by too few mycobacteria in CSF in the early stages of infection. False-positive results result from cross-contamination with amplified DNA products in the laboratory (Lin et al., 1995).

In the absence of demonstrating the organism in smear or culture of CSF, finding a site of extrameningeal tuberculous infection supports the diagnosis of tuberculous meningitis. A chest radiograph should be obtained as part of the diagnostic evaluation of tuberculous meningitis. Radiographic evidence of pulmonary tuberculosis, specifically hilar adenopathy or an upper lobe infiltrate, is found in less than 50% of cases of tuberculous meningitis in adults. The Mantoux intradermal tuberculin skin test is helpful when positive. The test is interpreted 48 hours after placement, and is considered positive if the amount of induration is more than 5 mm. The test can, however, be falsely negative, even in the absence of immunosuppression and in association with a positive reaction to the common antigens used to determine anergy.

The most common neuroimaging abnormalities in tuberculous meningitis are hydrocephalus and leptomeningeal enhancement postcontrast administration. In addition, evidence may be seen of medium or small vessel infarction (Fig. 26-4), and tuberculomas can develop during therapy.

Treatment

Treatment of tuberculous meningitis in adults is initiated with a combination of isoniazid (300 mg/day), rifampin (10 mg/kg/day, up to 600 mg/day), and pyrazinamide (25–35 mg/kg/day) for 2 months, followed by isoniazid and rifampin for an additional 7 to 10 months of therapy. Pyridoxine (50 mg daily) is added to this regimen to avoid peripheral neuropathy caused by isoniazid-induced pyridoxine deficiency. Monthly liver function studies should be obtained in adults receiving isoniazid and rifampin. The risk of hepatotoxicity from isoniazid is approximately 1%. This risk doubles with the addition of rifampin (Leonard and Des Prez, 1990). In patients with a high

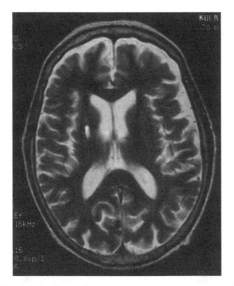

FIG. 26-4. Cranial magnetic resonance scan in patient with tuberculous meningitis demonstrating right posterior limb internal capsule infarction.

probability of a drug-resistant strain of *M. tuberculosis*, therapy is initiated with a combination of isoniazid, rifampin, pyrazinamide, and either streptomycin (1 g daily by intramuscular injection) or ethambutol (15–25 mg/kg/day) for 2 months. This is followed by isoniazid and rifampin, to complete a 9- to 18-month course of therapy. Patients at risk for drug-resistant strains of tuberculosis are those who have had inadequate treatment for pulmonary tuberculosis either because of an irregular drug supply, inappropriate regimens, or poor compliance (Pablos-Mendes et al., 1998). The chief toxicity of ethambutol is optic neuritis, which occurs in as many as 3% of patients receiving 25 mg/kg/day, but is very rare at a dose of 15 mg/kg/day (Leonard and Des Prez, 1990). If ethambutol is required for long-term therapy because the organism is resistant to isoniazid, ethambutol 25 mg/kg/day is given for 1 to 2 months, and 15 mg/kg/day thereafter. Table 26-5 summarizes the antimicrobial therapy of tuberculous meningitis, including the adverse effect of antituberculous agents and the management of these complications.

The Infectious Disease Society of America recommends the use of corticosteroid therapy in patients with tuberculous meningitis (McGowan et al., 1992). Corticosteroid therapy improves the outcome for patients with tuberculous meningitis (Dooley et al., 1997). Dexamethasone (8–12 mg/day) or the equivalent of prednisone is recommended and corticosteroid therapy is tapered over 6 to 8 weeks (Dooley et al., 1997).

BRAIN ABSCESS

A brain abscess is a focal, suppurative process within the brain parenchyma.

Epidemiology in Older Adults

A brain abscess in the older adult can be caused by either bacteria or opportunistic pathogens such as *Toxoplasma gondii*, *Aspergillus* species, *Nocardia asteroides*, or mycobacterial or fungal species reviewed above. A brain abscess can also be caused by *Taenia solium* (neurocysticercosis).

A bacterial brain abscess can develop from direct spread from a contiguous site of infection (e.g., the paranasal sinuses), otitis media, mastoiditis or from dental infections. A brain abscess can follow head trauma or be a complication of a neurosurgical pro-

TABLE 26-5. *Antimicrobial therapy of tuberculous meningitis*

Antituberculous agent	Adult dose	Adverse effect	Recommended action
Isoniazid	300 mg/d single oral dose	Hepatotoxicity Peripheral neuropathy	Monthly LFT Pyridoxine
Rifampin	10 mg/kg/d maximal daily dose—600 mg	Hepatotoxicity Turns urine orange brownish color	Monthly LFT Warn patient this will happen
Pyrazinamide	25–35 mg/kg/d	Hepatotoxicity Hyperuricemia	Monthly LFT Monitor uric acid
Streptomycin	1 g/d intramuscularly	Nephrotoxicity	Monthly creatinine; will need to decrease dose in renal insufficiency
		Vestibulotoxicity	Reassure patient this will improve after therapy
Ethambutol	15–20 mg/kg/d	Optic neuritis	Monthly eye examination

LFT, liver function tests.

TABLE 26-6. *Etiologic organisms of a brain abscess*

Predisposing condition	Etiologic organism
Paranasal sinusitis	Microaerophilic and anaerobic streptococci *Haemophilus* species *Bacteroides* species (non-*fragilis*) *Fusobacterium* species
Otitis media and mastoiditis	*Bacteroides* species (including *B. fragilis*) Streptococci *Pseudomonas aeruginosa* Enterobacteriaceae
Dental infections	Streptococci *Bacteroides fragilis*
Endocarditis	*Viridans streptococci* *Staphylococcus aureus*
Pyogenic lung infection	*Streptococcus* sp. *Actinomyces* sp. *Fusobacterium* sp.
Urinary sepsis	Enterobacteriaceae Pseudomonaceae
Intraabdominal source	*Streptococcus* sp. Enterobacteriaceae Anaerobes
Neurosurgical procedure	Staphylococci Enterobacteriaceae Pseudomonaceae
Immunocompromised	*Aspergillus* sp. (multiple abscesses) *Nocardia asteroides* (single abscess) *Toxoplasma gondii* (multiple abscesses) Mycobacteria *Cryptococcus neoformans* *Histoplasma capsulatum*

Adapted from Calfee DP, Wispelwey B. Brain abscess. *Semin Neurol* 200;20:353–360, with permission.

cedure. A brain abscess can be a complication of infective endocarditis or the hematogenous spread of bacteria from a pyogenic lung infection, the urinary tract, or an intraabdominal infection. Table 26-6 lists the most likely etiologic organisms of a brain abscess, based on predisposing or associated conditions.

Clinical Presentation

The most common symptom of a brain abscess is a headache. The headache is often characterized as a constant, dull, aching sensation that is either hemicranial or generalized, and refractory to analgesic therapy. Fever is present in only 50% of patients at the time of diagnosis, and the absence of fever should not exclude the diagnosis. New onset focal or generalized seizure activity is a common presenting sign, as is a focal neurologic deficit. The latter predicts the location of the brain abscess. Hemiparesis is the most common localizing sign of a frontal lobe abscess. A temporal lobe abscess can present with a disturbance of language or an upper homonymous quadrantanopsia. A cerebellar abscess presents with nystagmus, difficulty with coordination, and ataxia. As the brain abscess evolves and is surrounded by edema, signs of increased ICP develop, including papilledema, nausea and vomiting, and drowsiness. Meningismus is not present unless the abscess has ruptured into the ventricle or the infection has spread to the subarachnoid space.

Diagnosis

The diagnosis of a brain abscess is made by CT or MRI. CT has the advantage of being easy to do in acutely ill patients, but MRI is better able to demonstrate the abscess in the early (cerebritis) stage, and is superior to CT for identifying cerebellar abscesses. Neuroimaging studies should be obtained without and then with contrast. The initial workup should also include a search for the primary site of infection. Sinusitis is well visualized on MRI. Blood cultures, an echocardiogram, urinalysis and urine culture, and chest radiograph should be obtained. Approximately 90% of patients with a nocardia brain abscess have pulmonary involvement (Maccario et al., 1998). Serology should be performed to detect antibodies to *Toxoplasma gondii*. Most patients with aspergillus brain abscess have evidence of pulmonary disease on chest radiography.

The microbiological diagnosis of a brain abscess is made by stain and culture of abscess material obtained by stereotactic needle aspiration.

Treatment

Antimicrobial therapy of a brain abscess is initially based on the source of infection, and then modified when the results of stain and culture of abscess material and antimicrobial susceptibility tests are known (Table 26-7). Prophylactic anticonvulsant therapy is recommended for at least 3 months after resolution of the abscess. The decision to discontinue anticonvulsant therapy is based on findings on electroencephalogram (EEG). If the EEG is abnormal, anticonvulsant therapy should be continued. If the EEG is normal, anticonvulsant therapy can be slowly withdrawn.

Steroids are not given routinely to patients with a brain abscess. Intravenous dexamethasone therapy (10 mg every 6 hours) is reserved for patients with mass effect caused by brain abscess edema and ICP.

TABLE 26-7. *Antimicrobial therapy of brain abscess*

Organism	Total daily adult dose (dosing interval)
Streptococcus sp.	Penicillin G 20–24 million U/d (every 4 h)
	OR
	Cefotaxime 12 g/d (every 4 h)
Bacteroides sp.	Metronidazole 2,000 mg/d (every 6 h)
Fusobacterium sp.	Metronidazole 2,000 mg/d (every 6 h)
Haemophilus sp.	Ceftriaxone 4 g/d (every 12 h)
Pseudomonas aeruginosa	Ceftazidime 6 g/d (every 8 h)
Staphylococci	
Methicillin-sensitive	Nafcillin 9–12 g/d (every 4 h)
Methicillin-resistant	Vancomycin 2 g/d (every 6 h)
Aspergillus sp.	Liposomal amphotericin B 5 mg/kg/d
Nocardia asteroides	Trimethoprim 15–20 mg/kg/d–Sulfamethoxazole 75–100 mg/kg/d
Toxoplasma gondii	Trimethoprim 15–20 mg/kg/d–Sulfamethoxazole 75–100 mg/kg/d

Serial CT or MRI scans should be obtained on a monthly or bimonthly basis to document resolution of the abscess (Roos and Tyler, 2000).

INFECTIOUS CAUSES OF STROKE

Table 26-8 provides the recommended studies on CSF to be performed to rule out an infectious cause of a stroke in the older adult. Bacterial and fungal causes of stroke are discussed under their own subsections in this chapter. Syphilitic meningovasculitis can cause a stroke in an older adult. The classic CSF abnormalities in syphilitic meningovasculitis are a lymphocytic pleocytosis—an elevated protein concentration and a reactive CSF venereal disease research laboratory (VDRL) test. A reactive CSF VDRL result confirms the diagnosis of neurosyphilis, except when the CSF is blood-tinged. Blood in the CSF can give a false-positive CSF VDRL results. A nonreactive CSF fluorescent treponemal antibody absorption test or microhemagglutination-*T. pallidum* test excludes the diagnosis; however, a reactive CSF fluorescent treponemal antibody absorption test or a reactive microhemagglutination *T. pallidum* does not establish the diagnosis.

INFECTIOUS CAUSES OF DEMENTIA

Table 26-9 lists the CSF studies for infectious causes of dementia. In every patient with signs of dementia, it is hoped that a reversible cause can be detected and treated. In reality, however, few infectious causes of dementia exist. Patients with viral, fungal, or tuberculous meningitis can be confused, but their confusion should not be mistaken for dementia. With an increased awareness of sporadic Creutzfeldt-Jakob disease and new variant Creutzfeldt-Jakob disease, this disease is included in the differential diagnosis of dementia, raising the question of which are the best diagnostic studies to perform to rule this out. At least six genotypic variants of Creutzfeldt-Jakob disease are known (Zerr et al., 2000). When dementia is associated with myoclonus, ataxia and the classic EEG appearance of periodic sharp and slow wave complexes, the diagnosis of Creutzfeldt-Jakob disease can be made clinically. In the absence of myoclonus, ataxia, and a characteristic EEG pattern of Creutzfeldt-Jakob disease, CSF can be sent for 14.3.3 protein testing. The detection of the 14.3.3 protein in CSF has been suggested as a marker for prion disease; however, false-negative and false-positive findings have been

TABLE 26-8. *Cerebrospinal fluid studies for infectious etiologies of stroke in the older adult*

Cell count
Glucose concentration
Gram's stain and bacterial culture
Latex agglutination
Limulus amebocyte lysate assay
Venereal Disease Research Laboratory (test)
India ink and fungal culture
Acid-fast bacilli and *Mycobacterium tuberculosis*
   culture

TABLE 26-9. *Cerebrospinal fluid studies for infectious etiologies of dementia*

Cell count
Glucose concentration
Fungal smear and culture
Acid-fast smear and *Mycobacterium tuberculosis*
   culture
Cryptococcal polysaccharide antigen
Histoplasma polysaccharide antigen
Coccidioides immitis complement fixation antibodies
14.3.3 protein
Venereal Disease Research Laboratory (test)

reported to be associated with herpes simplex virus encephalitis, hypoxic encephalopathy, acute stroke, and other conditions that induce acute neuronal damage (Mastrianni and Roos, 2000). A definitive diagnosis can only be made by brain biopsy. Currently, no specific treatment is available for this disease.

CONCLUSIONS

Every older adult with unrelenting headache should have a CT scan or MRI, followed by examination of the CSF. A number of tables in this chapter are provided to guide the clinician in diagnostic studies on CSF. Similarly, every febrile older adult with a stroke should have CSF analysis to rule out an infectious cause of the stroke. Bacterial, fungal, and tuberculous meningitis are all treatable with antimicrobial agents, but delays in treatment lead to complications, including seizures, stroke, and hydrocephalus, that may not be reversible. Patients with fungal and tuberculous meningitis who develop hydrocephalus should have shunting procedures, as untreated hydrocephalus is a major contributor to mortality in these diseases. The most important way to prevent pneumococcal meningitis in the older adult is by vaccination, and neurologists should routinely remind their patients to be certain they are revaccinated every 5 years.

REFERENCES

Bacterial Meningitis

McIntyre PB, Berkey CS, King SM, et al. Dexamethasone as adjunctive therapy in bacterial meningitis. *JAMA* 1997;278:925–931.

National Committee for Clinical Laboratory Standards. *Performance standards for antimicrobial susceptibility testing.* Villanova, PA: National Committee for Laboratory Standards; 1994.

Quagliarello VJ, Scheld WM. Treatment of bacterial meningitis. *N Engl J Med* 1997;336:708–716.

Tauber MG, Moser B. Cytokines and chemokines in meningeal inflammation: biology and clinical implications. *Clin Infect Dis* 1999;28:1–12.

Fungal Meningitis

Davis LE. Fungal infections of the central nervous system. *Neurol Clin* 1999;17:761–781.

Gottfredsson M, Perfect JR. Fungal meningitis. *Semin Neurol* 2000;20:307–322.

Park MK, Hospenthal DR, Bennett JE. Treatment of hydrocephalus secondary to cryptococcal meningitis by use of shunting. *Clin Infect Dis* 1999;28(3):629–633.

Stevens DA. Coccidioidomycosis. *N Engl J Med* 1995;332:1077–1081.

Wheat LJ, Kohler RB, Tewari RP, et al. Significance of Histoplasma antigen in the cerebrospinal fluid of patients with meningitis. *Arch Intern Med* 1989;149:302–304.

Yoshikawa TT. Epidemiology and unique aspects of aging and infectious diseases. *Clin Infect Dis* 2000;30:931–933.

Tuberculous Meningitis

Dooley DP, Carpenter JL, Rademacher S. Adjunctive corticosteroid therapy for tuberculosis: a critical reappraisal of the literature. *Clin Infect Dis* 1997;25:872–887.

Leonard JM, Des Prez RM. Tuberculous meningitis. *Infect Dis Clin North Am* 1990;4:769–787.

Lin JJ, Harn HJ, Hsu YD, et al. Rapid diagnosis of tuberculous meningitis by polymerase chain reaction assay of cerebrospinal fluid. *J Neurol* 1995;242:147–152.

McGowan JE, Chesney PJ, Crossley KB, et al. Guidelines for the use of systemic glucocorticosteroids in the management of selected infections. *J Infect Dis* 1992;165:1–13.

Pablos-Mendez A, Raviglione MC, Laszlo A, et al. Global surveillance for antituberculosis-drug resistance 1994–1997. *N Engl J Med* 1998;338:1641–1649.

Traub M, Colchester ACF, Kingsley DPE, et al. Tuberculosis of the central nervous system. *Q J Med* 1984;53:81–100.

Udani PM, Parekh UC, Dastur DK. Neurological and related syndromes in CNS tuberculosis: clinical features and pathogenesis. *J Neurol Sci* 1971;14:341–357.

Brain Abscess

Maccario M, Tortorano AM, Ponticelli C. Subcutaneous nodules and pneumonia in a kidney transplant recipient. *Nephrol Dial Transplant* 1998;13:796–798.

Roos KL, Tyler KL. Bacterial meningitis, brain abscess, empyema and suppurative thrombophlebitis. In: Braunwald E, Fauci AS, Kasper DL, et al., eds. *Harrison's principles of internal medicine*, 15th ed. New York: McGraw-Hill, 2000.

Infectious Causes of Dementia

Mastrianni JA, Roos RP. The prion diseases. *Semin Neurol* 2000;20:337–352.

Zerr I, Schulz-Schaeffer WJ, Giese A, et al. Current clinical diagnosis is Creutzfeldt-Jacob disease: identification of uncommon variants. *Ann Neurol* 2000;48:323–329.

SUGGESTED READINGS

Gottfredsson M, Perfect JR. Fungal meningitis. *Semin Neurol* 2000;20:307–322.

Garcia-Monco JC. Central nervous system tuberculosis. *Neurol Clin* 1999;17:737–759.

Mastrianni JA, Roos RP. The prion diseases. *Semin Neurol* 2000;20:337–352.

Roos KL. *Meningitis: 100 maxims in neurology.* New York: Arnold, London and Oxford University Press, 1996:1–208.

Roos KL, Tunkel AR, Scheld WM. Acute bacterial meningitis in children and adults. In: Scheld WM, Whitley RJ, Durack DT, eds. *Infections of the central nervous system*, 2nd ed. Philadelphia: Lippincott-Raven, 1997:335–401.

Viral Illnesses in the Nervous System
of the Elderly

Robert W. Schabbing and John R. Corboy

INTRODUCTION

In both animals and humans, morbidity and mortality caused by cancer, infection, and possibly autoimmunity, increase with age. Viral infections in the nervous system contribute to this morbidity and mortality. Viral infections can directly cause disease in the elderly, as with shingles, or may be more indirect, as with the postpolio syndrome. Older patients can be more susceptible to complications of viral illnesses. Also, viruses are purported to be associated with a variety of brain tumors and degenerative conditions commonly occurring in the elderly, such as Alzheimer's disease and Parkinson's disease.

Deterioration of the immune system with aging, *immunosenescence*, is believed to be an important contributor to this morbidity and mortality. All aspects of the immune system can be affected by immunosenescence, but dysregulated T-cell function may play a critical role. Factors that can contribute to T-cell immunosenescence include hematopoietic stem cell defects, thymic involution, defects in antigen presentation, aging of resting T cells, disruption of activation of T cells, or disturbance of clonal expansion (Pawalec et al., 1999).

Most tests of T-cell function are depressed in the elderly, and good T-cell function is associated with longevity (Roberts-Thomson et al., 1974; Murasko et al., 1988; Wayne et al., 1990). Paradoxically, aging also is associated with an increased production of autoantibodies. Although these do not appear to include disease-associated antibodies (Candore et al., 1997), a small number of autoimmune disorders appear to be more common in the elderly (Burns and Goodwin, 1997). Thus, immunosenescence more appropriately can be thought of as a state of immune dysregulation, the complete nature of which remains to be determined.

The incidence and severity of some nervous system infections are increased in the elderly. For example,

although rates of asymptomatic infection with St. Louis encephalitis virus are similar across all age groups, the rates of nervous system invasion and mortality are significantly elevated in individuals above 55 years of age (Marfin et al., 1993). Determination of an association between a specific alteration of immune function and any disease state in the elderly, however, is more difficult (Voetes et al., 1997). An exception is the age-associated increase in reactivation of varicella-zoster virus (VZV), shingles, which is associated with a decrease in the frequency of VZV-specific T cells which produce interferon-γ (Berger et al., 1981; Zhang et al., 1994). Thus, the precise role immunosenescence plays in most viral infections in the nervous system is unknown.

NEUROPATHIES AND NEURONOPATHIES

Varicella-Zoster Virus and Neurologic Disease

Herpes zoster, or shingles, is a relatively common viral-mediated illness affecting the elderly. Its annual incidence is approximately 5 to 6.5/1,000 at age 60, increasing to 8 to 11/1,000 at age 70 (Donahue et al., 1995). In the elderly, postherpetic neuralgia (PHN) is a common complication of herpes zoster infection. The elderly may also be predisposed to other complications from shingles (Galil et al., 1997). Zoster virus infection and its sequelae pose a significant diagnostic and therapeutic challenge in geriatric neurology.

Varicella-zoster virus is a double-stranded DNA virus in the family of human herpesviruses. The typical initial infection in childhood results in chickenpox, after which the virus becomes latent in sensory and cranial ganglia. In some individuals, VZV reactivates and causes herpes zoster, or shingles. An immunocompromised state, primary infection during infancy, and old age are risk factors for the development of shingles (Gilden et al., 2000). Immunosenescence may explain this increased risk in the elderly. In the elderly who are not immunosuppressed, reactivation is generally limited to a single or a few adjacent dermatomes. Vesicular eruptions containing infectious viral particles develop within this restricted area. Herpes zoster most frequently occurs in the thoracic dermatomes, and somewhat less in the trigeminal dermatomes. Multiple dermatomes or a generalized infection are more likely to be involved in immunosuppressed patients, for example, patients with a hematologic malignancy or iatrogenic immunosuppression. The eruptions are nearly always associated with pain, itching, and alterations in sensation, including dysesthesias, paresthesias, and hypesthesia. During an episode of acute zoster infection, oral narcotics are frequently required. This pain and alteration in sensation, referred to as neuralgia, can precede the eruption or persist long after its resolution. In a few patients, dermatomal pain has occurred in the absence of rash or a structural cause (e.g., degenerative spine changes) and been attributed to VZV reactivation. This rare condition is termed "zoster sine herpete." Polymerase chain reaction (PCR) has confirmed the presence of virus in cerebrospinal fluid in some of these patients (Gilden et al., 1994). This does not appear to be a common cause of unexplained unilateral pain (McKendrick et al., 1999).

Persistence of pain for several weeks or longer following the onset of rash defines PHN. The pain can be severe and debilitating. The occurrence of PHN is closely associated with age. It is rare in patients younger than 50 years of age, but is seen in up to 40% of patients older than 60 years of age, although the incidence can be significantly lower (de Moragas and Kierland, 1957; Helgason et al., 2000). The cause of PHN is unclear, although it may be related to ongoing, low-level viral replication in the ganglia. Interleukin-8, an inflammatory cytokine, is elevated in the cerebrospinal fluid of patients with PHN, and inflammatory changes have been reported in a postmortem study (Kijuchi et al., 1999; Watson et al., 1991). Treatment of zoster infection with antiviral medications is aimed primarily at avoidance of PHN. Therefore, treatment with antiviral medications may be un-

necessary if the patient is immunocompetent and younger than 50 years of age. Presently, it is common practice to use oral antiviral agents for the treatment of elderly patients with zoster (Table 27-1). However, studies of the efficacy of oral antiviral agents in preventing PHN have produced conflicting results. If initiated within 72 hours following the onset of rash, a 1-week course of oral antiviral treatment may hasten resolution of PHN (Jackson et al., 1997; Wood et al., 1996). Studies have shown famciclovir (500 mg three times daily) and valacyclovir (1,000 mg three times daily) to be as effective as acyclovir (800 mg five times daily) in preventing PHN, while requiring significantly less frequent dosing (Tyring et al., 1995; Tyring, 1996; Beutner et al., 1995). However, their cost is substantially greater. Some authors have suggested, however, that treatment is cost effective (Tyring et al., 1995; Huse et al., 1997; Grant et al., 1997; Gruger and Backhouse, 1997; Tyring et al., 2000). Longer treatment does not confer a significant advantage (Wood et al., 1994). No studies have been done on intravenous antiviral therapy in immunocompetent patients for the prevention of PHN. The addition of glucocorticoids to treatment with oral antiviral medication has not been shown to be superior to antiviral medications alone (Wood et al., 1994; Whitley et al., 1996; Esmann et al., 1987). Treatment with a tricyclic antidepressant at the onset of rash, with antiviral medication, may also prevent PHN (Bowsher, 1997). For the treatment of intractable PHN (Table 27-2), tricyclic antidepressants (amitriptyline, nortriptyline, or desipramine 25 to 75 mg daily), gabapentin (up to 3,600 mg total daily dose), capsaicin cream, and a lidocaine transdermal patch have been demonstrated to be beneficial in partially relieving pain (Volmink et al., 1996; Watson et al., 1998; Kirshore-Kumar et al., 1990; Rowbotham et al., 1998; Bernstein et al., 1989; Watson et al., 1993; Rowbotham et al., 1996). An acetylsalicylic acid patch might also be effective (Tajti et al., 1999). Oral narcotics remain an alternative, although the elderly are more susceptible to complications such as sedation, cognitive impairment, and constipation (Watson et al., 1998). Intrathecal methylprednisolone has also

TABLE 27-1. *Oral antiviral medications for the prevention of postherpetic neuralgia*

Medication	Dose	Frequency	Duration	Cost[a]
Acyclovir	800 mg	5 times daily	7 days	119.37
Famciclovir	500 mg	3 times daily	7 days	142.67
Valacyclovir	1,000 mg	3 times daily	7 days	134.67

[a]Treatment cost calculated for a complete 7-day course, based on retail prices at a university hospital pharmacy in 2001.

TABLE 27-2. *Medications for the treatment of chronic postherpetic neuralgia*

Tricyclic antidepressants (amitriptyline, nortriptyline, desipramine)
Gabapentin
Capsaicin topical cream
Lidocaine transdermal patch
Acetylsalicylic acid patch
Sustained release oral narcotics (OxyContin)
Intrathecal methylprednisolone

been demonstrated to be effective in a clinical trial (Kotani et al., 2000).

A variety of complications may result from shingles. When associated with the ophthalmic division of the trigeminal nerve, zoster infection can result in keratitis and is a potential cause of blindness. Oral acyclovir and valacyclovir are effective in reducing complications (Cobo et al., 1986; Neoh et al., 1994; Colin et al., 2000). Evaluation of these patients should include a prompt referral to an ophthalmologist for a slit-lamp examination. Ophthalmic involvement is frequent in patients with nasal lesions (Hutchinson's sign). Numerous reports have been made of hemorrhagic and ischemic stroke following ophthalmic zoster infection in both immunocompetent and immunocompromised hosts, occurring weeks to several months later. Immunocompetent patients tend to develop a large vessel vasculitis or granulomatous arteritis, associated with a cerebrospinal fluid pleocytosis, oligoclonal bands, and intrathecal immunoglobulin synthesis (Gilden et al., 2000). Viral spread through trigeminal branches innervating intracranial and extracranial arteries has been proposed as the mechanism, with viral presence in areas of arterial inflammation confirmed microscopically and by PCR (MacKenzi et al., 1981; Doyle et al., 1983; Melanson et al., 1996). Similarly, restricted regions of strokes have been reported following zoster infection in other cranial nerve and in cervical distributions. A small vessel arteritis or encephalitis has been described in immunocompromised hosts, characterized by ischemic and hemorrhagic strokes in cortical and subcortical gray matter, and in white matter. This sometimes has a demyelinating appearance, and can occur in the absence of a preceding rash (Gilden et al., 2000). Facial nerve involvement may be associated with facial weakness (Bell's Palsy) and external auditory canal cutaneous or palatal mucosal eruptions (Ramsey-Hunt syndrome). Other cranial nerve palsies, sometimes multiple, have also been reported. Limb weakness can occur in patients with cervical or lumbosacral in-

volvement, and has been termed "zoster paresis." Myelitis may also be present, which may be associated with localized leptomeningitis and vasculitic necrosis of the dorsal and ventral spinal roots, as well as demyelination and gray-matter necrosis (Hogan and Krigman, 1973). Myelitis appears to be more common in immunocompromised hosts. Several case reports advocate the use of intravenous acyclovir for the treatment of zoster paresis, although no clinical trials have been performed to confirm the benefit of this treatment.

Acute Paralytic Poliomyelitis and the Postpolio Syndrome

Poliovirus is the cause of acute paralytic poliomyelitis. Postpolio syndrome, a disorder of progressive weakness, can occur several years later in polio survivors. Acute paralytic poliomyelitis is now eradicated in the Americas. Therefore, the postpolio syndrome is seen nearly exclusively in the elderly because of the aging population of polio survivors, and the long delay in developing postpolio syndrome.

Poliovirus (enteroviruses 1, 2, and 3) belongs to the RNA virus family *Picornaviridae*, and is the cause of acute paralytic poliomyelitis. Acute paralytic polio is characterized by flaccid paresis of the limbs, trunk, and bulbar musculature. Of individuals infected with poliovirus, 1% or less develop this neurologic syndrome (Dalakas, 1995). Many develop typical symptoms of a viral illness, or remain completely asymptomatic. Respiratory and gastrointestinal secretions transmit the infection. The virus enters through the gastrointestinal tract, with subsequent spread to local lymph nodes and then the bloodstream. The selective vulnerability of lower motor neurons to poliovirus may result from production of a viral receptor by these cells, although involvement of the central nervous system is more diffuse than simply the lower motor neurons. The human poliovirus receptor (*h*PVR) has been localized to the motor endplate. Skeletal muscle injury may play a role in allowing retrograde transport of the poliovirus to lower motor neurons. This provides a mechanism for selective eradication of a neuronal subpopulation, lower motor neurons (anterior horn cells) in the spinal cord and bulbar nuclei. The *h*PVR gene is probably a member of the immunoglobulin superfamily. The gene product mRNA gives rise to two secretory and two membrane-bound glycoproteins. Although a murine homolog of this gene has been identified, mice do not develop acute paralytic poliomyelitis. However, a similar syndrome, both clinically and pathologically, can be experimentally produced in *h*PVR-transgenic mice (Gromeier et al., 1995; Gromeier and Wimmer, 1998).

It has been estimated that 50% of an individual's motor neurons can be partially or completely damaged during acute paralytic poliomyelitis, and yet a full clinical recovery can occur. In approximately 25% of individuals with a history of acute paralytic poliomyelitis, a chronic progressive illness characterized by lower motor neuron dysfunction develops years later (Dalakas, 1995). This syndrome, originally termed an "overuse phenomenon," was first reported by Raymond and Charcot in 1875 (Raymond, 1875). They described a young man who had acute paralytic poliomyelitis at age 6 months, who developed unilateral arm and leg weakness at age 19 years. Sporadic cases with similar descriptions of new, progressive weakness in patients with remote poliomyelitis continued to be reported, sometimes with associated upper motor neuron findings and suggestions of an association with amyotrophic lateral sclerosis (ALS). In 1972, Anderson et al. (1972) described paralytic poliomyelitis survivors with diminished endurance caused by orthopedic deformities and associated arthralgias and myalgias. That same year, Mulder et al. (1972) described 32 patients with well-documented histories of acute paralytic poliomyelitis who many years later developed progressive weakness, not attributable to orthopedic deformities, and distinguishable from ALS. In these patients was seen a paucity of upper motor neuron findings, and a slower rate of deterioration. The observations of Anderson and Mulder were essential in the establishment of clinical criteria for postpolio syndrome (Dalakas, 1995).

Postpolio syndrome is a clinical diagnosis made in patients with a history of documented acute paralytic poliomyelitis. The acute illness is followed by partial recovery of motor function and functional stability or apparent recovery for several years. New symptoms of weakness or fatigue then develop. In a subset of these patients, the symptoms are caused by musculoskeletal deformities, as described by Anderson et al. (1972). Poliomyelitis survivors are predisposed to compression neuropathies and plexopathies from long-term use of wheelchairs, crutches, and braces. Pain, disuse atrophy, and diminished endurance can result from posture changes and joint deformities. These produce further deterioration and functional decline. Another subset, sometimes overlapping with the first, will develop new weakness and atrophy, typically but not exclusively in previously involved limbs. This is a lower motor neuron disease characterized by progressive muscular atrophy (Dalakas, 1995). Specific symptoms relate to the region or regions affected. Bulbar involvement is frequent, even in patients lacking a history of bulbar involvement during acute poliomyelitis. This can lead to dysphagia or respiratory insufficiency, as in other motor neuron diseases. Sleep apnea can also occur. The origin of the sleep apnea may be central, obstructive, or a combination of these (Dean et al., 1998; Hsu and Staats, 1998).

A variety of causes for postpolio syndrome have been considered. Histopathologic and electrophysiologic data indicate that a chronic state of ongoing denervation and reinnervation exists in patients following acute paralytic poliomyelitis. It has been postulated that a combination of unaffected and affected but partially or fully recovered neurons coexists in the postpolio bulbar motor nuclei and spinal cord. Recovery results from two predominant mechanisms: (*a*) recovered function in the injured neurons and (*b*) reinnervation of denervated muscle fibers by remaining motor neurons. The latter process results in group typing on muscle biopsy, and in large amplitude, long duration motor units on electromyelogram (EMG). Some neurons may be ineffective in maintaining sprouts to reinnervated fibers, leaving scattered denervated fibers. Others may succumb to premature cell death, leaving larger numbers of denervated fibers. When the balance of denervation outweighs reinnervation, weakness ensues (Dalakas, 1995). This progression in weakness is very slow. Some authors have shown that a statistical progression in weakness cannot be appreciated over a period of 3 years, but can be seen after 10 years (Dalakas, 1995).

Epidemiologic data suggest age is not a direct factor in the development of postpolio syndrome, but rather it is the length of time following acute poliomyelitis. This finding detracts from normal aging and motor neuron senescence as a cause of postpolio syndrome. High IgM GM-1 antiganglioside antibodies have been found in acute poliomyelitis and in postpolio syndrome, but a causal role for these antibodies has not been established. Limited endomysial and spinal cord inflammation has also been reported. Antibody and PCR studies have demonstrated evidence of persistent poliovirus infection in a minority of patients, leading to the hypothesis that persistent infection with mutated poliovirus may be the cause (Dalakas, 1995). However, it seems unlikely that ongoing viral replication and resultant cell death is the cause of postpolio syndrome.

A specific diagnostic test is lacking. Nerve conduction studies and needle EMG should be performed to exclude entrapment neuropathies, confirm the presence of a motor neuron disease, and exclude rare conditions such as multifocal motor neuropathy. Needle EMG changes are nonspecific. Fasciculation potentials and abnormal spontaneous activity (fibrillations and positive sharp waves) should be present, with superimposed changes of chronic denervation. These changes can be seen in all survivors of paralytic poliomyelitis, not simply those with postpolio syndrome. The presence of abnormal spontaneous activity does not establish a diagnosis of postpolio syndrome (Dalakas, 1995). Similar changes can also be seen in radiculopathies and in other motor neuron diseases. Single fiber EMG demonstrates increased jitter, which is consistent with a disorder of neuromuscular junction transmission and endplate instability (Dalakas, 1995). The serum creatinine kinase may be mildly to moderately elevated, as in many motor neuron diseases. The postpolio syndrome is distinguished from ALS by the history of acute paralytic polio, the relative paucity of upper motor neuron findings, and the slow rate of progressive weakness.

Clinical management of the postpolio syndrome centers on an exercise strengthening program, energy conservation, and attention to orthopedic and bracing issues as noted above. No medication has been shown to be effective in the direct treatment of progressive weakness. Moderate exercise has been shown to increase strength and endurance, and to reduce fatigue. Excessive exercise, however, can exacerbate symptoms (Agre et al., 1997; Agre, 1995). Although initially promising, amantadine, acetyl cholinesterase inhibitors, and prednisone have been shown to be ineffective in the treatment of postpolio syndrome (Stein et al., 1995; Trojan et al., 1999; Dinsmore et al., 1995). Specific neuropsychiatric abnormalities have not been demonstrated in patients with postpolio syndrome (Grafman et al., 1995). However, many patients have significant anxiety associated with their symptoms of fatigue, weakness, and atrophy. Attention to these concerns, sometimes with appropriate psychiatric treatment, is an essential part of overall treatment.

The clinical similarities of acute poliomyelitis and the postpolio syndrome have raised conjecture that sporadic ALS may have a viral etiology. Most studies do not support an association between poliovirus and ALS (Karpati and Dalakas, 2000). Other enteroviruses have been associated with acute paralytic disease, including echovirus and Coxsackie virus infections. However, their association with more chronic forms of motor neuron disease, such as ALS, has yet to be established. A recent study by Berger et al. (2000) found a highly significant correlation between the presence of enterovirus viral RNA and ALS, as studied by *in situ* reverse transcriptase PCR (RT-PCR) on postmortem spinal cords (Karpati and Dalakas, 2000). However, Walker et al. (2001), also using RT-PCR, found no evidence of echovirus RNA in postmortem spinal cord and motor cortex samples. This will likely be an ongoing area of research.

VIRAL INFECTIONS AND BRAIN TUMORS

Although brain tumors are seen in young and old, many (e.g., glioblastomas) are more common in the elderly. The cause of brain tumors remains unknown in most cases, and epidemiologic studies have failed to identify any relevant environmental factors associated with the production of brain tumors. Simian virus 40 (SV40), a papovavirus family member, can transform neural hamster cells and induce brain tumors after intracerebral inoculation (Duigou et al., 1990; Walsh et al., 1986). Genetic sequences from SV40 have been found in a number (35%) of brain tumors (Martini et al., 1996; Butel and Lednicky, 1999; Ohgaki et al., 2000). The SV40 large tumor antigen (Tag) may be found in even higher numbers of several brain tumors, and Tag complexes with tumor suppressor gene products can be found in a high percentage of these same tumors (Zhen et al., 1999). These findings suggest a possible link of SV40 with brain tumors in humans.

Polio vaccine used in the middle portion of the 20th century, however, was contaminated with SV40, prompting the question whether this contamination accounts for the association noted above. In Finland, where the contaminated vaccine was not used, SV40 DNA sequences are not seen in brain tumors, whereas 25% to 56% of brain tumors in Switzerland, which used the contaminated vaccine, do contain the SV40 sequences (Ohgaki et al., 2000). No selective increase in brain tumors is seen in countries where SV40-contaminated vaccine was used (Carbone et al., 1997). Thus, the relationship of SV40 to brain tumors remains unproved to date.

NEURODEGENERATIVE DISORDERS

Alzheimer's Disease

Alzheimer's disease is a chronic neurodegenerative disease of the elderly manifested by progressive decline in multiple areas of cognitive function. The cause of the disease is not known. Both spontaneous, acquired forms and inherited forms are seen, which are similar clinically except that age of onset tends to be younger in the inherited forms. Development of Alzheimer's disease has recently been linked to homozygous status of the apolipoprotein epsilon 4 (APOe4) gene (Roses, 1998). APOe4, a carrier of cholesterol, is found in neurons and other cells in the brain. Its function in the pathogenesis of Alzheimer's disease is incompletely understood, but may be linked to deposition of amyloid, a characteristic feature in the brains of patients with the disease.

The possibility of an environmental cause for sporadic Alzheimer's disease, including potential roles for aluminum toxicity and head trauma, has been explored in some detail, but no firm conclusions have been drawn (see Chapter 20). The possibility of aluminum toxicity has been raised and rejected, and head trauma appears to play a limited role.

Several of the human herpes viruses are known to infect neurons in the brain and to persist in neurons. Thus, they have been considered candidate viruses in Alzheimer's disease. In 1990, using *in situ* hybridization techniques, herpes simplex virus type 1 (HSV-1) RNA was detected significantly more often in the trigeminal ganglia of patients with Alzheimer's disease than in controls. However, no evidence of viral RNA was seen in the hippocampus of patients with extensive changes consistent with Alzheimer's disease (Deatly et al., 1990). Using the more sensitive technique of PCR, researchers have found viral DNA in the hippocampus and temporal cortex of two thirds of patients with Alzheimer's disease (Jamieson et al., 1992). Similarly, viral DNA can be detected in a variety of locations in the about 60% to 65% of brains of control patients, including the medulla, pons, olfactory bulbs, gyrus rectus, amygdala (Baringer and Pisani, 1994), and frontal temporal cortex (Jamieson et al., 1992). VZV DNA cannot be found in the brain with similar techniques (Lin et al., 1997).

The role of HSV-1 and its relationship to APOe4 has been further explored in a PCR study of patients with Alzheimer's disease and controls. The APOe4 allele frequency was significantly higher in patients with Alzheimer's disease positive for HSV-1 (53%) than in the HSV-1-negative group (10%), the HSV-1-positive non-Alzheimer's disease group (3.6%), or the HSV-1 negative non-Alzheimer's disease group (6.3%) (Itzhaki et al., 1997). This suggests the combination of HSV-1 and APOe4 is a strong risk factor for development of Alzheimer's disease, but the role either plays in the pathogenesis remains unclear.

One possible role for HSV-1 is implicated by significant homology of glycoprotein B (gB) of HSV-1 to carboxyl-terminal region of the A-beta peptide that accumulates in diffuse and neuritic plaques in Alzheimer's disease. This gB fragment forms beta-pleated sheets, self-assembles into thioflavin-positive fibrils indistinguishable from A-beta, accelerates the formation of A-beta fibrils *in vitro*, and is toxic to primary cortical neurons at doses comparable to those of A-beta (Cribbs et al., 2000). Other pathogenic possibilities remain to be explored. Thus, although the potential relationship of HSV-1 to Alzheimer's disease is unclear, this remains an active area of research.

Parkinson's Disease

The possibility of a viral etiology for Parkinson's disease was originally raised after the pandemic of von Economo's disease, so-called "encephalitis lethargica." Beginning in 1917, it was followed months to years later by an illness similar to Parkinson's disease. The etiology of von Economo's disease was never actually determined, but is assumed to be viral, based on the clinical syndrome, the presence of oligoclonal bands in the cerebrospinal fluid, and autopsy changes consistent with viral infection. The influenza A pandemic that followed von Economo's disease was a separate phenomenon, however, and was not clearly related to parkinsonism (Casals et al., 1998). Studies looking for evidence of an excess amount of influenza A antibodies in the postencephalitic patients with Parkinson's disease have been negative (Marttila and Rinne, 1976). Since von Economo's pandemic, only sporadic cases of a Parkinson's-like illness have been associated with viral illness (Casals et al., 1998; Marttila and Rinne, 1976; Wang et al., 1993; Peatfield, 1987; Picard et al., 1996). Measles infection in childhood has been associated with a decreased risk of developing Parkinson's disease, although the significance of this finding is unclear (Sasco and Paffenbarger, 1985).

More direct studies looking for evidence of a viral etiology of Parkinson's disease have also been pursued. Early attempts to visualize viral particles (Schwartz and Elizan, 1979) or detect viral DNA from influenza A or HSV-1 (Wetmur et al., 1979) in brains of those with Parkinson's disease were unsuccessful. One report identified possible antibodies to coronaviruses in the cerebrospinal fluid of patients with the disease (Fazzini et al., 1992). Antibodies to cytoplasmic dynein, however, have been shown to bind to neuronal cytoplasm and to the pathological Lewy bodies seen in patients with Parkinson's disease (Yamada et al., 1996). The significance of this in isolation is unclear. Overall, the evidence actually supporting the role of any virus is Parkinson's disease is sparse.

For more information on Parkinson's disease, see Chapter 22.

ACKNOWLEDGMENTS

The authors would like to thank Ms. Karen Klick for editorial assistance.

REFERENCES

Agre JC, Rodriquez AA, Franke TM. Strength, endurance, and work capacity after muscle strengthening exercise in postpolio subjects. *Arch Phys Med Rehabil* 1997;78: 681–686.

Agre JC. The role of exercise in the patient with post-polio syndrome. *Ann NY Acad Sci* 1995;753:321–334.

Anderson AD, Levine SA, Gellert H. Loss of ambulatory ability in patients with old anterior poliomyelitis. *Lancet* 1972;2:1061–1063.

Baringer JR, Pisani P. Herpes simplex virus genomes in human nervous system tissue analyzed by polymerase chain reaction. *Ann Neurol* 1994;36:823–829.

Berger MM, Kopp N, Vital C. Detection and cellular localization of enterovirus RNA sequences in spinal cord of patients with ALS. *Neurology* 2000;54:20–25.

Berger R, Florent G, Just M. Decrease of the lymphoproliferative response to varicella-zoster virus antigen in the aged. *Infect Immunol* 1981;32: 24–27.

Bernstein JE, Korman NJ, Bickers DR, et al. Topical capsaicin treatment of chronic postherpetic neuralgia. *J Am Acad Dermatol* 1989;21:265–270.

Beutner KR, Friedman DJ, Forszpaniak C, et al. Valacyclovir compared with acyclovir for improved therapy for herpes zoster in immunocompetent adults. *Antimicrob Agents Chemother* 1995;39:1546–1553.

Bowsher D. The effects of preemptive treatment of postherpetic neuralgia with amitriptyline: a randomized, double-blind, placebo-controlled trial. *J Pain Symptom Manage* 1997;13:327–331.

Burns EA, Goodwin JS. Immunodeficiency of aging. *Drug Aging* 1997;11:374–397.

Butel JS, Lednicky JA. Cell and molecular biology of simian virus 40: implications for human infections and disease. *J Natl Cancer Inst* 1999;91:119–134.

Candore G, Dilorenzo G, Mansueto P, et al. Prevalence of organ-specific and non organ-specific autoantibodies in healthy centenarians. *Mech Ageing Dev* 1997;94: 183–190.

Carbone M, Rizzo P, Pass HI. Simian virus 40, polio vaccines and human tumors: a review of recent developments. *Oncogene* 1997;15:1877–1888.

Casals J, Elizan TS, Yahr MD. Postencephalitic parkinsonism—a review. *J Neural Transm* 1998;105:645–676.

Cobo LM, Foulks GN, Liesegang T, et al. Oral acyclovir in the treatment of acute herpes zoster ophthalmicus. *Ophthalmology* 1986;93:763–770.

Colin J, Prisant O, Cochener B, et al. Comparison of the efficacy and safety of valacyclovir and acyclovir for the treatment of herpes zoster ophthalmicus. *Ophthalmology* 2000;107:1507–1511.

Cribbs DH, Azizeh BY, Cotman CW, et al. Fibril formation and neurotoxicity by a herpes simplex virus glycoprotein B fragment with homology to the Alzheimer's A beta peptide. *Biochemistry* 2000;39:5988–5994.

Dalakas MC. Pathogenetic mechanisms of post-polio syndrome: morphological, electrophysiological, virological, and immunological correlations. *Ann NY Acad Sci* 1995; 753:167–185.

Dalakas MC. Post-polio syndrome 12 years later. How it all started. *Ann NY Acad Sci* 1995;753:11–18.

Dalakas MC. The post-polio syndrome as an evoked clinical entity. Definition and clinical description. *Ann NY Acad Sci* 1995;25:68–80.

de Moragas JM, Kierland RR. The outcome of patients with herpes zoster. *Arch Dermatol* 1957;75:193–196.

Dean AC, Graham BA, Dalakas M, et al. Sleep apnea in patients with postpolio syndrome. *Ann Neurol* 1998;43: 661–664.

Deatly AM, Haase AT, Fewster PH, et al. Human herpes virus infections and Alzheimer's disease. *Neuropathol Appl Neurobiol* 1990;16:213–223.

Dinsmore S, Dambrosia J, Dalakas MC. A double-blind, placebo-controlled trial of high-dose prednisone for the treatment of post-poliomyelitis syndrome. *Ann NY Acad Sci* 1995;753:303–313.

Donahue JG, Choo PW, Manson JE, et al. The incidence of herpes zoster. *Arch Intern Med* 1995;155:1605–1609.

Doyle PW, Gibson G, Dohlman CL. Herpes zoster ophthalmicus with contralateral hemiplegia: identification of cause. *Ann Neurol* 1983;14:84–85.

Duigou GJ, Walsh JW, Oeltgen J, et al. Alterations in SV40 DNA integration patterns are associated with acquisition of the invasive phenotype in hamster brain tumors. *Anticancer Res* 1990;10:1683–1692.

Esmann V, Geil JP, Kroon S, et al. Prednisolone does not prevent post-herpetic neuralgia. *Lancet* 1987;2:126–129.

Fazzini E, Fleming J, Fahn S. Cerebrospinal fluid antibodies to coronavirus in patients with Parkinson's disease. *Mov Disord* 1992;7:153–158.

Galil K, Choo PW, Donahue JG, et al. The sequelae of herpes zoster. *Arch Intern Med* 1997;157:1209–1213.

Gilden DH, Kleinschmidt-DeMasters BK, LaGuardia JJ, et al. Neurologic complications of the reactivation of varicella-zoster virus. *N Engl J Med* 2000;342:635–645.

Gilden DH, Wright RR, Schneck SA, et al. Zoster sine herpete, a clinical variant. *Ann of Neurol* 1994;35:530–533.

Grafman J, Clark K, Richardson D, et al. Neuropsychology of post-polio syndrome. *Ann NY Acad Sci* 1995;753: 103–110.

Grant DM, Mauskopf JA, Bell L, et al. Comparison of valacyclovir and acyclovir for the treatment of herpes zoster in immunocompetent patients over 50 years of age: a cost-consequence model. *Pharmacotherapy* 1997;17:333–341.

Gromeier M, Lu HH, Wimmer E. Mouse neuropathogenic poliovirus strains cause damage in the central nervous system distinct from poliomyelitis. *Microb Pathog* 1995; 18:253–267.

Gromeier M, Wimmer E. Mechanism of injury-provoked poliomyelitis. *J Virol* 1998;72:5056–5060.

Gruger J, Backhouse ME. Economic evaluation of antiviral therapy for the treatment of herpes zoster in immunocompetent adults. *Pharmacoeconomics* 1997;11: 262–273.

Helgason S, Petursson G, Gudmundsson S, et al. Prevalence of postherpetic neuralgia after a first episode of herpes zoster: prospective study with long term follow-up. *BMJ* 2000;321:794–796.

Hogan EL, Krigman MR. Herpes zoster myelitis. Evidence for viral invasion of spinal cord. *Arch Neurol* 1973;29: 309–313.

Hsu AA, Staats BA. "Postpolio" sequelae and sleep-related disordered breathing. *Mayo Clin Proc* 1998;73:216–224.

Huse DM, Schainbaum S, Kirsch AJ, et al. Economic evaluation of famciclovir in reducing the duration of postherpetic neuralgia. *Am J Health Syst Pharm* 1997;54: 1880–1884.

Itzhaki RF, Lin WR, Shang D, et al. Herpes simplex virus type 1 in brain and risk of Alzheimer's disease. *Lancet* 1997;349:241–244.

Jackson JL, Gibbons R, Meyer G, et al. The effect of treating herpes zoster with oral acyclovir in preventing postherpetic neuralgia. A meta-analysis. *Arch Intern Med* 1997;157:909–912.

Jamieson GA, Maitland NJ, Wilcock GK, et al. Herpes simplex virus type 1 DNA is present in specific regions of brain from aged people with and without senile dementia of the Alzheimer type. *J Pathol* 1992;167:365–368.

Karpati G, Dalakas MC. Viral hide-and-seek in sporadic ALS. A new challenge. *Neurology* 2000;54:6–7.

Kijuchi A, Kotani N, Takamura K, et al. A comparative therapeutic evaluation of intrathecal versus epidural methylprednisolone for long-term analgesia in patients with intractable postherpetic neuralgia. *Reg Anesth Pain Med* 1999;24:287–293.

Kirshore-Kumar R, Max MB, Schafer SC, et al. Desipramine relieves postherpetic neuralgia. *Clin Pharmacol Ther* 1990;47:305–312.

Kotani N, Kushikata T, Hashimoto H, et al. Intrathecal methylprednisolone for intractable postherpetic neuralgia. *N Engl J Med* 2000;343:1514–1519.

Lin WR, Casas I, Wilcock GK, et al. Neurotropic viruses and Alzheimer's disease: a research for varicella zoster virus DNA by the polymerase chain reaction. *J Neurol Neurosurg Psychiatry* 1997;62:586–589.

MacKenzi RA, Forbes GS, Karnes WE. Angiographic findings in herpes zoster arteritis. *Ann Neurol* 1981;10: 458–464.

Marfin AA, Bleed DM, Lofgren JP, et al. Epidemiologic aspects of a St. Louis encephalitis epidemic in Jefferson County Arkansas 1991. *Am J Trop Med Hyg* 1993;49: 30–37.

Martini F, Iaccheri L, Lazzarin L, et al. SV40 early region and large T antigen in human brain tumors, peripheral blood cells, and sperm fluids from healthy individuals. *Cancer Res* 1996;56: 4820–4825.

Marttila RJ, Halonen P, Rinne UK. Influenza virus antibodies in Parkinsonism. Comparison of postencephalitic and idiopathic Parkinson patients and matched controls. *Arch Neurol* 1977;34:99–100.

Marttila RJ, Rinne UK. Arteriosclerosis, heredity, and some previous infections in the etiology of Parkinson's disease. A case-control study. *Clin Neurol Neurosurg* 1976;79: 46–56.

McKendrick MW, Care CC, Kudesia G, et al. Is VZV reactivation of a common cause of unexplained unilateral pain? Results of a prospective study of 57 patients. *J Infect* 1999;39:209–212.

Melanson M, Chalk C, Georgevich L, et al. Varicella-zoster virus DNA in CSF and arteries in delayed contralateral hemiplegia: evidence for viral invasion of cerebral arter-

ies. *Neurology* 1996;47:569–570.

Mulder DW, Rosenbaum RA, Layton DD. Late progression of poliomyelitis or forme fruste amyotrophic lateral sclerosis? *Mayo Clin Proc* 1972;47:756–761.

Murasko DM, Weiner P, Kaye D. Association of lack of mitogen-induced lymphocyte proliferation with increased mortality in the elderly. *Aging: Immunology and Infectious Disease.* 1988;1:1–23.

Neoh C, Harding SP, Saunders D, et al. Comparison of topical and oral acyclovir in early herpes zoster ophthalmicus. *Eye* 1994;8:688–691.

Ohgaki H, Huang H, Haltia M, et al. More about: cell and molecular biology of Simian Virus 40: implications for human infections and disease. *J Nat Cancer Inst* 2000;92: 495–497.

Okumura H, Kurland, LT, Waring SC. Amyotrophic lateral sclerosis and polio: is there an association? *Ann NY Acad Sci* 1995;753:245–256.

Pawelec G, Effros RB, Caruso C, et al. T cells and aging. *Front Biosci* 1999;4:D216–D269.

Peatfield RC. Basal ganglia damage and subcortical dementia after possible insidious Coxsackie virus encephalitis. *Acta Neurol Scand* 1987;76:340–345.

Picard F, de Saint-Martin A, Salmon E, et al. Postencephalitic stereotyped involuntary movements responsive to L-dopa. *Mov Disord* 1996;11:567–570.

Raymond M. Paralysie essentielle de l'enfance, atrophie musculaire consecutive. *Soc Biol* 1875;27:158.

Roberts-Thomson IC, Whittingham S, Youngchaiyud U, et al. Ageing, immune response and mortality. *Lancet* 1974; 2:368–370.

Roses AD. A new paradigm for clinical evaluations of dementia: Alzheimer disease and apolipoprotein E genotypes. *Genetics of Alzheimer Disease* 1998;37–66.

Rowbotham M, Harden N, Stacy B, et al. Gabapentin for the treatment of postherpetic neuralgia: a randomized controlled trial. *JAMA* 1998;280:1837–1842.

Rowbotham MC, Davies PS, Verkempinck C, et al. Lidocaine patch: double-blind controlled study of a new treatment method for post-herpetic neuralgia. *Pain* 1996;65: 39–44.

Sasco AJ, Paffenbarger RS Jr. Measles infection and Parkinson's disease. *Am J Epidemiol* 1985;122:1017–1031.

Schwartz J, Elizan TS. Search for viral particles and virus-specific products in idiopathic Parkinson disease brain material. *Ann Neurol* 1979;6:261–263.

Stein DP, Dambrosia JM, Dalakas MC. A double-blind, placebo-controlled trial of amantadine for the treatment of fatigue in patients with the post-polio syndrome. *Ann NY Acad Sci* 1995;753:296–302.

Tajti J, Szok D, Vecsei L. Topical acetylsalicylic acid versus lidocaine for postherpetic neuralgia: results of a double-blind comparative clinical trial. *Neurobiology* 1999;7: 103–108.

Trojan DA, Colet JP, Shapiro S, et al. A multicenter, randomized, double-blinded trial of pyridostigmine in postpolio syndrome. *Neurology* 1999;53:1225–1233.

Tyring S, Barbarash RA, Nahlik JE, et al. Famciclovir for the treatment of acute herpes zoster: effects on acute disease and postherpetic neuralgia. A randomized, double-blind, placebo-controlled trial. Collaborative famciclovir herpes zoster study group. *Ann Intern Med* 1995;123: 89–96.

Tyring SK, Beutner KR, Tucker BA, et al. Antiviral therapy for herpes zoster: randomized, controlled clinical trial of valacyclovir and famciclovir therapy in immunocompetent patients 50 years and older. *Arch Fam Med* 2000; 9:863–869.

Tyring SK. Efficacy of famciclovir in the treatment of herpes zoster. *Semin Dermatol* 1996;15:27–31.

Voets AJ, Tulner LR, Ligthart GJ. Immunosenescence revisited. Does it have any clinical significance? *Drugs Aging* 1997;11:1–6.

Volmink J, Lancaster T, Gray S, et al. Treatments for postherpetic neuralgia—a systematic review of randomized controlled trials. *Fam Pract* 1996;13:84–91.

Walker MP, Schlaberg R, Hays AP. Absence of echovirus sequences in brain and spinal cord of amyotrophic lateral sclerosis patients. *Ann Neurol* 2001;49:249–253.

Walsh JW, Zimmer SG, Oeltgen J, et al. Invasiveness in primary intracranial tumors. Part 1. An experimental model using cloned SV40 virus-produced hamster brain tumors. *Neurosurgery* 1986;19:185–200.

Wang WZ, Fang XH, Cheng XM, et al. A case-control study on the environmental risk factors of Parkinson's disease in Tianjin, China. *Neuroepidemiology* 1993;12:209–218.

Watson CP, Babul N. Efficacy of oxycodone in neuropathic pain: a randomized trial in postherpetic neuralgia. *Neurology* 1998;50:1837–1841.

Watson CP, Tyler KL, Bickers DR, et al. A randomized vehicle-controlled trial of topical capsaicin in the treatment of postherpetic neuralgia. *Clin Ther* 1993;15:510–526.

Watson CP, Vernich L, Chipman M, et al. Nortriptyline versus amitriptyline in postherpetic neuralgia: a randomized trial. *Neurology* 1998;51:1166–1171.

Watson CPN, Deck JH, Morshead C, et al. Post-herpetic neuralgia: further post-mortem studies of cases with and without pain. *Pain* 1991;44:105–117.

Wayne SL, Rhyne RL, Garry PJ, et al. Cell-mediated immunity as a predictor of morbidity and mortality in subjects over 60. *J Gerontol* 1990;45:45–48.

Wetmur JG, Schwartz J, Elizan TS. Nucleic acid homology studies of viral nucleic acids in idiopathic Parkinson's disease. *Arch Neurol* 1979;36:462–464.

Whitley RJ, Weiss H, Gnann JW, et al. Acyclovir with and without prednisone for the treatment of herpes zoster. A randomized, placebo-controlled trial. The National Institute of Allergy and Infectious Disease Collaborative Antiviral Study Group. *Ann Intern Med* 1996;125: 376–383.

Wood MJ, Johnson RW, McKendrick MW, et al. A randomized trial of acyclovir for 7 days or 21 days with and without prednisolone for treatment of acute herpes zoster. *N Engl J Med* 1994;330:896–900.

Wood MJ, Kay R, Dworkin RH, Soong SJ, et al. Oral acyclovir therapy accelerates pain resolution in patients with herpes zoster: a meta-analysis of placebo-controlled trials. *Clin Infect Dis* 1996;22:341–347.

Yamada T, Yamanaka I, Nakajima S. Immunohistochemistry of a cytoplasmic dynein (MAP 1C)-like molecule in rodent and human brain tissue: an example of molecular mimicry between cytoplasmic dynein and influenza A virus. *Acta Neuropathol (Berl)* 1996;92:306–311.

Zhang Y, Cosyns M, Levin MJ, et al. Cytokine production in varicella zoster virus-stimulated limiting dilution lymphocyte cultures. *Clin Exp Immunol* 1994;98: 128–133.

Zhen HN, Zhang X, Bu XY, et al. Expression of the simian virus 40 large tumor antigen (Tag) and formation of Tag-p53 and Tag-pRb complexes in human brain tumors. *Cancer* 1999;86:2124–2132.

28

Neuro-Oncology of the Elderly

Julie E. Hammack

INTRODUCTION

Cancer is the second leading cause of death in persons over 60 years of age. In 1997, more than 430,000 Americans over 60 years of age died of this disease. With the shift in demographics to a larger percentage of elderly and with improved prevention and treatment of heart disease and stroke, elderly patients with cancer will become even more prevalent in the new century. As many as 20% to 25% of patients with systemic cancer harbor intracranial metastases at the time of death and 5% of patients with systemic cancer develop epidural cord compression during the course of their illness. Applying these percentages to the statistics noted above indicates a very large number of patients presenting to their physicians with neurologic signs and symptoms directly related to their systemic malignancies.

Although primary brain tumors currently account for less than 2% of all malignancies in the elderly, their frequency has increased steadily over the last three decades. Some studies have estimated the increase in incidence in those over 65 years of age from 15% to 500% over periods ranging from 9 to 20 years (Blumenthal and DeAngelis, 1998; Lowry et al., 1998). The increased incidence is particularly pronounced in the extreme elderly (≥85 years). The cause of this troubling increase is unclear. It may be caused, at least partially, by the widespread availability of sophisticated neuroimaging and increased access to specialized medical care for the elderly over the last 30 years. These advances alone, however, do not fully account for this trend. The incidence of primary malignant brain tumors started to rise even before the introduction of computed tomography (CT) scanning in the early 1970s and the trend continues to increase even since the 1980s, when CT scanning capability became standard in most medical facilities (Werner et al., 1995).

Neuro-oncology is the study of cancer's effects on the central and peripheral nervous system. This includes direct involvement of the nervous system by tumor and so-called "remote effects," which broadly include paraneoplastic disorders, cerebrovascular complications, infections, and toxic or metabolic disorders that can be secondary effects of cancer or its treatment. Table 28-1 lists the various categories of neurologic illness seen in patients with cancer.

This chapter focuses on the primary and metastatic tumors of the brain and spinal cord most commonly seen in the older adult. A section in this chapter outlines the well-described, although rare, paraneoplastic neurologic disorders.

CLASSIFICATION

Brain and spinal tumors can be broadly classified as either primary (tumor arising from cells of the brain and spinal cord or their coverings) or metastatic (tumor spread from other primary sites within the body). By definition, metastatic tumors are always malignant. Primary tumors can be benign or malignant, depending on the underlying histopathology. Overall, metastatic brain tumors are those brain tumors most commonly seen in elderly patients. Although in a patient presenting with a new, solitary brain neoplasm and no history of systemic cancer, a primary tumor is the more likely diagnosis.

Among primary brain tumors, most series suggest that meningioma is most common, followed by malignant (high-grade) glioma, pituitary adenoma, schwannoma (including acoustic neuroma), low-grade glioma, and primary central nervous system (CNS) lymphoma (PCNSL).

METASTATIC TUMORS

Brain Metastases

Among older adults, metastatic tumors are more common than primary brain tumors, occurring in 20% to 25% of all patients dying of cancer, based on autopsy series (Pickren et al., 1983; Posner and Chernik, 1978). Virtually any systemic tumor can metastasize to the brain. Breast and lung cancers are

TABLE 28-1. *Neurologic illnesses in patients with cancer*

Direct tumor involvement	Brain or cord parenchymal metastases
	Meningeal metastases
	Dural metastases
	Epidural metastases
	Plexus metastases
	Peripheral nerve metastases
Toxic metabolic disorders	Liver or renal disease
	Electrolyte disturbances (SIADH)
	Hypercalcemia
	Hypomagnesemia
	Hypothyroidism
	Chemotherapy toxicity
	Opioid toxicity
	Corticosteroid toxicity
Vascular disorders	Nonbacterial thrombotic endocarditis
	Disseminated intravascular coagulation
	Hyperviscosity syndrome
	Thrombocytopenia
	Hypercoagulable state
	Dural sinus thrombosis
	Tumor embolus
	Tumor hemorrhage
Infection	*Listeria monocytogenes*
	Cryptococcus neoformans
	Aspergillus fumigatus
	Mucor
	Herpes zoster
	JC virus
	Cytomegalovirus
	Toxoplasmosis
Adverse effects of therapy	Radiation encephalopathy
	Radiation myelopathy
	Radiation plexopathy/radiculopathy
	Chemotherapy-induced encephalopathy
	Chemotherapy-induced neuropathy
	Steroid psychosis
	Steroid myopathy
	Phantom limb syndrome
	Postmastectomy pain syndrome
	Postthoracotomy syndrome
Paraneoplastic syndromes	Lambert-Eaton myasthenic syndrome
	Myasthenia gravis
	Paraneoplastic cerebellar degeneration
	Paraneoplastic limbic encephalitis
	Paraneoplastic sensory neuropathy
	Opsoclonus-myoclonus syndrome
	Polymyositis/dermatomyositis

SIADH, syndrome of inappropriate antidiuretic hormone.

the commonest systemic tumors and, therefore, account for most brain metastases. Some less common malignancies have a special proclivity to metastasize to the brain. Thus, although melanoma accounts for only 1% of systemic tumors, it has accounted for as much as 10% of brain metastases and as many as 40% of patients with melanoma were found to harbor brain metastases at autopsy (Amer et al., 1978). Small cell lung cancer is more than twice as likely to metastasize to the brain as other types of lung cancer.

Some evidence indicates that the incidence of metastatic brain tumors is increasing (Pickren et al., 1983; Posner and Chernik, 1978). This is likely caused by a combination of factors: (*a*) Sophisticated neuroimaging allows diagnosis of brain metastases even at an asymptomatic stage; (*b*) improved treatment of the systemic cancer means that patients are living longer and have more opportunities to develop brain metastases; and (*c*) the CNS appears to be a "sanctuary" from the effects of chemotherapy, allowing brain metastases to grow, even when systemic tumor is controlled.

The pathogenesis is hematogenous tumor spread in most patients. In more than 50% of cases, the lesions are multiple. The "watershed" region of the cerebral hemispheres is the most likely site of metastases, and the corticomedullary junction the most common point of origin (Delattre, Krol et al., 1988). These pathologic data suggest that arterial tumor microemboli lodge in the distal capillary arcades of the cerebral arteries. Supratentorial metastases are distinctly more common than infratentorial (90% vs. 10%) in patients with breast and lung cancer. The metastases are more evenly divided between the supra- and infratentorial compartment in patients with colon cancer and uterine cancer. This suggests a possible role of metastasis via Batson's venous plexus, although some studies refute that hypothesis (Delattre, Krol et al., 1988; O'Neill et al., 1994).

Clinical Presentation

Most brain metastases (80%) occur in patients in whom the diagnosis of systemic malignancy is already established. The clinical presentation varies considerably among individuals and largely depends on the location of the brain metastasis or metastases. In younger patients, the most common symptoms are headache and seizure. Among elderly patients, focal deficits (e.g., hemiparesis and aphasia) and cognitive changes are distinctly more common, perhaps because older brains have more atrophy and room to accommodate an expanding mass lesion. It is not clear why elderly patients are less likely to present with seizures. Perhaps the seizure threshold of the elderly brain is higher.

Not infrequently, elderly patients with brain metastases are misdiagnosed as having a "stroke." This is especially common in patients who do not have a previous diagnosis of a primary tumor or in those who present with very acute symptomatology. Focal seizure or tumor hemorrhage can both masquerade clinically as a stroke. The diagnosis usually is not difficult if a careful history is taken and neuroimaging used appropriately.

Diagnosis

A CT of the head with contrast is sufficient in most cases to make the diagnosis of brain metastases. It is less expensive than magnetic resonance imaging (MRI) and easier to perform on a patient who is confused or uncooperative. In patients whose condition is deteriorating rapidly, CT is adequate to diagnose secondary conditions such as obstructive hydrocephalus and tumor hemorrhage. Extra care must be taken in elderly patients to ensure that their renal function is adequate to handle the iodinated contrast. Approximately 5% of patients will have an allergic reaction to the contrast dye, which can precipitate focal seizures in as many as 15% of patients with brain metastases. MRI with contrast is more sensitive, particularly for small brain metastases. It is also more expensive and requires more patient cooperation.

Both CT and MRI demonstrate enhancing lesions, typically with central necrosis. Metastases are usually multiple, which can be better appreciated on MRI when the lesions are tiny. Typically in brain metastases, the lesions are well circumscribed and have a disproportionate amount of edema than expected for the size of the enhancing lesion (Fig. 28-1). These features distinguish them radiographically from primary brain tumors, which tend to be more diffuse and have a pattern of edema that more closely approximates the area of enhancement. Rarely, brain abscess mimics the appearance of metastases.

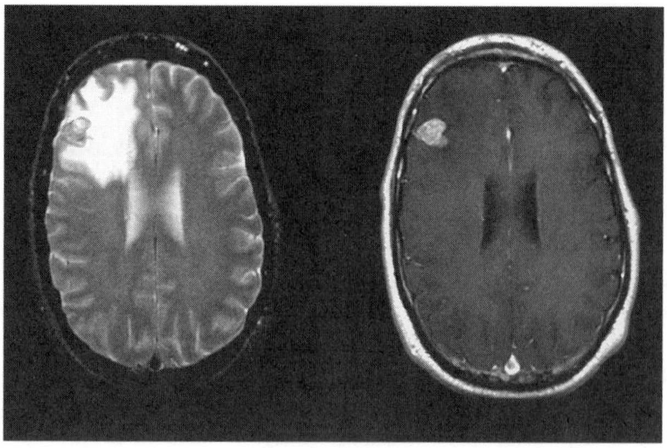

FIG. 28-1. Brain metastasis. Axial magnetic resonance image of the head: T_2-weighted image (**left**) and T_1-weighted image with gadolinium contrast (**right**). Note the large amount of edema, compared to the lesion's size.

In patients who have known metastatic systemic cancer, the diagnosis is generally made radiographically and pathologic confirmation may not be required before treatment. The situation is more problematic in patients without a known primary malignancy. If the radiographic picture is suggestive of metastatic tumor, a careful search for systemic malignancy should be undertaken. This begins with a thorough physical examination, followed by appropriate blood tests and imaging procedures. Lung, breast, skin, and the gastrointestinal system are the most common sources of a primary malignancy in these cases. If no primary tumor can be found, then surgical biopsy or resection of one of the brain lesions is appropriate to make a diagnosis.

Treatment

Although the approach to treatment can vary, depending on the individual patient and type of malignancy, some interventions apply to all. Corticosteroids reduce peritumoral edema and can significantly reduce headache from raised intracranial pressure and may improve neurologic deficits produced by tumor mass effect. Approximately 30% to 40% of patients with brain metastases will have seizures at some point in their illness. This figure is higher among patient with hemorrhagic metastases and those with metastatic melanoma, in whom it is greater than 50% (Byrne et al., 1983). Any patient who has had a seizure should receive anticonvulsants, as should those patients with metastatic melanoma. Otherwise, prophylactic anticonvulsants are best avoided as they interact with corticosteroids and various chemotherapy agents. Both phenytoin and carbamazepine can cause Stevens-Johnson syndrome, particularly in those receiving whole brain radiation therapy (WBRT) (Delattre, Safai et al., 1988). Moreover, no significant reduction in the incidence of seizures has been seen in patients who received prophylactic anticonvulsants (Glantz et al., 1996).

Surgery

In patients with multiple lesions, surgery is limited to those who lack a known primary tumor. In this situation, biopsy without resection is appropriate to make a pathologic diagnosis. More extensive surgery is indicated in selected situations. For instance, in a patient with a large cerebellar metastasis obstructing the fourth ventricle, a resection of the offending metastasis may be life saving and allow the patient to tolerate WBRT without brain herniation. Data suggest that patients who have a surgically accessible solitary metastasis (as proved on enhanced MRI) and limited systemic cancer survive longer with less neurologic disability if they have resection of their metastasis (Patchell et al., 1990; Vecht et al., 1993). Surgery is a further consideration in patients with a recurrent metastasis after WBRT has been administered or in those with tumors that are known to be radiation resistant.

Radiation Therapy

WBRT is the mainstay of treatment for most patients with brain metastases. It prolongs survival but is not considered curative. Most patients with brain metastases will die of progressive systemic cancer, not brain disease. The treatment is given to ports encompassing the whole brain, to a total dose of 2,000 to 3,000 cGy in 10 to 15 fractions. More accelerated radiation schedules may be appropriate in very frail patients with a short life expectancy. WBRT is usually well tolerated. Radiation-induced tumor swelling is best managed with corticosteroids. If they survive more than 6 to 12 months, elderly patients can be particularly susceptible to develop radiation encephalopathy. This is characterized by subcortical dementia with gait apraxia and urinary incontinence. CT and MRI demonstrate cortical atrophy, hydrocephalus *ex vacuo*, and diffuse white matter changes. More localized radiation, including gamma knife and stereotactic linear accelerator therapy, is probably best reserved for small recurrent brain metastases. The role of these latter therapies in the primary treatment of brain metastases remains to be determined.

Chemotherapy

Most chemotherapy agents do not penetrate the blood–brain barrier well. With rare exception, chemotherapy agents have little efficacy in the treatment of brain metastases.

Prognosis

Once brain metastases have developed, the patient's cancer, with rare exception, has reached an incurable stage. Without treatment, life expectancy is usually less than 4 to 6 weeks and most patients die from their neurologic disease. With radiation therapy, survival extends to a median of 3 to 6 months. Most treated patients will die of progressive systemic cancer, not of brain metastases. Long-term survival (>1 year) is exceedingly rare among elderly patients.

Epidural Cord Compression

Tumor in the epidural space usually has spread from the adjacent vertebra. Vertebral metastases are common, occurring in 25% to 70% of patients with metastatic cancer (Galasko, 1981). The thoracic spine is particularly susceptible, as it makes up the largest bony mass of the spine. The solid tumors that most commonly metastasize to the vertebra, are lung, breast, prostate, renal, and thyroid cancer. Myeloma is the most common hematopoietic tumor to produce epidural cord compression. Tumor can invade the epidural space through the intervertebral foramen, without direct invasion of bone. The latter mechanism is seen in lymphomas arising from the paraspinal lymph nodes. Clinical signs of epidural cord or cauda equina compression can develop in as many as 5% to 10% of patients with metastatic cancer.

Clinical Presentation

Pain, the most common initial symptom, is present in 95% of patients at presentation to the physician (Portenoy et al., 1987). The pain can derive from the bony vertebral involvement or from compression of spinal roots. Vertebral pain is usually sharp or dull and localized over the involved vertebra and worse with activities that stress the spine, such as standing and twisting. Bone pain is typically worse at night. Radicular pain is sharp and lancinating and is distributed along the root's cutaneous dermatome. Radicular pain can also be worse with movement and with Valsalva maneuvers. Bone and radicular pain often precede neurologic deficits by weeks or months.

Neurologic deficits can develop acutely or subacutely and depend on the spinal level of involvement. Epidural tumor in the cervical and thoracic region will produce a myelopathy with spastic limb weakness, sensory level to pain and temperature and loss of bowel, bladder, and sexual function. Lhermitte's phenomenon may occur in patients with epidural tumors in the cervical or thoracic region. Compression of the thecal sac below L2 will produce a cauda equina syndrome with flaccid paraparesis, saddle distribution sensory loss, and loss of bowel, bladder and sexual function. Epidural cord and cauda equina compression constitutes a neurologic emergency. Once neurologic function is lost, it may not be regained, despite appropriate treatment. Diagnosis and treatment, therefore, should proceed as quickly as possible.

Diagnosis

Although a plain x-ray study of the spine can identify the vertebral lesion in approximately 80% to 90%

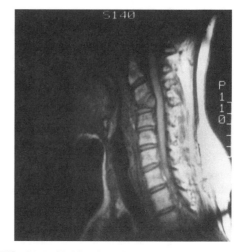

FIG. 28-2. Epidural cord compression from vertebral metastasis (lung primary). Sagittal magnetic resonance image of the cervical spine: T$_1$-weighted image without contrast showing malignant involvement of C3 vertebra with compression fracture and extension of tumor into the epidural space with compression of the cord.

of patients with epidural tumor (Portenoy et al., 1989), it does not visualize the epidural space. MRI of the spine is superior in this regard and has largely replaced myelography, except for cases in which MRI cannot be performed (i.e., patients with cardiac pacemakers). MRI will demonstrate the level of vertebral and epidural involvement and confirm the presence of cord or cauda equina compression (Fig. 28-2). In addition to the spinal level of clinical interest, it is generally recommended that the entire spine be visualized with sagittal MRI views to rule out other levels of subclinical epidural involvement. As many as 30% of patients may have other levels of epidural involvement on MRI that are not suspected clinically (Schiff et al., 1998).

Treatment

If epidural cord or cauda equina compression is clinically suspected, the patient should immediately be given high dose intravenous corticosteroids. Dexamethasone (100 mg) is the treatment of choice. This reduces tumor swelling and spinal cord edema. It may prevent neurologic deterioration while the patient is awaiting diagnostic procedures and more definitive treatment. Side effects of high dose steroids include manic psychosis, insomnia, and hyperglycemia. Hiccoughs are extremely common. If the dexamethasone is given as an i.v. bolus, 50% of patients will experience intense but short-lasting perineal burning (Baharav et al., 1986). This effect is self-limited, but patients should be warned before the steroids are given as a bolus.

In those patients with a histologically proved primary malignancy, emergent radiation therapy to the spine is the most appropriate treatment, in most instances. Generally, the treatment is given in 10 to 15 fractions to a maximum dose of 2,000 to 3,000 cGy. The radiation ports usually encompass two levels above and below the area of epidural tumor. Most patients should continue to receive corticosteroids during the radiation therapy on a tapering schedule. Surgical intervention may be appropriate in patients without a tumor diagnosis, those who have received previous radiation to the spine, and those with radiation-resistant tumors. Surgical procedures to remove epidural tumor are often extensive, requiring vertebral resection and spinal fusion. Not surprisingly, these aggressive procedures are often not appropriate for frail, elderly patients. Patients with recurrent or progressive epidural tumor in a previously radiated area may be candidates for a second course of radiation, if surgery is not feasible. In this instance, repeat radiation appears to carry a minimal risk of radiation myelopathy (Schiff et al., 1995).

Prognosis

The presence of bony metastases implies advanced cancer and most patients will die within 6 to 12 months of their systemic malignancy. The presence of epidural tumor will not usually hasten death unless the patient develops a complication of paralysis, such as deep venous thrombosis and pulmonary embolus, urosepsis from neurogenic bladder, or sepsis from decubitus ulcers. Timely diagnosis and treatment of epidural cord compression will reduce the likelihood that the patient will spend his or her remaining days wheelchair bound and dependent on others. If treatment is given before the development of severe neurologic dysfunction, the prognosis for neurologic recovery or maintenance of function is good. If treatment is not begun until after the patient is paraplegic and incontinent, then it is highly unlikely that steroids and radiation will bring recovery of function.

Leptomeningeal Metastases

Leptomeningeal metastases are much less common than intraparenchymal brain and epidural cord metastases, but they still account for significant neurologic morbidity. The tumors that most commonly invade the leptomeninges are leukemia (particularly acute lymphoblastic leukemia), lymphoma, breast, lung, and melanoma. The incidence of leptomeningeal metastases has declined in leukemias and lymphomas, coincident with the use of "prophylactic" intrathecal chemotherapy. Data suggest that the incidence may be increasing in patients with solid tumors (e.g., breast and lung). The most likely reason for this is improved systemic chemotherapy, which allows patients to live longer, but which does not penetrate the blood–brain barrier, allowing a sanctuary for tumor cells. The most likely mode of entry is hematogenous, although tumor cells can enter the cerebrospinal fluid (CSF) from intraparenchymal brain metastases adjacent to the pial or ependymal surface of the brain.

Clinical Presentation

Leptomeningeal tumor can involve the CNS at the supratentorial, posterior fossa, or spinal level and may involve all three levels simultaneously. Within the supratentorial compartment and posterior fossa, typical signs and symptoms include headache, cognitive decline, visual loss, diplopia, facial pain and anesthesia, dysarthria, hearing loss and tinnitus, dysphagia, and ataxia. Papilledema may be present, either as a result of hydrocephalus and raised intracranial pressure or from direct optic nerve infiltration. At the spinal level, multiple painful radiculopathies are common, occasionally with evidence of a myelopathy. The basal meninges of the brain and cauda equina are most commonly involved, presumably because gravity causes the cancer cells to settle in the most dependent CSF spaces.

Diagnosis

A contrasted MRI of the clinically involved area is the most useful imaging procedure. It often demonstrates diffuse or nodular linear enhancement of the basal meninges, surface of the spinal cord, and spinal roots (Fig. 28-3). Communicating hydrocephalus may be present, caused by obstruction of CSF egress in the basal meninges or arachnoid granulations. A normal contrast MRI of the head or spine does not exclude the diagnosis.

The definitive diagnostic procedure is examination of the CSF for malignant cells. Multiple lumbar punctures may be required to isolate malignant cells on cytologic examination (Balm and Hammack, 1996; Wasserstrom et al., 1982). Virtually all patients will have some abnormality in the CSF: elevated opening

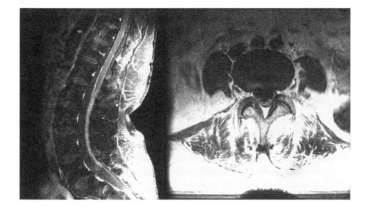

FIG. 28-3. Leptomeningeal metastases (breast primary). Sagittal and axial magnetic resonance image of the lumbar spine: T_1-weighted images with gadolinium contrast demonstrating diffuse pial enhancement of the cord and enhancement and thickening of the lumbosacral roots.

pressure, elevated protein level, low glucose, elevated nucleated cell count, or CSF tumor marker (i.e., carcinoembryonic antigen). If lymphoma is suspected, the CSF cytologic examination should include T- and B-cell surface markers to look for a monoclonal population of B cells, which is typical of lymphoma. The lumbar puncture will help exclude other disorders (e.g., fungal and tubercular meningitis) and granulomatous diseases that can present in a similar fashion.

Treatment

Although spread of lymphoma and leukemia to the leptomeninges is a poor prognostic indicator, occasionally it is possible to clear the CSF of cancer cells with a combination of intra-CSF chemotherapy (methotrexate or cytosine arabinoside [AraC]) and radiation therapy. In patients with carcinoma, however, treatment is considered palliative. Most patients with leptomeningeal carcinoma also have advanced systemic malignancy. Generally, it is appropriate to administer radiation therapy to the symptomatic areas only, in the hope of improving or maintaining neurologic function. Attempting to radiate the entire neuraxis will not rid the CSF of tumor cells, and will produce significant myelosuppression. Some patients with leptomeningeal carcinoma may benefit from the addition of intra-CSF chemotherapy (methotrexate, AraC, or thiotepa) given either by lumbar puncture or Ommaya reservoir. Usually, this treatment is best reserved for patients with limited systemic cancer and good performance status.

Prognosis

When carcinomas spread to the meninges, it portends a very poor prognosis. Without treatment, survival is usually less than 1 month. About one half of these patients die from complications of their neurologic illness, such as aspiration pneumonia and pulmonary embolus. The other half die from progression of their systemic cancer. Most patients with leptomeningeal carcinoma have extensive systemic tumor at the time the neurologic disease is diagnosed. Even with radiation or intra-CSF chemotherapy, the median survival is only 3 to 6 months from the onset of neurologic symptoms in most patients (Balm and Hammack, 1996).

PARANEOPLASTIC NEUROLOGIC SYNDROMES

Paraneoplastic neurologic disease refers to disorders seen in association with systemic malignancy that are not caused by direct tumor involvement or by other toxic or metabolic, infectious, and vascular complications of cancer. Most of these disorders affect the central or peripheral nervous system in a specific clinical pattern and are believed to be of autoimmune origin. These are rare disorders that occur in less than 1% of patients with systemic cancer. It is important to rule out metastatic tumor and other neurologic complications of cancer before making the diagnosis of a paraneoplastic syndrome. It is important to include the possibility of paraneoplastic disease in the differential diagnosis of patients with cancer and neurologic disease and even to consider these disorders in patients without a history of cancer. As many as 60% of patients with paraneoplastic neurologic disease do not have a previous diagnosis of malignancy. In these patients, the neurologic syndrome heralds the diagnosis of cancer.

This section deals with the most common and best described paraneoplastic syndromes, including paraneoplastic cerebellar degeneration (PCD), paraneoplastic encephalomyelitis/paraneoplastic sensory neuronopathy (PEM/PSN), paraneoplastic opsoclonus myoclonus (POM), and Lambert Eaton myasthenic syndrome (LEMS). Much overlap exists between these syndromes and many patients present with clinical features of two or more syndromes.

Most patients with these disorders have an identifiable antineuronal antibody specific to their paraneoplastic syndrome. In one disorder, LEMS, the antibody (anti-VGCC) is known to be pathogenic. In the other syndromes, the antibodies serve as a marker for the underlying tumor but have not been shown to produce the syndrome when transferred to laboratory animals. In each of these disorders, it is believed that the systemic tumor cell expresses an "onconeural antigen," which produces an immune response in the patient. This onconeural antigen shares similarities to antigens normally expressed by specific neural tissue. The host immune response (cell-mediated and humoral) then attacks both the tumor and the specific neural tissue that shares antigenic similarity. This theory is strengthened by the fact that patients' tumors often share antigenic similarities with neural tissue and by the frequent observation that patients with paraneoplastic neurologic disease often have limited or no metastatic disease and small primary tumors. The latter observation suggests that the immune response to tumor may be particularly strong in these patients.

Paraneoplastic Cerebellar Degeneration

PCD is the best described and possibly the most common autoimmune paraneoplastic disorder. Clinically, it is characterized by the subacute onset of pancerebellar and brainstem signs and symptoms. Vertigo, nausea, gait and limb ataxia, dysarthria, nystagmus, and diplopia evolving over days or weeks are the most common clinical features. At the time of diagnosis, the patient is usually severely disabled and nonambulatory. Occasionally, PCD overlaps with some of the other paraneoplastic syndromes, and evidence of limbic encephalitis, LEMS, opsoclonus, and sensory neuronopathy may be present.

Most commonly seen in women, PCD is associated with breast, ovarian, uterine, and fallopian tube cancers. PCD is also seen in association with small cell lung cancer, Hodgkin's lymphoma, and a host of other malignancies (Posner, 1995). Pathologically, PCD is characterized by diffuse severe loss of Purkinje's cells in the cerebellar cortex with associated astrocytic gliosis. Inflammatory changes are rarely seen, but may be present in the meninges or deep cerebellar nuclei.

Diagnosis

Early in the course of the illness, CT and MRI of the head may be normal. These studies are essential to exclude other causes of cerebellar dysfunction, including tumor, abscess, infarct, and demyelinating disease. After several months, marked cerebellar atrophy is usually present in patients with PCD (Fig. 28-4). CSF is abnormal in 50% of patients showing nonspecific abnormalities, including lymphocytic pleocytosis and elevated protein (Hammack et al., 1990).

The presence of antineuronal antibodies in the serum and CSF is extremely helpful in making the diagnosis of PCD. These antibodies are highly specific for the presence of an underlying tumor, but their absence does not exclude the possibility of a paraneoplastic cause. Anti-Yo (APCA) is found in the serum and CSF of patients with breast and gynecologic malignancies and PCD. This antibody is specific for the cytoplasm of the Purkinje's cell and appears to bind to proteins that regulate DNA transcription and protein synthesis. Anti-Yo has been shown to react with patients' own tumors but not with similar tumors from patients without PCD (Furneaux et al., 1990). Anti-Hu (ANNA-1) is an antibody seen in patients with PCD and small cell lung cancer (see below). Anti-Tr is an antibody reactive with Purkinje's cell cytoplasm seen in some patients with Hodgkin's disease and PCD. These antibodies have not been shown to be pathogenic and should be considered as markers for their underlying tumors. They are extremely helpful, when present in the serum or CSF, in confirming the

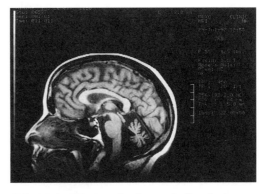

FIG. 28-4. Paraneoplastic cerebellar degeneration. Sagittal magnetic resonance image of the head: T$_1$-weighted image without gadolinium demonstrating marked cerebellar atrophy.

diagnosis of PCD and leading the search for the underlying malignancy if it is unknown.

If PCD is suspected, a complete search for underlying cancer is warranted. A complete medical history and physical examination are appropriate starting points. Investigations may include a CT of the chest, abdomen, and pelvis, and in women, a mammogram.

Treatment and Results

Unfortunately, no good treatment currently exists for PCD. Immunosuppressive therapy with corticosteroids, plasma exchange, intravenous immunoglobulin (IVIG), and cyclophosphamide has been largely unsuccessful. Occasionally, treating the underlying malignancy produces improvement, but this too is rare, which may be because injury and death of Purkinje's cells is rapid and probably completed by the time the diagnosis is made. Most patients are permanently and severely disabled by this syndrome and, thus, derive little benefit from the observation that their tumors are often less aggressive than expected (Hetzel et al., 1990).

Paraneoplastic Encephalomyelitis/Paraneoplastic Sensory Neuronopathy

PEM/PSN is a disorder that encompasses several syndromes affecting different areas of the nervous system, including the cerebellum, brainstem, cerebral hemispheres, spinal cord, and dorsal root ganglia. Pathologically, it is characterized by perivascular and parenchymal inflammation within multiple areas of the CNS. PEM/PSN is most commonly associated with lung carcinoma (particularly small cell), but has been reported with numerous other malignancies as well. As with PCD, the neurologic syndrome precedes the diagnosis of cancer in most patients (Lucchinetti et al., 1998).

The clinical manifestations depend on the area of involvement and a given patient often develops signs and symptoms reflecting multifocal involvement of the nervous system. Limbic encephalopathy with subacute dementia, mood changes, and seizures is common, as is a pancerebellar syndrome, which can be clinically identical to that seen with PCD. Another clinical presentation is a rapidly ascending myelopathy with evidence of upper and lower motor neuron dysfunction, incontinence, and rising sensory level. Patients with dorsal root ganglionitis present with severe sensory ataxia, pseudoathetosis, painful paresthesiae, and signs of autonomic dysfunction. A small percentage of patients with PEM/PSN will also develop LEMS.

Diagnosis

The results of neuroimaging are usually normal, although some patients have been reported to have nonspecific T_2 signal abnormalities, with minimal or no enhancement within the temporal lobes, brainstem, or spinal cord. The CSF usually shows nonspecific inflammation with a lymphocytic pleocytosis and elevated protein level, but it may be normal. In patients with limbic encephalopathy, the electroencephalogram may show epileptiform changes, diffuse slowing, or both. Nerve conduction studies will show markedly reduced or absent sensory nerve action potentials in patients with PSN. Occasionally, reduction is seen in the compound muscle action potentials (CMAP) and evidence of denervation on needle examination.

The anti-Hu (ANNA-1) antibody is present in the serum and CSF of some patients with PEM/PSN. The antibody indicates that the patient likely harbors a bronchogenic carcinoma (usually small cell) (Dalmau et al., 1992). Anti-Yo, anti-Ri, and anti-Ta, other antibodies that may be present in PEM/PSN, indicate underlying gynecologic, breast, and testicular tumors, respectively. Many patients with PEM/PSN will not have serum or CSF antibodies, and their absence does not exclude the possibility of paraneoplastic disease.

A careful search for malignancy is required in any patient in whom PEM/PSN is suspected. If one of the specific antibodies is present, this will guide the search. If the patient is seronegative, a CT of the chest, abdomen, and pelvis is indicated in all patients. In men, a testicular ultrasound is advisable and women should have a mammogram.

Treatment and Results

With most patients, the PEM/PSN disorder will progress rapidly over a period of weeks, to the point of severe disability, and then stabilize. Some patients may die of complications of their neurologic illness such as aspiration and pulmonary embolus. Most patients will not respond to immunosuppressive therapy or plasmapheresis. Rarely, clinical improvement will occur if the underlying malignancy is discovered and treated. This seems to be particularly true in patients with PEM and testicular cancer.

Paraneoplastic Opsoclonus Myoclonus

POM, a rare but fascinating disorder, presumedly is caused by an autoimmune injury to the brainstem pause cells controlling conjugate ocular movement.

Affected patients have spontaneous, chaotic, conjugate vertical, and horizontal eye movements that are worse with fixation. These movements persist during sleep and eye closure. Cerebellar ataxia, myoclonus, and evidence of more diffuse CNS involvement may be present with dementia or altered sensorium. In adults, this syndrome is most commonly associated with small cell lung cancer and breast cancer. Most patients develop the neurologic syndrome before the diagnosis of cancer.

As with other paraneoplastic syndromes, the neuroimaging and CSF examination are either normal or nonspecifically abnormal. Patients with small cell lung cancer usually have anti-Hu antibody in the serum, CSF, or both and patients with breast cancer are typically seropositive for anti-Ri. A careful search for malignancy is warranted, as these patients seem more likely to improve neurologically with treatment of their cancers than other patients with paraneoplastic syndromes. As with other paraneoplastic syndromes, immunosuppressive therapy does not appear to be effective.

Lambert Eaton Myasthenic Syndrome

LEMS is the only neurologic paraneoplastic disorder in which circulating antibodies have been demonstrated to produce clinical disease. The antibodies are directed against the voltage-gated calcium channel (VGCC) on the presynaptic motor nerve terminal. These calcium channels are involved in the release of acetylcholine at the neuromuscular junction, and their blockade results in muscle weakness that improves somewhat with repeated muscle contraction (facilitation). Acetylcholine release at other sites (muscarinic and nicotinic) in the peripheral nervous system is affected, resulting in autonomic dysfunction with dry eyes and mouth, incontinence, erectile dysfunction, postural hypotension, gastroparesis, and reduced sweating. LEMS is most closely associated with small cell lung cancer, although only 50% to 60% of patients with LEMS harbor an underlying cancer.

The usual clinical presentation of LEMS is with proximal limb weakness, sometimes with myalgias and autonomic dysfunction. Ocular and pharyngeal weakness is relatively rare. The deep tendon reflexes are usually absent or markedly reduced.

Diagnosis

The diagnosis is confirmed with nerve conduction studies, which demonstrate low compound muscle action potentials (CMAP) with low frequency repetitive stimulation that repair with exercise and with rapid repetitive stimulation. Ninety percent will have anti-VGCC antibodies in the serum. The titer of the antibody does not correlate with disease severity. A careful search for bronchogenic carcinoma should be made in all patients with LEMS, particularly if they are or have been smokers.

Treatment and Results

The only paraneoplastic neurologic disorder that responds to immunosuppressive treatment is LEMS. However, in patients who are found to have an underlying cancer, the first step in treatment is to treat the malignancy. Some patients will experience remission with treatment of their underlying cancer. Guanidine hydrochloride and 3, 4-diaminopyridine improve neuromuscular transmission by enhancing the release of acetylcholine. Pyridostigmine, an acetylcholinesterase inhibitor, is moderately helpful and can be used in conjunction with these medications. Immunosuppressive therapy, including IVIG, plasma exchange, corticosteroids, and azathioprine, may be used but should be reserved for patients who have not improved despite treatment of their malignancy. Most patients will have some persistence of signs and symptoms despite maximal treatment.

PRIMARY BRAIN TUMORS

As alluded to in the introduction to this chapter, primary brain tumors make up a small percentage of cancer in the elderly. The incidence of malignant glioma and primary CNS lymphoma has been steadily increasing over the last 20 years in the elderly for reasons that remain unclear. The most common primary brain tumors in the elderly are meningioma, glioma, vestibular schwannoma, pituitary adenoma, and primary CNS lymphoma. This section focuses on meningioma, glioma, and CNS lymphoma as the management and prognosis of these tumors in elderly patients clearly differs from younger patients.

Meningioma

Histologically, the most common primary brain tumor in the elderly is meningioma. Depending on the series cited, they account for as many as 50% of brain tumors diagnosed in the elderly (Kuratsu and Ushio, 1997). In autopsy series, this tumor was seen in as many as 1% to 2% of individuals (Nakasu et al., 1987; Rausing et al., 1970). Meningiomas are more common in women by a factor of 3:1. Although, they can occur at any age they are most commonly diagnosed in the sixth and seventh decades.

Meningiomas derive from the arachnoid cap cells of the arachnoid granulations. They are most commonly seen along the cerebral convexities, along the falx cerebri, at the skull base, and in the thoracic spinal canal. Ten percent to 15% may have multiple meningiomas. Although the cause of meningioma is unknown, they are more common in patients with type 2 neurofibromatosis, breast cancer, and those who have been exposed to cranial ionizing radiation (Black, 1993). Most meningioma cells express progesterone receptors and, to a lesser extent, estrogen and androgen receptors. This feature may account for their preponderance in women and the increased incidence seen in women with a history of breast cancer. Meningiomas are almost always benign tumors. Atypical or "malignant" meningiomas account for less than 5% of cases (Jaaskelainen et al., 1986).

Clinical Presentation

As many as one third of all meningiomas are asymptomatic at the time of their discovery (Kuratsu and Ushio, 1997). They are discovered when CT or MRI is performed for unrelated symptoms. In those patients with symptomatic meningioma, headache, focal neurologic deficits, and seizure are the most common presenting signs and symptoms. As in the case of metastatic tumors, elderly patients may be *less* likely to present with signs of raised intracranial pressure and *more* likely to present with symptoms of cognitive decline and personality change. The classic bifrontal falcine or skull base meningioma commonly presents in this fashion. As meningioma is a slow growing tumor in most cases, the symptoms have often been present for many months before being diagnosed.

Diagnosis

CT and MRI are the most useful diagnostic procedures. Without contrast, CT often shows a calcified extraaxial, dural-based mass, with compression of the underlying brain, sometimes associated with peritumoral edema. With contrast, the tumor will enhance homogenously and the presence of a "dural tail" of enhancement may be noted (Fig. 28-5). On noncontrast MRI, the tumor is relatively isointense with brain on T_1- and T_2-weighted images. With contrast, the tumor brightly enhances and the aforementioned dural tail may be seen. MRI offers the advantage of visualizing the tumor in different planes and assessing the patency of any adjacent dural sinus, which meningiomas are likely to invade and occlude. The tumor compresses but remains well demarcated from the underlying brain. Invasion of the underlying brain may suggest the presence of an atypical or malignant meningioma or an alternative diagnosis such as a dural metastasis from carcinoma or lymphoma.

Treatment

It is often best to observe small, asymptomatic tumors if serial CT or MRI of the head show no evidence of tumor growth. This is particularly true in frail elderly patients where perioperative morbidity can be high (Kuratsu and Ushio, 1997), particularly in those with skull base lesions. In symptomatic meningiomas, surgical resection is appropriate for patients with tumors of the convexity, anterior cranial fossa, anterior falx cerebri, foramen magnum, and spinal canal. In these areas, complete resection is often possible with low risk to the surrounding neural structures. In patients with tumors in the sphenoid wing, cavernous sinus, clivus, cerebellopontine angle, and posterior falx with involvement of the superior sagittal sinus, an attempt at an aggressive resection carries

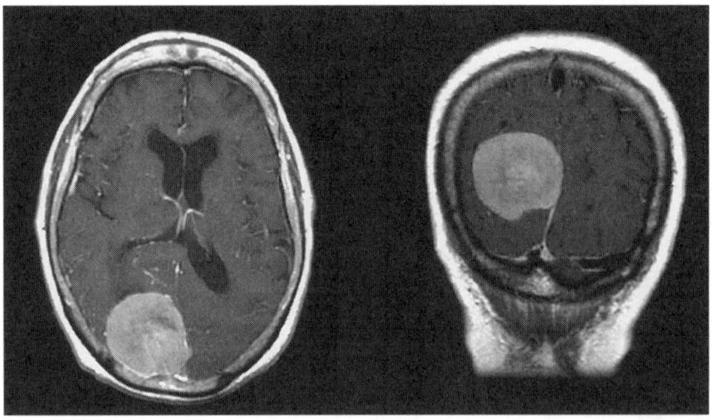

FIG. 28-5. Falcine meningioma. Axial and coronal magnetic resonance image of the head: T_1-weighted images with gadolinium contrast demonstrating a large, homogeneously enhancing mass arising from the falx with compression of adjacent brain. Note the enhancement of the adjacent dura on the coronal view (the dural "tail").

a high risk of cranial nerve deficits and brain injury. In these patients, either a less aggressive approach or nonsurgical treatment may be indicated. It is important to keep in mind that elderly patients have a higher risk of surgical morbidity and mortality from medical complications than younger patients (Awad et al., 1989; Djindjian et al., 1988).

External beam radiation therapy may be an alternative to surgery in some symptomatic patients, particularly in those patients felt to be poor operative candidates, either because of the location of the tumor or the patient's medical condition. Postoperative radiation may be required in cases of a large amount of residual tumor or if the tumor recurs after surgery. Local control of tumor with radiation in these instances appears to be good (Mesic et al., 1986; Taylor et al., 1988). Adjuvant radiation therapy is indicated in patients with atypical or malignant meningiomas. Radiosurgery with stereotactic linear accelerator or gamma knife appears to offer similar results, with less risk of radiation toxicity to the surrounding brain (Kondziolka et al., 1991).

The role of chemotherapy in meningioma is not well defined. The antiprogestin, mifepristone (RU-486), has not yet been shown to be useful in the treatment of meningioma. Some preliminary evidence indicate that hydroxyurea, an inhibitor of DNA synthesis, may be a helpful adjuvant in the treatment of unresectable or recurrent meningioma, although these results have yet to be duplicated (Schrell et al., 1997).

Glioma

Gliomas are tumors derived from the neuroglial cells: astrocytes, oligodendrocytes, and ependymal cells. A variety of classification systems exist, although these tumors are basically divided into *low grade* and *high grade*, depending on the presence of various histologic features, including pleomorphism, mitoses, necrosis, and vascular proliferation. Tumor cellular morphology and grading is important in predicting survival and selecting treatment. The factors most important in determining prognosis are patient age, tumor histology, and performance status. Extent of tumor resection can also be important prognostically. Of these factors, age appears to be paramount; patients above 60 years of age generally fare worse do than younger patients with the same tumor histology and performance status. In elderly patients, the most common glioma is a malignant glioma, including the glioblastoma multiforme, anaplastic astrocytoma,

anaplastic oligodendroglioma, and anaplastic mixed glioma. Glioblastoma, the most common form, carries the worst prognosis. Low-grade gliomas are rare in older patients. When they occur, their behavior is often more aggressive than that seen in younger patients.

The cause of glioma is unknown. An increased risk is seen of glioma development many years after receiving ionizing radiation to the head. Some evidence links large environmental exposures to electromagnetic fields and some chemicals and glioma (Wrensch et al., 1993). Some heritable syndromes have a higher risk of glioma, including Turcot's syndrome, Li-Fraumeni syndrome, and neurofibromatosis, although these usually present with brain tumors in younger adults. In most elderly patients, gliomas are entirely sporadic occurrences.

Clinical Presentation

Similar to metastatic tumors, the most common presenting symptoms of glioma in elderly patients are mental status changes, seizure, and focal neurologic deficits. Headache and other symptoms of raised intracranial pressure are distinctly less common than in younger patients, but do occur. Elderly patients generally have some degree of brain atrophy and, thus, are better able to accommodate an expanding mass without early signs and symptoms of raised intracranial pressure. It is extremely common for the symptoms of glioma in the elderly to be initially mistaken for stroke or degenerative dementia.

Diagnosis

The diagnostic studies of choice are CT or MRI of the head with contrast. Both will demonstrate edema and mass effect. Glioblastoma almost always enhances with contrast and typically has an area of central necrosis (Fig. 28-6). Low-grade gliomas are less likely to enhance. Unlike brain metastases, gliomas are usually solitary and have a more infiltrative appearance of edema and contrast enhancement. Gliomas commonly spread along white matter tracts and cross the corpus callosum.

A definitive diagnosis requires surgery. Although aggressive resection has been generally recommended in patients with both low- and high-grade glioma, the benefit in patients over 65 years of age is not clear (Kelly and Hunt, 1994). Certainly, in the extreme elderly (80+ years), aggressive resection is probably best replaced by a simple biopsy.

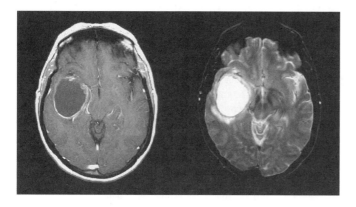

FIG. 28-6. Malignant glioma. Axial magnetic resonance image of the head: T_1-weighted image with gadolinium contrast and T_2-weighted image. Note the large area of central necrosis, the enhancing rim, and the relatively small amount of surrounding edema.

Treatment and Results

Biopsy is necessary to make a definitive diagnosis. As noted, more aggressive resection, which improves survival in younger patients, does not appear to do so in the elderly. Kelly and Hunt (1994) noted that patients over 65 years of age who had aggressive resection of their malignant gliomas survived a mean of only 13 weeks longer than similar aged patient who had only biopsy and similar postoperative therapy.

Radiation therapy is appropriate for most patients and does prolong survival to a modest degree. The standard therapy is 60 Gy external beam radiation in 30 to 33 fractions to encompass the postoperative tumor volume as seen on MRI or CT, with a margin of several centimeters. In elderly patients with malignant glioma and a poor performance status whose survival is expected to be particularly limited, a shortened course of radiation with larger fractions may be as effective (Bauman et al., 1994). The incidence of radiation-induced leukoencephalopathy with cognitive changes is higher in elderly patients. As survival is limited in most patients, however, this is not usually a major clinical concern.

The response to chemotherapy in elderly patients is even more disappointing than that of radiation therapy. Even in younger patients, only about 20% will respond to chemotherapy and the percentage is probably lower in elderly patients. Standard chemotherapy is with nitrosoureas (carmustine or lomustine). These are alkylating agents that penetrate the blood–brain barrier. Carmustine is given intravenously and lomustine is administered orally. The main, dose-limiting side effects are bone marrow suppression and pulmonary fibrosis. Other drugs shown to have some activity against glioblastoma include temozolomide, procarbazine, cisplatin, and etoposide.

Even with aggressive surgery, radiation, and chemotherapy, malignant glioma is virtually always fatal. The median survival is less than 1 year and very few longer term survivors are seen, particularly among patients over 60 years of age.

Primary Central Nervous System Lymphoma

The human immunodeficiency virus infection and chronic immunosuppression necessitated by organ transplantation, autoimmune disease, and cancer chemotherapy are factors that directly increase the risk of developing primary CNS lymphoma (PCNSL)— a relatively rare neoplasm. The incidence of this malignancy is on the rise even in patients who are immunocompetent (Eby et al., 1988). In this latter group, advanced age appears to be the common factor. Most patients who are immunocompetent who develop PCNSL are 50 years of age or older. Latent Epstein-Barr infection is implicated as a cause of PCNSL in patients who are immunocompromised, but not in those who are immunocompetent.

Primary CNS lymphoma is usually of B cell origin and can develop anywhere within the CNS. The tumor is often multifocal and has a proclivity to the periventricular white matter and basal ganglia. Leptomeningeal spread occurs in approximately 10% of patients and as many as 10% to 20% of patients will have involvement of the vitreous humor of the eye (Hochberg and Miller, 1988).

Clinical Presentation

Progressive focal neurologic deficits and neuropsychiatric dysfunction are the most common presenting symptoms (Tomlinson et al., 1995). Headache and seizures do occur but are less common, particularly in the elderly. In those with ocular involvement, visual obscuration or visual loss can occur; in those with leptomeningeal involvement, cranial neuropathies and spinal polyradiculopathies are common.

Diagnosis

In patients with PCNSL, head CT and MRI with contrast will demonstrate one or more homogeneously enhancing lesions, usually involving deep white matter or the basal ganglia (Fig. 28-7). The lesions tend to abut the ventricular surface. MRI is superior in defining the presence of leptomeningeal deposits and spinal cord involvement. PCNSL in patients who are immunocompromised often shows central necrosis with ring enhancement. This imaging pattern is distinctly unusual in patients who are immunocompetent.

If PCNSL is suspected, MRI of the entire neuraxis is indicated for staging purposes. CSF examination may reveal lymphomatous involvement in 10% to 20% of patients. Obviously, lumbar puncture is contraindicated in those with significant supratentorial or posterior fossa mass effect and impending herniation. Slit lamp examination of the eyes is necessary for staging and, occasionally, vitreous aspiration and cytologic examination yield the diagnosis.

Approximately 4% of patients presenting with brain lymphoma will be found to have occult systemic lymphoma (O'Neill et al., 1995). These patients have metastatic systemic lymphoma and not PCNSL. To exclude this possibility, CT of the chest, abdomen,

and pelvis; bone marrow examination; and, in men, testicular ultrasound are indicated as part of the staging process.

Assuming no systemic disease is found, the vitreous is clear of cells, and CSF cytology is negative, diagnostic stereotactic biopsy of the brain lesion is indicated. Aggressive resection of PCNSL is not recommended. Extent of resection is not a prognostic variable and attempts at resection often lead to disabling or fatal brain hemorrhage.

If PCNSL is suspected, it is best to avoid the preoperative use of corticosteroids, unless the patient is in imminent danger of herniation. Corticosteroids exert a tumor-lytic effect on lymphoma. Treatment with corticosteroids before biopsy can produce a rapid and dramatic tumor response and render the biopsy nondiagnostic. If the patient must receive corticosteroids, the biopsy should proceed as quickly as possible, assuming the targeted lesion is present on reimaging.

Pathologic examination of the tumor will usually reveal atypical lymphocytes in a perivascular location. Immunohistochemistry will reveal these to be monoclonal B cells, sometimes with reactive T cells intermixed. Epstein-Barr viral genome is commonly found within lymphoma cells in patients who are immunocompromised but not in the sporadic PCNSL found in those who are immunocompetent.

Treatment and Results

As in malignant glioma, age and performance status are important prognostic factors in patients with PCNSL. Among patients older than 60 years, the median survival is less than 1 year, even with maximal therapy (Corry et al., 1998). Moreover, few long-term survivors are seen in this group of patients.

Previously, radiation was considered the primary therapy for PCNSL. More recently, chemotherapy has been found to have a clear role in treatment. The approach in patients who are immunocompetent is to treat with chemotherapy first and then proceed with whole-brain radiation therapy immediately after or at the time of tumor recurrence. A variety of chemotherapy agents appear to be effective in treating PCNSL, although high-dose intravenous methotrexate is used most often, with or without the addition of those combination chemotherapies known to be active in systemic lymphomas. These latter agents include AraC, cyclophosphamide, doxorubicin, vincristine, and dexamethasone, among others. Whole brain radiation (WBRT) in the range of 45 Gy in 25 fractions is standard. Usually, radiation is given after chemotherapy to lessen the risk of leukoencephalopathy. The latter is

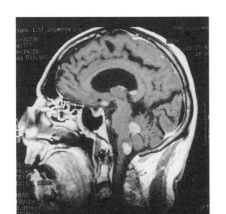

FIG. 28-7. Primary central nervous system lymphoma. Sagittal magnetic resonance image of the head: T_1-weighted image with gadolinium contrast. Note the multiple enhancing lesions in the brainstem, fourth ventricle, corpus callosum, thalamus, and infundibulum.

particularly common if methotrexate is administered after radiation therapy. The orbits are included in patients with ocular disease. Radiation can be given to local symptomatic areas of the spine. Leptomeningeal spread is best treated either with high-dose intravenous methotrexate or intra-CSF methotrexate via Ommaya reservoir.

Although PCNSL often responds well to chemotherapy and radiation, it virtually always recurs and survival is rarely more than a year in the elderly patient. Treatment-related neurotoxicity is common in those patients who do survive more than a year. Leukoencephalopathy with subcortical dementia, gait apraxia, and incontinence is more common in the elderly than in younger patients who have received WBRT, with or without chemotherapy (Blumenthal and DeAngelis, 1998).

In frail elderly patients with poor performance status, the expectations from treatment in PCNSL are limited. In these patients, it may be appropriate to advise supportive care only. Some benefit and little risk may be seen in giving pulse doses of corticosteroids (1 g intravenous methylprednisolone monthly) (O'Neill et al., 1999) to these patients at high risk of developing treatment-related toxicity from other modalities.

CONCLUSION

The diagnosis and care of elderly patients with primary and metastatic tumors of the nervous system and neurologic complications of systemic cancer is challenging. These disorders can present differently in elderly patients and, as with other neurologic disorders, elderly patients generally fare worse than their younger counterparts. Some cancer treatments are less effective or have greater toxicity in the elderly. The expanding numbers of older patients and the increasing incidence of brain tumors specific to this population requires that the practicing neurologist be aware of the diagnostic and therapeutic issues unique to these patients.

REFERENCES

Amer MH, Al-Sarraf M, Baker LH, et al. Malignant melanoma and central nervous system metastases: incidence, diagnosis, treatment, and survival. *Cancer* 1978; 42:660–668.

Awad IA, Kalfas I, Hahn JF, et al. Intracranial meningiomas in the aged: surgical outcome in the era of computed tomography. *Neurosurgery* 1989;24:557–560.

Baharav E, Harpaz M, Mittelman M, et al. Dexamethasone-induced perineal irritation. *N Engl J Med* 1986;314: 515–516.

Balm M, Hammack J. Leptomeningeal carcinomatosis. Presenting features and prognostic factors. *Arch Neurol* 1996;53(7):626–632.

Bauman GS, Gaspar LE, Fisher BJ, et al. A prospective study of short-course radiotherapy in poor prognosis glioblastoma multiforme. *Int J Radiat Oncol Biol Phys* 1994;29:835–839.

Black PM. Meningiomas. *Neurosurgery* 1993;32:643–657.

Blumenthal DT, DeAngelis LM. Aging and primary central nervous system neoplasms. *Neurol Clin North Am* 1998;16:671–686.

Byrne TN, Cascino TL, Posner JB. Brain metastasis from melanoma. *J Neurooncol* 1983;1:313–317.

Corry J, Smith JG, Wirth A, et al. Primary central nervous system lymphoma: age and performance status are more important than treatment modality. *Int J Rad Oncol Biol Phys* 1998;41(3):615–620.

Dalmau J, Graus F, Rosenblum MK, et al. Anti-Hu-associated paraneoplastic encephalomyelitis/sensory neuronopathy. A clinical study of 71 patients. *Medicine* 1992;71: 59–72.

Delattre J-Y, Krol G, Thaler HT, et al. Distribution of brain metastases. *Arch Neurol* 1988;45:741–744.

Delattre J-Y, Safai B, Posner JB. Erythema multiforme and Stevens-Johnson syndrome in patients receiving cranial irradiation and phenytoin. *Neurology* 1988;38: 194–198.

Djindjian M, Caron JP, Athayde AA, et al. Intracranial meningiomas in the elderly (over 70 years old): a retrospective study of 30 surgical cases. *Acta Neurochir* 1988; 90:121–123.

Eby NL, Grufferman S, Flannelly CM, et al. Increasing incidence of primary brain lymphoma in the US. *Cancer* 1988;62:2461–2465.

Furneaux HM, Rosenblum MK, Dalmau J, et al. Selective expression of Purkinje cell antigens in tumor tissue from patients with paraneoplastic cerebellar degeneration. *N Engl J Med* 1990;322:1844–1851.

Galasko CSB. The anatomy and pathways of skeletal metastases. In: Weiss L, Gilbert HA, eds. *Bone metastasis.* Boston: GK Hall & Co, 1981:49–63.

Glantz M, Cole BF, Friedberg MH, et al. A randomized, blinded placebo-controlled trial of anticonvulsant prophylaxis in adults with newly diagnosed brain tumors. *Neurology* 1996;46 (4):985–991.

Hammack JE, Kimmel DW, O'Neill BP, et al. Paraneoplastic cerebellar degeneration: a clinical comparison of patients with and without Purkinje cell cytoplasmic antibodies. *Mayo Clin Proc* 1990;65:1423–1431.

Hetzel DJ, Stanhope R, O'Neill BP, et al. Gynecologic cancer in patients with subacute cerebellar degeneration predicted by anti-Purkinje cell antibodies and limited in metastatic volume. *Mayo Clin Proc* 1990;65: 1558–1563.

Hochberg FH, Miller DH. Primary central nervous system lymphoma. *J Neurosurg* 1988;68: 835–853.

Jaaskelainen J, Haltia M, Servo A. Atypical and anaplastic meningiomas: radiology, surgery, radiotherapy and outcome. *Surg Neurol* 1986;25:233–242.

Kelly PJ, Hunt C. The limited value of cytoreductive surgery in elderly patients with malignant gliomas. *Neurosurgery* 1994;34(1):62–67.

Kondziolka D, Lunsford LD, Coffey RJ, et al. Stereotactic radiosurgery of meningiomas. *J Neurosurg* 1991;74: 552–559.

Kuratsu J, Ushio Y. Epidemiological study of primary intracranial tumors in elderly people. *J Neurol Neurosurg Psychiatry* 1997;63:116–118.

Lowry JK, Snyder JJ, Lowry PW. Brain tumors in the elderly. *Arch Neurol* 1998;55:922–928.

Lucchinetti CF, Kimmel DW, Lennon VA. Paraneoplastic and oncologic profiles of patients seropositive for type 1 antineuronal nuclear autoantibodies. *Neurology* 1998;50:652–657.

Mesic JB, Hanks GE, Doggett RL. The value of radiation therapy as an adjuvant to surgery in intracranial meningiomas. *Am J Clin Oncol* 1986;9:337–340.

Nakasu S, Hirano A, Shimura T, et al. Incidental meningiomas in autopsy study. *Surg Neurol* 1987;27:319–322.

O'Neill BP, Buckner JC, Coffey RJ, et al. Brain metastatic lesions. *Mayo Clin Proc* 1994;69:1062–1068.

O'Neill BP, Dinapoli RP, Kurtin PJ, et al. Occult systemic non-Hodgkin's lymphoma (NHL) in patients initially diagnosed as primary central nervous system lymphoma (PCNSL): how much staging is enough? *J Neurooncol* 1995;25(1):67–71.

O'Neill BP, Haberman TM, Witzig TE, et al. Prevention of recurrence and prolonged survival in primary central nervous system lymphoma (PCNSL) patients treated with adjuvant high-dose methylprednisolone. *Med Oncol* 1999;16(3):211–215.

Patchell RA, Tibbs PA, Walsh JW, et al. A randomized trial of surgery in the treatment of single metastases to the brain. *N Engl J Med* 1990;322:494–500.

Pickren JW, Lopez G, Tsukada Y, et al. Brain metastases: an autopsy study. *Canc Treat Symp* 1983;2:295–313.

Portenoy RK, Galer BS, Salamon O, et al. Identification of epidural neoplasm: radiography and bone scintigraphy in the symptomatic and asymptomatic spine. *Cancer* 1989;64:2207–2213.

Portenoy RK, Lipton RB, Foley KM. Back pain in the cancer patient: an algorithm for evaluation and management. *Neurology* 1987;37(1):134–138.

Posner JB, Chernik NL. Intracranial metastases from systemic cancer. *Adv Neurol* 1978;19:575–587.

Posner JB. Paraneoplastic syndromes. *Neurologic complications of cancer*. Contemporary neurology series. Philadelphia: FA Davis, 1995.

Rausing A, Ybo W, Stenflo J. Intracranial meningioma. A population study of ten years. *Acta Neurol Scand* 1970;46:102–110.

Schiff D, Shaw EG, Cascino TL. Outcome after spinal reirradiation for malignant epidural spinal cord compression. *Ann Neurol* 1995;37(5):583–589.

Schiff D, O'Neill BP, Wang CH, et al. Neuroimaging and treatment implications of patients with multiple epidural spinal metastases. *Cancer* 1998;83(8):1593–1601.

Schrell UM, Rittig MG, Anders M, et al. Hydroxyurea for treatment of unresectable and recurrent meningiomas. II. Decrease in the size of meningiomas in patients treated with hydroxyurea. *J Neurosurg* 1997;86(5):840–844.

Taylor BW, Marcus RB, Friedman WA, et al. The meningioma controversy: postoperative radiation therapy. *Int J Radiat Oncol Biol Phys* 1988;15:299–304.

Tomlinson FH, Kurtin PJ, Suman VJ, et al. Primary intracerebral malignant lymphoma: a clinicopathological study of 89 patients. *J Neurosurg* 1995;82(4):558–566.

Vecht CJ, Haaxma-Reiche H, Noordijk EM, et al. Treatment of single brain metastasis: radiotherapy alone or combined with neurosurgery? *Ann Neurol* 1993;3:583–590.

Wasserstrom W, Glass JP, Posner JB. Diagnosis and treatment of leptomeningeal metastases from solid tumors: experience with 90 patients. *Cancer* 1982;49:759–772.

Werner MH, Phuphanich S, Lyman GH. The increasing incidence of malignant gliomas and primary central nervous system lymphoma in the elderly. *Cancer* 1995;76:1634–1642.

Wrensch M, Bondy ML, Wiecke J, et al. Environmental risk factors for primary malignant brain tumors: a review. *J Neurooncol* 1993;17(1):47–64.

WEB SITES

American Brain Tumor Association: *http://www.abta.org*

National Cancer Institute: *http://www.nci.nih.gov*

29

Introduction: Neurological Manifestations of Systemic Disease

Although Neurology, as a field, has grown as an independent specialty with separate clinical services, the nervous system does not operate in a vacuum. A considerable relationship exists between the nervous system and other organ systems that causes a multitude of neurologic manifestations of systemic disease and a number of systemic problems secondary to neurologic illnesses. This chapter surveys the common neurologic manifestations of systemic disease that commonly occur in the older adult.

29.1

Neurological Manifestations of Systemic Disease: Cardiology and Pulmonary

Lori H. Travis

A great many cardiac and pulmonary disease states can have an impact on the nervous system. These conditions range from those seen almost every day by the practicing neurologist, to those seen only once or twice in a career. Several conditions are extremely common, and may be easily treatable. This chapter reviews some of the most frequently seen cardiac and pulmonary conditions that cause neurologic dysfunction.

NEUROLOGIC MANIFESTATIONS OF CARDIAC DISEASE

Cardiac disease affects many members of the US population, particularly the elderly. Several cardiac conditions can cause neurologic symptoms or pathology. Embolism to the central nervous system (CNS) is associated with several cardiac conditions, including atrial fibrillation, the sick sinus syndrome, myocardial infarction, cardiac valvular disease, mitral annular calcification (MAC), mitral valve prolapse (MVP), cardiac valve replacement, left atrial myxoma, dilated cardiomyopathy, and patent foramen ovale (PFO).

Cardiac surgery, particularly coronary artery bypass grafting (CABG), also prevalent in the older US population, can cause neurologic complications.

Neurologic symptoms can also result from endocarditis (infective and nonbacterial thrombotic) and hypoperfusion states (systemic hypoperfusion, as well as the subclavian steal syndrome).

Cardiogenic Embolism

An embolus can dislodge from the heart and travel to the blood vessels supplying the brain (Fig. 29-1). If it occludes one of these vessels, stroke can occur. A cardioembolic source was found in 19% of ischemic strokes recorded in the Stroke Data Bank (Sacco et al., 1989).

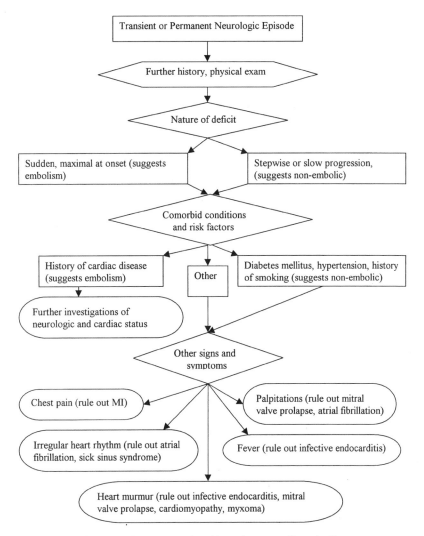

FIG. 29-1. Diagnosis algorithm chart: cardioembolism.

The most common cause of cardiogenic emboli is *atrial fibrillation*, a cardiac arrhythmia characterized by irregular heart rhythm and often associated clinically with symptoms of palpitations. Atrial fibrillation is present in approximately 6% of the population above 65 years of age (Feinberg et al., 1995). Untreated, atrial fibrillation increases the risk of stroke by about 5% per year (Fauci et al., 1998). It is recommended that those with sustained atrial fibrillation receive anticoagulation with warfarin for stroke prophylaxis, unless otherwise contraindicated.

Other arrhythmias can also contribute to thrombus formation, leading to embolus to the brain. The *sick sinus syndrome* is one example. Fluctuations in heart rate from bradycardia to tachycardia and, at times, even si-

nus pauses or atrial fibrillation are characteristic of this syndrome. Even after pacemaker insertion, patients with sick sinus syndrome can experience stroke.

Another common cause of cardiogenic embolism is *myocardial infarction*. Embolic stroke occurs in approximately 1% of hospitalized patients with myocardial infarction (Bradley et al., 2000). The types of myocardial infarction that carry the highest risk of thrombus or embolus formation are transmural, apical, and anterolateral. This risk is increased in those with a history of emboli and congestive heart failure. Stroke, in this setting, often occurs within the first week after myocardial infarction, but those who survive the first week without stroke continue to carry an increased risk of stroke for the next 3 months.

Cardiac valvular disease can lead to embolism. Rheumatic mitral valvular disease produces the highest incidence of systemic emboli, especially in association with atrial fibrillation in the elderly. However, total numbers with rheumatic heart disease in the US population are decreasing. If evidence of embolus or atrial fibrillation is seen, the recommended treatment is long-term anticoagulation with warfarin (Salem et al., 1998).

MAC is also associated with an increased incidence of embolus; the risk of stroke in MAC is twice that of controls (Benjamin et al., 1992). MAC is a syndrome defined by evidence of calcification around the mitral valve, but is also associated with mitral stenosis and regurgitation, and atrial fibrillation. One study showed that the prevalence of MAC can be as high as 35% in older men (Aronow et al., 1997a).

Emboli in MAC appear to be composed at times of fibrin, although they can also be composed of calcium. Currently, anticoagulation with warfarin is recommended in patients with MAC who also have evidence of systemic, noncalcific emboli or atrial fibrillation (Salem et al., 1998).

MVP, although usually not associated with cerebral embolism, can cause emboli and subsequent stroke. MVP is a common form of valvular disease, present in approximately 6% of women and 4% of men (Salem et al., 1998). It is sometimes associated with emboli and stroke, but the risk factors that predispose to these complications are unclear. Currently, antithrombotic therapy (aspirin) is recommended when evidence exists of unexplained transient ischemic attacks in the patient with MVP, and anticoagulation with warfarin is recommended with evidence of embolus, recurrent events on aspirin, or coexisting atrial fibrillation (Salem et al., 1998).

A common cardiac cause of embolism is valve replacement with mechanical valves. Presumably, prosthetic valves provide a surface upon which thrombus forms. The treatment is prophylactic anticoagulation in those with mechanical heart valve replacements; the exact international normalized ratio recommendations vary with the type of mechanical valve used.

Cardiac emboli can also form in patients with *left atrial myxoma*. This slow-growing cardiac tumor initially presents with cerebral embolism; the typical patient's age is in the 50s. Less commonly, the tumor fragments can continue to grow in the CNS, causing local mass effect, or can create arterial aneurysms at the site of embolism. Evaluation for suspected myxoma is best initiated with echocardiography. Surgery is often the best treatment option (Giuliani et al., 1996).

Those with *dilated cardiomyopathy* are at increased risk for emboli to the cerebral vasculature. The prevalence of dilated cardiomyopathy was found in one study to be 1% in older men (Aronow et al., 1997a). Embolic risk presumably results from hypokinesis of the left ventricle, with subsequent thrombus formation.

Emboli can arise distal to the heart, but gain access to the cerebral circulation via a cardiac route; such is the case with PFO. A PFO is a small opening connecting the right and left atria. It is a remnant of fetal circulation, which closes in most people after birth, but remains open in approximately 25% of the population (Barnett et al., 1998). The thrombus can originate in the deep veins of the legs, or within the heart. In either case, the thrombus passes through the PFO on its way from the right atrium to the left and, subsequently, to the brain.

Although PFO may be a more common route of embolus in the young than the old, it should nevertheless be considered in the older patient with stroke of unknown cause, especially when other cerebrovascular risk factors are absent. The most sensitive test to detect PFO is a transesophageal echocardiogram (TEE) with contrast. Once a PFO is found, options for treatment vary. As aforementioned, PFO is present in a large percentage of the population and, although it is a potential route of embolic transmission, the mere presence of a PFO in an individual does not confirm its role in stroke.

It is currently unclear whether medical or surgical management of PFO is best in the older patient. Evidence of large PFO size, right to left shunting, presence of an atrial septal aneurysm, or evidence of deep venous thrombosis more likely indicate that the PFO is related to stroke in a given individual, and make more aggressive management justifiable. In these patients, some advocate long-term therapy with warfarin, although others feel that surgical closure is best. In cases in which long-term anticoagulation is contraindicated, antiplatelet therapy may be adequate (Salem et al., 1998).

Cardiac Surgical Complications

Cardiac surgeries can have neurologic sequelae. The most frequently performed cardiac surgery is CABG, with approximately 400,000 CABG procedures performed annually in the United States and Canada (Brillman, 1993). The CABG procedure involves the bypass of diseased segments of the coronary arteries, to optimize perfusion of the heart tissue. Some CABG procedures involve the use of cardiopulmonary bypass (CPB). CPB uses tubing to connect the ascending aorta to the right atrium. The ascending aorta is cross-clamped and cardiac asystole is induced. During this time, blood flow is maintained through the tubing by a machine.

CPB surgery increases the likelihood of neurologic complications, including stroke and global cerebral hypoperfusion (Sila, 1998). Stroke occurs in 2% to 5% of surgeries; risk of stroke related to surgery also increases with advancing age (Sila, 1998). Stroke is a known complication of cardiac valvular surgery as well, but is much less common in cardiac catheterization and percutaneous transluminal coronary angioplasty.

Other common complications of cardiac surgery are postoperative encephalopathy and cognitive dysfunction, which occur in approximately 3% to 12% of cardiac surgeries (Breuer et al., 1983). The cause of encephalopathy may be related to microembolism or to cerebral hypoxia, and it tends to occur more frequently when intraaortic balloon pumps or pressors have been used (Sila, 1998). Newman et al. (2001) found that postoperative cognitive decline, including memory difficulties, is prevalent (at discharge, 53% of patients having CABG) and may persist for years postoperatively (42% at 5 years). Factors associated with persistent cognitive decline were older age, lower level of education, and evidence of cognitive decline at hospital discharge.

Other, less common complications of cardiac surgery include intracerebral hemorrhage, brachial plexopathy, and coma.

Endocarditis

Infective endocarditis used to be most common in those with rheumatic heart disease, but is now more common, in the United States, in intravenous drug users. The approximate incidence of endocarditis is 1.7 to 4/100,000 (Scheld and Sande, 1995). It is characterized by growth of infective vegetations on the heart valves, which can dislodge and produce emboli, some of which may gain access to the cerebral circulation. The causative organism is most commonly *Staphylococcus aureus*. However, although less common, the vegetations produced by group B streptococci, *Haemophilus* species, and *Pseudomonas aeruginosa* appear to be more susceptible to embolus propagation.

Signs and symptoms of acute bacterial endocarditis (ABE) include acute onset of high fever, rigors, malaise, and new heart murmur. Headache and mental status changes are common manifestations. Signs and symptoms of subacute bacterial endocarditis include insidious onset of malaise, anorexia, weight loss, and heart murmur.

The prevalence of embolism in endocarditis is between 12% and 40% (Salem, 1998). Emboli to the brain are more common in ABE and with mitral valve involvement. Embolus formation appears to be decreased more effectively by initiation of antibiotic therapy than by anticoagulation and, therefore, anticoagulation is generally not recommended in cases of native valve endocarditis (Paschalis et al., 1990). Emboli tend to occur most commonly at presentation or within 2 days of initiation of antibiotic therapy (Cunha et al., 1996).

In mechanical prosthetic valve endocarditis, it is recommended that anticoagulation not be interrupted after the diagnosis, although the patient must be informed that the risk of cerebral hemorrhage will be increased (Salem, 1998).

Infective emboli in the cerebral vasculature can produce mycotic aneurysms, which carry the risk of rupture, producing subarachnoid hemorrhage. This complication occurs in approximately 10% of cases of ABE (Cunha et al., 1996). The symptoms include severe headache and mental status changes, and should be evaluated by emergent brain imaging and neurosurgical consultation, followed by angiography. Other neurologic complications of endocarditis include meningitis, brain abscess formation, and diffuse encephalopathy.

Investigations that aid in the diagnosis of endocarditis are blood cultures, electrocardiogram, TEE, and erythrocyte sedimentation rate. Neurologic investigations include computed tomography (CT) scan of the head, especially to rule out intracerebral hemorrhage or infarction. If CT scan is unrevealing in the face of neurologic deficit or suspicion of neurologic complications, magnetic resonance imaging (MRI) of the head may prove more helpful. MRI is superior to CT for microabscesses within the brain parenchyma. Cerebrospinal fluid examination may show evidence of pleocytosis if meningitis is present.

Therapy for endocarditis includes prompt initiation of appropriate antibiotic therapy. Penicillin G and nafcillin with an aminoglycoside may be an appropriate initial regimen, although the exact causative organism identified should guide antibiotic choice (Cunha et al., 1996).

Nonbacterial thrombotic endocarditis (NBTE) is caused by vegetations on the heart valves, without evidence of a causative infectious organism. This syndrome occurs more commonly in older individuals, and is often associated with neoplasia, disseminated intravascular coagulation, or chronic illness. The primary neurologic complication of NBTE is embolism, which occurs in approximately 42% of cases (Lopez et al., 1987). Diagnosis of NBTE is often difficult, and involves a search for infectious causes with blood cultures and TEE. CT scan or MRI of the head is useful in cases of cerebral embolism. Treatment is aimed at control of the underlying condition. Anticoagulation with heparin is recommended if embolism has occurred, but can also be considered even in cases without embolism (Salem, 1998).

Hypoperfusion

Systemic hypotension can produce cerebral or spinal cord hypoperfusion. The areas of hypoperfusion are anatomically correlated to the areas of the brain and spinal cord that are on the border between vascular territories (watershed regions). These regions include the parietooccipital and parietotemporal regions, as well as the region around the area of the central sulcus. Hypoperfusion-related infarctions in the cerebral hemispheres tend to be bilateral.

In the spinal cord, the thoracic region is typically affected by hypoperfusion. Hypoperfusion results from many causes including systemic hypotension, aortic surgery, or aortic dissection. Thoracic cord hypoperfusion can present with paraplegia, a thoracic spine sensory level, and hyperreflexia. Treatment of the underlying cause of hypoperfusion is the best method of correcting the cerebral or cord ischemia. If ischemia has progressed to infarction, however, it may be impossible to salvage the involved regions in time to regain function (Goetz and Pappert, 1999).

A well-known hypoperfusion condition, the *subclavian steal syndrome*, is characterized by transient symptoms, including limb claudication, headaches, vertigo, nausea, and unsteadiness of gait. These episodic symptoms are often precipitated by arm use. Frequently, the cause of the symptoms is atherosclerotic stenosis of the subclavian artery (more frequently the left than the right), which causes blood-flow direction to reverse in the vertebral arteries. Blood flows from the brain to the upper limb on the affected side, causing relative vertebrobasilar insufficiency. Suspicion of subclavian steal can be substantiated by a low blood pressure or weak pulse in the affected arm, and confirmed by angiography. Treatment, if necessary, is surgical. However, patients with this relatively benign syndrome are fre-

quently asymptomatic, and do not require further treatment.

NEUROLOGIC MANIFESTATIONS OF PULMONARY DISEASE

Pulmonary conditions commonly affect older individuals, and can produce neurologic sequelae (Fig. 29-2). The following may be encountered in neurologic practice: sleep apnea, hypoxia, hypercapnia, hyperventilation, and high-altitude sickness (HAS).

Sleep Apnea

Obstructive sleep apnea (OSA) is a clinical syndrome of recurrent total or partial cessation of airflow during sleep. Usually, these apneas occur because of increased compliance of the upper airway, with reduced functional space for airflow. Apneas often last for more than 10 seconds, and cause a brief awakening, at which time the patient is able to restore airflow. The patient often falls back to sleep, and is unaware of having awakened. Although the absolute number of apneas and hypopneas varies during sleep, most agree that at least five episodes per hour of sleep are needed for the diagnosis. Patients with OSA often awaken feeling unrefreshed, and experience daytime somnolence. Other symptoms of OSA (e.g., memory deficits and morning headaches) may be related to relative cerebral hypoxia at night.

Typically, OSA occurs in overweight, middle-aged men with a history of loud snoring, often accompanied by a history of alcohol consumption. OSA is common, occurring in 2% of middle-aged women, and 4% of middle-aged men (Fauci et al., 1998). The diagnosis of OSA can be confirmed by overnight oximetry or, more reliably, by overnight polysomnography. Conservative treatment includes weight reduction, decreased alcohol intake, and sleeping in positions other than on the back. Other therapies that may be of benefit include aminophylline, progesterone, protriptyline, clomipramine (Tobin et al., 1983). More aggressive treatments include surgery to increase functional space within the airway (uvulopalatopharyngoplasty), nocturnal continuous positive airway pressure to aid in maintenance of airway patency, and, at the extreme, tracheostomy. However, the success rates for these therapies have not been well established, and although aggressive surgical treatments are available, their efficacy may be limited (Goldman and Bennett, 2000).

Central sleep apneas can occur as well, although often they occur in combination with obstructive ap-

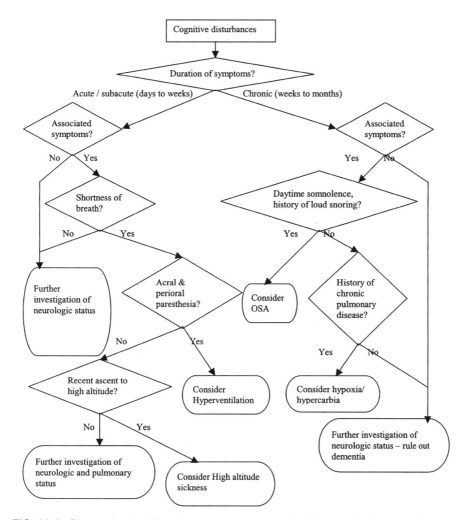

FIG. 29-2. Diagnosis algorithm chart: neurologic manifestations of pulmonary disease.

nea, rather than in isolation. Central apneas are also characterized by recurrent apneas during sleep, but the cause, unlike that of OSA, is a reduced ventilatory drive. Symptoms are similar. See Chapter 13, Sleep in the Older Person, for more information on this topic.

Hypoxia and Hypercapnia

Pulmonary disease also causes neurologic symptoms if it is severe enough to produce hypoxemia or hypercapnia. *Hypoxemia* is described as a reduction in arterial oxygen tension (P_{O_2}) below the normal range of 80 – 100 mmHg. *Hypercapnia* is an increase in arterial tension of carbon dioxide (P_{CO_2}) above the normal range of 35 to 45 mmHg. These derangements

cause an increase in cerebral blood flow and vasodilation, which are frequently well tolerated because of compensatory mechanisms and cerebral autoregulation. However, acute onset of respiratory difficulties, or prolonged hypoxemia or hypercapnia can cause symptoms such as headache, memory disturbances, sleep difficulties, and daytime sleepiness. In more severe disease, signs and symptoms include decreased level of consciousness, papilledema, and asterixis.

Pulmonary conditions that can cause hypoxemia and hypercapnia include asthma and chronic obstructive pulmonary disease. An electroencephalogram may show diffuse slowing in the theta and delta range, with slowing of the alpha rhythm. Other helpful investigations related primarily to the underlying cause of hypoxemia include arterial blood gas determination, pulmonary function tests, and chest radiograph. Treatment of encephalopathic symptoms is directed toward correction of the underlying process, and focuses on ventilation and gas exchange.

Hyperventilation

An additional derangement of pulmonary status that frequently leads to neurologic symptoms is hypocapnia, or a reduction in arterial tension of carbon dioxide (PCO_2) below the normal range of 35 to 45 mmHg. This situation is often induced by hyperventilation, be it conscious or unconscious. The cerebral response to hyperventilation is vasoconstriction and reduced cerebral blood flow. Hyperventilation is triggered by a wide variety of situations, including pulmonary emboli, congestive heart failure, pain, pregnancy, fever, prolonged conversation, and anxiety.

Symptoms of hyperventilation include shortness of breath, dizziness, visual changes, and paresthesias of the hands, feet, and mouth. Although they often pose no real health risk, these symptoms are frequently distressing for the patient. The best treatment involves ascertaining the underlying condition producing hyperventilation, and targeting that condition with the best medical therapy.

High-Altitude Sickness

HAS is a syndrome that occasionally occurs after an individual has rapidly reached a high altitude. It occurs more frequently in those who are overweight, but other predictive features are lacking. HAS typically consists of headache, decreased concentration, dizziness, and sleep disturbances, often hours to days after reaching a high altitude. Occasionally, HAS progresses in severity to coma.

Treatment for the mild form includes an arrest of ascent to higher altitude until symptoms completely subside. Acetazolamide has been suggested, but its efficacy is not yet established (Sutton et al., 1979). For more severe forms of HAS, the patient may need to be urgently removed to lower altitudes and provided with supplemental oxygen.

SUMMARY

Thus, the intimate relationship between cardiac, pulmonary, and neurologic disease is readily appreciated. The neurologist can expect to encounter patients with cardiac and pulmonary disease. An understanding of those cardiac and pulmonary conditions that commonly cause CNS symptoms is a great asset to the practicing neurologist.

REFERENCES

Aranow WS, Ahn C, Kronzon I. Prevalence of echocardiographic findings in 554 men and in 1,243 women aged >60 years in a long-term health facility. *Am J Cardiol* 1997a;79:379–380.

Aranow WS, Tresch D, Rich MW. Congestive heart failure in older adults. *J Am Geriatr Soc* 1997;45(8): 968–974.

Barnett HJM, Mohr JP, Stein BM, et al., eds. *Stroke pathophysiology, diagnosis, and management*, 3rd ed. New York: Churchill Livingstone, 1998.

Benjamin EJ, Plehn JF, D'Agostino RB, et al. Mitral annular calcification and the risk of stroke in an elderly cohort. *N Engl J Med* 1992;327(6):374–379.

Bradley WG, Daroff RB, Fenichel GM, et al., eds. *Neurology in clinical practice*, Vol. II, 3rd ed. Boston: Butterworth-Heinemann, 2000.

Breuer AC, Furlan AJ, Hanson MR, et al. Central nervous system complications of coronary artery bypass graft surgery: prospective analysis of 421 patients. *Stroke* 1983;14(5):682–687.

Brillman J. Central nervous system complications in coronary artery bypass graft surgery. *Neurol Clin* 1993;11: 475–495.

Cunha BA, Gill MV, Lazar JM. Acute infective endocarditis. *Infect Dis Clin North Am* 1996;10(4):811–834.

Fauci AS, Braunwald E, Isslebacher KJ, et al, eds. *Harrison's principles of internal medicine*, 14th ed. New York: McGraw-Hill, 1998.

Feinberg W, Blackshear J, Laupacis A, et al. Prevalence, age distribution, and gender of patients with atrial fibrillation. *Arch Intern Med* 1995;155:469–473.

Giuliani ER, Gersh BJ, McGoon MD, et al., eds. *Mayo Clinic practice of cardiology*, 3rd ed. St. Louis: Mosby, 1996.

Goetz CG. *Textbook of clinical neurology*, 1st ed. Philadelphia: WB Saunders, 1999.

Goldman L, Bennett J, eds. *Cecil textbook of medicine*, 21st ed. Philadelphia: WB Saunders, 2000.

Lopez JA, Ross RS, Fishbein MC, et al. Nonbacterial thrombotic endocarditis: a review. *Am Heart J* 1987;113: 773–784.

Newman M, Kirchner J, Phillips-Bute B, et al. Longitudinal assessment of neurocognitive function after coronary artery bypass surgery. *N Engl J Med* 2001:344(6): 395–402.

Paschalis C, Pugsley W, John R, et al. Rate of cerebral embolic events in relation to antibiotic and anticoagulant therapy in patients with bacterial endocarditis. *Eur Neurol* 1990;30:87.

Podrid PJ. Cardiovascular disease in the elderly. *Cardiol Clin* 1999;17(1):173–187.

Sacco RL, Ellenberg JH, Mohr JP, et al. Infarcts of undetermined cause: the NINCDS stroke data bank. *Ann Neurol* 1989;25(4):382–390.

Salem DN, Levine HJ, Pauker SG, et al. Antithrombotic therapy in valvular heart disease. *Chest* 1998;114(5): 590–601.

Scheld WM, Sande MA. Endocarditis and Intravascular Investigations. In: Mandell GL, Bennett JE, Dolin R, eds. *Mandell, Douglas, and Bennett's principles and practice of infectious diseases,* 4th ed. New York: Churchill Livingstone, 1995:740–783.

Sila CA. Neurologic complications of vascular surgery. *Neurol Clin* 1998;16(1):10–20.

The Stroke Prevention in Atrial Fibrillation Investigators. Predictors of thromboembolism in atrial fibrillation. *Ann Intern Med* 1992;116(1):1–12.

Sutton JR, Houston CS, Mansell AL, et al. Effect of acetazolamide on hypoxemia during sleep at high altitude. *N Engl J Med* 1979;301:1329.

Tobin MJ, Cohn MA, Sackner MA. Breathing abnormalities during sleep. *Arch Intern Med* 1983;143:1221.

29.2

Neurological Complications of Systemic Disease: GI and Endocrine

Vicki Shanker

GASTROINTESTINAL DISTURBANCE AND NEUROLOGIC DISEASE

Gastrointestinal dysfunction can often manifest as cerebral impairment in the older adult. Changes can be as subtle as short-term memory loss or difficulty with concentration. Often, these signs are the initial or only presentation of a gastrointestinal disturbance. To achieve a rapid diagnosis, it is valuable for the primary care physician to be alert and aware of these presentations. This chapter provides a brief overview of the major gastrointestinal disturbances associated with neurologic complications in the elderly.

Hepatic Encephalopathy

Hepatic encephalopathy is a neuropsychiatric syndrome that can occur secondary to hepatocellular failure. Hepatitis, cirrhosis, and portal-systemic shunting are common causes. The clinical presentation of hepatic encephalopathy has been categorized in the literature into four separate stages (Table 29-1).

The first stage is notable for subtle neuropsychiatric impairment and changes in the patient that may only be recognizable by close family and friends. Symptoms include extreme mood disturbances, decreased attention span, slurred speech, and mild con-fusion. Intellectual function is preserved. The presence of asterixis, involuntary flapping hand movements with wrist extension, may be noted on physical examination.

As the disease process continues, intellectual and motor function is impaired and basic activities of daily life become challenging. Consciousness may fluctuate. Signs on examination include hypotonia, hyporeflexia, and a positive Babinski sign. Comatose states dominate endstage hepatic encephalopathy. Neurologic examination in endstage disease is significant for increased deep tendon reflexes.

The pattern of encephalopathy described is similar to that seen in other metabolic disturbances. However, some signs have been identified as more specific to liver dysfunction. These include a parkinsonian-like tremor, monotonous speech, dyskinesia, hypokinesia, bradykinesia, diminished facial expression (hypomimia), and increased muscle tone (Jones and Weissenborn, 1997).

Encephalopathic changes emerge over a period of days to weeks. In most patients, the disease does not develop past the first two stages. However, for cases in which it does, the course is not necessarily a direct route to severe impairment. The disease course can fluctuate between levels of impairment or it can steadily worsen. Depending on the cause, the course

TABLE 29-1. *Hepatic encephalopathy: characteristics of encephalopathic stages*

Grade	Level of consciousness	Personality/behavioral changes	Neurologic signs
0	Alert	None	Absent May have subtle abnormalities in psychometric testing if subclinical course
1	Alert; decreased attention	Mood changes Mild confusion Mild agitation	Asterixis Hypoactive reflexes Dysarthria
2	Lethargic	Overt personality changes Inappropriate behavior Fluctuating orientation to time	Asterixis Hyperactive reflexes Loss of sphincter tone
3	Somnolent but arousable	Episodes of rage Continuous disorientation to time and/or place	Asterixis Hyperactive reflexes Increased muscle tone
4	Comatose	Comatose	Decerebrate

From Riorda SM, Williams, R. Treatment of hepatic encephalopathy. *N Engl J Med* 1997;337:473–479, with permission.

of the disease can be acute, subacute, or chronic. A precipitating factor is often identified in an acute presentation but occurs variably in chronic forms (Table 29-2). When the causative factor is identified and then eliminated or treated, resolution of the symptoms usually follows. In the absence of a precipitating event, prognosis is poor.

Diagnosis

Diagnosis is based primarily on history, physical examination, and a strong clinical suspicion. The workup focuses on evidence of hepatocellular insufficiency and mental impairment. Test results are consistent with, but not specific to hepatic encephalopathy. Laboratory tests such as elevated liver function tests, increased prothrombin time, and raised ammonia levels may show signs of hepatic dysfunction. Of note, ammonia levels are not always elevated with hepatic dysfunction. When ammonia levels are elevated,

they do not consistently correlate with the degree of hepatic encephalopathy. Brain imaging is also nonspecific. Computed tomography (CT) is useful in these cases to rule out other considerations in the differential diagnosis. The main magnetic resonance imaging findings are symmetric pallidal hyperintensity in T_1-weighted images. The nigral substance area and the dentate cerebellar nucleus may show similar abnormalities. Electroencephalograph findings of triphasic waves are commonly found but are nonspecific. A referral to a neuropsychologist is valuable in further assessment of mental dysfunction in hepatic encephalopathy.

Treatment

Treatment focuses largely on reduction of systemic ammonia and on inhibition of γ-aminobutyric acid (GABA) receptor activation. Both have been identified as contributors to the pathophysiology of hepatic encephalopathy. Elevated ammonia levels have been shown to augment GABA-mediated neurotransmission, increasing neuronal inhibition.

Dietary protein restriction is a common approach to reducing intestinal production of ammonia. Patients are restricted to 20 g/day of protein. The dosage is increased 10 g for 3 to 5 days, until a tolerance threshold is reached. If tolerance is less than 1g/kg, vegetable protein is recommended as the primary source of protein because of its high fiber content. Fiber aids in improved food motility through the gastrointestinal system, decreasing the opportunity for protein absorption.

TABLE 29-2. *Common precipitators of hepatic encephalopathy*

Azotemia
Constipation
Excessive protein intake
Gastrointestinal hemorrhage
Hepatoma
Hypokalemia
Placement of portosystemic shunt
Progressive damage to hepatic parenchyma
Systemic alkalosis

Nonabsorbable disaccharides (e.g., lactulose and lactitol) are used to osmotically remove ammonia from the body. The estimated daily dose ranges from 30 to 60 g. The dose is titrated to produce two to four soft acidic (pH <6) stools per day. In an acute episode, the recommended starting dose is 30 to 45 mL at 1- to 2-hour intervals until a laxative effect is observed. Elderly patients taking lactulose should be monitored closely for fluid and electrolyte loss with chronic use, because they are more susceptible to neurologic impairment associated with dehydration and electrolyte loss than are younger patients.

Neomycin (6 g/day) and metronidazole (800 mg/day), inhibitors of urease-producing bacteria, are used to reduce ammonia. In the geriatric population, serum concentrations of these medications tend to be elevated as total clearance is reduced. Thus, elderly patients are more likely to suffer from side effects, including ototoxicity, nephrotoxicity, and gastrointestinal disturbance. Rifaximin (1,200 mg/day) is a nonabsorbable alternative to neomycin and metronidazole. The question of an additive effect of lactulose with antibiotics is currently under investigation. However, stool pH has been noted to increase, suggesting that disaccharide-metabolizing bacteria are killed by the antibiotic (Weber, 1994). Absence of these bacteria reduces the effectiveness of lactulose.

Other approaches to reducing ammonia levels include eradication of *Helicobacter pylori*, if present, because of its contribution to serum ammonia levels. Ornithine aspartate, an enzyme that converts ammonia to urea, is effective in serum ammonia reduction and can be taken orally. Benzoate or phenylacetate treatment reacts with glycine and glutamine, respectively, to increase metabolic conversion to form hippurate and phenacetylglutamine. Zinc is a necessary cofactor in two of the five enzymes in the urea cycle. Supplementation is recommended for those who are zinc deficient. Studies have explored the role of flumazenil, a benzodiazepine antagonist, in hepatic encephalopathy. Some have proposed that binding to the benzodiazepine receptor by substances not normally present in the brain plays an important role in hepatic encephalopathy. Flumazenil has had mixed results in clinical studies (Grimm et al., 1988; Bansky et al., 1989).

Liver transplantation is preferable to medical management in most patients with endstage cirrhosis, regardless of age. However, other medical problems may limit the utility of this option. The surgical creation of portal-systemic shunts, especially the transjugular intrahepatic portal-systemic shunt, is a frequently used procedure in those awaiting transplant.

However, patients above 65 years of age are significantly more likely to develop hepatic encephalopathy after this procedure.

Nutritional and Vitamin Deficiency

As the body ages, the efficiency of the gastrointestinal system remains remarkably intact. However, in the presence of disease, an older adult's ability to extract necessary nutrients and vitamins from the diet becomes impaired. To further compound the risk of nutritional deficiency, dietary intake in this population is often inadequate (Buchman, 1996).

A decrease in gastric acid production is among the most common changes in the aging gastrointestinal system. The presence of hypochlorhydria or achlorhydria facilitates the atrophy of the stomach mucosa. Lack of gastric acid production leads to bacterial overgrowth in the upper intestinal tract and malabsorption. Vitamin B_6, vitamin B_{12}, and folate are most notably affected by these changes. However, despite folate malabsorption, serum folate levels are often elevated because of an increase in the number of folate-synthesizing bacteria in the small intestine. Estimates of atrophic gastritis in the geriatric population range from 11% to 50% (Hurwitz et al., 1997; Saltzman and Russell, 1998). The most common cause of gastritis in this population is *H. pylori* infection in the gut. Table 29-3 summarizes the age-related changes, neurologic presentation, and treatment of the most common vitamin deficiencies seen in the elderly.

Vitamin B_{12} deficiency is reported to occur in approximately 30% of people above 60 years of age (Krasinski et al., 1986). The neurologic manifestations of the deficiency are well known and reported. The Schilling test is often used in diagnosis. The test is often separated into three separate stages. In the first phase of the test, the patient is given an oral dose of radiolabeled vitamin B_{12} followed by an intramuscular injection 2 hours later. The purpose of this is to saturate the body's B_{12} binding sites. The absorbed oral B_{12} cannot bind to the already saturated transcobalamine proteins and will be excreted in the urine by glomerular filtration. A percentage of the administered dose excreted in the urine over 24 hours is calculated. In patients with pernicious anemia or intestinal malabsorption, the urinary excretion is usually less than 6%, compared with the normal value, which is greater than 9%. Phase II is performed in a manner similar to the first test, with the exception that intrinsic factor is given with the oral dose of B_{12}. Pernicious anemia is suggested

TABLE 29-3. *Vitamin deficiencies*

Nutritional deficiency	Changes with aging	Neurologic presentation	Recommended treatment[a]
Vitamin B_6 (Pyridoxine) Vitamin B_{12}	Decreased serum levels Decreased levels of protein bound	Grand mal seizures Carpal tunnel syndrome Peripheral neuropathy Subacute combined systemic degeneration Dementia Psychosis Depression Irritability Apathy	2.0–2.2 mg/d men 1.6–2.0 mg/d women 2 µg/d men 1.6 µg/d women In deficiency, intramuscular injections of vitamin B_{12} (1,000 µg) for 5 days followed by 300 µg every 3 months
Folate	Decreased absorption	Depression	10 mg alpha-tocopherol equivalent for men 8 mg alpha-tocopherol equivalent for women
Thiamine		Wernicke's encephalopathy Korsakoff's syndrome "Dry" beri-beri Disorientation	1.2 mg/d men 1.0 mg/d women 10 mg/d thiamine is the corrective treatment in deficiency states If Wernicke's is suspected, 50 mg/d intramuscular injection for several days; then, 2.5–5 mg/d orally
Vitamin E		Spinocerebellar degeneration Peripheral axonopathy	50–100 IU/d

[a]Recommended daily allowance ≥51 years of age.

when the patient has an abnormal result in phase I followed by a normal test in phase II. If the first two tests produce abnormal results, the patient is treated with 2 weeks of tetracycline for possible bacteria overgrowth. Phase III of the Schilling test is performed after a 2-week course of antibiotic. The test is the same as the second phase. If the test is normal, it can be deduced that bacterial overgrowth caused the vitamin deficiency. Of note, the test results can be normal in elderly patients with atrophic gastritis, despite deficiency, because these patients malabsorb only protein-bound vitamin B_{12}.

Folate is found in leafy green vegetables and is supplemented in many foods. Folate deficiency is not generally associated with impairment of the nervous system. It has been identified as a source of depressive mood disorders and patients with low levels of serum folate have poorer responses to antidepressant medication (Hutto, 1997).

One mistake commonly made in treatment is masking *cobalamin deficiency* with folate supplementation. Lack of adequate amounts of either vitamin impairs DNA synthesis, resulting in a megaloblastic anemia. When large doses of folate are taken, the megaloblastic anemia is ameliorated (Grinblat, 1985). However, the underlying neurologic dam-

age persists and is able to advance. This is why both cobalamin and folic acid should be assessed when a megaloblastic anemia is suspected.

Pyridoxine deficiency is reported to be present in 32% of independent American elderly (Manore et al., 1989). It is usually associated with poor diet. Use of isoniazid or L-dopa can cause a pyridoxine deficiency as well.

Folate, vitamin B_6, and vitamin B_{12} are all cofactors involved in *homocysteine* metabolism (Stabler et al., 1997). Elevated levels of homocysteine are associated with atherosclerosis and increased risk of stroke.

Thiamine deficiency is rarely encountered, except in those with a history of alcoholism (Griffiths et al., 1967). Studies in Britain have found an incidence of thiamine deficiency in the elderly population ranging from 22% to 40% in an institutionalized population and between 8% and 31% in noninstitutionalized elderly (Vir and Love, 1997). Two disease states that can arise from thiamine deficiency are Wernicke-Korsakoff's psychosis and dry beriberi. "Dry" beriberi is a peripheral neuropathy usually identified by complaints of symmetric distal weakness, paresthesias, and pain. Hyporeflexia is usually seen on examination. The main characteristics of Wernicke-Korsakoff include nystagmus, ophthalmoplegia, ataxia, and global mental confusion. Motor deficits may also be present.

Finally, patients with problems absorbing fat and those with abetalipoproteinemia are susceptible to developing a vitamin E deficiency. Low levels of vitamin E have been associated with neuronal degeneration in the spinocerebellar tract, Clark's columns, and nuclei of Goll and Burdach.

In summary, the elderly are susceptible to neurologic changes produced by an underlying gastrointestinal disturbance. Most of these disturbances are reversible and often easily treated. Physicians with a heightened awareness of the various neurologic presentations may rapidly proceed to treatment of the underlying disorder, preventing further complications.

ENDOCRINE DISTURBANCE AND NEUROLOGIC DISEASE

Disturbances in the endocrine system often lead to metabolic imbalances. Diabetes mellitus type II, which presents in more than 14 million Americans, is the most well known of these imbalances. The nervous system responds to fluctuations of glucose in the body and it is impaired in patients suffering from diabetes mellitus over an extended period of time. This section addresses some of these changes and highlights some of the neurologic presentations and complications associated with other endocrine disturbances in the elderly.

Thyroid

Hypothyroidism

Hypothyroidism is a clinical syndrome produced by thyroid hormone deficiency. The prevalence of hypothyroidism in the elderly population has been estimated to fall in the range of 0.9% to 17.5% (Griffen, 1990; Hanson et al., 1975). The incidence of hypothyroidism in women is greater than in men, at all ages.

Hashimoto's thyroiditis is the most common cause of hypothyroidism in the elderly. Other common sources of hypothyroidism in the elderly include a history of radioactive iodine ablation therapy for Graves' disease, previous thyroidectomy, subacute thyroiditis, and use of drugs such as lithium and amiodarone (Wallace and Hofmann, 1998).

Hypothyroidism typically has an insidious onset in the elderly (Hurley and Gharib, 1995). Common clinical symptoms in the general population include depression, weight gain, hair loss, dry skin, cold intolerance, constipation, and muscle cramps. However, elderly patients often do not present with these classic symptoms. Instead, they may complain of anorexia and weight loss, incontinence, mental confusion, decreased mobility, and a recent history of falls. Frequently noted mental status changes include impaired concentration, word fluency, attention capabilities, and psychomotor slowing. Additionally, hypothyroidism can mask itself as obstructive sleep apnea, myopathy, carpal tunnel syndrome, or cerebellar ataxia. Of note, elderly patients, especially those with hypothermia, are more likely to develop myxedema coma (Khaira and Franklyn, 1999).

On examination, patients often show impairment in learning, word fluency, attention, and motor speed tests. Delayed relaxation of the ankle reflex, a common finding in hypothyroidism, is often difficult to observe in geriatric patients because many have diminished ankle reflexes as a normal change associated with aging. Decreased radial and biceps reflexes are more sensitive for this finding in the elderly.

Diagnostic evaluation of hypothyroidism should include laboratory measurements of thyroid-stimulating hormone (TSH), free T_4, and T_3U (Barzel, 1995). Elevated levels of TSH, in combination with depressed T_4 values, are characteristic of the disorder.

Many elderly patients will show TSH values between 10 and 20 $\mu IU/L$ with a normal serum T_4. This subset is diagnosed with subclinical hypothyroidism, most of whom are clinically asymptomatic. Prevalence estimates of subclinical hypothyroidism in the elderly have ranged from 7% to 17% of the ambulatory elderly population. Management of these patients is controversial. Some clinicians support treatment because approximately one fifth of the subclinical population will experience progression to overt hypothyroidism within 1 year of laboratory findings. The goal is to prevent development of symptoms. Others recommend therapy in all of these patients with thyroidal peroxidase antibodies (Braverman, 1999). This argument supports regular testing of thyroid hormone and TSH levels to identify patients at risk. However, many physicians have questioned the benefit of hormone replacement in patients without overt clinical symptoms.

L-thyroxine is the standard medical treatment for hypothyroidism. The synthetic hormone has a long half-life and can convert to T_3 *in vivo*. In older patients, the recommended starting dose is 0.025 mg/day. The medication can be gradually titrated upward every 4 to 6 weeks, until laboratory values of TSH are within normal limits. Because clearance of T_4 is reduced in the elderly, it is not necessary to check TSH levels more often than every 3 to 4 weeks. It is estimated that an effective dose of L-thyroxine in the elderly ranges between 0.075 and 0.125 mg/day.

Hyperthyroidism

The prevalence of hyperthyroidism in older persons is reported to range between 0.5% and 2.3% (Bagchi et al., 1990). Grave's disease and toxic multinodular goiter are the most common causes of hyperthyroidism in all age ranges. Patients taking thyroid hormone supplementation for an extended period of time may also develop hyperthyroidism in later years because of decreased metabolic clearance of thyroid hormone.

Common characteristics including heat intolerance, diaphoresis, palpitations, tremulousness, nervousness, restlessness, and weight loss are reported in only one fourth of all elderly with hyperthyroidism. Subtle complaints that may warrant further workup for hyperthyroidism in this population include chronic fatigue, emotional lability, muscle weakness, and wasting of the proximal muscles. Depression, lethargy, agitation, dementia, and confusion are common psychiatric manifestations.

Diagnosis can be confirmed with laboratory results of an elevated T_4 (or T_3 in cases where T_4 is normal) and a decreased TSH. Other findings may include an elevated alkaline phosphatase, mildly increased serum calcium, and decreased serum cholesterol.

Radioactive ablation is the recommended treatment in the elderly because of the operative risks associated with surgery. Medication therapy is not recommended because of the danger of toxicity as well as the difficulty in maintaining the extensive regimen required.

Adrenal Gland

The aging process is not associated with changes in cortisol production from the adrenal cortex. Both Cushing's disease and adrenal insufficiency are rare in the elderly (Winger and Hornick, 1996). However, because adrenal dysfunction is both a serious and often treatable condition, it should be considered in situations of unexplained hypotension or shocklike conditions. Neurologic complaints in those with excess cortisol include impotence and psychiatric problems. Cushing's syndrome can be confirmed with the dex-

amethasone test. The test is significant if, after receiving a 1-mg dose of oral dexamethasone given at 11 p.m. the previous evening, the fasting cortisol value is greater than 5 µg/dL the following morning. Affective disorders and Alzheimer's disease can produce false-positive results in the overnight dexamethasone suppression test (DST) (Miller et al., 1994). It is hypothesized that this occurs as a result of glucocorticoid receptor down-regulation in regions of the brain that usually inhibit glucocorticoid or cell loss (Sapolsky and Plotsky, 1990). The 2-day, low-dose DST is a more sensitive test, but more inconvenient to perform. Twenty-four hour urine cortisol is abnormal if greater than 150 g/dL. Serum corticotropin is measured to help differentiate the source of cortisol excess.

A common cause of adrenal insufficiency in the elderly is hemorrhage in the adrenal glands (Ackermann, 1994). This is usually seen in those taking coumadin. Elderly patients with adrenal insufficiency may present with delirium or dementia. Serum cortisol response to a corticotropin analog is the standard test. The corticotropin stimulation test should not be done if acute adrenal collapse is suspected. In these instances, serum cortisol is measured and the patient is rapidly administered 100 mg hydrocortisone intravenously (i.v.), followed by 10 mg/hour of hydrocortisone i.v. until the cortisol level is known. CT of the adrenal gland may indicate a metastatic, granulomatous, or atrophic process. Treatment is cortisol maintenance doses of 20 mg in the morning and 10 mg at night. Dexamethasone or prednisone is an alternative treatment favored because both drugs have longer half-lives and do not require biotransformation. Some patients will need mineralocorticoid treatment as well.

Parathyroid

Hypoparathyroidism is a recognized cause of secondary parkinsonism. Physiologically, calcium channels are involved in dopaminergic regulation. When the calcium channels are blocked, dopamine levels fall and parkinsonian symptoms emerge. Treatment is aimed at resolution of the hypocalcemic state.

Pancreas

Hyperglycemia

As the body ages, several changes occur that increase the risk of developing type 2 diabetes mellitus.

The modifications include decreased glucose tolerance, increased adipose tissue, and increased insulin resistance. The age of the patient not only increases the risk of having type 2 diabetes mellitus but also the risk of developing complications from the disease.

Neurologic complications of diabetes are more common than is often recognized by both the patient and the clinician. Although only 15% of patients with diabetes present with symptoms and signs of neurologic deficits, it is estimated that half of all patients with diabetes mellitus manifest neuropathic symptoms or show nerve conduction abnormalities. One multicenter study estimated 28.5% of the diabetic population has a neuropathy (Young et al., 1993). Factors that increase the risk of developing a neuropathy include (*a*) extended disease duration (12.5–13.5 years); (*b*) age >50; and (*c*) longstanding hyperglycemia secondary to poor diabetic control (Valensi et al., 1997; Young et al., 1993).

The underlying cause of both focal and multifocal diabetic neuropathy is thought to be ischemia to the vasa nervorum, the blood supply to the nerves. Diabetes mellitus can affect the nervous system in a multitude of ways. The most common neurologic presentation is a distal polyneuropathy that is primarily sensory in nature. Although most sensory changes in diabetic patients are painless, 7.5% report unpleasant sensations and pain. Sensory complaints manifest themselves in many forms, including numbness and tingling, hyperesthesias, and dysesthesias. When patients complain of pain, it is often described as lightening stabs, shooting, prickling, aching, or burning. The pain often worsens at night. Sensory changes are most often localized bilaterally in the feet and lower legs. The hands are usually affected in more severe cases. The presenting pattern is identified as "stocking glove" because of its classic distribution. The anterior chest and abdominal area can be involved as well.

Acute, painful neuropathy is a rare syndrome characterized by intense pain, predominantly in the distal lower extremities. The syndrome primarily appears in men who are diabetic. Patients complain of a burning sensation, with notable dysesthesias. Other symptoms include weight loss, depression, insomnia, and impotence. Sensory examination findings may be normal or show mild impairment in pain and temperature sensations. Motor examination findings may be significant for a mild foot weakness; however, normal examination results are not atypical. If nerve conduction study findings are abnormal, they will show decreased amplitude or absent sensory nerve action potentials. If sural nerve biopsy is performed, axonal degeneration is noted (Ross, 1993).

Impairment of sensory function can have adverse effects. For example, patients with diabetes mellitus are more likely to have silent myocardial infarctions. Additionally, distal sensory neuropathy decreases the patient's ability to detect foot trauma and increases the risk of infection and limb amputation (O'Connor et al., 1998). Older adults are especially susceptible to these risks. One English study found that 65% of diabetic amputees were above 65 years of age (Deerochanawong et al., 1992).

Mononeuropathies and radiculopathies can also occur, although much less frequently. Both tend to occur in older patients with undiagnosed or mild diabetes. Although any nerve can be affected, third and sixth nerve palsies are the most common (Moster, 1999). Isolated peripheral nerves can be affected as well. Femoral and sciatic nerves are most commonly affected in these instances. Thoracoabdominal neuropathy typically occurs in patients with longstanding diabetes. This truncal neuropathy, most often noted in patients over 50 years of age, is a condition in which the patient experience hyperpathic pain on the chest in a T3 through T12 distribution. Half of these patients have significant weight loss. Electromyography may show denervation in the intercostal and abdominal muscles.

Diabetic amyotrophy, an often ambiguously used term, is distinctive because it mostly targets people over 50 years of age. The term describes a syndrome involving both sensory and motor impairment (Riddle, 1990). Motor examination shows moderate to severe weakness and atrophy in the pelvifemoral muscles. Sensory abnormalities are described as aching or burning sensations in the back, hip, and thigh, with preserved sensation in these regions on physical examination. Both motor and sensory abnormalities have an asymmetric distribution. Onset can be acute or subacute. Prognosis for recovery is good, with a reported 60% of patients showing good recovery within 1 to 2 years.

The initial focus for treatment is alleviation of sensory complaints and neuropathic pain. The most common effective treatments include analgesics, tricyclic antidepressants, and antiepileptic medication (Table 29-4). However, in the elderly, problematic side effects often emerge (Table 29-4). Physical and occupational therapy have been shown to be effective for the relief of predominantly motor neuropathies.

Estimates indicate that 20% to 40% of patients with diabetes suffer from autonomic nervous system

TABLE 29-4. *Common medications used in painful diabetic neuropathy*

Classification	Dosage comments	Drugs	Changes specific to older populations
Analgesics	Recommend to start with half normal adult dose Monitor carefully	Ibuprofen Naproxen	The steady state concentration of the medication can be doubled in an older population
Antiepileptic drugs	Begin at subtherapeutic dosage and slowly titrate up to lowest possible effective dose	Gabapentin (NNT 3.8, NNH not available) Carbamezapine (NNT 3.3, NNH 1.9) Phenytoin (NNT 2.1, NNH 9.5)	In clinical studies, patients >65 years of age showed a side effect profile similar to that of younger populations Increased risk of developing SIADH, urinary retention, bradycardia, atrioventricular block, confusion, and agitation in the elderly Metabolized slower with an elevated risk of serum concentration toxicity in elderly
Tricyclic antidepressants	Start at 25 mg/d at bedtime, the dosage can be adjusted upward as needed or tolerated	Amitriptyline (NNT 2.1, NNH 9.7) Desipramine (NNT 2.2, NNH 20)	Increased sensitivity to anticholinergic, sedative, and hypotensive effects Less anticholinergic effects than other tricyclics

NNH, number needed to harm; NNT, number needed to treat; SIADH, syndrome of inappropriate antidiuretic hormone.

Data based on Nash, TP. Treatment options in painful diabetic neuropathy. *Acta Neurol Scand* 1999;173(Suppl): 36–42; and the United States Pharmacopeial Convention; 1999.

(ANS) dysfunction. The cardiovascular, gastrointestinal, and genitourinary systems are all at risk for damage (Table 29-5). Of note, one of the most detrimental effects of ANS impairment is the loss of a sympathetic response to hypoglycemic states. This loss usually occurs within the first 5 to 10 years after developing diabetes. Postural hypotension is especially common and problematic in the elderly because of an increased risk of falls. The elderly population is more likely to have complications from falls and, thus, the presence of postural hypotension increases the morbidity and mortality rates of older patients. Some of the major ANS complaints and common presentations consistent with these dysfunctions are discussed in Table 29-5.

History and neurologic examination are usually sufficient for diagnosis. Additional tests can be useful for specific problems. If postural hypotension is suspected, The American Diabetes Association recommends a battery of five tests: heart rate changes, performing the Valsalva maneuver during lying, standing, and deep breathing, as well as blood pressure changes after standing and sustained hand grip (Belmin and Valensi, 1996).

Several strategies have emerged to help combat the effects of diabetes on the ANS. Postural hypotension can be treated with the use of elastic stockings, elevation of the head when lying down, and increased salt in the diet. Fludrocortisone, a medication with the ability to increase plasma volume and arterial tone, is sometimes used in cases of postural hypotension.

Medications that increase the tone of the inferior esophageal sphincter and increase esophageal contraction have been used to improve gastric emptying in patients with gastroparesis. The medications include metoclopramide, cisapride, and domperidone. Although metoclopramide has been used successfully in younger populations, it can produce severe side effects, including delirium, parkinsonism, sedation, and urinary retention. For this reason, it is usually avoided in treatment of geriatric populations. Some studies have reported that erythromycin is useful for improving gastric motility in patients with gastroparesis (Jassens et al., 1990). Tetracycline has been found to be an effective treatment in some cases of diabetic diarrhea.

Patients with a neurogenic bladder should be advised to empty the bladder every 3 hours. In more severe cases, the patients can be taught to perform manual abdominal compression with urination or to self-catheterize. Parasympathomimetics are sometimes helpful in treatment. Follow-up with a urologist should be encouraged in all cases of neurogenic bladder and sexual dysfunction.

Several studies have addressed the prevention of diabetic neuropathy. The only current conclusive statement is that good glycemic control translates into less fre-

TABLE 29-5. *Summary of autonomic nervous system impairment*

Autonomic nervous system impairment	Neurologic dysfunction	Common symptoms/signs
Cardiovascular	Postural hypotension	Light-headedness Weakness Impaired vision Syncopal episodes
	Impaired heart rate	Resting tachycardia Loss of sleep, bradycardia Fixed heart rate
Gastrointestinal	Esophageal dysfunction	
	Gastroparesis	Epigastric discomfort Anorexia Nausea/vomiting
	Constipation	
	Diarrhea	Watery; often nocturnal or postprandial
Genitourinary	Erectile dysfunction	Insidious onset with gradual progression; impotence present in 35% of all diabetic men
	Neurogenic bladder	Begins with decreased urinary frequency Late problems of urinary retention with overflow incontinence Recurrent urinary tract infections
Other impairment	Thermoregulatory dysfunction	Distal anhydrosis Heat intolerance Gustatory sweating
	Pupillary constriction with impaired light response	
	Failure to respond to hypoglycemic states	Risk of hypoglycemic coma

quent and less severe neuropathies (Partanen et al., 1995). For this reason, maintenance of serum glucose should be closely monitored and kept as close to normal limits as possible.

Hypoglycemia

Hypoglycemia is a significant problem in the elderly population suffering from diabetes. Missing the diagnosis can lead to severe consequences, including coma and death. Typically, the disease presents insidiously. Patients often appear confused and disoriented. They may complain of transient neurologic deficits and their neurologic examination findings may fluctuate. The elderly are more susceptible to falls and hypothermia during these episodes. Diabetic medications should be closely monitored in these patients and oral hypoglycemic agents should be stopped or maintained on the lowest possible dose.

CONCLUSION

It is important for the general physician to take into account that typical diseases often do not present typ-ically in the older adult, especially in cases of endocrine dysfunction. Often, neurologic changes are vastly different from those seen in a younger patient with the same disease. The classic signs or symptoms of a disease may not be evident on history or physical examination. Screening should be done often to prevent missing a diagnosis and delaying treatment. Failure to identify these diseases can lead to serious morbidity and mortality.

REFERENCES

Ackermann RJ. Adrenal disorders: know when to act and what tests to give. *Geriatrics* 1994;49:32–37.

Bagchi N, Brown TR, Parish RF. Thyroid dysfunction in adults over the age of 55 years. A study in an urban U.S. community. *Arch Intern Med* 1990;150:785–787.

Bansky G, Meier PJ, Riederer E, et al. Effects of the benzo-diazepine receptor antagonist flumazenil in hepatic encephalopathy in humans. *Gastroenterology* 1989;97: 744–750.

Barzel US. Hypothyroidism. *Clin Geriatr Med* 1995;11: 239–249.

Belmin J, Valensi P. Diabetic neuropathy in elderly patients. *Drugs Aging* 1996;8:416–429.

Braverman LE. Subclinical hypothyroidism and hyperthyroidism in elderly subjects: should they be treated. *J Endocrinol Invest* 1999;22:1–3.

Buchman A. Vitamin supplementation in the elderly: a critical evaluation. *Gastroenterologist* 1996;4:262–265.

Deerochanawong C, Home PD, Alberti KG. A survey of lower limb amputation in diabetic patients. *Diabet Med* 1992;9:942–946.

Griffen J. Review: hypothyroidism in the elderly. *Am J Med Sci* 1990;299:344–345.

Griffiths LL, Brocklehurst JC, Sott DL, et al. Thiamine and ascorbic acid level in the elderly. *Gerontol Clin* 1967;9: 1–10.

Grimm G, Ferenci P, Katzenshlager R, et al. Improvement of hepatic encephalopathy treatment with flumazenil. *Lancet* 1988;2:1392–1394.

Grinblat J. Folate status in the aged. *Clin Geriatr Med* 1985; 1:711–728.

Hansen J, Skovsted L, Siersbok-Nielsen K. Age dependent changes in iodine metabolism and thyroid function. *Acta Endocrinol* 1975;79:60–65.

Hurley DL, Gharib H. Detection and treatment of hypothyroidism and Graves' disease. *Geriatrics* 1995;50: 41–44.

Hurwitz A, Brady DA, Schaal E, et al. Gastric acidity in older adults. *JAMA* 1997;278:659.

Hutto BR. Folate and cobalamin in psychiatric illness. *Compr Psychiatry* 1997;28:305–314.

Janssens J, Peters TL, Vantrappen G, et al. Improvement of gastric emptying in diabetic gastroparesis by erythromycin. *N Engl J Med* 1990;322:1028–1031.

Jones EA, Weissenborn K. Neurology and the liver. *J Neurol Neurosurg Psychiatry* 1997; 63:279–293.

Khaira JS, Franklyn JA. Thyroid conditions in older patients. *The Practioner* 1999;243:214–221.

Krasinski SD, Russel RM, Samloff IM, et al. Fundic atrophic gastritis in an elderly population. Effect on hemoglobin and several serum nutritional indicators. *J Am Geriatr Soc* 1986;34:800–806.

Manore MM, Vaughan LA, Carroll SS, et al. Plasma pyridoxal 58phosphate concentration and dietary vitamin B-6 intake in free-living, low-income elderly people. *Am J Clin Nutr* 1989;50:339–345.

Miller AH, Sastry GS, Speranza AJ, et al. Lack of association between cortisol hypersecretion and nonsuppression on the DST in patients with Alzheimer's disease. *Am J Psychiatry* 1994;151:267–270.

Moster ML. Neuro-ophthalmology of diabetes. *Current Opinion in Ophthalmology* 1999;10:376–381.

Nash TP. Treatment options in painful diabetic neuropathy. *Act Neurol Scand* 1999;173(Suppl):36–42.

O'Connor PJ, Spann SJ, Woolf SH. Care of adults with type 2, diabetes mellitus. *J Fam Pract* 1998;47: S13–S22.

Partanen J, Niskanen L, Lehtinen J, et al. Natural history of peripheral neuropathy in patients with non-insulin dependent diabetes mellitus. *N Engl J Med* 1995;333: 89–94.

Riddle, MC. Diabetic neuropathies in the elderly: management update. *Geraitrics* 1990;45:32–36.

Riordan SM, Williams R. Treatment of hepatic encephalopathy. *N Engl J Med* 1997;337:473–379.

Ross MA. Neuropathies associated with diabetes. *Med Clin North Am* 1993;77:111–124.

Saltzman JR, Russell RM. The aging gut. Nutritional issues. *Gastroenterol Clin North Am* 1998;27:309–324.

Samuels MH. Subclinical thyroid disease in the elderly. *Thyroid* 1998;8:803–813.

Sapolsky RM, Plotsky PM. Hypocortisolism and it possible neural base. *Biol Psychiatry* 1990;27:937–952.

Stabler SP, Lindenbaum J, Allen RH. Vitamin B-12 deficiency in the elderly: current dilemmas. *Am J Clin Nutr* 1997;66: 741–749.

United States Pharmacopeial Convention. USPDI 19th ed. Taunton, MA: Micromedex Inc., 1999.

Valensi P, Giroux C, Seeboth-Ghalayini B, et al. Diabetic peripheral neuropathy: effects of age duration of diabetes, glycemic control, and vascular factors. *J Diabetes Complications* 1997;11:27–34.

Vir S, Love A. Thiamine status of institutionalized and noninstitutionalized aged. *Int J Vitam Nutr Res Suppl* 1997; 47:325–335.

Wallace K, Hofmann MT. Thyroid dysfunction: how to manage overt and subclinical disease in older patients. *Geriatrics* 1998;53:32–41.

Weber FL Jr. Combination therapy with lactulose or lactitol and antibiotics. In: Conn HO, Bircher J, eds. *Hepatic encephalopathy: syndromes and therapies.* Bloomington, IL: Medi-Ed Press, 1994:285–297.

Winger JM, Hornick MD. Age-associated changes in the endocrine system. *Endocrine Disorders* 1996;31: 827–844.

Young MJ, Boulton AJM, Macleod AF, et al. A multicentre study of the prevalence of diabetic peripheral neuropathy in the United Kingdom hospital clinical population. *Diabetolgia* 1993;36:150–154.

WEB SITES

American Association of Clinical Endocrinologists: *www.aace.com*

Centers for Disease Control: *www.cdc.gov/health/diseases*

Centers for Disease Control: *www.cdc.gov/health/seniors*; American Diabetes Association: *www.diabetes.org*

Endocrinology Public Resource Service: *www.endocrinology.com*

National Institutes of Health: *www.nih.gov/health*

29.3

Neurological Manifestations of Systemic Disease: Disturbances of the Kidneys, Electrolytes, Water Balance, Rheumatology, Hematology/Oncology, Alcohol, and Iatrogenic Conditions

Kevin M. Biglan

NEUROLOGIC COMPLICATIONS OF RENAL DISEASE

Acute and chronic renal failure has a variety of deleterious effects on the nervous system. The mechanism is multifactorial and represents a combination of uremia, disturbances of electrolytes and water balance, impaired drug metabolism, anemia, associated comorbid illness, and the effects of hemodialysis. The incidence of chronic renal failure increases with increasing age (Andreoli et al., 1993), and uremia accounts for 10% of delirium in the elderly (Lipowski, 1994).

Acute Complications of Renal Failure

Uremic Encephalopathy

Encephalopathy or delirium is common in renal failure. Given the increased risk of delirium in the elderly (Flacker and Marcantonio, 1998), encephalopathy is nearly universal in the elderly patient who develops acute deterioration in renal function. Clinically, uremic encephalopathy is similar to delirium from other metabolic derangements (Raskin and Fishman, 1976, 143–148). Table 29-6 summarizes the clinical manifestations of this condition (Raskin, 1976; Burn and Bates, 1998). Early in the course, fatigue, apathy, difficulty with attention and concentration, and subtle motor signs predominate. Later, frank delirium that can progress to coma and seizures occurs (Raskin and Fishman, 1976, 143–148; Burn and Bates, 1998). Upper motor neuron signs may be seen, but generally they are symmetric.

The level of uremia correlates poorly with the degree of impairment. Azotemia only confirms that a patient has renal dysfunction and does not confirm

the cause of the delirium. The rapidity of renal deterioration is important in the development of encephalopathy (Burn and Bates, 1998). It can occur in the setting of decompensated chronic renal failure and acute renal failure. It is less likely to occur in well-compensated chronic renal failure, although it can predispose such patients to delirium from other causes (Flacker and Marcantonio, 1998).

Computed tomography (CT) and magnetic resonance imaging (MRI) can reveal nonspecific changes but should be performed in patients receiving hemodialysis (see complications of hemodialysis). Electroencephalography (EEG) can be useful in determining if superimposed seizures are contributing to a patient's confusion. In such cases, the EEG is abnormal, showing generalized slowing in the theta and delta range (Raskin and Fishman, 1976, 143–148; Burn and Bates, 1998). Caution must be used in interpreting the EEG, as spike and wave complexes can be seen in up to 14% of patients without clinical seizure activity (Burn and Bates, 1998).

Treatment of uremic encephalopathy entails correcting the underlying renal disease and, possibly, hemodialysis. Correction of an underlying anemia can

TABLE 29-6. *Clinical manifestations of uremic encephalopathy*

Fatigue
Motor abnormalities: clumsiness, ataxia, paratonia, hyperreflexia, Babinski's signs
Frontal lobe release signs
Delirium
Asterixis/myoclonus
Postural and kinetic tremor
Seizures

further improve cognitive function in some patients (Pickett et al., 1999). Seizures should be treated appropriately. Caution must be used with certain anticonvulsants (i.e., phenytoin and valproic acid) (Anderson, 1998), because of the reduced protein binding in renal failure secondary to hypoalbuminemia (Raskin and Fishman, 1976, 143–148).

Chronic Complications of Renal Failure

Uremic Neuropathy

Neuropathy occurs in 70% of patients with chronic renal failure. It is more common in older patients and men (Burn and Bates, 1998). It is a distal, symmetric, sensorimotor axonal polyneuropathy (Burn and Bates, 1998; Raskin and Fishman, 1976, 204–210). The severity and course are variable and, in mild cases, may resolve or improve with dialysis. Successful renal transplantation results in a dramatic improvement in the neuropathy (Burn and Bates, 1998).

Clinically, patients complain of burning paresthesias and distal motor weakness. Findings on physical examination are diminished or absent reflexes, muscle atrophy, and a stocking-glove sensory loss. Restless legs syndrome, a frequent accompaniment (Trenkwalder et al., 1995), is a condition characterized by abnormal sensations in the legs and arms accompanied by a desire to move the legs. Standing or walking relieves the symptoms, whereas rest exacerbates them. The symptoms are more severe in the evening or at night (Walters, 1995). Dopamine agonists (i.e., pramipexole or ropinirole) (Trenkwalder et al., 1995; Ondo, 1999), given at night, are useful for ameliorating the symptoms.

Myopathy

Myopathy in renal failure is multifactorial. Proximal muscle weakness and atrophy associated with bone pain make up the clinical picture. Neurophysiologic studies reveal a myopathic pattern, whereas muscle histology is nonspecific. Rarely, a fulminant painful myopathy associated with necrosis occurs (Burn and Bates, 1998).

Complications of Dialysis

Dialysis Dysequilibrium Syndrome

The elderly are at high risk for developing dysequilibrium, a complication of dialysis. It can occur during or shortly after peritoneal or hemodialysis. It occurred more commonly before 1970 when patients were rapidly dialyzed over a short period of time, but this syndrome is rarely seen today (Burn and Bates, 1998; Raskin and Fishman, 1976, 204–210).

A wide variety of symptoms may be seen, from the mild (headaches, myalgias, restlessness) to the severe (coma and seizures). Symptoms begin at the end of dialysis or shortly thereafter. Dialysis dysequilibrium is believed to occur secondary to large osmotic gradients between the brain and plasma, resulting in large fluid shifts into the brain parenchyma. Clinically, this results in increased intracranial pressure and obtundation from cerebral edema (Burn and Bates, 1998; Raskin and Fishman, 1976, 204–210).

Prevention is the key to managing this problem. Slow dialysis, every 1 to 2 days, and the use of osmotically active solutes have largely eliminated this complication.

Dementia

Impaired cognition is common in endstage renal disease (Lass et al., 1999). A significantly higher percentage of patients on dialysis will have dementia compared with age-matched controls (Lass et al., 1999). Although the cause is unclear, it may be related to ischemic disease in some patients (Lass et al., 1999). Also, cerebral atrophy is seen in patients with renal failure on dialysis and the degree of atrophy correlates with duration of dialysis (Kamata et al., 2000).

In addition, a specific syndrome has been associated with chronically dialyzed patients. It is commonly referred to as *dialysis dementia, dialysis encephalopathy, or progressive myoclonic dialysis encephalopathy* (O'Hare et al., 1983). This is a progressive and potentially fatal disorder characterized by progressive cognitive decline (Burn and Bates, 1998). Disorders of speech—a slowness and hesitancy of speech and paraphasia—occur commonly and early in the course of this disorder (Burn and Bates, 1998; O'Hare et al., 1983). Some cases progress to an overt expressive aphasia, whereas others may represent an apraxia of speech (O'Hare et al., 1983). Myoclonus is ubiquitous and ataxia and apraxias can occur. Changes in personality, with psychosis and hallucinations, occur in more advanced cases. Seizures occur late in as many as 60% to 100% of patients (Burn and Bates, 1998; O'Hare et al., 1983).

Frontal intermittent rhythmic delta activity is the most characteristic finding on EEG (Burn and Bates, 1998; O'Hare et al., 1983). Generalized slowing, triphasic waves and spike and wave activity may also be seen on EEG (O'Hare et al., 1983). Neuroimaging and cerebrospinal fluid (CSF) examination are useful in ruling out other causes of the patient's deterioration (Burn and Bates, 1998).

This dementing disorder has been linked to aluminum concentrations in dialysate water supply (Mach et al., 1988; Davison et al., 1982). The use of deionized water with low aluminum levels has nearly eliminated this condition (Davison et al., 1982). However, sporadic cases do occur and may be associated with aluminum-containing, phosphate-binding agents used in this population (Burn and Bates, 1998). Treatment consists of the use of aluminum free water in the dialysate and aluminum chelating agents (desferrioxamine). Paradoxically, a period of clinical worsening may occur at the initiation of therapy (Burn and Bates, 1998).

Subdural Hematoma

SDH can occur in 1% to 3% of patients receiving hemodialysis in the absence of trauma (Burn and Bates, 1998). The cause is multifactorial, and likely reflects a combination of cerebral atrophy, large fluid shifts during dialysis, coagulopathies, and the use of anticoagulants during dialysis. Signs and symptoms include diminished level of consciousness, headache, and focal neurologic deficits. However, bilateral SDH are common and can present with confusion, lethargy, and gait dysfunction. Therefore, a high index of suspicion must be maintained for this complication. All patients on dialysis who develop an alteration in mental status should have a CT scan to rule out the possibility of SDH. Conservative treatment, with close clinical follow-up, may be all that is needed in some patients; however, surgical drainage may also be required.

DISTURBANCES OF SODIUM AND WATER BALANCE

Dehydration

Dehydration is the most common fluid disturbance in the elderly (Lavizzo-Mourey et al., 1988). Dehydration accounts for 1.5% of hospital admissions of the elderly and frequently complicates other illnesses (Reyes-Ortiz, 1997). In addition, dehydration is a major risk factor for the development of delirium in the inpatient setting (Inouye, 2000). Table 29-7 summarizes the major risk factors for dehydration in elderly nursing home patients (Lavizzo-Mourey et al., 1988).

Treatment of dehydration requires removing any offending drugs and hydration with isotonic saline until the patient is hemodynamically stable. Subsequently, 0.45% saline solution can be used until the water deficit is corrected. Caution must be used in us-

ing hypotonic solutions as they may precipitate hyponatremia.

Hyponatremia

In general, water balance is strictly maintained such that the serum sodium concentrations range between 138 and 142 mmol/L (Kumar and Berl, 1998). Deficits in the ability of the kidney to dilute the urine, coupled with increased fluid intake, results in hyponatremia.

Neurologic complications of hyponatremia are dependent on the severity of the hyponatremia and the rate that it evolved. Rapid development (<48 hours) can precipitate cerebral edema and result in obtundation, leading to coma and seizures (Kumar and Berl, 1998; Delanty et al., 1998). When hyponatremia is known to have developed in less than 48 hours and the patient has neurologic symptoms, then rapid correction is warranted (Kumar and Berl, 1998). This can be achieved by the infusion of hypertonic saline (3% NaCl) in combination with a loop diuretic (Kumar and Berl, 1998). Electrolytes must be followed closely.

When the duration of hyponatremia is unknown, it must be corrected with extreme caution because of the risk of central pontine myelinolysis (CPM) (Kumar and Berl, 1998; Laureno and Karp, 1997). The rate of sodium replacement should not exceed 0.55 mmol/L/hour and not more than 12 mmol/L in the first 24 hours of treatment (Sterns et al., 1994). Frequent and close monitoring is needed in these patients. Clinical symptoms in chronic hyponatremia can be nonexistent; in this circumstance, immediate treatment is not warranted (Kumar and Berl, 1998).

Hypernatremia

Hypernatremia is less common than hyponatremia, however, central nervous system (CNS) manifestations are frequently more prominent (Kumar and Berl, 1998). Also, the elderly are more susceptible to hypernatremia than other age groups (Ayus and Arieff, 1996). Symptoms of delirium, with alterations in level of consciousness and seizures, can occur (Kumar and Berl, 1998; Delanty et al., 1998). Focal

TABLE 29-7. *Risk factors for dehydration*

Age >85 yr
Chronic or acute diseases >4
Medications >4
Winter season
Requires assistance with feeding
Immobility

deficits may reflect subdural hemorrhage if the change in sodium levels occurred rapidly (Aminoff, 2000). In the most common setting, hypernatremia reflects a hypovolemic state and treatment is as outlined for dehydration.

Central Pontine Myelinolysis

CPM is a catastrophic disorder associated with the rapid correction of hyponatremia. The term CPM is misleading as extrapontine white matter is frequently involved. Pathologically, extensive and symmetric white matter dysmyelination is out of proportion to neuronal loss. Clinical presentations vary, depending on the degree and location of myelinolysis, although more than 90% of patients will have the classic findings of spastic quadriparesis and pseudobulbar palsy. Prognosis varies from death to complete recovery. MRI of the brain reveals symmetric areas of T2 hyperintensity in the pontine and extrapontine white matter. Caution must be used in interpreting scans too early, as the characteristic changes may delay the clinical presentation of CPM by 2 weeks (Laureno and Karp, 1997; Charness, 1993).

The only treatment is prevention, and the hyponatremia must be corrected cautiously. However, CPM has been reported to develop despite *safe* correction of hyponatremia (Laureno and Karp, 1997). Therefore, correcting the hyponatremia with the associated potential of myelinolysis must outweigh the risks of illness from hyponatremia.

DISTURBANCES OF POTASSIUM BALANCE

Hypokalemia

Hypokalemia is common in elderly patients admitted to the hospital (Judge, 1968). In its mildest forms, it is associated with myalgias and proximal muscle weakness; in severe cases, profound weakness, rhabdomyolysis, and tetany can occur (Aminoff, 2000). Rarely, this will occur acutely and be associated with thyrotoxicosis (Akhter and Wiede, 1997; van Dam et al., 1996). Potassium replacement is effective in treating the symptoms (Aminoff, 2000).

Hyperkalemia

Hyperkalemia causes a profound, rapidly progressive, flaccid quadriplegia sparing the cranial nerve musculature (Aminoff, 2000; Evers et al., 1998). Paresthesias are sometimes seen. Drugs or renal failure are common causes (Evers et al., 1998). Mortal-

ity is related to cardiovascular complications (Aminoff, 2000). Aggressive reduction of the serum potassium results in resolution of the symptoms (Evers et al., 1998).

DISTURBANCES OF CALCIUM BALANCE

Hypocalcemia

Hypocalcemia is an abnormally low concentration of ionized calcium. It is usually the result of hypoparathyroidism (Finkelstein et al., 1993, 538–546) and is a well-recognized complication of thyroid or parathyroid surgery (Aminoff, 2000). Tetany associated with perioral and limb paresthesia is the most common manifestation (Aminoff, 2000; Finkelstein et al., 1993, 538–546). Seizures and psychosis can also occur (Delanty et al., 1998; Aminoff, 2000). Chvostek's sign (i.e., spasm of the facial muscles with percussion of the facial nerve) and Trousseau's sign (i.e., spasm of the hand after inflation of a blood pressure cuff above the systolic blood pressure) are positive (Finkelstein et al., 1993, 538–546). Symptoms correct with calcium replacement (Aminoff, 2000).

Hypercalcemia

Hypercalcemia, which is more common than hypocalcemia, may be the result of hyperparathyroidism, malignancy, or drugs (Finkelstein et al., 1993, 538–546; Hanagan, 1982). Delirium can occur but seizures are rare. Muscle weakness and fatigability are peripheral manifestations (Aminoff, 2000). Therapy is based on the underlying cause and clinical symptoms (Hanagan, 1982). Intravenous hydration, loop diuretics, glucocorticoids, and calcitonin can be used nonspecifically to reduce serum calcium levels while the underlying cause is being investigated (Finkelstein et al., 1993, 538–546).

DISTURBANCES OF MAGNESIUM BALANCE

Hypomagnesemia

Hypomagnesemia results from poor dietary intake or absorption or through increased magnesium loss via renal mechanisms (Berkelhammer and Bear, 1985). It is frequently associated with hypocalcemia and the clinical symptoms are similar (Aminoff, 2000; Berkelhammer and Bear, 1985). Hypomagnesemia must always be suspected when a patient with hypocalcemia fails to respond to calcium replacement (Aminoff, 2000). Treatment with oral magnesium supplementation is usually sufficient.

Hypermagnesemia

Hypermagnesemia is rarely relevant clinically and is usually associated with renal failure (Finkelstein et al., 1993, 530–538). Somnolence, confusion, and weakness associated with reduced or absent reflexes are the neurologic manifestations (Aminoff, 2000). Treatment consists of dialysis in renal failure or intravenous administration of 100 to 200 mg of calcium (Finkelstein et al., 1993, 530–538).

NEUROLOGIC COMPLICATIONS OF CANCER

The incidence of cancer increases with age. The elderly, therefore, are at an increased risk of developing neurologic complications from cancer. In addition, besides routine chemotherapy, neurologic symptoms are the most common reason for hospitalization of individuals with known cancer (Gilbert and Grossman, 1986). Neurologic disease in cancer occurs via four separate mechanisms: (*a*) metastatic involvement of brain parenchyma, meninges, or spinal cord; (*b*) direct extension into neural structures (e.g., lumbosacral plexus); (*c*) remote involvement (i.e., paraneoplastic syndromes); and (*d*) neurotoxic effects of cancer therapy (Gilbert and Grossman, 1986; Clouston et al., 1992; Jaeckle et al., 1985; Goldberg et al., 1982). This section briefly discusses the first three mechanisms (see Chapter 28 for additional information on these topics), focusing primarily on the toxic effects of cancer therapy.

Metastatic Disease

Metastasis can occur in any portion of the nervous system, although the brain is the most common region involved (Clouston et al., 1992). Spinal cord involvement occurs through vertebral body metastasis and subsequent extension into the epidural space with cord compression (Clouston et al., 1992). Less commonly, metastasis to the meninges can occur (Clouston et al., 1992; Grossman and Krabak, 1999), presenting with symptoms of increased intracranial pressure, multiple cranial neuropathies, and multiple radiculopathies. Leptomeningeal metastases have a poor prognosis without aggressive therapy (Grossman and Krabak, 1999). In terms of overall numbers, tumors of the lung and breast most commonly metastasize to the nervous system (Clouston et al., 1992; Grossman and Krabak, 1999).

Direct Invasion

Pancoast tumors of the lung may extend into the brachial plexus, causing plexopathies that affect the muscles of the lower cord of the brachial plexus and a Horner's syndrome (Jones and Detterbeck, 1998). Pelvic tumors can extend into the lumbosacral plexus, resulting in a disabling plexopathy (Jaeckle et al., 1985; Pettigrew et al., 1984). Finally, tumors of the nasopharynx can invade through the skull base, causing cranial neuropathies, pneumoencephalos and death (Peterson and Heim, 1991; Kiu et al., 1996). Treatment depends on the tumor type, but commonly consists of a combination of chemotherapy, radiation therapy, and surgery.

Paraneoplastic Syndromes

Neurologic paraneoplastic syndromes affect less than 1% of all cancer patients, however they have a significant impact on the patient's quality of life and can precede the cancer diagnosis in 50% of cases (Nath and Grant, 1997). Table 29-8 summarizes the

TABLE 29-8. *Summary of paraneoplastic syndromes*

Syndrome	Antibody	Tumor types
Cerebellar degeneration	Anti-Yo	Ovary, breast, lung
Limbic encephalitis/myelitis	Anti-Hu	Small cell lung
Opsoclonus-myoclonus	Anti-Ri	Breast (adults)
Sensory neuronopathy	Anti-Hu	Small cell lung
AIDP/CIDP	Anti-GM1/MAG[a]	Hodgkins, osteosclerotic myeloma
Lambert-Eaton myasthenic syndrome	Anti-voltage gated calcium channel (NMJ)	Small cell lung, prostate, cervix

AIDP, acute inflammatory demyelinating polyneuropathy; CIDP, chronic inflammatory demyelinating neuropathy; NMJ, neuromuscular junction.
[a]Anti-MAG antibodies are associated with a pure motor polyneuropathy.

more common paraneoplastic syndromes (Nath and Grant, 1997; Posner, 1995, 353–385; Ropper and Gorson, 1998).

COMPLICATIONS OF CANCER TREATMENT

Chemotherapeutic Agents

Neurologic side effects of cancer treatments are common and frequently add to the confusion surrounding neurologic symptoms in these patients. Many chemotherapeutic agents have neurotoxic side effects (Kaplan and Wiernik, 1982).

Methotrexate

Intrathecal methotrexate (MTX) causes an acute meningeal reaction approximately 2 to 4 hours after administration. Meningismus, headache, nausea, lethargy, and spinal fluid pleocytosis are common (Kaplan and Wiernik, 1982). No long-term sequelae of this manifestation occur and it resolves spontaneously in days (Goldberg et al., 1982; Kaplan and Wiernik, 1982). However, it must be distinguished from bacterial meningitis, which can cause delays in treatment.

A subacute reaction to MTX can occur after multiple intrathecal injections (Goldberg et al., 1982). This reaction results in clinical signs of a spinal cord lesion with paraplegia, and sensory level and bladder dysfunction. The condition gradually improves over days to months, and recovery is variable (Kaplan and Wiernik, 1982).

Encephalopathies associated with long-term MTX use have been identified independent of the method of delivery. Patients are confused, lethargic, and ataxic and may have seizures. A delayed necrotizing encephalopathy is also seen years after treatment with intrathecal or intravenous MTX (Goldberg et al., 1982; Kaplan and Wiernik, 1982). This condition begins insidiously, progressing to dementia. It has been associated with high doses of MTX combined with cranial irradiation (Kaplan and Wiernik, 1982).

Cytosine Arabinoside

Cytosine arabinoside (AraC) can cause a reversible cerebellar syndrome peaking after 2 to 3 days of onset. Most patients recover completely after cessation of the drug. Age above 50 years appears to be the greatest risk factor for this complication (Posner, 1995b). AraC given intrathecally can cause a chemical meningitis and myelopathy similar to that seen with methotrexate (Kaplan and Wiernik, 1982).

Platinum

Platinum-based drugs (cisplatin) have long been associated with ototoxicity, causing symptoms of tinnitus and hearing loss (Goldberg et al., 1982; Kaplan and Wiernik, 1982). A distal symmetric, predominantly sensory, axonal neuropathy is also seen (Goldberg et al., 1982; Kaplan and Wiernik, 1982). The neuropathy is dose-dependent, and synergistic toxicity is seen with doxorubicin, vindesine, and etoposide (Sahenk, 1987).

Vinca Alkaloids

The use of vinca alkaloids is limited by its ubiquitous involvement of the nervous system (Goldberg et al., 1982; Kaplan and Wiernik, 1982). Peripheral neuropathy occurs early in nearly all patients receiving vinca alkaloids (e.g. vincristine) (Goldberg et al., 1982; Kaplan and Wiernik, 1982; Argov and Mastaglia, 1979). The neuropathy is a distal symmetric sensorimotor axonal polyneuropathy. Motor manifestations resolve with discontinuation of the drug but sensory manifestations persist (Goldberg et al., 1982). Vincristine has been associated with an autonomic neuropathy that preferentially affects the gastrointestinal tract, causing constipation. Cranial neuropathies are also seen and must be distinguished from carcinomatous involvement of the meninges (Goldberg et al., 1982; Kaplan and Wiernik, 1982).

Hexamethylmelamine

Hexamethylmelamine causes a peripheral neuropathy similar to vincristine (Goldberg et al., 1982). It has also been associated with a wide variety of CNS effects from parkinsonism to ataxia (Kaplan and Wiernik, 1982).

Fluorouracil

Fluorouracil causes an acute cerebellar syndrome 2 weeks to 6 months into treatment (Goldberg et al., 1982; Kaplan and Wiernik, 1982). The incidence of this complication appears to be dose-related (Kaplan and Wiernik, 1982). This syndrome is reversible with discontinuation of the drug, however, it rapidly recurs if the drug is reintroduced (Goldberg et al., 1982; Kaplan and Wiernik, 1982). Metastasis to the cerebellum constitutes the major differential diagnosis and must be ruled out if this condition occurs.

The combination of fluorouracil with levamisole has been associated with a multifocal inflammatory leukoencephalopathy. Symptoms begin within a few months of initiating treatment and are characterized by confusion and focal neurologic signs. MRI reveals multiple gadolinium-enhancing white matter lesions. Discontinuation of the drug and treatment with corticosteroids may result in improvement (Posner, 1995b).

Taxol

Taxol is one of the newer chemotherapeutic agents to be approved for the treatment of resistant ovarian cancers. Taxol causes a distal, predominantly sensory, axonal neuropathy (Sahenk et al., 1994).

Radiation Therapy

Radiation can have a negative impact on the nervous system by direct toxic effects of radiation on neural tissues or by damaging the vasculature that supplies neural tissue (Palmer, 1972; DeAngelis et al., 1989; Dropcho, 1991; Rottenberg et al., 1977; Murros and Toole, 1989). Secondary tumors of the nervous system occur as a result of irradiation received as a child and, therefore, do not generally have an impact on the elderly receiving therapeutic radiation for cancer (Dropcho, 1991).

Radiation-induced injury to the nervous system occurs when the neural tissue lies within the field of radiation. This can occur as incidental radiation (radiation to head and neck tumors with incidental brain radiation) or directly (whole brain radiation for metastatic tumors). Direct injury to the spinal cord can be divided into transient myelopathy, delayed progressive myelopathy, or motor neuron syndrome. Radiation injury to the brain can be acute, early delayed, or delayed (Dropcho, 1991). The peripheral nervous system (PNS) is also susceptible to radiation injury and radiation-induced plexopathy is a well-recognized complication of radiation therapy (Pettigrew et al., 1984; Harper et al., 1989).

Spinal Cord Injury

A transient myelopathy associated with incidental radiation to the spinal cord is the most common spinal cord complication of radiation treatments (Dropcho, 1991). The symptoms, which are relatively mild, develop several months after treatment. Symptoms consist mainly of paresthesia and Lhermitte's sign. Objective neurologic findings are wholly lacking. The symptoms resolve over 1 to 9 months (Dropcho, 1991).

Delayed progressive myelopathy is a more feared complication of radiation involving the spinal cord. The symptoms can occur as early as a few months after treatment or as long as 5 years (Dropcho, 1991). Sensory complaints of paresthesia and anesthesia are the earliest manifestations (Palmer, 1972; Dropcho,

1991). The condition is progressive, resulting in disabling weakness and bladder dysfunction (Palmer, 1972; Dropcho, 1991). The motor and sensory level corresponds anatomically with the level radiated. A Brown-Sequard pattern of involvement may be seen (Palmer, 1972; Dropcho, 1991). Neuroimaging with MRI can help distinguish this condition from other causes of myelopathy, particularly metastatic disease.

An isolated lower motor neuron syndrome has been reported in individuals who have received spinal radiation. The lumbosacral spine is preferentially involved in this condition (Dropcho, 1991).

Cerebral Injury

In cerebral injury, an acute reaction to brain irradiation occurs within days of radiotherapy. Symptoms include headache, lethargy, and nausea. Cerebral edema is the believed cause and treatment with dexamethasone prophylactically is recommended for individuals with a large tumor burden or who are receiving a large dose of radiation (Dropcho, 1991).

Early delayed encephalopathy is a self-limited complication occurring a few months after irradiation and lasting several weeks before resolving. Headache and lethargy are the prominent symptoms. Dexamethasone is sometimes used. Neuroimaging may show worsening edema and be indistinguishable from tumor recurrence. Stereotactic biopsy may be necessary to rule out treatment failures (Dropcho, 1991).

Delayed cerebral necrosis can occur months to years after direct or incidental brain radiation (Dropcho, 1991). Dementia, seizures, headache, personality changes, or focal neurologic signs are common (DeAngelis et al., 1989; Dropcho, 1991; Rottenberg et al., 1977). Imaging may reveal focal abnormalities indistinguishable from tumor or diffuse abnormalities in the deep white matter and cerebral atrophy (DeAngelis et al., 1989; Dropcho, 1991). DeAngelis et al. (1989) recommend a trial of steroids and consideration of ventriculoperitoneal shunting.

Cerebrovascular disease of the intracranial and extracranial vessels is another cause of delayed cerebral injury (Dropcho, 1991; Murros and Toole, 1989). The cerebrovascular disease manifests itself by transient ischemic attacks and, rarely, strokes. This condition is believed to represent accelerated atherosclerosis (Dropcho, 1991; Murros and Toole, 1989).

Peripheral Injury

As mentioned, plexopathy can result from radiation injury (Harper et al., 1989). This condition is frequently difficult to distinguish from tumor involvement of the plexus. Myokymia clinically and electrophysiologically may be more common in radiation injury (Harper et al., 1989). MRI of the plexus may be useful in distinguishing the two entities.

NEUROLOGIC COMPLICATIONS OF HEMATOLOGIC ILLNESS

Thrombotic Thrombocytopenic Purpura

Thrombotic thrombocytopenic purpura is a severe multisystem disease characterized by fever, thrombocytopenia, microangiopathic hemolytic anemia, neurologic symptoms, and impaired renal function (Eldor, 1998). It tends to affect a younger population, but can be seen in any age group. Table 29-9 reviews the common conditions where thrombotic thrombocytopenic purpura is seen (Eldor, 1998).

Neurologic complications can be secondary to ischemia in the small blood vessels or hemorrhage, resulting in permanent neurologic deficits. Transient and fluctuating neurologic signs without permanent deficits are more common. These can include headache, delirium, motor and sensory deficits, seizures, and even coma (Eldor, 1998).

Plasma exchange is the mainstay of treatment. Corticosteroids, antiplatelet medications, and immunosuppressants can be used as adjuvant therapy. Splenectomy is reserved for patients who are refractory to other treatments (Eldor, 1998).

Disseminated Intravascular Coagulation

Disseminated intravascular coagulation (DIC) is a syndrome of widespread intravascular coagulation. Clinically, patients develop widespread ischemia followed by bleeding. Multiple causes exist for DIC, including infection, trauma, cancer, and vascular diseases. Treatment is geared toward the underlying cause. Additionally, supportive care is frequently nec-

essary. Fluid resuscitation, fresh frozen plasma, and platelet transfusions are useful. The neurologic complications are related to CNS ischemia (stroke) and hemorrhage (Frewin et al., 1997).

NEUROLOGIC MANIFESTATIONS OF RHEUMATOLOGIC DISEASE AND SYSTEMIC VASCULITIDES

Epidemiology of Rheumatic Disease in the Elderly

Spinal osteoarthritis and spondylosis are nearly universal consequences of aging. Other rheumatic diseases are much less common. Although most rheumatic diseases begin in young to mid adulthood, they can also affect the older adult population. Notable exceptions include rheumatoid arthritis and giant cell arteritis, which actually have an increasing prevalence with increasing age (Rosenbaum et al., 1996). Improved therapies have allowed many young individuals with rheumatologic disease to live longer. Therefore, the more common rheumatic disorders primarily affecting the aged are discussed in this section. Table 29-10 provides information on the epidemiology of these disorders (Rosenbaum et al., 1996; Nakamura, 1997; Sigal, 1987; Steen and Medsger, 1990; Harris and Pierangeli, 1997; Jennette and Falk, 1997; Okada et al., 1991; Lafitte, 2000; Averbuch-Heller et al., 1992; Reich et al., 1990; Caselli et al., 1988; Scott, 1993; Dreyer and Boden, 1999).

The incidence of neurologic complications of rheumatologic diseases varies from the exceedingly rare (e.g., the sensory neuronopathy of Sjögrens disease) (Rosenbaum et al., 1996; Font et al., 1990) to the very common (e.g., headache in giant cell arteritis) (Caselli and Hunder, 1997). However, these neurologic complications may be the initial manifestation of the disease (Guillevin et al., 1997) and are frequently associated with high morbidity and mortality. For these reasons, this subgroup of disorders deserves special attention.

Osteoarthritis

Osteoarthritis is ubiquitous in the elderly. It is a common cause of neurologic disease and disability. The most common complaint associated with osteoarthritis is pain. Low back pain is one of the most common reasons patients seek medical attention (Rosenbaum et al., 1996). Frank neurologic dysfunction secondary to radiculopathy, mononeuropathy, and myelopathy are common consequences of degenerative disease of the joints. Infrequently, osteoarthri-

TABLE 29-9. *Conditions that may precipitate thrombotic thrombocytopenic purpura*

Bacterial infections: shigella, *Escherichia coli*, salmonella, *Campylobacter jejuni, yersinia*, pneumococcus
Viral infections: coxsackie B, echovirus, influenza, Epstein-Barr virus, herpes simplex virus
Cancer: adenocarcinoma, lymphoma
Drugs: penicillin, sulfa, quinine, ticlopidine, cyclosporin, FK 506, chemotherapy
Bone marrow transplantation

TABLE 29-10. *Epidemiology of rheumatic diseases*

Disease	Prevalence (per 100,000)	Incidence (per million per year)	Female: male ratio	Age at onset	Neurologic involvement (% with)
Rheumatoid arthritis	0.2–2.0	300	2–3:1	40–60	7–13 (excluding pain)
Systemic lupus erythematosus	0.0005–0.04	46–74	7–9:1	15–30	36
Systemic sclerosis	4×10^{-6}–0.007	6.3–18.7	3–15:1	30–50	6–40
Primary Sjögrens			9:1	40–50	20
Sarcoidosis		40–100	3:2	20–40	5
Giant cell arteritis (age >50)	0.13–0.24	30–200	3:1	>60	10–40
Polyarteritis nodosa group	0.7–6.3	9	1:2	40–60	PAN/CSS = 50–75 MPA = 14–36
Wegener's granulomatosis		4	1:2	30–45	22–54
Cryoglobulinemic vasculitis			2:1	50–65	40

CSS, Churg-Strauss syndrome; MPA, microscopic polyangiitis; PAN, polyarteritis nodosa.

tis can impair cerebral blood flow, producing symptoms of cerebral ischemia (George and Laurian, 1989).

Osteoarthritis is characterized by the slow, steady, progression of articular pain. The pain worsens with use, is relieved with rest, and has little associated morning stiffness. Physical examination reveals a painful enlarged joint with a limited range of motion. Rarely, is peripheral osteoarthropathy a cause of neurologic dysfunction. However, entrapment neuropathy at the carpal tunnel may be related to osteophyte formation and bony hypertrophy (Dray and Jablon, 1987).

Osteoarthritis of the spine associated with spondylosis of the intervertebral discs is a much more common cause of neurologic morbidity. Spondylosis refers to the desiccation and degeneration of the intervertebral disc associated with aging (Rosenbaum et al., 1996). Spondylosis is also commonly used to refer to the combination of osteoarthritis of the intervertebral joints and degeneration of the fibrocartilaginous discs (Truumees and Herkowitz, 2000). The two conditions invariably coexist, and disc desiccation and loss of disc height associated with aging are likely causative factors in osteoarthritis of intervertebral joints (Truumees and Herkowitz, 2000).

Radiculopathy

Radiculopathies can result from two different mechanisms. Encroachment of the neural foramina by osteophytes and bony spurs is the most common cause of radiculopathy in the elderly. The foraminal narrowing usually remains quiescent until a minor trauma results in symptoms (Truumees and Herowitzet, 2000). Less common in the older population is acute disc herniation with resultant foraminal narrowing.

Clinically, radiculopathy is characterized by pain with radiation in a radicular pattern. Weakness and numbness in the distribution of the nerve root involved can also occur. Excessive mobility of the neck or back will exacerbate the symptoms, as will Valsalva maneuvers (Truumees and Herowitz., 2000). In the cervical spine, the C6-C7 followed by the C5-C6 disk spaces are most commonly involved. In the lumbosacral spine the L4-L5 and L5-S1 disks are usually involved (Rosenbaum et al., 1996). Table 29-11 outlines the clinical symptoms seen with radiculopathy by the nerve root involved (Rosenbaum et al., 1996; Brazis et al., 1996).

A variety of examination maneuvers are useful in making the diagnosis of radiculopathy. *Spurling's maneuver*, where the head is extended and rotated toward the symptomatic side resulting in worsening of radicular symptoms, is helpful in confirming the diagnosis of cervical radiculopathy. The *compression test* entails pushing down on the head with resultant foraminal narrowing and exacerbation of the patient's symptoms. Abduction of the arm on the affected side results in pain diminishment in cervical radiculopathy (Truumees and Herkowitz, 2000). Lumbar radiculopathy can be similarly elicited. The *straight leg raising sign* is positive if the patient reports pain radiating down the posterior aspect of the leg into the calf or foot when the hip is flexed greater than 20 degrees while the knee is maintained in extension. A positive *crossed straight leg raising maneuver* is more specific for radiculopathy but less sensitive. In this maneuver, pain is elicited in the opposite leg from the one raised (Rosenbaum et al., 1996).

Electrodiagnostic studies are useful in confirming suspected radiculopathy. Electromyography (EMG) shows abnormalities in the muscles supplied by the nerve root involved, whereas sensory nerve conduc-

TABLE 29-11. *Signs and symptoms of radiculopathy*

Disc level	Spinal root	Muscles	Sensory loss	Deep tendon reflexes
C2–C3	C3	Levator scapulae	Lateral neck Lower occiput	None
C3–C4	C4	Rhomboids' diaphragm	Lower neck	None
C4–C5	C5	Deltoid	Lateral forearm	Biceps
C5–C6	C6	Biceps	Thumb and index finger	Biceps/brachioradialis
C6–C7	C7	Triceps	Third and fourth fingers	Triceps
C7–T1	C8	Intrinsic hand muscles	Medial forearm fifth finger	Finger flexors

Disc level	Spinal root (medial disc)[a]	Muscles	Sensory loss	Deep tendon reflexes
L2–L3	L3	Hip flexors, quadriceps	Anterior thigh	Patellar
L3–L4	L4	Quadriceps	Knee and medial leg	Patellar
L4–L5	L5	Hip adductors, extensor great toe	Lateral leg, great toe	None
L5–S1	S1	Hip extension, plantar flexors	Lateral foot, sole of foot	Ankle jerk

[a]Lateral disc herniations affect the nerve root above the disc level (e.g., the T12–L1 disc space effects the T12 spinal root). Symptoms correspond to the spinal root affected.

tion studies are normal (Wilbourne and Aminoff, 1988). Electrodiagnostic studies can be particularly useful in differentiating causes of disability in the elderly who may have multiple pathologic conditions.

Plain radiographs of the cervical spine have a high false-positive rate in the elderly, frequently showing degenerative findings in asymptomatic individuals (Truumees and Herkowitz, 2000; Monro and Uttley, 1989). Therefore, plain radiographs are not recommended in the evaluation of radiculopathy. Myelograms, CT scans, or MRI readily show the anatomic relationship of the spinal roots, intravertebral disks, and neural foramina. Each study has similar sensitivity and specificity (Larrson et al., 1989), although MRI better reveals nerve root and cord compression (Kriss and Kriss, 2000). In addition, MRI can rule out more serious causes of radiculopathy in the elderly (e.g., metastatic cancer and epidural infections).

Although radiologic evaluation is important in the evaluation of possible radiculopathy, careful correlation of imaging results with patient history and physical examination findings is essential. When abnormal radiologic findings are seen in the absence of supportive historical, clinical, and EMG findings, other causes of the patient's symptoms must be sought.

The natural history of radiculopathy tends to be benign. Most individuals have complete or partial resolution of their symptoms (Truumees and Herkowitz, 2000). Therefore, conservative therapy is recommended initially. Medical therapy consists of nonsteroidal anti-inflammatory drugs (NSAID) (Tru-

umees and Herkowitz, 2000; Kriss and Kriss, 2000). Caution should be exercised when using these agents in the elderly who are particularly susceptible to developing NSAID-associated peptic ulcers, and hepatic and renal dysfunction (Sager and Bennett, 1992; Monro and Uttley, 1989). Soft collars can be useful in relieving pain. Exercise, initially under the guidance of a physical therapist, should be encouraged. Surgical decompression should be considered in an individual with disabling pain and weakness that persists for more than 3 months (Truumees and Herkowitz, 2000).

Spinal Stenosis

The degenerative changes of the spine that occur with aging can also cause progressive narrowing of the spinal canal (Truumees and Herkowitz, 2000; Garfin et al., 2000). Symptoms arising from degenerative spinal stenosis occur at an average age of 73 years in women and at a slightly younger age in men (Garfin et al., 2000). Depending on the location and degree of the narrowing, various symptoms can occur. Narrowing of the cervical spinal canal causes myelopathy, whereas narrowing below the conus medullaris causes signs and symptoms of nerve root compression.

Unlike cervical radiculopathy, pain is not a common feature of cervical myelopathy. Symptoms are varied and include weakness, clumsiness, anesthesia, paresthesia, balance and gait difficulties, urinary frequency, and incontinence (Truumees and Herkowitz,

2000). Upper motor neuron signs predominate below the level of stenosis. These include spasticity, hyperreflexia, Hoffman's signs (i.e., spontaneous flexion of the thumb and other fingers when the third digit is rapidly flicked into extension (Truumees and Herkowitz, 2000), and extensor plantar reflexes (Babinski's sign). Lower motor neuron signs (i.e., atrophy and hyporeflexia) may be seen at the level of stenosis because of involvement of the anterior horn cells and spinal roots. Lhermitte's sign refers to an electric shock that radiates down the spine into the extremities with neck flexion (Truumees and Herkowitz, 2000; Kriss and Kriss, 2000). This phenomenon is a sensitive marker of cervical spine pathology. In the elderly, Lhermitte's sign should prompt the search for a compressive lesion of the cervical spine.

Spinal stenosis of the lumbar spine causes compression of multiple nerve roots of the cauda equina. The condition progresses insidiously, usually beginning with low back pain. The classic signs and symptoms of cauda equina are outlined in Table 29-12 (Brazis et al., 1996; Garfin et al., 2000; Hall et al., 1985).

Pseudoclaudication, also known as "neurogenic claudication," occurs in 94% of patients with lumbar spinal stenosis (Hall et al., 1985). This condition refers to leg pain or paresthesia associated with walking or extension of the low back. Unlike true vascular claudication, it is relieved within minutes of resting or changing postures. Individuals with pseudoclaudication can walk long distances if bent at the waist and may bicycle without difficulties. This is in contrast to vascular claudication, where pain in the legs is elicited by any leg exercise (Rosenbaum et al., 1996). The straight leg raising sign is uncommon, being positive in only 10% of patients (Garfin et al., 2000; Hall et al., 1985).

Unlike radiculopathy, electrodiagnostic studies are less useful in the evaluation of spinal stenosis, although these studies can be useful in ruling out peripheral neuropathy or amyotrophic lateral sclerosis as a cause of the patient's symptoms. Although EMG can suggest or support the diagnosis of lumbar spinal stenosis, MRI is the study of choice (Garfin et al., 2000). Plain radiographs, however, should not be ignored. Flexion and extension views of the spine can give valuable information about spine stability. CT imaging is not recommended, especially in the elderly. CT often misses multilevel disease and more ominous causes of stenosis (e.g., tumors, fractures, and infections). MRI is essential in the elderly to distinguish these causes of spinal stenosis from degenerative causes. CT myelography can be useful in individuals for whom MRI is contraindicated (Garfin et al., 2000).

In general, spinal stenosis progresses in a stepwise manner over years. It begins insidiously with pain or intermittent paresthesia and can progress to a severely disabling condition (Truumees and Herkowitz, 2000). Patients with mild symptoms (i.e., those that do not interfere with daily function) have the best prognosis (Truumees and Herkowitz, 2000). In one study, two thirds of patients continued to have only mild impairment over 20 years with nonsurgical management (Nurick, 1972).

Conservative therapy, focusing on education and a well-designed exercise program, can be useful in individuals with only mild impairment (Truumees and Herkowitz, 2000). Surgery is indicated when spinal stenosis interferes with performance of daily activities and quality of life or evolves over a short period of time (Truumees and Herkowitz, 2000; Garfin et al., 2000). Patients need to be educated regarding the realistic outcomes of surgical decompression. Relief of back pain is not an indication for surgery. Surgical treatment is aimed at preventing progressive disability and relieving symptoms of neurogenic claudication and gait impairment (Okada et al., 1991; Truumees and Herkowitz, 2000; Garfin et al., 2000; Hall et al., 1985). Medical comorbidity has a negative impact on recovery after surgery, although older age itself is not a contraindication for surgery (Garfin et al., 2000). In fact, when the history, physical examination, and MRI studies are consistent; surgery is an excellent option in this patient population.

TABLE 29-12. *Signs and symptoms of the cauda equina syndrome*

Symptoms	Signs
Early asymmetric radicular pain	Asymmetric sensory loss
Pain relieved with back flexion	Asymmetric weakness
Asymmetric numbness and paresthesia	Absent or decreased reflexes
Asymmetric weakness	
Late sphincter involvement	
Pseudoclaudication	

Rheumatoid Arthritis

Rheumatoid arthritis is the second most common rheumatologic disorder, after osteoarthritis. Unlike most immune-mediated rheumatologic diseases, it has a predilection for an older population and its incidence increases with age (Rosenbaum et al., 1996). It is a chronic, inflammatory, symmetric polyarthritis (Rosenbaum et al., 1996; Chang and Paget, 1993). It is a disease of the small joints of the hands and feet, and unlike osteoarthritis, is associated with morning stiffness. It classically affects the metacarpophalangeal, proximal interphalangeal, wrist, and metatarsophalangeal joints (Harris, 1990). Extra articular complications occur in 10% to 20% of patients, with neurologic complications being very common (Chang and Paget, 1993).

Neurologic manifestations of rheumatoid arthritis are rarely if ever the presenting symptom, occurring late or in the presence of active articular or systemic disease. Carpal tunnel syndrome is the most common neurologic manifestation of rheumatoid arthritis. Atlantoaxial subluxation with spinal cord compression at the C1-C2 disc space is, however, the most ominous cause of neurologic morbidity (Rosenbaum et al., 1996; Dreyer and Boden, 1999; Monro and Uttley, 1989; Chang and Paget, 1993; Gurley and Bell, 1997). Peripheral neuropathy (Schneider et al., 1985; Bekkelund et al., 1999; Sivri and Guler-Uysal, 1998), myopathy (Wegelius et al., 1969), and rarely CNS involvement (Jackson et al., 1984; Markenson et al., 1979) have also been reported.

Cervical Subluxation

Cervical subluxation is caused by chronic inflammation of the synovial joints of the cervical spine, resulting in weakening of the ligaments, cartilage, and bone of these joints (Monro and Uttley, 1989; Chang and Paget, 1993). The destructive influence of this process results in intervertebral subluxation. The ligaments that maintain the odontoid process in position relative to the atlas bone and cranium are particularly susceptible, and atlantoaxial subluxation is the most common abnormality of the cervical spine in rheumatoid arthritis (Rosenbaum et al., 1996; Monro and Uttley, 1989; Chang and Paget, 1993; Gurley and Bell, 1997). Radiographic evidence of cervical spine disease is seen in most patients (Dreyer and Boden, 1999; Neva et al., 2000), however, only 7% to 13% develop neurologic symptoms (Dreyer and Boden, 1999). Long disease duration, positive rheumatoid factor, male sex, and erosive peripheral joint disease increase the risk of developing this complication (Chang and Paget, 1993). The elderly are potentially at high risk as well, because of the superimposition of spondylotic changes with rheumatoid changes in the neck (Monro and Uttley, 1989).

Complaints referable to atlantoaxial subluxation can be vague or even nonexistent (Chang and Paget, 1993).

Neck pain and headache are nearly universal in individuals with rheumatoid arthritis and cervical spine disease (Rosenbaum et al., 1996; Gurley and Bell, 1997). When symptoms are present, they are similar to those described for cervical spinal stenosis from osteoarthritis. However, compression of the medulla or vertebral arteries may elicit complaints of paroxysmal loss of consciousness, vertigo, dysarthria, balance difficulties, and visual disturbances (Dreyer and Boden, 1999; Chang and Paget, 1993).

Neurologic findings are difficult to elicit in the patient with rheumatoid arthritis. Weakness and atrophy can be related to disuse, secondary to painful involvement of peripheral joints. Severe joint disease or peripheral neuropathy can mask hyperreflexia (Dreyer and Boden, 1999). Although hyperreflexia is the most common neurologic finding in these patients (Stevens et al., 1971), neurologic findings often correlate poorly with radiographic findings (Rosenbaum et al., 1996). In addition, the absence of neurologic findings is not necessarily predictive of a neurologic prognosis (Dreyer and Boden, 1999).

Despite the presence or lack of symptoms and signs, rheumatoid arthritis involvement of the cervical spine is potentially serious and life threatening. Mikulowski et al. (1975) found 10 of 104 deaths associated with rheumatoid arthritis to be attributable to medullary compression secondary to severe atlantoaxial subluxation. Neurologic symptoms in these patients were relatively sparse. Therefore, a high index of suspicion must be maintained to identify those patients at risk for this complication.

Treatment decisions in rheumatoid cervical spine disease are complex and controversial (Gurley and Bell, 1997). Individuals with neurologic deficits or intractable pain associated with cervical spine subluxation are candidates for surgical intervention (Dreyer and Boden, 1999). More challenging is identifying individuals at high risk for neurologic complications and death and avoiding unnecessary surgery in asymptomatic individuals. Figure 29-3 outlines a potential algorithm to assist in making these treatment decisions (Dreyer and Boden, 1999; Boden et al., 1994).

Entrapment Neuropathies

Peripheral nerve involvement is common in rheumatoid arthritis, with entrapment neuropathies at the carpal tunnel and tarsal tunnel making up most of the peripheral nerve injuries (Chang and Paget, 1993). *Carpal tunnel syndrome* results from compression of the median nerve at the carpal tunnel in the wrist. Common clinical symptoms include nocturnal paresthesias

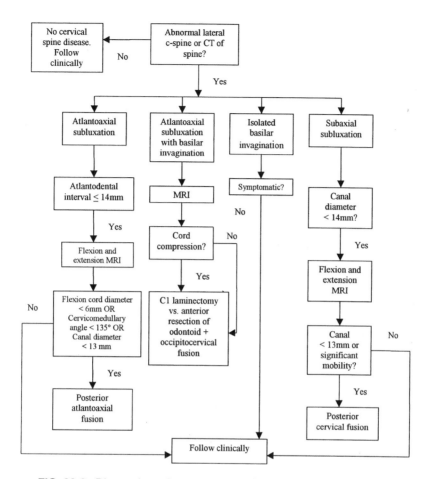

FIG. 29-3. Diagnosis and management of rheumatoid spine disease.

in the first three digits of the hand, anesthesia in the median distribution of the hand, and later weakness of the abductor pollicis brevis. *Tarsal tunnel syndrome* results from compression of the posterior tibial nerve as it passes under the medial malleolus in the medial aspect of the ankle. Paresthesia and pain on the plantar surface of the foot are common symptoms. Conservative therapy with anti-inflammatory medications and wrist splints are frequently adequate. Surgical decompression can be considered in individuals who develop motor impairment (Chang and Paget, 1993).

Peripheral Neuropathy

Patients with rheumatoid arthritis also develop diffuse peripheral neuropathy, the incidence of which appears to be associated with disease severity (Rosenbaum et al., 1996; Chang and Paget, 1993).

Early studies evaluating outpatients suggest a low incidence of this complication (Rosenbaum et al., 1996). However, in one study that surveyed 70 patients with disease severe enough to require hospital admission, signs and symptoms of a diffuse polyneuropathy were found in 64% of these patients (Good et al., 1965). Two major types of peripheral neuropathy can be seen: a symmetric predominantly sensory neuropathy and a more severe sensorimotor mononeuritis multiplex (Chang and Paget, 1993).

The predominantly *sensory neuropathy* is a distal symmetric neuropathy involving the small fiber sensory modalities of pain and temperature. Its onset is insidious, presenting with distal anesthesia and burning paresthesia. Physical examination shows the expected stocking-glove sensory loss, with relative preservation of vibration and position sense, and with little evidence of motor involvement (Chang and

Paget, 1993). The prognosis in this condition is variable, with some individuals reporting spontaneous improvement and others' condition remaining stable for years (Rosenbaum et al., 1996). In general, no specific treatment is warranted, although amitriptyline or gabapentin can be useful in alleviating the burning pain sometimes associated with this condition. It should be noted that gold therapy for rheumatoid arthritis has also been associated with a reversible neuropathy (Ben-Ami et al., 1999).

The *mixed sensorimotor neuropathy* is usually associated with a systemic vasculitis and presents as a mononeuritis multiplex (Chang and Paget, 1993; Schneider et al., 1985; Sivri and Guler-Uysal, 1998). It can appear rarely as a diffuse polyneuropathy (Chang and Paget, 1993), which likely represents the confluence of a mononeuritis multiplex. The appearance of mononeuritis multiplex often heralds a systemic vasculitis. It can present acutely and progress rapidly, distinguishing it from mononeuropathy secondary to entrapment. It is frequently associated with active rheumatoid arthritis, palpable purpura, skin ulcers, anemia, leukocytosis, high rheumatoid factor titers, hypocomplementemia, constitutional symptoms, ischemia in other organ systems, and proteinuria (Chang and Paget, 1993; Schneider et al., 1985).

Prognosis in these patients is poor, with a 40% to 63% mortality rate (Chang and Paget, 1993; Chang et al., 1984). For fulminant cases, aggressive treatment is mandatory and consists of a combination of high dose pulse steroids (1 g methylprednisolone, intravenous) and cyclophosphamide (0.5 g/m^2) (Chang and Paget, 1993). Plasmapheresis has been used in the past, but has recently fallen out of favor because it lacks efficacy (Clark et al., 1999). Oral cyclophosphamide and prednisone have been advocated for less severe disease. Treatment of systemic vasculitis is discussed in the section *Systemic Vasculitides*.

Myopathy

Although muscle weakness is a common complaint in rheumatoid arthritis, its cause is multifactorial. Disuse atrophy and drugs, especially steroids, have been implicated. Muscle enzyme levels are normal (Rosenbaum et al., 1996; Chang and Paget, 1993). Muscle biopsies show type II atrophy, without evidence of inflammation, necrosis, regeneration, or vasculitis (Haslock et al., 1970).

Central Nervous System Involvement

As previously alluded, CNS involvement in rheumatoid arthritis is extraordinarily rare. Isolated case reports have suggested that CNS vasculitis, meningitis, and rheumatoid nodule formation within the CNS can all occur (Jackson et al., 1984; Markenson et al., 1979; Ramos and Mandybur, 1975).

Systemic Lupus Erythematosus

Systemic lupus erythematosus is a disease primarily of young women (Rosenbaum et al., 1996; Sigal, 1987) and is rarely if ever seen in the elderly.

Systemic Sclerosis

Systemic sclerosis or scleroderma is a rare disorder characterized by excessive fibrosis, microvascular disease, and autoimmune phenomena (Rosenbaum et al., 1996). Raynaud's phenomenon is the most common presenting symptom, occurring in more than 90% of patients. Additional findings include characteristic fibrosis and thickening of the skin, symptoms of gastrointestinal dysmotility, abnormal pulmonary function, and an inflammatory arthritis and tenosynovitis (Rosenbaum et al., 1996; Generini et al., 1999). Antinuclear antibodies (ANA) titers are frequently elevated (Rosenbaum et al., 1996). PNS involvement in the form of neuropathy and myopathy can be seen in upward of 40% of patients (Averbuch-Heller et al., 1992). CNS involvement is rare, although encephalopathy secondary to end-organ failure (e.g., renal crisis) can be seen (Sigal, 1987; Norton and Nardo, 1970).

The peak incidence of the disease occurs during the fourth and fifth decades (Steen and Medsger, 1990). A 50% mortality rate is seen at 10 years (Steen and Medsger, 1990); therefore, this disease is seen uncommonly in the older population. However, onset of the disease after 50 years of age is associated with a worse survival rate than in younger patients (Steen and Medsger, 1990). The disease tends to progress most rapidly in the first 5 to 10 years from diagnosis and then remain quiescent (Steen and Medsger, 1990).

Peripheral Nervous System Involvement

Myopathy is the most common neurologic involvement in systemic sclerosis (Averbuch-Heller et al., 1992; Generini et al., 1999). An indolent chronic myopathy has been reported in 60% to 80% of patients (Generini et al., 1999). In this group, muscle enzyme levels may be normal or only mildly elevated, EMG finding is benign and muscle biopsies show subtle histologic changes. A smaller, but still substantial, population will have evidence of an inflammatory myopathy (Averbuch-Heller et al., 1992; Generini et al., 1999; Hietaharju et al., 1993). In these cases, marked elevation is seen of muscle enzymes (aldolase more so than creatinine kinase). EMG study shows low amplitude polyphasic motor units. Muscle biopsy can be consistent with either a polymyositis or even inclusion body myositis (Averbuch-Heller et al., 1992; Generini et al., 1999). In the indolent and more benign form of myopathy, no specific treatment is necessary. More aggressive forms can be successfully treated with prednisone (60 mg/day) (Averbuch-Heller et al., 1992).

Peripheral nerve involvement is common and falls into three categories: polyneuropathy, cranial neuropathies (usually the trigeminal nerve), and entrapment neuropathies (usually the median nerve at the carpal tunnel) (Sigal, 1987; Averbuch-Heller et al., 1992; Generini et al., 1999; Mondelli et al., 1995). The polyneuropathy associated with systemic sclerosis is an axonal mixed sensorimotor neuropathy (Cerinic et al., 1996). Frequently, the neuropathy is subclinical (Mondelli et al., 1995). Trigeminal neuropathy occurs in 4% of the patients (Farrell and Medsger, 1982), and begins with gradual sensory loss in a trigeminal distribution and spares the motor portion of the nerve. The symptoms frequently become painful. Gabapentin or amitriptyline can be useful for neuropathic pain associated with this condition.

Primary Sjögren's Syndrome

Sjögren's syndrome can be seen as a component of another connective tissue disease, namely rheumatoid arthritis. In that circumstance, the neurologic complications are the same. This section discuss the less frequent circumstance where Sjögren's syndrome exists in the absence of another connective tissue disease (i.e., primary Sjögren's syndrome) (Rosenbaum et al., 1996).

The diagnostic criteria for this disorder are debated among rheumatologists (Fox and Saito, 1994; Alexander, 1992). Using the strictest criteria, the diagnosis of Sjögren's syndrome requires the presence of destruction of the exocrine portion of the lacrimal and salivary glands in association with evidence for a systemic autoimmune process (Fox and Saito, 1994; Oxholm, 1992). Applying these criteria, Sjögren's syndrome is a rare disorder. However, with a more liberal criterion requiring only the presence of salivary and lacrimal gland dysfunction, it has an overall prevalence of 2% (Alexander, 1993). Despite this controversy, it is likely that Sjögren's syndrome is under recognized in the elderly (Alexander, 1992).

The hallmark of the disease is the presence of the "sicca syndrome," xerophthalmia (dry eyes) and xerostomia (dry mouth). Xerophthalmia can be documented with the *Schirmer's test*. A drop of topical anesthetic is applied to the eye and then a strip of filter paper is applied to the lateral lower eyelid for 5 minutes. Individuals with dry eyes will wet less than 5 mm of the filter strip (Rosenbaum et al., 1996). Aging and drugs are common causes of the sicca syndrome (Rosenbaum et al., 1996); therefore, one must exercise caution in making the diagnosis of Sjögren's syndrome in the elderly based on exocrine dysfunction alone. Evidence for autoimmunity is demonstrated by either showing a mononuclear infiltrate in a biopsy of the lacrimal or salivary glands or via the presence of autoantibodies in the sera of affected patients. ANA, anti-Ro (SS-A) and anti-La (SS-B), are the autoantibodies most commonly elevated in Sjögren's syndrome (Alexander et al., 1994; Harley et al., 1986).

Neurologic involvement is common, with a preference for the PNS (Font et al., 1990; Alexander et al., 1982; Mellgren et al., 1989). In fact, Sjögren's original description included a patient with bilateral VII nerve palsies (Lafitte, 2000). CNS manifestations have only been reported within the last two decades (Alexander, 1992); however, recent reports suggest the incidence of CNS involvement may be as high as 20% in some tertiary referral centers (Alexander et al., 1986).

Peripheral Nervous System Involvement

A pure sensory polyneuropathy is widely recognized as being associated with Sjögren's syndrome (Font et al., 1990; Alexander et al., 1994). The cause is secondary to lymphocytic infiltration of the dorsal root ganglia (Malinow et al., 1986). Dorsal column function (vibration and joint position sense) is preferentially affected. Trigeminal sensory neuropathies can coexist. A sensory neuropathy may be the first manifestation of Sjögren's syndrome, even in the absence of more classic symptoms (Font et al., 1990). Therefore, an evaluation for Sjögren's syndrome should be pursued in any patient presenting with a pure sensory neuropathy. This condition can present subacutely (Malinow et al., 1986) with asymmetric sensory loss and painful paresthesia. Treatment consists of the use of corticosteroids, but results have been equivocal (Rosenbaum et al., 1996).

Although sensory neuronopathy is the classic PNS abnormality associated with Sjögren's, a diverse group of disorders of the PNS can occur. Among those reported are mixed sensorimotor neuropathies (Alexander et al., 1982; Mellgren et al., 1989), chronic relapsing inflammatory neuropathies (Gross, 1987), entrapment neuropathies (e.g., carpal tunnel syndrome) (Alexander et al., 1982), cranial neuropathies (Rosenbaum et al., 1996; Alexander et al., 1982), myopathies (Alexander, 1993; Guttman et al., 1985), and hypokalemic periodic paralysis (secondary to renal tubular acidosis) (Christensen, 1985). A trigeminal sensory neuropathy, the prototypical cranial neuropathy encountered, can be unilateral or bilateral. Loss of sensation in the maxillary and mandibular distributions, with sparing of the orbital division, is common (Rosenbaum et al., 1996).

Central Nervous System Involvement

Until recently, CNS involvement in Sjögren's syndrome was thought to be uncommon, but it has been associated with a wide variety of CNS manifestations from seizure and stroke to aseptic meningitis and myelitis (Alexander, 1992; Bragoni et al., 1994; Alexander and Alexander, 1983). The most common clinical presentation is a relapsing-remitting CNS disease that is similar to multiple sclerosis. MRI examination of the brain may reveal areas of subcortical T2 hyperintensity that may be dismissed as ischemic disease from other causes in the elderly (Alexander, 1992). CSF examination reveals a mild mononuclear pleocytosis, elevated protein, elevated IgG index, and oligoclonal banding (Alexander et al., 1986). Rarely, CNS involvement can present as either a cortical and subcortical dementia. This dementia is potentially reversible with corticosteroid treatment, suggesting that Sjögren's syndrome should be considered as a possible cause of reversible dementia (Alexander, 1992).

Treatment

No standardized therapeutic strategy exists for treating individuals with CNS Sjögren's. Therapy should be geared toward the subset of patients who develop cumulative neurologic impairment over time. The mainstay of treatment is the use of corticosteroids. This may not be successful in all patients, necessitating the use of cyclophosphamide in those individuals who continue to deteriorate neurologically. Alexander (1992) recommends intravenous pulse cyclophosphamide monthly for a minimum of 12 months in conjunction with oral corticosteroids for these patients.

Sarcoidosis

Sarcoidosis is a rare, multisystem, granulomatous disease of unknown cause. Lung is the most common organ system involved, affecting more than 90% of patients (Johns and Michele, 1999). The diagnosis is based on a compatible clinical presentation involving at least two distinct organ systems, with pathologic evidence of noncaseating granulomas, in the absence of evidence for other granulomatous diseases (e.g., mycobacterial or fungal disease) (Johns and Michele, 1999).

It occurs in any ethnic group, however, in North America it is 10 times more common in blacks. It affects predominantly young adults in their 20s and 30s, however, it can affect any age group. Neurologic involvement is uncommon, occurring in only 5% of all patients with sarcoidosis (Stern, 1985). When neurologic involvement does occur, it is the presenting manifestation of the illness in 50% of cases. In addition, neurologic involvement is associated with high morbidity and mortality rates and can be difficult to diagnose and treat (Johns and Michele, 1999).

As with many of the diseases discussed in this section, sarcoidosis can affect the entire neuraxis. Cranial nerve involvement is the most common neurologic manifestation (Stern et al., 1985; Sharma and Sharma, 1991; Delaney, 1977). Other common features include a meningitis, pituitary or hypothalamic dysfunction, polyneuropathy, and myopathy (Stern et al., 1985; Delaney, 1977; Sharma, 1997, 220–228; Oksanen, 1986; Chapelon et al., 1990). Seizures, strokelike episodes, and even intracranial mass lesions have all been reported (Alexander, 1993; Sharma, 1997, 220–228; Oksanen, 1986).

Cranial Neuropathies

Cranial nerve VII palsies occur in two thirds of individuals with neurosarcoidosis (Sharma and Sharma, 1991). The facial palsy associated with sarcoidosis is indistinguishable from Bell's palsy. It can be bilateral in up to one third of the cases (Sharma and Sharma, 1991). The presence of bilateral facial palsy must always raise the suspicion of a secondary cause, such as sarcoidosis. The optic nerve is commonly involved (Sharma and Sharma, 1991; Delaney, 1977; Oksanen, 1986). Clinically, patients have decreased visual acuity and color vision and may have restricted visual fields. Frequently, trigeminal and vestibulocochlear nerves are also involved, and the involvement can be bilateral (Stern et al., 1985; Oksanen, 1986).

Neuromuscular Involvement

Involvement of the peripheral nerves and muscle in sarcoidosis is common and varied (Stern, 1985; Sharma, 1997, 220–228; Oksanen, 1986; Chapelon et al., 1990; Lynch et al., 1998). Peripheral nerve involvement can have a variety of forms, from mononeuropathy to the Guillain-Barré syndrome (Delaney, 1977; Sharma, 1997). Asymptomatic involvement of muscle can occur in more than 50% of patients with sarcoidosis (Delaney, 1977; Lynch et al., 1998). In this circumstance, muscle biopsy reveals granulomas surrounded by normal tissue. Symptomatic myopathy associated with myalgias, proximal weakness, and elevated muscle enzymes occurs in a minority of patients, but can be disabling (Lynch et al., 1998).

Central Nervous System Involvement

Meningitis is one of the more common CNS complications of sarcoidosis (Johns and Michele, 1999; Oksanen, 1986; Chapelon et al., 1990). It preferentially involves the basal meninges and hypothalamus. It can result in hydrocephalus, increased intracranial pressure, and hypothalamic and pituitary dysfunction (Delaney, 1977; Oksanen, 1986). Seizures are also common and may reflect granulomatous lesions of the cortex or intracranial mass lesions.

Diagnostic Evaluation

Neuroimaging reveals increased contrast uptake in the meninges. Spinal fluid analysis may reveal a mononuclear pleocytosis, elevated protein, and low glucose (Johns and Michele, 1999). Serum and CSF angiotensin-converting enzyme levels can be elevated, which is specific for sarcoidosis, but relatively insensitive (Scott, 1993; Oksanen, 1986). Gallium scanning, on the other hand, is sensitive for the detection of extraneural sarcoid but nonspecific (Sulavik et al., 1990). However, the combination of uptake of gallium in the lacrimal and salivary glands (panda sign) with uptake in the hilar lymph nodes (lambda sign) is found almost exclusively in sarcoidosis (Sulavik et al., 1990).

Treatment

Most patients will respond in the short term to treatment with corticosteroids although relatively high doses (40–80 mg/day of prednisone) are needed (Johns and Michele, 1999; Sharma, 1997, 1–3). The exact duration of treatment is not known. Johns and Michele (1999) recommend starting with 40 mg/day of prednisone for 2 weeks and then gradually reducing the dose over 8 weeks. Patients are then maintained on 10 to 15 mg daily for 8 months, after which they are weaned

gradually over 4 months until off the medications. Relapses occur in one third of individuals (Scott, 1993), requiring an increase in the prednisone dose. Occasionally, methotrexate, azathioprine, chlorambucil, thalidomide, and cyclosporine have been used successfully in steroid-resistant cases (Sharma, 1997, 1–3).

Systemic Vasculitides

The vasculitides are a group of disorders that share in common the histologic features of inflammation directed against blood vessels (Moore and Cups, 1983). This inflammation can be secondary to one of the rheumatic diseases previously discussed, or the vascular inflammation can be the primary event. The nervous system is involved to varying degrees in all of the systemic vasculitides (Moore and Cups, 1983). The pathophysiology of neurologic involvement is primarily related to ischemia from occluded vessels or hemorrhage from weakened blood vessel walls (Rosenbaum et al., 1996).

Many of the systemic vasculitides affect the elderly. They are characterized by evidence of multiorgan disease, constitutional symptoms, multiple ischemic events in multiple vascular distributions, and a variety of organ-specific syndromes (Rosenbaum et al., 1996). This section reviews a few of the relatively more common systemic vasculitic syndromes that primarily involve the older population.

Temporal (Giant Cell) Arteritis

Temporal arteritis is a systemic granulomatous vasculitis of medium to large vessels, involving primarily branches of the carotid artery. It is a disease of the elderly, with more than 95% of cases occurring in those over 50 years of age (Rosenbaum et al., 1996). Clinically, patients complain of headache, malaise, arthralgias, myalgias, scalp tenderness, and jaw claudication (Keltner, 1982). Physical examination reveals a tender, indurated temporal artery with a diminished or absent pulse (Keltner, 1982). Headache is the most frequent symptom, occurring in 70% to 90% of patients (Silberstein et al., 1998). Temporal arteritis should be suspected in all elderly patients with a new onset headache or change in the pattern of a previous headache (Silberstein et al., 1998). Laboratory examination reveals an elevated erythrocyte sedimentation rate and an anemia of chronic disease (Keltner, 1982). Table 29-13 summarizes the American College of Rheumatology criteria for diagnosing temporal arteritis (Keltner, 1982). For a more detailed discussion of temporal arteritis, see Chapter 11.

TABLE 29-13. *American College of Rheumatology criteria for the diagnosis of temporal arteritis*[a]

Age ≥50 yrs
New onset localized headache
Decreased pulse or tenderness of the temporal artery
Erythrocyte sedimentation rate ≥50 mm/h
Arterial biopsy showing a necrotizing arteritis or a granulomatous process

[a]The presence of 3+ criteria has a specificity of 91% and a sensitivity of 93.5%.

Polyarteritis Nodosa Group

The polyarteritis nodosa group (PAN) is the prototypical systemic vasculitis (Rosenbaum et al., 1996). The group of disorders consists of PAN, Churg-Strauss syndrome, and microscopic polyangiitis (MPA) (Guillevin et al., 1997). They are defined by symptoms of multiorgan involvement secondary to panarteritis of medium and small vessels (Jennette and Falk, 1997; Guillevin et al., 1996). The absence of glomerulonephritis or vasculitic involvement of the small arterioles, venules and capillary beds distinguishes PAN. Churg-Strauss syndrome is an eosinophilic inflammation of the respiratory tract associated with asthma. MPA affects the smallest vessels and, therefore, glomerulonephritis is common (Jennette and Falk, 1997; Gross, 1995). Perinuclear antineutrophil cytoplasmic antibodies may be found in MPA and Churg-Strauss (Jennette and Falk, 1997; Gross, 1995). This group of disorders occurs in all ages throughout adulthood, with the mean incidence in the fifth and sixth decades. Neurologic involvement occurs in all subtypes (Sigal, 1987; Jennette and Falk, 1997).

PNS involvement is the most common manifestation of these protean disorders (Sigal, 1987). Mononeuritis multiplex is the classic pattern of peripheral nerve involvement. Almost any peripheral nerve can be involved; peroneal involvement is the most common, resulting in a foot drop (Chang et al., 1984). CNS involvement can occur in as many as 50% of cases and should not be overlooked, as it is a leading cause of mortality in this population (Sigal, 1987). CNS manifestations tend to occur late in the course of the disease in the setting of prominent systemic symptoms. CNS symptoms include ischemic events, hemorrhage, and encephalopathy.

Treatment entails aggressive immunosuppression. Generally, a combination of corticosteroids and cyclophosphamide are recommended. Intravenous pulse administration of methylprednisolone (15 mg/kg every 24 hours for 3 days) is used as initial treatment secondary to its rapid onset of effectiveness and relative safety (Guillevin et al., 1996). Following pulse corticosteroids, oral prednisone (1 mg/kg daily) is given and can later be tapered as the patient improves. The addition of cyclophosphamide further improves the prognosis (Fauci et al., 1979), although evidence indicates that steroids are sufficient in a subset of patients (Guillevin et al., 1996). Cyclophosphamide is given as an intravenous pulse ($0.6\ g/m^2$) monthly for 12 months (Guillevin et al., 1996).

Wegener's Granulomatosis

Wegener's granulomatosis is characterized by a granulomatous inflammation of the upper and lower respiratory tract, associated with a focal glomerulonephritis and a systemic necrotizing vasculitis of small vessels (Jennette and Falk, 1997). Most patients will have a central antineutrophil cytoplasmic antibody (Gross, 1995). Again, neurologic involvement is common (Jennette and Falk, 1997; Nishino et al., 1993).

Peripheral neuropathy, in the form of a mononeuritis multiplex, is the most common neurologic manifestation (Nishino et al., 1993). CNS involvement has also been reported (Nishino et al., 1993; Bajema et al., 1997). Ischemic strokes and seizures are the most common CNS manifestations (Nishino et al., 1993). Unique to Wegener's is CNS involvement by direct invasion of granulomatous inflammatory tissue through the paranasal sinuses into the brain (Sigal, 1987).

Treatment is similar to that outlined for PAN, however, recurrences can be more frequent (Rosenbaum et al., 1996). Also, methotrexate (20 mg/week) may be a useful and less toxic alternative to cyclophosphamide (Fauci et al., 1979).

Cryoglobulinemic Vasculitis

Cryoglobulinemic vasculitis is caused by the deposition of cryoglobulins in vessel walls and the subsequent inflammatory reaction this incites (Jennette and Falk, 1997). Up to 90% of cases are associated with hepatitis C virus infection (Lamprecht et al., 1999). The most common clinical manifestations are purpura, arthralgias, and glomerulonephritis (Jennette and Falk, 1997; Lamprecht et al., 1999). Polyneuropathy is commonly seen, and electrophysiologic evidence of neuropathy may be seen in 80% of patients (Lamprecht et al., 1999). Less commonly, the CNS is involved.

Treatment for acute exacerbations or rapidly progressive cryoglobulinemic vasculitis is similar to that outlined for other systemic vasculitides. However, during clinical remission, maintenance treatment with interferon alpha is suggested (Lamprecht et al., 1999).

ALCOHOL AND THE NERVOUS SYSTEM

Epidemiology of Alcohol Use in the Elderly

Recreational and problematic use of alcohol in the elderly is common. One study revealed that 62% of subjects between 60 and 94 years of age regularly drank alcohol (Mirand and Welte, 1996). Of men, 13% and of women, 2% were considered heavy drinkers (more than two drinks per day). Overall, approximately 6% of all older adults are heavy drinkers. Alcohol use also places a significant burden on the healthcare system. Of all hospitalizations in the elderly, 1% are directly related to alcohol use or an alcohol-related disease (Adams et al., 1993). An increase of 50% in the number of elderly alcoholics is believed to have occurred from 1970 to 2000 (Anonymous, 1996).

Neurologic sequelae of alcohol use are common. Alcoholic psychosis (i.e., alcoholic dementia, delirium, amnestic syndrome, and withdrawal hallucinosis) is the third most common alcohol-related admission diagnosis in the elderly (Adams et al., 1993). The alcohol-related neurologic disorders compromise a diverse group of illnesses that can affect every level of the nervous system, from cortex to muscle (Table 29-14). As the population continues to grow older and the number of elderly alcoholics increases, a dramatic increase can be expected in neurologic complications of alcohol use.

Acute Effects of Alcohol Use

Alcohol is a CNS depressant. Paradoxically, the initial effects of intoxication are excitation of the cortex. Slowing of motor and cognitive functioning soon follow as a result of direct toxic effects of alcohol on neurons. As serum alcohol levels increase, consciousness is progressively impaired and coma can occur (Scheepers, 1997).

The elderly are particularly vulnerable to the effects of alcohol intoxication. The reduction in lean body mass in the elderly results in a relatively increased peak alcohol concentration for any given alcohol dose compared with younger individuals (Rigler, 2000). Older adults are also particularly predisposed to falls. Alcohol intoxication impairs coordination and balance, slows motor reaction, and can result in hypotension, greatly increasing the risk of falling (Rigler, 2000). Individuals who chronically use alcohol can develop neuropathy, myopathy, and cerebellar degeneration, as well as impaired cognition and judgment, further increasing the risk of falling while intoxicated. This may account for the high incidence of fractures (Anonymous, 1996) and SDH in this population.

Rarely, acute alcohol intoxication can cause seizures (Freedland and McMicken, 1993). In the elderly population, symptomatic causes of seizures (e.g. SDH, strokes, or tumors) must be aggressively sought. More commonly, seizures are the result of alcohol withdrawal (Earnest and Yarnell, 1976).

The treatment of acute alcohol intoxication is supportive, although the complications of chronic alcoholism should always be considered and treated accordingly. Patients should be observed, injuries resultant from intoxication treated, fluid balance maintained, and a safe environment maintained during recovery (Marco and Kelen, 1990).

TABLE 29-14. *Alcohol related nervous system disease*

Acute effects	Chronic effects
Altered mood	Wernicke's encephalopathy
Impaired cognition	Korsakoff's syndrome
and judgement	Dementia
Cerebellar dysfunction	Cerebellar degeneration
Ataxia	Central pontine myelinolysis
Incoordination	Neuropathy
Dysarthria	Myopathy
Vestibular dysfunction	Alcohol withdrawal
Nystagmus	syndrome
Impaired balance	Delirium tremens
Hypothermia	Seizures
Coma	
Seizures	

Chronic Effects of Alcohol Use

Wernicke's Encephalopathy

Wernicke's encephalopathy is a potentially devastating and preventable disorder caused by thiamine deficiency (Victor et al., 1989). Most cases occur in alcoholic patients, although any malnourished individual is at increased risk. Thiamine deficiency in alcoholics is multifactorial and related to an inadequate diet, impaired gastrointestinal absorption, and impaired hepatic storage.

The classic clinical triad consists of encephalopathy or delirium, ophthalmoplegia, and ataxia. This classic triad is rarely seen or recognized clinically

(Harper, 1983; Torvik et al., 1982) and, therefore, a high index of suspicion must be maintained to make the diagnosis. Oculomotor abnormalities are nearly universal (Victor et al., 1989), but can be subtle; they include nystagmus, adduction palsies, and conjugate gaze palsies. Gait ataxia, which occurs in approximately 87% of patients, results from cerebellar and vestibular injury (Victor et al., 1989). Autopsy studies looking at clinical symptoms retrospectively, found the classic triad in only 10% of patients (Harper, 1983; Torvik et al., 1982). Caine et al. (1997) found that the presence of two of the following four signs was specific for the diagnosis: (a) dietary deficiencies, (b) oculomotor abnormalities, (c) cerebellar dysfunction, and (d) an altered mental state or mild memory impairment. MRI can aid in making the diagnosis, showing a high intensity signal on T2 around the cerebral aqueduct and third ventricle (Gallucci et al., 1990; Antunez et al., 1998).

Treatment

Rapid and appropriate treatment is essential as patients can quickly progress through stupor to coma and even death (Victor et al., 1989). Treatment regimens for Wernicke's vary (Hope et al., 1999). Victor et al. (1989) recommend immediate administration of 100 mg intravenous thiamine per day for at least 5 days. Oral supplementation of thiamine should be continued thereafter. Treatment usually results in rapid resolution of oculomotor abnormalities, followed by improvement in ataxia, and finally confusion. Permanent sequelae are common, especially in alcoholics. These complications range from mild nystagmus to ataxia to the disabling amnestic disorder—Korsakoff's syndrome. Importantly, glucose should never be administered without concurrent thiamine in an alcoholic, confused, or potentially malnourished patient, as this can unmask underlying thiamine deficiency and result in an acute Wernicke's dementia (Victor et al., 1989; Watson et al., 1981).

Korsakoff's Syndrome

Of alcoholics recovering from Wernicke's encephalopathy, 80% will exhibit an amnestic disorder consistent with the Korsakoff's syndrome (Victor et al., 1989). Clinically, selective anterograde and retrograde memory loss with relative preservation of other cognitive functions characterize the syndrome. Confabulation is common. Although the disorder is generally thought to reflect the sequelae of thiamine deficiency, it rarely occurs in patients without alcoholism recovering from Wernicke's (Homewood and Bond, 1999). This suggests that the cause of Korsakoff's syndrome is multifactorial, including alcohol abuse, thiamine deficiency, and genetic predisposition (Matsushita et al., 2000). Pathologic and quantitative MRI studies of patients with the Korsakoff's syndrome reveal damage to the anterior and midline thalamic nuclei, which correlates with memory impairment. Recovery is variable and independent of treatment, although alcohol abstinence and thiamine supplementation are recommended. Approximately 20% of patients will recover completely or nearly so (Victor et al., 1989).

Alcoholic Dementia

Dementias in the elderly alcoholic represent a wide spectrum of underlying diseases, from the aforementioned Korsakoff's syndrome to Alzheimer's disease. Neuropsychological tests show impairment in 50% to 70% of alcoholics, and this number is probably higher in elderly alcoholics. Considerable debate occurs whether alcohol itself is neurotoxic or the dementia in alcoholics is secondary to other causes. Victor et al. (1989) believe that the dementia seen in alcoholics is related solely to the Wernicke-Korsakoff syndrome. He believes that this syndrome can contribute to broader cognitive deficits than the isolated memory disturbances commonly reported. The distinction is likely academic, and Oslin et al. (1998) have recently proposed diagnostic criteria for alcoholic-related dementia

TABLE 29-15. *Criteria for alcohol-related dementia*

Probable alcohol-related dementia	Features that cast doubt on the diagnosis
Diagnosis of dementia associated with significant alcohol use	The presence of aphasia
Clinical or radiologic evidence of other alcohol-related end organ or neurologic disease	Clinical evidence of neurologic focality (other than ataxia or neuropathy)
Improvement or stabilization of dementia after alcohol cessation	Radiologic evidence of infarction, subdural hematoma, or other focal brain disease

Adapted from Oslin D, Atkinson RM, Smith DM, et al. Alcohol related dementia: proposed clinical criteria. Int J Geriatr Psychiatry 1998;13:203–212, with permission.

that includes the Wernicke-Korsakoff syndrome. An abbreviated list of criteria is found in Table 29-15.

In an elderly alcoholic it is important not to dismiss the cause of dementia solely to the toxic affects of alcohol. Searching for reversible causes of dementia is as essential, if not more so, in the alcoholic patient. Nutritional deficits and focal causes of dementia may be more common in these patients and should be aggressively sought. Neurodegenerative dementias, such as Alzheimer's disease, should also be identified, as these dementias are more amenable to symptomatic therapy with acetylcholinesterase inhibitors. (See Chapter 21.2 *Dementia Disorders* for information on evaluating the patient with dementia.)

Treatment of alcohol-related dementia consists of alcohol abstinence. Nutritional supplementation, particularly with thiamine, should also be considered.

Cerebellar Degeneration

Isolated cerebellar degeneration secondary to Purkinje cell loss was first associated with alcohol use in 1959 (Victor et al., 1959). The prominent involvement of midline cerebellar structures (i.e., anterior and superior vermis) accounts for the clinical picture of gait ataxia and truncal titubation with minimal appendicular involvement (Victor et al., 1989). The abnormalities seen grossly and pathologically are similar to those seen in Wernicke's encephalopathy, suggesting a common pathophysiology (Victor et al., 1959; Mancall and McEntee, 1965). The disorder tends to occur after years of alcohol use and is gradually progressive (Mancall and McEntee, 1965). The diagnosis is based on a history of chronic alcohol use, neurologic examination, and neuroimaging showing midline cerebellar atrophy (Charness, 1993). As with most alcoholic nervous system disorders, treatment consists of alcohol cessation and nutritional supplementation. Physical therapy with gait training can ameliorate some of the ambulation difficulties.

Central Pontine Myelinolysis

Central pontine myelinolysis (CPM) is an acute neurologic disorder of cerebral white matter with potentially devastating effects. It is an iatrogenic condition associated with the rapid correction of hyponatremia. It is most commonly seen in alcoholics, which suggests some underlying predisposition in these patients (Charness, 1993). However, it can occur in any patient population, and is discussed in detail under disorders associated with alterations of electrolytes and water balance.

Alcoholic Neuropathy

Peripheral nerve disorders in alcoholic patients are common. Polyneuropathy is the most common manifestation (Charness et al., 1989). More than half of all alcoholic patients in one study had clinical evidence of peripheral nerve injury (Behse and Buchthal, 1977). However, mononeuropathies of the radial nerve caused by compression injury can also be seen, the so-called "Saturday night palsy." This occurs when the arm is draped over a chair or hard surface for prolonged periods while the individual is unconscious or intoxicated and results in a wrist drop and loss of sensation over the posterolateral aspect of the hand (Carlson and Logigian, 1999).

Polyneuropathy of alcoholism, as with most disorders of the nervous system associated with alcohol use, probably represents a combination of the direct toxic effects of alcohol and nutritional deficits (Behse and Buchthal, 1977; Wohrle et al., 1998). It is a gradually progressive disorder involving sensory, motor, and autonomic nerves. Common symptoms include anesthesia, paresthesia, burning dysesthesia, and weakness (Behse and Buchthal, 1977). The physical examination reveals loss of deep tendon reflexes, stocking-glove sensory loss, and distal weakness (Behse and Buchthal, 1977).

Prognosis is variable, although some patients show improvement or stabilization after alcohol cessation. Nutritional causes of peripheral neuropathy should be sought, particularly of the B vitamins (see Gastrointestinal Nutrition section and Chapter 25). There is no specific treatment other than nutritional supplementation and the cessation of alcohol.

Alcoholic Myopathy

Myopathy is an important cause of weakness in alcoholics. Approximately half of alcoholic patients show weakness on physical examination, about one third complain of muscle weakness and myalgias (Urbano-Marquez et al., 1989). In one study, 46% of alcoholics had biopsy evidence of myopathy. Also, a correlation was found between weakness and lifetime alcohol use (Urbano-Marquez et al., 1989). Because muscle mass decreases with age (Hubbard and Squier, 1989), elderly patients who abuse alcohol are more likely to develop clinical symptoms associated with myopathy.

Usually, the onset is insidious, occurring over weeks to months. Rarely, an acute myopathy can occur in association with binge drinking. Clinically, patients develop weakness, pain, and muscle tenderness and swelling over hours to days. Muscle necrosis and myoglobinuria can occur. In the elderly patient, aggressive hydration, electrolyte determination, and cardiac monitoring are essential to prevent renal failure and cardiac arrhythmias (Haller and Knochel, 1984). Ultimately, treatment for both acute and chronic myopathies entails alcohol abstinence. Recovery is gradual and can be complete (Charness, 1993).

Alcohol Withdrawal Syndrome

As noted, alcohol abuse is common among the elderly. In addition, alcoholism is frequently missed in hospitalized elderly patients (Beresford et al., 1988). It stands to reason that the abrupt cessation of alcohol that is associated with hospitalization might result in alcohol withdrawal in a substantial number of hospitalized elderly. In fact, 10% of elderly alcoholics admitted to the hospital develop delirium associated with alcohol withdrawal (Finlayson et al., 1988). The elderly are particularly susceptible to delirium, and alcohol withdrawal should always be considered in the differential diagnosis of acute confusional states. In general, alcohol withdrawal is associated with minor symptoms, however, it can develop into a very serious and even fatal condition (Charness, 1993). It is essential to recognize alcohol withdrawal in elderly patients and treat it aggressively and promptly.

Table 29-16 outlines the common characteristics of alcohol withdrawal. An irregular, fast postural and kinetic tremor of the hands is the most common manifestation (Neiman et al., 1990). Hallucinations, illusions, autonomic hyperactivity, nausea and vomiting, delirium, and tonic-clonic seizures are also seen (Charness, 1993; Neiman et al., 1990). Delirium tremens, a condition characterized by severe confusion, agitation, insomnia, severe generalized tremor, hallucinations and delusions, and autonomic hyperactivity, is the most serious condition associated with alcohol withdrawal (Charness, 1993; Neiman et al., 1990).

Figure 29-4 outlines two approaches to managing alcohol withdrawal. The fixed schedule regimen entails giving fixed doses of prophylactic medications around the clock to patients at risk for developing alcohol withdrawal. The symptom-triggered approach requires close monitoring of patients at risk and intervening when symptoms of alcohol withdrawal become apparent. Both approaches have been shown to be equally effective in reducing withdrawal symptoms, however, the symptom triggered approach results in the administration of lower dosages of medication and a shorter duration of therapy (Mayo-Smith, 1997). This is an especially important consideration in elderly patients, who are more sensitive to the sedative effects of benzodiazepines. Another consideration in this group is the use of long-acting versus short-acting benzodiazepines. It can be useful to use shorter acting agents in the elderly for the same reasons, as long-acting agents can produce excessive sedation. However, it is important to realize that, despite these drawbacks, longer acting agents are associated with smoother withdrawal and a lower risk of breakthrough symptoms and seizures (Mayo-Smith, 1997).

Benzodiazepines should be used as first-line agents in managing withdrawal in all populations. In fact, monotherapy with benzodiazepines is usually sufficient to suppress withdrawal. The use of beta-blockers, carbamazepine, and neuroleptics has been studied in alcohol withdrawal but should not be used as first-line agents or as monotherapy. Beta-blockers should be reserved for those patients with comorbid disease, particularly coronary artery disease, and significant autonomic hyperactivity. Carbamazepine can be used in those patients with seizures and has been shown to have some anti-withdrawal properties. In general, neuroleptic use should be avoided as they can precipitate seizures. However, these agents can be useful when dealing with a severely agitated and hallucinating patient. Finally, all patients with suspected alcohol abuse should be treated with thiamine supplementation (Mayo-Smith, 1997).

IATROGENIC NEUROLOGIC COMPLICATIONS

Iatrogenic illness refers to the unintended deleterious consequences of medical diagnostic or therapeutic interventions. The remainder of this section reviews some common neurologic complications of medical interventions.

TABLE 29-16. *Clinical characteristics of alcohol withdrawal*

Tremor—postural hand to generalized axial and
   appendicular
Nausea/vomiting
Delirium
Hallucinations/illusions
Agitation
Autonomic hyperactivity
Generalized tonic-clonic seizures

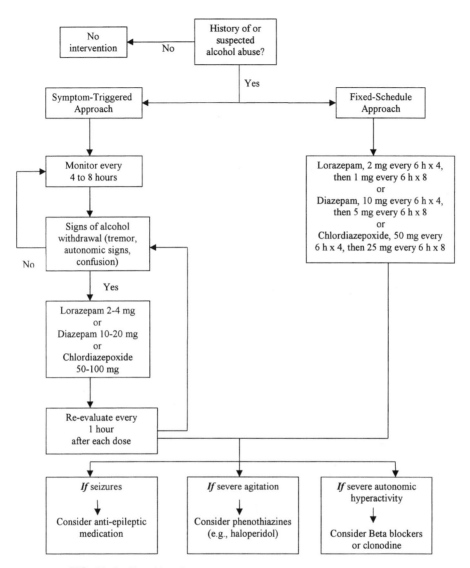

FIG. 29-4. Algorithm for the management of alcohol withdrawal.

NEUROLOGIC COMPLICATIONS OF ORGAN TRANSPLANTATION

Complications of Immunosuppressive Medications

Cyclosporin

Cyclosporine is the most common immunosuppressant agent used in transplantation (Patchell, 1994). Neurologic complications occur in 15% to 40% of patients (Kahan, 1989). Table 29-17 summarizes factors associated with an increased risk of neurologic side effects from cyclosporine (Kahan, 1989; Walker and Brochstein, 1988).

Tremor is the most common neurologic complication, occurring early and diminishing over time (Wijdicks et al., 1995). Delirium occurs in approximately 5% of patients and presents with two distinct clinical syndromes (Patchell, 1994). Lethargy, confusion, cortical blindness, and visual hallucinations characterize the first syndrome. The second syndrome consists of cerebellar findings, focal weakness, and delirium. Fo-

TABLE 29-17. *Risk factors for central nervous system toxicity from cyclosporine*

Cranial irradiation
Hypocholesterolemia
Hypomagnesemia
Beta-lactam antibiotic therapy
High-dose steroids
Hypertension
Uremia

cal or generalized seizures can occur and are associated with high serum levels of the drug (Patchell, 1994).

FK 506

Fine tremor of the hands and paresthesias are the most common complications of the potent immunosuppressant, FK 506 (Burkhalter et al., 1994). In addition, this drug has been associated with a wide variety of other neurologic complications. Delirium is the most common serious complication, occurring in 16% of patients in one series (Burkhalter et al., 1994). Other complications observed include coma, seizures, CPM, sleep disturbances, and nightmares (Burkhalter et al., 1994; Eidelman et al., 1991; Wijdicks et al., 1994). Most side effects are reversible with a reduction in the dose or elimination of this drug (Patchell, 1994).

OKT3 Monoclonal Antibody

The major neurologic complications of OKT3 are an aseptic meningitis and an acute encephalopathy. The meningitis occurs early after the drug is initiated, prompting an evaluation for an infectious cause. However, the meningeal symptoms are self-limited and resolve within a few days and should not prompt discontinuation of the drug. The encephalopathy can be severe, with obtundation, myoclonus, and seizures. As with the meningitis, this condition is self-limited, whether or not the medication is discontinued. However, it is slow to clear and can take weeks (Patchell, 1994).

Corticosteroids

Steroid myopathy, which occurs in most patients on chronic steroids, is the result of type II fiber atrophy. Clinically, patients have proximal muscle weakness that is most severe in the pelvic girdle. The myopathy resolves with discontinuation of the drug (Patchell, 1994).

Steroid psychosis is a complex and variable constellation of clinical signs and symptoms (Wolkowitz et al., 1997). Depression, mania, anxiety, irritability, insomnia, restlessness, and fatigue can all be seen. The exact frequency of this complication is unknown, occurring in 2% to 57% of patients. Increasing age and steroid dose are the strongest predictors of this complication. Withdrawal of the steroids can precipitate an acute worsening of the symptoms. Prevention is the key to treatment. Using the lowest possible dose or every-other-day dosing can be useful. Valproic acid and carbamazepine can be useful as prophylactic agents. Neuroleptics and benzodiazepines are used to treat agitation and anxiety, respectively. Finally, when tapering steroids, a very slow taper is recommended.

Central Nervous System Infections

CNS infections occur in 5% to 10% of transplant patients at some point (Conti and Rubin, 1988). CNS infections are frequently life threatening with mortality rates of 44% to 77% (Conti and Rubin, 1988). *Listeria monocytogenes*, *Cryptococcus neoformans* and *Aspergillus fumigatus* account for 80% of CNS infections in this population (Conti and Rubin, 1988). Other important pathogens are *Toxoplasma gondii* and JC polyomavirus, which is responsible for progressive multifocal leukoencephalopathy (Patchell, 1994).

The familiar signs of CNS infection (fever, meningismus) are frequently lacking in these patients because of their use of strong immunosuppressant medications (Patchell, 1994). Therefore, a high index of suspicion must be maintained to diagnosis these infections.

Complications of the Specific Transplant Procedure

Renal Transplant

Compression injuries of the femoral nerve or lateral femoral cutaneous nerve are common complications of renal transplant surgery (Patchell, 1994). Femoral nerve injury causes weakness of knee extension, with preservation of hip adduction. Sensory changes can occur along the anterolateral aspect of the leg or on the lateral aspect of the thigh, respectively. Caudal spinal cord ischemia rarely occurs as a result of the surgery (Patchell, 1994).

Bone Marrow Transplantation

The procedure for delivering the donor's bone marrow is benign and not associated with any neurologic sequelae. Although acute graft-versus-host disease (GVHD) is not associated with neurologic complications, chronic GVHD is fraught with a variety of autoimmune disorders. Polymyositis and myasthenia gravis, which have been reported in association with GVHD, respond to immunosuppression (Nelson and McQuillen, 1988).

Cardiac Transplantation

Heart transplantation causes neurologic morbidity secondary to complications of cardiac bypass and the development of blood and air emboli. Up to 50% of patients show evidence of cerebral infarction or diffuse hypoxic-ischemic injury after transplantation (Patchell, 1994). This increased risk of stroke continues after the surgery as a result of cardiac arrhythmias. Mechanical injuries to the brachial plexus also occur from the retraction of the chest wall during the surgery (Patchell, 1994).

Liver Transplantation

Of liver transplant patients, 12% to 20% will experience neurologic complications, most during the first week following surgery (Mazariegos et al., 1999). The most unusual of these is CPM (see the section on electrolytes for a detailed description), found in 7% to 13% of patients at autopsy (Patchell, 1994; Mazariegos et al., 1999). In addition, encephalopathy is common, with the elderly being at the highest risk (Mazariegos et al., 1999).

IATROGENIC COMPLICATIONS OF CRITICAL CARE

Delirium

Delirium is common in the hospitalized elderly, especially in the critical care setting (Flacker and Marcantonio, 1998). In these patients, the cause of the confusional state is usually multifactorial. Iatrogenic influences, namely medications, play a large role (Flacker and Marcantonio, 1998). Table 29-18 summarizes the medications that can contribute to delirium in the critical care setting.

Critical Illness Polyneuropathy

Critical illness polyneuropathy is a common condition in critically ill patients, complicating 70% of

TABLE 29-18. *Drugs that may contribute to delirium*

Benzodiazepines
Barbiturates
Opioid narcotics
Antiemetics
Anticonvulsants
H_2 receptor antagonists
Ciprofloxacin
Digoxin
Diphenhydramine
Lidocaine

coma-producing septic encephalopathies (Young, 1995). It frequently becomes manifest as the patient begins to recover but is unable to be weaned from the ventilator (Young, 1995; Zochodne et al., 1987). It is characterized by profound distal greater than proximal weakness and hypo-areflexia (Young, 1995; Zochodne et al., 1987). A facial diplegia can occur, although other cranial nerves are spared (Zochodne et al., 1987). Electrophysiologic studies reveal an axonal neuropathy with evidence of denervation (Young, 1995; Zochodne et al., 1987). Treatment is supportive. Patients who survive their underlying illness have an excellent prognosis, although recovery can take many months. Proposed risk factors are summarized in Table 29-19 (Young, 1995; Wijdicks et al., 1994).

Critical Illness Myopathy

Critical illness myopathy, an acute myopathy, occurs in intubated individuals receiving high-dose corticosteroids and vecuronium (Young, 1995). Clinically, it is similar to the neuropathy previously discussed. Patients have a quadriparesis and difficulty weaning from the ventilator. Pathologic studies have revealed a loss of myosin filaments in the muscle (Young, 1995).

TABLE 29-19. Risk factors for the development of critical illness polyneuropathy

Sepsis
Multiorgan failure
Corticosteroids
Nondepolarizing neuromuscular blocking agents (vecuronium, pancuronium)

TABLE 29-20. *Drugs associated with seizures*

Phenothiazines
Atypical antipsychotics: clozapine
Tricyclic antidepressants-associated with overdose
Bupropion
Selective serotonin reuptake inhibitors: in combination
 with monoamine oxidase inhibitors or other
 serotonergic medications
Theophylline
Salicylate overdose
Chemotherapy: etoposide, ifosfamide, cisplatin
Antimicrobials: penicillin, metronidazole, isoniazid[a]
Benzodiazepine, barbiturate or narcotic withdrawal

[a]Treat with vitamin B_6 replacement.

MISCELLANEOUS NEUROLOGIC COMPLICATIONS OF MEDICATIONS

Medications Associated with Seizures

A variety of drugs have been implicated in causing seizures. Table 29-20 summarizes common medications associated with seizures (Delanty et al., 1998; Snavely and Hodges, 1984).

Medications that Affect Neuromuscular Transmission

The list of drugs that affect neuromuscular transmission and, therefore, cause signs and symptoms of weakness is long. Most of these medications do not cause weakness in healthy patients. However, they can unmask evidence of a neuromuscular disease in asymptomatic patients and should be used cautiously in those with known neuromuscular diseases (Howard, 1990). Only D-penicillamine, which is known to cause a myasthenic syndrome, should be absolutely avoided in patients with diseases of the neuromuscular junction (Howard, 1990). Table 29-21

TABLE 29-21. *Drugs that may impair neuromuscular transmission*

Aminoglycoside antibiotics
Miscellaneous antibiotics: penicillin, sulfa,
 tetracyclines, fluoroquinolones
Beta-blockers
Quinine/quinidine
Procainamide
Nondepolarizing neuromuscular blocking agents
 >polarizing
Phenothiazines
Chloroquine
D-penicillamine
Lidocaine/procaine: intravenously
Phenytoin

TABLE 29-22. *Drug-induced movement disorders*

Phenomenology	Drugs
Tremor	Amphetamines
	Theophylline
	Lithium
	Valproic acid
	Levothyroxine
	Tricyclic antidepressants
	Cyclosporine
	FK506
Chorea	Levothyroxine
	Dopamine agonists
	Amantadine
	Phenytoin
	Estrogen
	Monoamine oxidase inhibitors
	Neuroleptics/neuroleptic derived antiemetics[a]
Dystonia	Neuroleptics/neuroleptic derived antiemetics
	Levodopa
	Dopamine agonists
Myoclonus	Amphetamines
	Selective serotonin reuptake inhibitors
	Levodopa
	Dopamine agonists
Parkinsonism	Neuroleptics
	Atypical antipsychotics
	Reserpine/tetrabenazine
	Methyldopa
	Lithium
Akathisia	Neuroleptics
	Selective serotonin reuptake inhibitors
	Tricyclic antidepressants
	Lithium
	Estrogens
Restless leg syndrome	Neuroleptics
	Selective serotonin reuptake inhibitors
	Phenytoin

[a]Chorea occurs as a component of the tardive dyskinesia syndrome and is a delayed complication of using this class of drugs.

summarizes the medications associated with impaired neuromuscular transmission (Howard, 1990).

Medications Associated with Movement Disorders

Drugs have been associated with every type of movement disorder. The elderly are particularly susceptible to neuroleptic-induced parkinsonism and tardive dyskinesia. Therefore, these drugs should be used cautiously in the elderly (Jankovic, 1981). Table 29-22 outlines the more common drug-induced movement disorders (Jankovic, 1981; Sachdev and Loneragran, 1991; Kraus et al., 2000; Sanz-Fuentenebro et al., 1996; Drake, 1988).

REFERENCES

Adams WL, Yuan Z, Barboriak JJ, et al. Alcohol-related hospitalizations of elderly people. Prevalence and geographic variation in the United States [published erratum appears in *JAMA* 1993;270(17):2055]. *JAMA* 1993;270(10):1222–1225.

Akhter J, Wiede LG. Thyrotoxic periodic paralysis; a reversible cause of paralysis to remember. *S D J Med* 1997;50(10):357–358.

Alexander E. Central nervous system disease in Sjögren's syndrome: new insights into immunopathogenesis. *Rheum Dis Clin North Am* 1992;18(3):637–673.

Alexander EL, Alexander GE. Aseptic meningoencephalitis in primary Sjögren's syndrome. *Neurology* 1983;33(5):593–598.

Alexander EL, Malinow K, Lejewski JF, et al. Primary Sjögren's syndrome with central nervous system disease mimicking multiple sclerosis. *Ann Intern Med* 1986;104(3):323–330.

Alexander EL, Provost TT, Stevens MB, et al. Neurologic complications of primary Sjögren's syndrome. *Medicine* 1982;61(4):247–257.

Alexander EL, Ranzenbach MR, Kumar AJ, et al. Anti-Ro(SS-A) autoantibodies in central nervous system disease associated with Sjögren's syndrome (CNS-SS): clinical, neuroimaging and angiographic correlates. *Neurology* 1994;44(5):899–908.

Alexander EL. Neurologic disease in Sjögren's syndrome: mononuclear inflammatory vasculopathy affecting central/peripheral nervous system and muscle. A clinical review and update of immunopathogenesis. *Rheum Dis Clin North Am* 1993;19(4):869–908.

Aminoff MJ. Neurologic complications of systemic disease in adults. In: Bradley WG, Daroff RB, Fenichel GM, et al., eds. *Neurology in clinical practice.* Boston: Butterworth-Heinemann, 2000:1029–1030.

Anderson GD. A mechanistic approach to antiepileptic drug interactions. *Ann Pharmacother* 1998;32:554–563.

Andreoli TE, Evanoff GV, Ketel BL, et al. Chronic renal failure. In: Andreoli TE, Bennett JC, Carpenter CCJ, et al., eds. *Cecil's essentials of medicine.* Philadelphia: WB Saunders, 1993:244–254.

Anonymous. Alcoholism in the elderly. Council on Scientific Affairs, American Medical Association [see comments]. *JAMA* 1996;275(10):797–801.

Antunez E, Estruch R, Cardenal C, et al. Usefulness of CT and MRI imaging in the diagnosis of acute Wernicke's encephalopathy. *AJR* 1998;171(4):1131–1137.

Argov Z, Mastaglia FL. Drug-induced peripheral neuropathies. *BMJ* 1979;1:663–666.

Averbuch-Heller L, Steiner I, Abramsky O. Neurologic manifestations of progressive systemic sclerosis. *Arch Neurol* 1992;49(12):1292–1295.

Ayus JC, Arieff AI. Abnormalities of water metabolism in the elderly. *Semin Nephrol* 1996;16(4):277–288.

Bajema IM, Hagen EC, Weverling-Rijnsburger AW, et al. Cerebral involvement in two patients with Wegener's granulomatosis [review]. *Clin Nephrol* 1997;47(6):401–406.

Behse F, Buchthal F. Alcoholic neuropathy: clinical, electrophysiological, and biopsy findings. *Ann Neurol* 1977;2(2):95–110.

Bekkelund SI, Torbergsen T, Husby G, et al. Myopathy and neuropathy in rheumatoid arthritis. A quantitative controlled electromyographic study. *J Rheumatol* 1999;26(11):2348–2351.

Ben-Ami H, Pollack S, Nagachandran P, et al. Reversible pancreatitis, hepatitis, and peripheral polyneuropathy associated with parenteral gold therapy. *J Rheumatol* 1999;26(9):2049–2050.

Beresford TP, Blow FC, Brower KJ, et al. Alcoholism and aging in the general hospital. *Psychosomatics* 1988;29:61–72.

Berkelhammer C, Bear RA. A clinical approach to common electrolyte problems: 4. Hypomagnesemia. *CMAJ* 1985;132(4):360–368.

Boden SD, Dodge LD, Bohlman HH, et al. Rheumatoid arthritis of the cervical spine. A long-term analysis with predictors of paralysis and recovery. *J Bone Joint Surg Am* 1994;75(9):1282–1297.

Bragoni M, Di Piero V, Priori R, et al. Sjögren's syndrome presenting as ischemic stroke. *Stroke* 1994;25(11):2276–2279.

Brazis PW, Masdeu JC, Biller J. *Localization in clinical neurology*, 3rd ed. Boston: Little, Brown and Company, 1996.

Burkhalter EL, Starzl TE, Van Thiel DH. Severe neurological complications following orthoptic liver transplantation in patients receiving FK 506 and prednisone. *J Hepatol* 1994;21:572–577.

Burn DJ, Bates D. Neurology and the kidney. *J Neurol Neurosurg Psychiatry* 1998;65(6):810–821.

Caine D, Halliday GM, Kril JJ, et al. Operational criteria for the classification of chronic alcoholics: identification of Wernicke's encephalopathy. *J Neurol Neurosurg Psychiatry* 1997;62(1):51–60.

Carlson N, Logigian EL. Radial neuropathy. *Neurol Clin* 1999;17(3):499–523.

Caselli RJ, Hunder GG, Whisnant JP. Neurologic disease in biopsy-proven giant cell (temporal) arteritis. *Neurology* 1988;38(3):352–359.

Caselli RJ, Hunder GG. Giant cell (temporal) arteritis. *Neurol Clin* 1997;15(4):893–902.

Cerinic MM, Generini S, Pidnone A, et al. The nervous system in systemic sclerosis (scleroderma). *Rheum Dis Clin North Am* 1996;22(4):879–893.

Chang DJ, Paget SA. Neurologic complications of rheumatoid arthritis. *Rheum Dis Clin North Am* 1993;19(4):955–973.

Chang RW, Bell CL, Hallett M. Clinical characteristics and prognosis of vasculitic mononeuropathy multiplex. *Arch Neurol* 1984;41(6):618–621.

Chapelon C, Ziza JM, Piette JC, et al. Neurosarcoidosis: signs, course and treatment in 35 confirmed cases [review]. *Medicine* 1990;69(5):261–276.

Charness ME, Simon RP, Greenberg DA. Ethanol and the nervous system [see comments] [review]. *N Engl J Med* 1989;321(7):442–454.

Charness ME. Brain lesions in alcoholics. *Alcohol Clin Exp Res* 1993;17(1):2–11.

Christensen KS. Hypokalemic paralysis in Sjögren's syndrome secondary to renal tubular acidosis. *Scand J Rheumatol* 1985;14(1):58–60.

Clark WF, Rock GA, Buskard N, et al. Therapeutic plasma exchange: an update from the Canadian Apheresis Group [see comments]. *Ann Intern Med* 1999;131(6):453–462.

Clouston PD, DeAngelis LM, Posner JB. The spectrum of neurologic disease in patients with systemic cancer. *Ann Neurol* 1992;31:268–273.

Conti DJ, Rubin RH. Infection of the central nervous system in organ transplant recipients. *Neurol Clin* 1988;6(2): 241–260.

Davison AM, Walker GS, Oli H, et al. Water supply and aluminum concentration, dialysis dementia, and effect of reverse-osmosis water treatment. *Lancet* 1982;2(8302): 785–787.

DeAngelis LM, Delattre JY, Posner JB. Radiation-induced dementia in patients cured of brain metastases. *Neurology* 1989;39:789–796.

Delaney P. Neurologic manifestations in sarcoidosis: review of the literature, with a report of 23 cases [review]. *Ann Intern Med* 1977;87(3):336–345.

Delanty N, Vaughan CJ, French JA. Medical causes of seizures. *Lancet* 1998;352(9125):383–390.

Drake M. Restless legs with antiepileptic drug therapy. *Clin Neurol Neurosurg* 1988;90(2):151–154.

Dray GJ, Jablon M. Clinical and radiologic features of primary osteoarthritis of the hand. *Hand Clin* 1987;3(3): 351–369.

Dreyer SJ, Boden SD. Natural history of rheumatoid arthritis of the cervical spine [review]. *Clin Orthop* 1999;(366): 98–106.

Dropcho EJ. Central nervous system injury by therapeutic irradiation. *Neurol Clin* 1991;9(4):969–987.

Earnest MP, Yarnell PR. Seizure admissions to a city hospital: the role of alcohol. *Epilepsia* 1976;17:387–393.

Eidelman BH, Abu-Elmagd K, Wilson J, et al. Neurologic complications of FK 506. *Transplant Proc* 1991;23(6): 3175–3178.

Eldor A. Thrombotic thrombocytopenic purpura: diagnosis, pathogenesis and modern therapy. *Bailliere's Clin Haematol* 1998;11(2):475–495.

Evers S, Engelien A, Karsch V, et al. Secondary hyperkalaemic paralysis. *J Neurol Neurosurg Psychiatry* 1998;64(2):249–252.

Farrell DA, Medsger TA Jr. Trigeminal neuropathy in progressive systemic sclerosis. *Am J Med* 1982;73(1):57–62.

Fauci AS, Katz P, Haynes BF, et al. Cyclophosphamide therapy of severe systemic necrotizing vasculitis. *N Engl J Med* 1979;301(5):235–238.

Finkelstein JS, Mitlak BH, Slovik DM. Normal physiology of bone and bone minerals. In: Andreoli TE, Bennett JC, Carpenter CCJ, et al. eds. *Cecil's essentials of medicine.* Philadelphia: WB Saunders, 1993:530–538.

Finkelstein JS, Mitlak BH, Slovik DM. The parathyroid glands, hypercalcemia, and hypocalcemia. In: Andreoli TE, Bennett JC, Carpenter CCJ, et al., eds. *Cecil's essentials of medicine.* Philadelphia: WB Saunders, 1993: 538–546.

Finlayson RE, Hurt RD, Davis LJ Jr, et al. Alcoholism in elderly persons: a study of the psychiatric and psychosocial features of 216 inpatients. *Mayo Clin Proc* 1988;63(8): 761–768.

Flacker JM, Marcantonio ER. Delirium in the elderly. Optimal management. *Drugs Aging* 1998;13(2):119–130.

Font J, Valls J, Cervera R, et al. Pure sensory neuropathy in patients with primary Sjögren's syndrome: clinical, immunological, and electromyographic findings. *Ann Rheum Dis* 1990;49(10):775–778.

Fox RI, Saito I. Criteria for the diagnosis of Sjögren's syndrome. *Rheum Dis Clin North Am* 1994;20(2):391–407.

Freedland ES, McMicken DB. Alcohol-related seizures. Part 1: pathophysiology, differential diagnosis, and evaluation. *J Emerg Med* 1993;11:463–473.

Frewin R, Henson A, Provan D. ABC of clinical haemotology: haemotological emergencies. *BMJ* 1997;314(7090): 1333–1336.

Gallucci M, Bozzao A, Splendiani A, et al. Wernicke encephalopathy: MR findings in five patients. *Am J Neuroradiol* 1990;11(5):887–892.

Garfin SR, Herkowitz HN, Mirkovic S. *Spinal stenosis.* Instructional Course Lectures, 2000;49:361–374.

Generini S, Fiori G, Moggi P, et al. Systemic sclerosis. A clinical overview [review]. *Adv Exp Med Biol* 1999;455: 73–83.

George B, Laurian C. Impairment of vertebral artery flow caused by extrinsic lesions. *Neurosurgery* 1989;24(2): 206–214.

Gilbert MR, Grossman SA. Incidence and nature of neurologic problems in patients with solid tumors. *Am J Med* 1986;81(6):951–954.

Goldberg ID, Bloomer WD, Dawson DM. Nervous system toxic effects of cancer therapy. *JAMA* 1982;247(10): 1437–1441.

Good AE, Christopher RP, Koepke GH. Peripheral neuropathy associated with rheumatoid arthritis: a clinical and electrodiagnostic study of 70 consecutive rheumatoid arthritis patients. *Ann Intern Med* 1965;63:87.

Gross M. Chronic relapsing inflammatory polyneuropathy complicating sicca syndrome. *J Neurol Neurosurg Psychiatry* 1987;50(7):939–940.

Gross WL. Antineutrophil cytoplasmic autoantibody testing in vasculitides. *Rheum Dis Clin North Am* 1995;21(4): 987–1003.

Grossman SA, Krabak MJ. Leptomeningeal carcinomatosis. *Cancer Treat Rev* 1999;25(2):103–119.

Guillevin L, Lhote F, Gayraud M, et al. Prognostic factors in polyarteritis nodosa and Churg-Strauss syndrome. A prospective study in 342 patients. *Medicine* 1996;75(1): 17–28.

Guillevin L, Lhote F, Gherardi R. Polyarteritis nodosa, microscopic polyangiitis, and Churg-Strauss syndrome: clinical aspects, neurologic manifestations, and treatment. *Neurol Clin* 1997;15(4):865–866.

Gurley JP, Bell GR. The surgical management of patients with rheumatoid cervical spine disease. *Rheum Dis Clin North Am* 1997;23(2):317–332.

Guttman L, Govindan S, Riggs JE, et al. Inclusion body myositis and Sjögren's syndrome. *Arch Neurol* 1985;42 (10):1021–1022.

Hall S, Bartleson JD, Onofrio BM, et al. Lumbar spinal stenosis. Clinical features, diagnostic procedures, and results of surgical treatment in 68 patients. *Ann Intern Med* 1985;103:271–275.

Haller RG, Knochel JP. Skeletal muscle disease in alcoholism. *Med Clin North Am* 1984;68(91):103.

Hanagan JR. Hypercalcemia in malignant disease. *Clin Ther* 1982;5(2):102–112.

Harley JB, Alexander EL, Bias WB, et al. Anti-Ro (SS-A) and anti-La (SS-B) in patients with Sjögren's syndrome. *Arthritis Rheum* 1986;29(2):196–206.

Harper C. The incidence of Wernicke's encephalopathy in Australia—a neuropathological study of 131 cases. *J Neurol Neurosurg Psychiatry* 1983;46:593–598.

Harper CM, Thomas JE, Cascino TL, et al. Distinction between neoplastic and radiation-induced brachial plexopathy, with emphasis on the role of EMG. *Neurology* 1989; 39(502):506.

Harris ED Jr. Rheumatoid arthritis. Pathophysiology and implications for therapy. *N Engl J Med* 1990;322(18): 1277–1289.

Harris EN, Pierangeli S. Antiphospholipid antibodies and cerebral lupus. *Ann NY Acad Sci* 1997;823:270–278.

Haslock DI, Wright V, Harriman DG. Neuromuscular disorders in rheumatoid arthritis. A motor-point muscle biopsy study. *Q J Med* 1970;39(155):335–358.

Hietaharju A, Jaaskelainen S, Kalimo H, et al. Peripheral neuromuscular manifestations in systemic sclerosis (scleroderma). *Muscle Nerve* 1993;16(11):1204–1212.

Homewood J, Bond NW. Thiamin deficiency and Korsakoff's syndrome: failure to find memory impairments following nonalcoholic Wernicke's encephalopathy. *Alcohol* 1999;19(1):75–84.

Hope LC, Cook CC, Thomson AD. A survey of the current clinical practice of psychiatrists and accident and emergency specialists in the United Kingdom concerning vitamin supplementation for chronic alcohol misusers. *Alcohol Alcohol* 1999;34(6):862–867.

Howard JF Jr. Adverse drug effects on neuromuscular transmission. *Semin Neurol* 1990;10(1):89–102.

Hubbard BM, Squier MV. The physical ageing of the neuromuscular system. In: Tallis R, ed. *The clinical neurology of old age.* Oxford: John Wiley and Sons, 1989:3–26.

Inouye SK. Prevention of delirium in hospitalized older patients: risk factors and targeted intervention strategies. *Ann Med* 2000;32(4):257–263.

Jackson CG, Chess RL, Ward JR. A case of rheumatoid nodule formation within the central nervous system and review of the literature. *J Rheumatol* 1984;11(2): 237–240.

Jaeckle KA, Young DF, Foley KM. The natural history of lumbosacral plexopathy in cancer. *Neurology* 1985;35:8–15.

Jankovic J. Drug-induced and other orofacial-cervical dyskinesias. *Ann Intern Med* 1981;94:788–793.

Jennette JC, Falk RJ. Small-vessel vasculitis [see comments] [review]. *N Engl J Med* 1997;337(21):1512–1523.

Johns CJ, Michele TM. The clinical management of sarcoidosis. A 50-year experience at the Johns Hopkins Hospital. *Medicine* 1999;78(2):65–111.

Jones DR, Detterbeck FC. Pancoast tumors of the lung. *Curr Opin Pulm Med* 1998;4(4):191–197.

Judge TG. Hypokalaemia in the elderly. *Gerontol Clin* 1968; 10:102–107.

Kahan BD. Cyclosporine. *N Engl J Med* 1989;321: 1725–1738.

Kamata T, Hishida A, Takita T, et al. Morphologic abnormalities in the brain of chronically hemodialyzed patients without cerebrovascular disease. *Am J Nephrol* 2000;20:27–31.

Kaplan RS, Wiernik PH. Neurotoxicity of antineoplastic drugs. *Semin Oncol* 1982;9(1):103–130.

Keltner JL. Giant-cell arteritis. Signs and symptoms. *Ophthalmology* 1982;89(10):1101–1110.

Kiu MC, Wan YL, Ng SH, et al. Pneumocephalus due to nasopharyngeal carcinoma: case report. *Neuroradiology* 1996;38(1):70–72.

Kraus T, Schuld A, Pollmacher T. Periodic leg movements in sleep and restless legs syndrome probably caused by olanzapine. *J Clin Pharmacol* 2000;19(5):478–479.

Kriss TC, Kriss VM. Neck pain. Primary care work-up of acute and chronic symptoms. *Geriatrics* 2000;55(1): 47–48.

Kumar S, Berl T. Sodium. *Lancet* 1998;352(9123):220–228.

Lafitte C. Neurological manifestations in Sjögren syndrome. *Arch Neurol* 2000;57(3):411–413.

Lamprecht P, Gause A, Gross WL. Cryoglobulinemic vasculitis. *Arthritis Rheum* 1999;42(12):2507–2516.

Larrson EM, Holtas S, Cronquist S, et al. Comparison of myelography, CT myelography and magnetic resonance imaging in cervical spondylosis and disk herniation. Pre and postoperative findings. *Acta Radiol* 1989;30(3): 233–239.

Lass P, Buscombe JR, Harber M, et al. Cognitive impairment in patients with renal failure is associated with multiple-infarct dementia. *Clin Nucl Med* 1999;24(8):561–565.

Laureno R, Karp B. Myelinolysis after correction of hyponatremia. *Ann Intern Med* 1997;126(1):57–62.

Lavizzo-Mourey R, Johnson J, Stolley P. Risk factors for dehydration among elderly nursing home residents. *J Am Geriatr Soc* 1988;36:213–218.

Lipowski ZJ. Acute confusional states (delirium) in the elderly. In: Albert ML, Knoefel JE, eds. *Clinical neurology of aging.* Oxford: Oxford University Press, 1994:347–362.

Lynch JP, Sharma OP, Baughman RP. Extrapulmonary sarcoidosis [review]. *Semin Respir Infect* 1998;13(3): 229–254.

Mach JR, Korchik WP, Mahowald MW. Dialysis dementia. *Clin Geriatr Med* 1988;4(4):853–867.

Malinow K, Yannakakis GD, Glusman SM, et al. Subacute sensory neuronopathy secondary to dorsal root ganglionitis in primary Sjögren's syndrome. *Ann Neurol* 1986; 20(4):535–537.

Mancall EL, McEntee WJ. Alterations of the cerebellar cortex in nutritional encephalopathy. *Neurology* 1965;15:303–313.

Marco CA, Kelen GD. Acute intoxication. *Emerg Med Clin North Am* 1990;8(4):731–748.

Markenson JA, McDougal JS, Tsairis P, et al. Rheumatoid meningitis: a localized immune process. *Ann Intern Med* 1979;90(5):786–789.

Matsushita S, Kato M, Muramatsu T, et al. Alcohol and aldehyde dehydrogenase genotypes in Korsakoff syndrome. *Alcohol Clin Exp Res* 2000;24(3):337–340.

Mayo-Smith MF. Pharmacological management of alcohol withdrawal. A meta-analysis and evidence-based practice guideline. American Society of Addiction Medicine Working Group on Pharmacological Management of Alcohol Withdrawal [see comments]. *JAMA* 1997;278(2):144–151.

Mazariegos GV, Molmenti EP, Kramer DJ. Early complications after orthoptic liver transplantation. *Surg Clin North Am* 1999;79(1):109–129.

Mellgren SI, Conn DL, Stevens JC, et al. Peripheral neuropathy in primary Sjögren's syndrome. *Neurology* 1989; 39(3):390–394.

Mikulowski P, Wollheim FA, Rotmil P, et al. Sudden death in rheumatoid arthritis with atlanto-axial dislocation. *Acta Medica Scandinavica* 1975;198(6):445–451.

Mirand AL, Welte JW. Alcohol consumption among the elderly in a general population, Erie County, New York. *Am J Public Health* 1996;86(7):978–984.

Mondelli M, Romano C, Della P, et al. Electrophysiological evidence of "nerve entrapment syndromes" and subclinical peripheral neuropathy in progressive systemic sclerosis (scleroderma). *J Neurol* 1995;242(4):185–194.

Monro P, Uttley D. Spinal cord and spinal root disease, secondary to diseases of the spine. In: Tallis R, ed. *The clinical neurology of old age.* Oxford: John Wiley and Sons, 1989:251–283.

Moore PM, Cupps TR. Neurological complications of vasculitis. *Ann Neurol* 1983;14(2):155–167.

Murros KE, Toole JF. The effect of radiation on carotid arteries. *Arch Neurol* 1989;46:449–455.

Nakamura RM. Neuropsychiatric lupus. *Rheum Dis Clin North Am* 1997;20(1):379–393.

Nath U, Grant R. Neurological paraneoplastic syndromes. *J Clin Pathol* 1997;50(12):975–980.

Neiman J, Lang AE, Fornazzari L, et al. Movement disorders in alcoholism: a review [see comments] [review]. *Neurology* 1990;40(5):741–746.

Nelson KR, McQuillen MP. Neurologic complications of graft-versus-host disease. *Neurol Clin* 1988;6(2):389–403.

Neva MH, Kaarela K, Kauppi M. Prevalence of radiologic changes in the cervical spine—a cross sectional study after 20 years from presentation of rheumatoid arthritis. *J Rheumatol* 2000;27(1):90–93.

Nishino H, Rubino FA, DeRemee RA, et al. Neurological involvement in Wegener's granulomatosis: an analysis of 324 consecutive patients at the Mayo Clinic. *Ann Neurol* 1993;33(1):4–9.

Norton WL, Nardo JM. Vascular disease in progressive systemic sclerosis (scleroderma) [review]. *Ann Intern Med* 1970;73(2):317–324.

Nurick S. The natural history and the results of surgical treatment of the spinal cord disorder associated with cervical spondylosis. *Brain* 1972;95(1):101–108.

O'Hare JA, Callaghan NM, Murnaghan DJ. Dialysis encephalopathy. Clinical, electroencephalographic and interventional aspects. *Medicine* 1983;62(3):129–141.

Okada K, Shirasaki N, Hayashi H, et al. Treatment of cervical spondylotic myelopathy by enlargement of the spinal canal anteriorly, followed by arthrodesis. *J Bone Joint Sur Am* 1991;73(3):352–364.

Oksanen V. Neurosarcoidosis: clinical presentations and course in 50 patients. *Acta Neurol Scand* 1986;73(3): 283–290.

Ondo W. Ropinirole for restless legs syndrome. *Mov Disord* 1999;14(1):138–140.

Oslin D, Atkinson RM, Smith DM, Hendrie H. Alcohol related dementia: proposed clinical criteria. *Int J Geriatr Psychiatry* 1998;13:203–212.

Oxholm P. Primary Sjögren's syndrome—clinical and laboratory markers of disease activity. *Semin Arthritis Rheum* 1992;22(2):114–126.

Palmer JJ. Radiation myelopathy. *Brain* 1972;95:109–122.

Patchell RA. Neurological complications of organ transplantation. *Ann Neurol* 1994;36:688–703.

Peterson IM, Heim C. Inverted squamous papilloma with neuro-ophthalmic features. *Journal of Clinical Neuro-Ophthalmology* 1991;11(1):35–38.

Pettigrew LC, Glass JP, Maor M, et al. Diagnosis and treatment of lumbosacral plexopathy in patients with cancer. *Arch Neurol* 1984;41(1282):1285.

Pickett JL, Theberge DC, Brown WS, et al. Normalizing hematocrit in dialysis patients improves brain function. *Am J Kidney Dis* 1999;33(6):1122–1130.

Posner JB. Paraneoplastic syndromes. In: Posner JB, ed. *Neurologic complications of cancer.* Philadelphia: FA Davis, 1995a:353–385.

Posner JB. Side effects of chemotherapy. In: Posner JB, ed. *Neurologic complications of cancer.* Philadelphia: FA Davis, 1995b.

Ramos M, Mandybur TI. Cerebral vasculitis in rheumatoid arthritis. *Arch Neurol* 1975;32(4):271–275.

Raskin NH, Fishman RA. Neurologic disorders in renal failure (first of two parts). *N Engl J Med* 1976;294(3):143–148.

Raskin NH, Fishman RA. Neurologic disorders in renal failure (second of two parts). *N Engl J Med* 1976;294(4):204–210.

Reich KA, Giansiracusa DF, Stongwater SL. Neurologic manifestations of giant cell arteritis. *Am J Med* 1990;89: 67–72.

Reyes-Ortiz CA. Dehydration, delirium and disability in elderly patients. *JAMA* 1997;278(4):287–288.

Rigler SK. Alcoholism in the elderly [review]. *Am Fam Physician* 2000;15;61(6):1710–1716.

Ropper AH, Gorson KC. Neuropathies associated with paraproteinemia. *N Engl J Med* 1998;338(22):1601–1607.

Rosenbaum RB, Campbell SM, Rosenbaum JT. *Clinical neurology of rheumatic diseases.* Boston: Butterworth-Heinemann, 1996.

Rottenberg DA, Chernik NL, Deck MDF, et al. Cerebral necrosis following radiotherapy of extracranial neoplasms. *Ann Neurol* 1977;1:339–357.

Sachdev P, Loneragran C. The present status of akathisia. *J Nerv Ment Dis* 1991;179(7):381–389.

Sager DS, Bennett RM. Individualizing the risk/benefit ratio of NSAIDs in older patients. *Geriatrics* 1992;47(8): 24–31.

Sahenk Z, Barohn R, New P, et al. Taxol neuropathy. Electrodiagnostic and sural nerve biopsy findings. *Arch Neurol* 1994;51:726–729.

Sahenk Z. Toxic neuropathies. *Semin Neurol* 1987;7(1): 9–17.

Sanz-Fuentenebro FJ, Huidobro A, Tejadas-Rivas A. Restless legs syndrome and paroxetine. *Acta Psychiatr Scand* 1996;94(6):482–484.

Scheepers BD. Alcohol and the brain. *British Journal of Hospital Medicine* 1997;57(11):548–551.

Schneider HA, Yonker RA, Katz P, et al. Rheumatoid vasculitis: experience with 13 patients and review of the literature. *Semin Arthritis Rheum* 1985;14(4):280–286.

Scott TF. Neurosarcoidosis: progress and clinical aspects [review]. *Neurology* 1993;43(1):8–12.

Sharma OP, Sharma AM. Sarcoidosis of the nervous system. A clinical approach [review]. *Arch Intern Med* 1991;151 (7):1317–1321.

Sharma OP. Neurosarcoidosis: a personal perspective based on the study of 37 patients. *Chest* 1997;112(1):220–228.

Sharma OP. Treatment of sarcoidosis. If not corticosteroids, then what? *Pulmonary Perspectives* 1997;1:1–3.

Sigal LH. The neurologic presentation of vasculitic and rheumatologic syndromes. A review [review]. *Medicine* 1987;66(3):157–180.

Silberstein SD, Lipton RB, Goadsby PJ. *Headache in clinical practice,* 1st ed. Oxford: Isis Medical Media, 1998.

Sivri A, Guler-Uysal F. The electroneurophysiological evaluation of rheumatoid arthritis patients. *Clin Rheumatol* 1998;17(5):416–418.

Snavely SR, Hodges GR. The neurotoxicity of antibacterial agents. *Ann Intern Med* 1984;101:92–104.

Steen VD, Medsger TA Jr. Epidemiology and natural history of systemic sclerosis. *Rheum Dis Clin North Am* 1990;16 (1):1–11.

Stern BJ, Krumholz A, Johns C, et al. Sarcoidosis and its neurological manifestations [review]. *Arch Neurol* 1985; 42(9):909–917.

Sterns RH, Cappuccio JD, Silver SM, et al. Neurologic sequelae after treatment of severe hyponatremia; a multicenter perspective. *J Am Soc Nephrol* 1994;4(8):1522–1530.

Stevens JC, Cartlidge NE, Saunders M, et al. Atlanto-axial subluxation and cervical myelopathy in rheumatoid arthritis. *Q J Med* 1971;40(159):391–408.

Sulavik SB, Spencer RP, Weed DA, et al. Recognition of distinctive patterns of gallium-67 distribution in sarcoidosis. *J Nucl Med* 1990;31(12):1909–1914.

Torvik A, Lindboe CF, Rogde S. Brain lesions in alcoholics: a neuropathological study with clinical correlations. *J Neurol Sci* 1982;56:233–248.

Trenkwalder C, Stiasny K, Pollmacher T, et al. L-dopa therapy of uremic and idiopathic restless legs syndrome: a double-blind, crossover trial. *Sleep* 1995;18(8):681–688.

Truumees E, Herkowitz HN. *Cervical spondylotic myelopathy and radiculopathy.* Instructional Course Lectures 2000;49:339–360.

Urbano-Marquez A, Estruch R, Navarro-Lopez F, et al. The effects of alcoholism on skeletal and cardiac muscle [see comments]. *N Engl J Med* 1989;320(7):409–415.

van Dam GM, Reisman Y, van Wieringen K. Hypokalemic thyrotoxic periodic paralysis: case report and review of an Oriental syndrome. *Neth J Med* 1996;49(2):90–97.

Victor M, Adams RD, Collins GH. *The Wernicke-Korsakoff syndrome and related neurological disorders due to alcoholism and malnutrition*, 2nd ed. Philadelphia: FA Davis, 1989.

Victor M, Adams RD, Mancall EL. A restricted form of cerebellar cortical degeneration occurring in alcoholic patients. *Arch Neurol* 1959;71:579–688.

Walker RW, Brochstein JA. Neurologic complications of immunosuppressive agents. *Neurol Clin* 1988;6(2):261–278.

Walters AS. Toward a better definition of the restless legs syndrome. The international restless legs syndrome study group. *Mov Disord* 1995;10(5):634–642.

Watson AJ, Walker JF, Tomkin GH, et al. Acute Wernicke's encephalopathy precipitated by glucose loading. *Ir J Med Sci* 1981;150(10):301–303.

Wegelius O, Pasternack A, Kuhlback B. Muscular involvement in rheumatoid arthritis. *Acta Rheumatologica Scandinavica* 1969;15(4):257–261.

Wijdicks EFM, Litchy WJ, Harrison BA. The clinical spectrum of critical illness polyneuropathy. *Mayo Clin Proc* 1994;69(10):955–959.

Wijdicks EFM, Wiesner RH, Dahlke LJ, et al. FK506-induced neurotoxicity in liver transplantation. *Ann Neurol* 1994;35(4):498–501.

Wijdicks EFM, Wiesner RH, Krom RAF. Neurotoxicity in liver transplant recipients with cyclosporin immunosuppression. *Neurology* 1995;45:1962–1964.

Wilbourn AJ, Aminoff MJ. AAEE minimonograph:32: the electrophysiologic examination in patients with radiculopathies. *Muscle Nerve* 1988;11(11):1099–1114.

Wohrle JC, Spengos K, Steinke W, et al. Alcohol-related acute axonal polyneuropathy: a differential diagnosis of Guillain-Barré syndrome. *Arch Neurol* 1998;55(10):1329–1334.

Wolkowitz OM, Reus VI, Canick J, et al. Glucocorticoid medication, memory and steroid psychosis in medical illness. *Ann NY Acad Sci* 1997;823:81–96.

Young GB. Neurologic complications of systemic critical illness. *Neurologic Critical Care* 1995;13(3):645–658.

Zochodne DW, Bolton CF, Wells GA, et al. Critical illness polyneuropathy. A complication of sepsis and multiple organ failure. *Brain* 1987;110:819–842.

30

Acute and Chronic Seizures in the Older Adult

Joseph I. Sirven

INTRODUCTION

Epilepsy, one of the oldest recorded conditions, is characterized by repeated spontaneous seizures affecting 1.5 to 3 million people in the United States annually. After an initial peak in the first years of life, the incidence of epilepsy remains stable for decades before increasing after the age of 65 to a higher incidence peak than that found in childhood (Fig. 30-1) (Hauser, 1992; Hauser et al., 1993). Despite the high prevalence of epilepsy in older adults, it is commonly misperceived as a rare occurrence and, therefore, unimportant. Furthermore, medical management of the older patient with epilepsy is often based on information extrapolated from younger patients without consideration for the unique problems and issues associated with a geriatric population. The causes of epilepsy in older adults are unique to this population and affect the approach to treatment strategies (Fig. 30-2). Moreover, the psychosocial effects of seizures in old age can have profound consequences on quality of life. Because little literature is available regard-ing this problem and no clear consensus exists concerning its management, this chapter reviews the diagnosis and treatment of epilepsy, with an emphasis on new therapies.

EPIDEMIOLOGY

Seizures and recurrent seizures (epilepsy) occur more frequently in the elderly because they are often secondary to conditions that present more commonly in patients above 60 years of age. These conditions include strokes, hemorrhages, infections, and degenerative diseases such as dementia. Therefore, to gain a clear understanding of the incidence of epilepsy in people over the age of 60 years, distinctions must be made between acute symptomatic seizures and epilepsy. *Acute symptomatic seizures* or *provoked seizures* occur in the context of an acute metabolic disturbance or at the time of an acute insult to the central nervous system (CNS). *Epilepsy*, or *repeated unprovoked seizures*, is commonly a long-term complication from a CNS lesion.

Acute Seizures

Acute symptomatic seizures include seizures occurring in the context of an acute metabolic disturbance and at the time of an acute insult to the CNS, which distinctly differs from epilepsy, or chronic unprovoked seizures. The incidence of acute seizures in those above 60 years of age has been estimated to be 100/100,000, which increases linearly with each decade of advancing age (Hauser, 1992; Hauser et al., 1993; Luhdorf et al., 1989; Sanders et al., 1990; Loiseau et al., 1990; Tallis et al., 1991; Annegers et al., 1995). One recent British study has shown that 24% to 30% of incident cases in the United Kingdom occur in individuals above 65 years of age (Sanders et al., 1990). When these values are extrapolated to the US population, it is predicted that 50,000 older Americans will have an acute seizure each year (Annegers et al.,

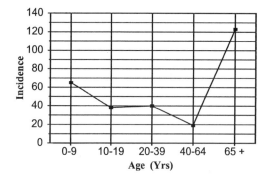

FIG. 30-1. Age-specific average annual incidence of epilepsy per 100,000 population. Adapted from Hauser WA et al. Incidence of epilepsy and unprovoked seizures in Rochester, Minnesota, 1934–1984. *Epilepsia* 1993;34: 453–468.

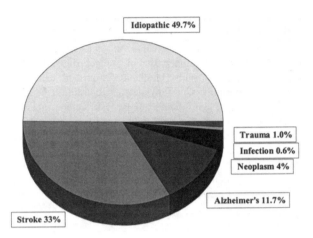

FIG. 30-2. Cause of epilepsy in the elderly.

1995). In the Sanders et al. study (1990), most of these seizures were secondary to cerebrovascular disease, particularly hemorrhage, followed by metabolic abnormalities, trauma, alcohol withdrawal, toxicity, and CNS infections (Sanders et al., 1990; Tallis et al., 1991; Annegers et al., 1995; Kilpatrick et al., 1992; So et al., 1996; Giroud et al., 1994; Lancsman et al., 1993; Hauser et al., 1984; Ettinger and Shinnar, 1993; Hauser et al., 1994; Hauser, 1997). Moreover, 30% of acute seizures in older adults presented as status epilepticus, which is twice the incidence of status epilepticus in the general population (Hauser et al., 1994; Hauser, 1997; Towne et al., 1994). This statistic is of concern because status epilepticus requires emergency care. Furthermore, because status epilepticus can present as a confusional state without overt generalized tonic clonic activity, misdiagnosis often delays treatment, contributing to the high mortality rate associated with it in this age group (Towne et al., 1994).

Acute symptomatic seizures arising from metabolic conditions are common in older adults and are likely to be seen in both the ambulatory and hospital settings. Several conditions can precipitate seizures. Hypoglycemia associated with insulin use and nonketotic hyperglycemia are often reported causes of seizures in patients with diabetes (Malouf and Brust, 1985; Singh et al., 1973). Hyponatremia, uremia, and hypocalcemia are also associations well represented in the literature (Loiseau, 1997). Abrupt discontinuation of sedative and anxiolytic drugs is a prominent cause of seizures in this age group. All barbiturates and benzodiazepines present a risk of withdrawal seizures (Messing et al., 1984; Zaccara et al., 1990; Thomas et al., 1993). The use of medications that lower the seizure threshold is an important cause of acute seizures. Drugs such as phenothiazine, tricyclic antidepressants, and theophylline; antibiotics such as new generation quinolones; and certain pain medications such as meperidine can lead to seizures (Messing et al., 1984; Zaccara et al., 1990; Thomas et al., 1993; Remick and Fine, 1979). Both CNS and systemic infections (e.g., meningitis, pneumonia, and urosepsis) can also promote seizures (Loiseau, 1997; Annegers et al., 1988). Acute trauma and embolic stroke are also common causes of acute seizures. See Hauser (1992, 1997) for a more detailed discussion regarding acute seizures.

Chronic Seizures—Epilepsy

Recurrent, unprovoked seizures or epilepsy also has a peak incidence in older age groups. The annual incidence of epilepsy is 134/100,000 in those 65 years of age or older (Hauser, 1992; Hauser et al., 1993; Luhdorf et al., 1989; Sanders et al., 1990; Loiseau et al., 1990; Tallis et al., 1991). In contrast, the incidence of Alzheimer's type dementia is 123/100,000 (Hauser, 1997). The following were identified as the major causes of epilepsy in the older adult in an Olmsted County population study: cerebrovascular disease (33%), dementia (11.7%), neoplasm (4%), infection (0.6%), and trauma (1%) (Hauser, 1997). In the remaining 50% of the older patient with epilepsy, no definitive cause was found (Hauser, 1997). For all of the listed conditions, the risk of epilepsy is highest in the first year after the occurrence of the CNS insult (Hauser, 1997).

DIAGNOSTIC EVALUATION

One obstacle in the treatment of epilepsy in older adults is misdiagnosis. Older patients are more likely to experience seizures of partial rather than generalized onset, but the manifestations of those seizures differ in older patients from those of a younger age. One suggested reason is that the epileptic focus in older adults involves the frontal and parietal lobes rather than the temporal lobe (Ramsey and Pryor, 2000). Thus, these patients are less likely to experience auras such as *déjà vu* and other symptoms classically associated with temporal lobe epilepsy. Rather, these patients will complain of dizziness, posturing, paresthesias, and other symptoms related to frontal and parietal lobe function. Thus, it becomes difficult to differentiate these symptoms from other common conditions.

The presentation of partial seizures can be diagnosed incorrectly as nonspecific confusional states. Indeed, nonconvulsive status epilepticus can present with acute behavioral changes that range from mutism to hallucinations (Tinuper, 1997). Delirium, a common syndrome in the older adult, may be secondary to nonconvulsive seizures or status epilepticus. Moreover, the fluctuating mental status associated with these seizures may be attributed to dementia or other recurrent confusional states and, thus, delay appropriate treatment. Lastly, the postictal period can last for days in the older adults, further contributing to the difficulty in diagnosis.

Several types of transient episodes that mimic seizures can occur in the elderly, which confounds diagnosis. Syncope, transient ischemic attacks, transient global amnesia, and vertigo are common at this age but can present similarly to seizures (Tinuper, 1997). Diagnosis requires a detailed and accurate history, and this is often lacking in older adults because of either poor patient memory or lack of witnesses. Table 30-1 lists common discriminators of these

events and seizures. Although these variables may be helpful, they remain nonspecific.

The initial evaluation of older patients with seizures is similar to that of younger patients. A thorough history must be obtained from both the patient and family. Carefully detailed questions about the episodes and about epilepsy risk factors, including minor or major head trauma and concomitant medications, must be asked. In many cases, the history will not be accurate because of poor memory or a lack of witnesses, and diagnostic evaluations including electroencephalography (EEG), electrocardiography, neuroimaging, and serum electrolytes will be necessary.

Electroencephalogram

Evaluating older patients with epilepsy using EEG does not differ from the process in younger patients. However, EEG changes occurring with age are often mentioned in official EEG reports, but are not indicative of epilepsy. These changes include both slowing and a decrease in amplitude of the resting background, alpha rhythm, whereas slow EEG frequencies such as theta and delta can increase with age in both a diffuse or focal manner. Slowing of the background and slow EEG frequencies are often nonspecific when they occur diffusely but can implicate a CNS structural lesion if they occur focally. EEG patterns of uncertain significance can emerge with age, for example, small sharp spikes or subclinical rhythmic electrical discharges of adulthood, the latter occurring exclusively in older adults (Lee and Pedley, 1997; Otomo, 1966; Roubicek, 1977; Silverman et al., 1955; Westmoreland and Klass, 1981; Westmoreland, 1990; White et al., 1977).

TABLE 30-1. *Variables that distinguish between common spells in the elderly*

Variable	Seizure	Syncope	TIA	TGA	Vertigo
Warning/aura	Sometimes	Faint feeling	None	None	None
Duration	1–2 minutes	Seconds to minutes	Minutes to hours	Minutes to hours	Minutes to days
Effect of posture	None	Variable	None	None	Variable
Spell symptoms	Tonic-clonic movement, but variable	Loss of tone/brief clonic jerks	Deficits along a vascular pattern	Confusion/ amnesia	Nausea, ataxia, tinnitus
Incontinence	Variable	Variable	None	None	None
Heart rate	Increased	Irregular/decreased	Variable	No effect	Variable
Postspell symptoms	Confusion, sleep	Alert	Alert	Alert	Alert
EEG during effect event	Epileptiform pattern	Diffuse slowing	Focal slowing	Rare slowing	No

EEG, electroencephalogram; TGA, transient global amnesia; TIA, transient ischemic attack.

Epileptiform transients (e.g., sharp or spike waves), which are commonly seen in patients with seizures, occur less frequently in older than younger individuals (Ramsey and Pryor, 2000; Drury and Beydoun, 1998). Only 26% to 37% of older patients with epilepsy demonstrated epileptiform abnormalities on routine EEG (Ramsey and Pryor, 2000; Drury and Beydoun, 1998). Thus, the absence of epileptiform abnormalities on an EEG should not exclude the diagnosis of seizures or epilepsy. The presence of epileptiform transients, however, may be seen in patients with diseases other than epilepsy (e.g., dementia, stroke, neoplasms, and prion diseases) (Drury and Beydoun, 1998; Ehle and Johnson, 1977; Muller and Kral, 1967; Chatrian et al., 1964). Nevertheless, capturing epileptiform transients on an EEG strongly suggests epilepsy. The "gold standard" of diagnosing seizures on EEG is the actual recording of a seizure. New technologies can now make recording a seizure feasible by the use of video EEG recording or ambulatory EEG. Therefore, when the diagnosis of seizures or epilepsy is in question, prolonged video EEG or ambulatory monitoring should be pursued. Situations warranting prolonged monitoring include repeated episodes of impaired consciousness, and dizziness or paroxysmal movements where the diagnosis is uncertain.

Imaging

Imaging studies (magnetic resonance imaging [MRI]/computed tomography [CT]) should be performed as part of the initial evaluation of all older patients with epilepsy to identify and treat causes such as CNS hemorrhage, tumor, and abscess. MRI is the procedure of choice because it is superior to CT in detecting all pathologic processes except subarachnoid hemorrhage (Zimmerman, 1997). CT should be used only in emergent situations or when MRI is contraindicated. Contrast enhancement should be used for both modalities because it improves detection of tumors and infections such as abscess.

Similar to EEG, age-related changes are commonly seen on MRI. These findings include diffuse atrophy, defined as cerebral volume loss manifesting as dilation of ventricles and sulci (Zimmerman, 1997; Drayer, 1988). Periventricular hyperintensity (unidentified bright objects) is noted commonly and is associated with hypertension and atherosclerosis (Zimmerman, 1997; Drayer, 1988; Zimmermann et al., 1986). Dilatations of the Virchow Robbins spaces and poor differentiation between gray and subcortical white matter are also observed (Heier, et al., 1989;

Heier, 1992; Bradley et al., 1984; Awad et al., 1986). When any of these radiologic signs are found, be careful not to attribute the cause of epilepsy to these nonspecific findings. Rather, these findings can implicate longstanding hypertension or small vessel atherosclerosis. In summary, imaging should not be considered in isolation when seeking the cause of epilepsy but should be weighed with the overall clinical picture.

Which Tests Should Be Ordered?

Because toxic or metabolic problems are common causes of acute symptomatic seizures, every patient with a new onset of seizure requires a complete blood count, including differential white cell and platelet count; standard clinical chemistry, including electrolytes, calcium; and tests of liver and renal function, as well as a routine urinalysis. An EEG should also be performed to confirm the diagnosis or to classify epilepsy type because this may influence treatment. If laboratory evaluation is nonspecific, imaging with MRI or CT with contrast enhancement should be obtained, particularly because cerebrovascular disease and tumor are common causes of epilepsy in older adults. A lumbar puncture will not be obtained routinely unless the seizure occurred in the setting of a fever or meningitis is suspected.

TREATMENT

When Should Antiepileptic Drugs Be Initiated?

The main reason for prescribing antiepileptic drug (AED) therapy is to prevent further seizures. Thus, such therapy is recommended when a reasonable chance exists that seizures will recur (Sperling et al., 1997). A single seizure with an obvious precipitating cause does not imply an underlying tendency toward seizure recurrence requiring AED treatment. For example, if an individual had seizures caused by a new medication or electrolyte disturbance, AED do not have to be initiated; rather, the offending medication is discontinued, or the underlying electrolyte imbalance is corrected. Current information is inadequate to make evidence-based decisions concerning treatment of an idiopathic seizure in older adults. No studies have investigated the risks of no treatment versus adverse effects of AED. Therefore, treatment should be started in cases of a strong likelihood of seizure recurrence.

Several factors are associated with an increased risk of seizure recurrence in younger patients that also may be applicable to this population: partial seizures, postictal paralysis, a family history of epilepsy, an EEG showing an epileptiform pattern, and an abnormal neurologic examination. All these findings are associated with a higher risk of recurrence (Sperling et al., 1997; Hopkins et al., 1988; Berg and Shinnar, 1991; Annegers et al., 1986). One factor that affects seizure recurrence unique to older adults is age. Older patients are more likely to have a seizure recurrence as compared with younger patients (Hopkins et al., 1988). This should not be construed to suggest that older patients should immediately be placed on AED after a first seizure. Rather, more investigation is needed to better identify those risk factors that most likely will lead to seizure recurrence in this population. As a general guideline, any individual who has had a seizure and has a structural cortical lesion (i.e., tumor, encephalomalacia from a stroke or trauma) has a higher risk of seizure recurrence and would benefit from AED. However, a patient with a new stroke or tumor does not need to be placed routinely on prophylactic antiepileptic medication unless a seizure occurs (Glantz et al., 2000).

Specific Antiepileptic Drugs

During the past several decades, seizures and epilepsy have been treated with drugs that had been used for decades, including phenytoin (Dilantin), carbamazepine (Tegretol), valproic acid (Depakote, Depakene), primidone (Mysoline), phenobarbital (Luminal), ethosuximide (Zarontin), and clonazepam (Klonopin). These drugs are effective, but they are limited by adverse effects and complicated pharmacokinetics. Table 30-2 summarizes all AED, their indications, risks, and costs. Since 1993, however, several novel AED have been introduced to overcome the limitations of traditional therapy (Table 30-3). Several reviews have discussed the older AED in relation to their use in older adults (Cloyd et al., 1994; Leppik, 1992; Wilmore, 1996; Thomas, 1997; Cameron and Macphee, 1995; Haider et al., 1996; Tallis, 1990); however, few have discussed new drugs. The new antiepileptic compounds—felbamate, gabapentin, lamotrigine, levetiracetam, oxcarbazepine, topiramate, tiagabine, and zonisamide—are currently available by prescription in the United States. All of the new drugs are chemically unique, structurally unrelated to standard AED (except in the case of oxcarbazepine, which is related to carbamazepine) and different from one another. Table 30-4 outlines the potential advantages and disadvantages of the new AED compared with standard therapy for the older population (Haider et al., 1996; Tallis, 1990; Sirven and Liporace, 1997; McLean, 1997). As is the case

TABLE 30-2. *Current antiepileptic drugs*

Antiepileptic drug	Indication	Risks	Cost/month
Carbamazepine	SPS, CPS, 2 GTC	Diplopia, dizziness, idiosyncratic aplastic anemia, rash, hyponatremia, osteoporosis	<$50.00
Diazepam	Acute seizures	Hypotension, respiratory depression, sedation, tolerance	N/A
Clonazepam	Myoclonic, atonic, GTC	Hypotension, respiratory depression, sedation, tolerance	N/A
Ethosuximide	Absence	Sedation, GI distress	<$50.00
Felbamate	SPS, CPS, 1–2 GTC, atonic, absence	Dizziness, headache Idiosyncratic hepatic failure or aplastic anemia, insomnia, weight loss	>$100.00
Gabapentin	SPS, CPS, 2 GTC	Fatigue, transient GI distress	>$100.00
Lamotrigine	SPS, CPS, 1–2 GTC	Dizziness, headache, rash	>$100.00
Levetiracetam	SPS, CPS, 1–2 GTC	Somnolence, coordination difficulties	>$100.00
Oxcarbazepine	SPS, CPS, 1–2 GTC	Dizziness, diplopia, ataxia, hyponatremia	>$100.00
Phenobarbital	SPS, CPS, 1–2 GTC	Cognitive effects, respiratory depression, sedation	<$50.00
Phenytoin	SPS, CPS, 1–2 GTC	Ataxia, gingival hyperplasia, hirsutism, lymphadenopathy, nystagmus, osteoporosis	<$50.00
Primidone	SPS, CPS, 1–2 GTC	Sedation, depression, dizziness	<$50.00
Tiagabine	SPS, CPS, 1–2 GTC	GI distress, cognitive effects	>$100.00
Topiramate	SPS, CPS, 1–2 GTC	Impaired memory, weight loss, word finding difficulty	>$100.00
Zonisamide	SPS, CPS, 1–2 GTC	Somnolence, dizziness, agitation, difficulty concentrating, weight loss	>$100.00
Valproic acid	SPS, CPS, 1–2 GTC, atonic, absence	Tremor, thrombocytopenia, increased NH4	<$100.00

CPS, complex partial seizure; GI, gastrointestinal; GTC, primary generalized tonic-clonic seizure; 2-GTC, secondarily generalized seizure; SPS, simple partial seizure.

TABLE 30-3. *New antiepileptic medications*

Medication	Metabolic route	Hepatic enzyme	Adverse effects (common)	Adverse effects (idiosyncratic)
Felbamate	Hepatic	Yes[a]	Anorexia, weight loss, insomnia, nausea, headache	Aplastic anemia, hepatic failure
Gabapentin	Renal excretion	No	Drowsiness, nausea, fatigue	None reported
Lamotrigine	Hepatic	No	Rash, tremor, nausea, dizziness, headache, weight gain	Severe rash
Levetiracetam	Hepatic	No	Somnolence, dizziness, coordination difficulty, agitation	None reported
Oxcarbazepine	Hepatic	Yes	Dizziness, diplopia, ataxia, tremor, dyspepsia	Hyponatremia
Tiagabine	Hepatic	No	Dizziness, tremor, confusion, drowsiness	None reported
Topiramate	Renal with minimal hepatic	Yes (minimal)	Dizziness, drowsiness, confusion, ataxia, paresthesias, weight loss	Renal stones
Zonisamide	Hepatic	No	Somnolence, dizziness, nausea, agitation, concentration difficulty, weight loss	Allergic reaction in patients allergic to sulfa drugs, renal stones

[a]Enzyme-inducing properties *in vitro,* but may inhibit metabolism of valproate, phenytoin, phenobarbital, and carbamazepine epoxide and dosage of those medications needs to be reduced when administered with felbamate.

with traditional AED, systematic investigation of these drugs in older adults has not been performed (Cameron and Macphee, 1995).

Which Antiepileptic Drug? Traditional Versus New

Although many choices now exist for treatment of epilepsy, few clinical trials have compared new and old AED directly for various seizure types, much less by age (Tallis, 1997). Moreover, newer AED were subjected to placebo-controlled trials before US Food and Drug Administration approval, whereas the older

AED did not have to undergo this type of clinical trial (Tallis, 1997; Stolarek et al., 1995). Therefore, meaningful conclusions regarding differences in efficacy or tolerability between old and new drugs do not exist. Ongoing trials will be comparing these drugs in older adults. One such trial is comparing gabapentin, carbamazepine, and lamotrigine in a Veterans Administration facility population (Rowan et al., 1997). Similar trials will be necessary to answer these important questions. For now, however, individual decisions based on a patient's history and the side effects and pharmacology profiles of AED will determine which medications can be used safely.

TABLE 30-4. *Advantages and disadvantages of new antiepileptic drugs*

Antiepileptic drug	Advantages	Disadvantages
Felbamate	Broad spectrum of coverage, efficacy	Serious idiosyncratic side effects, expensive
Gabapentin	Few side effects, no drug interactions, easy to dose, renal excretion	Limited efficacy, multiple daily doses, expensive
Lamotrigine	Broad spectrum of coverage, well tolerated, twice daily dosing	Slow to initiate, rash, expensive
Levetiracetam	Twice daily dosing, easy to initiate, efficacy at low doses	Relatively unknown medication, expensive
Oxcarbazepine	Absence of hematologic effects, twice daily dosing	Hyponatremia, expensive
Topiramate	Broad spectrum of coverage, twice daily dosing, limited drug interactions, mostly renal metabolism	Cognitive adverse effecfts, expensive, weight loss
Tiagabine	Well tolerated, limited drug interactions	Multiple daily doses, cognitive adverse effects, expensive
Zonisamide	Well tolerated	Weight loss, cognitive adverse effects, expensive

TABLE 30-5. *Paradigm for antiepileptic drug choice by seizure type*

Seizure type	First choice	Second choice
Simple partial, complex partial, secondarily generalized	Carbamazepine, phenytoin, lamotrigine, levetiracetam, oxcarbazepine, topiramate	Gabapentin, felbamate, primidone, phenobarbital, tiagabine, valproic acid, zonisamide
Absence	Ethosuximide	Lamotrigine, valproic acid
Myoclonic	Valproic acid	Clonazepam, zonisamide
Primary generalized tonic-clonic	Valproic acid, phenytoin	Felbamate, lamotrigine, phenobarbital, topiramate, zonisamide
Atonic	Valproic acid, clonazepam	Felbamate

Some concrete guidelines may help to guide the clinician to the AED that should be used (Table 30-5). Carbamazepine, lamotrigine, oxcarbazepine, phenytoin, and topiramate are first-line agents in most patients with partial seizures. Levetiracetam, valproic acid, tiagabine, gabapentin, and zonisamide are reasonable alternatives if the first-line agents fail. Although equally effective, phenobarbital and primidone are used less often because of cognitive side effects. Seizures in the generalized epilepsies usually respond to valproic acid. Valproic acid is also the drug of choice for treating absence seizures. In patients with generalized tonic clonic seizures, phenytoin, carbamazepine, and valproic acid are the drugs of choice; however, lamotrigine, topiramate, zonisamide, and phenobarbital may also be helpful. In an acute seizure emergency (e.g., status epilepticus), diazepam or lorazepam are the drugs of choice, followed by fosphenytoin. An economic issue to consider in the decision is that all of the new medications are much more costly than their traditional counterparts.

Drug Interactions

One of the more important considerations regarding choice of AED is drug interaction. A recent study surveying medication use among the older patient population in the metropolitan Minneapolis-St. Paul area showed that two thirds of adults over 60 years of age take prescription medications with an individual taking 7 drugs at one time and up to 13 per year (Cloyd et al., 1994). The interactions resulting from multiple drug therapy can lead to significant adverse effects.

Two broad types of drug interactions occur: pharmacokinetic and pharmacodynamic. Pharmacokinetic drug interactions are defined as those interactions altering absorption, distribution, metabolism, or elimination. The most common pharmacokinetic drug interaction is an alteration in hepatic metabolism. Drugs that induce or inhibit hepatic metabolism of other drugs can either increase toxicity or reduce the effectiveness of other medications. For example, macrolide antibiotics (e.g., erythromycin) inhibit hepatic enzyme induction. So, if erythromycin is used concomitantly with carbamazepine, this can easily result in carbamazepine toxicity. In contrast, pharmacodynamic interactions are defined as those when medications have mechanisms of action that are either synergistic or antagonistic. For example, both benzodiazepines and barbiturates have an additive effect when combined because both affect the γ-aminobutyric acid$_A$ binding site. Therefore, choosing an AED with a unique mechanism of action with limited hepatic metabolism may be most beneficial in the older patient. Thus, all of the new AED may be better choices for older adults with seizures. For a detailed discussion regarding AED drug interaction, see the chapter by McLean (1997).

Serum Antiepileptic Drug Levels

Measuring AED concentrations is important in adjusting epilepsy management for two reasons: assessment of compliance and ascertaining toxicity. This monitoring of AED levels becomes even more important in the older population because older patients may have problems with memory, making compliance with a drug regimen difficult. The pharmacokinetic changes associated with advancing age of decreased drug clearance and reduced metabolism can contribute to toxicity, which may be prevented with a check of serum concentration (Cloyd et al., 1994). However, problems are seen in using the published serum level ranges for antiepileptic medications because these levels are based on younger patients and, therefore, may not be applicable to older patients. Evidence suggests that older adults are more sensitive to the sedative and cognitive effects of benzodiazepines than younger patients with similar drug concentration. Thus, older adults may have a narrow therapeutic window, which can place them at greater risk for toxicity. Factors contributing to the narrow therapeutic window include the lower protein binding seen in older age resulting in a high free level of medication. Thus, concentrations of highly protein bound AED (e.g., phenytoin, carbamazepine, valproic acid) should be monitored as free unbound plasma concentrations. However, most of the new AED do not yet have defined serum concentrations. Thus, checking serum concentrations may not be helpful in determining *therapeutic levels*, but it may be helpful in determining the patient's own therapeutic level rather than ascertaining toxicity.

OTHER THERAPIES

Vagal Nerve Stimulator

Vagal nerve stimulation has been approved for use in the treatment of epilepsy. In this procedure, the carotid sheath is opened and two spiral electrodes are wrapped around the vagus nerve and connected to an infraclavicular generator pack. In experienced surgical hands, the procedure lasts less than 2 hours. The implanted device is a programmable stimulator, either with the stimulation programmed in advance or so that patients can turn the device on or off at any time by placing a magnet against the implant site.

The mechanism of the antiepileptic effect of the vagal nerve stimulator is not known. The efficacy of this procedure compares favorably with medications. The average seizure reduction is 31% at 3 months, with 50% to 60% of patients achieving at least a 50% reduction by 1 year (Sirven et al., 2000). Adverse effects were found to be few, consisting of hoarseness, coughing, and paresthesias. No clinically significant episodes of bradycardia were reported postoperatively. Vagal nerve stimulation is a promising treatment that merits further study. As with all novel epilepsy treatments, no systematic studies have been done on the use of this device in older persons. However, a retrospective study examining these issues found no unique adverse effects (Sirven et al., 2000) in older adults. Thus, in this population, individuals should not be biased against using this therapy based solely on the patient's age.

Epilepsy Surgery

In about 30% to 40% of all patients with epilepsy, seizures are not completely controlled by medical therapy. Some of these patients may be candidates for surgical treatment. Temporal lobectomy, the most common surgical procedure for epilepsy, has proliferated recently since its efficacy and safety has become well-documented (Sperling et al., 1996). However,

few studies have included older surgical patients (McLachlan et al., 1992; Sirven et al., 2000; Malamut et al., 1998; Cascino et al., 1991; Tallis, 1996). Three studies have investigated epilepsy surgery in older patients specifically, and all found that this treatment could be successful in older patients without significant declines in memory and intelligence quotients (McLachlan et al., 1992; Sirven et al., 2000; Malamut et al., 1998; Cascino et al., 1991). Thus, although more studies are needed, older adults should not be excluded from surgical consideration based solely on age. Rather, exclusion criteria should be similar to those for younger patients, which would include lack of a definite epileptic focus or a seizure focus in an inoperable location such as the motor strip or areas of language or memory functioning.

Which Treatment? Medications Versus Surgery

Figure 30-3 illustrates an algorithm for management of seizures in the older adult. Treatment is initi-

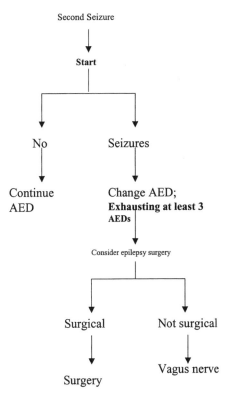

FIG. 30-3. An algorithm for the treatment of epilepsy in older adults. Please note that the first seizure is often not treated if no specific cause for the seizure is found. Treatment begins after the second seizure.

ated after the second seizure. If seizures persist despite a trial of antiepileptic medication with documentation of a therapeutic level or adverse effects, then other AED are tried. Once three antiepileptic medications have been tried and seizures persist, then surgery should be considered. Surgery should only be pursued in individuals in whom an improvement in the quality of life is likely or in a patient with injurious seizures. Thus, an older adult living in a nursing home with dementia and seizures would not be an appropriate candidate for surgery. In sum, the benefits must outweigh the risks. If the patient is not a candidate for surgery or fails to respond to surgery, then vagus nerve stimulation would be an appropriate option.

PSYCHOSOCIAL IMPLICATION OF SEIZURES IN OLDER ADULTS

Seizures can have an impact on the lives of older adults in many ways. However, quality-of-life issues in epilepsy remain largely neglected in the medical literature, particularly in this age group. A brief synopsis of what is currently known in this domain is presented here. The postictal recovery time in older adults can be prolonged (Tallis et al., 1991). Seizures can lead to falls and subsequent fractures (Tallis, 1996; Vestergaard et al., 1999), which can have profound consequences in an older individual's life, such as injuries leading to immobility and dependence (Tallis, 1996). Several investigations have validated the impact of falls in older adults (Tinnetti and Williams, 1997; Tinnetti et al., 1988; O'Loughlin et al., 1993; Blake et al., 1988). Tinetti et al. recently demonstrated that falls are a strong predictor of placement in a skilled nursing facility, with the accompanying loss of independence, privacy, and financial issues associated with institutionalization (Tinnetti and Williams, 1997).

Social issues are also a particular concern. In all age groups, seizures can lead to revocation of driving privileges and a loss of independence. Six states (California, Delaware, Nevada, New Jersey, Oregon, and Pennsylvania) now require mandatory reporting of a seizure to their state motor vehicle bureau. In other states, it is up to the individual physician to report a patient with a seizure. The loss of driving privileges can be as devastating to older as to younger patients. One may argue that younger individuals are more distressed by the loss of the ability to drive, but active older persons are equally affected, particularly when adequate public transportation is lacking.

SUMMARY

Epilepsy in older adults is a major public health problem with large pathologic, psychosocial, and economic burdens on society. The impact of epilepsy and its new treatments have not been investigated as systematically in older patients as in younger patients. Future research into the pathophysiology of the aging brain and, in particular, its relation to epilepsy, as well as treatments of epilepsy in older adults, is fundamental to adequately treat the burgeoning aged population in the next century.

REFERENCES

Annegers JF, Hauser WA, Lee JR, et. al. Incidence of acute symptomatic seizures in Rochester, Minnesota 1935–1984. *Epilepsia* 1995;36:327–333.

Annegers JF, Nocolosi A, Beghi E, et al. The risk of unprovoked seizures after encephalitis and meningitis. *Neurology* 1988;38:1407–1410.

Annegers JF, Shirts SB, Hauser WA, et al. Risk of seizure recurrence after an initial unprovoked seizure. *Epilepsia* 1986;27:43–50.

Awad IA, Spetzler RF, Hodak JA, et al. Incidental subcortical lesions in the elderly. Correlation with age and cerebral vascular risk factors. *Stroke* 1986;6:1084–1090.

Berg AT, Shinnar S. The risk of seizure recurrence following a first unprovoked seizure: a quantitative review. *Neurology* 1991;41:965–972.

Blake AJ, Morgan K, Bendall MJ, et al. Falls by elderly people at home: prevalence and associated factors. *Age Ageing* 1988;17:365–372.

Bradley WG, Waluch V, Brandt-Zawadski M, et al. Patchy periventricular white matter lesions in the elderly: a common observation during NMR imaging. *Noninvasive Medical Imaging* 1;1:35–41.

Cameron H, Macphee GJ. Anticonvulsant therapy in the elderly—a need for placebo controlled trials. *Epilepsy Res* 1995;21:149–157.

Cascino GD, Sharbrough FW, Hirschorn KA, et al. Surgery for focal epilepsy in the older patient. *Neurology* 1991; 41:1415–1417.

Chatrian GE, Shaw CM, Leffman H. The significance of periodic lateralized epileptiform discharges in EEG. An electrographic, clinical, and pathological study. *Electroencephalogr Clin Neurophysiol* 1964;17:177–193.

Cloyd JC, Lackner TE, Leppik IE. Antiepileptics in the elderly. Pharmacoepidemiology and pharmacokinetics. *Arch Fam Med* 1994;3:589–598.

Drayer BP. Imaging of the aging brain. Part I. Normal findings. *Radiology* 1988;166:785–796.

Drury I, Beydoun A. Interictal epileptiform activity in elderly patients with epilepsy. *Electroencephalogr Clin Neurophysiol* 1998;106:369–373.

Ehle AL, Johnson PC. Rapidly evolving EEG changes in a case of Alzheimer's disease. *Ann Neurol* 1977;34:1: 593–595.

Ettinger AB, Shinnar S. New-onset seizures in an elderly hospitalized population. *Neurology* 1993;43:489–492.

Giroud M, Gras P, Fayolle H, et al. Early seizures after acute stroke: a study of 1,640 cases. *Epilepsia* 1994;35(5): 959–964.

Glantz MJ, Cole BF, Forsyth PA, et al. Practice parameter: anticonvulsant prophylaxis in patients with newly diagnosed brain tumor: report of the Quality Standards Subcommittee of the American Academy of Neurology. *Neurology* 2000;54(10):1886–1893.

Haider A, Tuchek J, Haider S. Seizure control: how to use the new antiepileptic drugs in older patients. *Geriatrics* 1996;51:42–45.

Hauser WA, Annegers JF, Kurland LT. Incidence of epilepsy and unprovoked seizures in Rochester, Minnesota: 1935–1984. *Epilepsia* 1993;34:453-468.

Hauser WA, Cascino GD, Annegers JF, et al. Incidence of status epilepticus and associated mortality. *Epilepsia* 1994;(Suppl 8)33.

Hauser WA, Ramirez-Lassepas M, Rosenstein R. Risk for seizures and epilepsy following cerebrovascular insults. *Epilepsia* 1984;26:666(abst).

Hauser WA. *Epidemiology of seizures and epilepsy in the elderly.* Boston: Butterworth-Heinemann, 1997:7–18.

Hauser WA. Seizure disorders: the changes with age. *Epilepsia* 1992;(Suppl 4)33:S6–S14.

Heier LA, Bauer CJ, Schwartz L, et al. Large Virchow-Robin spaces: MR-clinical correlation. *AJNR* 1989;10 929–936.

Heier LA. White matter disease in the elderly: vascular etiologies. *Neuroimaging Clin N Am* 1992;2:441–445.

Hopkins A, Garman A, Clarke C. The first seizure in adult life: value of clinical features, electroencephalography and computerized tomographic scanning in prediction of seizure recurrence. *Lancet* 1988;1:721–726.

Kilpatrick CJ, Davis SM, Tress BM, et al. Early seizures after acute stroke. Risk of late seizures. *Arch Neurol* 1992; 49:509–511.

Lancsman ME, Golimstok A, Norscini J, et al. Risk factors for developing seizures after a stroke. *Epilepsia* 1993;34 (1):141–143.

Lee K, Pedley T. Electroencephalography and seizures in the elderly. In: Rowan AJ, Ramsay RE, eds. *Seizures and epilepsy in the elderly.* Boston: Butterworth-Heinemann, 1997:139–158.

Leppik IE. Metabolism of antiepileptic medications: newborn to elderly. *Epilepsia* 1992;(Suppl 4)33:S32–S40.

Loiseau J, Loiseau P, Duche B, et al. A survey of epileptic disorders in southwest France: seizures in elderly patients. *Ann Neurol* 1990;27:233–237.

Loiseau P. Pathologic processes in the elderly and their association with seizures. In: Rowan AJ, Ramsey RE, eds. *Seizures and epilepsy in the elderly.* Boston: Butterworth-Heinemann, 1997:63–68.

Luhdorf K, Jensen LK, Plesner AM. Epilepsy in the elderly: incidence, social function, and disability. *Epilepsia* 1989;30:389–399.

Malamut BL, Cloud B, Sirven JI, et al. Neuropsychological and psychosocial outcome after unilateral temporal lobectomy over age 45. *Neurology* 1998;(Suppl 4)50:A202 (abst).

Malouf R, Brust JCM. Hypoglycemia: causes, neurologic manifestations, and outcomes. *Ann Neurol* 1985;17: 421–430.

McLachlan RS, Chovaz CJ, Blume WT, et al. Temporal lobectomy for intractable epilepsy in patients over age 45 years. *Neurology* 1992;42:662–665.

McLean MJ. New antiepileptic medications: pharmacokinetic and mechanistic considerations in the treatment of seizures and epilepsy in the elderly. In: Rowan AJ, Ram-

sey RE, eds. *Seizures and epilepsy in the elderly.* Boston, Butterworth-Heinemann 1997:239–307.

Messing RO, Closson RG, Simon RP. Drug-induced seizures: a 10-year experience. *Neurology* 1984;34:1582–1586.

Muller HF, Kral VA. The EEG in advanced senile dementia. *J Am Geriatr Soc* 1967;15:415–426.

O'Loughlin JL, Robitaille Y, Boivin JF, et al. Incidence of and risk factors for falls and injurious falls among the community-dwelling elderly. *Am J Epidemiol* 1993;137: 342–354.

Otomo E. Electroencephalography in old age: dominant alpha rhythm. *Electrencephalogr Clin Neurophysiol* 1966; 21:489–491.

Ramsey RE, Pryor F. Epilepsy in the elderly. *Neurology* 2000;(Suppl 1)55:S9–S14.

Remick RA, Fine SH. Antipsychotic drugs and seizures. *J Clin Psychiatry* 1979;40:78–80.

Roubicek J. The electroencephalogram in the middle aged and the elderly. *J Am Geriatr Soc* 1977;25:145–152.

Rowan AJ, Ramsey RE, Collins JF, et al. Treatment of seizures in the elderly population. A new DVA cooperative study. *Epilepsia* 1997;(Suppl 8)38:89(abst).

Sanders JWA, Hart YM, Johnson AL, et al. Natural general practice study of epilepsy: newly diagnosed epileptic seizures in general population. *Lancet* 1990;336: 1267–1270.

Silverman AJ, Busse EW, Barnes RH. Studies in the process of aging: electroencephalographic findings in 400 elderly subjects. *Electroencephalogr Clin Neurophysiol* 1955;7: 67–77.

Singh BM, Gupta DR, Strobos RJ. Nonketotic hyperglycemia and epilepsia partialis continua. *Arch Neurol* 1973;29:187–190.

Sirven JI and VNS in the Elderly Group. Vagus nerve stimulation therapy for epilepsy in older adults. *Neurology* 2000;54(5):1179–1182.

Sirven JI, Liporace JD. New antiepileptic drugs. Overcoming the limitations of traditional therapy. *Postgrad Med* 1997;102:147–162.

Sirven JI, Malamut BL, O'Connor MJ, et al. Temporal lobectomy outcome in older versus younger adults. *Neurology* 2000;54 (11):2166–2170.

So EL, Annegers JF, Hauser WA, et al. Population-based study of seizure disorders after cerebral infarction. *Neurology* 1996;46:350–355.

Sperling MR, Bucurescu G, Kim B. Epilepsy management. Issues in medical and surgical treatment. *Postgrad Med* 1997;102:102–118.

Sperling MR, O'Connor MJ. Saykin AJ, et al. Temporal lobectomy for refractory epilepsy. *JAMA* 1996;276: 470–475.

Stolarek JH, Brodie A, Brodie MJ. Management of seizures in the elderly: a survey of UK geriatricians. *J R Soc Med* 1995;88:686–689.

Tallis R, Hall G, Craig I, et al. How common are epileptic seizures in old age? *Age Ageing* 1991;20:442–448.

Tallis R. Antiepileptic drug trials in the elderly: rationale, problems, and solutions. In: Rowan AJ, Ramsey RE. *Seizures and epilepsy in the elderly.* Boston: Butterworth-Heinemann, 1997:311–320.

Tallis R. Epilepsy in old age. *Lancet* 1990;336:295–296.

Tallis R. Treatment of epilepsy in the elderly patient. In: Shorvon S, Dreifuss D, Fish D, et al., eds. *The treatment of epilepsy.* London: Blackwell Science Ltd., 1996: 227–237.

Thomas P, Lebrun C, Chatel M. De novo absence status epilepticus as a benzodiazepine withdrawal syndrome. *Epilepsia* 1993;34:355–358.

Thomas RJ. Seizures and epilepsy in the elderly. *Arch Intern Med* 1997;157:605–617.

Tinnetti ME, Speechley M, Ginter SF. Risk factors for falls among elderly persons living in the community. *N Engl J Med* 1988;319:1701–1707.

Tinnetti ME, Williams CS. Falls, injuries due to falls, and the risk of admission to a nursing home. *N Engl J Med* 1997;337:1279–1284.

Tinuper P. The altered presentation of seizures in the elderly. In: Rowan AJ, Ramsey RE, eds. *Seizures and epilepsy in the elderly*. Boston: Butterworth-Heinemann, 1997:123–130.

Towne AR, Pellock JM, Ko D, Delorenzo RJ. Determinants of mortality in status epilepticus. *Epilepsia* 1994;5:27–34.

Vestergaard P, Tigaran S, Rejnmark L, et al. Fracture risk in epilepsy. *Acta Neurol Scand* 1999;99:269–275.

Westmoreland BF, Klass DW. A distinctive rhythmic EEG discharge of adults. *Electroencephalogr Clin Neurophysiol* 1981;51:186–191.

Westmoreland BF. Benign variants and patterns of uncertain clinical significance. In: Daly DD, Pedley TA, eds. *Current practice of clinical electroencephalography*, 2nd ed. New York: Raven Press, 1990:243–252.

White JC, Langston JW, Pedley TA. Benign epileptiform transients of sleep: clarification of the small sharp spike controversy. *Neurology* 1977;27:1061–1068.

Wilmore LJ. Management of epilepsy in the elderly. *Epilepsia* 1996;(Suppl 6)37:S32–S33.

Zaccara G, Muscas GC, Messori A. Clinical features, pathogenesis and management of drug-induced seizures. *Drug Saf* 1990;5:109–151.

Zimmerman R. Diagnostic methods II: imaging studies. In: Rowan AJ, Ramsay RE, eds. *Seizures and epilepsy in the elderly*. Boston: Butterworth-Heinemann, 1997:159–177.

Zimmermann RD, Fleming CA, Lee BC, et al. Periventricular hyperintensity as seen by magnetic resonance: prevalence and significance. *AJNR* 1986;7:13–20.

SUGGESTED READING

Rowan AJ, Ramsay RE, eds. *Seizures and epilepsy in the elderly*. Boston: Butterworth-Heinemann, 1996.

WEB SITES

American Epilepsy Society: *www.aesnet.org*
Epilepsy Foundation of America: *www.efa.com*

GLOSSARY OF ABBREVIATIONS

AED   Antiepileptic drugs

CNS   Central nervous system

CPS   Complex partial seizures

CT   Computed tomography

EEG   Electroencephalography

EKG   Electrocardiography

IQ   Intelligence Quotient

MRI   Magnetic Resonance Imaging

PLED   Periodic lateralized epileptiform discharges

1-2 GTC   Primary and secondarily generalized seizures

2 GTC   Secondary generalized seizures

SPS   Simple partial seizures

SE   Status epilepticus

SREDA   Subclinical rhythmic epileptiform discharges of adults

TGA   Transient global amnesia

TIA   Transient ischemic attack

UBO   Unidentified bright objects

UK   United Kingdom

VNS   Vagus nerve stimulation

31

Recognition and Management of Late Life Mood Disorders

James M. Ellison and Gary L. Gottlieb

INTRODUCTION

Aging is not inevitably accompanied by a disturbance of mood, yet depressive symptoms among elderly women and men are common and disabling. Most depressed elderly patients who seek treatment do so in a primary care setting, where detection is often poor and treatment frequently inadequate. Individuals confined in long-term care facilities rely on primary care clinicians for treatment or referral to a mental health specialist, with the result that many go untreated. Elderly sufferers of depression or of mania, which is less prevalent, consume disproportionately large amounts of medical healthcare resources (Unutzer et al., 1997; Bartels et al., 2000) and die excessively early of medical causes (Rovner, 1993; Bartels et al., 2000) or suicide (Conwell et al., 1996). For those who survive, the functional impairment associated with a mood disorder can exhaust caregivers and tip the balance from independent living toward an early need for institutional care. Improved recognition and management of late life mood disorders can alleviate suffering, reduce functional impairment, decrease mortality, and spare caregivers a substantial burden. This chapter reviews the syndromes most frequently seen among the elderly, focusing on their clinical and epidemiologic characteristics and summarizing current approaches to management.

DIAGNOSIS OF LATE LIFE DEPRESSION

Depressive symptoms fall into several characteristic syndromes. The American Psychiatric Association's *Diagnostic and Statistical Manual of Mental Disorders*, 4th Edition (American Psychiatric Association, 2000) defines *major depressive episodes* as requiring five or more core symptoms present during a 2-week period, not attributable to the use of a substance or a medical illness. One of the symptoms must be depressed mood or loss of interest or plea-

sure, whereas others can be drawn from the following list: weight loss, insomnia or hypersomnia, psychomotor agitation or retardation, fatigue or loss of energy, worthlessness or guilt, diminished concentration, and recurrent thoughts of death or suicide. Psychotic features such as delusions, hallucinations, or severe disturbance of motor function (stupor or agitation) may also be present. *Dysthymic disorder,* a less florid depressive state, is diagnosed when depressed mood has been accompanied by two or more of the depressive symptoms listed above for an extended period of time (present more days than not for at least 2 years) (American Psychiatric Association, 2000). The presence of fewer, milder, or briefer symptoms is termed *minor depression* or *subsyndromal depression*.

In assessing elderly patients, the diagnosis of depression is made more challenging by muted or obscure expression of signs and symptoms. In contrast with younger patients, the depressed elderly often place less emphasis on a sad or depressed mood; instead, anger, irritability, anxiety, cognitive difficulties, or somatic concerns may be the focus of attention. Somatic symptoms associated with known medical illnesses affect most of the depressed elderly. Medically explainable symptoms are often magnified by the presence of depression and confounded by the presence of additional symptoms that are not medically explainable. Although psychological symptoms of depression are present in most depressed elderly (Simon et al., 1999), their detection requires attentive investigation. When cognitive impairment is prominent, mood symptoms are even less likely to be reported. Deterioration of activities of daily living and deterioration of interpersonal interactions may then provide the strongest clue to the presence of a mood disorder.

Among depressed elderly patients who present with prominent cognitive symptoms, the diagnosis of *dementia syndrome of depression* (DSD) may be made. Formerly termed *pseudodementia* because of the cognitive improvement associated with successful resolution of depression, this syndrome can lead to an erroneous diagnosis of primary dementia, resulting in a missed opportunity to treat depression (Kiloh, 1961). Ample follow-up evidence now demonstrates that DSD, although responsive to antidepressant treatment in the short run, often presages the later onset of a primary dementia (Kaszniak and Christenson, 1997; Reifler, 2000). Features that help to differentiate DSD from a primary dementia include the more likely presence of an autonomous mood disorder, lengthier symptom duration before seeking treatment, more rapid progression of symptoms, greater patient awareness of and complaint regarding cognitive symptoms, and previous psychiatric history. In addition to these features, on neuropsychological assessment the patient may show poorer effort in attempting to perform tasks, greater intactness of recognition memory, better performance with prompting, and more variable performance on similarly difficult tasks (Kaszniak and Christenson, 1997).

DEMOGRAPHICS AND RISK FACTORS

Many clinicians and patients assume that mood disorders are more prevalent among the elderly than among young adults, given the recognized losses and stresses associated with aging, but epidemiologic data consistently contradict such an assertion. With the possible exception of the oldest old (Zonderman and Costa, 1991; cited in Blazer, 1994), evidence suggests that mood disorders are no more prevalent among the elderly than among younger adults (Blazer, 1994). Data from the Epidemiologic Catchment Area studies estimated 1-year prevalences among community-dwelling elderly of 2.7% for major depression (Weissman et al., 1991). By contrast, subsyndromal depression affects a large number, an estimated 8% to 15%, of community-dwelling elderly persons (Blazer, 1994).

In contrast to the general population of community-dwelling elderly, specific subgroups have been shown to suffer higher prevalences of depression. Borson et al., (1986) detected major depression in 10% of an elderly population with chronic medical illnesses. In a primary care clinic setting, a prevalence of 5.6% was measured for major depression among the elderly patients, and an additional 7.9% had probable or masked depression (Barrett et al., 1988). In long-term care facilities, the only mental disorder more common among the elderly than depression is dementia. The prevalence of major depression in nursing homes is estimated as between 6% and 25%, with 30% to 50% of nursing home residents suffering

subsyndromal symptoms (Katz and Parmelee, 1994). The annual rate of new cases of major depression is as high as 9.4%, and each year an additional 7.4% develop new minor depressions (Parmelee et al., 1992).

Among the risk factors linked to late life depression, a higher prevalence is associated with female gender (Blazer, 1994); lower levels of educational attainment; a history of childhood poverty, sexual assault, parental separation or divorce; lower income and occupational attainments; widowhood or other unmarried states; lack of integration into a supportive social network; chronic financial or medical stresses; acute provoking events (George, 1994); and a history of heavy alcohol consumption (Saunders et al., 1991). Neither race nor ethnicity appears to be an important risk factor for late life depression (Myers et al., 1984).

Depression and aging are themselves risk factors for suicide, an all too frequent complication of late life depression. The rate of completed suicide increases significantly with advancing age, notably among white men (McIntosh et al., 1994). Among the elderly, depression is strongly correlated with the risk of either suicide attempts (Lyness et al., 1992; Nieto et al., 1992) or completion (Barraclough, 1971; Conwell, 1994; Conwell et al., 1996). The increased prevalence of depression in various medical illnesses (e.g., multiple sclerosis, epilepsy, Huntington's disease, traumatic spinal lesions, cranial trauma, peptic ulcer disease, rheumatoid arthritis, cardiopulmonary diseases, renal disease requiring chronic hemodialysis, and chronic pain) may explain the increased suicide risk among patients with these illnesses (Mackenzie and Popkin, 1987).

DETECTION

Studies of service utilization indicate that the elderly with mood disorders are seriously undertreated. Most of the mentally ill elderly receive no services specifically for their psychiatric diagnoses. A recently published study of elderly patients treated in four primary care health maintenance organization (HMO) clinics, for example, found that only 7% of the depressed patients received treatment for depression in 1993 and only 11% to 22% of these saw a psychiatrist (Unutzer et al., 2000). In long-term care facilities, undertreatment is particularly sparse. As recently as 1985, the National Nursing Home Survey determined that fewer than 10% of the institutionalized elderly received services for their psychiatric diagnoses (Gottlieb, 1994). Underrecognition and undertreatment are perpetuated by both provider and patient factors.

Primary care clinicians deliver most of the psychiatric care received by elderly adults. Although nearly 85% of older adults visit a primary care physician at least once a year, those with mood disorders frequently elude detection. Primary care clinicians may lack the time to thoroughly evaluate mood-related symptoms or the training and interest required for successful diagnosis and treatment. Psychotropic medications are frequently prescribed in primary care, but most of these medications are sedatives and hypnotics rather than antidepressants (Burns and Taube, 1990). Unutzer et al. (1999) raised the possibility that elderly patients receive different care from that provided to younger adults. They found that depressed patients above 60 years of age receiving care from an HMO were less likely than younger depressed adults to receive adequate antidepressant doses within the first 90 days of treatment. The elderly patients were also less likely to have more than two primary care visits for depression within the first 12 weeks after a new antidepressant was prescribed, or specialty mental healthcare within the first 6 months after the antidepressant prescription. The underprescribing of psychotherapy is highlighted by the observation that most older adults treated for a psychiatric diagnosis in primary care receive only psychotropic drugs (Burns and Taube, 1990).

In addition to these provider factors, some patient factors interfere with effective treatment of depression in this population. Elderly patients may fail to recognize in themselves the symptoms of a depression, or shame prevents them from divulging complaints perceived as stigmatizing. When psychiatric referral is offered, refusal is common (Waxman et al., 1984). The high cost of medications, not currently covered by Medicare, provides another powerful disincentive for accepting treatment. Even when treatment is begun, adherence to a treatment regimen is often limited. One to two thirds of the elderly do not comply or only partially comply with a prescribed medication regimen (Tideiksaar, 1984).

Detection of depression in the elderly can be facilitated by use of screening tools that are self-administered or rely on clinician assessments. Among the self-administered tools, the Beck Depression Inventory is validated in elderly patients. The clinician-administered Hamilton Depression Scale (HAM-D or HRDS) relies heavily on somatic symptoms, weakening its usefulness in medically ill elderly patients. The Geriatric Depression Scale (GDS) is brief, easily administered, and focuses minimally on somatic symptoms. The Cornell Scale, which focuses on depressive behaviors, is suitable for rating of depressed patients with or without dementia, but requires more time to administer because interviews with both the patient and the caregiver are required (Applegate et al., 1990).

Depression must be differentiated from medical illnesses, especially those characterized by fatigue or apathy; from the effects of sedating or mood-altering medications and substances; and from other behavioral disturbances, including bereavement, anxiety disorders, and psychotic disorders. Many medical causes of depression can be detected by a limited evaluation. A minimal workup for depression in an elderly patient must include a comprehensive history, which may need to be supplemented or validated by another informant; review of relevant records and prior treatments, and a physical examination. A mental status examination with screening of cognitive functions (e.g., with the Mini-Mental State Examination [MMSE]) is also required. And, finally, laboratory tests, including complete blood count, erythrocyte sedimentation rate, electrolytes, calcium, glucose, thyroid-stimulating hormone, renal and liver functions, B_{12} and folate levels, and rapid plasma reagin (RPR). An electrocardiogram is required before prescribing a tricyclic antidepressant and establishes a useful baseline measure even for treatment with agents of lesser potential cardiotoxicity.

An imaging study, such as computed tomography or magnetic resonance imaging (MRI) is of greatest diagnostic and prognostic value when cognitive symptoms accompany depressive symptoms. In many such cases, an MRI will reveal subcortical white matter hyperintensity on T2-weighted images. Although these findings are not specific for depression, their presence in depressed individuals is associated with older age, later age at onset, and less frequent family history of mental illness (Krishnan et al.,1997). Executive dysfunction seen in this syndrome is correlated with greater risk of relapse, recurrence, and residual depressive symptoms (Alexopoulos et al., 2000).

TREATMENT

Psychotherapy

Although often neglected in the treatment of late life depression, *psychotherapy* is increasingly regarded as an effective intervention. A metaanalysis of studies that included several different approaches to psychotherapy found psychotherapeutic treatment more effective than placebo or no treatment (Scogin and McElreath, 1994). *Interpersonal therapy* (IPT), developed as a time-limited intervention for midlife depression, has been useful in treating older patients as well because it focuses on highly relevant issues including grief, loss, and role transitions (Weissman and Markowitz, 1994). *Cognitive-behavior therapy* provides another brief and effective approach, aimed at helping patients identify and correct distorted thoughts that perpetuate depression while introducing more pleasurable activities into their lives (Thompson, 1996). Psychodynamic group approaches have been evaluated in the elderly in comparison with cognitive behavioral approaches and found to be of similar efficacy (Steuer et al., 1984), although a need exists for further studies to clarify the relative advantages of these different approaches. Other types of psychotherapy reported to be helpful have included *reminiscence/life review*, *psychoeducation*, and *relaxation-meditation*. Individuals who are intolerant of medication and electroconvulsive therapy (ECT) or who prefer a psychosocial approach to treatment can be referred to a mental health specialist for a trial of psychotherapy in individual or group format. Family conflict, stressful life events, or poor social supports might be appropriate indications for inclusion of psychotherapy in a treatment plan (Niederehe, 1994). Psychotic or bipolar features, heightened suicidal risk, or substance abuse should, when possible, prompt the involvement of a mental health specialist to address the more complex and risky treatment courses associated with these attributes.

Antidepressant Medication

Antidepressant treatment of late life depression, provided more frequently than psychotherapy, is the subject of several thorough and informative recent reviews (Roose and Suthers, 1998; Finkel, 1996; Newhouse, 1996; Gerson et al., 1999). No specific agent or antidepressant class emerges as the clear preference, but medications are concluded to be significantly better than placebo treatment. Pharmacotherapy of late life depression is complicated by age-related pharmacodynamic and pharmacokinetic factors. In particular, the elderly show an increased sensitivity to anticholinergic and antidopaminergic side effects. These pharmacodynamic vulnerabilities are combined with the pharmacokinetic changes of delayed drug absorption, reduced oxidative metabolism, and diminished glomerular filtration and drug secretion. The net effects are slower attainment of steady-state kinetics, higher peak and steady-state serum drug levels, and consequently greater likelihood of adverse drug effects (Zubenko and Sunderland, 2000). Several of the newer antidepressants are inhibitors or substrates of the hepatic microsomal enzyme systems that interact also with commonly coadministered treatments for medical illnesses. Paroxetine, fluoxetine, and, to a

lesser extent, sertraline inhibit the CYP 2D6 enzyme, potentially interfering with clearance of such coadministered medications as tricyclic antidepressants, selegiline, donepezil, dextromethorphan, codeine, meperidine, oxycodone, tramadol, encainide, flecainide, lidocaine, mexiletine, propafenone, metoprolol, propranolol, and timolol, among others. Nefazodone and fluvoxamine are significant inhibitors of the CYP 3A4 enzyme, potentially interfering with clearance of several coadministered antidepressants, alprazolam, clonazepam, diazepam, midazolam, triazolam, buspirone, carbamazepine, lamotrigine, donepezil, acetaminophen, codeine, clarithromycin, erythromycin, ketoconazole, astemizole, tamoxifen, amiodarone, disopyramide, lidocaine, quinidine, calcium channel blockers, lovastatin, steroids, caffeine, and omeprazole, among others. Fluvoxamine also inhibits the CYP IA2 enzyme, potentially limiting clearance of drugs including clozapine and warfarin (Zubenko and Sunderland, 2000).

Table 31-1 lists the antidepressants and their dosages for use in late life depression. Many clinicians now initiate treatment with one of the selective serotonin reuptake inhibitors (SSRI) or other newer serotonergic or nonserotonergic agents, citing data that support claims of their equal efficacy, more tolerable side effect profiles (fewer anticholinergic, cardiac, and cognitive adverse effects), lower drop-out rates, and better overall effect on quality of life. In contrast, other clinicians continue to initiate treatment preferentially with a tricyclic antidepressant, usually nortriptyline. They cite the greater unit costs of the newer agents, their low response rates in some studies, their pharmacokinetic interactions with commonly coadministered medications, and the existence of some comparison data favoring nortriptyline as more effective than fluoxetine (Roose et al., 1994) or sertraline (Oslin et al., 2000).

Among the serotonergic medications, fluoxetine was shown in a large multicenter placebo-controlled, double-blind trial to be well-tolerated in a group of patients 60 years of age and older (Tollefson and Holman, 1993), although the percentage of patients rated on the Hamilton Rating Scale for Depression (HAM-D) as responders to 20 mg/day after 6 weeks was somewhat low (36% vs. 27% with placebo). The remission rate was 21% for fluoxetine and 13% for placebo in the intent-to-treat analysis, and the discontinuation and adverse effects rates for fluoxetine and placebo were similar. A large open study in which elderly depressed patients again received fluoxetine (20 mg/day) showed a remission rate of 35% in the intent-to-treat analysis (Mesters et al., 1993). At higher doses (20–80 mg/day), the efficacy of fluoxetine was equiv-

TABLE 31-1. *Selected antidepressants for use in late life depression*

Generic name	Trade name	Starting dose— range (mg/d)	Treatment dose— range (mg/d)	Notes
Tricyclic antidepressants (TCA)				
Nortriptyline	Pamelor Aventyl	10–25	25–100	TCA with least postural hypotension Follow plasma levels: therapeutic window 50–150 ng/mL
Desipramine	Norpramin	10–25	25–150	TCA with least anticholinergic effect
Selective serotonin reuptake inhibitors (SSRI)				
Fluoxetine	Prozac Prozac Weekly	10 90 once weekly	10–40	Liquid preparation available Initiate after establishment of daily dose regimen of 20 mg/d, waiting 1 week after last daily dose
Sertraline	Zoloft	25	50–200	Oral suspension available
Paroxetine	Paxil	10	10–40	Possesses mild anticholinergic effects
Citalopram	Celexa	10	10–40	
Fluvoxamine	Luvex	25	50–200	
Serotonin antagonist and reuptake inhibitors (SARI)				
Nefazodone	Serzone	50 b.i.d.	100–500	Sedating for many patients
Trazodone	Desyrel	25–50	25–200	Dose range applies to trazodone's common use, as a hypnotic agent often combined with another antidepressant
Serotonin norepinephrine reuptake inhibitor (SNRI)				
Venlafaxine	Effexor	25	50–225	Blood pressure elevation associated with higher dose range
	Effexor XR	37.5	50–225	
Norepinephrine dopamine reuptake inhibitor (NDRI)				
Bupropion	Wellbutrin	75	100–300	Contraindicated with eating disorders, caution with seizure disorders
	Wellbutrin SR	100	100–300	
Noradrenergic and specific serotonergic antidepressant (NaSSA)				
Mirtazapine	Remeron	7.5–15	15–45	
Monoamine oxidase inhibitors (MAOI)				
Phenelzine	Nardil	15	15–45	Requires restrictions of diet and coadministered medications
Tranylcypromine	Parnate	10	10–40	
Stimulants				
Methylphenidate	Ritalin	2.5	10 b.i.d. ⎫	Slow release preparations
Dexedrine	Dextrostat	2.5	10 b.i.d. ⎭	also available

b.i.d., twice daily.
Antidepressant classification system is from Stahl SM. *Essential psychopharmacology,* 2nd ed. New York: Cambridge University Press, 2001, with permission.
Chart is modified from Kennedy GJ. *Geriatric mental health care.* New York: Guilford Press, 2000.

alent to that of doxepin, and its side effects better tolerated, in a group of elderly depressed outpatients (Feighner and Cohn, 1985). A reduced dosage of fluoxetine is not recommended in the elderly, although treatment can be started at 10 mg/day to reduce the risk of overwhelming the patient with initial side effects. Fluoxetine's side effects, similar to those of other serotonergic antidepressants, include nausea and other gastrointestinal symptoms, headache, al-

tered sleep, and sexual dysfunction. Weight loss has been cited as a clinical concern in particular with fluoxetine, but Goldstein et al. (1997) reported that this is associated with pretreatment high body mass index. Hyponatremia, an uncommon complication of SSRI antidepressants, is believed to be more common among elderly patients.

In a double-blind comparison to fluoxetine (20–40 mg/day), sertraline (50–100 mg/day) produced a similar drop in mean HAM-D score after 12 weeks in a group of outpatients with a mean age of 74 years. Sertraline was claimed superior on the basis of greater cognitive improvement on one of three administered tests; better improvement on the Physical Health and Psychological Health subscale of the Quality of Life Enjoyment and Satisfaction Questionnaire; and nonsignificant statistical trends toward a higher rate of remissions and a lower number of drop outs (Finkel et al., 1999). Sertraline's linear kinetics (Newhouse, 1996), its lack of an active, long-acting metabolite, and its lesser inhibition of hepatic microsomal enzymes (Rothschild, 1996) are considered advantageous properties in treating the elderly. Treatment can be initiated at 25 or 50 mg/day in the elderly and titrated up to 100 to 150 mg/day.

The other SSRIs, too, have each been reported effective antidepressants in the elderly. Citalopram's half-life is long enough to justify once daily dosing and its capacity for sedation, gastrointestinal side effects, or sexual dysfunction appear on a par with the other selective serotonergic agents. In comparison with mianserin (30–60 mg/day), citalopram (20–40 mg/day) achieved similar rates of response in a group of elderly patients with and without dementia (Karlsson et al., 2000). Fluvoxamine has been compared with the heterocyclic dothiepin, moclobemide, mianserin, and imipramine. Its efficacy has been reported as similar to these agents. Gastrointestinal side effects were the most common adverse effects and cardiac effects were not significant (Newhouse, 1996). Paroxetine's anticholinergic properties, nonlinear kinetics, and association with discontinuation symptoms can be considered relative drawbacks to its use.

Venlafaxine is a blocker of norepinephrine, serotonin, and dopamine reuptake that lacks anticholinergic, antihistaminergic, and antiadrenergic side effects. Several open series (Khan et al., 1995; Dierick, 1996; Amore et al., 1997; Zimmer et al., 1997; Tsolaki et al., 2000) and one double-blind comparison study (Mahapatra and Hackett, 1997) attest to its efficacy and safety in the elderly. The double-blind comparison was of venlafaxine (50–150 mg/day) with dothiepin (50–150 mg/day). Response to therapy was seen in 60% of each group, and discontinuation as a result of adverse reactions was low with both venlafaxine (7%) and dothiepin (8%). Venlafaxine's side effect profile is similar to that of SSRIs. In addition, it is known to increase diastolic blood pressure in some patients (Rothschild, 1996), but appeared not to increase it in old more than in young patients in an open trial that included both age groups (Zimmer et al., 1997). Treatment in the elderly can be initiated at 37.5 mg/day.

Nefazodone, a serotonin reuptake blocker with 5-HT_2 antagonism, has not been specifically studied in groups of elderly depressed patients, but is sometimes advocated as useful on the basis of its anxiolytic and sedative properties. Its lack of alteration of sleep architecture may be an advantage (Armitage et al., 1994), but safety concerns were recently aroused by a report of three cases of subfulminant liver failure associated with this medication (Aranda-Michel et al., 1999). In using nefazodone in the elderly, treatment should be initiated at half the usual starting dose for younger adults (i.e., 50 mg twice daily). Because of nefazodone's inhibition of the hepatic microsomal enzyme 3A4, care must be taken with concurrent use of triazolam or alprazolam (Rothschild, 1996).

Bupropion, a norepinephrine and dopamine reuptake inhibitor, is available in both immediate release and slow release formulations. A 7-week double-blind, placebo-controlled comparison of immediate release bupropion with imipramine in depressed patients ranging from 55 to 80 years of age showed significant superiority of bupropion over placebo and equivalent efficacy to imipramine. Bupropion's adverse effects were mild (Branconnier et al., 1983). A similar 4-week comparison also revealed bupropion to have a lower incidence of orthostatic hypotension than imipramine (Kane et al., 1983). Immediate release bupropion was found to be safe in elderly patients with left ventricular impairment, ventricular arrhythmias, or conduction defects even at high doses (mean 445 mg/day) in a follow-up study of 36 patients by (Roose et al., 1991). The slow release form of bupropion (100–300 mg/day) was compared with paroxetine (10–40 mg/day) in a 6-week randomized, double-blind comparison study among depressed elderly 60 years of age or older (Weihs et al., 2000). Mean HAM-D and HAM-A scores decreased similarly with either drug and the only significant difference among adverse events was the greater presence of somnolence and diarrhea in the paroxetine group. Immediate release bupropion is associated with an increased risk of seizures and should be avoided in patients who have other predisposing factors to seizures. Risk is decreased by administering the medication on a three times daily regimen, with no more than 450 mg immediate release daily dose or 400 mg/day slow release daily dose and no single dose exceeding 200 mg. The elderly are predisposed to accumulate bupropion and its metabolites (Sweet et al., 1995). Bupropion's side effects typically include headache, somnolence, insomnia, agitation, dizziness, diarrhea, dry mouth, and nausea. An unusual side effect reported in several elderly patients on bupropion was the tendency to fall backward (Szuba and Leuchter, 1992).

Among currently available antidepressants, mirtazapine possesses a unique mechanism that joins antagonism of presynaptic noradrenergic α_2 presynaptic autoreceptors and heteroreceptors with antagonism of H_1, 5-HT_2, and 5-HT_3 receptors. The resulting clinical effect is a depression-reducing increase in synaptic norepinephrine and serotonin levels, accompanied by sedation, appetite-enhancement, and minimal nausea, a combination that might be anticipated to help anxious, insomniac, anorexic elderly depressed patients. The two available controlled trials provide some support for mirtazapine's use in the elderly. A comparison of mirtazapine (15–45 mg/day) with amitriptyline (30–90 mg/day) in a 6-week, double-blind comparison among elderly depressed patients (60–85 years of age) yielded evidence of similar reduction of HAM-D and MADRS scores, but less improvement on the Clinical Global Impression-Global Improvement Scale and more cognitive disturbance (Hoyberg et al., 1996). The incidence of anticholinergic effects in both groups was similar. A placebo-controlled, double-blind trial comparing mirtazapine (mean dose 20.1 mg/day) with trazodone (mean dose 151.1 mg/day) in outpatients above 55 years of age showed both to be more effective than placebo. A significantly higher incidence of appetite increase was reported with mirtazapine than with trazodone (24% vs. 6%), and both active treatments were frequently associated with dry mouth and somnolence. Mirtazapine treatment can be initiated at 7.5 to 15 mg at bedtime in the elderly and titrated cautiously to doses ranging between 30 and 45 mg/day.

In a series of studies of late life depression, trazodone was shown effective. It was associated with fewer side effects than the tertiary amine tricyclics (Salzman, 1994); however, its wide dosage range and capacity to cause orthostatic hypotension, priapism, sedation, confusion, and memory disturbances have relegated it to a subsidiary antidepressant role (Rothschild, 1996). It continues to be used frequently as a treatment for agitation in demented elderly patients (Sultzer et al., 1997) and as an aid for insomnia.

The relative role for SSRIs versus the tricyclics, especially nortriptyline, is a matter of continuing debate. An early comparison of fluoxetine with nortriptyline in melancholic elderly patients showed nortriptyline's efficacy to be superior, although the comparison was not carried out in parallel, double-blind groups (Roose et al., 1994). In comparisons with amitriptyline and doxepin, fluoxetine performed with similar efficacy and had fewer side effects (Newhouse, 1996). Comparisons of sertraline with amitriptyline and nortriptyline, although not guided by serum levels, reported sertraline to produce similar improvements in depression and

greater improvements in quality of life and cognitive performance with a lower rate of adverse effects (Newhouse, 1996; Finkel et al., 1999; Finkel, 1996). A recent contemporaneous comparison of open-label sertraline (mean dose 83.1 mg/day) with double-blind nortriptyline treatment, however, showed nortriptyline (mean dose 49.0 mg/day) to be more efficacious in cognitively intact frail elderly. On the other hand, a low-dose regimen of nortriptyline (mean dose 9.25 mg/day) was superior to sertraline in treating depressed cognitively impaired frail elderly. The numbers of study completers were not significantly different between agents (Oslin et al., 2000). Paroxetine has been compared with doxepin, clomipramine, amitriptyline (Newhouse, 1996), or nortriptyline (Mulsant et al., 1999). In each of these reports, paroxetine was claimed to produce equal efficacy with similar or fewer adverse events. A double-blind comparison of citalopram (20–40 mg/day) with amitriptyline (50–100 mg/day) in elderly depressed patients showed equivalent antidepressant efficacy and fewer adverse effects (Kyle et al., 1998).

Of the heterocyclic antidepressants comprising the tricyclic agents and the tetracyclic drug maprotiline, nortriptyline is the most extensively studied agent. Although nortriptyline possesses significant anticholinergic properties, it produces only limited orthostatic hypotension but its use can be optimized by monitoring serum levels (Roose and Suthers, 1998). A study of older patients with major depressive disorder in which the nortriptyline level was appropriately monitored showed a 60% remission rate in the intent-to-treat analysis. By the end of the fifth week, 89% of those who would achieve remission had done so (Flint and Rifat, 1996). In a study that combined IPT with a therapeutic nortriptyline serum level, the intent-to-treat remission rate was even higher (78%), with only a 12% dropout rate (Reynolds et al., 1996). Roose and Suthers (1998) caution that nortriptyline treatment is associated with significant anticholinergic effects, an increase in heart rate, and less improvement in quality of life than sertraline in one comparison study.

Two studies attest to nortriptyline's usefulness in patients above 70 years of age. Katz et al. (1990) treated 30 nursing home patients (mean age 84 years) with placebo or nortriptyline (25–50 mg/day) and noted much improvement in 58.3% of the nortriptyline-treated patients but only in 9.1% of those on placebo. One third of patients dropped out because of side effects. Finkel et al. (1999) treated 37 patients (mean age 75 years) with nortriptyline and compared them with a similar group treated with sertraline. The response rate and measurements of quality of life were higher in the sertraline group, and those treated with sertraline were less likely to discontinue treatment for adverse effects (12.8% vs. 24.3%). In neither of these studies were nortriptyline serum levels monitored, a factor that may have prevented optimal use of nortriptyline.

With the exception of desipramine, the use of which is supported by a small number of studies, the other heterocyclic antidepressants are less frequently recommended for use in the elderly. Desipramine, although associated with greater orthostatic hypotension than nortriptyline, remains a useful and effective agent. Both nortriptyline and desipramine are converted to toxic hydroxy-metabolites that require renal clearance—a factor of importance in the renally impaired patient (Salzman, 1994). Use of heterocyclic antidepressants can be accompanied by side effects, including sedation, confusion, urinary retention, exacerbation of glaucoma, blurred vision, increase in heart rate, delayed ventricular conduction, dry mouth, constipation, fatigue, dizziness, atrial fibrillation, orthostatic hypotension, falls, and gait disturbance. Compared with the serotonergic agents, heterocyclic antidepressants are more dangerous in overdose. Their quinidinelike property of slowing cardiac conduction renders them undesirable for treatment of patients with bundle branch disease.

The currently available monoamine oxidase inhibitors, although found to be effective agents (Salzman, 1994), have come to occupy a secondary role in the treatment of late life depression. Their associated side effects of orthostatic hypotension, anticholinergiclike properties, and need for careful monitoring of diet and other medications to avoid hypertensive interactions make them riskier drugs for use in the elderly when compared with newer agents (Rothschild, 1996).

Despite the frequency of their use, only limited controlled data are available to support the efficacy of stimulants among the depressed elderly (Satel and Nelson, 1989). Methylphenidate, in particular, is advocated on the basis of one controlled trial among medically ill, depressed geriatric patients (Wallace et al., 1995) and other uncontrolled clinical series (Kaplitz, 1975; Katon and Raskind, 1980; Askinazi et al., 1986; Pickett et al., 1990) that indicate significant response rates and limited adverse reactions. Factors that justify a stimulant trial for the treatment of depression typically include apathy or psychomotor retardation, concurrent medical illness, intolerance of standard antidepressants, and the need for a rapid response. Dexedrine is considered similarly useful, although clinicians may avoid it because of concerns about misuse (Murray and Cassem, 1998).

Electroconvulsive Therapy

ECT is a powerful and accepted intervention in the treatment of late life depression. One California survey found its use in adults 65 years of age and older to be more than three times as frequent as among the general adult population (Kramer, 1985). Despite the recent availability of newer and safer antidepressants, some elderly patients nonetheless fail to respond to medications as robustly as to ECT. Others fulfill alternative indications for the use of ECT, such as preference for that treatment modality, a history of prior good response to ECT, or need for a rapid clinical response because of acutely life-threatening illness or complications (American Psychiatric Association, 1990). No comparison has shown an antidepressant to have a response rate superior to that obtained with ECT, although the methodologies of such studies have been criticized (Sackeim, 1994). Not only response rates but also remission rates (asymptomatic state) are claimed to be superior with ECT (Hamilton, 1982). Delusions or psychomotor retardation are considered predictors of response to ECT (Katona, 1994). Prior medication resistance, but not increasing age, is considered a predictor of poorer response to ECT (Sackeim, 1994). Although the treatment is safe enough for use with frail elderly patients, an increased risk of complications is associated with factors such as increased intracranial pressure, unstable cardiac function, recent intracerebral hemorrhage, concurrent use of medications for medical conditions, or increased risk for undergoing anesthesia. Many patients know that ECT can adversely affect memory and resist the recommendation for this treatment on that basis, but memory effects are often mild and time-limited. Retrograde amnesia appears and clears rapidly after each seizure, whereas a longer-lasting difficulty in retaining newly learned information often resolves within several weeks after ECT is concluded (Sackeim, 1994). ECT has been used successfully even among patients with concurrent dementia, although the likelihood of transient postictal confusion is heightened by preexisting cognitive impairment (Nelson and Rosenberg, 1991).

Delusions, defined as fixed, false, beliefs, are a frequent concomitant of late life depression (Meyers and Greenberg, 1986). Treatment of delusional depression in the aged, however, is impeded by the greater difficulty that elderly patients have in tolerating the side effects associated with a sufficiently high level of antipsychotic medication. Evidence of the efficacy of ECT in treating delusional depression, combined with the frequency of intolerance of adequate combined pharmacotherapy in elderly patients, makes ECT a reasonable early choice in treating this syndrome. In younger patients, the newer antipsychotic, olanzapine, has already been shown to be effective in both prospective (Konig et al., 2001) and retrospective studies (Rothschild et al., 1999). Controlled studies of olanzapine and the other atypical antipsychotics may in time justify their preferred use in treating late life delusional depression.

TREATMENT RESISTANT DEPRESSION

Several different approaches have been reported for addressing treatment-resistant depression in the elderly. Lithium augmentation, the best-documented option, is often successful at blood levels between 0.4 and 0.8 mmol/L (Katona, 1994). Bupropion has safely been used in medically frail elderly patients as an augmenter to serotonergic agents (Spier, 1998). In postmenopausal depressed elderly women, Schneider et al. (1997) demonstrated an augmenting effect when estrogen replacement therapy (ERT) was added to fluoxetine (20 mg/day). In one report, a brief pulse of dexamethasone aided treatment of two elderly patients with resistant depression (Bodani et al., 1999). These interventions are best reserved for partial responders, with a switch to a different antidepressant when no response has occurred to an antidepressant trial adequate in dose and duration.

TREATMENT OF DEPRESSION IN DEMENTED PATIENTS

Depressive disorders are estimated to affect a mean of 19% of patients with Alzheimer's disease (Wragg and Jeste, 1989). The prevalence of depression among patients who have vascular dementia may be even higher than among those with Alzheimer's disease (Newman, 1999). The GDS remains a valid and reliable instrument in patients with MMSE scores as low as 15 (McGivney et al., 1994) and other instruments, too, may be useful in patients with mild to moderate dementia (Katz, 1998). Caregivers of demented patients tend to report more depressive symptoms than are detected on clinical interviews, a phenomenon that could reflect the increased variability of mood and other depressive symptoms in demented patients, leading to overreporting by caregivers and underrecognition by clinicians (Katz, 1998). Apathy, passivity, decreased initiative, and poor concentration are symptoms associated with dementia and, therefore, are less use-

ful than mood symptoms themselves in diagnosing depression in demented patients.

In three of the five placebo-controlled antidepressant trials, significant benefits were seen with antidepressant treatment of depressed demented patients. Minaprine (a serotonergic, dopaminergic, procholinergic antidepressant), clomipramine, and moclobemide were the agents in the successful trials, whereas studies of imipramine and maprotiline failed to demonstrate drug versus placebo differences (Katz, 1998). Whichever agent is chosen, a heightened vulnerability to adverse medication effects would be expected in demented patients.

PROGNOSIS AND MAINTENANCE TREATMENT

Although the rate of response to treatment of depression in the elderly was high in a study that involved well-monitored and adequate treatment, 90% of the patients placed on placebo maintenance after successful treatment experienced a recurrence of depression (Reynolds et al., 1999a). Because adequate treatment of late life depression is the exception rather than the rule, the actual prognosis for depressed elderly patients, therefore, would seem to be poor under naturalistic conditions. Data consistent with the bleaker appraisal come from a metaanalysis of outcomes for elderly subjects in the community and primary care, which indicated after 24 months that only one third of the subjects were well, whereas one third were depressed, and 21% had died (Cole et al., 1999). It is becoming clear that late life depression contributes to excess mortality, not merely from suicide but also by increasing the mortality associated with some medical illnesses. In a recent longitudinal, 4-year study of 2,847 men and women aged 55 to 85 years, the presence of major depression increased by threefold the risk of cardiac death, whereas the presence of minor depression was associated with a risk increase approximately half as large (Penninx et al., 2001). Similarly, depression can increase the risk for cerebrovascular disease (Krishnan, 2000) and depressive symptoms 1 month after a cerebrovascular accident and increase the risk of mortality at 12 and 24 months (House et al., 2001).

Maintenance pharmacotherapy and psychotherapy have been shown in several studies to reduce the risk of recurrence. In the largest of these, the Pittsburgh study, a group of recovered late life depressed patients was randomized to one of three treatment conditions and followed for 3 years. The patients who received combined IPT and maintenance nortriptyline

(80–120 ng/mL level) did best, with a recurrence rate of only 20%. Patients who received nortriptyline without IPT did less well, with a recurrence rate of 43%, which was less than half the recurrence rate among placebo subjects (Reynolds et al., 1999a). A subsequent report on this study indicated that patients maintained on a higher plasma level of nortriptyline (80–120 ng/mL) experienced more constipation but fewer residual depressive symptoms than patients maintained on a lower level (40–60 ng/mL) of nortriptyline (Reynolds et al., 1999b). Although some patients with milder baseline levels of depression and excellent remission during acute and continuation therapy stages did well on maintenance IPT alone, a high baseline level of depression (Hamilton score ≥ 20) was a strong predictor of relapse (Taylor et al., 1999). Full-dose antidepressant maintenance has gained further support from the recent report by Flint and Rifat (2000) of the efficacy of full-dose antidepressant medication, supplemented in some cases with adjunctive lithium, in a 4-year follow-up study of patients 60 years of age and older that showed a cumulative probability of remaining well without recurrence during that period to be 70%.

BIPOLAR DISORDER IN LATE LIFE

Compared with accumulating knowledge about late life depression, much less is understood about the characteristics of bipolar disorder in the elderly. Diagnosis of bipolar disorder requires current or past manic or hypomanic symptomatology. The diagnosis of a manic episode requires the presence of at least three of the following symptoms, in addition to an elevated mood, or at least four of the symptoms, in addition to an irritable mood: grandiosity, decreased need for sleep, pressure to keep talking, flight of ideas, distractibility, increased activity, or excessive involvement in potentially risky pleasurable pursuits (e.g., inappropriate spending or sexual behavior) (American Psychiatric Association, 2000). Current or previous hypomanic or manic behavior determines a bipolar diagnosis even when the predominant presenting clinical picture is depressive. The individual with both manic and depressive episodes is diagnosed *bipolar 1*, whereas a syndrome of hypomanic and depressive episodes is termed *bipolar II* (American Psychiatric Association, 2000).

Bipolar depression, diagnosed when depressive symptoms occur with concurrent or prior manic or hypomanic symptoms, is often treated with antidepressants. Increasingly, this is regarded as a hazardous approach because accumulating evidence indicates such treatment is associated with induction of manic episodes, increased cycling, development of treatment resistance, and ineffective prophylaxis of subsequent episodes (Altshuler et al., 1995; Wehr et al., 1988; Quitkin et al., 1981). Mood stabilizing medications and their dosages are presented in Table 31-2. Lithium salts, although they have received less attention in elderly populations (Bowden, 1998), remain a first-line agent. An oft-cited but very small study in younger adults suggested that bupropion, in comparison with desipramine, was less frequently associated with induction of manic episodes during 1 year of prospective follow-up (Sachs et al., 1994).

Mania is uncommon among community-dwelling elderly, with approximately 0.1% of individuals above 65 years of age meeting diagnostic criteria for bipolar disorder type I and 0.7% for bipolar disorder type II (Weissman et al., 1988; Weissman et al., 1991). This group, nonetheless, constitutes 5% to 19% of the elderly who seek treatment for mood disorders (Young, 1992). In long-term care facilities, the prevalence of bipolar disorders may be as high as 9.0% (Chen et al., 1998). As a group, elderly patients with bipolar disorder show more severe symptoms, greater impairment in community-living skills, increased use of mental health services (psychiatric partial hospitalization or hospitalization, skills-training services, or case-management services), and greater cognitive impairment than a comparison group with unipolar depression (Bartels et al., 2000). In addition, greater frequency of episodes has been demonstrated in the bipolar elderly (Chen et al., 1998).

Mania with first onset in late life has been a matter of particular interest, because late onset is associated with an increased presence of medical (including metabolic, infectious, and neoplastic disorders), neurologic (including vascular lesions, brain injury, and degenerative disorders), or medication-related causes (including antidepressant treatment, steroids, sympathomimetics). Furthermore, late onset mania is characterized by a lower rate of bipolar family history, a possibly increased vulnerability to relapse, and a mortality rate even higher than that among the elderly who are depressed (Young, 1992; Krauthammer and Klerman, 1978; Shulman and Tohen, 1994; Chen et al., 1998). An increase in the number of subcortical hyperintensities on MRI has been demonstrated in a group of late onset manic patients (McDonald and Nemeroff, 1996).

Treatment

Guidelines for the treatment of mania in the elderly derive from uncontrolled studies and extrapolation from findings in younger adults. Acute treatment of

TABLE 31-2. *Selected mood stabilizers for use in late life mood disorders*

Generic name	Trade name	Starting dose—range (mg/d)	Treatment dose—range (mg/d)	Notes
Lithium salts				
Lithium carbonate	Eskalith	300	300–1,500	Follow blood level, target
Lithium controlled release	Lithobid	300	300–1,500	therapeutic range is 0.4–1.0
	Eskalith CR	450	450–1,800	mEq/L
Lithium citrate		150	300–1,500	Liquid preparation
Anticonvulsants				
Divalproex sodium	Depakote	250	250–2,000	Enterically coated, less gastrointestinal intolerance. Therapeutic range usually within blood level limits of 50–100 μg/mL
Valproic acid	Depakene	250	250–2,000	Therapeutic level usually within blood level limits of 50–100 μg/mL
Carbamazepine	Tegretol	100	200–1,000	Cytochrome P-450 enzyme inducer. Therapeutic level usually within range of 4–12 μg/mL
Lamotrigine	Lamictal	12.5	25–200	Slow titration is required to minimize risk of adverse reaction (Stevens-Johnson syndrome)
Topiramate	Topamax	25	25–200	Use is associated with weight loss
Gabapentin	Neurontin	100	200–2,000	

Chart is modified from Kennedy GJ. *Geriatric mental health care.* New York: Guilford Press, 2000, with permission.

mania in younger adults often employs antipsychotic agents, particularly when concurrent psychotic symptoms are present, but these may be more problematic in older adults because of the increased likelihood of adverse effects, including orthostatic hypotension, sedation, and extrapyramidal symptoms, including tardive dyskinesia. The atypical antipsychotics, associated with fewer extrapyramidal symptoms, merit further exploration in the acute treatment of late life mania. They have not been specifically studied in the elderly with bipolar disorder, but in younger patient groups clozapine, risperidone, olanzapine, and quetiapine have each been shown beneficial (Umapathy et al., 2000). Information about the antipsychotic agents for use in late life mood disorders is presented in Table 31-3.

Lithium salts are regarded as first-line agents in treating geriatric acute mania (Young, 1998). Available as lithium carbonate or as the liquid lithium citrate, lithium salts have not been studied in the elderly under double-blind conditions but have been investigated in open trials. In the elderly, lithium salts are known to be toxic at lower levels than in younger adults, justifying use of levels as low as 0.4 to 0.8 mEg/L (Bowden, 1998). The presence of cog-

nitive impairment or preexisting tremor further increases the likelihood of a toxic reaction. The side effects of lithium include polyuria, tremor, mental slowing and memory difficulties, sinus node dysfunction, peripheral edema, hypothyroidism or nontoxic goiter; a worsening of arthritis, nausea, diarrhea, and acne or psoriasis. These can become intolerable, even at serum levels below those regarded as toxic in younger adults. Lithium's serum level can be raised by many nonsteroidal anti-inflammatory drugs and by thiazide diuretics. In the elderly, reduced renal clearance and hepatic metabolism, respectively, can increase the serum levels of lithium or divalproex sodium (McDonald and Nemeroff, 1996).

Valproic acid, an anticonvulsant shown effective in treating acute mania in younger adults, is modestly effective and well tolerated in elderly manic patients (McFarland et al., 1990; Risinger et al., 1994). Among a mixed age population studied retrospectively, lithium refractory patients and those with neurologic abnormalities were a particularly responsive group for treatment with valproic acid (Stoll et al., 1994). In addition, younger patients with mixed states (concurrent depressive and manic symptoms) re-

TABLE 31-3. *Selected antipsychotic agents for use in late life mood disorders*

Generic name	Trade name	Starting dose— range (mg/d)	Treatment dose— range (mg/d)	Notes
Typical antipsychotic agents (high potency)				
Haloperidol	Haldol	0.5	2–10	Available as liquid, i.m. injection, i.v. injection
	Haldol decanoate	12.5 i.m. q14–28d	50–200 i.m. q28d	Depot injectable preparation
Perphenazine	Trilafon	2	4–32	Available as liquid, i.m. injection
Fluphenazine	Prolixin	0.5	2–10	Available as liquid, i.m. injection
	Prolixin decanoate Prolixin enanthate	12.5 i.m. q7–14d	12.5–50 i.m. q14–21d	Depot injectable preparation
Atypical antipsychotic agents				
Risperidone	Risperdal	0.25	0.5–6	Available as liquid
Olanzapine	Zyprexa	2.5	2.5–15	
Quetiapine	Seroquel	25	50–500	Sedative
Clozapine	Clozaril	6.25	25–200	Anticholinergic, low in EPS
Ziprasidone	Geodon	20	20–60 b.i.d.	Monitoring of QTc suggested

b.i.d., twice daily; EPS, extrapyramidal symptoms; i.m., intramuscularly; i.v., intravenously.
Chart is modified from Kennedy GJ. *Geriatric mental health care.* New York: Guilford Press, 2000.

spond better to valproic acid than to lithium (Bowden, 1998). Serum levels between 50 and 150 µg/mL are often effective. Valproic acid is an inhibitor of cytochrome P450 enzymes, which can increase the levels of many coadministered drugs. Sedation, weight gain, nausea, transient hair loss, hyperammonemia, and rare severe reactions (aplastic anemia, pancreatitis, hepatic failure) have been associated with treatment (Bowden, 1998; McDonald and Nemeroff, 1996).

Other anticonvulsants have been used in elderly bipolar patients but as yet without support from controlled studies. Carbamazepine, problematic because of its side effects and drug interactions, has largely been superseded by valproic acid. Several newer anticonvulsants have aroused interest, including gabapentin, topiramate, vigabatrin, and lamotrigine. Lamotrigine has attracted particular attention as a treatment for bipolar depression, for which it is effective in younger adults (Calabrese et al., 1999), but no studies yet attest to its safety in the treatment of elderly bipolar patients.

As with depression, ECT remains an important intervention in the acute treatment of late life bipolar episodes, whether depressive or manic, especially in those patients who are resistant to medication or who require a rapid symptomatic resolution. Most responders can then be switched to pharmacotherapeutic maintenance. The combination of ECT with lithium, which has been associated with confusional reactions, is to be avoided (Young, 1998).

Regarding maintenance treatment and prevention of subsequent episodes of mania or depression in bipolar elderly, little information is available (Young 1997). Valproic acid or lithium, demonstrated effective in younger populations, are commonly used in the elderly as well. Maintenance ECT is an option for patients whose depressive or manic bipolar symptoms respond poorly to maintenance medication regimens (Umapathy et al., 2000; McDonald, 2000).

SUMMARY

As our population of elderly continues to grow, the importance of recognizing and properly treating the mood disorders of late life will continue to increase. Detection, differential diagnosis, aggressive and comprehensive treatment, maintenance therapy, and vigorous follow-up are necessary to achieve success in the management of late life disorders. Optimal treatment will benefit patients and their families by reducing a major source of morbidity in late life and deferring the need for caregiver support. Society's benefit, moreover, will be apparent in patients' increased productivity, sustained autonomy, and lesser use of healthcare resources.

REFERENCES

Alexopoulos GS, Meyers BS, Young RC, et al. 'Vascular depression' hypothesis. *Arch Gen Psychiatry* 1997;54: 915–922.

Alexopoulos GS, Meyers BS, Young RC, et al. Executive dysfunction and long-term outcomes of geriatric depression. *Arch Gen Psychiatry* 2000;57:285–290.

Altshuler LI, Post RM, Leverich GS, et al. Antidepressant-induced mania and cycle acceleration: a controversy revisited. *Am J Psychiatry* 1995;152:1130–1138.

American Psychiatric Association. *Diagnostic and statistical manual of mental disorders*, 4th ed., text revision. Washington, DC: American Psychiatric Association, 2000.

American Psychiatric Association (APA Task Force on ECT). *The practice of electroconvulsive therapy: recommendations for treatment, training, and privileging.* Washington, DC: American Psychiatric Press, 1990.

Amore M, Ricci M, Zanardi R, et al. Long-term treatment of geropsychiatric depressed patients with venlafaxine. *J Affect Disord* 1997;46:293–296.

Applegate WB, Blass JP, Williams TF. Instruments for the functional assessment of older patients. *N Engl J Med* 1990;322:1207–1214.

Aranda-Michel J, Koehler A, Bejarano PA, et al. Nefazodone-induced liver failure: report of three cases. *Ann Intern Med* 1999;130(4 Pt 1):285–288.

Armitage R, Rush AJ, Trivedi M, et al. The effects of nefazodone on sleep architecture in depression. *Neuropsychopharmacology* 1994;10:123–127.

Askinazi C, Weintraub RJ, Karamouz N. Elderly depressed females as a possible subgroup of patients responsive to methylphenidate. *J Clin Psychiatry* 1986;47:467–469.

Barraclough BM. Suicide in the elderly. *Br J Psychiatry* 1971;6(Suppl):87–97.

Barrett JE, Barrett JA, Oxman TE, et al. The prevalence of psychiatric disorders in a primary care practice. *Arch Gen Psychiatry* 1988;45:1100–1106.

Bartels SJ, Forester B, Miles KM, et al. Mental health service use by elderly patients with bipolar disorder and unipolar major depression. *Am J Geriatr Psychiatry* 2000; 8(2):160–166.

Blazer DG. Epidemiology of late-life depression. In: Schneider LS, Reynolds CF 3rd, Lebowitz BD, et al. eds. *Diagnosis and treatment of depression in late life*. Washington, DC: American Psychiatric Press, Inc., 1994:9–19.

Bodani M, Sheehan B, Philpot M. The use of dexamethasone in elderly patients with antidepressant-resistant depressive illness. *J Psychopharmacol* 1999;13:196–197.

Borson S, Bames RA, Kukull WA, et al. Symptomatic depression in elderly medical outpatients. I. Prevalence, demography, and health service utilization. *J Am Geriatr Soc* 1986;34:341–347.

Bowden CL. Anticonvulsants in bipolar elderly. In: Nelson JC, ed. *Geriatric psychopharmacology*. New York: Marcel Dekker, 1998:285–299.

Branconnier RJ, Cole JO, Ghazvinian S, et al. Clinical pharmacology of bupropion and imipramine in elderly depressives. *J Clin Psychiatry* 1983;44(5 Sect 2):130–133.

Burns BJ, Taube CA. Mental health services in general medical care and in nursing homes. In: Fogel BS, Furino A, Gottlieb GL, eds. *Mental health policy for older Americans: protecting minds at risk*. Washington, DC: American Psychiatric Press, 1990:63–83.

Calabrese JR, Bowden CL, Sachs GS, et al. A double-blind placebo-controlled study of lamotrigine monotherapy in outpatients with bipolar I depression. *J Clin Psychiatry* 1999;60:79–88.

Chen ST, Altshuler LL, Spar JE. Bipolar disorder in late life: a review. J Geriatr Psychiatry Neurol 1998;11:29–35.

Cole MG, Bellavance F, Mansour A. Prognosis of depression in elderly community and primary care populations: a systematic review and meta-analysis. *Am J Psychiatry* 1999;156:1182–1189.

Conwell Y. Suicide in the elderly patients. In: Schneider LS, Reynolds III CF, Lebowitz BD, et al., eds. *Diagnosis and treatment of depression in late life*. Washington, DC: American Psychiatric Press, 1994:397–418.

Conwell Y, Duberstein PR, Cox C, et al. Relationships of age and axis I diagnoses in victims of completed suicide: a psychological autopsy study. *Am J Psychiatry* 1996; 153:1001–1008.

Diereck M. An open-label evaluation of the long-term safety of oral venlafaxine in depressed elderly patients. *Ann Clin Psychiatry* 1996;8:169–178.

Feighner JP, Cohn JB. Double-blind comparative trials of fluoxetine and doxepin in geriatric patients with major depressive disorder. *J Clin Psychiatry* 1985;46(3, Sec 2):20–25.

Finkel SI. Efficacy and tolerability of antidepressant therapy in the old-old. *J Clin Psychiatry* 1996;57(Suppl5):23–28.

Finkel SI, Richter EM, Clary CM, et al. Comparative efficacy of sertraline vs. fluoxetine in patients age 70 or over with major depression. *Am J Geriatr Psychiatry* 1999; 7:221–227.

Flint A, Rifat S. The effect of sequential antidepressant treatment on geriatric depression. *J Affect Disord* 1996;3 6:95–105.

Flint AJ, Rifat SL. Maintenance treatment for recurrent depression in late life. *Am J Geriatr Psychiatry* 2000;8: 112–116.

George LK. Social factors and depression in late life. In: Schneider LS, Reynolds III CF, Lebowitz BD, et al., eds. *Diagnosis and treatment of depression in late life*. Washington, DC: American Psychiatric Press, 1994: 131–153.

Gerson S, Belin TR, Kaufman A, et al. Pharmacological and psychological treatments for depressed older patients: a meta-analysis and overview of recent findings. *Harvard Rev Psychiatry* 1999;7:1–28.

Goldstein DJ, Hamilton SH, Masica DN, et al: Fluoxetine in medically stable, depressed geriatric patients: effects on weight. *J Clin Psychophannacol* 1997;17:365–369.

Gottlieb GL. Barriers to care for older adults with depression. In: Schneider LS, Reynolds CF 3rd, Lebowitz BD, et al., eds. *Diagnosis and treatment of depression in late life*. Washington, DC: American Psychiatric Press, 1994: 377–396.

Hamilton M. The effect of treatment on the melancholias (depression). *Br J Psychiatry* 1982;140:223–230.

House A, Knapp P, Bamford J, et al. Mortality at 12 and 24 months after stroke may be associated with depressive symptoms at 1 month. *Stroke* 2001;32:696–701.

Hoyberg OJ, Maragakis B, Mullin J, et al. A double-blind multicentre comparison of mirtazapine and amitriptyline in elderly depressed patients. *Acta Psychiatr Scand* 1996; 93:184–190.

Kane JM, Cole K, Sarantakos S, et al. Safety and efficacy of bupropion in elderly patients: preliminary observations. *J Clin Psychiatry* 1983;44(5, Sect 2):134–136.

Kaplitz SE. Withdrawn, apathetic geriatric patients responsive to methylphenidate. *J Am Geriatr Soc* 1975;23: 271–276.

Karlsson 1, Godderis J, Augusto De Mendonca Lima C, et al. A randomised, double-blind comparison of the efficacy and safety of citalopram compared to mianserin in elderly, depressed patients with or without mild to moderate dementia. *Int J Geriatr Psychiatry* 2000;15: 295–305.

Kaszniak AW, Christenson GD. Differential diagnosis of dementia and depression. In: Storandt M, VandenBos GR, eds. *Neuropsychological assessment of dementia and depression in older adults: a clinician's guide.* Washington, DC: American Psychological Association, 1997:81–117.

Katon W, Raskind M. Treatment of depression in the medically ill elderly with methylphenidate. *Am J Psychiatry* 1980;137:963–965.

Katona CLE. The management of depression in old age. *Depression in old age.* Chichester, England: John Wiley & Sons, 1994;93–121.

Katz IR. Diagnosis and treatment of depression in patients with Alzheimer's disease and other dementias. *J Clin Psychiatry* 1998;59(Suppl 9):38–44.

Katz IR, Simpson GM, Curlik SM, et al. Pharmacologic treatment of major depression for elderly patients in residential care settings. *J Clin Psychiatry* 1990;51(Suppl 7): 41–47.

Katz IR, Parmelee PA. Depression in elderly patients in residential care settings. In: Schneider LS, Reynolds III CF, Lebowitz BD, et al., eds. *Diagnosis and treatment of depression in late life.* Washington, DC: American Psychiatric Press, 1994:437–461.

Khan A, Rudolph R, Baumel B, et al. Venlafaxine in depressed geriatric outpatients: an open label clinical study. *Psychopharmacol Bull* 1995;31:753–788.

Kiloh LG. Pseudo-dementia. *Acta Psychiatr Scand* 1961;37: 336–351.

Koenig HG, Meador KG, Cohen HJ, et al. Depression in elderly hospitalized patients with medical illness. *Arch Intern Med* 1988; 148:1929–1936.

Konig F, von Hippel C, Petersdorff T, et al. First experiences in combination therapy using olanzapine with SSRIs (citalopram, paroxetine) in delusional depression. *Neuropsychobiology* 2001;43:170–174.

Kramer BA. Use of ECT in California, 1977–1983. *Am J Psychiatry* 1985;142:1190–1192.

Krauthammer C, Klerman GL. Secondary mania: manic syndromes associated with antecedent physical illness or drugs. *Arch Gen Psychiatry* 1978;35:1333–1339.

Krishnan KRR. Depression as a contributing factor in cerebrovascular disease. *Am Heart J* 2000;140(Suppl 4):70–76.

Krishnan KRR, Hays JC, Blazer DG. MRI-defined vascular depression. *Am J Psychiatry* 1997;154:497–501.

Kyle CJ, Peterson BE, Overo KF. Comparison of the tolerability and efficacy of citalopram and amitriptyline in elderly depressed patients treated in general practice. *Depress Anxiety* 1998;47–53.

Lyness JM, Conwell Y, Nelson JC. Suicide attempts in elderly psychiatric inpatients. *J Am Geriatr Soc* 1992;40:320–324.

Mackenzie TB, Popkin MK. Suicide in the medical patient. *Int J Psychiatry Med* 1987;17:322.

Mahapatra SN, Hackett D. A randomised, double-blind, parallel-group comparison of venlafaxine and dothiepin in geriatric patients with major depression. *Int J Clin Pract* 1997;51:209–213.

McDonald WM. Epidemiology, etiology, and treatment of geriatric mania. *J Clin Psychiatry* 2000;61(Suppl 13): 3–11.

McDonald WM, Nemeroff CB. The diagnosis and treatment of mania in the elderly. *Bull Menninger Clinic* 1996;60: 174–196.

McFarland BH, Miller MR, Straurnflord AA. Valproate use in the older manic patient. *J Clin Psychiatry* 1990;51: 479–481.

McGivney SA, Mulvihill M, Taylor B. Validating the GDS depression screen in the nursing home. *J Am Geriatr Soc* 1994;42:490–492.

McIntosh JL, Santos JF, Hubbard RW, et al. *Elder suicide: research, theory and treatment.* Washington DC, American Psychological Association, 1994.

Mesters P, Cosyns P, Dejaiffe G, et al. Assessment of quality of life in the treatment of major depressive disorder with fluoxetine, 20 mg, in ambulatory patients aged over 60 years. *Int Clin Psychohannacol* 1993;8:337–340.

Meyers BS, Greenberg R. Late-life delusional depression. *J Affect Disord* 1986;11:133–137.

Mulsant BH, Pollock BG, Nebes RD, et al. A double-blind randomized comparison of nortriptyline and paroxetine in the treatment of late-life depression: 6-week outcome. *J Clin Psychiatry* 1999;60(Suppl 20):16–20.

Murray GB, Cassem E. Use of stimulants in depressed patients with medical illness. In: Nelson JC, ed. *Geriatric Psychopharmacology.* New York: Marcel Dekker, 1998: 245–257.

Myers JK, Weissman MM, Tischler GL, et al. Six-month prevalence of psychiatric disorders in three communities. *Arch Gen Psychiatry* 1984;41:959–970.

Nelson JP, Rosenberg DR. ECT treatment of demented elderly patients with major depression: a retrospective study of efficacy and safety. *Convulsive Therapy* 1991;7: 157–165.

Newhouse PA. Use of serotonin selective reuptake inhibitors in geriatric depression. *J Clin Psychiatry* 1996;57(Suppl 5):12–22.

Newman SC. The prevalence of depression in Alzheimer's disease and vascular dementia in a population sample. *J Affect Disord* 1999;52:169–176.

Niederehe GT. Psychosocial therapies with depressed older adults. In: Schneider LS, Reynolds III CF, Lebowitz BD, et al., eds. *Diagnosis and treatment of depression in late life.* Washington, DC: American Psychiatric Press, 1994; 293–315.

Nieto E, Vieta E, Lazaro L, et al. Serious suicide attempts in the elderly. *Psychopathology* 1992;25:183–188.

Oslin DW, Streim JE, Katz IR, et al. Heuristic comparison of sertraline with nortriptyline for the treatment of depression in frail elderly patients. *Am J Geriatr Psychiatry* 2000;8:141–149.

Parmelee PA, Katz IR, Lawton MP. Incidence of depression in long term care settings. *J Gerontol* 1992;47: MI89–MI96.

Penninx BWJH, Beekman ATF, Honig A, et al. Depression and cardiac mortality. Results from a community-based longitudinal study. *Arch Gen Psychiatry* 2001;58: 221–227.

Pickett P, Masand P, Murray GB. Psychostimulant treatment of geriatric depressive disorders secondary to medical illness. *J Geriatr Psychiatry Neurol* 1990;3:146–151.

Quitkin FM, Kane JM, Rifkin A, et al. Lithium and imipramine in the prophylaxis of unipolar and bipolar III depression: a prospective, placebo-controlled comparison. *Psychophannacol Bull* 1981;17:142–144.

Reifler BV. A case of mistaken identity: pseudodementia is really predementia. *J Am Geriatr Soc* 2000;48:593–594.

Reynolds CF 3rd, Frank E, Kupfer D. Treatment outcome in recurrent major depression: a post hoc comparison of elderly ("young old") and midlife patients. *Am J Psychiatry* 1996;153:1288–1292.

Reynolds CF 3rd, Frank E, Perel JM, et al. Nortriptyline and interpersonal psychotherapy as maintenance therapies for recurrent major depression: a randomized controlled trial in patients older than 59 years. *JAMA* 1999a;281:39–45.

Reynolds CF 3rd, Perel JM, Frank E, et al. Three-year outcomes of maintenance nortriptyline treatment in late-life depression: a study of two fixed plasma levels. *Am J Psychiatry* 1999b;156:1177–1181.

Risinger RC, Risby ED, Risch SC. Safety and efficacy of divalproex sodium in elderly bipolar patients. *J Clin Psychiatry* 1994;55;215.

Roose SP, Dalack GW, Glassman AH, et al. Cardiovascular effects of bupropion in depressed patients with heart disease. *Am J Psychiatry* 1991;148:512–516.

Roose SP, Glassman AH, Attia E, et al. Comparative efficacy of selective serotonin reuptake inhibitors and tricyclics in the treatment of melancholia. *Am J Psychiatry* 1994;151:1735–1739.

Roose SP, Suthers KM. Antidepressant response in late-life depression. *J Clin Psychiatry* 1998;59(Suppl 10):4–8.

Rothschild AJ. The diagnosis and treatment of late-life depression. *J Clin Psychiatry* 1996;57:(Suppl 5):5–11.

Rothschild AJ, Bates KS, Boehringer KL, et al. Olanzapine response in psychotic depression. *J Clin Psychiatry* 1999; 60:116–118.

Rovner BW. Depression and increased risk of mortality in the nursing home patient. *Am J Med* 1993;94(5A):19S–22S.

Sachs GS, Lafter B, Stoll AL, et al. A double-blind trial of bupropion versus desipramine for bipolar depression. *J Clin Psychiatry* 1994;55:391–393.

Sackeim HA. Use of electroconvulsive therapy in late-life depression. In: Schneider LS, Reynolds III CF, Lebowitz BD, et al., eds. *Diagnosis and treatment of depression in late life*. Washington, DC: American Psychiatric Press, 1994:259–277.

Salzman C. Pharmacological treatment of depression in elderly patients. In: Schneider LS, Reynolds III CF, Lebowitz BD, et al., eds. *Diagnosis and treatment of depression in late life*. Washington, DC: American Psychiatric Press, 1994;181–244.

Satel SL, Nelson JC. Stimulants in the treatment of depression: a critical overview. *J Clin Psychiatry* 1989;50: 241–249.

Saunders PA, Copeland JR, Dewey ME, et al. Heavy drinking as a risk factor for depression and dementia in elderly men. Findings from the Liverpool longitudinal community study. *Br J Psychiatry* 1991;159:213–216.

Schneider LS, Small GW, Hamilton SH, et al. Estrogen replacement and response to fluoxetine in a multicenter geriatric depression trial. *Am J Geriatr Psychiatry* 1997; 5:97–106.

Scogin F, McElreath L. Efficacy of psychosocial treatments for geriatric depression: a quantitative review. *J Consult Clin Psychol* 1994;62;69–74.

Shulman KI, Tohen M. Unipolar mania reconsidered: evidence from an elderly cohort. *Br J Psyhciatry* 1994; 164:547–549.

Simon GE, VonKorff M, Piccinelli M, et al. An international study of the relation between somatic symptoms and depression. *N Engl J Med* 1999;341:1329–1335.

Spier SA. Use of bupropion with SRIs and venlafaxine. *Depress Anxiety* 1998;7:73–75.

Steuer JL, Mintz J, Hammen CL, et al: Cognitive-behavioral and psychodynamic group psychotherapy in treatment of geriatric depression. *J Consult Clin Psychol* 1984;52: 180–189.

Stoll AL, Banov M, Kolbrener M, et al. Neurologic factors predict a favorable valproate response in bipolar and schizoaffective disorders. *J Clin Psychopharmacology* 1994;14:311–13.

Sultzer DL, Gray KF, Gunay I, et al. A double-blind comparison of trazodone and haloperidol for treatment of agitation in patients with dementia. *Am J Geriatr Psychiatry* 1997;5:60–69.

Sweet RA, Pollock BG, Kirshner M, et al. Pharmacokinetics of single- and multiple-dose bupropion in elderly patients with depression. *J Clin Pharmacol* 1995;35:876–884.

Szuba MP, Leuchter AF. Falling backward in two elderly patients taking bupropion. *J Clin Psychiatry* 1992;53: 157–159.

Taylor MP, Reynolds III CF, Frank E, et al. Which elderly depressed patients remain well on maintenance interpersonal psychotherapy alone? Report from the Pittsburgh study of maintenance therapies in late-life depression. *Depress Anxiety* 1999;10:55–60.

Thompson LW. Cognitive-behavioral therapy and treatment for late-life depression. *J Clin Psychiatry* 1996;57(Suppl 5):29–37.

Tideiksaar R. Drug noncompliance in the elderly. *Hospital Physician* 1984;20:92–93,96–98,101.

Tollefson GD, Holman SL. Analysis of the Hamilton Depression Rating Scale factors from a double-blind, placebo-controlled trial of fluoxetine in geriatric major depression. *Int Clin Psychopharmacology* 1993;8: 253–259.

Tsolaki M, Fountoulakis KN, Nakopoulou E, et al. The effect of antidepressant pharmacotherapy with venlafaxine in geriatric depression. *Int J Geriatric Psychopharmacology* 2000;2:83–85.

Umapathy C, Mulsant BH, Pollock BG. Bipolar disorder in the elderly. *Psychiatric Annals* 2000;30:473–480.

Unutzer J, Simon G, Belin TR, et al. Care for depression in HMO patients aged 65 and older. *J Am Geriatr Soc* 2000; 48:871–878.

Unutzer J, Katon W, Russo J, et al. Patterns of care for depressed older adults in a large-staff model HMO. *Am J Geriatr Psychiatry* 1999;7:235–243.

Unutzer J, Patric DL, Simon G, et al. Depressive symptoms and the cost of health services in HMO patients aged 65 years and older. A 4-year prospective study. *JAMA* 1997; 277:1618–1623.

Wallace AE, Kofoed LL, West AN. Double-blind, placebo-controlled trial of methylphenidate in older, depressed, medically ill patients. *Am J Psychiatry* 1995;152: 929–931.

Waxman HM, Carner EA, Klein M. Underutilization of mental health professionals by community elderly. *Gerontologist* 1984;24:23–30.

Wehr TA, Sack DA, Rosenthal NE, et al. Rapid cycling affective disorder: contributing factors and treatment responses in 51 patients. *Am J Psychiatry* 1988;145: 179–184.

Weihs KL, Settle EC, Batey SR, et al. Bupropion sustained release versus paroxetine for the treatment of depression in the elderly. *J Clin Psychiatry* 2000;61:196–202.

Weissman MM, Leaf PJ, Tischler GL, et al. Affective disorders in five United States communities. *Psychol Med* 1988;18:141–153.

Weissman MM, Bruce NEL, Leaf PF, et al. Affective disorders. In: Robbins LN, Regier DA, eds. *Psychiatric disorders in America.* New York: Free Press, 1991:53–80.

Weissman MM, Markowitz JC. Interpersonal psychotherapy. Current status. *Arch Gen Psychiatry* 1994;51: 599–606.

Wragg RE, Jeste D. Overview of depression and psychosis in Alzheimer's disease. *Am J Psychiatry* 1989;146: 577–587.

Young RC. Use of lithium in bipolar disorder. In: Nelson JC, ed. *Geriatric psychopharmacology.* New York: Marcel Dekker, 1998:259–272.

Young RC. Geriatric mania. *Clin Geriatr Med* 1992;8: 387–99.

Young RC. Bipolar mood disorders in the elderly. *Psychiatr Clin North Am* 1997;20:121–136.

Zimmer B, Kant R, Zeiler D, et al. Antidepressant efficacy and cardiovascular safety of venlafaxine in young vs old patients with comorbid medical disorders. *Int J Psychiatry Med* 1997;27:353–364.

Zonderman AB, Costa PT. The absence of increased levels of depression in older adults: evidence from a national representative study. Paper presented at the annual meeting of the American Psychological Association, San Francisco, CA, 1991; cited in Blazer, DG. Epidemiology of late-life depression. In: Schneider LS, Reynolds III CF, Lebowitz BD, et al., eds. *Diagnosis and treatment of depression in late life.* Washington, DC: American Psychiatric Press, 1994;9–19.

Zubenko, GS, Sunderland T. Geriatric psychopharmacology. Why dose age matter? *Harvard Rev Psychiatry* 2000;7: 311–333.

SUGGESTED READINGS

Katona CLE. *Depression in old age.* Chichester: John Wiley & Sons, Ltd. 1994.

Kennedy GJ, ed. *Suicide and depression in late life.* New York: John Wiley & Sons, 1996.

Nelson JC, ed. *Geriatric psychopharmacology.* New York: Marcel Dekker, 1998.

Salzman C, ed. *Clinical geriatric psychopharmacology,* 3rd ed. Baltimore: Williams & Wilkins, 1998.

Schneider LS, Reynolds III CF, Lebowitz BD, et al, eds. *Diagnosis and treatment of depression in late life.* Washington, DC: American Psychiatric Press, 1994.

WEB SITES OF INTEREST FOR PATIENT SUPPORT

National Depressive & Manic-Depressive Association (educational materials and supportive peer groups for patients and their support systems): *www.ndmda.org*

Dr. Ivan Goldberg's A Depression Central (information for clinicians, patients and their support systems): *www.psycom.net/depression.central.html*

Dr. Peter Brigham's Bipolar Disorders Web page (current therapeutic information): *http://people.ne.mediaone.net/pmbri/BP_pharm.html*

NAMI (information about mental illness and about advocacy for the mentally ill): *www.nami.org*

American Foundation for Suicide Prevention (support groups for bereaved survivors of others' suicides): *www.afsp.org*

Depression Caregiver Support (message board offering support and interaction for caregivers): *www.members.tripod.com/garyicare/*

National Association of Geriatric Care Managers (locate a professional care manager in your area): *www.caremanager.org*

32

Somatization in Older Adults

Jennifer J. Bortz and Amy S. Schultz

"Care more particularly for the individual patient than for the special features of the disease."
—William Osler, 1899

As with the confluence of color and form in an impressionist's landscape, the boundaries of medicine and psychiatry inextricably blur with advancing age. Dynamic changes in physical, neurochemical, metabolic, emotional, and behavioral functioning are virtually inseparable. Clarity and therapeutic direction often require a broadened perspective to appreciate the multiplicity of older patients' physical complaints, which is certainly true of symptoms falling within the spectrum of *somatoform* disorders in older adults.

Late life psychiatric disorders are a common, although complex, source of excess functional disability. The prevalence of severe depressive symptoms in individuals 65 to 79 years of age is approximately 15%. More than 20% of persons 80 years of age and older have similarly severe manifestations of depression (Older Americans 2000). In a collaborative study conducted under the auspices of the World Health Organization, somatization was considered to be common across cultures and associated with "significant (health) problems and disability" (Gurege et al., 1997). Psychiatric symptoms in older adults are associated with increased medical utilization, longer duration of inpatient hospitalization, diminished quality of life, and declines in functional independence. Although less is empirically known about somatization in older adults, somatization occurrence is considered widespread and its effects insidious and costly. Among patients presenting in primary care settings, Smith (1994) found a ninefold increase in healthcare utilization expenditures among older patients with concomitant somatization. Costs to patients and their families are likely inestimable.

This chapter begins with an overview of classification schemes used in the differential diagnosis of somatoform disorders, followed by a brief epidemiology review. Biological, psychological, and psychosocial mechanisms are then discussed as inseparable sources of somatization behavior in older adults. Theoretical

bases of unconscious symptom production are described and further exemplified in discussions of psychogenic movement disorders, nonepileptic seizures, and psychogenic pain disorders. The final discussions relate to common treatment barriers, therapeutic approaches of benefit to older adults, and recommendations for future research.

CLASSIFICATION SCHEMES

Within the diagnostic classification of *somatoform disorders*, the *Diagnostic and Statistical Manual of Mental Disorders*, 4th edition (DSM-IV) delineates seven categorical entities:

1. Conversion disorder
2. Hypochondriasis
3. Somatization disorder
4. Pain disorder
5. Undifferentiated somatoform disorder
6. Body dysmorphic disorder
7. Somatoform disorder not otherwise specified

The unifying trait of disorders falling within the somatoform classification is that patients present for evaluation of somatic complaints for which a physical reason is not the primary cause. By definition, a physiologic cause has either been ruled out or *independently* does not explain symptom severity, frequency, or associated degree of functional disability.

Of particular relevance to this chapter, DSM-IV omitted *organic* rule-out differentials from its classification scheme. This term appeared throughout earlier versions but was eliminated in recognition of both known and highly suspected biological substrates of primary psychiatric disorders (Spitzer, 1992). The phrase "due to a general medical disorder" appears in its place. The classification "Mental Disorders Due to a General Medical Condition" is also new to this edition. Such revisions underscore the "physical" versus "mental" distinction as an anachronistic perspective in modern medicine.

The defining feature of somatization is that covert psychological factors are presumed to play a major role in symptom production. Importantly, this role is not feigned or otherwise consciously produced. Such symptoms fall within the distinct categories of *factitious disorders* or *malingering*, which are not addressed in this chapter. DSM-IV criteria for somatoform disorders most commonly seen in older adults are presented in Tables 32-1 through 32-5.

Inspection of this classification scheme reveals serious flaws as applied to everyday clinical practice and to scientific research efforts. Many patients seen in primary care settings do not meet the symptom threshold required for major diagnostic classification, yet clearly present with excess symptom production and functional impairment (e.g., Hiller et al., 1995). For example, Fink et al. (1999) recently published a study involving 191 consecutive patients seen in family practice settings. Most patients either met criteria for somatization disorder, not otherwise specified or undifferentiated somatization disorder (29.93% and 27.3%, respectively). The prevalence of major DSM-IV somatoform diagnoses, in contrast, was relatively small, ranging between 1.0% and 8.1%. Thus, although somatization as a symptom is common, relatively few patients actually meet diagnostic criteria for major classification.

In response, alternative classification schemes have been devised. Considered overly inclusive in clinical and research settings, several authors propose abandoning *undifferentiated somatoform disorder* in favor of *multisomatoform* disorder (MSD) (Kroenke et al., 1998). MSD criteria consists of (*a*) a history of three or more currently bothersome unexplained physical complaints, and (*b*) unexplained symptoms, more days than not, for at least 2 years. In a study of 1,000 patients seen in primary care settings, MSD classification was associated with a higher number of self-reported disability days, more clinic visits, and greater clinician-perceived patient difficulty relative to patients with primary mood and anxiety disorders (Koenig, 1998). Although MSD has not been widely used, it foreshadows the need for clinically meaningful and useful diagnostic terms in an aging populace.

Finally, Lipowski (1988) is credited with early conceptualization of somatization reactions as occurring along a clinical continuum. The diagnostic and clinical utility of somatization as a spectrum disorder is greatly enhanced by this dynamic framework. In all, older individuals inherently present with more complex clinical, medical, and pharmacologic histories than younger-aged patients for whom DSM-IV or MSD frameworks were designed. Multiple symptom involvement is considered the rule rather than the exception in this population. As reviewed by Blazer (1996), geriatricians routinely manage complex disease presentations, not only with traditional medical intervention, but also via patient education, nutrition, and promotion of emotional and psychosocial well-being. To this end, diagnostic and treatment strategies are guided by attention to *geriatric syndromes* rather than specific diagnostic entities. The syndrome approach underscores the fact that competent care must address (*a*) multiple causes of symptom clusters; (*b*) functional impairment derived from or concomitant with presenting symptoms; and (*c*) the need for interdisciplinary input to improve health-related quality of life and prevent frailty. Merits of this approach are many, including promotion of evidence-based management strategies and generation of quantitative outcome and cost-effectiveness measures. Perhaps of greatest importance, however, is that the *syndromal* approach provides a more realistic understanding of psychological distress in older adults as intertwined with physical and psychiatric illness.

TABLE 32-1. *Diagnostic criteria for conversion disorder*

A. One or more symptoms or deficits affecting voluntary motor or sensory function that suggest a neurological or other general medical condition.
B. Psychological factors are judged to be associated with the symptom or deficit because the initiation or exacerbation of the symptom or deficit is preceded by conflicts or other stressors.
C. The symptom or deficit is not intentionally produced or feigned (as in factitious disorder or malingering).
D. The symptom or deficit cannot, after appropriate investigation, be fully explained by a general medical condition, or by the direct effects of a substance, or as a culturally sanctioned behavior or experience.
E. The symptom or deficit causes clinically significant distress or impairment in social, occupational, or other important areas of functioning or warrants medical evaluation.
F. The symptom or deficit is not limited to pain or sexual dysfunction, does not occur exclusively during the course of somatization disorder, and is not better accounted for by another mental disorder.

From American Psychiatric Association. *Diagnostic and statistical manual of mental disorders,* 4th ed. Washington, DC, 1994, with permission.

TABLE 32-2. *Diagnostic criteria for hypochondriasis*

A. Preoccupation with fears of having, or the idea that one has, a serious disease based on the person's misinterpretation of bodily symptoms.
B. The preoccupation persists despite appropriate medical evaluation and reassurance.
C. The belief in criterion A is not of delusional intensity (as in delusional disorder, somatic type) and is not restricted to a circumscribed concern about appearance (as in body dysmorphic disorder).
D. The preoccupation causes clinically significant distress or impairment in social, occupational, or other important areas of functioning.
E. The duration of the disturbance is at least 6 months.
F. The preoccupation is not better accounted for by generalized anxiety disorder, obsessive-compulsive disorder, panic disorder, a major depressive episode, separation anxiety, or another somatoform disorder.

From American Psychiatric Association. *Diagnostic and statistical manual of mental disorders,* 4th ed. Washington, DC, 1994, with permission.

TABLE 32-3. *Diagnostic criteria for pain disorder*

A. Pain in one or more anatomical sites is the predominant focus of the clinical presentation and is of sufficient severity to warrant clinical attention.
B. The pain causes clinically significant distress or impairment in social, occupational, or other important areas of functioning.
C. Psychological factors are judged to have an important role in the onset, severity, exacerbation, or maintenance of the pain.
D. The symptom or deficit is not intentionally produced or feigned (as in factitious disorder or malingering).
E. The pain is not better accounted for by a mood, anxiety, or psychotic disorder and does not meet criteria for dyspareunia.

From American Psychiatric Association. *Diagnostic and statistical manual of mental disorders,* 4th ed. Washington, DC, 1994, with permission.

TABLE 32-4. *Diagnostic criteria for somatization disorder*

A. A history of many physical complaints beginning before age 30 years that occur over a period of several years and result in treatment being sought or significant impairment in social, occupational, or other important areas of functioning
B. Each of the following criteria must have been met, with individual symptoms occurring at any time during the course of the disturbance:
  1. Four pain symptoms: a history of pain related to at least four different sites or functions (e.g., head, abdomen, back joints, extremities, chest, rectum, during menstruation, during sexual intercourse, or during urination)
  2. Two gastrointestinal symptoms: a history of at least two gastrointestinal symptoms other than pain (e.g., nausea, bloating, vomiting other than during pregnancy, diarrhea, or intolerance of several different foods)
  3. One sexual symptom: a history of at least one sexual or reproductive symptom other than pain (e.g., sexual indifference, erectile or ejaculatory dysfunction, irregular menses, excessive menstrual bleeding, vomiting throughout pregnancy)
  4. One pseudoneurological symptom: a history of at least one symptom or deficit suggesting a neurological condition not limited to pain (conversion symptoms such as impaired coordination or balance, paralysis or localized weakness, difficulty swallowing or lump in throat, aphonia, urinary retention, hallucinations, loss of touch or pain sensation, double vision, blindness, deafness, seizures, dissociative symptoms such as amnesia; or loss of consciousness other than fainting)
C. Either (1) or (2):
  1. After appropriate investigation, each of the symptoms in Criterion B cannot be fully explained by a known general medical condition or the direct effects of a substance (e.g., a drug of abuse, a medication)
  2. When there is a related general medical condition, the physical complaints or resulting social or occupational impairment are in excess of what would be expected from the history, physical examination, or laboratory findings
D. The symptoms are not intentionally produced or feigned (as in factitious disorder or malingering)

From American Psychiatric Association. *Diagnostic and statistical manual of mental disorders,* 4th ed. Washington, DC, 1994, with permission.

TABLE 32-5. *Diagnostic criteria for undifferentiated somatoform disorder*

A. One or more physical complaints (e.g., fatigue, loss of appetite, gastrointestinal or urinary complaints)
B. Either (1) or (2):
  1. After appropriate investigation, the symptoms cannot be fully explained by a known general medical condition or the direct effects of a substance (e.g., a drug of abuse, a medication)
  2. When there is a related general medical condition, the physical complaints or resulting social or occupational impairment are in excess of what would be expected from the history, physical examination, or laboratory findings.
C. The symptoms cause clinically significant distress or impairment in social, occupational, or other important areas of functioning.
D. The duration of the disturbance is at least 6 months.
E. The disturbance is not better accounted for by another mental disorder (e.g., another somatoform disorder, sexual dysfunction, mood disorder, anxiety disorder, sleep disorder, or psychotic disorder).
F. The symptoms are not intentionally produced or feigned (as in factitious disorder or malingering)

From American Psychiatric Association. *Diagnostic and statistical manual of mental disorders,* 4th ed. Washington, DC, 1994, with permission.

EPIDEMIOLOGY

Estimates regarding the overall prevalence of somatoform disorders vary widely, owing to differences in diagnostic criteria, sample characteristics, and even to discrepancies in determining what is considered a medical disease and what is not. In primary care settings, the prevalence of somatoform disorders was estimated to be between 22% to 58% (Fink et al., 1999). Community surveys have shown an "exaggerated concern about health" in approximately 10% of older adults (Blazer, 1996). Somatization is recognized not only as the presence of somatic symptoms without a known or sole physiologic cause, but also entails complaints made to a health professional, taking medications, or making significant life-style alterations because of a symptom burden (Pribor et al., 1994).

The literature provides conflicting information regarding demographic characteristics of late life somatization; while some researchers report that gender, education, age, depression, socioeconomic status, and social activity covary with somatization symptoms, other studies show no relation between it and gender, ethnicity, situational stress, recent bereavement, retirement, or physical disability (Barsky, 1992; Monopoli and Vaccaro, 1998). In terms of age-related factors, Pribor et al. found no age-related differences in symptom frequency, number of surgeries, medical hospitalizations, or psychiatric hospitalizations in their study of 353 women meeting DSM-V criteria for somatization disorder (Pribor et al., 1994). Only 10% of their sample, however, were above 65 years of age. Sheehan and Banerjee (1999) again underscore the difficulty of estimating the prevalence of late life somatization in this population because of discrepancies in defining clinical populations, the sampling procedures, and the diversity of measurement instruments.

MECHANISMS OF SOMATIZATION IN OLDER ADULTS

Biological Foundations

The discovery of neurologic, genetic, and biochemical links to somatization and other psychiatric conditions is advancing at a rapid pace. A Medline search restricted to the past 10 years yielded 4,867 articles identified with the keywords "psychiatric," "brain," and "imaging" or "neuroimaging." Approximately two thirds of these articles (i.e., 3,294) were published within the past 5 years.

Although in its infancy, neuroimaging techniques have recently been used to investigate metabolic correlates of conversion symptoms, such as functional hemiplegia (Marshall et al., 1997), amnesia (Yasuno et al., 2000), and gait disorders (Yazici and Kostakoglu, 1998). These preliminary studies reveal cerebral perfusion changes that suggest shared neuroanatomic pathways between symptoms of organic and functional origin. Similar techniques with more extensive histories of investigation add to our understanding of structural and functional correlates of major depression (Sato et al., 1999), anxiety disorders (Rauche et al., 2000; Soars and Mann, 1997), depression in older adults (Steffens et al., 2000), and acquired late-onset obsessive-compulsive disorder (Chacko et al., 2000).

Twin and other familial studies reveal possible genetic predispositions for somatization. For example, up to half of the stable variance in self-report of somatization symptoms resulted from genetic factors in the absence of familial-environmental effects in the "Virginia 30,000" twin-family sample (Kendler et al., 1995). In a recent study of risk factors associated with psychogenic nonepileptic seizures (PNES), families of patients with PNES reported significantly more health problems, distress, and criticism than families of patients with true epilepsy (Wood et al., 1998). Bieinvenu et al. (2000) found a higher incidence of somatoform disorders in family members of patients with hypochondriasis or other *obsessive-compulsive spectrum disorders* compared with first-degree relatives of case control probands. Similarly, Locke et al. (2000) documented a significant relationship between patients' report of irritable bowel syndrome and dyspepsia and first-degree relatives' report of abdominal pain or bowel problems. No such relationship was evidenced between patients' symptoms and spouses' report of abdominal pain or bowel problems. As in the former two studies, however, it is unclear whether familial associations indicate exposure to similar environments, reporting bias due to increased familial awareness of target symptoms, or a genetic inheritance. At any rate, neuroimaging and genetic advances provide evidence that unconscious symptom production involves biological substrates. This does not, of course, diminish the role of other important factors such as psychological conflict and psychosocial mechanisms.

Psychological Foundations

The expression of unresolved or repressed psychological conflict in physical form has long been considered a major, if not sole, basis for somatization behavior at any age. Based on the early works of Briquet, Charcot, Freud, Breuer, and Janet, somatization is understood to reflect painful psychological turmoil translated into a more acceptable and concrete (i.e., physical) form.

> ... In hysteria the unbearable idea is rendered innocuous by the quantity of excitation attached to it being transmitted into some bodily

form of expression ... conversion may be either total or partial, and it proceeds along the line of the motor or sensory innervation that is more or less intimately related to the traumatic experience." Freud, 1953.

Sadavoy (1999) provides a useful theoretic understanding of psychiatric disorders in the context of developmental changes in late life. According to this conceptualization, as impulse and action-oriented defenses diminish with normal aging, other responses to affective states become increasingly evident. Expression of these inner states, in turn, often mimics symptoms associated with axis I disorders. The expression of distress is further tied to unique personality traits, characterological adjustment, and external stressors. A list of stress reactions commonly occurring in late life is presented in Table 32-6. Thus, personality structure and both internal and external stressors are considered to mediate excess symptom production in older adults.

Relatedly, major authors in the field have emphasized the contribution of interpersonal and psychosocial factors to late life somatization. According to symptom perception models, attention and related cognitive resources once directed toward others may become progressively drawn inward (Gottlieb, 1989), promoting a greater awareness of, and focus on, bodily functioning. Selective attention, thus, serves to amplify a patient's awareness and sensitivity to changes in physical status, which in turn facilitates symptom reporting (vanWijk and Kolk, 1997). Research on symptom reporting in conditions of bodily focused and distracted attention for hypochondriacal patients (Haenen et al., 1997) and panic patients (Kroeze et al., 1996), indicates that heightened somatic awareness contributes to more reports of per-

TABLE 32-6. *Stress reactions occurring in late life*

Stresses	Psychological reactions
Social status and friendship pattern changes	Impotence, lost self-esteem, lost productivity
Physical change: beauty, strength	Narcissistic assault
Illness or infirmity	Dependency conflicts
Cognitive decline	Ego deficits or impaired affect control
Sexual decline	Shame
Bereavement	Abandonment conflicts
Economic stress	Uncertainty or lost control
Loss of stature (e.g., retirement)	Impotence, lost self-esteem, lost productivity
Relocation to institution	Forced intimacy or separation anxiety
Awareness of mortality	Death anxiety
Social status and friendship pattern changes	Separation or individuation
Family changes (e.g., parenting rolls)	Dominance and intimacy conflicts

From Sadavoy J. *Handbook of counseling and psychotherapy with older adults.* New York: John Wiley & Sons, 1999, with permission.

ceived symptoms and sensations. Difficulty meeting personal and social expectations (Blazer, 1996) or perceived inadequacies in social or personal domains (Gottlieb, 1989) are also hypothesized to underlie such functional complaints.

Alternatively, with the death of a spouse, same-age family members, or friends, a growing sense of isolation can pave the way for physical illness to become a primary means of interpersonal communication (Blazer, 1996). The opportunity for increased social interaction can incidentally or explicitly reinforce somatization behavior. Obtaining help for physical problems typically consists of contact with friends or family to provide transportation to or from the doctor's office, social connections with office staff, and repeated visits with the physician that focus on the isolated individual's life and problems. Although intended to clarify and reduce physical symptoms, such interactions simultaneously provide increased social interaction and support. Kouzis and Eaton (1998), for example, found that high distress combined with low social support in an adult community sample resulted in a fourfold increase in medical service utilization.

In summary, somatization in older adults is facilitated by a combination of biological, psychological, and psychosocial mechanisms. It is unlikely that these factors operate in isolation. Instead, they appear to interact in some weighted measure that is *individual-specific* to produce excess functional, physical, and emotional disability.

In the next section, we review theoretic considerations and common presentations of conversion in patients presenting with neurologic complaints.

COMMON FORMS OF CONVERSION DISORDERS

By definition, conversion manifests as a physical abnormality in the absence of primary central or peripheral nervous system dysfunction, and can present as virtually any neurologic sign, symptom, or syndrome. In this context, neurologic symptoms emerge as signs of extreme emotional distress or psychological conflict that cannot otherwise be adequately expressed. The defining feature of conversion is that symptoms are distanced from knowledge regarding their realm of origin; that is, such symptoms result from processes effectively barred from conscious awareness. Little is known regarding the nature of conversion in late life. The following overview of psychogenic imitators of seizures and movement and pain disorders is intended to provide some insight into somatization symptoms occurring in the context of common imitators of neurologic disease.

Psychogenic Seizure Disorders

The highest incidence of new onset seizures is now among individuals more than 65 years of age. Approximately 30% of seizures in this population are idiopathic. Cerebrovascular disease and tumor account for 30% to 50% and approximately 16% of seizures in this cohort, respectively (Eisenschenk and Gilmore, 1999). To our knowledge, no studies have been published regarding PNES in the older adult population, although this form of conversion disorder does occur in late life. Up to 40% of patients admitted to comprehensive epilepsy center for diagnostic workup of intractable seizures are found to have psychiatric imitators of epilepsy (Gates and Mercer, 1995). In younger populations, established risk factors of PNES include a history of childhood sexual or physical abuse and female gender. Links between trauma histories and conversion are well documented (Alper et al., 1993).

In any clinical arena, separating PNES from true epileptic seizures is a difficult, time, and resource-consuming endeavor. The degree of sign and symptom overlap with true epilepsy is considerable, as PNES can mimic virtually any type of seizure disorder. Further, a significant number of patients with NES have concomitant histories of neurologic insult, including seizures and other nonspecific electroencephalographic (EEG) abnormalities (Lelliot and Fenwick, 1991). Inpatient 24-hour video-EEG monitoring is required to establish the diagnosis of psychogenic seizures with relative confidence. In this setting, PNES is diagnosed when all other causes of events have been ruled out and when the patient's typical events occur, either spontaneously or via placebo induction, during the course of normal EEG recordings. The likelihood of seizures that can escape scalp EEG detection, specifically ictal discharges arising from areas deep within the brain, must also be considered unlikely in arriving at a diagnosis of PNES.

Psychogenic Movement Disorders

Psychogenic movement disorders similarly mimic almost any behavioral symptom associated with central or peripheral motor symptoms, including tremor, balance and gait disturbance, myoclonus, dyskinesias, and tics (Williams et al., 1995). Tremor and postural instability are relatively common presenting problems in older adults, and as such are discussed in greater detail below.

The incidence of psychogenic movement disorders is unknown and diagnosis continues to depend on exclusion of all other causes as well as ruling in criteria associated with non-neurologic signs and symptoms. Problems related to diagnostic classification have emerged as well. Fahn and Williams' classification system (1988), as described below, is frequently used to identify the degree of diagnostic certainty ascribed to various types of motor conversion disorders.

Tremor

Psychogenic tremor is based on exclusion of all other causes as well as the presence of atypical clinical presentations (Consensus Statement of the Movement Disorder Society on Tremor, 1998). Atypical clinical features include a complex mixture of resting, postural, and action features marked by a fluctuating course, spontaneous remission, or changing characteristics. Psychogenic tremor is typically associated with abrupt onset, abrupt remission, or both clinical features. Amplitude is often diminished during periods of distraction. Common markers of functionality are entrainment during motor coordination tasks and presence of the coactivation sign (i.e., resistance to passive movement in testing for rigidity). Psychogenic tremor can also appear in the contralateral limb on forced restraint of the involved limb.

In the largest published series of patients with psychogenic tremor, Kim et al. (1999) conducted a 10-year retrospective medical chart and videotape review in an attempt to identify clinical characteristics of this disorder. Patients were classified according to Fahn and Williams' (1988) categories of diagnostic certainty: (*a*) documented, (*b*) clinically established, (*c*) probable, and (*d*) possible. *Documented* classification required symptom improvement with psychotherapy, suggestion, placebo, or evidence of symptom remission when left alone. Patients considered to be *clinically established* evidenced movements that were inconsistent or incongruent with organic tremor, in the context of either other definite psychogenic neurologic signs, multiple somatizations, or obvious psychiatric disturbance. These two groups were merged to form the *clinically definite* group. Less stringent criteria were present in probable and possible categories, and both of these diagnostic groups were subsequently excluded from the study.

A total of 46 women and 24 men fulfilled *clinically definite* criteria. Disappearance or marked suppression of tremor when concentrating on other motor or mental tasks occurred in 80% of patients. In 88% of patients, variability in frequency, direction, amplitude, or site of tremor was evidenced. Of patients, 39% had other concomitant psychogenic movement disorders: 48% had psychogenic myoclonus, 41%

dystonia, 7% parkinsonism, and movements which were so unusual that they could not be classified occurred in 22% of these patients. Seven patients (10%) had more than one concomitant psychogenic movement disorder. The authors conclude that psychogenic tremor can be differentiated from neurologic tremor on the basis of characteristic clinical and historical features and not solely on the basis of exclusion. They acknowledge, however, that the diagnosis often requires extended or repeated observation. As with other conversion symptoms, a concomitant neurologic disorder may be present. In such cases, separating neurologic from psychogenic tremor can be an extremely difficult if not impossible task.

Gait and Balance Disorders

Although prevalence is unknown, functional gait and balance disorders perhaps are of greatest concern to the older adult population. Postural disturbances are similarly worrisome in late life, owing to the significance of increased risk of falls and related complications. Of 147 million injury-related emergency department visits from 1992 to 1995, falls were the leading cause of external injury (24%) (Burt, 1998) (Fingerhut, 1998). Among persons 75 years of age and older, falls account for 70% of accidental deaths (Sattin, 1992), with the injury rate for falls highest among persons 85 years of age and older (Tibbits, 1996). Compared with age peers admitted for other reasons, hospital stays are more than twice as long for elderly patients admitted after a fall (Dunn et al., 1992). These patients experience greater functional decline and are at greater risk for institutionalization (Kiel et al., 1991; Tinetti et al., 1993). The risk of falls and associated morbidity caused by psychogenic gait and balance disorders is unknown, but it would appear that such symptoms would inherently place individuals at greater risk compared with older adults with no history of gait or balance abnormality.

Characteristics of psychogenic gait include abrupt buckling of the knees, swaying with eyes closed, foot-dragging in the absence of leg circumduction, hyperreflexia, and Babinski sign. Rapid postural adjustment is often preserved in psychogenic gait disturbance. Inability to turn or walk when leg movements are preserved while lying down is a well-documented sign of conversion, termed *astasia-abasia.* However, ataxia caused by central cerebellar lesions and frontal gait disorders can manifest a similar dissociation (Keane, 1989). As in other motor conversion disorders, distraction can improve gait and balance dysfunction (Lempert et al., 1991).

Psychogenic Pain Disorders

The prevalence of pain disorders in older adults suggests that somatization behavior can contribute to excess functional disability in late life. Of individuals above 65 years of age, 80% to 85% experience some form of medical problem that predisposes them to pain (Gallagher et al., 2000). In general, high levels of either somatization behavior or diagnosable somatization disorder have been documented in people with chronic pain (Bacon et al., 1994), as well as in medical conditions with well-defined neuropathology. A recent examination of trends in chronic pain research reported an increase in the number of studies involving chronic pain in older adults (Norton et al., 1999). In one such study, more symptoms of somatization and major depression were documented in older adults with postherpetic neuralgia than in age-matched adults with nonpainful, but highly aversive conditions of medically explained chronic vertigo (Clark et al., 2000).

Rheumatologic disorders are particularly common in older adults. As reviewed by Michet et al. (1995), approximately 80% of individuals who have reached retirement age are afflicted with some form of rheumatologic disease, including polymyalgia rheumatica, crystalline arthropathies, degenerative joint disease, and fibromyalgia. Unique challenges in the diagnosis and management of rheumatologic conditions in this population include atypical presenting symptoms, nonspecific complaints, a relatively high number of comorbid conditions, and increased incidence of adverse drug effects. It follows that such uncertainty would increase the risk of misdiagnosis or delayed diagnosis and treatment, as well as the risk of both over- and underrecognition of related somatization behaviors in older adults.

In contrast with rheumatologic diseases of known origin, pain syndromes that do not have pathognomonic markers are often flagged as somatoform in nature. Fibromyalgia, for example, is characterized by chronic diffuse muscle pain and affects approximately 8% to 9% of patients over age 60 (Gowin, 2000; Wolfe et al., 1995). Fibromyalgia in older adults is typically a chronic condition that has been present to varying degrees over a span of many years, and rarely presents *de novo* in late life. An association between fibromyalgia and other medical conditions with somatization features (e.g., chronic fatigue and irritable bowel syndromes) has been identified (Sperber et al, 1999; Goldenberg, 1996). Relatedly, patients with fibromyalgia have been found to exhibit more somatization behaviors compared with patients with rheumatoid arthritis, osteoarthritis, and low back pain (Krag et al., 1995; Wolfe and Hawley, 1999). Diseases such as rheumatoid arthritis and fibromyalgia, characterized by a systemic pain experience, can be influenced by such psychological factors as neuroticism (Affleck et al., 1992) and self-efficacy (Keefe et al., 1997). Moreover, standard treatment recommendations include educational and therapeutic efforts directed toward improvement of stress and chronic pain management skills (Bradley and Alberts, 1999). Still, the cause of fibromyalgia remains unknown and further research is required to fully clarify whether it is a unique pain disorder or a syndrome that disseminates into the spectrum of psychogenic pain disorders.

COMORBID PSYCHOLOGICAL CONDITIONS

Late life somatoform disorders rarely occur in isolation (Fink et al., 1999). Somatization, depression, and anxiety show an excess comorbidity that is much more common than would be expected based on prevalence rates alone (Maier and Falkai, 1999). Losses inherent to advancing age are reflected in progressive declines in physical status, activity level, socialization, personal relationships, and independence. In this context, it is not surprising that depression facilitates excess functional disability in older adults (Barsky, 1992; Monopoli and Vaccaro, 1998). Anxiety is similarly considered a common pathway to increased somatic reactivity in older adults (Sheehan and Banerjee, 1999).

Depression

As with younger adults, depression is the most common emotional disorder occurring in late life (Butler et al., 1991). Almost 20 % of community dwelling older adults have significant depressive symptoms, although only 3% meet criteria for major depression (Pollock and Reynolds, 2000). Few longitudinal studies investigating the course of late-life depression have been conducted. According to the National Institute of Mental Health (NIMH) Epidemiological Catchment Area study, advanced age, changes in health status and disability, sleep disturbance, and availability of formal support services significantly affect onset and chronicity of depressive symptoms in older adults (Kennedy et al., 1991).

Complicating diagnostic and treatment efforts, depressed elderly are more likely to suffer from somatization disorders than are their peers who are not depressed (Sheehan and Banerjee, 1999) and, as the other side of the "chicken-vs.-egg dilemma," older adults are more likely to express depressive symptoms through somatic complaints (Gallo et al., 1997; Gottleib, 1989). Vegetative signs of depression include decreased or increased appetite, hypersomnia or insomnia, psychomotor agitation or retardation, and fatigue (DSM-IV, 1994). Thus, equally plausible differentials for physical complaints without a known physiologic cause include depression, somatization, other psychiatric disorders, or any combination thereof. Similar to the complexity of parsing out various contributors of somatization behavior in older adults, differential diagnosis of depression in late life is complicated by an extensive overlap between signs of normal aging, primary affective disorders, adverse reactions to medications, and neurologic disease (Brown et al., 1994; Jenike, 1988).

Unique to late life depression is the high rate of completed suicide in this age cohort. In 1988, the completed suicide rate was 26.5/100,000 in individuals between 80 and 84 years of age, more than twice the rate documented in the general population (Conwell et al., 1990; National Institutes of Health (NIH) Consensus Panel, 1992). A particularly sobering statistic is that 70% of these patients saw their primary care physician within 1 month before death and were neither treated nor apparently recognized as severely depressed by their doctor (Conwell, 1994). In recognition of such concerns, the NIMH is currently funding research to test the efficacy of depression intervention education in primary care clinics (NIMH, 2000).

Improving the detection of suicidal intent by itself may not alter morality statistics in this age group. Uncapther and Arean (2000) found that primary care physicians surveyed in this study were able to recognize depression and suicidal risk in vignettes that featured both adult and geriatric patients. However, these physicians reported less willingness to treat older patients, indicating that they believed suicidal ideation was both rational and normal in this group. Not only were physicians less willing to initiate therapeutic measures themselves, but they were also not optimistic that mental health professionals could significantly help older patients. If such attitudes were extrapolated to treatment efforts directed toward other psychiatric disorders of late life, somatization may similarly persist as an unfortunate consequence of recalcitrant agism.

Anxiety

Anxiety disorders are also common in later life, yet are among the least studied and clinically recognized of the psychiatric syndromes in this population (Sadavoy and LeClair, 1997). The 6-month prevalence rate of all anxiety disorders occurring in individuals 65 years of age and older is 19.7% (Blazer et al., 1991). Among medically ill older patients, 10% to 20% have clinically significant symptoms of anxiety (Hocking and Koenig, 1995). Moreover, prognosis, illness duration, and antidepressant response in major psychiatric syndromes are significantly related to anxiety (Flint, 1994).

Anxiety, similar to somatization and depressive symptoms, can be indirectly expressed through a multitude of physical symptoms, including fatigue, disturbed sleep, nausea, diarrhea, and dysphasia (DSM-IV, 1994). Masked anxiety can serve to facilitate medical treatment seeking in older adults because older adults more likely viewed these symptoms as signs of medical illness. However, anxiety can also produce significant medical complications in older adults, including cardiac arrhythmias and insomnia (Sheikh, 1994). It is important to recognize and treat all clinically significant problems presenting in late life, regardless whether a clear demarcation is possible between psychological and primary medical disorders.

TREATMENT

William Osler's quote at the beginning of this chapter speaks to the topic of treatment for somatization in older adults. If the individual takes precedence over "the special features of the disease," treatment of symptoms that increase functional disability and diminish the patient's quality of life is no less a charge than that imposed on treatment of well-defined medical conditions. In fact, it could be argued that the certainty of diagnosis is relatively low in many medical conditions for which various types of treatment are routinely initiated.

Barriers To Treatment

Although numerous barriers to treatment of somatization exist, at least four major obstacles are seen to therapeutic delivery and efficacy in older adults:

1. Identifying psychiatric problems in need of attention
2. Generating recommendations for treatment by physicians and related healthcare providers
3. Facilitating patients' willingness to pursue treatment
4. Obtaining appropriate therapy and treatment services

To some extent, such issues have been raised in earlier parts of this chapter. These four treatment obstacles are specifically discussed below.

Medically unexplained physical symptoms are common, with only 10% to 25% of symptoms such as chest pain, dizziness, and fatigue attributed to primary organic disease (Fink et al., 1999). Although the numbers are declining, statistics reflecting the failure of primary care physicians to recognize psychological disorders in older adults are unacceptably high (Rogers et al., 1993). Patients' reluctance to complain about emotional distress, as previously described, occurs in the context of widespread misunderstanding and stigma about psychiatric illness in general. Thus, patients' deliberate or unconscious masking of psychological distress by more socially acceptable complaints of physical illness and disability notably contributes to underdetection of these psychiatric disorders (Gottlieb, 1989; Waxman, 1986), particularly with regard to somatization in older adults.

Once identified, psychological disorders are undeniably undertreated in this population. Bridging the seemingly monumental gap between diagnosis and treatment in older patients with less clearly defined symptoms appears both rare and difficult. Undertreatment of psychiatric symptoms in primary care settings has been attributed to multiple factors, including limited training and awareness of contemporary advances in treatment options. Overreliance on biomedical models of psychological disorders and attitudinal biases further hinders promotion of more comprehensive therapeutic intervention (Alexopoulous, 1992; Callahan et al., 1992). In a recent study in the United Kingdom, only 10% of older adults with depression were prescribed antidepressants, although this group consulted primary and secondary healthcare providers far more frequently than cohorts who were not depressed cohorts (Livingston et al., 1997).

Individual attitudes, beliefs, and biases further complicate treatment considerations. Concomitant psychiatric disorders, which frequently have the greater impact on daily functioning, are often readily dismissed—or worse, considered an acceptable burden of normal aging. Consider the sentiment echoed in the following public address by a prominent writer in the field:

> ...(regarding hypochondriacal symptoms in older adults) "therapeutic interventions .... should be modest and only aim to produce limited improvement...simple benign, old-fashioned interventions are most helpful, such as hot water bottles and heating pads..."

One must ask the question how often in medicine the stated goal is "to produce limited improvement"

in an otherwise treatable disorder. Medical utilization and epidemiologic data suggest this is not acceptable. Haas et al. (1999) examined the degree of psychopathology in a sample of older health maintenance organization patients with high utilization records. High-utilizing patients evidenced significantly more psychopathology, perceived their health status as worse than that of other medial subpopulations, and utilized approximately 40% more visits to medical providers. According to the Global Burden of Disease study (Murray and Lopez, 1996) as the world population ages and infectious diseases are controlled, psychiatric and neurologic conditions are projected to increase from 10.5% of total burden to almost 15% in 2020. The impact of an ever-shrinking healthcare system that defines cost efficiency in terms of seeing more patients for less time is no less accountable for this problem.

Once barriers associated with recognition and intention to treat are overcome, problems associated with initiating treatment must be addressed. Such problems occur in the form of patients' resistance to treatment and in the availability of appropriate treatment and services to individuals with late-life somatization.

INTERVENTION ISSUES

As a psychological disorder, the underlying need or purpose driving excess symptom production cannot be successfully treated with pharmacologic intervention alone (Barsky, 1992). Medication is often an invaluable adjunct to treatment, particularly in patients with masked depression or anxiety. However, psychotherapy is considered the treatment of choice for primary somatization disorders. Smith et al. (2000) prospectively studied 4,401 consecutive inpatient referrals to adult consultation-liaison psychiatry services affiliated with two major teaching hospitals. Of 127 patients diagnosed with somatoform disorders, psychiatrists recommended additional laboratory tests for 14%, additional medical or surgical consultations for 11%, and an increased vigor of medical treatment of 13%. Medications recommended for patients included antidepressants (40%), anxiolytics (18%), sedatives (18%), and antipsychotics (10%). Psychological therapy was recommended for 76% of patients diagnosed with somatoform disorders.

An often omitted, although crucial step, in initiating therapeutic treatment with older adults is assessment of cognitive integrity. A high degree of overlap exists among signs of normal aging, affective disorders, and neurologic illness in this cohort. Memory complaints, for example, are inherent to emotional distress and are positively correlated with age. In a community sample of 810 adults, Bassett and Folstein (1993) found 43% of participants 65 to 74 years of age complained of memory impairment as did 88% of those 85 and older. A higher prevalence of memory complaints occurred in individuals with affective disturbance, anxiety, and adjustment disorders. Multivariate analysis revealed age, emotional distress, and physical illness to be independent predictors of memory complaint. The frequency of concomitant emotional and behavioral sequelae in patients with neurologic disease is similarly high. For example, mood and personality disorders are often the earliest signs of Huntington's disease (Mendez, 1994); depression, apathy and behavior dyscontrol are known concomitants of stroke and frontal lobe insult (Starkstein et al., 1993; Stuss et al., 1992); depression is seen in approximately 40% of patients with Parkinson's disease, and in approximately 17% to 29% of patients in early stages of Alzheimer's disease.

Concomitant dementia, brain injury, or psychiatrically based memory impairment present unique challenges in treating psychiatric illness in older adults. Therapeutic intervention is guided by comprehensive diagnostic assessment that includes review of relevant clinical history, psychosocial resources, and cognitive status. The primary goals of neuropsychological evaluation in this context are to delineate the individual's cognitive strengths and weaknesses; to use qualitative and quantitative findings in identifying relevant clinical syndromes; and to develop realistic treatment recommendations based on integration of clinical, psychological, and cognitive data (Bortz and O'Brien, 1995; LaRue, 1992).

In the absence of cognitive impairment, traditional psychotherapeutic approaches require minimal, if any, fundamental modification in their application to healthy older adults. However, issues that can affect treatment efficacy include a potential need to use age-relevant examples, to attend to complications caused by primary sensory deficits, and to minimize the impact of attitudinal barriers on the working alliance and therapeutic process. Furthermore, because psychological problems are often perceived by older adults to be somatic in nature, initial treatment targeting somatic features of emotional disorders may be better tolerated than those that primarily focus on the patient's affective experience. Targeting select somatic symptoms (e.g., insomnia), which can be nonspecific signs of emotional distress, has been shown to be an effective and nonthreatening means of estab-

lishing a therapeutic relationship (Friedman et al., 1991; see review by Engle-Friedman et al., 1992).

No controlled treatment studies specifically targeting somatization in older adults have been published (Sheehan and Banerjee, 1999). Recent treatment outcome studies of late life depression indicate that 80% of older adults improve after receiving appropriate medication, psychotherapy, or both (Little et al., 1998). In fact, a combination of antidepressant medication and psychotherapy has been shown to be more effective at reducing depressive recurrence over a 3-year period than either treatment alone (Reynolds et al., 1999).

SUMMARY AND DIRECTIONS FOR FUTURE RESEARCH

In conclusion, recognition of somatization in late life remains a challenging endeavor. Limitations imposed by adherence to strict diagnostic criteria are considerable, and it appears more useful to conceptualize somatization in terms of individual-specific syndromes or symptoms. Somatization in older adults is likely the product of a combination of biological, psychological, and social factors. Recognition that somatization is truly caused by unconscious symptom production, not unlike more common neurologic deficits accompanied by impaired awareness, cannot be overemphasized. Reciprocal relationships between depression, anxiety, and late life somatization are considered common. Finally, awareness of unique treatment barriers affecting older adults, the persistence of agism, and risks associated with not treating somatization in this population provide a basis for moving forward in both diagnostic and treatment arenas.

As for future research, empirical questions and answers necessarily emerge from fundamental bodies of scientific knowledge. In this regard, development of a core knowledge base regarding somatization in older adults is in its infancy. Diagnostic clarity and consensus are yet to be realized. Education and use of effective screening measures provide some promise of improving recognition of somatization in primary care settings (Kroenke et al., 1998). However, it is discouraging to find that even when somatization is identified, such recognition may have little to no impact on subsequent treatment (Katona and Livingston, 2000). Means of effectively lowering treatment barriers clearly require further development. Systematic advancement of methods to assess neurologic and other forms of pathologic comorbidity is essential, given their prevalence and related treatment implications in this cohort. Further exploration of hypotheses regarding common final pathways between primary neurologic and somatization disorders is needed, as are efforts to discover genetic predispositions to psychiatric imitators of neurologic illness. Thus, collaborative works by experts in the fields of neuroscience, geriatric medicine, psychiatry, primary care, and social sciences will undoubtedly produce a higher yield of answers to basic, but key, empirical questions regarding the complex nature and treatment of late life somatization.

REFERENCES

Affleck G, Urrows S, Tennen H, et al. Daily coping with pain from rheumatoid arthritis: Patterns and correlates. *Pain* 1992;51(2):221–229.

Alexopoulous GS. Geriatric depression reaches maturity. *Int J Geriatr Psychiatry* 1992;7:305–362.

American Psychiatric Association. *Diagnostic and statistical manual of mental disorders, 4th ed. Washington, DC: American Psychiatric Association, 1994.*

American Psychological Association. What practitioners should know about working with older adults. Washington, DC: American Psychological Association, 1997.

Bacon NM, Bacon SF, Atkinson JH, et al. Somatization symptoms in chronic low back pain patients. *Psychosom Med* 1994;56(2):118–127.

Barsky AJ. The diagnosis and management of hypochondriacal concerns in the elderly. *J Geriatr Psychiatry* 1992;25(1):129–141.

Bassett SS, Folstein MF. Memory complaint, memory performance, and psychiatric diagnosis: a community study. *J Geriatr Psychiatry Neurol* 1993;6(2):105–111.

Bienvenu OJ, Samuels JF, Riddle MA, et al. The relationship of obsessive-compulsive disorder to possible spectrum disorders: results from a family study. *Biol Psychiatry* 2000;48(4):287–293.

Blazer D. Geriatric psychiatry. In: Hales R, Yudofsky S, eds. *The American Psychiatric Press textbook of psychiatry.* Washington, DC: American Psychiatric Press, 1996.

Blazer D, George LK, Hughes D. The epidemiology of anxiety disorders: an age comparison. In: Saltzman C, Lebowitz BD, eds. *Anxiety in the elderly.* New York: Springer, 1991.

Bortz JJ, O'Brien KP. Psychotherapy with older adults: theoretical issues, empirical findings, and clinical applications. In: Nussbaum PD, ed. *Handbook of neuropsychology and aging.* New York: Plenum Press, 1995.

Bradley LA, Alberts KR. Pain management in the rheumatic diseases. *Rheum Dis Clin North Am* 1999;25(1):215–232.

Brown RG, Scott LD, Bench CJ, et al. Cognitive function in depression: its relationship to the presence and severity of intellectual decline. *Psychol Med* 1994;2(4):829–847.

Burt CW. Injury visits to hospital emergency departments: United States, 1992–95. *Vital Health Stat* 1998;13:1–76.

Butler RN, Lewis MI, Sutherland T. *Aging and mental health: positive psychosocial and biomedical approaches* 4th ed. Columbus, OH: Charles E. Merrill, 1991.

Callahan CM, Nienaber NA, Hendrie HC, et al. Depression of elderly outpatients: primary care physicians' attitudes and practice patterns. *J Gen Intern Med* 1992;7 (1):26–31.

Chacko RC, Corbin MA, Harper RG. Acquired obsessive-compulsive disorder associated with basal ganglia lesions. *J Neuropsychiatry Clin Neurosci* 2000;12(2):269–272.

Clark MR, Heinberg LJ, Haythornthwaite JA, et al. Psychiatric symptoms and distress differ between patients with postherpetic neuralgia and peripheral vestibular disease. *J Psychosom Res* 2000;48:51–57.

Conwell Y, Rotenberg M, Caine ED. Completed suicide at age 50 and over. *J Am Geriatr Soc* 1990;38(6):640–644.

Conwell Y. Suicide in elderly patients. In: Schneider L, Reynolds III C, Lebowitz B, et al., eds. *Diagnosis and treatment of depression in late life.* Washington, DC: American Psychiatric Press, 1994.

Dunn JE, Rudberg MA, Furner SE, et al. Mortality, disability, and falls in older persons: the role of underlying disease and disability. *Am J Public Health* 1992;82:395–400.

Eisenschenk S, Gilmore R. Adult-onset seizures: clinical solutions to a challenging patient work-up. *Geriatrics* 1999;54(11):18–28.

Engle-Friedman M, Bootzin RR, Hazelwood L, et al. An evaluation of behavioral treatments for insomnia in the older adult. *J Clin Psychol* 1992;48(1):77–90.

Fahn S, Williams DT. Psychogenic dystonia. *Adv Neurol* 1988;50:431–455.

Fink P, Sorensen L, Engberg M, et al. Somatization in primary care: prevalence, health care utilization, and general practitioner recognition. *Psychosomatics* 1999;40(4):330–338.

Flint AJ. Epidemiology and comorbidity of anxiety disorders in the elderly. *Am J Psychiatry* 1994;151(5):640–649.

Freud S. *The defense neuro-psychoses.* In: Collected papers. Vol. 1. London: Hogarth, 1953:59–75.

Friedman L, Bliwise DL, Yesavage JA, et al. A preliminary study comparing sleep restriction and relaxation treatments for insomnia in older adults. *J Gerontol* 1991; 46(1):P1–P8.

Gallo JJ, Rabins PV, Iliffe S. The "research magnificent" in late life: psychiatric epidemiology and the primary health care of older adults. *Int J Psychiatry Med* 1997;27(3):185–204.

Goldenberg DL. Controversies in fibromyalgia and related conditions. *Rheum Dis Clin North Am* 1996;22(2):393–406.

Gottlieb GL. Hypochondriasis: a psychosomatic problem in the elderly. *Adv Psychosom Med* 1989;19:67–84.

Gureje O, Simon GE, Ustun TB, et al. Somatization in cross cultural perspective: a World Health Organization study in primary care. *Am J Psychiatry* 1997;154(7):989–995.

Haas LJ, Spendlove DC, Silver MP, et al. Psychopathology and emotional distress among older high-utilizing health maintenance organization patients. *Journal of Geropsychology* 1999;54A(11):M577–M582.

Haenen AM, Schmidt AJ, Schoenmakers M, et al. Suggestibility in hypochondriacal patients and healthy control subjects: an experimental case-control study. *Psychosomatics* 1997;38(6):543–547.

Hiller W, Rief W, Fichter MM. Further evidence for a broader concept of somatization disorder using the somatic symptom index. *Psychosomatics* 1995;36(3):285–294.

Hocking LB, Koenig HG. Anxiety in medically ill older patients: a review and update. *Int J Psychiatry Med* 1995; 25(3):221–238.

Jenike MA. Psychoactive drugs in the elderly: antidepressants. *Geriatrics* 1988;43(11):43–57.

Keane JR. Hysterical gait disorders: 60 cases. *Neurology* 1989;39:586–589.

Keefe FJ, Lefebvre JC, Maixner W, et al. Self-efficacy for arthritis pain: relationship to perception of thermal laboratory pain stimuli. *Arthritis Care and Research* 1997; 10(3):177–184.

Kendler KS, Walters EE, Truett KR, et al. A twin-family study of self-report symptoms of panic-phobia and somatization. *Behav Genet* 1995;25(6):499–515.

Kennedy GJ, Kelman HR, Thomas C. Persistence and remission of depressive symptoms in late life. *Am J Psychiatry* 1991;148(2):174–178.

Kiel DP, O'Sullivan P, Teno JM, et al. Health care utilization and functional status in the aged following a fall. *Med Care* 1991;29:221–228.

Kim YJ, Pakiam S-I, Lang AE. Historical and clinical features of psychogenic tremor: a review of 70 cases. *Can J Neurol Sci* 1999;26:190–195.

Kouzis AC, Eaton WW. Absence of social networks, social support, and health services utilization. *Psychol Med* 1998;28:1301–1310.

Krag NJ, Norregaard J, Hindberg I, et al. Psychopathology measured by established self-rating scales and correlated to serotonin measures in patients with fibromyalgia. *European-Psychiatry* 1995;10(8):404–409.

Kroenke K, Spitzer RL, deGruy FV, et al. A symptom checklist to screen for somatoform disorders in primary care. *Psychosomatics* 1998;39(3):263–272.

Kroeze S, van den Hout M, Haenen MA, et al. Symptom reporting and interoceptive attention in panic patients. *Percept Mot Skills* 1996;82(3):1019–1026.

LaRue A. *Aging and neuropsychological assessment.* New York: Plenum, 1992.

Lipowski ZJ. Somatization: The concept and its clinical application. *Am J Psychiatry* 1988;145(11):1358–1368.

Little JT, Reynolds CF, Dew MA, et al. How common is resistance to treatment in recurrent, nonpsychotic geriatric depression? *Am J Psychiatry* 1998;155(8):1035–1038.

Livingston G, Manela M, Katona C. Cost of community care for older people. *Br J Psychiatry* 1997;171:56–59.

Locke GR, Zinsmeister AR, Talley NJ, et al. Familial association in adults with functional gas disorders. *Mayo Clin Proc* 2000;75(9):907–912.

Maier W, Falkai P. The epidemiology of comorbidity between depression, anxiety disorders and somatic diseases. *Int Clin Psychopharmacol* 1999;14(2):S1–S6.

Marshall JC, Halligan PW, Fink GR, et al. The functional anatomy of a hysterical paralysis. *Cognition* 1997;64(1):B1–B8.

Mendez MF. Huntington's disease: update and review of neuropsychiatric aspects. *Int J Psychiatry Med* 1994;24 (3):189–208.

Michet CJ, Evans JM, Fleming KC, et al. Common rheumatologic diseases in elderly patients. *Mayo Clin Proc* 1995;70(12):1205–1214.

Monopoli A, Vaccaro A. Depression, hypochondriasis, and demographic variables in a non-institutionalized elderly sample. *Clinical Geropsychologist* 1998;19(3):75–79.

Morrison J. Managing somatization disorder. *Dis Month* 1990;36(10):537–591.

Murray CJL, Lopez AD, eds. The global burden of disease and injury series. Vol. I: *A comprehensive assessment of mortality and disability from diseases, injuries, and risk factors in 1990 and projected to 2020.* Cambridge, MA: Harvard School of Public Health on behalf of the World Health Organization and the World Bank, Harvard University Press. (NIH Publication No. 01-4586), 1996.

National Institute of Mental Health. *Older adults: depression and suicide facts.* (NIH Publication No. 01-4593). Rockville, MD: Author, 2000. IQ17

National Institutes of Health (NIH) Consensus Panel, 1992.

Norton PJ, Asmundson GJ, Norton GR, et al. Growing pain: ten-year research trends in the study of chronic pain and headache. *Pain* 1999;79(1):59–65.

Pollock BG, Reynolds CF. Depression late in life. *Harvard Mental Health Letter* 2000;17(3):3–5.

Pribor EF, Smith DS, Yutzy SH. Somatization disorder in elderly patients. *Am J Geriatr Psychiatry* 1994:109–117.

Rauche et al, 2000.

Reynolds CF, Frank E, Perel JM, et al. Nortriptyline and interpersonal psychotherapy as maintenance therapies for recurrent major depression: a randomized controlled trial in patients older than 59 years. *JAMA* 1999;281(1): 39–45.

Rogers WH, Wells KB, Meredith LS, et al. Outcomes for adult outpatients with depression under prepaid or fee-for-service financing. *Arch Gen Psychiatry* 1993;50(7): 517–525.

Sadavoy J. *Handbook of counseling and psychotherapy with older adults.* New York: John Wiley & Sons, 1999.

Sadavoy J, LeClair JK. Treatment of anxiety disorders in late life. *Can J Psychiatry* 1997;42(1):28S–34S.

Sato R, Bryan RN, Fried LP. Neuroanatomic and functional correlates of depressed mood: the Cardiovascular Health Study. *Am J Epidemiol* 1999;150(9):919–929.

Sattin RW. Falls among older persons: a public health perspective. *Annu Rev Public Health* 1992;13:489–508.

Sheehan B, Banerjee S. Review: somatization in the elderly. *Int J Geriatr Psychiatry* 1999;14:1044–1049.

Smith GC, Clarke DM, Handrinos D, et al. Consultation-liaison psychiatrists' management of somatoform disorders. *Psychosomatics* 2000;41(6):481–499.

Smith GR. The course of somatization and its effects on utilization of health care resources. *Psychosomatics* 1994;35(3):263–267.

Smith SL, Sherrill KA, Colenda CC. Assessing and treating anxiety in elderly persons. *Psychiatr Serv* 1995;46(1): 36–59.

Soars and Mann, 1997.

Sperber AD, Atzmon Y, Neumann L, et al. Fibromyalgia in the irritable bowel syndrome: studies of prevalence and clinical implications. *Am J Gastroenterol* 1999;94(12):3541–3546.

Starkstein SE, Federoff JP, Price TR, et al. Apathy following cerebrovascular lesions. *Stroke* 1993;24(11):1625–1630.

Steffens DC, Byrum CE, McQuoid DR, et al. Hippocampal volume in geriatric depression. *Biol Psychiatry* 2000;48 (4):301–309.

Stuss DT, Gow CA, Hetherington CR. "No longer Gage": frontal lobe dysfunction and emotional changes. *J Consult Clin Psychol* 1992;60(3):349–359.

Tibbits GM. Patients who fall: how to predict and prevent injuries. *Geriatrics* 1996;51:24–31.

Tinetti ME, Liu WL, Claus EB. Predictors and prognosis of inability to get up after falls among elderly persons. *JAMA* 1993;269:65–70.

Uncapher H, Arean PA. Physicians are less willing to treat suicidal ideation in older patients. *J Am Geriatr Soc* 2000;48(2):188–192.

van Wijk CM, Kolk AM. Sex differences in physical symptoms: The contribution of symptom perception theory. *Soc Sci Med* 1997;45(2):231–246.

Waxman HM. Community mental health care for the elderly—a look at the obstacles. *Public Health Rep* 1986; 101(3):294–300.

Williams DT, Ford B, Fahn S. Phenomenology and psychopathology related to psychogenic movement disorders. *Adv Neurol* 1995;65:231–257.

Wolfe F, Hawley DJ. Evidence of disordered symptom appraisal in fibromyalgia: increased rates of reported comorbidity and comorbidity severity. *Clin Exp Rheumatol* 1999;17(3)297–303.

Wood BL, McDaniel S, Burchfiel K, et al. Factors distinguishing families of patients with psychogenic seizures from families of patients with epilepsy. *Epilepsia* 1998;39 (4):432–437.

Yasuno F, Nishikawa T, Nakagawa Y, et al. Functional anatomical study of psychogenic amnesia. *Psychiatry Res* 2000;99(1):43–57.

Yazici KM, Kostakoglu L. Cerebral blood flow changes in patients with conversion disorder. *Psychiatry Res* 1998; 83(3):163–168.

SUGGESTED READING

Allum JH, Shepard NT. An overview of the clinical use of dynamic posturography in the differential diagnosis of balance disorders. *J Vestib Res* 1999;9(4):223–252.

Anooshian J, Streltzer J, Goebert D. Effectiveness of a psychiatric pain clinic. *Psychosomatics* 1999;40(3): 226–232.

Backman L, Almkyist O, Nyberg L, et al. Functional changes in brain activity during priming in Alzheimer's disease. *J Cogn Neurosci* 2000;12(1):134–141.

Barsky AJ, Orav EJ, Ahern DK, et al.. Somatic style and symptom reporting in rheumatoid arthritis. *Psychosomatics* 1999;(40(5):396–403.

Bellack, eds. *The clinical psychology handbook* , 2nd ed. Elmsford, NY: Pergamon Press, 19xx:430–464.

Binzer M, Andersen PM, Kullgren G. Clinical characteristics of patients with motor disability due to conversion disorder: a prospective control group study. *J Neurol Neurosurg Psychiatry* 1997;63(1):83–88.

Binzer M, Kullgren G. Motor conversion disorder: a prospective 2- to 5-year follow-up study. *Psychosomatics* 1997;39(6):519–527.

Black JL, Allison TG, Williams DE, et al. Effect of intervention for psychological distress on rehospitalization rates in cardiac rehabilitation patients. *Psychosomatics* 1998;39(2):134–143.

Black JL, Barth EM, Williams DE, et al. Stiff-man syndrome: results of interviews and psychologic testing. *Psychosomatics* 1998;39(1):38–44.

Bostwick JM, Masterson BJ. Psychopharmacological treatment of delirium to restore mental capacity. *Psychosomatics* 1998;39(2):112–117.

Burvill PW, Stampfer H, Hall W. Does depressive illness in the elderly have a poor prognosis? *Aust N Z J Psychiatry* 1986;20(4):422–427.

Copeland JRM. Comparative epidemiology of psychiatric disorders in older age: prevalence and incidence. In: Stefanis C, Hippius H, Muller-Spahn F, eds. *Neuropsychiatry in old age: an update*. Seattle: Hogrefe & Huber, 1996.

Crimlisk HL, Bhatia K, Cope H, et al. Slater revisited: six year follow up study of patients with medically unexplained motor symptoms. *BMJ* 1998;316(7131):582–590.

Crow SJ, Collins J, Justic M, et al. Psychopathology following cardioverter defibrillator implantation. *Psychosomatics* 1998;39(4):305–310.

de Beurs E, Beekman AT, van Balkom AJ, et al. Consequences of anxiety in older persons: its effect on disability, well-being and use of health services. *Psychol Med* 1999;29(3):583–593.

Deuschl G, Bain P, Brin M. Consensus statement of the Movement Disorder Society on tremor: ad hoc scientific committee. *Mov Disord* 1998;13(Suppl 3):2–23.

Epstein SA, Kay G, Clauw D, et al. Psychiatric disorders in patients with fibromyalgia: A multicenter investigation. *Psychosomatics* 1999;40(1):57–63.

Factor SA, Podskalny GD, Molho ES, et al. Psychogenic movement disorders: frequency, clinical profile, and characteristics. *J Neurol Neurosurg Psychiatry* 1995;59(4): 406–412.

Foong J, Ridding M, Cope H, et al. Corticospinal function in conversion disorder. *J Neuropsychiatry Clin Neurosci* 1997;9(2):302–303.

Fulop G, Strain JJ, Fahs MC, et al. A prospective study of the impact of psychiatric comorbidity on length of hospital stays of elderly medical-surgical inpatients. *Psychosomatics* 1998;39(3):273–280.

Gowin KM. Diffuse pain syndromes in the elderly. *Rheum Dis Clin North Am* 2000;26(3):673–683.

Halligan PW, Athwal BS, Oakley DA, et al. Imaging hypnotic paralysis: implications for conversion hysteria. *Lancet* 2000;18:986–987.

Hargrave R, Rafal R. Depression in corticobasal degeneration. *Psychosomatics* 1998;39(5):481–482.

Haut MW, Petros TV, Frank RG, et al. Speed of processing within semantic memory following severe closed head injury. *Brain Cogn* 1991;17(1):31–41.

Heckers S, Anick D, Boverman JF, et al. Priapism following olanzapine administration in a patient with multiple sclerosis. *Psychosomatics* 1998;39(3):288–290.

Jackson JL, O'Malley PG, Kroenke K. Clinical predictors of mental disorders among medical outpatients: validation of the "S4" model. *Psychosomatics* 1998;39(5):431–436.

Johnson SK, DeLuca J, Natelson BH. Assessing somatization disorder in the chronic fatigue syndrome. *Psychosom Med* 1996;58:50–57.

Kente RL. Elements of neuroticism in relation to headache symptomatology. *Psychol Rep* 1997;80(1):227–235.

Kishi Y, Kathol RG. Integrating medical and psychiatric treatment in an inpatient medical setting: the type IV program. *Psychosomatics* 1999;40(4):345–355.

Kroenke K, Spitzer RL, deGruy FV, et al. Multisomatoform disorder: an alternative to undifferentiated somatoform disorder for the somatizing patient in primary care. *Arch Gen Psychiatry* 1997;54(4):352–358.

Kunkel EJ, Bakker JR, Myers RE, et al. Biopsychosocial aspects of prostate cancer. *Psychosomatics* 2000;41(2):85–94.

Lenze EJ, Mulsant BH, Shear MK, et al. Comorbid anxiety disorders in depressed elderly patients. *Am J Psychiatry* 2000;157(5):722–728.

Lipton RB, Goadsby P, Silberstein SD. Classification and epidemiology of headache. *Clinical Cornerstone* 1999;1 (6):1–10.

Lydiard RB, Brawman-Mintzer O. Anxious depression. *J Clin Psychiatry* 1998;59(18):10–17.

Maruff P, Velakoulis D. The voluntary control of motor imagery: imagined movements in individuals with feigned motor impairment and conversion disorder. *Neuropsychologica* 2000;38(9):1251–1260.

Moene FC, Hoogduin KA, Van Dyck R. The inpatient treatment of patients suffering from (motor) conversion symptoms: A description of eight cases. *International Journal of Clinical Experimental Hypnosis* 1998;46(2):171–190.

Monday K, Jankovic J. Psychogenic myoclonus. *Neurology* 1993;43(2):349–352.

Nicholson NL, Blanchard EB Appelbaum KA. Two studies of the occurrence of psychophysiological symptoms in chronic headache patients. *Behav Res Ther* 1990;28(3): 195–203.

Okasha A, Ismail MK, Khalil AH, et al. A psychiatric study of nonorganic chronic headache patients. *Psychosomatics* 1999;40(3):233–238.

Sadavoy J. Integrated psychotherapy for the elderly. *Can J Psychiatry* 1994;39(8):19–26.

Sadavoy J, Leszcz M. *Treating the elderly with psychotherapy: the scope for change in later life.* Madison, CT: International Universities Press, 1987.

Scarrabelotti M, Carroll M. Awareness of remembering achieved through automatic and conscious processes in multiple sclerosis. *Brain Cogn* 1998;38(2):183–201.

Schneider G, Kruse A, Nehen HG, et al. The prevalence and differential diagnosis of subclinical depressive syndromes in inpatients 60 years and older. *Psychother Psychosom* 2000;69(5):251–260.

Shaibani A, Sabbagh MN. Pseudoneurologic syndromes: recognition and diagnosis. *Am Fam Phys* 1998;57(10):1–10.

Sloane PD, Hartman M, Mitchell CM.. Psychological factors associated with chronic dizziness in patients 60 and older. *J Am Geriatr Soc* 1994;42:847–852.

Smith BB. Treatment of dementia: healing through cultural arts. *Pride Institute Journal of Long Term Home Health Care* 1992;11:37–45.

Spence SA, Crimlisk HL, Cope H, et al. Discrete neurophysiological correlates in prefrontal cortex during hysterical and feigned disorder of movement. *Lancet* 2000; 355(9211):1243–1244.

Tachibana H, Miyata Y, Takeda M, et al. Event-related potentials reveal memory deficits in Parkinson's disease. *Brain Res Cogn Brain Res* 1999;8(2):165–172.

Teasell R, Shapiro A. Chronic conversion disorders. *Arch Phys Med Rehabil* 1998;79(11):1482–1483.

Terao T, Collinson S. Imaging hypnotic paralysis. *Lancet* 2000;8:162–163.

Umapathy C, Ramchandani D, Lamdan RM, et al. Competency evaluations on the consultation-liaison service: some overt and covert aspects. *Psychosomatics* 1999;40 (1):28–33.

Watanabe TK, O'Dell MW, Togliatti TJ. Diagnosis and rehabilitation strategies for patients with hysterical hemiparesis: a report of four cases. *Arch Phys Med Rehabil* 1998; 79(6):709–714.

Wolfe F, Ross K, Anderson IJ, et al. The prevalence and characteristics of fibromyalgia in the general population. *Arthritis Rheum* 1995;38(1):19–28.

Woodman CL, Tabatabai F. New-onset panic disorder after right thalamic infarct. *Psychosomatics* 1998;39(2): 165–167.

33

Neurorehabilitation

Jonathan L. Fellus

INTRODUCTION

Among all of the subspecialties in the field of neurology, most practitioners are probably least familiar with *neurorehabilitation*. This chapter covers the field of rehabilitation following the three most common or important clinical neurologic entities seen in rehabilitation facilities. They are cerebral infarct (CI), acquired brain injury (ABI), which includes traumatic brain injury (TBI), and spinal cord injury (SCI). Focus is on the clinical approach to the elderly patient who sustains injuries requiring neurorehabilitation rather than the aging patient with remote onset of a disabling neurologic event. Discussion begins with a description of the rehabilitation process (i.e., the nature of recovery and how patients flow through various levels of care). The diagnosis and management of the most common problems associated with CI, ABI, and SCI are presented next. Finally, important syndromes that overlap different diagnostic groups are presented. Although rehabilitation can and should begin in the acute care setting, focus here is on the physician's role during the inpatient rehabilitation stay.

DEFINITION AND BACKGROUND

Traditionally, neurologists have concerned themselves with system impairment at the level of the organ and descriptions of the natural history of a disease or syndrome by observation over long periods of time. However, with recent research trends focusing on outcomes and quality-of-life measures, neurologists are increasingly faced with the challenge of not just diagnosing a clinical entity but minimizing an individual's dysfunction as a result of disease. Moreover, with shortened acute care encounters, more neurologists are following their patients into the rehabilitation arena where length of stay is still, relatively speaking, long. At the same time, practitioners of physical medicine and rehabilitation or physiatrists

who focus on a person's functioning are moving toward a greater emphasis on the underlying mechanism of disease because of increased pharmacologic interventions and the economic imperative of shortened lengths of stay. Therefore, the two fields find themselves moving rapidly toward each other.

The field of neurorehabilitation concerns itself ultimately with maximizing functional recovery after a neurologic insult. Rehabilitation after neurologic injury requires clinical attention to the patient as a whole and in the context of that person's various societal roles. Neurologists can and should provide principal care (distinguished from primary care which is rendered to a healthy population) for persons with disabilities secondary to traumatic and nontraumatic processes. Neurologists who understand the rehabilitation process following an acute neurologic event are better positioned to provide more comprehensive and effective services as the patient moves through the continuum of care. This role as principal medical caregiver entails delivering basic medical care, coordinating appropriate consultations, and acting as the final common pathway to the patient (Alexander, 1996). Rehabilitation specialists are vigilant for, and are able to treat, the consequences of comorbid illnesses and common complications seen in persons with impaired mobility, cognition, self-care, or communication.

Following a patient through rehabilitation, therefore, represents a unique opportunity to build strong doctor-patient ties and influence future health decision-making, outcome, and appropriate follow-up. Because the inpatient rehabilitation stay probably represents the single longest continuously monitored time period, a rare chance exists to observe the evolution of disease and healing, document rare syndromes, and conduct clinical research. Because of the inherent variability of recovery from neurologic injury, the timing of interventions remains particularly challenging. When, how, and how much to intervene in the natural recovery process can confound even the most experienced clinician. Nevertheless, the field of neurorehabilitation offers ample excitement because of the increasingly varied and effective interventions available.

THE INTERDISCIPLINARY TEAM

The unique composition and role of the group of professionals responsible for coordinated care stands as the single most distinguishing feature of rehabilitation. This group approach is also the most important feature of rehabilitation having an impact on the patient's recovery. Whereas a multidisciplinary team functions as a group of individual caregivers independently approaching the patient from their own discipline's viewpoint, each member considers perspectives of other team members through ongoing dialogue, and incorporating mutual goals, strategies, and recommendations (e.g., determining a successful reward system to modulate agitation following TBI). No other specialty in medicine views the patient through this particular paradigm. This approach results in achieving patient-centered functional goals in the most comprehensive and expedient manner.

Typically, the rehabilitation team includes a physical therapist who works toward maximizing mobility; an occupational therapist to address activities of daily living (ADL), related cognitive tasks, and improvement in upper limb function; and a speech-language pathologist or therapist who facilitates optimal communication and language-based cognitive function, given the patient's limitations. Rehabilitation nurses, the only professionals in 24-hour contact with the patient, maintain continuity of care and reinforce skills learned in therapies. They also play a major role in skin care, nutrition, monitoring for secondary complications, safety management, psychological support, and reestablishing continence or bowel-bladder regimens. A psychologist or, more often, a neuropsychologist helps patients adjust to disability, monitors for and treats emotional reactions, coordinates team behavioral management, and administers tailored psychometric tests to guide the emphasis of ongoing or subsequent cognitive therapies. A social worker or nurse case manager begins discharge planning even before the patient's arrival and secures benefits from payors, according to patients' needs, trying to reconcile the team's recommendations with the particulars of an individual's coverage and the desires and resources of patient and family.

The Committee on Accreditation of Rehabilitation Facilities also requires a dietitian to monitor the patient's nutritional needs and status. Recreational therapists, a recommended addition to the team, can show patients how to maintain quality of life through avocational pursuits.

The rehabilitation neurologist may first encounter the patient in acute care, thus beginning a long-term commitment to care at a time when many questions are raised about the process ahead. During this period or on initial presentation to the rehabilitation facility, the physician establishes confidence with patient and family, begins the education process, and shares the treatment plan and prognosis. Understanding that the patient and those around the patient are in extended crisis, the physician must balance hope with reality, provide guidance and direct interventions, and be supportive and compassionate. No one is, therefore, better equipped to balance these needs than the rehabilitation neurologist familiar with both the mechanism of injury and the natural history of the illness, as well as the multitiered period of therapy punctuated by potential setbacks over the ensuing months. Spending additional time on the front end of the patient encounter will return the dividends of trust and bonding, smoothing the way for a productive relationship across arduous terrain. Long-term cooperation is especially important because of the chronic disability in this population, and few sustained, comprehensive doctor-patient relationships are forged during such life-altering situations. This is why this time holds the potential for such significant influence on the course of recovery ahead.

The physician with rehabilitation expertise (e.g., neurologist or physiatrist) leads this core team who meets at least once per week for involved patients—otherwise every 2 weeks—to discuss the treatment plan, obstacles, progress, short- and long-range goals and the projected timeframe in which goals can be realistically achieved. The evolution of these team meetings, combined with factors such as resources and the home situation, will determine where and how a patient will receive subsequent rehabilitation along the continuum of care.

Team members can consult other specialists and should establish close working relationships with representatives from these fields who understand the unique needs of the population in need of neurorehabilitation. Frequently consulted disciplines include otorhinolaryngologists for vestibular or vocal dysfunction, gastroenterologists for percutaneous endoscopy gastrostomy placement, orthopedists for spasticity management, cardiologists for cardiovascular fitness assessment, (neuro) psychiatrists for neuroaffective disorders, and orthotists to fabricate and fit a leg brace, for example. Other consultants that should be readily accessible to the core team may come from the fields of audiology, rehabilitation engineering, vocational rehabilitation, substance abuse or addiction counseling, or chaplaincy.

The physician leading the rehabilitation team should also be aware of and perhaps even establish satellite clinics, which can focus more resources on unusually difficult sequelae, or complex patient needs. Interdisciplinary subgroups can form clinics for spasticity, swallowing, vision, motor control, gait, wheelchair, and brace assessment.

PHILOSOPHY OF REHABILITATION

The paradigm of neurorehabilitation is uniquely centered on functional activities required for daily living. No other field of medicine is more concerned with how the individual can achieve maximal freedom from the effects of disease than precisely how that individual came to illness. Inpatient neurorehabilitation addresses basic ADL, including dressing, washing, eating, grooming, communication, and mobility. For the patient to transition back to the community, the team places more emphasis on the impact of the neurologic disability on recreational pursuits and domestic and vocational roles. Early in the process, the team identifies the patient's strengths and weaknesses, exploits those strengths where possible, and circumvents deficits through remediation, compensatory strategies, or assistive devices. Strengths not only refer to individual qualities (e.g., motivation), but also to the support system in place. Together with a realistic discharge plan, these factors determine if a given patient is a good rehabilitation candidate for a particular level of care. In striving for the maximal level of functioning, neurorehabilitation is concerned with promoting spontaneous recovery, adaptation, compensation and preventing secondary medical (e.g., decubiti), physiologic (e.g., spasticity), or psychological (e.g., depression) complications.

The terms used to describe functional limitations in the rehabilitation population were formalized and adopted by the World Health Organization in 1980. *Impairment* describes altered function or structure at the level of the organ. Common examples of impairment include those system deficits found on neurologic examination such as sensorimotor loss, dysphasia, spasticity, inattention, incoordination, and memory and visual field loss. *Disability* is defined as that which a person cannot accomplish as a result of impairment (e.g., ADL, mobility, socializing, or communicating), therefore, disability concerns a functional ability at the level of the person. For example, a woman with ataxia

cannot feed herself or a patient with paraplegia who cannot ambulate. *Handicap* has an impact at the level of society and indicates a compromise of one's functioning within various social roles. Therefore, handicap reflects a disadvantage resulting from disability or impairment for which the community fails to accommodate based on particular cultural factors or the nature of occupational and family responsibilities.

Clinically, neurorehabilitation can be viewed as a process of learning that seeks to restore function whenever possible, speed recovery from impairment, minimize disability or handicap, and maximize community reintegration to reestablish quality of life. Four types of rehabilitative processes are blended to achieve these goals: remediation, compensation, prevention of secondary complications, and maintenance of function.

Remediation

Remediation begins immediately after injury and directly aims to limit neurologic impairment. Neuronal structures can recover by several mechanisms: reversal of ischemia, resolution of edema, recruitment of secondary or primitive pathways, dendritic arborization, and synaptogenesis (Alexander, 1998). How much neuroplasticity the older adult brain can demonstrate is unclear, yet positron emission tomography and functional magnetic resonance imaging increasingly reveal neurophysiologic patterns of cortical and subcortical reorganization (Ricker et al., 2001; Levy et al., 2001).

One caveat borne out by several studies examining the effects of excitotoxicity is that healing nerve tissue can be overly taxed by the metabolic demands and free radical generation of aggressive, early rehabilitation therapy. A major recent focus of neurorehabilitation is the importance of facilitating optimal *neurorecovery* by avoiding certain drugs that lead to slowed or reduced outcome. Feeney and Goldstein's work has done much to elucidate this phenomenon, showing that medications commonly (and unnecessarily, as discussed below) prescribed after central nervous system (CNS) injuries can permanently affect progress, even after single dose administration (Goldstein et al., 1990; Feeney et al., 1982). Conversely, some studies demonstrate how psychostimulants, for example, likely potentiate recovery from damage. Future discoveries, it is hoped, will yield pharmacologic treatments directly facilitating neurophysiologic recovery. Although the various therapeutic disciplines have long sought interventions that directly remediate impairments through shaping CNS repair, studies proving this have been weak and few. One exciting new therapy demonstrating significant, often dramatic clinical benefit is *constraint induced therapy* (CIT) or forced use paradigms (Blanton and Wolf, 1999; Dromerick et al., 2000; Van der Lee et al., 1999), discussed in the common problems section below.

Compensation

When remediation incompletely restores function, patients must adapt psychologically and physically to new circumstances. Neurorehabilitation applies practical strategies to compensate for evolving deficits. Durable medical equipment, including assistive devices (e.g., braces or grabbers); Fresnel Prism lenses for hemianopsia; and cognitive strategies (e.g., memory books or repetition) help accommodate to a new functional status. Counseling and realistic goal setting will guide which daily or leisure activities are pursued and determine the necessary level of assistance to ensure safety.

Prevention of Secondary Complications

Not only are medical and neurologic complications following CNS impairment to be expected, but comorbid disease in the elderly usually amplifies the risk and severity of such clinical events. The neurorehabilitationist must understand the natural history of recovery, always be vigilant for common, late-developing sequelae, and institute prompt treatment to limit further functional deterioration. This can be especially challenging when following this elderly population long term, because of progressive and nonspecific, age-related functional decline. Again, it is just as important to consider certain preventive interventions as it is to remove offending factors or medications, which can induce clinical complications. For instance, a hemiparetic, somnolent stroke survivor arrives in a rehabilitation facility with a painful shoulder and at risk for aspiration pneumonia. The neurosurgeon who clipped the aneurysm and evacuated the hematoma initiated phenobarbital for seizure prevention. After tapering and stopping the anticonvulsant, the patient's shoulder pain resolved (illustrating phenobarbital rheumatism) (Taylor and Posner, 1989) and arousal improved, reducing aspiration risk and enabling participation in all therapies.

Maintenance of Function

Instructing patients and their caregivers how to manage disability, reduce self-injury, and carry out an appropriate exercise or stretching regimen remains a cornerstone or major goal of rehabilitation, continuing long beyond traditional hands-on therapy. This approach emphasizes the belief that neurorehabilitation is a lifelong process. Formal inclusion of lay persons—usually called "family training"—in the process of recovery is important, because insurers rarely cover "maintenance" therapy.

REHABILITATION PROCESS IN THE OLDER ADULT

Disability

Of those elderly living in the community, more than 75% report no limitation of ADL. Functional deficits in 23% of respondents were for walking (19%), getting outside (10%), bathing (10%), getting in and out of bed (8%), dressing (6%), toileting (4%), and eating (2%). Notably, only 10% of this disabled group were assisted with functional activities (Department of Health and Human Services, 1987). With increasing age, the need for assistance rises so that of those above 80 years of age, 40% require help (Williams, 1986).

Optimizing function through neurorehabilitation of the older adult depends on significant understanding of basic principles of geriatric medicine. Premorbid health and functional status becomes as important or more important than any single principle of rehabilitation in directing the effort of the team and apportioning resources. Comorbidity such as arthritis, neuropathy, diabetes, cardiovascular, and pulmonary disease can dominate the clinical picture, significantly limiting a given intervention's efficacy. Age-associated cognitive and sensory dysfunction and generalized decreased functional reserves usually affect severity of deficits and treatment goals (Weber et al., 1995). Nevertheless, results of studies on whether the elderly can tolerate and benefit from formal, interdisciplinary rehabilitation are positive (Cifu and Lorish, 1994).

Assessment

The complex process of assessing candidacy for a given course of rehabilitation in the elderly requires attention to several unique factors (Gershkoff, 1993). Obtaining a clear picture of premorbid medical issues and functional status is basic and critical. Specific goal setting will flow from an understanding of biophysiologic reserves and, in turn, determine the setting and structure of the rehabilitation program.

Therefore, the patient's primary care physician should be consulted and any recommendations for management incorporated into the therapy program.

Likewise, team members should contact those who previously cared for or knew the patient so that expectations, intentions, and goals can all be reconciled. This is often the first step toward a comprehensive exploration of the formal and informal support systems that comprise an individual's social network (Alexander, 1998). Informal support systems include friends, family, and community or religious organizations. Other determinants that assume increasing importance with age are the role in the family structure, advance directives, role of organized religion or spirituality, and interdependence of significant other.

Understanding funding sources for medical care is a key component of goal setting and discharge planning. Benefits for various levels of rehabilitation services vary widely among providers. However, Medicare, a federally run program, provides uniform coverage and is the sole form of insurance coverage for 98% of the elderly in the United States. Recently, managed care Medicare has further eroded rehabilitation coverage, as many enrollees opt for less coverage to cut costs, underestimating the need for such care. Further, rehabilitation services are not covered by secondary or copayment insurance. Medicaid programs insure the medically indigent population and are administered by individual states whose criteria for eligibility and coverage for inpatient and outpatient rehabilitation services vary significantly. Although, notably, Medicaid funds more than 85% of all nursing home care in the United States.

Settings

Rehabilitation services can be provided at any level along the classic continuum of care (Fig. 33-1). Multiple factors will determine where the individual receives therapies but several key determinants are more heavily weighted. The intensity of services must strike a balance between family wishes and patient's readiness. Therefore, medical stability or need for frequent medical treatment follow-up (e.g., radiation therapy or hemodialysis) will determine whether the patient is more appropriately rehabilitated in an acute hospital care setting or inpatient therapy in a freestanding rehabilitation facility. Prognosis for, and timing of, expected recovery might mean that subacute rehabilitation is more appropriate, for instance, for someone slow to emerge from coma or who is to remain non-weight-bearing for 6 weeks because of bilateral leg fractures. It follows that severity of deficits likewise affects disposition. Although the ideal journey through the spectrum of rehabilitation services seems appropriately geared to the average patient, the neurorehabilitationist should always explore creative solutions, especially when working with payors, not simply employing a top-down strategy but occasionally a bottom-up approach when the clinical situation dictates. In other words, goals are fluid and the patient in subacute who responds favorably to a psychostimulant intervention or the discontinuation of sedative drugs or who regains weight-bearing potential after fractures have healed, should be considered for the acute care setting.

Generally, patients must meet certain criteria as candidates for the most intensive level of rehabilitation. They should possess:

1. A new disability or an acute worsening of baseline status
2. An ability to participate in and tolerate a minimum of 3 hours of therapy daily
3. A workable support system to facilitate transition to the goal-determined, least restrictive environment
4. An appropriate funding source

Occasionally, the predetermined plan from acute care is to schedule a lower functioning ("low level") patient for a 2-week trial in acute rehabilitation, with the understanding that if progress is not sufficiently apace to justify treatment at that level, therapy would then continue at a lower intensity (e.g., subacute care). The acute setting trial, if successful, may achieve the goal of minimizing multiple, potentially disruptive reorientation by the team and patient alike, thus maintaining continuity. Other goals include comprehensively assessing the likely need for specialized devices or delivery, by a highly trained team, of uncommon interventions not available in lower settings that can often make a greater impact during earlier recovery stages. Through greater and more specialized vigilance, the patient is spared the development of medical or neurologic complications. Finally, this early assessment team can focus on putting in place preventive measures to address expected sequelae and follow-up with education as less experienced caregivers take over.

An often overlooked ancillary component of the rehabilitation process, family training, facilitates what is commonly known as a day pass but is best thought of as a "therapeutic home visit." Such visits help caregivers and patients comprehend the burden of care and can accelerate the long process of reassessing short- and long-term goals, in general, and discharge

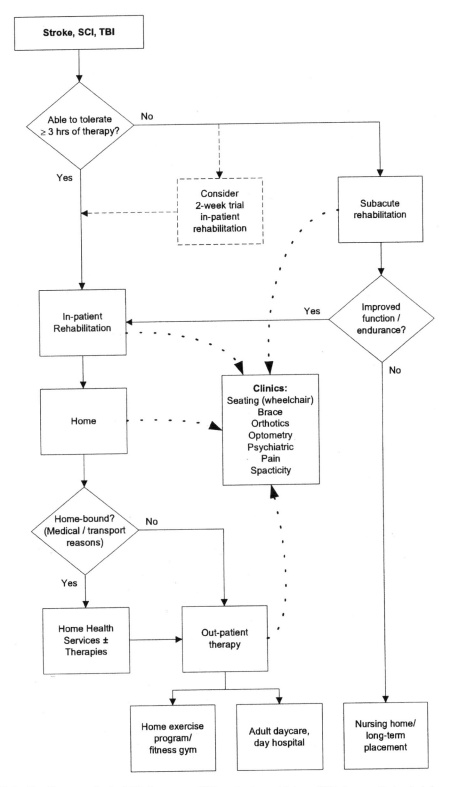

FIG. 33-1. Continuum of rehabilitation care. SCI, spinal cord injury; TBI, traumatic brain injury.

plans specifically. Conversely, discharge location will also dictate the degree of active caregiver involvement. Less hands-on time will be spent on ADL, for example, if goals are set for discharge to long-term care. The team, in turn, monitors the family's acquisition of skills needed both to allow the patient the chance to maximize independence and to maintain safety. Thus, the outcome of family training may well have a reciprocal effect on discharge planning or may result in lengthening or even shortening an inpatient stay. The timing of such training, therefore, is pivotal to maintaining an efficient and dynamic team, preparing all parties involved for the realities ahead.

Other practical forces, in the near future, will exert influence on placement issues. Currently, Medicare's prospective payment system is being informally implemented by rehabilitation facilities, with a target launch date of January 2002. Until that time, such facilities had been exempted from the strict, diagnosis related group-type driven lengths of stay, which reshaped acute care over the past two decades (Melvin, 1999). Inevitably, this mandate for change will have a profound effect, on both treatment intensity and goal setting, but will cause rehabilitation facilities to be ever more discriminating in their assessment of inpatient candidacy. Although already a critical factor in the decision-making process, a sound discharge plan will likely become the keystone of successful movement of the elderly patient through rehabilitation settings.

IMPACT OF GENERAL MEDICAL HEALTH AND COMORBIDITY

A discussion of common medical problems found in the elderly is beyond the scope of this chapter. However, certain basic principles apply and should be revisited by the treatment team, particularly when progress proves slow, erratic, or out of the ordinary. Such relative treatment failures may signal the interaction of an underlying medical condition. Because rehabilitation usually occurs immediately following an acute event, less dramatic signs and symptoms of disease are frequently overlooked or mistakenly attributed to the index event. The situation is compounded by the patient's frequent inability to accurately communicate subjective concerns during recovery from neurologic injury. Moreover, especially in the case of trauma but often with CNS vascular disease, an overrepresentation is seen of those who have neglected routine medical screening and follow-up. Priorities must be established in addressing medical needs so not to compete for the elderly

patient's limited energy, keeping in mind, too, that sending patients out for testing or treatment frequently interferes with therapy sessions. However, the clinician must also balance a patient's immediate rehabilitation needs against the likelihood that medical follow-up will be sought. Because successful rehabilitation is predicated on fitness, maintaining safety and preventing both loss of function and recurrent disease, postdischarge medical monitoring will help achieve these goals, sustaining gains made in therapy. In the ideal case, the patient's primary care physician should be consulted for comanagement.

Comorbidity, therefore, can intensify newly acquired deficits (e.g., neuropathy in a hemiplegic); become newly acquired or discovered during rehabilitation stays (e.g., seizure disorders); or have an impact on the recovery process through inadequate postacute management (e.g., uncontrolled stroke risk factors resulting in recurrent infarcts). Additionally, because of the dynamic interaction between the rehabilitation process and the underlying medical condition, the team must examine the physical, cognitive, and physiologic consequences of injury on self-care. For example, consider the previously independent man who is diabetic who develops hemiplegia and is unable to draw his own insulin or perform a blood sugar fingerstick. Cognitively, he may be unable to determine the appropriate number of units and will likely need more units anyway because he is less active. Or perhaps he may require less insulin if he makes gains, becomes more physically active than before the stroke, and adopts better exercise habits. Alternatively, spasticity can eventually develop, thereby increasing metabolic demand which, in turn, leads to lower insulin requirements. Avoiding hypo- or hyperglycemia is essential to CNS attempts to heal. By anticipating such medical-rehabilitation interactions, clinicians will prevent secondary insult, thereby achieving another ideal of neurorehabilitation.

TRAUMATIC AND OTHER ACQUIRED BRAIN INJURIES

TBI is arguably the most common cause of neurologic mortality and morbidity in the United States (Kurtzke and Kurland, 1987). Although many studies show that age at injury has a powerful effect on recovery (Carlsson et al., 1968; Vollmer et al., 1991; Vollmer, 1993; Lokkeberg and Grimmes, 1984; Teasdale et al., 1979; Hernesniemi, 1979; Pentland et al., 1986; Braakman et al., 1980), a more recent study concluded that age has a potent yet complex effect on recovery, particularly beyond age 40 years, where outcomes worsen. Epidemiologically, the incidence of TBI in the geriatric population remains incompletely defined, although statistics have long demonstrated a bimodal age cohort risk peaking for males aged 15 to 24 years and the elderly above 75 years of age. Most recent estimates are that 50,000 TBI per year occur in the elderly or an incidence of 200/100,000, half that of the most at-risk (16–34 years of age) group. Overall, males outnumber females 2:1, but in the subset over 80 years of age, the female to male ratio is 3:2 (Wilson, 1987; Goodman and Englander, 1992; Amacher and Bybee, 1979; Sosin et al., 1989).

Because the systematic improvements in trauma care, driven by organized emergency care networks and widespread dissemination of evidence-based guidelines, increasingly larger percentages of accident victims are surviving to enter the rehabilitation system. Thus, the prevalence of trauma-induced disability rises with each year. However, signs indicate that more effective prevention strategies and safety features may counter this statistic.

Falls account for the most common cause of TBI in persons over 65 years of age. When motor vehicles are involved, the elderly are more often the pedestrian and it should not be surprising that most fatalities occur as a result. Alcohol is frequently associated, especially in men, and indeed is correlated with worse outcomes. Uncompleted suicide, again more common in men, and elder abuse are being recognized as causes of growing importance and should not be overlooked as explanations in cases in which the cause of TBI is cryptic or undetermined (CDC, 1996). Finally, because of the combined effect of pre- and postmorbid risk factors resulting from cognitive, behavioral, motoric, and vestibular impairments, TBI can be characterized as a relapsing-remitting disease in need of chronic risk reduction and management to maximize potential for recovery, maintain functional gains, and prevent recurrent events.

Pathology and Mechanism of Injury

Traumatic brain injuries are categorized as either closed or penetrating, depending on whether protective structures have been breached directly by an object. Three major categories of CNS damage can follow directly from a physical force exerted on the craniocervical structures and their contents. *Focal insults*, such as cortical contusions, most commonly of the frontal and temporal lobes, occur when the brain collides with the inner table of the skull or grinds across the fossae's bony ridges. *Focal parenchymal damage* occurs along the tract of a penetrating missile-type foreign body. Mass lesions, such as *subdural hematomas* (SDH) or *intraparenchymal hemorrhages* (IPH), can evolve at almost any rate, requiring close monitoring. In matching the mechanism to pathology in cases of ambiguous cause, typical focal bleeding will localize to dorsolateral brainstem and corpus callosum. Diffuse axonal injury (DAI) requires acceleration-deceleration forces sufficient to disconnect neural fibers directly (i.e., "shearing forces"); or after a delay of up to 24 to 48 hours, as the disrupted cytoskeleton causes axonal transport to malfunction, leading to ballooned segments that ultimately rupture, resulting in retraction balls. Depending on severity, brain scans may reveal petechial hemorrhages as the only associated *early* macroscopic sign of underlying DAI. Brain atrophy (with associated *ex vacuo* changes) from the neural dropout that ensues represents a late manifestation of this process.

Secondary or delayed factors are equally important to consider and may even account for a greater proportion of morbidity and mortality if not properly handled. Particularly in assessing prognosis and potential to benefit from rehabilitation services, sustained raised intracranial pressure must be documented. Similarly, herniation syndromes, superimposed anoxic-ischemic events (to be suspected in prolonged accident scene extrication), prolonged hyperpyrexia, electroconvulsive events, and hydrocephalus can further stress an already compromised organ. At a more fundamental level, excitotoxicity and associated metabolic cascades contribute to loss of neural elements, but are currently less amenable to clinical intervention. Any or all above examples of pathophysiologic disruption can coexist.

Grading Severity

A basic appreciation of the more commonplace scales and prognostic indicators will assist the clinician with more efficient use of resources. Table 33-1 shows the general relationship between length of coma (LOC)—sometimes synonymous with alteration of consciousness for milder degrees of severity—and posttraumatic amnesia (PTA), also called "anterograde amnesia." PTA is essentially defined as the period of time it takes the person with TBI to regain functional, day-to-day recall for basic facts or events. This is sometimes called "carryover" by treating members of the team. More formally, when the patient on two consecutive days scores more than 75 on the Galveston Orientation Amnesia Test, PTA has resolved.

TABLE 33-1. *Severity of traumatic brain injury*

Degree	Length of coma (LOC)	Posttraumatic amnesia
Mild	Up to minutes	Minutes to hours
Moderate	Up to 24 hours	Hours to days
Severe	Up to 1 week	Days to one week
Very severe	Weeks	Several weeks
Extremely severe	Weeks to months	Months

Clinical Course

After moderate to severe TBI, LOC is roughly proportional to severity or degree of DAI unless other mechanisms conspire to delay regaining of consciousness. Katz's update of the familiar Ranchos Los Amigos Scale (Table 33-2) provides a generic map with which to shepherd a patient through progressive levels of recovery. Note, however, that recovery after TBI is often nonlinear, punctuated by complications, setbacks, and the evolution through stages of maladaptive behaviors or syndromes of variable duration. The postacute period, therefore, is best conceptualized as a highly dynamic and individualized process—a moving target—in which not all "healing" is necessarily positive. It is also not uncommon for seemingly new behaviors or disabilities to emerge as states of arousal evolve or as the patient encounters novel situations, stimuli, and challenges.

Management

Depending on the referring hospital or trauma center, the person with TBI can arrive with a bewildering array of variably controlled, active medical problems along with whatever premorbid medical history the elderly typically carry. Deconditioning, anemia, nutritional depletion, respiratory compromise, autonomic instability, arrhythmia, endocrine dysfunction, pain, dysphagia, coagulopathy, infection, incontinence, and emotional disturbance are but a few of the most commonly encountered medical problems. Consider the case study below followed by typical admission orders to an inpatient brain injury unit.

A 74-year-old man, living alone, with hypertension and early, untreated Parkinson's disease was found unconscious at the bottom of a flight of stairs. Glasgow Coma Score was 7, blood pressure was 170/90 and he was intubated in the field. His alcohol level equaled 0.07 mg/dL. Battle's sign was present and brain computed tomography scan showed bifrontal contusions, petechial hemorrhages, left temporoparietal IPH and left basal skull fracture. He suffered a 90-second generalized tonic-clonic seizure on day 2 and his phenytoin level was 6.8. Because LOC was 10 days, a tracheostomy was performed and a gastrostomy tube and Greenfield filter placed. At time of transfer from acute care 3 weeks from injury, he was intermittently agitated with sleep-wake cycle inversion, still in PTA; he had dysconjugate gaze and decreased blink to right superior threat. He had receptive greater than expressive aphasia, was taking nothing orally, and was dually incontinent with indwelling catheter. He also had gross right hemiparesis with action-induced equinovarus posturing of the right foot; hyperactive reflexes throughout except at the left ankle; and pain with right shoulder ranging but otherwise good pain lo-

TABLE 33-2. *Recovery from traumatic brain injury*

Coma: eyes closed, unresponsive
Vegetative state: gross wakefulness with sleep-wake cycles reestablished, but no cognitive responsiveness
Minimally conscious state: semipurposeful wakefulness and responds at times reliably to environmental stimuli; usually still mute
Confusional state: labile state changes from hyperaroused (agitated) to hypoaroused with recovering speech and severe attentional deficits, in ongoing PTA
Postconfusional, evolving independence: resolving PTA with improvement in cognition and social interaction. Achieving independence in self-care/ADL and developing independence at home
Social competence, community reentry: recovering cognitive abilities with goal-directed behavior, social skills and appropriate personality traits. Developing community independence with return to academic or vocational pursuits

ADL, activities of daily living; PTA, posttraumatic amnesia.
Adapted from Mills V, Cassidy J, Ratz D, eds. *Neurologic rehabilitation.* Blackwell Science1997: 116.

calization. He required moderate assistance of two to sit at the edge of bed but was totally dependent for all ADL. Nystagmus was noted with Hall-Pike maneuver. Attention, arousal, and endurance were poor. A course of antibiotics for urinary tract infection and aspiration pneumonia was to continue. Stage two sacral skin breakdown with necrotic center was dressed. Tachycardia was noted and phenobarbital level was 21, phenytoin having been stopped because of liver function test elevation and rash 1 week previously.

The patient was examined after a thorough review of transfer records and discussion with family members about premorbid status, personality, and clinical course. To illustrate some approaches to management, medical issues will be addressed first. (Treatment choices are meant to demonstrate a typical clinical point rather than represent the only correct answer). The patient is weaned from oxygen to humidified room air, maintaining pulse oximetry and downsizing tracheostomy, as indicated. An ear nose throat consult could be ordered, if needed, to evaluate hearing loss with basal skull fracture, hemotympanum, tinnitus, and vestibulopathy. Anemia may require erythropoietin if iron supplementation is insufficient. Complete antibiotics, follow leukocytosis, and consider urine and sputum culture or chest film if tachycardia continues or fever rises. Occult deep venous thrombosis less often is the source of fever and tachycardia; if respiratory distress develops, then pulmonary embolism must be swiftly investigated. Bouts of dysautonomia can be spontaneous or triggered by occult infection or painful stimulus. Beta-blockers are often used for prominent and disruptive bursts of autonomic activity. Consider plain films of the right shoulder and left knee to evaluate possible occult fractures which, according to one study, approach 11% prevalence in the rehabilitation setting (Garland and Bailey, 1981). Gastric feeding ideally runs from after daytime therapies to breakfast time with a noon bolus to simulate lunch, so as not to interfere with therapy sessions. Water bolus (200–250 mL) three or four times daily. Order a video fluoroscopic swallowing study; remove urinary catheter after antibiotic completion, checking postvoid residuals ultrasonographically. Time-void patient at regular intervals, preferably just before therapies to avoid interruptions. Turn patient off sacrum, add vitamin C and zinc sulfate to promote skin healing, and apply medicated cream to decubitus to break down necrosis. Assess for signs of deep vein thrombosis (DVT) and provide prophylaxis with compression stockings and low–molecular-weight heparin (LMWH) until the patient is ambulatory.

To maximize participation in therapies, quickly reestablish sleep-wake cycle with trazodone or low-dose zolpidem. Use physical or chemical restraints extremely sparingly when controlling agitation (see section on behavior below). Treat pain with the least sedating medication and begin a gradual taper of phenobarbital for several reasons discussed below under the section on seizures. One important, underappreciated side effect termed "phenobarbital rheumatism" may account for the right shoulder pain. As communication improves, neurooptometry can evaluate diplopic, blurred vision, and other special senses should be tested, especially olfaction. If anosmia exists, patients discharged to home must be cautioned to use smoke detectors. Subjective hypothermia and delayed, undesirable weight gain are two common, yet poorly understood, sequelae that can have an impact on quality of life and maintenance costs when patients return home. Intranasal vasopressin, one squirt per nostril daily for one month, effectively reduces subjective hypothermia but the mechanism is unknown (Eames, 1997).

Movement disorders, often delayed by months or years, can appear as a result of TBI or preexisting disorders typically may worsen. In the case presented above, symptoms of Parkinson's disease eventually required treatment with a dopamine agonist—bromocriptine—chosen because of numerous reports in the literature of a beneficial effect on initiation (Echiverri et al., 1988; Drubach et al., 1995). This syndrome, termed "abulia," is frequently encountered with bifrontal lesions, particularly the cingulate region, and individuals display variable levels of reduced drive, motivation, interest, and spontaneity not dissimilar to some features of parkinsonism. Furthermore, because a precipitous decline in cerebrospinal fluid (CSF) dopamine metabolites is well documented, potentiation of dopaminergic pathways following TBI is frequently attempted and is thought to be a key factor in modulating mood, behavior, and cognition.

This patient also developed hypertonia of the right foot, which required botulinum toxin injection to facilitate orthotic fitting and functional ambulation. Electromyography with nerve conduction testing confirmed a left peroneal traumatic neuropathy, which later developed into neuropathic pain syndrome requiring trials of antiepileptic drugs (AED), tricyclic antidepressants, corticosteroids, and multiple modalities in physical therapy. Fluidotherapy involves inserting a distal limb into a chamber where warm corn husks are blown around, which is theorized to stimulate and desensitize hyperpathic and allodynic skin regions involved by complex regional pain syndrome, formerly called "reflex sympathetic dystrophy."

When the patient was no longer on phenobarbital, arousal, mood, cognition, and attention improved noticeably. However, these gains reached a plateau 2 weeks later (now 2 months post-TBI), so methylphenidate was added, resulting in modest improvement in attention, initiation, fatigue, and aphasia. Occasional recurrence of urinary incontinence and slight worsening of balance when ambulating prompted CT brain imaging. The results revealed posttraumatic hydrocephalus, necessitating ventricular shunting, following which the patient continued to make steady gains in most areas.

SEIZURE RISK AND MANAGEMENT

Posttraumatic seizures (PTS) occur in up to 20% of older persons, with more than half of these within the first postinjury week. Most PTS are self-limited and focal unless exacerbating factors such as fever or electrolyte disturbance coexist. Therefore, even with higher risk patients (i.e., those with IPH, SDH, or penetrating head injury) evidenced-based practice parameters issued by the American Academy of Neurological Surgeons and the American Board of Physical Medicine and Rehabilitation recommend discontinuation of preventive anticonvulsants after the first week (Yablon, 1993; Bullock, 1995; Brain Injury Special Interest Group of the American Academy of Physical Medicine and Rehabilitation, 1998). Moreover, no evidence supports the common belief that suppressing seizures for any given time period post-TBI will prevent the ultimate development of a posttraumatic seizure disorder. Similar evidenced-based guidelines were recently issued by the American Academy of Neurology concerning anticonvulsant drug use in persons with newly diagnosed brain tumors. The task force cited the relative risk of side effects versus any measurable benefit. Elderly patients recovering from brain tumor excision frequently have rehabilitation on brain injury units. Referring physicians who transfer patients on AED should be advised that maximizing potential recovery dictates that such patients should have AED discontinued.

Therefore, one of the most important early clinical decisions is to discontinue (or in the case of barbiturates and benzodiazepines, wean) patients from AED. Not only are severe reactions frequently first encountered in the rehabilitation setting (e.g., the classic rash of phenytoin 2–3 weeks following initiation), but the very disabilities addressed by rehabilitation techniques are caused or exacerbated by common AED

TABLE 33-3. *Medications which potentially impede neurorecovery after brain injury*

Dopamine receptor antagonists (neuroleptics)
Alpha$_2$ agonists (clonidine)
Benzodiazepines (γ-aminobutyric acid potentiation, inhibitory)
Anticonvulsants (phenobarbital and phenytoin worst offenders)
Alpha$_1$ adrenergic antagonists (e.g., prazosin)
Cholesterol-lowering agents

side effects. Ataxia, diplopia, cognitive dysfunction, fatigue, dizziness, and tremor are all commonly associated with TBI itself or AED use. Equally as important, prospective studies in the animal literature and mostly retrospective analyses of human data over the last decade have shown that certain medications can both slow the pace of neurorecovery and even permanently reduce overall outcome (Table 33-3) (Feeney et al., 1982; Goldstein et al., 1990).

Rehabilitation clinicians, therefore, should search for acts of commission interfering with recovery before attempting to treat common posttraumatic deficits. If compelling reasons exist to sustain AED use following TBI, every effort should be made to exploit secondary indications in an attempt to parsimoniously treat several syndromes with a single agent. For instance, when neuropathic or central pain is present, an option might be gabapentin, carbamazepine, or lamotrigine. When a history of migraine predominates, choose valproate. Gabapentin should be used with severe hepatic disease. When neuropsychiatric or neurobehavioral disorders dominate the clinical picture, AED play an even more prominent role, as discussed in following sections.

INTERPLAY OF BEHAVIOR, AFFECT, AND COGNITION

At either end of the neurobehavioral spectrum lie the prototypes of the hypo- and hyperkinetic states: abulia and agitation, respectively. Although they are not classically placed among the list of posttraumatic cognitive dysfunctions, they have a direct impact on cognition and, in fact, share certain features (e.g., attention). Similarly, initiation, communication, and speed of processing are all categorized as cognitive domains, but overlap with the neurobehavioral deficits in question. Affective changes, too, can confound the clinician. Depression, for example, is frequently encountered post-TBI and can be manifested either by vegetative or by positive features (e.g., as in an agitated depression). Such concurrent neuropsychiatric states must be accounted for and often may be parsimoniously treated with a single agent, which is the ultimate achievement.

Guidelines of Psychopharmacology

Both pharmacologic and classic and evolving neuropsychological approaches have been extensively studied in the treatment of behavioral dysfunction. Yet few if any such strategies are proved to be of such widespread benefit as to be considered the standard of care. Therefore, neurorehabilitationists, practicing much in the sphere of the art of medicine, must choose from a palette of options and paint the best picture of a successful outcome. As compelling testimony to the lack of certainty in this area of medicine, most pharmacologic indications mentioned here are off-label. An additional confound is sorting out the relative contribution of spontaneous recovery versus an intervention—pharmacologic or otherwise.

General principles concerning this patient population bear emphasizing. Response to any given agent is often state-dependent (i.e., arousal) and unpredictable. Response to single or brief dosing may differ from longer term treatment. The dictum of geriatric pharmacology applies doubly to the brain-injured patient: start with low dosages and titrate slowly. The injured brain is more sensitive and susceptible to dose-related side effects, and idiosyncratic effects are more difficult to monitor for in this unpredictable population. Knowledge of which drugs can actually impair recovery is critical (Table 33-3). If drugs must be used, change to a less detrimental drug as soon as possible, constantly reassess the risk-to-benefit ratio, or both. Before instituting an agent aimed at a target behavior, rigorously assess the potential that an existing medication is the cause. That is, before remedying an act of omission, address acts of commission. Avoid overtreatment, which can lead to a behavioral state equally disruptive to the rehabilitation process. The ultimate goal, whenever possible, is always to stabilize the situation with medications and establish nonpharmacologic interventions during this window of opportunity. A timely drug holiday is always indicated to assess if the intervention is still required. Knowledge of drugs' secondary effects facilitates pharmacologic parsimony.

The Abulic State

For the purposes of this discussion, focus turns to the patient who has clearly emerged from coma and who is generally awake and alert. The phenomenology and treatment of posttraumatic mental or physical fatigue will not be addressed, although shared features with abulia are apparent. An overlap also exists with the clinical phenomenon of labile arousal post-TBI, wherein patients suddenly *shut down* in the middle of tasks, presumably because (after metabolic or medication effects have been ruled out) of failure of tonic arousal via the ascending reticular activating system. Also carefully assess sleep patterns and promptly treat commonly encountered posttraumatic sleep-wake cycle inversion before blaming reduced effort by the patient. Give careful consideration to the possible coexistence of psychiatric disease (e.g., catatonia), especially given its higher incidence in the TBI population.

Characteristics seen in abulia minor include mental slowness, distractibility, reduced vigor or energy, inertia, disinterestedness, decreased enthusiasm, and poverty of movement with brady-, oligo-, and hypokinesia. The pure syndrome, therefore, presents as a global reduction of all action, ideation, and emotion and slowed cortical activity is general or uniform rather than selective. In the clinical setting, however, wide variation is seen in the degree to which any combination of these components may exist. Less dramatic states of abulia, therefore, can be identified as the clinician becomes attuned to the range of abulic features, especially when the pathology on imaging corresponds to the phenomenology.

A dopamine-producing cell population distinct from the substantia nigra exists in the midbrain in the ventral tegmental area and projects widely to cortical structures, especially to the cingulate gyrus. This pathway has been termed the "mesencephalofrontal activating system." Damage to the source, tract, or target structures causes variable degrees of decreased initiation, motivation, or drive. When minor, this manifests clinically as apathy; when severe, as akinetic mutism. Because it is difficult to modify akinetic mutism, the behavioral spectrum is preferably sequenced: eukinesia, apathy, abulia minor, and (most severely) abulia (Fisher, 1983).

Pharmacotherapy for Abulic States

Studies to date have mostly demonstrated an effect with catecholaminergic upregulation or potentiation (Table 33-4). More specific benefit has been linked to dopaminergic augmentation in the form of L-dopa (Drubach et al., 1995), dopamine agonists, amantadine, or reuptake inhibition. Because of the relative prominence of D1 receptors in the cortex versus D2 receptors found subcortically, it appears that the

TABLE 33-4. Medications used to treat various neurobehavioral syndromes

Classic stimulants	Dextroamphetamine	Methylphenidate	Pemoline	Modafinil
Purported mechanism of action	Direct release DA/NE CAT reuptake blockade Reduced CAT turnover	Similar to d-amphetamine, except increase CAT, turnover	Unclear, possible Release of DA, decreased CAT turnover	Distinct site of action from classic stimulants; GABA antagonism-glutamate augmentation
Dose range (mg/d)	5–60	10–80	56.25–112.5	200–400
Time → peak effects	2–4 h	1–2 h	Days–weeks	Hours
Pharmacological halflife (h)	7–10	2–4	12	15
Initial monitoring required	Tachycardia, HTN, anorexia, dysphoria, insomnia	Tachycardia, HTN, anorexia, dysphoria, insomnia	Anorexia, hepatotoxicity	None

CAT, catecholamine transferase; DA, dopamine; GABA, g-aminobutyric acid; HTN, hypertension; NE, norepinephrine.

older, less specific dopamine agonists (i.e., bromo-criptine) are better choices because the newer dopaminergics are designed more specifically to target the D_2 receptors concentrated in the basal ganglia (Zafonte, 2000).

Certain antidepressants should be chosen over others because of their relative activating properties or target neurotransmitter. Fluoxetine and protripty-line are the most activating of the selective serotonin reuptake inhibitors (SSRI) and tricyclics, respectively. Bupropion would be chosen for its putative mechanism of norepinephrine and dopamine reuptake inhibition.

Hyperaroused States

The most recent accepted definition of agitation (Mysiew and Sandel, 1997) categorizes it as a subtype of delirium, occurring during the period of PTA. Yet, considerable overlap still confounds the study of the discrete state. Common descriptions of such excess of behavior include aggression, akathisia, emotional lability, irritability, anger, destructive, maladaptive, or antisocial behavior. Perhaps reflecting the disagreement over terminology, little consensus exists over the pathophysiologic and anatomic correlates of agitated behavior. Therefore, no further attempt will be made here to resolve the controversy.

One paradigm of agitation equates the condition with either inadequate suppression or overexcitation. Fisher (1983) found it useful to identify regions of the brain along an anterior-posterior axis that tend to activate or restrain. He pointed out that frontal lesions more often result in reduced activity (because of unopposed, posterior cerebral-driven restraint) and vice-versa. Thus, for example, parietal lesions leading to acute agitated delirium or acute confusional state (Mori et al., 1987) and the agitated patient with cortical blindness or Wernicke's aphasia leave frontal activation areas unopposed.

Pharmacotherapy for Agitated States

For this discussion, assume that pharmacologic therapies are used only after less invasive measures (e.g., behavioral techniques or even physical restraints) fail. A brief discussion of each category of medication follows, highlighting common clinical factors influencing the choice of specific drugs. Emphasis is also on treating overlapping or coexisting syndromes with a single agent.

Beta-Blockers

Propranolol is the beta-blocker most frequently cited in studies of episodic dyscontrol, rage, and aggression. It is the most lipophilic and, therefore, crosses the blood–brain barrier most effectively. Dosages can begin at 30 mg/day to a maximum of 720 mg/day, because peripheral beta-receptors are fully inhibited at 300–400 mg/day. A convenient long-acting form is available. Nadolol can also be given once daily. Pindolol avoids bradycardic side effects.

Tricyclics

Generally, tricyclics are not considered first-line medications because of anticholinergic and cardiac side effects potential as well as lowered seizure threshold. However, a tricyclic antidepressant can be an excellent parsimonious choice if also aiming to treat posttraumatic migraine, myofascial pain, emotional incontinence or depression, and insomnia (for instance, consider amitriptyline). Desipramine is among the least anticholinergic.

Clonidine

A central adrenergic agonist, clonidine is not favored because of its association with reduced motor outcome but it can be chosen for concurrent treatment of spasticity and central or reflex sympathetic dystrophy-like pain syndromes. Abrupt withdrawal can cause hypertensive crisis or psychosis.

Buspirone

An orphan anxiolytic, buspirone can be initiated at 5 to 10 mg twice daily to a maximum of 60 mg/day. Evidence supports its use when agitation is associated with hostility, irritability, or anger, or with features of obsessive compulsive disorder (Stanislav et al., 1994). Desirable features include negligible side effects, drug-drug interactions, sedation, or addiction potential. Drawbacks include the delay to response and lack of efficacy as an acute intervention.

Serotonergics

Serotonergics are useful when agitation coexists with depression (unclear if the term "agitated depression" applies) or with anxiety. SSRI also appear effective in the treatment of anger. However, overtreatment can lead to apathy. Trazodone is a frequent choice when prominent insomnia accompanies agitation and, possibly, in sundowning, but priapism is a concern.

Amantadine

Amantadine potentiates dopamine by various mechanisms. It should not be a first-line choice, however, in the elderly; when psychosis is present (tends to induce hallucinations); when a risk of seizure predominates; or when orthostasis is a prominent concern. Dosages are initially 50 mg twice daily or 7 a.m. and 2 p.m., increasing by 50 mg/day every 5 to 7 days to a maximum of 400 mg/day.

Anticonvulsants

Because so many patients present to the brain injury unit on AED and at precisely the time when evolving through periods of agitation, upstream care providers should at least take the time to change over from the ubiquitous phenytoin to one of the AED with behavior or mood-stabilizing properties. Psychiatrists have used mostly carbamazepine or valproate and, more recently, gabapentin and lamotrigine to modulate behavior and mood (Wroblewski et al., 1997). All can be effective in controlling agitation. Furthermore, gabapentin is well appreciated for its analgesic properties and lack of drug interaction. Lamotrigine is said to be the least sedating AED and may even be activating. Carbamazepine and valproate, in particular, should be monitored for blood levels. One caveat is that the newest AED (e.g., topiramate) are too sedating or cognitively suppressing for common usage.

Neuroleptics

Classic, older antipsychotics are to be used only as a last resort, especially during the acute phase of recovery (first 6 months). This recommendation stems from the convincing evidence (Feeney et al., 1982) that dopamine-blocking agents have a detrimental effect on neural recovery. If psychotic ideation accompanies agitation, a lower threshold exists to use these drugs. When antipsychotics must be used, the newer, more specific (*atypicals*) are preferred. Risperidone works quickly. Olanzapine can be parsimoniously chosen when reestablishment of sleep is desired, but weight gain can be enormous (potentially a plus with concomitant anorexia) with its use. Quetiapine is the third atypical drug to consider. Clozapine can be the most dopamine receptor-specific but is a last resort because of bone marrow aplasia. The usual concerns are doubly feared in the setting of TBI: haloperidol-like drugs lower seizure threshold and their anticholinergic properties exert undesirable effects on cognition (e.g., memory).

Benzodiazepines

Benzodiazepines are not first-line drugs, except in extreme situations (or when concomitant anxiety or sleep disturbances are prominent) because patients are often rendered overly sedated and at increased fall risk. Amnestic properties negate rehabilitation carryover of learned tasks. Paradoxic reactions are not uncommon, especially in elderly. Obvious problems exist with habituation and withdrawal symptoms (i.e., seizures). Bias clinical use toward a shorter acting lorazepam or oxazepam.

Psychostimulants

Components of attention deficit disorders can overlap with agitation. Occasionally, posttraumatic agitation is almost entirely related to overstimulation and, therefore, is best pharmacologically approached as an attention deficit: hyperactivity-like disorder.

Ample literature supports use of the classic psychostimulants in TBI, independent of premorbid disease. Perhaps best known for maintaining tonic arousal, psychostimulants can have a known antidepressant effect as well. Strong evidence indicates that these play a role in potentiating motor recovery after ABI (Goldstein et al., 1990; Walker, Batson, et al., 1995). The common sequelae of posttraumatic mental and physical fatigue respond well to psychostimulant intervention (Elovic, 2000).

Common Posttraumatic Neuropsychiatric Scenarios

Reference was made above, in various contexts, to the use of antidepressants and the overlap of affective and behavioral conditions. Early on, depression must be differentiated from abulia, catatonia, posttraumatic stress disorder, appropriate bereavement or adjustment disorder, and medication or metabolic effect. Depression is also commonly coincident with the clearing of trauma-induced anosognosia. Therefore, closely monitor long-term for its emergence.

Depression should be distinguished from emotional incontinence (untriggered affective display) and emotional lability (inappropriately easily triggered affect) by asking the patient or family. Crying is much more common than laughter in all ABI. Document mood-incongruent states and comment on whether the patient (family) desires treatment of symptoms. Treat inappropriate affective states with SSRI or tricyclic antidepressant. Venlafaxine has the added benefit of noradrenergic effects. Decreased libido and anorgasmia are frequent limiting factors in all serotonergic potentiators. Avoid this with the use of bupropion, which is dopaminergic, noradrenergic, and highly activating, and can reduce nicotine craving. Reported epileptogenic risk is not borne out in clinical practice.

Posttraumatic mania is uncommon and almost always transient, mainly associated with temporal lobe contusions. Use mood-stabilizing AED (carbamazepine, valproate, lamotrigine), then atypical antipsychotics followed by lithium (Ichim et al., 2000).

The SSRI or buspirone may address anxiety, with more severe symptoms treated with benzodiazepines or atypical antipsychotics.

Posttraumatic mental and physical fatigue is poorly understood and even more poorly researched. Treatment approaches are borrowed from patients with multiple sclerosis, chronic fatigue syndrome, narcolepsy, and obstructive sleep apnea, using psychostimulants described above (Table 33-4; Elovic, 2000).

STROKE

Because stroke is overwhelmingly a disease of the elderly, background information about its cause, mechanism, and pathology can be found in other chapters. Unlike TBI, rehabilitation of CNS vascular disease has a growing body of evidence-based guidelines, several examples of which are highlighted here. One clinical reality deserves special mention before discussing classic rehabilitation interventions. Because neurorehabilitation occurs downstream from acute care, the quality and uniformity of referring physicians' knowledge of the relevant literature varies widely. Thus, the neurorehabilitationist is well positioned to reduce risk of recurrent infarcts and this reduction of associated morbidity stands as a major goal of the rehabilitation process.

Selected areas addressed by evidence-based guidelines put out by the Agency for Health Care Policy and Research (Langhorne et al., 1993) are summarized in an effort to alert the clinician that these factors are key to good outcomes. However, even though such a review attempts to capture the state of the art, bear in mind that most neurorehabilitation relies more heavily on the art of medicine without absolute, rigorously tested standards of care on which to rely when treating a specific individual patient or problem.

- Following acute CNS vascular disease, care should be rendered in dedicated stroke units where clinicians coordinate interventions (including early rehabilitation services), leading to better functional outcomes and reduced mortality (Jorgensen et al., 1995; Indredavik et al., 1998, Indredavik et al., 1999; Leira and Adams, 1999). Although not explicitly stated, it follows that dedicated stroke rehabilitation units should achieve outcomes more expeditiously and with greater success.

- Stroke complications and significant risk factors for recurrent events must be vigorously monitored while initiating disease-specific health promotion in this captive audience. When previously not or inappropriately addressed, explore indications for warfarin, surgery, or antiplatelet agents, especially when additional history (e.g., about compliance) reveals salient facts such as whether the infarct represents a true failure of premorbid preventive strategies (Halar, 1999; Kelly-Hayes and Phipps, 1999). Medical comorbidity usually accompanies stroke in the elderly and substantial energy is often exerted in aggressively managing these—a task made more challenging when neurorehabilitation occurs in a free-standing facility without on-site diagnostics. For reasons related to the stroke itself as well as the resultant functional consequences, many such comorbid illnesses will require reassessment of self-care or caregiver burden.

- Risk of DVT rises after 70 years of age, trauma, major surgery with anesthesia longer than 30 minutes, prior DVT, and in association with obesity, malignancy, or congestive heart failure. Therefore, a low threshold exists for obtaining duplex sonograms of the extremities. Compression hose, LMWH and warfarin can be used for prevention, the latter two to prevent progression as well.

- Depression following stroke occurs in between 30% and 50% of patients and clearly slows recovery and magnifies disability, both cognitive and physical (Alexander, 1998). At 2 years poststroke, patients who are not depressed still perform ADL better (Parikh et al., 1990). Mechanisms of depression can be primary (neuropsychiatric), secondary (reactive), or both. Factors making the diagnosis of poststroke depression particularly challenging include atypical symptomology in the elderly, dysphasia, and differentiating mood-incongruent affect (lability). Neurorehabilitationists should become comfortable with first-line treatments for depression (Knapp et al., 2000) and good responses are especially rewarding when latent functional ability is unmasked. Resolution of pseudodementia provides a dramatic example of such success.

- Bowel and bladder dysfunction commonly interferes with rehabilitation on many levels and should be comprehensively managed. Particularly with physical disability and lower staff-to-patient ratios found in rehabilitation settings, practical factors (e.g., reaching the call bell or the bathroom in time) combine with neurophysiologic sequelae to exacerbate the clinical picture. Although seemingly labor intensive, a simple practical approach, *timed voiding*, actually represents efficient staff use when taking into account soiled linens and lost billable time in therapy.

- Constipation, common in the elderly, often worsens because of poor hydration, dietary change, including reduced fiber, and decreased activity levels. Preventive strategies include basic dietary changes, early mobilization, and a pharmacologic bowel program.
- Swallowing problems can commonly lead to malnutrition, dehydration, or aspiration pneumonia. Nursing and speech and occupational therapists provide table-side monitoring, but videofluoroscopy is the gold standard in these cases.
- Maintaining skin integrity depends on all team members in some way. Unchanged diapers will lead to macerated skin; rough transfers from bed to other surfaces causes shear, especially to the elderly person's skin, which is lacking in subcutaneous fat. Nutritional support is essential (vitamin C and Zinc supplementation assist wound healing) and repositioning at least every 2 hours reduces pressure or decubitus ulceration.
- Fall risk assessment consumes significant attention on the ward, primarily because of the need to document indications for physical restraints. Before acquiring neurologic illness, the elderly already face an elevated risk of falling and suffer proportionally greater morbidity as a result of falls. Particularly when poor judgment, insight, balance, strength, and vision conspire to raise baseline fall risk, a multidisciplinary strategy is needed. Two commonly overlooked factors are excessive use of sedative-hypnotics and postural hypotension (often a medication side effect as well).

Finally, prognosis after inpatient stroke rehabilitation relates to discharge disposition. One recent study of 239 persons over 65 years of age found that 81% were discharged to home, 10% to a skilled nursing facility, 7% to acute care secondary to complications, and 2% died on the rehabilitation unit (Alexander, 1998).

SPINAL CORD INJURY

Few neurologic entities present a more dramatic clinical picture than the often sudden and severe disabling consequences of SCI. Any and all body systems can suffer from the effects of SCI, triggering medical, emotional, social, and economic aspects of disability. Regardless of age (Yarkony et al., 1988; Sibbarae et al., 1987), appropriate rehabilitative interventions improve life expectancy, quality of life, and level of independent living (McKinley et al., 1996). Nevertheless, life-threatening complications, mortality, hospital stays, and monetary concerns remain significantly greater for the older person with SCI (Lovasik, 1999; Cifu et al., 1999).

In the United States, prevalence of SCI exceeds 200,000, with 11,500 new cases each year (Lasfargues et al., 1995); paraplegia and quadriplegia are equally represented. Causes of SCI clearly differentiate along age groups (Roth et al., 1992) and the association with underlying medical illness in the elderly further distinguishes the clinical rehabilitation course. Degenerative spondylosis, rheumatoid arthritis, and compressive or invasive malignant processes commonly lead to spinal cord compromise and the need for postoperative rehabilitation services. Falls are the most common cause of traumatic SCI in the elderly (Spivak et al., 1994), followed by motor vehicle accidents and violence. Even when a traumatic SCI results from relatively minor forces, underlying problems (e.g., stenosis, osteophytic change, disc disease) frequently magnify the effects of those physical forces.

Diagnosing the causes appropriately occurs in acute care. Specifically characterizing the clinical syndrome with a carefully documented sensorimotor and autonomic assessment along American Spinal Injury Association guidelines aids accurate communication across disciplines and functional level prognosis. Central cord syndrome is particularly prominent in the geriatric population (Penrod, 1990). Especially with myelopathy secondary to cervical stenosis, the workup for subacute combined degeneration should be documented. Also unique to SCI, delayed symptom progression should be worked up for syringomyelia, most commonly seen in the cervical cord. The enlarging cavity presents with capelike, dissociated (spinothalamic tract) sensory loss, and rapid progression or painful transformation is an indication for shunting.

Three SCI-specific, common sequelae (Teasell and Allatt, 1991) are highlighted next and more complications are discussed under the section on managing clinical syndromes that span various rehabilitation diagnoses.

- Pain can originate in neurologic or musculoskeletal structures, the latter often resulting from redistribution of body weight and maladaptive joint alignments. Tendinitis and bursitis commonly present. After aggravating factors are corrected, where possible, nonsteroidal anti-inflammatory drugs, phonophoresis, heat, massage, and although rarely required, steroid injection can control symptoms.

- Neuropathic pain, either chronic or paroxysmal, can be triggered by radiculopathy or cord distraction itself. Typical descriptions include burning, lancinating, tingling, pulling, squeezing, or electrical sensations. Despite a potential for effects on arousal, cognition, gastrointestinal, and urinary functioning, tricyclic antidepressants, anticonvulsants (gabapentin, carbamazepine, lamotrigine, phenytoin), and benzodiazepines are traditionally used. Transcutaneous nerve stimulation and counterirritant therapy can work alone or augment pharmacologic strategies. New or sudden escalation of pain should prompt investigation of a new lesion or systemic pathology.

- Neurogenic bowel and bladder syndromes, among the most common complications of SCI, are successfully managed with practical, multimodal, and team-coordinated approaches (Madersbacher and Oberwalder, 1987). Particularly in the elderly, premorbid physiology and anatomy combine to complicate diagnosis. Various patterns of urgency, frequency, incontinence, and retention can coexist. Detrusor sphincter dyssynergia is diagnosed by urocystometrogram. Intermittent catheterization is taught to reduce infection risk, urolithiasis, and hydronephrosis. Urinary tract infections are constantly suspected. Beyond timed voiding and external (condom or Texas) catheters to minimize therapy disruptions, regular schedules frequently establish an automatic neural rhythm of voiding. Medication options consist of cholinergics (bethanechol) to stimulate bladder wall contraction; alpha-adrenergic medication (e.g. terazosin) to relax the internal sphincter; anticholinergics (propantheline, oxybutynin, tolterodine) for detrusor relaxation. Lioresal, by relaxing the pelvic floor, can limit outflow resistance.

- Constipation (with resultant impaction and obstruction) and fecal incontinence can have devastating effects on skin integrity, wound hygiene, physiologic homeostasis, and social functioning, among others. Planned evacuation every other day generally avoids either extreme. Graduated bowel programs rely on adequate fluid intake, high fiber diet, stool softeners, laxatives, and disimpaction, paired with suppositories. The individual's daily needs must be matched to timing of interventions.

- Autonomic dysreflexia follows disruption of sympathetic outflow pathways and the concomitant inability to modulate responses to often minor noxious or non-noxious stimuli originating below the lesion. Basic, yet common, triggers include overdis-

tended bladder, pain, decubitus ulcer or ingrown toenail.

Diaphoresis, anxiety, and (of greatest concern) hypertension can ensue with systolic readings above 300 mmHg, leading to risk of intracranial hemorrhage. Treatment involves remedying the offending stimulus, immediate elevation of the head and lowering of the legs, and, if necessary, topical nitrates.

Educational programs initiated in the acute rehabilitation setting remain the backbone of functional and health maintenance. Patients are taught monitoring strategies to prevent late-developing complications of the renal, musculoskeletal, cardiovascular, and integumentary systems (Bergman et al., 1997).

MANAGEMENT OF SELECTED PROBLEMS ACROSS DIAGNOSTIC CATEGORIES

Spasticity

A disorder of motor function, spasticity, is most often described as a velocity-dependent, increased resistance to passive joint movement, but can also manifest as involuntary spasms at rest or be action induced. Decreased motor control and hyperreflexia usually coexist. The relevant pathophysiology is thought to involve impaired modulation of spinal reflex arcs by upper motor neuron circuitry.

Patterns include focal, regional, hemi-, para-, or generalized hypertonicity. Not all spasticity can or even should be treated. Mild spasticity can be assistive by facilitating weightbearing (if tone is extensor) or improving circulation with occasional spasms. Therefore, tone reduction is indicated only if spasticity interferes with some level of function, care, positioning, or comfort (Gormley et al., 1997). Goals will differ in the ambulatory versus the wheelchair- or bed-bound individual. When grading severity, the Ashworth scale (Table 33-5) facilitates objective clinical documentation and meaningful interdisciplinary communication. Even with aggressive treatment, however, many patients' spasticity will progress to some degree of joint contracture.

Efforts to reduce spasticity again begin with the cooperation of many team members. All work to identify and eliminate nociceptive triggers (e.g., bowel-bladder dysfunction, DU, heterotopic ossification, and anxiety). When conservative, classic therapy techniques (e.g., stretching, positioning, splinting, and serial casting) fall short, consider pharmacologic intervention. Most oral medications have intolerable effects on arousal, cognition, and uninvolved muscles, particularly in ABI and stroke. These effects are magnified in the elderly population. Dantrolene is the

TABLE 33-5. *Ashworth spasticity scale*

Score	Description
1	No increased tone
2	Slightly increased tone with a "catch" during flexion or extension
3	More marked increase with tone; however, joint or limb still ranged with ease
4	Significant increase in tone; passive movement very difficult
5	Affected muscles rigid or contracted in flexion or extension

one exception in terms of CNS side effects, because it acts peripherally on excitation-contraction uncoupling at the sarcoplasmic reticulum. Hepatotoxicity is a concern, however. Diazepam and baclofen use, in addition to weakness, prompts a warning of withdrawal seizures. These two drugs work on the γaminobutyric acid (GABA-B) receptors. Tizanidine, functionally related to clonidine, was developed specifically for hypertonicity and acts at multiple levels of the nervous system. Generally well tolerated if titrated very slowly, beginning with a nighttime dose, it can cause sedation, orthostasis, or dry mouth but does not usually result in weakness.

When fewer or more focal muscle groups are involved, oral medication use is discouraged. More localized interventions (e.g., botulinum toxin) are favored for several reasons. Specific muscles can be partially and temporarily chemodenervated and the therapy is also effective in the often overlapping condition of dystonia (further discussed below), which can follow TBI or stroke. When determining appropriate doses (typically ranging from 100–400 U type-A toxin currently available), consider severity of spasticity and muscle size, as recommended use is limited to 400 U every 3 months. More aggressive chemodenervation is performed with phenol injections whose effects last up to 6 months and carry more risk than botulinum when other than pure motor nerves (e.g., musculocutaneous and obturator) are injected. Mixed nerve injections can cause severe, potentially unremitting, painful paresthesiae as a complication.

The most invasive therapy, short of irreversible, orthopedic procedures (e.g., myotomy, tenotomy, tendon transfers) is placement of an intrathecal catheter attached to a surgically implanted programmable pump to deliver baclofen to the spinal CSF. Intrathecal baclofen (ITB) therapy is generally reserved for relatively severe tone in at least two limbs where chemodenervation is too impractical or has failed. The major advantages include avoiding cognitive side effects, programmability, and reversibility. Although relatively expensive, cost compares favorably to maximum dose botulinum toxin given every 3 months. Demonstrated surrogate benefits of ITB on ADL, bowel-bladder function, caregiver burden, hygiene, quality of life, pain, sexual function, gait, range of motion, and many other areas have been demonstrated in numerous studies. The US Food and Drug Administration approval of ITB in 1992 for spinal origin spasticity and in 1996 for cerebral origin spasticity has meant approved coverage by Medicare and Medicaid providers.

Deep Vein Thrombosis

Venous thromboembolism is perhaps one of the most common and feared complications seen in the rehabilitation setting. Immobility from TBI, SCI, or CI is the major risk factor. Risk of developing DVT increases with trauma (particularly to the lower extremities or pelvis), major surgery, obesity, age above 70 years, cancer, and prior DVT. Subtle signs such as low-grade fever, tachycardia, poorly circumscribed pain and mild leukocytosis may be the only clue. Appropriate prophylaxis in this high risk, elderly group, therefore, is critical. However, the clinical research is silent on strict guidelines for the various neurologic diagnoses. Most clinicians now use compression stockings and subcutaneous, LMWH as soon as is deemed clinically safe, although choices for treatment may be particularly complicated following CNS hemorrhagic events. Most believe that as long as the underlying cause of a hemorrhage (hypertension, traumatic SDH, aneurysm) has been addressed, anticoagulation can be safely initiated after about 2 weeks. Although not all cases of DVT are clinically significant, LMWH with changeover to coumadin for 2 to 4 months is usually the treatment because of the risk of clot propagation. Small DVT below the knee is the exception, especially if the patient is somewhat ambulatory. Negative finding on interim Doppler ultrasonography may shorten the course of treatment. Dynamic pumps are not used in the rehabilitation setting because when the patient goes to therapy, DVT can develop while the pumps are off and, in theory, would be propelled centrally when the compression restarts after pumps are reapplied in bed. A high index of suspicion and low threshold for workup of resultant pulmonary embolism should be on the minds of all team members, especially when a patient develops new onset dyspnea or desaturation. Ventilation-perfusion scans and venography remain the gold standard and should be pursued, particularly when the decision to anticoagulate needs to be weighed against the option of caval filter placement.

Movement Disorders

Just as spasticity represents a delayed and maladaptive attempt at healing by the CNS, so too do several other motor disorders. In fact, a large, relatively unknown body of literature deals with posttraumatic or postanoxic delayed onset movement disorders. A common reason for the elderly to present to acute rehabilitation following coronary artery bypass graft or similar surgery is the complication of hypoxic-ischemic injury (HII). Myoclonus, dystonia, tremor, and parkinsonism can ensue. Myoclonus may respond to benzodiazepines and use of wrist or ankle weights. 5-Hydroxytryptophan can be obtained from government research sources for particularly severe cases. Attempts to treat dystonia (usually action-induced and demonstrating co-contraction of agonists and antagonists with a rotational component) include anticholinergics or botulinum injections if more focal disability exists. The akinetic-rigid form of parkinsonism that follows acute HII, however, does not typically respond to conventional treatments used in Parkinson's disease. Nevertheless, dopamine agonists, anticholinergics, and amantadine may be of benefit to some patients. One feature of movement disorders following HII in the elderly that clearly distinguishes it from young populations is the time course to onset. Significantly less delay from injury (days to weeks as opposed to months to years) is seen in the elderly and this is thought to parallel the reduced neuronal reserve and plasticity of the older brain. Medications that contribute to symptom burden (e.g., antidopaminergic drugs) must be assiduously avoided in these cases.

Deconditioning and Fatigue

Both mental and physical fatigue are extremely common following stroke and ABI or TBI. Equipped with less physical reserve, the elderly—particularly those with a sedentary, chronically inactive lifestyle–are significantly more susceptible to the deconditioning and fatiguing effects of immobility following neurologic compromise. Elevated heart rate with decreased cardiac reserve is frequently evident. Loss of muscle mass and flexibility often coexist. Preventing complications resulting from immobility of the elderly should be a primary focus of the rehabilitation team. Even modest amounts of physical training in elderly persons have been shown to result in beneficial effects on health (Fiatatrone and Evans, 1993). If after conser-

vative measures (e.g., conditioning exercise) have not proved sufficiently beneficial, trials of the psychostimulants or wake-promoting agents in Table 33-4 may be attempted with the usual caveats about heart rate and blood pressure as well as unwanted behavioral side effects. Modafinil appears to have the lowest risk and indeed has shown promise in multiple sclerosis-associated fatigue, quickly replacing amantadine as the treatment of choice. Optimizing endurance allows patients to extract the most benefit from therapy sessions. Of course, the differential diagnostic considerations should include depression, sleep-wake cycle assessment, behavioral syndromes (i.e., abulia), and reversible metabolic causes (e.g., hypothyroidism).

Promising Newer Therapies

Body Weight-Supported Treadmill Training

For a significant subgroup of patients who cannot yet fully support their body weight when upright, body weight-supported treadmill training represents a potentially powerful tool with which to accelerate recovery (Hesse, 1995; Hesse, 1999). The patient is placed in a harness that is suspended by a frame which can be adjusted to unweight the person with a gait impairment. The apparatus can then be positioned over a treadmill allowing a focus on gait mechanics which, in turn, are triggered by the treadmill action. Improvement in areas such as gait speed and mechanics is thought to follow from exploitation of primitive spinal gait circuitry. Because of its labor intensity, however, therapists are often reluctant to use this therapeutic option. Other benefits such as limiting muscle atrophy and risk of DVT are likely to soon be shown in randomized trials.

Constraint-Induced Therapy

Repetitive practice in an affected limb is essential to restore function after CNS insult. CIT (sometimes called "forced-use" paradigm) attempts to reverse the tendency toward what has been termed "learned non-use," by restricting automatic compensatory use of the better functioning limb (Taub et al., 1993, 1996). Recently, more controlled trials of CIT (Van der Lee et al., 1999; Blanton and Wolf, 1999; Dromerick et al., 2000) have solidified it as an effective new therapy, particularly after stroke and, to a lesser proved degree, in TBI. The unaffected limb can be restrained with a standard sling, a shoulder immobilizer, an ace wrap, or even a mitten. To be eligible for current protocols, patients must generally possess greater than 10 degrees of finger and wrist extension. Initial studies mostly required a minimum of 6 hours per day of restraint; however, Page et al.

(2001, personal communication) have developed an effective modified CIT protocol that only requires 3 hours per day.

SUMMARY

Neurorehabilitation of the elderly continues to grow and prove ever more effective. It is a field that remains open and stimulating to the motivated neurologist. The increasingly valued quality-of-life issues remain at the heart of this field. However, recent changes in the primary funding source for this population raises new challenges for the rehabilitation team, forcing ever more efficient delivery of services and critical assessment of both goals and outcome measures. The interested clinician will more effectively navigate the system by anticipating common logistical, medical, rehabilitative, and psychosocial pitfalls discussed in this chapter. A creative approach is often rewarded in this field and, as such, the need for evidence-based guidelines remains a goal. Up-to-date knowledge of novel pharmacologic and non-pharmacologic interventions is critical to successfully caring for this patient population.

REFERENCES

Alexander DN. Geriatric neurorehabilitation. *Neurol Clin North Am* 1998;16(3):713–733.

Alexander DN. Neurorehabilitation. In: Sage JI, Mark MJ, eds. *Practical neurology of the elderly adult*. New York: Marcel Dekker, 1996.

Amacher AL, Bybee DE. Toleration of head injury by the elderly. *Neurosurgery* 1979;20:954.

Bergman SB, Yarkone GM, Stiens SA. Spinal cord injury rehabilitation. II. Medical complications. *Arch Phys Med Rehabil* 1997 Mar;78(3):53–58.

Blanton S, Wolf SL. An application of upper extremity constraint-induced movement therapy in a patient with subacute stroke. *Phys Ther* 1999;79:847–853.

Braakman R, Gelpke GJ, Habbema JDF, et al. Systematic selection of prognostic features in patients with severe head injury. *Neurosurgery* 1980;6:362–370.

Brain Injury Special Interest Group of the American Academy of Physical Medicine and Rehabilitation. Practice parameter: antiepileptic drug treatment of posttraumatic seizures. *Arch Phys Med Rehabil* 1998;79:594.

Bullock R, et al. *Guidelines for the management of severe head injury*. San Francisco: Brain Trauma Foundation, 1995.

Carlsson CA, von Essen C, Lofgern J. Factors affecting the clinical course of patients with severe head injuries. 1. Influence of biological factors. 2. Significance of posttraumatic coma. *J Neurosurg* 1968;29:242–251.

CDC: Suicide among older persons: United States, 1980–1992. *MMWR* 1996;46:1.

Cifu DX, Lorish TR. Stroke rehabilitation: stroke outcome. *Arch Phys Med Rehabil* 1994;75:56.

Cifu DX, Seel RT, Kruetzer JS, et al. A multicenter investigation of age-related differences in lengths of stay, hospital-

ization charges, and outcomes for a matched tetraplegia sample. *Arch Phys Med Rehabil* 1999;80(7):733–740.

Dromerick AW, Edwards DF, Hahn M. Does the application of constraint-induced movement therapy during acute rehabilitation reduce arm impairment after ischemic stroke? *Stroke* 2000;31:2984–2988.

Drubach DA, Zeilig G, Perez J, et al. Treatment of abulia with carbidopa/levodopa. *Journal of Neurological Rehabilitation* 1995;9(3):151–155.

Eames P. Feeling cold: an unusual brain injury symptoms and its treatment with vasopressin. *Journal of Neurosurgery and Psychiatry* 1997;62(2):198–199.

Echiverri HC, Tattum WO, Merens TA, et al. Akinetic mutism: pharmacologic probe of the dopaminergic mesencephalofrontal activating system. *Pediatr Neurol* 1988;4:228–230.

Elovic E. Use of Provigil for underarousal following TBI. *J Head Trauma Rehabil* 2000;15(4):1068.

Feeney D, Gonzalez A, Law W. Amphetamine, haloperidol, and experience interact to affect rate of recovery after motor cortex injury. *Science* 1982;217:855–857.

Fiatatrone MA, Evans WJ. The etiology and reversibility of muscle dysfunction in the aged. *J Gerontol* 1993;48:77–83.

Fisher CM. Abulia minor vs. agitated behaviour. *Clin Neurosurg* 1983;32:9–31.

Garland DE, Bailey S. Undetected injuries in head-injured adults. *Clin Ortho* 1981;155:162–165.

Gershkoff AM, Cifu DX, Means KM. Geriatric rehabilitation: social, attitudinal and economic factors. *Arch Phys Med Rehabil* 1993;74:402.

Goldstein LB, Matchar DB, Morgenlander JC, et al. The influence of drugs on the recovery of sensorimotor function after stroke. *Journal of Neurological Rehabilitation* 1990;4:137–144.

Goldstein LB. Pharmacologic modulation of recovery after stroke: clinical data. *Journal of Neurological Rehabilitation* 1991;5:129–140.

Goodman H, Englander J. Traumatic brain injury in elderly individuals. *Phys Med Rehabil Clin N Am* 1992;3:441.

Gormley ME Jr, O'Brien CF, Yablon SA. A clinical overview of treatment decisions in the management of spasticity. *Muscle Nerve* 1997;6:14–20.

Halar EM. Management of stroke risk factors during the process of rehabilitation. Secondary stroke prevention. *Phys Med Rehabil Clin N Am* 1999;10(4):839–856.

Hernesniemi J. Outcome following head injuries in the aged. *Acta Neurochir (Wien)* 1979;49:67–79.

Hesse S, Uhlenbrock D, Werner C, et al. A mechanized gait trainer for restoring gait in nonambulatory subjects. *Arch Phys Med Rehab* 2000;81(9):1158–1161.

Ichim L, Berk M, Brook S. Lamotrigine compared with lithium in mania: a double-blind randomized controlled trial. *Ann Clin Psychol* 2000;12:5–10.

Indredavik B, Bakke F, Slordahl SA, et al. Treatment in a combined acute and rehabilitation stroke unit: aspects are most important. *Stroke* 1999;30:917–923.

Indredavik B, Baake P, Slordahl SA, et al. Stroke unit treatment improves quality of life: a randomized controlled trial. *Stroke* 1998;29:895–899.

Jorgensen HS, Nakayama H, Raaschou HO, et al. The effects of stroke unit: reductions in mortality, discharge rate to nursing home, length of hospital stay, and cost. *Stroke* 1995;26:1178–1182.

Kelly-Hayes M, Phipps MA. Preventive approach to poststroke rehabilitation in older people. *Clin Geriatr Med* 1999;15(4):801–817.

Knapp P, Young J, House A, et al. Non-drug strategies to re-solve psycho-social difficulties after stroke. *Age Aging* 2000;29(1):23–30.

Kurtzke JF, Kurland LT. The epidemiology of neurologic disease. In: Baker AB, Joynt RJ, eds. *Clinical neurology.* New York: Harper & Row, 1987:1–143.

Langhorne P, Williams BO, Gilchrist W, et al. Do stroke units save lives? *Lancet* 1993;342:395–398.

Lasfargues JE, Custis D, Morrone F, et al. A model for esti-mating spinal cord injury prevalence in the United States. *Paraplegia* 1995;33:62–68.

Leira EC, Adams HP Jr. Management of acute ischemic stroke. *Clin Geriatr Med* 1999;15(4):701–720.

Levy CE, Nichols DS, Schmalbrock PM, et al. Functional MRI evidence of cortical reorganization in upper-limb stroke hemiplegia treated with constraint-induced move-ment therapy. *Am J Phys Med Rehabil* 2001;80(1):4–12.

Lokkeberg AR, Grimmes RM. Assessing the influence of non-treatment variables in a study of outcome from severe head injuries. *J Neurosurg* 1984;61:254–262.

Lovasik D. The older patient with a spinal cord injury. *Crit Care Nurs Q* 1999;22(2):20–30.

Madersbacher G, Oberwalder M. The elderly para- and tetraplegic: special aspects of the urological care. *Para-plegia* 1987;25(4):318–323.

Melvin JL. Impact of health care financing administration changes on stroke rehabilitation. *Phys Med Rehabil Clin N Am* 1999;10(4):943–955.

McKinley WO, Conti-Wyneken AR, Vokac CW, et al. Reha-bilitative functional outcome of patients with neoplastic spinal cord compressions. *Arch Phys Med Rehabil* 1996; 77(9):892–895.

Mori E, Yamadori A. Acute confusional state and acute agi-tated delirium: occurrence after infarction in the right middle cerebral artery territory. *Arch Neurol* 1987;44: 1139–1143.

Mysiw WJ, Sandel ME. The agitated brain injured patient. Part 2: Pathophysiology and treatment. *Arch Phys Med Rehabil* 1997;78:213–220.

National Center for Health Statistics. NCHS advance data (No 133). Department of Health and Human Services, Washington, DC, 1987.

Page SJ, Sisto SA, Johnston MV, et al. Modified constraint induced therapy: a case study. *Arch Phys Med Rehabil* (in press).

Page SJ, Sisto SA, Johnston MV, Levine P, Hughes M. Mod-ified constraint induced therapy: a randomized, feasibility and efficacy study. *J Rehabil Res Dev* 2001;38(5): 583–590.

Parikh RM, Robinson RG, Lipsey JR, et al. The impact of poststroke depression on recovery in activities of daily liv-ing over a 2-year follow-up. *Arch Neurol* 1990;47:785–789.

Pentland B, Jones PA, Roy CW, et al. Head injury in the el-derly. *Age Aging* 1986;15:193–202.

Ricker JH, Hillary FG, DeLuca J. Functionally activated brain imaging (O-15 PET and fMRI) in the study of learn-ing and memory after traumatic brain injury. *J Head Trauma Rehabil* 2001;16(2):191–205.

Roth EJ, Lovell L, Heinemann AW, et al. The older adult with a spinal cord injury. *Paraplegia* 1992;30(7):520–526.

Sibbarap KV, Nemchausky BA, Niekelski JJ, et al. Spinal cord dysfunction in older patients—rehabilitation out-comes. *Journal of American Paraplegia Society* 1987;10 (2):30–35.

Sosin DN, Sacks JJ, Smith SM. Head injury-associated deaths in the US from 1979–1986. *JAMA* 1989;282:2251.

Spivak JM, Weiss MA, Cotler JM, et al. Cervical spine injuries in patients 65 and older. *Spine* 1994;19(20):2302–2306.

Stanislav SW, Fabre T, Crismon ML, et al. Buspirone's effi-cacy in organic-injured aggression. *J Clin Psychophar-macol* 1994;14:126–130.

Taub E, Miller NE, Novack TA, et al. Technique to improve chronic motor deficit after stroke. *Arch Phys Med Reha-bil* 1993;74:347–354.

Taub E, Pidikiti RD, DeLuca SC, et al. Effects of motor re-striction of an unimpaired upper extremity and training on improving functional tasks and altering brain/behaviors. In: Toole J, ed. *Imaging neurologic rehabilitation.* New York: Demos Publications, 1996.

Taylor LP, Posner JB. Phenobarbital rheumatism in patients with brain tumor. *Ann Neurol* 1989;25:92–94.

Teasdale G, Skene A, Parker L, et al. Age and outcome of se-vere head injury. *Acta Neurochir (Wien)* 1979;28(Suppl): 140–143.

Teasell R, Allatt D. Managing the growing number of spinal cord-injured elderly. *Geriatrics* 1991;46(6);78, 83–85, 89.

Van der Lee JH, Wagenaar RC, Lankhorst GJ, et al. Forced use of the upper extremity in chronic stroke patients: re-sults from a single-blind randomized clinical trial. *Stroke* 1999;30:2369–2375.

Vollmer DG. Prognosis and outcome of severe head injury. In: Cooper PR, ed. *Head injury,* 3rd ed. Baltimore: Williams & Wilkins, 1993:553–581.

Vollmer DG, Torner JC, Jane JA, et al. Age and outcome fol-lowing traumatic coma: why do older patients fare worse? *Neurosurgery* 1991;75(Suppl):37–49.

Walker-Batson D, Smith P, Curtis S, et al. Amphetamine paired with physical therapy accelerates motor recovery after stroke: further evidence. *Stroke* 1995;26(12):2254–2259.

Weber DC, Fleming KC, Evans JM. Rehabilitation of geri-atric patient. *Mayo Clin Proc* 1995;70:1198.

Williams TF. The aging process: biological and psycho-so-cial considerations. In: Brody SJ, Ruff GE, eds. *Aging and rehabilitation: advances in the state of the art.* New York: Springer, 1986:13.

Wilson JA. The functional effects of head injury in the el-derly. *Brain Inj* 1987;1:183.

Wroblewski Ba, Joseph AB, Kupfer J, et al. Effectiveness of valproic acid on destructive and aggressive behaviours in patients with acquired brain injury. *Brain Inj* 1997;11: 37–47.

Yablon SA. Posttraumatic seizures. *Arch Phys Med Rehabil* 1993;74:983.

Yarkony GM, Roth EJ, Heinemann AW, et al. Spinal cord in-jury rehabilitation outcome: the impact of age. *J Clin Epi-demiol* 1988;41(2):173–177.

Zafonte RD, Lexell J, Cullen N. Possible applications for dopaminergic agents following traumatic brain injury: Part I. *Journal of Head Trauma Rehabilitation* 2000;15 (5):1179.

SUGGESTED READING

Dobkin BH, ed. *Neurologic rehabilitation.* Philadelphia: FA Davis, 1996.

Mills VM, Cassidy JW, Katz DI, eds. *Neurologic rehabilita-tion: a guide to diagnosis, prognosis, and treatment plan-ning.* Malden, MA: Blackwell Science, 1997.

Rosenthal M, Griffith ER, Kruetzer JS, et al., eds. *Rehabil-itation of the adult and child with traumatic brain injury,* 3rd ed. Philadelphia: FA Davis, 1999.

34

Long-Term Care Options for the Aging

Deborah W. Frazer

INTRODUCTION

The Definition of Long-Term Care

Long-term care refers to all residential and health services required to support individuals with chronic disease or disability. In contrast, *acute care* refers to health services provided for a limited period of time, generally until a specific health condition has resolved. Acute care is usually provided in hospitals or outpatient physician offices. It is generally paid for by private or public health insurance, such as Medicare. Long-term care can be provided in a variety of settings, including nursing homes, assisted living facilities, or private homes. No single payment system is widely used for long-term care.

The Need for Long-Term Care

The well-documented aging of the United States population is attended by two demographic corollaries: dramatic increase in the number of individuals with physical disabilities and those with mental disabilities such as Alzheimer's disease. These impairments are chronic and may be progressive as well.

The number of Americans 65 years of age and older is projected to increase from 12.8% of the population in 1995 to 20% of the population in 2050. Americans 85 years of age and older, who are the heaviest users of long-term care, are the fastest growing segment of the population. The over-85 age group is expected to increase fivefold by 2050 (US Bureau of the Census, 1996).

With advancing age comes increased physical frailty and dependence. The average nursing home resident is a woman in her 80s, with some cognitive impairment, and needing help with four of five activities of daily living (ADL), such as bathing, eating, dressing, transferring, and toileting. Alzheimer's disease and other dementias are associated with increasing age. With the neurologic losses of dementia come further declines in functional abilities. The Centers for Medicare and Medicaid Services estimates that two of five Americans will need long-term care at some point in their lives.

With these projections for an aging population with attendant physical and mental disability, it is clear why healthcare experts refer to long-term care as "the looming crisis" (American Health Care Association, 2000).

A Brief History of Long-Term Care

What did our grandparents do for long-term care? Why won't that work for us?

First, our grandparents did not have the same life expectancy. In 1940, the survival rate from age 65 to age 90 was 7%; in the year 2000, that rate has more than tripled to 26%. (Cutler, 2000). Only recently, do most people face the prospect of an extended *old age*, probably with one or more chronic disabilities.

Second, for those in earlier generations who did live into their seventh, eighth, or ninth decades of life, immediate and extended families were usually available for caregiving. In years past, women typically worked at home, providing homemaking and caregiving for children, elders, and other dependent family members. With the growth of women in the paid labor force, the increased mobility of US families, and the rising rate of divorce, family-based long-term care has been strained (Frazer, 1999).

Third, earlier versions of long-term care *did* include care sites that are used today, but they have been transformed. Many counties in the United States developed *county homes* or *poor houses* for the sick or disabled indigent. Similarly, churches and synagogues sponsored *homes for the aged* that contained a mix of skilled nursing and personal care services. Although many of these government and faith-sponsored "homes" still exist today, they have undergone radical changes to keep pace with funding and regulatory changes.

The three historical sources of long-term care—family, faith-sponsored, and government—persist to-day. However, these sources alone are unlikely to be able to meet the rapidly increasing demand for long-term care services in the future.

THE RISE AND FALL OF NURSING HOMES AS THE LONG-TERM CARE SITE OF CHOICE

When the Social Security Act was passed in the 1930s, no agreement existed on a national health care system. In the 1960s, in a partial move toward national health care, Congress passed legislation mandating government sponsorship of Medicare (acute healthcare for the elderly) and Medicaid (acute healthcare for the poor). Medicaid dollars (a mix of federal and state monies) also were designated for use by indigent nursing home residents.

The latter usage of Medicaid funds quickly became a major public healthcare expenditure. Nursing homes, as the only government-paid site for long-term care, grew rapidly. Middle class families learned to "spend down" an elder's resources to become eligible for a "MA" (Medicaid) bed. The state and federal governments watched with alarm as every bed certified by Medicaid was quickly filled, with no end to demand in sight. A nursing home industry arose, with for-profit and publicly traded companies joining an area previously dominated by faith organizations and county governments. By the 1980s, many states imposed a moratorium on new nursing home bed construction, and a lengthy *Certificate of Need* process was required to obtain authorization to build new nursing homes.

At the same time that demand for publicly funded nursing home beds was skyrocketing, a crisis was looming in the quality of care being provided. A landmark report from the Institute of Medicine in 1985 detailed the ominous conditions that existed in many nursing homes and prompted the Nursing Home Reform Act contained in the Omnibus Budget Reconciliation Acts of 1987, 1989, and 1990. These reforms required greatly increased regulation and monitoring of nursing homes, which in turn, increased costs.

By the early 1990s, with the demographic press of an aging population and crises in costs and quality in nursing homes, conditions were ripe to develop new alternatives for long-term care.

LOOKING FOR OPTIONS: GROWTH OF THE "CONTINUUM OF CARE"

The term "continuum of care" refers to the expansion of options for elder care sites. Rather than having to choose between "staying in my own home" or "being put in a nursing home," families and providers began to recognize that more options were possible (Table 34-1). Figure 34-1 portrays the relationship of frailty to the options for long-term care.

Home Care

A variety of services are now available to support elders in their own homes. Skilled services are prescribed by a physician and provided by licensed healthcare professionals. These can include medication monitoring, wound or catheter care, health education for the elder or family member, rehabilitation services, medical social work, nutritional assessment and counseling, and respiratory services.

In addition to these professional services, a variety of *home support* or *homemaker* services are available, including help with ADL (bathing, dressing, eating, toileting), or *instrumental* activities of daily living (IADL) (housekeeping, laundry, shopping, transportation). These activities can be performed by home health aides or homemakers, who may or may not be state-certified. They may work for public agencies, such as an Area Agency on Aging, or a private, for-profit or non-profit agency. Elders or their families can also hire a home caregiver directly. The range of in-home elder caregivers is analogous to the range of in-home child caregivers, where families are often confused by differing titles (nanny, mother's helper, sitter), training, certifications, costs, and supervision.

Unlike in-home child care, home care for elders at times is paid for by public funds. Medicare may pay for prescribed care for a limited period of time following a hospitalization. Medicaid, the state program for low-income individuals, will pay for home care in some states under some conditions (e.g., as an alternative to nursing home care). Some long-term care insurance policies pay for some aspects of home care, but coverage varies widely from policy to policy. Frequently, home care is paid for directly by the elder or family. Extensive home care services can cost as much as nursing home charges.

A recent development to help elders pay for care services while remaining in their homes is the *reverse mortgage*, now available through many banks. Many elders, having been in their homes for decades, find themselves "house-poor" (i.e., living in highly appreciated housing from which they get no financial benefit, yet for which they pay high property taxes). The reverse mortgage is one way to address the needs of elders in this situation. In essence, the bank takes ownership (but not possession) of the elder's home,

TABLE 34-1. Long-term care (LTC) options: a summary of characteristics

	Home care	Family care	Independent living community	Assisted-living community	Skilled nursing home	Continuing care retirement community
Cost	Modest, if covered by insurance; expensive, if not	Modest	Somewhat more than living at home	Expensive; paid privately	Expensive; can be covered by third party	Expensive; paid privately
Health insurance coverage	Yes	No	No	No	Yes, for acute conditions	Yes, but only for acute conditions
Medicare coverage	Yes	No	No	No	Yes, for acute conditions	Yes, but only for acute conditions
Medical assistance coverage	Yes	No	No	Experimentally, in one or two states	Yes	Generally not
Long-term care insurance coverage	Usually	No	No	Sometimes	Yes, with limits	Sometimes
Independence	Yes	No	Yes	Yes	No	Usually
Privacy	Yes	No	Usually	Usually	No	Usually
Flexibility to move	Yes	Yes	Yes	Yes	Not usually	Not usually
Lifetime security	No	Yes, if it is working out and resources are available	No	Not usually	Usually	Yes
Extensive nursing care	No	No	No	No	Yes	Yes
Federal regulations	Yes, under, Medicare	No	No	No	Yes	Yes
24-hour nursing supervision	No	No	No	A few have	Yes	Yes, in the Healthcare section

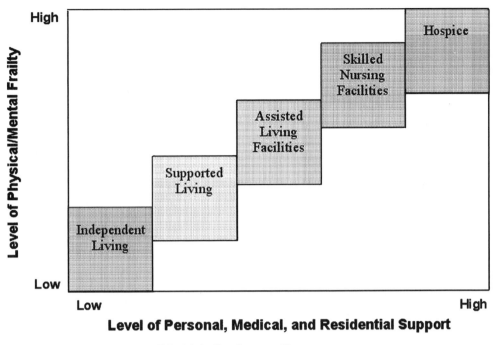

FIG. 34-1. Continuum of long-term care.

paying the elder a monthly *mortgage fee*, and allowing the elder to remain in the home. This boosts the elder's income, thus allowing the elder to benefit from appreciation in the home's value. This solution is attractive to those who wish to stay in their homes, but need extra money to pay for services.

Another recent development in home care is the concept of *life care at home*. Available only in selected geographical areas and paid for privately, this arrangement guarantees an individual or couple lifetime care, as much as possible in the elders' home. Typically, the elders are required to be in good physical and mental condition when entering the program. An entrance fee is charged and monthly fees begin immediately, even though no services may be necessary. Additional fees may be necessary as services are required in later years. Care is coordinated through a care manager, who conducts regular assessments and care plans. In essence, *life care at home* is a variant of long-term care insurance. Elders often find that it provides peace of mind and they enjoy the ongoing relationship with the care manager.

Elders and their families must be selective about home care providers. These are people who will be in the elder's private home, perhaps unsupervised. They may have access to everything from jewelry or cash to bank accounts and credit cards. Frail elders are vulnerable to psychological or physical abuse by caregivers. In the case of an elder who is physically or cognitively impaired, it is especially important to hire and monitor a competent and trustworthy caregiver. Help with referrals and selection is often provided through physicians, social workers, the local Area Agency on Aging, or a private geriatric care manager. Some referral sources, such as the Area Agency on Aging, cannot recommend a specific agency, but can delete an agency from their list in cases of significant complaints about an agency.

Physicians can provide a great service to elders and their families by helping them with home care decisions. Having a psychologist, social worker, or geriatric care manager as part of the office team (as staff or consultants) facilitates a seamless referral process for the elder and family, and helps the physician attend to the psychosocial aspects of care that are so intertwined with medical conditions. Such ancillary staff or consultants can do the extensive research necessary to identify high-quality local providers of home care services, and to match providers with the needs and financial resources of a physician's patients.

The elder or family (ideally, in conjunction with a professional) need to consider the following points regarding potential providers: how long they have been in business; how employees are selected, trained, and supervised; how they develop a plan or care; if and how care is documented; fees, billing, and funding sources; emergency procedures; complaint procedures; and references.

Family Care

Moving in with a sibling, daughter, or son is another variation on home care. The elder leaves his or her own home (and thus realizes the appreciated value of the home), and joins a relative's household. Savings are achieved by combining households, and many of the nonprofessional care services (ADL and IADL) can be provided by family members. Loneliness, a major problem of widowed or homebound elders, is alleviated. The chief disadvantages of this arrangement are loss of independence, autonomy, and privacy for elder and family, and the additional caregiver burden that may be placed on family members. To reduce the burden on families, any of the home care services mentioned above can also be provided in the family member's home.

Families often quickly move to *family care* arrangements because of the financial benefits, family tradition, and psychological factors such as love, obligation, or guilt. Although it is a satisfying arrangement for many families, it can very stressful for others. Families should be encouraged to have extensive discussions before reaching a decision, with all members present, and perhaps with a physician, social worker, or religious counselor facilitating the discussion. Especially in the case of a caregiving *child*, discussion should include how other siblings will concretely support the designated caregiving sibling, both emotionally and financially. The caregiving child should not underestimate the stress this arrangement can place on a busy household, especially in cases where a spouse and teenage children are at home. A trial period is strongly advised.

Respite Care

Respite care is the term used for an elder's short-term stay in an institutional setting (nursing home or assisted living) to provide respite for the caregiver. Perhaps, the caregiver is a spouse who must have surgery, or a middle-aged daughter who wants to vacation with her husband and children. Respite stays, typically 1 to 2 weeks, are paid privately. If taken in a pleasant, well-appointed assisted living facility, it can feel like a vacation for the elder. A nursing home respite stay would only be advisable for someone who needs skilled nursing services while the caregiver is away. Otherwise, it is more likely to feel *institutional* to the elder.

Some states provide respite care funds to family caregivers, recognizing the significant caregiving work that these families are doing and everyone's need for some time away. A local Area Agency on Aging will have information about public respite care funding.

Independent Living Communities

Independent living communities are facilities for older adults who do not need significant medical or personal care support, but who wish to live in a community designed for older adults. These are sometimes called "active adult communities" or "retirement communities."

Independent living communities include apartments, condominiums, and single family housing. They may be urban, suburban, or rural, and communities are available across the economic spectrum. The additional services that a community provides will reflect its location and the socioeconomic status of its members. Among the typical services are security (ranging from a security guard to a "gated" community); organized activities (trips, outings, in-house gatherings, classes and clubs); exercise opportunities (tennis, golf, exercise equipment or classes); and meal plans (often consisting of one meal per day in a restaurant-style dining center).

Most independent living communities are rental arrangements, although in some versions the members purchase their homes. Participation in these communities is typically on a private-pay basis, although some subsidized "senior housing" is available.

It should be noted that many elders enjoy living in *unofficial* independent living communities; these are usually apartment buildings with a high proportion of elderly residents. In gerontology, these are known as "naturally occurring retirement communities." Residents tend to watch out for each other and provide informal support to those who need temporary or modest amounts of assistance.

Independent living communities are often a transitional phase as elders seek freedom from the burdens of home ownership, but do not yet need health or personal care services. It is important to help elders and their families plan beyond this phase—to think through the options should more medical or personal care become necessary.

Adult Day Centers

Adult day centers provide a service variously referred to as *Adult Day Center*, *Adult Care Center*,

Adult Day Health Center, or *Adult Day Care Center*. What all these have in common is that they provide a place for elders to congregate during the day. The hours and services vary widely. All provide at least one meal (lunch), whereas some provide breakfast, snacks, and supper. All provide social and creative activities onsite; some may provide outings and trips off-site as well. A key differentiator is the extent to which the site provides professional healthcare services: skilled nursing, rehabilitation, medical social services, or medication management. Most have a nurse available. Some centers provide personal care, even including showers, nail care, and hairdressing. Many centers provide transportation.

The schedule of hours and days also varies widely, from as few as 4 hours per day to as many as 12 hours per day; and from a few days per week to 7 days. Some centers are targeted more to cognitively impaired individuals, whereas others are targeted to individuals with physical challenges.

Adult day centers provide a safe, social environment for elders. It can be an excellent adjunct or alternative to in-home care. Family members providing care may want their loved one to attend an outside program, especially if the family member works during the day. If the family member is not working outside the home, the adult day center can provide some hours each week of respite from the demands of caregiving. Typically, adult day centers are paid privately, although Medicare or other insurance may pay for some skilled professional services if the individual qualifies for the service.

PACE Programs

The acronym PACE stands for "Program of All-inclusive Care for the Elderly." At this writing, these programs are federally subsidized demonstration programs that have shown a high degree of success in delivering quality care to frail elders while maintaining them in their home settings, at a lower cost to taxpayers than nursing home placement.

The core feature of the PACE program is an adult day center that provides extensive direct services, as well as case management. Every participant enrolled in a PACE program is assigned to a case manager who coordinates all medical and social services, both at the site and at home. The case manager is responsible for cost management as well. The target group for PACE programs are elders who are frail enough to be nursing home eligible, but who wish to be, and can be, maintained at home with extensive and well-coordinated services.

If medical, quality of life, and financial outcomes continue for these programs, it is likely they will continue to expand, at least in urban low-income areas.

Assisted Living Communities

Assisted living communities vary widely from state to state, as they are regulated at the state level (versus nursing homes, which are regulated at the federal level) (General Accounting Office, 1999). In most states, the definition includes a residential facility that provides personal care as needed for ADL, and other supportive services (e.g., transportation). Typically, residents do not need extensive skilled medical care for an extended period of time. Some states (e.g., New Jersey and Florida) are permitting higher levels of nursing care to occur in assisted living settings. Many assisted living facilities have special units for individuals with Alzheimer's disease or related dementias. These units are often "secured" (locked) to prevent harm from wandering. Ideally, they should also provide higher staffing ratios and extensive activity or recreational programming.

The broad concept of assisted living includes group homes, personal care or boarding homes, and sheltered care homes. Sponsors of these facilities include churches, other non-profit agencies, local governmental agencies, or for-profit companies. Assisted living communities experienced phenomenal growth in the 1990s. Most of the expansion occurred in for-profit chains (perhaps even to the point of overexpansion, as indicated by some Chapter 11 filings). These companies brought in many concepts from the hospitality and hotel industry to serve individuals who formerly were served by the healthcare sector through nursing homes. Planners are hopeful that the expansion of assisted living choices will encourage individuals and families to use private pay dollars to purchase more consumer-oriented, *hospitality* residential services when only personal assistance is required. This establishes a continuum, so that nursing homes are used for skilled nursing and medical care, serving a more medically acute population. The assisted living facilities would be primarily paid privately, whereas public funds would be available for skilled nursing home care. Some states are experimenting with some use of public funds to support assisted living.

Monthly fees in assisted living facilities can range from about $1,500 to as much as $5,000, depending on size, location, and the extent of services and amenities. A minimal amount of personal care (1/2 to 1 hour daily) and two meals per day are usually included in a basic fee. More expensive services include continence management, medication management, and full meal service. At the highest end, assisted living communities may provide spa services, private dining facilities, limousine service to cultural events, libraries, and even an "open bar" during cocktail hour. The amount, level, and type of skilled nursing care that is available or permitted varies by state regulation and by facility.

SKILLED NURSING FACILITIES

Skilled nursing facilities (SNF) are also known as *nursing homes* or *convalescent centers*. SNF provide professional nursing care under the direction of a physician. The medical and nursing care is usually more intense than that provided in an assisted living facility, but less than that provided in a hospital. Much of the type of care that was only done in hospitals 10 or 15 years ago is now done in SNF, such as respiratory and catheter care, intravenous antibiotics, and rehabilitation services. Nursing homes can be used for short-term stays for respite, transitional care between hospital and home, or rehabilitation. They also are used for long-term care, including end-of-life care.

Nursing home costs can range from $4,000 to $6,000 per month. It often comes as a shock to individuals and families that Medicare may not cover these costs. Medical eligibility and financing for SNF care are complicated. For example, shorter stays may be covered by Medicare (for up to 90 days), but only if the individual has a *qualifying* hospital stay before SNF admission. Private health insurance may cover some or all of a short-term stay. However, neither Medicare nor private health insurance ever cover long-term care. Parts of a long-term stay may be covered by long-term care insurance. Indigent individuals are generally covered, if they meet the eligibility requirements, by the Medical Assistance program. Many people enter nursing homes paying with private funds and then switch to Medical Assistance when their personal funds are depleted. Individuals and their families should seek professional assistance to navigate the complexity of nursing home financing. Hospital social workers, Area Agencies on Aging, eldercare lawyers, and financial planners provide this type of financial counseling.

Hospice

Hospice care is reserved for those near the end of life, usually defined as within 6 months. Originally, and most typically, hospice was used for cancer pa-

tients. It is also used for patients with terminal acquired immunodeficiency syndrome (AIDS) and various other endstage diseases. Hospice is provided as Medicare benefit, under strict regulation. It requires that patients forego aggressive medical treatment to prolong life, in exchange for services designed to improve the quality of the end of life. Such services could be provided at home, in a hospice-specific facility, or within a nursing home. The services usually include home health aides, chaplaincy, social services, professional nursing, and pain management.

Although the number of recipients of hospice care doubled between 1992 and 1996, the average length of stay declined. This is attributed to physician confusion about the requirements of the program, and resulting hesitance to refer to it until an individual is very close to death. The Centers for Medicare and Medicaid Services is now encouraging physicians not to wait until a week or two before death to refer to hospice.

Continuing Care Retirement Communities

Continuing care retirement communities (CCRC) offer the entire continuum of care (independent living, assisted living, and skilled nursing) in one location. They provide companionship and freedom from the burdens of homeownership in the independent living section, accompanied by the security of guaranteed life-time care, on a financially predictable basis. It is a life-time contract for a residence, cleaning and maintenance, recreational opportunities, meals, personal care and skilled nursing care. Thus, CCRC are the financial equivalent to merging residential costs and long-term care insurance. CCRC are all privately paid, often requiring a substantial entrance fee (roughly equivalent to the cost of one's house), followed by lifelong monthly fees. They primarily serve middle to upper income individuals and couples.

The CCRC can have extended waiting lists, sometimes as much as 8 years. They typically require that elders be well enough to enter the independent living section. This extended time in independent living allows people to form important new friendships and explore the recreational and volunteer opportunities that are available. Many older adults report that CCRC feel something like a college campus and, indeed, some are located adjacent to college campuses.

This type of facility is an option that requires significant advance planning. Because of the legal and financial complexity of the contracts, it is always important to discuss this option (and specific contracts) with a lawyer, accountant, or financial planner.

Factors to Consider When Choosing Among Residential Care Options

Many factors need to be considered when choosing a long-term care option: preferences of the individual, couple, and family; current and predicted costs; matching care needs to provider capabilities; quality of care; and matching personal lifestyles to the environment of care (Fig. 34-2).

Preferences of the Individual, Couple, and Family

The first and perhaps most important preference is for geographical location. This decision can be complex and raise many sensitive issues in the family. Are Mom and Dad choosing to be near one child rather than another? Are they going to Florida, and expecting all the children to come as needed, despite the children's own family and job responsibilities? Do they really know what it will feel like to leave their friends, community, house of worship? Are they committing to an irreversible decision? How convenient is the nursing home or assisted living community to the home or workplace of the primary caregiving child? As with any other residential decision, the first thing to consider is: location, location, location!

A second and related decision is the decision to "stay in my own home" versus "moving to a new place." Most elders express a wish to "die in my own home"; however most will, in fact, die in a hospital or skilled nursing facility. For those who choose to stay in their homes, it is important to go over the costs, the potential burden to children, and the risks of being home alone. Many elders are happy at home until one member of a couple dies, leaving the remaining spouse grieving and lonely. Additionally, in many communities, the ability to drive a car is critical to maintain a comfortable quality of life: How will Dad get along when he can no longer drive? On the positive side, staying at home can be the best way to maintain dignity, privacy, and autonomy to the end of life. As always in long-term care, it is critical to discuss—in detail—preferences for end-of-life care with the family physician, and to execute the proper living will and durable power of attorney documents to ensure that those preferences are respected. These legal documents can include "do not hospitalize" provisions that make it more likely that the older adult's wishes to "die in my own home" are respected.

As mentioned, it is important when discussing preferences to include the issue of "burden to others." Elders frequently cite the fact that they do not want to

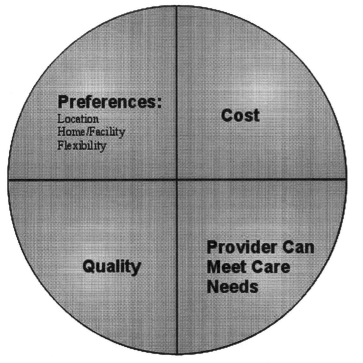

FIG. 34-2. Factors to consider when choosing long-term care.

be a burden to their children, but if the issues are not discussed openly among all family members, the elder may not understand correctly what feels burdensome to a child and what does not. Likewise, elders typically want to stay as independent as possible, but may not fully understand how different decisions would affect independence. Facilitating an open conversation about burden among family members is an excellent contribution the physician, nurse, or social worker can make.

Long-term care facilities and services are provided in the United States by for-profit, not-for-profit, religious, and governmental organizations. Examples are seen of excellent care and poor care in each ownership category, but elders should consider whether type of ownership is an important issue for them.

Finally, elders and their families should determine their preferences for commitment and security versus flexibility. For example, many assisted living facilities operate on a monthly rental agreement, with only 30 days notice required to leave (or to be asked to leave). At the other extreme are CCRC, which can require more than a $100,000 entrance fee that is not refundable after a 1 or 2 year period. The individual's tolerance for risk or desire for security should be a factor in decision-making, as well as the relative predictability of the health or disease status of the person.

Current and Expected Costs

Although no one has a crystal ball, physicians can be of great help to elders and their families in thinking through what future costs might be. For example, if a family member develops Alzheimer's disease at a relatively young age and has no comorbid conditions, the expected length of caregiving can exceed 10 years, with the final few years likely to require extensive personal care. Helping the family to envision gradually increasing personal care, at home or in a facility or both, is useful for them. On the other hand, an uncontrolled diabetic with high blood pressure and significant complications of the diabetes is likely to need skilled nursing care within a relatively short time frame, but is not likely to need care for the extended years that a well-controlled diabetic might. Having a rough estimate of the length of expected caregiving can help families with financial planning.

Understanding the type of care that will likely be needed also helps families with financial planning. If skilled care is likely, as in the case with a diabetic, then it is more likely to be covered by third party payors, at least for a limited time. If, however, the care is likely to be companion or personal care, it will not be covered, except by certain long-term care insurance policies. Encourage families to explore exactly what type of coverage they have and how it may or may not cover the expected care.

If an extended nursing home stay seems likely at some point in the future (even the distant future), the physician should encourage the elder and family to seek legal and financial planning advice about asset management, insurance coverage, and ways to reduce the risk of impoverishment.

Matching Care Need to Provider Capabilities

The most difficult type of long-term care to understand correctly is assisted living. The definition varies so widely that consumers are hard pressed to understand if this residential option will serve their or their parents' care needs. Consumers need answers to many questions about the facility and assistance provided by personnel, including the following:

Does the facility provide assistance with all ADL?

Is help available for toileting, including an every 2-hour continence management program?

Will they help with transferring from wheelchair to bed?

Will they help with IADL, such as transportation and shopping?

Are persons available to provide safe and professional financial management, such as bill-paying and mail management?

Will they supervise medications or actually administer them for a confused elder?

Are the people administering medications and other assistance with healthcare needs (insulin shots, eye drops, skin care) licensed and trained to deliver this care?

If an elder should need temporary skilled nursing care, can it be provided within the assisted living facility?

As skilled care needs increase, how would the facility handle it?

At what point do care needs exceed the assisted living facility's ability to meet them?

Quality of Care

Quality of care and maintaining quality of life are difficult to define and measure. Generally, elders and families should look for long-term care that maintains the highest level of independence, dignity, and respect; offers opportunities for intellectual, social, physical, and spiritual stimulation (but also the option to retreat from those); and fosters warm and caring interpersonal relationships among residents and between residents and staff. Happy and satisfied staff who are direct caregivers are often a marker of good quality care. Asking current residents whether they feel the above criteria are met is a good starting point for assessing quality.

Matching Personal Lifestyle to Environment of Care

In some ways, matching personal lifestyle to care environment is similar to the points raised above, but is closer to the concept of finding the right *match* between the personality of the elder and the *personality* of the environment of care. Has this elder always been reclusive, private, and suspicious or anxious around others? If so, an intensely social environment of care (e.g., a semiprivate room in a skilled nursing center) could be extremely stressful. Has this elder always been an extrovert who loves people, parties, and social occasions? Then being alone in a private home could be extremely stressful.

Another factor in finding the right fit between person and environment is the extent to which an individual only wants to be with others like himself or herself—with shared history, values, interests, food preferences, religious commitments, and so forth. Some elders prefer this type of homogeneous setting, whereas others thrive in a more religiously, culturally, racially, and socioeconomically diverse setting.

The final match characteristic goes back to location, location, location, but in terms of the *personality* of the location. Thought is especially needed when an elder is moving to be near a caregiving child to whether the move entails switching from an urban, suburban, or rural setting to a different setting. Equally important are regional differences found among the country's many diverse areas. Deeply ingrained regional styles can cause a distressing feeling of "not fitting in," especially when a frail elder does not have much reserve capacity to learn and adapt the new ways.

CONCLUSION

The United States currently has no system of long-term care. A fragmented patchwork of care is available which, in some cases, can provide what our el-

ders and families need. Until a comprehensive, accessible, coordinated system of long-term care is available, it is incumbent on all professionals, and most especially the physicians who are guiding patient care, to understand and help families to understand what options are available to them.

REFERENCES

American Health Care Association. *The looming crisis: long term health care.* Washington, DC: American Health Care Association, 2000.

Cutler NE. *Middle age & long-term care: the two meanings of "middle."* Conference presentation, "Long Term Care at the Crossroads," Center for Advocacy for the Rights and Interests of the Elderly. Philadelphia, September 2000.

Frazer DW. Family disruption: understanding and treating the effects of dementia onset and nursing home placement. In: Duffy M, ed. *Handbook of counseling and psychotherapy with older adults.* New York: John Wiley & Sons, 1999.

General Accounting Office. *Assisted living: quality-of-care and consumer protection issues in four states.* Washington, DC: General Accounting Office, April 1999.

US Bureau of the Census. *Current population reports.* Washington, DC: US Bureau of the Census, 1996.

SUGGESTED READINGS

All about hospice: a consumer's guide. Hospice Association of America, 1994. Choosing a quality nursing home. AAHSA, 2000. Washington, DC: AAHSA Publications, 901 E Street, NW, Suite 500, Washington, DC, 20004.

The consumers' directory of continuing care retirement communities. Washington, DC: AAHSA Publications, 2000.

The continuing care retirement community: a guidebook for consumers. Washington, DC: American Association of Homes and Services for the Aging (AAHSA) Publications, 1993, revision in process.

Your guide to choosing a nursing home. Washington, DC: Centers for Medicare and Medicaid Services (CMS), Department of Health and Human Services (HHS), 2001. Available by calling 1-800-MEDICARE.

WEB SITES

American Association of Homes and Services for the Aging: *www.aahsa.org*

American Association of Retired Persons: *www.aarp.org*

Assisted Living Federation of America: *www.alfa.org*

Administration on Aging: *www.aoa.dhhs.gov*

Health Care Financing Administration: *www.hcfa.gov*

U.S. Department of Health and Human Services/Healthfinder: *www.healthfinder.gov*

35

Ethical and Legal Issues in the Care of Elderly Patients with Neurological Illnesses

Bryan D. James and Jason H. T. Karlawish

INTRODUCTION

The care of elderly patients with neurologic illnesses includes managing a number of medical problems that include substantial ethical and legal issues. These issues are the result of morbidities caused by these illnesses. Neurodegenerative dementias typically impair a patient's ability to make a decision. Other people, such as their caregivers, must decide for them. Other neurologic illnesses such as epilepsy may not primarily affect a patient's cognition, but they do have a significant impact on the patient's ability to perform important tasks such as driving. Finally, in many chronic and progressive illnesses (e.g., amyotrophic lateral sclerosis) cures are not available. Hence, clinicians must have the skills to address matters of death and dying and discuss quality of life.

Unlike the other issues in this book that a physician addresses by applying the principles of medical science, ethical and legal issues require a physician to apply the principles of moral theory. Key principles are respect for autonomy (allowing a competent patient to voluntarily choose care), beneficence (minimizing interventions' risks and maximizing their benefits), and justice (treating equal people in an equal manner). At first inspection, applying these principles may seem to be matters of having a good character and knowing a good lawyer. But, as important as those matters are, a clinician needs to have skills similar to those used to diagnose and treat the diseases that raise these ethical and legal issues. These skills will allow the clinician to identify ethical and legal issues, categorize them, and find efficient ways to address them. The failure to master these skills can have a significant impact on the quality of patient care.

This chapter focuses on five key issues that physicians encounter in the care of elderly patients with neurologic illnesses. These are (*a*) competency and decision-making capacity; (*b*) advance care planning; (*c*) common challenges in end-of-life decision-mak-

ing, including terminal sedation and assisted suicide; (*d*) driving; and (*e*) elder abuse. The general structure of this chapter is to address the nature and scope of each issue and provide practical steps to identify and address it.

COMPETENCY AND DECISION-MAKING CAPACITY: THE FOUNDATION OF EFFECTIVE DECISION-MAKING

The concepts of *competency and decision-making capacity* are the foundations of effective decision-making. A physician should respect the choices made by competent patients and seek out a surrogate to make choices for those who are not competent. These concepts are operationalized in the practice of informed consent. This section presents definitions of the concepts, and outlines techniques to assess them and to make decisions when a patient is not competent. It also presents other models for decision-making.

Scope of the Problem

Many neurologic illnesses have an impact on cognition. The neurodegenerative dementias (e.g., Alzheimer's disease) are common causes of impairments. For example, among patients with mild to moderate Alzheimer's disease, fully 95% of them cannot adequately understand the information needed to know to make a treatment decision (Marson et al., 1995). This impairment can have dramatic impact on the patient's ability to make a competent treatment choice.

When Should a Physician Assess Decision-Making Capacity and Competency?

All adults are competent until shown otherwise. Several clinical situations are seen when it is prudent to assess a patient's decision-making capacity and competency. In general, these are situations when the patient faces choices that involve significant risks or uncertain benefits, or the patient refuses a low risk and high benefit intervention. For example, in the situation of a patient who accepts a low risk intervention, such as aspirin therapy for a transient ischemic attack, the physician would have little reason to carefully assess the patient's decision-making capacity. In contrast, the use of coumadin for this same problem should warrant a more careful assessment of the patient's decision-making capacity. This should be done regardless of the patient's decision to accept or decline the drug. In all of these conditions, the issue is not that the physician has reversed the assumption that the patient is competent. The issue is assuring that the physician has adequately taught the patient the key facts and engaged in a meaningful dialogue about the pros and cons of the physician's recommendation.

The Concepts of Competency and Decision-Making Capacity

Decision-making capacity and competency are distinct concepts. Decision-making capacity describes a person's ability to understand, appreciate, and rationally manipulate information (Appelbaum and Grisso, 1988). It is an individual quality akin to qualities such as intelligence, mood, or weight. In this way, decision-making capacity is a quality that can be measured just as intelligence is measured using tools, such as the Wechsler Adult Intelligence Scale, or weight using a scale calibrated in kilograms. In contrast, competency is a judgment about a person. Competent describes a person whose abilities to understand, appreciate, and rationally manipulate information are adequate to make a choice, given the risks, benefits, and alternatives of the decision (Appelbaum and Grisso, 1988).

How to Assess Competency and Decision-Making Capacity

To assess decision-making capacity, it is important to assess a patient's ability to understand, appreciate, and rationally manipulate the key information about a decision. Table 35-1 summarizes these abilities, with definitions and standard phrases to assess them. *Understanding* describes a patient's ability to know the meaning of the information. Assess this by asking the patient to say back in his or her own words the information disclosed. For example, ask a patient, "Can you tell me in your own words what are the reasons

TABLE 35-1. *The elements of decision making capacity—their definitions and standard ways to assess them*

Understanding: the ability to state the meaning of the relevant information (risks, benefits, indications, diagnosis, and options of care).
   Sample question to assess understanding: "Can you tell me in your own words what I just said about....?"

Appreciation: the patient's ability to recognize that the information applies to him or her.
   Sample question to assess appreciation of treatment: "Regardless of what your choice is, do you think that it is possible the medication can benefit you?" "Regardless of what your choice is, do you think that it is possible the medication can harm you?"
   Sample question to assess appreciation of diagnosis: "Can you tell me in your own words what you see as your medical problem?"

Rationally manipulating information: the abilities to compare information and infer consequences of choices.
   Sample question to assess comparative reasoning: "How is taking the medicine better than not taking it?"
   Sample question to assess consequential reasoning: "How might taking the medicine affect your everyday activities?"

for having the spinal tap?" Because understanding requires cognitive skills that include short-term memory and language, disease that impairs these cognitive functions can impair a patient's ability to understand.

Appreciation describes a patient's ability to recognize that the information applies to him or her. Assess this by asking the patient to set aside a decision and answer whether the patient thinks the facts apply to him or her. For example, ask a patient, "You may or may not want to have the spinal tap, we'll talk about that more in a minute. For now, I'd like to ask you about the risks and benefits of the procedure. Do you think that the spinal tap can benefit you?" Later, ask the patient, "Do you think that the spinal tap can harm you?" Then, ask a question to assess whether the patient thinks that he or she has the disease or problem under treatment. In all of these questions, the issue is whether the patient acknowledges that the information applies to him or her personally. Diseases can impair insight and judgment (e.g., a delusional disorder seen in schizophrenia, or Lewy body or frontal dementias) can impair a patient's ability to appreciate information.

Rationally manipulating information describes two capacities: *comparative* and *consequential reasoning*. Comparative reasoning describes a person's ability to examine options head-to-head. For example, ask the patient, "Can you tell me how not having the spinal tap is better than having it?" Consequential reasoning describes a person's ability to infer outcomes of the various options faced. For example, ask the patient, "What are some ways that having the spinal tap might affect your daily activities?"

The sample questions above are analogous to the questions a physician uses to assess a patient's chief complaint, such as headache or memory loss. In a clinical encounter, the issue of headache is raised. Physicians have concepts they want to assess: vascular headache, migraine, and so on. To do this, the physician has a set of well-rehearsed probe questions. Based on the patient's answers to these questions, the physician generates an assessment of the likelihood that the patient's headache is vascular, a migraine, or from some other cause. In the assessment of some complaints (e.g., depression), these questions can be standardized to the degree that they are collected into a scale. For example, the 15- or 30-item Geriatric Depression Scale asks a series of questions such as "Are you basically satisfied with your life?" (Yesavage et al., 1983). The patient's scores on each question are added up to generate an overall score of depressive symptoms. Although a score is not determinative of depression, the greater the patient's score, the more likely that the patient has depression.

In the case of decision-making capacity, measure the patient's ability to understand, appreciate, and rationally manipulate information. Ask standard questions and then assess the adequacy of the patient's answers. Efforts are made to correct deficiencies. After each answer, score the patient's performance (poor, good, excellent). The sum of these scores are then used to substantiate an assessment of how well the patient performs on each of the measures of decision-making capacity.

In addition to assessing these capacities, include an assessment of the patient's cognition and affect. These data are particularly useful because they will help to explain why deficits exist in a patient's decision-making capacity. Hence, assessing competency has not only an ethical warrant but also a clinical one. It may be the initial clue that a patient suffers from a clinically significant disorder in affect or cognition.

All adults are competent unless shown otherwise. Use data that describe a patient's decision-making capacity and the risks and benefits of the decision at hand to judge whether the patient is not competent. For example, a patient with mild Alzheimer's disease faces the decision whether to enroll in a clinical trial. In conversation, a physician may find that the patient appreciates the information and can reason about how the clinical trial will affect daily life but has considerable difficulty understanding all of the information

and comparing options. In such a case, the judgment whether the patient is competent will rely on the degree of the impairments in understanding and comparative reasoning. For example, the patient may not understand that the project is research and includes random assignment to drug or placebo. The physician must judge whether this misunderstanding, in the context of the risks and potential benefits of the research, means that the patient is not competent.

Other Models for Decision-Making

Competency and decision-making capacity are foundations of the principle of respect for autonomy. They derive from theories of rational decision-making that is operationalized in the doctrine of informed consent. In other words, they assume that people do and should "weigh the risks and benefits" before making a voluntary decision. Many patients do engage in this kind of decision-making and a physician should regard it as a key model to guide the role of doctor as teacher. However, a physician needs to respect that patients may not adhere to this same model.

Patients use other models for making decisions about clinical care and research. Chief among these models are decisions based on trust in other persons (e.g., family or physician) or trust in institutions (e.g., a university or pharmaceutical company) (Fost, 1975; McKneally and Martin, 2000). In a trust-based model, the person will cede the task of assessing the information or even making the decision to another person such as family member or physician. This other person is identified as *entrusted*. Although this model does differ from one that features rationally weighing information, it fits within the principle of respect for autonomy. It is reasonable for a person to cede authority to another, provided that decision to do so is voluntary and informed.

For a model based on trust to function ethically, the physician needs to recognize factors that can undermine trust. *Conflict of interest*, chief among these factors, is the term that describes a condition of two or more relationships that possess inherently contradictory commitments or obligations. For example, a physician who owns a for-profit testing facility and also prescribes testing at that facility is in a conflict of interest. Such a conflict can undermine or even negate the patient's trust. A physician has an obligation to disclose or even avoid the conflict.

ADVANCE CARE PLANNING

Advance care planning describes a competent person's preferences for future medical care. The physician's role in providing diagnosis and prognosis warrants a role in assisting the patient in this planning. Planning can take two forms: conversations that lead to considered plans or structured documents called "advance directives."

Advance Directives

An *advance directive* is a set of instructions indicating a competent person's preferences for future medical care. It is used to guide healthcare professionals in the event that the person should become unable to communicate personal wishes or competent to participate in medical decision-making. In general, an advance directive addresses ethically problematic decisions involving life-sustaining treatment for patients who are terminally ill or near death. Advance directives are intended to preserve patient autonomy by ensuring that patients are able to direct their future medical treatment and to help physicians avoid ethical dilemmas in treating incompetent patients.

Two kinds of advance directives exist: a living will and a durable power of attorney (DPA). *Living wills* are documents that instruct physicians proactively regarding the initiation, continuation or discontinuation, or withholding or withdrawal of particular forms of life-sustaining medical treatment (Furrow et al., 1991). A *DPA* for healthcare is a document that designates a person (also known as an "agent," "surrogate," "proxy," or "attorney-in-fact") to make medical decisions on a person's behalf should that person become unable to do so. A DPA allows for greater flexibility than a living will because the agent can make decisions, should certain circumstance arise. Authorities, such as the American Bar Association, recommend that a patient have both a living will and a DPA (Sabatino, 1994). Additionally, a patient's oral statements in conversations with relatives, friends, and healthcare providers are also recognized ethically and, in some states also legally, as advance directives, provided they are properly charted in the medical record. Table 35-2 lists a few good World Wide Web resources for more information on advance directives.

The authority of an advance directive has been tested by court cases including a Supreme Court decision (Furrow et al., 1991). All 50 states and the District of Columbia have laws recognizing the use of advance directives. Each state has a form based on the specifics of its laws. These legally binding documents take effect only when medical decisions must be made and the physician finds that the patient is not capable of making them. In some instances, the physician must also judge that the patient is in a terminal condition. A person can revoke or change the advance directive at any time. A physician who morally objects to a patient's advance directive may choose not to comply, but must facilitate the patient's transfer to another physician. The *Patient Self-Determination Act (PSDA)* is a federal law requiring healthcare facilities that receive Medicaid and Medicare funds to inform patients of their rights to execute advance directives. The requirements are to ask patients at admission if they have previously executed an advance directive, provide information about advance directives to patients and their proxies, and inform patients of their rights to execute advance directives if they wish (Furrow et al., 1991; Silverman et al., 1995).

Although the law has attempted to make information on advance directives more accessible to patients, few patients actually complete one (Emanuel et al., 1991; LaPuma et al., 1991; Gamble et al., 1991). Approximately 3% to 14% of the general adult population and 10% to 12% of hospitalized patients and nursing home residents have advance directives (Goodman et al., 1998). Rates of completion are higher among older patients and patients in poorer health than among patients who are relatively young and healthy (Miles et al., 1996; Gordon and Shade., 1999). Ethnic and cultural factors can also influence completion rates. Whites and Asians are more likely to complete advance directives than are blacks and Hispanics (Silverman et al., 1995; Rubin et al., 1994; Morrison et al., 1998). Education has also been

---

TABLE 35-2. *Web resources on advance directives*

American Association of Retired Persons (AARP)
 http://www.aarp.org/programs/advdir/home.html
Choice in dying (can download state-specific advance directive forms)
 http://www.choices.org/
Medline Plus: Death and Dying (links to many good sites)
 http://www.nlm.nih.gov/medlineplus/deathanddying.html
US Living Wills Registry
 www.uslivingwillregistry.com
An organized set of links to living will (advance directive) web pages.
 http://www.mindspring.com/~scottr/will.html

shown to be an independent predictor of completion (Silverman et al., 1995; Stelter et al., 1992).

A number of factors responsible for the low rate of completion of advance directives have been examined, including misconceptions of the role of clinicians or family members in end-of-life decisions and the perception that directives do not accomplish the goal of patient autonomy (Goodman et al., 1998; Teno et al., 1994). The latter concern may be justified as physicians are often unaware that a patient has an advance directive (Goodman et al., 1998) or careless about following a patient's wishes (Gregor and Dunn, 1995). Furthermore, studies suggest that advance directives have little effect on resuscitation decisions (Teno et al., 1997b; Teno et al., 1994), use of medical treatments in general (Schneiderman et al., 1992; Goodman et al., 1998), or costs (Schneiderman et al., 1992; Teno et al., 1997a; Teno et al., 1994). The ineffectiveness of advance directives is a major problem. If patients are to be encouraged to complete advance directives, they must be respected at the time they are intended to take effect.

Perhaps the greatest barrier to completion or following an advance directive is the lack of physician communication with patients. Although the PSDA mandates that advance directives must be discussed with patients, many physicians express concerns that these discussions take too much time or lead to patient suspicion that maximal care will not be provided (Rubin et al., 1994; Silverman et al., 1995). However, studies have shown that the latter concern may be unwarranted, as most patients surveyed expressed desires to have such discussions (Rubin et al., 1994; Edinger and Smucker, 1992; Lo et al., 1986). Concerns also exist that living wills are not specific enough to deal with certain clinical questions (Pantilat et al., 1999; Eisendrath and Jonsen, 1983; Teno et al., 1997b). A further concern is that an advance directive is ineffectual because physicians may not consider a patient "absolutely, hopelessly ill" during periods of diminished capacity, thus not executing the patient's directive (Teno et al., 1994). For advance directives to serve their purpose in preserving patient autonomy after losing competency and decreasing problematic clinical decision-making, physicians must educate patients about completing directives and attempt to better understand their patient's preferences for the use of life-sustaining treatment.

Physician-Patient Communication About Advance Care

Documents that describe advance care plans are only as useful as the degree that the people who will use them understand, appreciate, and reason through what the document says. In short, the documents do not obviate the need for communication between physicians and patients about patient values and goals. Such communication can occur during the physician-patient conversation about treatment decisions. If a patient has a serious chronic illness (e.g., amyotrophic lateral sclerosis), the physician should obtain explicit instructions about treatments that are likely to be needed in the future (Fischer et al., 2000). Aside from such likely scenarios, the focus of advance care communication should not simply be specific treatment decisions. In advance care conversations, physicians often discuss the easiest scenarios: few patients would wish to be kept alive if they were permanently unconscious with no hope of recovery, whereas most patients would desire aggressive treatment in a reversible situation (Tulsky et al., 1998). But such conversation will not be useful when faced with the more common uncertainty of end-of-life decisions.

To adequately assure that the physician's future actions respect the patient's autonomy, advance care conversations must go beyond preferences for specific treatment options and elicit the patient's deeper values, and goals. Patients asked about their goals for advance care planning, list influencing what interventions are done to them as only one of their goals. They also identify the goals of preparing for death, gaining a sense of control, strengthening relationships, and relieving burdens on others (Martin et al., 1999; Singer et al., 1998). Once the patient's values and goals are clarified, specific decisions can be easier to make. It is important for the physician not to hide behind technical aspects and avoid eliciting the patient's emotions. Patients' emotions and concerns are important when exploring their goals.

How can physicians explore patients' goals? The same technique they use in everyday clinical encounters can facilitate discussions about future care. In particular, open-ended questions and follow-up questions that incorporate the patient's own words are listed in Table 35-3.

Four important points can guide the physician-patient discussion. First, explicitly ask the patient about uncertainty. Patients often state that they would only want life-sustaining treatment if it will help them. This attitude is completely rational but does not take into account the reality that physicians are often uncertain about the outcome. Patients should be asked about such situations with questions such as, "What if we are not sure whether we will be able to get you off the breathing machine?" (Fischer et al., 2000). Sec-

TABLE 35-3. *Useful questions to prompt a discussion about end-of-life care*

[a]1. What concerns you most about your illness?
[a]2. How is treatment going for you (your family)?
[a]3. As you think about your illness, what is the best and the worst that might happen?
[a]4. What has been most difficult about this illness for you?
[a]5. What are your hopes (your expectations, your fears) for the future?
[a]6. As you think about the future, what is most important to you (what matters most to you?)
[b]7. Are there any situations in which you would not think life was worth living?
[b]8. What makes life worth living?

From [a]Lo B, Quill T, Tulsky J. Discussing palliative care with patients. *Ann Intern Med* 1999;130:744–749; and [b]Fischer GS, Arnold RM, Tulsky JA. Talking to the older adult about advance directives. *Clin Geriatr Med* 2000;16:239–254, with permission.

ond, ask whether reversibility of the condition would alter the patient's views. For example, if the patient states that he or she would never want to be placed on a ventilator, ask, "What if we could get you off in a short period of time?" (Fischer et al., 2000). Also ask whether the patient would want any treatment at all in "states worse than death" (Fischer et al., 2000). Controversial treatments such as artificial nutrition and hydration should be discussed here. Third, clarify what the patient means when using potentially vague and loaded terms such as "vegetable" or "quality of life" (Fischer et al., 2000). Finally, it is important to make sure throughout advance care planning that you and patient are communicating effectively. Do not dominate the conversation; spend as much time listening as talking. In short, many of the same principles described above in the section on assessing competency and decision-making capacity apply here. The principle to good communication is "ensuring that the patient *understands* the implications of his or her stated preferences and that the doctor *understands* the patient's values (emphasis ours)" (Fischer et al., 2000). Do everything possible to establish trust that everything possible will be done to meet the patient's goals and continue to respect the patient's autonomy.

Advance care planning is extremely important in the goal to respect the patient's autonomy and control over his or her future care. Studies have shown that most patients with chronic and fatal disease can express their preferences for life-extending or ameliorative care and, for most of these patients, these preferences remained stable over the course of their disease (Albert et al., 1999). Education and advance care planning can give

patients self-control over their future care should they no longer be able to express these preferences. This is particularly important because medical decisions are not simply driven by patient preferences but also by the preferences of their healthcare providers and the options available from the system in which they receive care (Pritchard et al., 1998). Hence, the physician must proactively elicit the patient's values.

COMMON CHALLENGES IN END-OF-LIFE DECISION-MAKING

Discussions with patients and their families can be high octane, emotionally charged events that address deeply personal issues and values. The steps and questions described above are designed to provide the physician with structure so that the conversations reach a conclusion and have focus. In the course of these conversations, ethically charged concepts and judgments may be used. These include distinctions between *withdrawing* versus *withholding* treatment, *extraordinary* versus *ordinary* treatment, requests for physician-assisted suicide or terminal sedation, and surrogate decision-making. It is important for physicians to know where medical ethics and the law stand on these potentially controversial topics.

Withdrawing versus Withholding Treatment

Physicians will often face the decision to withhold or withdraw treatment from a patient at the end of life. Many physicians feel justified in withholding treatments they have never started, but have reservations about withdrawing treatments they have already initiated. The withholding or withdrawing distinction draws heavily on the distinction between omission— not performing an action—and commission—performing an action (Bok, 1978). Not starting a procedure can be seen as abstaining from subjecting the patient to an overly invasive intervention. On the other hand, withdrawing a treatment that has already been started can be psychologically difficult, and this discomfort stems mostly from a sense of responsibility for action to bring about the patient's death. The act of withdrawing can also be seen as an act of abandonment or breach of expectations or promises. Although such a distinction is psychologically understandable, moral philosophers and the law view the distinction between withdrawing and withholding as untenable (Beauchamp and Childress, 1994; Bok, 1978; Meisel, 1991).

In the first place, the distinction between withholding as an omission and withdrawing as a commission is ambiguous. Withdrawing can happen through an omission such as not putting the infusion into a feeding tube, and withholding the next stage of treatment can be viewed as stopping treatment (i.e., withdrawing) (Beauchamp and Childress, 1994). More importantly, both starting and stopping treatment can be justified, depending on the circumstances; both can *cause* the death of a patient and both can *allow* the patient to die.

Crimes and moral wrongs can be committed by both omission and commission. The morality and legality does not and should not rest on the distinction but rather on the obligation the physician has to act in accordance with the patient's interests and wishes in the particular situation (Beauchamp and Childress, 1994). Adherence to the distinction can have unfortunate influences on patient care. It can lead to *overtreatment* when treatment is continued past the point where it is beneficial or desirable to the patient, and it can lead to *undertreatment* if patients and families worry about being trapped by treatment that once begun cannot be stopped (Meisel, 1991). Therefore, the distinction is morally suspect and can cause dangerous situations for patients. Treatment can always be permissibly withdrawn if it can be permissibly withheld.

Ordinary versus Extraordinary Treatment

Another distinction that has been invoked in care for patients at the end of life is that of ordinary versus extraordinary treatment. This distinction has its origins in Catholic moral theology and has become a widely used tenet in medical decision-making (Meisel, 1991; Bok, 1978; Beauchamp and Childress, 1994). The historical rule has been that ordinary treatments cannot legitimately be forgone, whereas extraordinary treatments can. Patient refusal of ordinary treatment has long been considered suicide, whereas refusal of extraordinary treatments has been accepted. In the same manner, physicians and families did not commit homicide by withdrawing or withholding extraordinary treatment. However, the main problem with this distinction is that no clear definition of the two terms is available and no meaningful difference is seen between them.

Ordinary has often been taken to mean "usual" or "customary" and extraordinary "unusual" or "uncustomary." This interpretation is difficult to apply in an age where the standard of care is constantly and rapidly changing. Furthermore, the customary treatment for a disease may not be appropriate for every patient. Whether the customary means of treatment

should be applied depends on the particular patient's wishes and conditions as a whole (Meisel, 1991; Beauchamp and Childress., 1994). Other proposed criteria for the distinction include whether the treatment is simple or complex, natural or artificial, noninvasive or highly invasive, inexpensive or expensive, and routine or heroic (Beauchamp and Childress, 1994). These criteria are firstly highly subjective, and they also do not capture certain deeper moral considerations. For example, if a complex treatment is available and in accordance with the patient's wishes and interests, why should it be morally distinguished from a simple treatment?

The distinction between ordinary versus extraordinary treatment misses the morally relevant issue in medical decision-making: the balance of benefits and burdens of any particular treatment when applied to a particular patient in a particular case. All treatments in any of the above scenarios can be beneficial or burdensome, depending on the particulars. Thus, the distinction between ordinary and extraordinary collapses into the balance between benefits and burdens for the patient (Meisel, 1991; Bok, 1978; Beauchamp and Childress, 1994). This should be the focus of discussion with patients or their surrogates, using the steps and techniques described in the previous two sections.

Physician-Assisted Suicide and Terminal Sedation

Strong arguments occur on both sides of the controversial debates over physician-assisted suicide and terminal sedation. Assisted suicide is "the practice of providing a competent patient with a prescription for medication for the patient to use with the primary intention of ending his or her own life" (Meier et al., 1998). Oregon is the only state in the nation to have legalized this practice. In the first year of implementation, 23 persons received prescriptions for lethal medications and 15 of them died after taking the medications (Chin et al., 1999). In contrast, terminal sedation is within the law of all states (*Vacco v Quill*, 1997; *Washington v. Glucksberg*, 1997). The term terminal sedation describes "the use of high doses of sedatives to relieve extremes of physical distress" (Quill and Byock, 2000). The focus of this section is on how to discuss these options for palliative care with the patient. Other references provide the techniques to perform these practices (Quill and Byock, 2000).

A discussion begins when the physician and the patient or surrogate accept that the patient is terminally ill. In providing assisted suicide, the patient must also possess decision-making capacity sufficient to be competent. A desire to escape interminable suffering is not necessarily irrational and, thus, the traditional medical view that the desire to end one's life is a sign of depression must be carefully examined in these circumstances (Tulsky et al., 2000). The elements of informed consent must be present according to the steps described in the first section of this chapter. Assess that the decision maker understands, appreciates, and reasons through the risks, benefits, and likely outcomes of assisted suicide, terminal sedation, and alternatives such as palliative care and voluntary cessation of eating and drinking (Tulsky et al., 2000). It is expected that these are emotional discussions.

Tulsky et al. describe useful phrases and probes to structure these discussions (Tulsky et al., 2000). Attend to the emotions of the patient and family through emphatic listening and asking appropriate open-ended questions. The emotions and values of the patient are very important because the core issue is deep suffering. Allow patients to share their thoughts and feelings fully. When a patient seems to be asking for assistance in dying, it is appropriate to address the request directly. For example, "I hear you saying that you might consider hastening your death. How were you hoping that I might be able to help you?" If the patient is more vague about the request, a response might be, "You've referred several times to wishing it were all over. Although you haven't quite said it, it sounds like you're thinking that there are alternatives to dying naturally. Can you share with me what you're thinking in that regard?" All alternatives to suicide such as palliative treatment and what can be reasonably expected from it should be discussed.

If the patient continues to request assisted suicide, physicians must assess their own values and beliefs about this practice. Physicians who are willing to participate may respond, "As you know, the law allows me to prescribe medications that you could use to end your life. There are situations in which I may be willing to do this to relieve your suffering. Let's talk more about this option." Physicians who are not willing to participate must let the patient know that the law allows such an option but they are personally unable to participate.

If a physician is comfortable in providing terminal sedation or cessation of eating and drinking, he or she can raise these options which are legal even in states where assisted suicide is illegal. If a physician considers all such activities unacceptable, a response could be, "My own conscience does not allow me to do that. I am sure that other physicians in our community would consider that possibility with you." A physician who is not willing to participate in assisted suicide must avoid any sense of abandonment.

Surrogate Decision-Making

A patient may not possess adequate decision-making capacity to participate in an informed consent or advance care planning. This is especially likely at the end of life when conditions such as delirium can impair cognitive function and is certainly common in the care of patients with neurodegenerative dementias. In these instances, the physician needs to turn to others known as *surrogates*. In general, surrogates are family members who have either acted informally as decision-makers or are authorized in a DPA. Many of the same steps and techniques described above in assessing decision-making capacity, and discussing end-of-life care apply to surrogates as they do to patients. However, some unique issues are seen.

When deciding for others, the patient's preferences, to the extent that they are known, and the patient's dignity and quality of life should guide the surrogate in making decisions. Using patient preferences is called a "substituted judgment." However, in many cases, preferences are unknown or, because of significant changes in the patient's health and well-being, they are not relevant to the decision at hand. In these circumstances, the focus is on the patient's dignity and quality of life; in other words, the patient's best-interests (Karlawish et al., 1999).

An additional challenge of surrogate decision-making is that the surrogate often has other roles, such as being the patient's caregiver, and has values and emotions that can influence decision-making. These roles, values, and emotions have two implications. First, the surrogate may have an understanding of the patient's illness that significantly differs from the physician's understanding. To practice effective decision-making, the physician needs to know this understanding. Before a decision is made, the physician should prompt the surrogate to narrate how he or she understands the patient's current situation. A useful open-ended question is, "I know I've cared for your Mom for many years, but a lot has happened. What's your understanding of how she got to this point and what's wrong?" The second implication of these roles, values, and emotions is that a caregiver's distress (or burden) and depression can have an impact on how that person assesses the patient's quality of life (Logsdon et al., 1999) and the value placed on disease course extension (Karlawish et al., 2000). Hence, screen the surrogate for distress and depression and, where appropriate, address these issues.

DRIVING LIMITATION AND CESSATION

The assessment of the older adult's ability to drive safely is an important issue for neurologists because many neurologic illnesses lead to an increased likelihood of sensory, motor, and cognitive deficits that can have an impact on the ability to drive. Although the law recognizes driving as a privilege and not a right, the ability to drive is an expression of liberty and independence, and provides a sense of self-esteem and control of one's everyday life. Most older Americans rely on the automobile as their primary means of transportation (Jette and Branch, 1992). Driving cessation often leads to decreased quality of life, loss of control, increased loneliness and isolation, and depression (Marattoli et al., 1997). However, physicians do have a duty to protect their patients' lives and maintain public safety. A physician must balance the autonomy and quality of life of their patient with the safety of their patient and society. Hence, a recommendation to limit or cease driving should be based on relevant criteria such as tests of functional competency.

As the population of Western countries ages, the percentage of older drivers is increasing (National Highway Traffic Safety Administration, 2000; Carr, 2000). Although older adults drive less than younger adults and, thus, account for fewer crashes, they are involved in a disproportionate number of crashes per mile driven (National Highway Traffic Safety Administration, 2000; Williams and Carsten, 1989; Jette and Branch, 1992). Additionally, older drivers suffer higher rates of injury and fatality in a crash than other age groups because of increasing fragility (Pasupathy and Lavizzo-Mourey, 2000).

Many relevant factors lead to this increased accident rate for older drivers, including an increased likelihood of visual and hearing deficits, as well as declines in motor and cognitive functions (National Highway Traffic Safety Administration, 1999; Underwood, 1992; Retchin et al., 1988; Gallo et al., 1999; Reuben, 1993; Reuben et al., 1988; Donnelly and Karlinsky, 1990; Foley et al., 1995; Colsher and Wallace, 1993; Marattoli et al., 1997; Pasupathy and Lavizzo-Mourey, 2000). Many central nervous system active medications commonly used by the elderly can affect driving ability (Pasupathy and Lavizzo-Mourey, 2000; Carr, 2000). Coexisting medical conditions prevalent in the elderly (e.g., seizure disorders, stroke, dementia, and Parkinson's disease) can also affect driving ability (National Highway Traffic Safety Administration, 1999; Carr et al., 1991; Carr, 2000; Reuben et al., 1988).

The condition that has received the most attention in studies of decreased driving ability in the elderly is dementia. Dementing illnesses can result in cognitive and behavioral changes that can impair the ability to drive. These changes include memory problems, visuospatial deficits, increased reaction time, impaired judgment, and attentional deficits (Donnelly and Karlinsky, 1990). Most notably, selective attention and perceptual-motor reaction time have been shown to lead to mistakes at intersections, traffic signals, or in changing lanes (Donnelly and Karlinsky, 1990). Of note, however, although drivers with later stages of Alzheimer's disease may pose a significant safety problem (Lucas-Blaustein et al., 1988), drivers with early dementia display driving impairment comparable to that tolerated in other segments of the driving population (Dubinsky et al., 2000; Hunt et al., 1993; Drachman and Swearer, 1993). Competency to drive is an expression of particular functional abilities and cannot be inferred automatically from a diagnosis of dementia (Donnelly and Karlinsky, 1990; Odenheimer, 1993; Trobe et al., 1996; Fitten et al., 1995; Drachman and Swearer, 1993).

Physicians cannot rely on age and diagnoses alone to assess a patient's ability to drive. Instead, they must assess the patient's driving history, specific functional abilities, and the significant risk factors listed above in making this determination. First, a history focusing on the driving task should be obtained from knowledgeable informants such as caregivers, family, or friends. The history should focus on new problems with driving such as "accidents, violations, near-misses, failure to yield, driving too slow, and routinely getting lost" (Carr et al., 1991; Donnelly and Karlinsky, 1990; Odenheimer, 1993). Also, recognize environmental factors that relate to injury risk such as driving frequency, distance, and patterns (difficult areas, congested hours, and nighttime are especially dangerous), and the type of vehicle driven (Carr et al., 1991; Pasupathy and Lavizzo-Mourey, 2000). To assess functional status, a focus on new activities of daily living (ADL) dependencies can reveal a breakdown in skills that had been overlearned and intact. These dependencies can reflect a decline in several areas of cognition and are more important than memory loss as indirect evidence for impaired driving skills (Carr et al., 1991; Odenheimer, 1993). The Mini-Mental Status Examination can also be indirect evidence if it reveals deficiencies in visuospatial skills and attention (Carr et al., 1991; Marattoli et al., 1997; Gallo et al., 1999; Pasupathy and Lavizzo-Mourey, 2000; Odenheimer, 1993). Tests of the driver's vision and motor function may reveal potential problems with the driving task (Pasupathy and Lav-izzo-Mourey, 2000). If the patient has any medical conditions or is on any medications that can affect driving ability, be aware of the potential for driving safety problems and, at the very least, bring these to the attention of the driver. Alcohol use is, of course, another significant risk factor and should be assessed.

If the presence of a driving-impaired condition is confirmed, perform another level of assessment to determine the patient's ability to drive. Gather more information about the condition or refer the patient to other professionals who can better determine the patient's ability to drive (Pasupathy and Lavizzo-Mourey, 2000). Occupational therapists can perform formal driving screens that include tests of perception, cognition, reaction time, and on-the-road evaluation (Pasupathy and Lavizzo-Mourey, 2000; Carr et al., 1991; Odenheimer, 1993). Furthermore, many states have laws requiring physicians to report patients with certain medical conditions that can impair driving ability to the Department of Transportation (Pasupathy and Lavizzo-Mourey, 2000). An extreme example is a California law requiring that all cases of dementia be reported (California Health & Safety Code § 103900). Physicians should be familiar with their state's laws on reporting, some of which are listed in Table 35-4. If reported, the patient will participate in a more complete evaluation.

A number of ways are seen to manage a patient's impaired ability to drive. Driving cessation is not the only option, and should only be considered for patients with significant and unmanageable impair-ments. The first step is to eliminate the conditions responsible for problems with driving, whether this be reducing medications, eliminating alcohol consumption, managing medical problems, or maximizing vision and hearing (Odenheimer, 1993). Environmental and behavioral patterns may also need to be changed, such as limiting driving frequency, driving on slower roadways, daytime driving, adapting the vehicle, or using another passenger as a navigator, depending on the specific problem (Carr et al., 1991; Odenheimer, 1993). Viable alternatives to driving (e.g., public transportation services) should also be discussed. The physician's decision to stop or restrict driving should be discussed openly with the patient and caregiver and appropriately documented.

ELDER ABUSE

Elder abuse, first described in the medical literature in 1975, is a recent domestic violence issue to gain public attention (Kleinschmidt, 1997; Lachs and Pillmer, 1995). Between one to two million, or 10%, of Americans over 65 years of age are the victims of abuse every year. Among these, nearly half (4%) may be victims of moderate to severe abuse (Kleinschmidt, 1997; Council on Scientific Affairs, 1987). This represents an increase of about 100,000 cases per year since 1981 (Council on Scientific Affairs, 1987). Furthermore, this abuse is frequent and recurring in up to 80% of cases (Council on Scientific Affairs, 1987). Unfortunately, only 1 of 14 cases of elder abuse is reported (Aravanis et al., 1992; Jones et al., 1988). These figures indicate that elder abuse is a significant threat to the health and well-being of elderly Americans and that physicians need to have the skills to identify, report, and intervene in situations of elder abuse. It is particularly important that physicians have these skills because most elderly persons are likely to have some encounter with a physician and most states require reporting of suspected abuse.

The increase in the prevalence of elder abuse has been attributed to a number of factors, most notably the vast growth of the elderly population (Kleinschmidt, 1997), a longer life expectancy, and a change in family structure (Council on Scientific Affairs, 1987). Despite this increase in prevalence, abuse of the elderly is difficult to quantify because of the many barriers to its identification and reporting. Both the victim and the abuser tend to downplay the seriousness of the abuse, and health professionals often do not accurately diagnose abuse because of disbelief, fear of accusation, or lack of awareness of the extent of problem (Council on Scientific Affairs,

TABLE 35-4. *Reporting requirements by state*

States that **require** physicians to report health conditions that are hazardous to driving to licensing agencies:
  Pennsylvania, New Jersey, Delaware, Georgia, Nevada, Oregon, California (requires reporting of dementia)
Immunity: In all seven states, reporting physicians have immunity from litigation.
States that **permit** physician reporting:
  Connecticut, Florida, Illinois, Maryland, Minnesota, Oklahoma, Rhode Island, Utah, North Dakota, Ohio
Immunity: All states *except* North Dakota and Ohio grant immunity to reporting physicians.
Other jurisdictions allow physician reporting only after the patient has refused to report himself or herself.

From National Highway Traffic Administration. Safe mobility for older people notebook. Washington, DC: US Department of Transportation, 1999.

1987). One of the largest obstacles to reliable research on the issue is the variation in terminology and lack of one accepted definition of elder abuse.

A review of 21 studies on elder abuse found 34 terms to describe elderly abuse (Kleinschmidt, 1997). This variation has made it difficult to compare and compile the data from different studies. However, all discussions of elder abuse share certain key elements and general descriptions of abuse types. The definition of elder abuse according to the American Medical Association (AMA) is "an act or omission which results in harm or threatened harm to the health and welfare of an elderly person" (American Medical Association, 1985). Most authors accept four basic categories of such acts or omissions. *Physical abuse* includes hitting, grabbing, pushing, and other acts that cause bodily injury. Some physical abuse definitions include sexual abuse and nonconsensual intimate contact, but some authors list this as a separate category. *Psychological abuse*, also called "emotional and verbal abuse," includes verbal and nonverbal insults, humiliation, infantilization, or threats (Kleinschmidt, 1997). Financial or material abuse includes theft, misappropriation of funds, and coercion (changing a will or deed) (Kleinschmidt, 1997). Neglect is the failure of the caregiver to provide appropriate care, usually in assistance with ADL (Kleinschmidt, 1997). Other recognized categories are self-neglect, which is conducted by the patient that threatens his or her own health or safety (Kleinschmidt, 1997); violation of personal rights (Jones et al., 1997); abandonment (American College of Physicians, 1998); and even miscellaneous (Kleinschmidt, 1997). A consensus on definitions and terms is needed to compare studies and findings.

Most risk factors for elder abuse deal with the social environment that the elder and abusive caregiver are placed within, such as stress, isolation, a family history of violence, and especially dependency. The dependence of the caregiver on the elder for financial and emotional support and the dependency of the elder on the caregiver for functional help with daily living are major sources of tension. Caregivers who are psychologically and emotionally unstable and abusing substances are at high risk of abusing those in their care.

The detection and assessment of elder abuse are difficult because, unlike most medical problems, patients and their caregivers are unlikely to report the problem spontaneously (Council on Scientific Affairs, 1987). The AMA recommends that physicians routinely ask geriatric patients about abuse, even if signs are absent (Aravanis et al., 1992). To identify abuse, look for certain observations that are indicative of abuse. These include delays between an injury or illness and the seeking of medical attention, frequent visits to the emergency room (despite a health plan), and presentation of a functionally impaired patient without a caregiver (Lachs and Pillemer, 1995). If a screen suggests abuse, this should be followed by a detailed history. Both the patient and caregiver should be interviewed together and separately. Hence, these questions can be integrated into a routine clinical encounter where a portion of the time is spent with the patient alone. Questions to elicit information about abuse include: "Are you afraid of anyone at home?" "Has anyone tried to harm you in any way?" "Have you been forced to use your money in a way you didn't want to?" (Kleinschmidt, 1997).

It is important that these interviews avoid confrontation and express empathy and understanding (Kleinschmidt, 1997; Lachs and Pillemer, 1995). Physicians need to have easily applicable skills to assess for caregiver stress, a common risk factor for abuse. A useful method is to ask about the presence of potentially stressful events (e.g., whether a patient with dementia repeats the same question over and over again). If this screen shows that the event occurs, the appropriate follow-up question is to determine how much distress the event causes. For example, "How bothersome is that?" The more bother that the caregiver reports for these events, the more stress he or she is experiencing. This assessment should be accompanied with a screen for depressive symptoms because clear links are seen between the distress (or burden) of caregiving and the incidence and severity of depressive symptoms (Vitaliano et al., 1991; Clyburn et al., 2000).

A physical examination may reveal injury indicative of abuse (Kleinschmidt, 1997; Lachs and Pillemer, 1995). If possible, a home assessment by a health professional can uncover important indicators of abuse (Council on Scientific Affairs, 1987). Finally, a physician should be familiar with the patient's social and financial resources, which can help in identifying a source of stress and conflict, suggest possible exploitation, and is important if an intervention is needed (Lachs and Pillemer, 1995).

If abuse is confirmed, the physician must intervene to stop the abusive situation. Physicians must know their state's laws on reporting elder abuse. Every state has such laws, and 46 states as well as the District of Columbia require mandatory reporting of abuse. Colorado, New York, Wisconsin, and Illinois have voluntary reporting laws (Jones et al., 1997). The goal of intervention is to provide the patient with more enjoyable and fulfilling life (Kleinschmidt, 1997). This is accomplished by ensuring the safety of the elderly patient while respecting the patient's autonomy (Lachs and Pillemer, 1995; Kleinschmidt, 1997). The focus should be preservation of the family and not the *rescue* of victims (Kleinschmidt, 1997). Ideally, a multidisciplinary team of caretakers from the medical, social service, mental health, and legal professions should be utilized (Council on Scientific Affairs, 1987). Interventions should be tailored to the specific situation. If the elderly person is in immediate danger, hospitalization may be justified (Lachs and Pillemer, 1995; Kleinschmidt, 1997). If a high burden of chronic disease is the cause of stress for the caregiver, home care or respite services may be appropriate (Lachs and Pillemer, 1995). If psychopathologic factors in the abuser are the cause of the problem, alternative living arrangements should be considered (Lachs and Pillemer, 1995). Supportive counseling and psychotherapy may be necessary for the abusive caregiver (Council on Scientific Affairs, 1987). When a competent patient insists on remaining in the abusive environment, the physician should emphasize the patient's other options and offer whatever interventions the patient will accept. For noncompetent patients, the court may need to appoint a guardian or conservator. If interventions do not stop the abuse, long-term care may be necessary.

CONCLUSION

The care of elderly patients with neurologic illnesses includes managing a number of medical problems that have substantial ethical and legal issues. This chapter focused on common issues that arise in the course of the doctor-patient relationship. In this intimate and largely private relationship, the physician has substantial power and responsibility. The steps and techniques described above allow a physician to properly exercise this power and responsibility. Specifically, they place the principles of beneficence, respect for autonomy, and justice in balance. This is especially important when addressing tough issues such as withdrawing treatment, providing terminal sedation, or reporting a case of elder abuse or driving impairment. The goal of this chapter is not to proscribe outcomes but to define methods so that all affected can accept the outcome and the process that led to the outcome.

REFERENCES

Albert SM, Murphy PL, Bene MLD, et al. A prospective study of preferences and actual treatment choices in ALS. *Neurology* 1999;53:278–283.

American College of Physicians. Management of elder abuse and neglect. *Ann Emerg Med* 1998;31:149–150.

American Medical Association. *Model elderly abuse reporting act.* Chicago: American Medical Association, 1985.

Appelbaum PS, Grisso T. Assessing patients' capacities to consent to treatment. *N Engl J Med* 1988;319:1635–1638.

Aravanis S, Adelman R, Breckman R, et al. *Diagnostic and treatment guidelines on elder abuse and neglect.* Chicago: American Medical Association, 1992.

Beauchamp TL, Childress JF. *Principles of biomedical ethics,* 4 ed. New York, Oxford: Oxford University Press, 1994.

Bok S. Death and dying: euthanasia and sustaining life: ethical views. In: Reich WT, ed. *Encyclopedia of bioethics.* Vol. I. New York: Free Press, 1978:268–278.

California Health & Safety Code § 103900 (West, 2000)

Carr D, Schmader K, Bergman C, et al. A multidisciplinary approach in the evaluation of demented drivers referred to geriatric assessment centers. *J Am Geriatr Soc* 1991;39: 1132–1136.

Carr DB. The older adult driver. *Am Fam Physician* 2000; 61:141–146, 148.

Chin AE, Hedberg K, Higginson GK, et al. Legalized physician-assisted suicide in Oregon. The first year's experience. *N Engl J Med* 1999;340:577–583.

Clyburn LD, Stones MJ, Hadjistavropoulos T, et al. Predicting caregiver burden and depression in Alzheimer's disease. *J Gerontol B Psychol Sci Soc Sci* 2000;55B:S2–S13.

Colsher PL, Wallace RB. Geriatric assessment and driver functioning. *Clin Geriatr Med* 1993;9:365–375.

Council on Scientific Affairs. Elder abuse and neglect. *JAMA* 1987;257:966–971.

Donnelly RE, Karlinsky H. The impact of Alzheimer's disease on driving ability: a review. *J Geriatr Psychiatry Neurol* 1990;3:67–72.

Drachman DA, Swearer JM. Driving and Alzheimer's disease: the risk of crashes. *Neurology* 1993;43:2448–2456.

Dubinsky RM, Stein AC, Lyons K. Practice parameter: risk of driving and Alzheimer's disease (an evidence-based review). *Neurology* 2000;54:2205–2211.

Edinger W, Smucker D. Outpatient's attitudes regarding advance directives. *J Fam Pract* 1992;35:650–653.

Eisendrath S, Jonsen A. The living will: help or hindrance? *JAMA* 1983;249:2054–2058.

Emanuel L, Barry M, Stoeckle J, et al. Advance directives for medical care: a case for greater use. *N Engl J Med* 1991;324:889–895.

Fischer GS, Arnold RM, Tulsky JA. Talking to the older adult about advance directives. *Clin Geriatr Med* 2000; 16:239–254.

Fitten LJ, Perryman KM, Wilkinson CJ, et al. Alzheimer and vascular dementias and driving. *JAMA* 1995;273: 1360–1365.

Foley DJ, Wallace RB, Eberhard J. Risk factors for motor vehicle crashes among older drivers in rural community. *J Am Geriatr Soc* 1995;43:776–781.

Fost NC. A surrogate system for informed consent. *JAMA* 1975;233:800–803.

Furrow BR, Johnson SH, Jost TS, et al. *Health law. Cases, materials, and problems.* American Casebook Series. St. Paul: West Publishing Co., 1991.

Gallo JJ, Rebok GW, Lesikar SE. The driving habits of adults aged 60 years and older. *J Am Geriatr Soc* 1999; 47:335–341.

Gamble E, McDonald P, Lichstein P. Knowledge, attitudes and behavior of elderly persons regarding living wills. *Arch Intern Med* 1991;151:277–280.

Goodman M, Tarnoff M, Slotman GJ. Effect of advance directives on the management of elderly critically ill patients. *Crit Care Med* 1998;26:701–704.

Gordon NP, Shade SB. Advance directives are more likely among seniors asked about end-of-life preferences. *Arch Intern Med* 1999;159:701–704.

Gregor J, Dunn D. Implementation of the Patient Self-Determination Act in a community hospital. *N Engl J Med* 1995;92:438–442.

Hunt L, Morris JC, Edwards D, et al. Driving performance in persons with mild senile dementia of the Alzheimer type. *J Am Geriatr Soc* 1993;41:747–753.

Jette AM, Branch LG. A ten-year follow-up of driving patterns among the community-dwelling elders. *Hum Factors* 1992;34:25–31.

Jones J, Dougherty J, Scheble D, et al. Emergency department protocol for the diagnosis and evaluation of geriatric abuse. *Ann Emerg Med* 1988;17:1006–1015.

Jones JS, Veenstra TR, Seamon JP, et al. Elder mistreatment: national survey of emergency physicians. *Ann Emerg Med* 1997;30:473–479.

Karlawish JHT, Klocinski J, Merz JF, et al. Caregivers' preferences for the treatment of patients with Alzheimer's disease. *Neurology* 2000;55:1008–1014.

Karlawish JHT, Quill T, Meier DE. A consensus-based approach to practicing palliative care for patients who lack decision-making capacity. *Ann Intern Med* 1999;130:835–840.

Kleinschmidt KC. Elder abuse: a review. *Ann Emerg Med* 1997;30:463–472.

Lachs MS, Pillemer K. Abuse and neglect of elderly persons. *N Engl J Med* 1995;332:437–443.

LaPuma J, Orentichler D, Moss R. Advance directives on admission: clinical implications and analysis of the Patient Self-determination Act of 1990. *JAMA* 1991;266:402–405.

Lo B, McLeod G, Saika G. Patient attitudes to discussing life-sustaining treatment. *Arch Intern Med* 1986;146:1613–1615.

Lo B, Quill T, Tulsky J. Discussing palliative care with patients. *Ann Intern Med* 1999;130:744–749.

Logsdon RG, Gibbons LE, McCurry SM, et al. Quality of life in Alzheimer's disease: patient and caregiver reports. *Journal of Mental Health and Aging* 1999;5:21–32.

Lucas-Blaustein MJ, Filipp L, Dungan C, et al. Driving in patients with dementia. *J Am Geriatr Soc* 1988;36:1087–1091.

Marattoli RA, Leon CFMd, Glass TA, et al. Driving cessation and increased depressive symptoms: prospective evidence from the New Haven EPESE. *J Am Geriatr Soc* 1997;45:202–206.

Marson DC, Ingram KK, Cody HA, et al. Assessing the competency of patients with Alzheimer's disease under different legal standards. *Arch Neurol* 1995;52:949–954.

Martin D, Thiel E, Singer P. A new model of advance care planning: observations from people with HIV. *Arch Intern Med* 1999;159:86–92.

McKneally MF, Martin DK. An entrustment model of consent for surgical treatment of life-threatening illness: perspective of patients requiring esophagectomy. *J Thorac Cadiovasc Surg* 2000;120:264–269.

Meier DE, Emmons C-A, Wallenstein S, et al. A national survey of physician-assisted suicide and euthanasia in the United States. *N Engl J Med* 1998;338:1193–1201.

Meisel A. Legal myths about terminating life support. *Arch Intern Med* 1991;151:1497–1502.

Miles S, Koepp R, Weber E. Advance end-of-life treatment planning: a research review. *Arch Intern Med* 1996;156:1062–1068.

Morrison SR, Zayas LH, Mulvihill M, et al. Barriers to completion of health care proxies: an examination of ethnic differences. *Arch Intern Med* 1998;158:2493–2497.

National Highway Traffic Safety Administration. *Safe mobility for older people notebook.* Washington, DC: US Department of Transportation, 1999.

National Highway Traffic Safety Administration. *Traffic safety facts 1999. Older population. http://www.nhtsa.dot.gov/people/ncsa/pdf/Older99.pdf.* Access date: November 15, 2000.

Odenheimer GL. Dementia and the older driver. *Clin Geriatr Med* 1993;9:349–364.

Pantilat SZ, Alpers A, Wachter RM. A new doctor in the house: ethical issues in hospitalist systems. *JAMA* 1999;282:171–174.

Pasupathy S, Lavizzo-Mourey R. The older driver. In: Forciea MA, Lavizzo-Mourey R, Schwab EP, eds. *Geriatric secrets*, 2nd ed. Philadelphia: Hanley and Belfus, 2000:115–120.

Pritchard RS, Fisher ES, Teno JM, et al. Influence of patient preferences and local health system characteristics on the place of death. *J Am Geriatr Soc* 1998;46:1242–1250.

Quill TE, Byock IR. Responding to intractable terminal suffering: the role of terminal sedation and voluntary refusal of foods and fluids. *Ann Intern Med* 2000;132:408–414.

Retchin SM, Cox J, Fox M, et al. Performance-based measurement among elderly drivers and nondrivers. *J Am Geriatr Soc* 1988;36:813–819.

Reuben DB. Assessment of older drivers. *Clin Geriatr Med* 1993;9:449–459.

Reuben DB, Silliman RA, Traines M. The aging driver: medicine, policy, and ethics. *J Am Geriatr Soc* 1988;36:1135–1142.

Rubin SM, Strull WM, Fialkow MF, et al. Increasing the completion of the durable power of attorney for health care: a randomized, controlled trial. *JAMA* 1994;271:209–212.

Sabatino CP. 10 Legal myths about advance directives. In: *Clearinghouse review: ABA Commission on Legal Problems of the Elderly*. Chicago: National Center on Poverty Law 1994;28:653–657.

Schneiderman L, Kronick R, Kaplan R. Effects of offering advance directives on medical treatments and costs. *Ann Intern Med* 1992;117:599–606.

Silverman HJ, Truma P, Schaeffer MH, et al. Implementation of the Patient Self-Determination Act in a hospital setting: an initial evaluation. *Arch Intern Med* 1995;155:502–510.

Singer P, Martin D, Lavery J, et al. Reconceptualizing advance care planning for a patient's perspective. *Arch Intern Med* 1998;158:879–884.

Stelter K, Elliott B, Bruno C. Living will completion in older adults. *Arch Intern Med* 1992;152:954–959.

Teno J, Lynn J, Connors Jr. A, et al. The illusion of end-of-life resource savings with advance directives. *J Am Geriatr Soc* 1997a;45:513–518.

Teno J, Lynn J, Phillips R, et al. Do formal advance directives affect resuscitations decisions and the use of resources for seriously ill patients? *J Clin Ethics* 1994;5: 23–30.

Teno J, Lynn J, Wegner N, et al. Advance directives for seriously ill hospitalized patients: effectiveness with the patient self-determination act and the SUPPORT intervention. *J Am Geriatr Soc* 1997b;45:500–507.

Trobe JD, Waller PF, Cook-Flannagan CA, et al. Crashes and violations among drivers with Alzheimer disease. *Arch Neurol* 1996;53:411–416.

Tulsky JA, Ciampa R, Rosen EJ. Responding to legal requests for physician-assisted suicide. *Ann Intern Med* 2000;132:494–499.

Tulsky JA, Fischer GS, Rose MR, et al. Opening the black box: how do physicians communicate about advance directives? *Ann Intern Med* 1998;129:441–449.

Underwood M. The older driver: clinical assessment and injury prevention. *Arch Intern Med* 1992;152:735–740.

Vitaliano PP, Russo J, Young HM, et al. The screen for caregiver burden. *Gerontologist* 1991;31:76–83.

Vacco v Quill, 117 S. Ct. 2293 (1997).

Washington v Glucksberg, 117 S. Ct. 2258 (1997).

Williams AF, Carsten O. Driver age and crash involvement. *Am J Public Health* 1989;79:326–327.

Yesavage J, Brink T, Rose T, et al. Development and validation of a geriatric depression screening scale: a preliminary report. *J Psychiatr Res* 1982–1983;17:37–49.

Appendix

RESOURCES

Although this list represents a comprehensive guide to organizations that address the clinical care needs of older people, it is not a resource of all social service agencies and organizations assisting older citizens. If you have questions that do not specifically relate to one of the following organizations, please contact your state or area agency on aging as listed by the Administration on Aging (AOA). These agencies provide information on, and refer callers to, local services for senior citizens. To locate state and area agencies on aging, visit the AOA Website at *http://www.aoa.dhhs.gov/agingsites/state.html* or call the Eldercare Locator service (1-800-677-1116) operated by the National Association of Area Agencies on Aging.

NOTE: The organizations on this list are arranged in categories in the following order:

General Aging
End-of-Life Issues
Education
Legal Issues and Elder Abuse
Resources on Specific Health Problems:
    Cancer
    Diabetes
    Nutritional Concerns
    Digestive Problems
    Head and Neck Problems
    Hearing Problems
    Heart and Circulation Problems
    Joint, Muscle, and Bone Problems
    Lung and Breathing Problems
    Memory and Thinking Problems
    Neurologic Problems
    Nutritional Concerns
    Pain
    Psychological Problems
    Sexuality and Sexual Concerns
    Sight Problems
    Skin Problems
    Urinary Problems

GENERAL AGING

Administration on Aging
330 Independence Avenue, SW
Washington, DC 20201
Tel: (202) 619-0724
Fax: (202) 401-7620
Website: *http://www.aoa.gov*
E-mail: *aoainfo@aoa.gov*

National Aging Information Center (NAIC)
(*A Service of the Administration on Aging*)
330 Independence Avenue, SW, Room 4656
Washington, DC 20201
Tel.: (202) 619-7501
TTY: (202) 401-7575
Fax: (202) 401-7620
Website: *http://www.aoa.gov/naic*
E-mail: *naic@aoa.gov*

Agency for Health Care Policy and Research
Clinical Practice Guidelines
Government Printing Office
Superintendent of Documents
Washington, DC 20402
Tel: (202) 512-1800
On-line retrieval: *http://www.ahcpr.gov*

Aging Network Services
440 East-West Highway
Bethesda, MD 20814
Tel: (301) 657-4329
Fax: (301) 657-3250
Website: *http://www.agingnets.com*
E-mail: *ans@agingnets.com*

Alliance for Aging Research
2021 K Street, NW, Suite 305
Washington, DC 20006
Tel: (202) 293-2856
Fax: (202) 785-8574
Website: *www.agingresearch.org*

American Academy of Home Care Physicians
P. O. Box 1037
Edgewood, MD 21040

Tel: (410) 676-7966
Fax: (410) 676-7980
Website: *www.aahcp.org*
E-mail: *aahcp@mindspring.com*

American Association of Homes & Services for the Aging

901 E Street, NW, Suite 500
Washington, DC 20004-2011
Tel: (202) 783-2242
Fax: (202) 783-2255
Website: *www.aahsa.org*
E-mail: *info@aahsa.org*

American Association of Retired Persons

601 E Street, NW
Washington, DC 20049
Tel: (800) 424-3410
Website: *www.aarp.org*
E-mail: *member@aarp.org*

American College of Health Care Administrators

1800 Diagonal Road, Suite 355
Alexandria, VA 22314
Tel: (703) 549-5822
Fax: (703) 739-7901
Toll free: (888) 888-ACHCA (2-2422)
Website: *www.achca.org*
E-mail: *info@achca.org*

American Federation for Aging Research

1414 Avenue of the Americas
New York, NY 10019
Tel: (212) 752-2327
Fax: (212) 832-2298
Website: *www.afar.org*
E-mail: *amfedaging@aol.com*

American Geriatrics Society

The Empire State Building
350 Fifth Avenue, Suite 801
New York, NY 10118
Tel: (212) 308-1414
Fax: (212) 832-8646
Website: *www.americangeriatrics.org*
E-mail: *info.amger@americangeriatrics.org*

American Health Care Association

1201 L Street, NW
Washington, DC 20005
Tel: (202) 842-4444
Fax: (202) 842-3860
Toll free for publications only: (800) 321-0343
Website: *www.ahca.org*

American Hospital Association

1 North Franklin
Chicago, IL 60606
Tel: (312) 422-3000
Fax: (312) 422-4796
Website: *www.aha.org*

American Medical Directors Association

10480 Patuxent Parkway, Suite 760
Columbia, MD 21044
Tel: (410) 740-9743
Toll free: (800) 876-2632
Fax: (410) 740-4572
Website: *www.amda.com*

American Occupational Therapy Association

P. O. Box 31220
Bethesda, MD 20824-1220
Tel: (301) 652-2682
Fax: (301) 652-7711
Website: *www.aota.org*

American Red Cross

Attn: Public Inquiry Office
431 18th Street NW
Washington, DC 20006
Tel: (202) 639-3520
Website: *www.redcross.org*

American Senior Fitness Association

P.O.Box 2575
New Smyrna Beach, FL 32170
Tel: (904) 423-6634
Fax: (904) 427-0613
Website: *www.seniorfitness.net*
E-mail: *sfa@ucnsb.net*

American Seniors Housing Association

1850 M Street, NW, Suite 540
Washington, DC 20036
Tel: (202) 974-2300
Fax: (202) 775-0112
Website: *www.nmhc.org*
E-mail: *info@nmhc.org*

American Social Health Association

Hotlines under the auspices of the ASHA
CDC National AIDS Hotline (English)—Toll free: (800) 342-AIDS
CDC National AIDS Hotline (Spanish)—Toll free: (800) 344-7432
CDC National AIDS Hotline —TTY Toll free: (800) 243-7889
CDC National STD Hotline —Toll free: (800) 227-8922

CDC National Immunization Information Hotline—
Toll free: (800) 232-2522
Website: *www.ashastd.org*

American Society on Aging
822 Market Street, Suite 511
San Francisco, CA 94103-1824
Tel: (415) 974-9600
Fax: (415) 974-0300
Website: *www.asaging.org*
E-mail: *info@asaging.org*

American Society of Consultant Pharmacists
1321 Duke Street
Alexandria, VA 22314-3516
Tel: (703) 739-1300
Fax: (703) 739-1321
Toll free: (800) 355-2727
Toll free fax: (800) 707-ASCP
Fast fax: (800) 220-1321
Website: *www.ascp.com*
E-mail: *info@ascp.com*

Assisted Living Federation of America
10300 Eaton Place, Suite 400
Fairfax, VA 22030
Tel: (703) 691-8100
Fax: (703) 691-8106
Website: *www.alfa.org*
E-mail: *info@alfa.org*

B'nai B'rith
1640 Rhode Island Avenue, NW
Washington, DC 20036-3278
Tel: (202) 857-6600
Fax: (202) 857-1099
Toll free: (888) 388-4224
Website: *www.bnaibrith.org*
Senior Housing
Tel: (202) 857-6581
Fax: (202) 857-0980
E-mail: *senior@bnaibrith.org*

Catholic Charities
1731 King Street, Suite 200
Alexandria, VA 22314
Tel: (703) 549-1390
Fax: (703) 549-1656
Website: *www.catholiccharitiesusa.org*

Children of Aging Parents
1609 Woodbourne Road, Suite 302-A
Levittown, PA 19057
Tel: (215) 945-6900
Fax: (215) 945-8720
Toll free information/referral: (800) 227-7294
Website: *www.careguide.net*

CDC National Prevention Information Network
For information on HIV, AIDS, STD, TB
P. O. Box 6003
Rockville, MD 20849-6003
Tel: (301) 562-1098
Toll free: (800) 458-5231
Toll free fax: (888) 282-7681
Toll free TTY: (800) 243-7012
Website: *www.cdcnpin.org*
E-mail: *info@cdcnpin.org*

Commission on Accreditation for Rehabilitation Facilities (CARF)
4891 East Grant Road
Tucson, AZ 85712
Tel: (520) 325-1044
Fax: (520) 318-1129
Website: *www.carf.org*

Department of Veteran Affairs
Office of Public Affairs
810 Vermont Avenue, NW
Washington, DC 20420
Tel: (202) 273-5700
Fax: (202) 273-6705
Website: *www.va.gov*

Disabled American Veterans
807 Maine Avenue, SW
Washington, DC 20024
Tel: (202) 554-3501
Fax: (202) 554-3581
Website: *www.dav.org*

Family Caregivers Alliance
69 Market Street
Suite 600
San Francisco, CA 94104
Tel: (415) 434-3388
Fax: (415) 434-3508
Website: *www.caregiver.org*
E-mail: *info@caregiver.org*

Gerontological Society of America
1030 15th Street, NW, Suite 250
Washington, DC 20005
Tel: (202) 842-1275
Fax: (202) 842-1150
Website: *www.geron.org*

Healthcare Information and Management Systems Society
230 East Ohio Street, Suite 500
Chicago, IL 60611-3269
Tel: (312) 664-4467
Fax: (312) 664-6143
Website: *www.himss.org*

Interfaith Caregivers Alliance
One West Armour Blvd., Suite 202
Kansas City, MO 64111
Tel: (816) 931-5442
Fax: (816) 931-5202
Website: *www.interfaithcaregivers.org*
E-mail: *info@interfaithcaregivers.org*

Joint Commission on Accreditation of Healthcare Organizations (JCAHO)
One Renaissance Boulevard
Oakbrook Terrace, IL 60181
Tel: (630) 792-5000
Fax: (630) 792-5005
Website: *www.jcaho.org*

Medicare Hotline
Toll free English and Spanish: (800) MEDICARE (633-4227)
Website: *www.medicare.gov*

National Adult Day Services Association
409 Third Street, SW
Washington, DC 20024
Tel: (202) 479-6682
Fax: (202) 479-0735
Website: *www.ncoa.org/nadsa*
E-mail: *nadsa@ncoa.org*

National Asian Pacific Center on Aging
Melbourne Tower, Suite 914
1511 Third Avenue
Seattle, WA 98101
Tel: (206) 624-1221
Fax: (206) 624-1023
Website: *www.napca.com*

National Association of Area Agencies on Aging
927 15th Street NW, 6th Floor
Washington, DC 20005
Tel: (202) 296-8130
Fax: (202) 296-8134
Website: *www.n4a.org*
E-mail: *rseay@n4a.org*
Toll free eldercare locator: Operated as a cooperative partnership of the Administration on Aging, the National Association of Area Agencies on Aging, and the National Association of State Units on Aging: (800) 677-1116.

National Association of Directors of Nursing Administration
10999 Reed Hartman Highway, Suite 233
Cincinnati, OH 45242
Tel: (513) 791-3679
Fax: (513) 791-3699

Toll free: (800) 222-0539
Website: *www.nadona.org*
E-mail: *info@nadona.org*

National Association for Home Care
228 7th Street, SE
Washington, DC 20003
Tel: (202) 547-7424
Fax: (202) 547-3540
Website: *http://www.nahc.org*

National Association of Professional Geriatric Care Managers
1604 North Country Club Road
Tucson, AZ 85716
Tel: (520) 881-8008
Fax: (520) 325-7925
Website: *www.caremanager.org*

National Association for the Support of Long Term Care
1321 Duke Street, Suite 304
Alexandria, VA 22314
Tel: (703) 549-8500
Fax: (703) 549-8342
Website: *www.NASL.org*

National Caucus and Center on Black Aged, Inc.
1424 K Street, NW
Washington, DC 20005
Tel: (202) 637-8400
Fax: (202) 327-0895
Website: *www.ncba-blackaged.org*
E-mail: *ncba@aol.com*

National Citizens' Coalition for Nursing Home Reform
1424 16th Street, NW, Suite 202
Washington, DC 20036-2211
Tel: (202) 332-2275
Fax: (202) 332-2949
Website: *www.nccnhr.org*
E-mail: *nccnhrl@nccnhr.org*

National Council on the Aging
409 3rd Street, SW
Washington, DC 20024
Tel: (202) 479-1200
Fax: (202) 479-0735
Website: *www.ncoa.org*
E-mail: *info@ncoa.org*

National Council on Patient Information and Education
4915 Saint Elmo Avenue, Suite 505
Bethesda, MD 20814-6053
Tel: (301) 656-8565

Fax: (301) 656-4464
Website: *www.talkaboutrx.org*
E-mail: *ncpie@erols.com*

National Family Caregivers Association
10400 Connecticut Avenue, #500
Kensington, MD 20895-3944
Tel: (301) 942-6430
Fax: (301) 942-2302
Toll free: (800) 896-3650
Website: *www.nfcacares.org*
E-mail: *info@nfcacares.org*

National Health Information Center
P. O. Box 1133
Washington, DC 20013-1133
Tel: (301) 565-4167
Toll free: (800) 336-4797
Fax: (301) 884-4256
Website: *http://nhic-nt.health.org*
E-mail: *nhicinfo@health.org*

National Indian Council on Aging
10501 Montgomery Blvd. NE, Suite 210
Albuquerque, NM 87111-3846
Tel: (505) 292-2001
Fax: (505) 292-1922
Website: *www.nicoa.org*
E-mail: *dave@nicoa.org*

**National Institute on Aging Information
  Clearinghouse**
P. O. Box 8057
Gaithersburg, MD 20898-8057
Toll free tel: (800) 222-2225

National Institute on Aging
Building 31, Room 5C27
31 Center Drive, MCS 2292
Bethesda, MD 20892-2292
Tel: (301) 496-1752
Fax: (301) 496-1072
Website: *www.nih.gov/nia*

**National Institute on Disability and
  Rehabilitation Research ABLEDATA**
8630 Fenton Street, Suite 930
Silver Spring, MD 20910
Tel: (301) 608-8998
Fax: (301) 608-8958
Toll free: (800) 227-0216
Website: *www.abledata.com*
E-mail: *adaigle@macroint.com*

National Rehabilitation Information Center
1010 Wayne Avenue, Suite 800
Silver Spring, MD 20910

Toll free: (800) 346-2742
Fax: (301) 562-2401
Website: *www.naric.com/naric*

National Subacute Care Association
7315 Wisconsin Avenue, Suite 424E
Bethesda, MD 20814
Tel: (301) 961-8680
Fax: (301) 961-8681
Website: *www.nsca.net*
E-mail: *nsca@tiac.net*

Projecto Ayuda
1452 West Temple Street, Suite 100
Los Angeles, CA 90026
Tel: (213) 487-1922
Fax: (213) 202-5905

United Seniors Health Cooperative
1331 H Street, NW
Washington, DC 20005
Tel: (202) 393-6222
Fax: (202) 783-0588
Website: *www.ushc-online.org*

Visiting Nurse Associations of America
11 Beacon Street, Suite 910
Boston, MA 02108
Tel: (617) 523-4042
Fax: (617) 227-4843
Website: *www.vnaa.org*

Well Spouse Foundation
610 Lexington Avenue, Suite 208
New York City, NY 10022
Tel: (212) 644-1241
Fax: (212) 644-1338
Toll free: (800) 838-0879
Website: *www.wellspouse.org*
E-mail: *wellspouse@aol.com*

END-OF-LIFE ISSUES

Americans for Better Care of the Dying
2175 K Street, NW, Suite 820
Washington, DC 20037
Tel: (202) 530-9864
Fax: (202) 467-2271
Website: *www.abcd-caring.com*
E-mail: *caring@erols.com*

Center to Improve Care of the Dying
Rand Corporation
Tel: (703) 413-1100

Choice in Dying, Inc.
1035 30th Street, NW

Washington, DC 20007
Tel: (202) 338-9790
Fax: (202) 338-0242
Toll free: (800) 989-WILL (9455)
Website: *www.choices.org*

Compassion in Dying
6312 SW Capital Highway, PMB 415
Portland, OR 97201
Tel: (503) 221-9556
Fax: (503) 228-9160
Website: *www.compassionindying.org*
E-mail: *info@compassionindying.org*

GriefNet
Internet Address: *www.rivendell.org*

Hospice Association of America
228 Seventh Street, SE
Washington, DC 20003
Tel: (202) 546-4759
Fax: (202) 547-9559
Website: *www.hospice-america.org*

Hospice Education Institute
190 Westbrook Road
Essex, CT 06426-1510
Tel: (860) 767-1620
Fax: (860) 767-2746
Toll free for publications: (800) 331-1620
Hospice link referral service—Toll free:
    (800) 331-1620
Website: *www.hospiceworld.org*
E-mail: *hospiceall@aol.com*

Hospice Foundation of America
2001 S Street NW, Suite 300
Washington, DC 20009
Tel: (202) 638-5419
Toll free: (800) 854-3402
Fax: (202) 638-5312
Website: *www.hospicefoundation.org*
E-mail: *hfa@hospicefoundation.org*

The Last Acts Campaign
Barksdale Ballard & Co.
1951 Kidwell Drive, Suite 205
Vienna, VA 22182
Tel: (703) 827-8771
Fax: (703) 827-0782
Website: *www.lastacts.org*

Life with Dignity
1744 Riggs Place NW, Suite, 300
Washington, DC 20009
Tel: (202) 986-0118
Website: *http://members.aol.com/lwdfdn*
E-mail: *lwdfdn@aol.com*

**National Hospice and Palliative Care
    Organization**
1700 Diagonal Road, Suite 300
Alexandria, VA 22314
Tel: (703) 837-1500
Website: *www.nhpco.org*
E-mail: *info@nhpca.org*

EDUCATION

Association for Gerontology in Higher Education
1030 15th Street NW, Suite 240
Washington, DC 20005-1503
Tel: (202) 289-9806
Fax: (202) 289-9824
Website: *www.aghe.org*

Association of American Medical Colleges
2450 N Street NW
Washington, DC 20037-1126
Tel: (202) 828-0400
Fax: (202) 828-1125
Website: *www.aamc.org*

Legal Issues and Elder Abuse
Legal Services for the Elderly
130 West 42nd Street, 17th Floor
New York, NY 10036
Tel: (212) 391-0120
Fax: (212) 719-1939
E-mail: *hn4923@handsnet.org*

National Academy of Elder Law Attorneys
1604 North Country Club Road
Tucson, AZ 85716
Tel: (520) 881-4005
Fax: (520) 325-7925
Website: *www.naela.org*
E-mail: *info@naela.com*

National Center on Elder Abuse
A consortium of the following six partners with
    NASUA, the lead agency:
National Association of State Units on Aging
    (NASUA)
Commission on Legal Problems of the Elderly of the
    American Bar Association (ABA)
The Clearinghouse on Abuse and Neglect of the
    Elderly of the University of Delaware (CANE)
The San Francisco Consortium for Elder Abuse
    Prevention of the Goldman Institute on Aging
    (GIOA)
The National Association of Adult Protective
    Services Administrators (NAAPSA)
The National Committee to Prevent Elder Abuse
    (NCPEA)

National Association of State Units on Aging
1225 I Street, Suite 725
Washington, DC 20005
Tel: (202) 898-2578
Fax: (202) 898-2583
Website: *www.nasua.org*
E-mail: *info@nasua.org*

National Clearinghouse on Elder Abuse
Literature
University of Delaware
College of Human Resources, Education and Public
Policy
Department of Consumer Studies
211 Allison Annex
Newark, DE 19716
Tel: (302) 831-3525
Fax: (302) 831-6081

National Committee for Prevention of Elder Abuse
Research
Institute on Aging
UMASS Memorial Health Care
119 Belmont Street
Worcester, MA 01605
Tel: (508) 334-6166
Fax: (508) 334-6906
Website: *www.preventelderabuse.org*

National Senior Citizens Law Center
1101 14th Street, NW, Suite 400
Washington, DC 20005
Tel: (202) 289-6976
Fax: (202) 289-7224
Website: *www.nsclc.org*

RESOURCES ON SPECIFIC HEALTH
PROBLEMS

Cancer

American Cancer Society, Inc.
National Headquarters
1599 Clifton Road, NE
Atlanta, GA 30329
Tel: (404) 320-3333
Fax: (404) 329-5787
Toll free National Cancer Information Center: (800)
227-2345
Website: *www.cancer.org*

National Cancer Institute
Public Inquiries Office
Building 31, Room 10A31
31 Center Drive, MSC 2580
Bethesda, MD 20892-2580
Tel: (301) 435-3848

Toll free: (800) 4-CANCER(422-6237)
Website: *www.nci.nih.gov*

Diabetes

American Diabetes Association
Attn: Customer Service
1701 North Beauregard Street
Alexandria, VA 22311
Tel: (703) 549-1500
Fax: (703) 549-6995
Toll free: (800) DIABETES (232-3472)
Website: *www.diabetes.org*
E-mail: *customerservice@diabetes.org*

National Diabetes Information Clearinghouse
1 Information Way
Bethesda, MD 20892-3560
Tel: (301) 654-3327
Fax: (301) 907-8906
Website: *www.niddk.nih.gov*
E-mail: *ndic@info.niddk.nih.gov*

Digestive Problems

American Liver Foundation
75 Maiden Lane, Suite 603
New York, NY 10038
Toll free: (800) GO LIVER (465-4837)
Website: *www.liverfoundation.org*
E-mail: *webmail@liverfoundation.org*

National Digestive Disease Information
Clearinghouse
2 Information Way
Bethesda, MD 20892-2480
Tel: (301) 654-3810
Website: *www.niddk.nih.gov*
E-mail: *nddic@info.niddk.nih.gov*

United Ostomy Association
19772 MacArthur Boulevard, Suite 200
Irvine, CA 92612-2405
Tel: (949) 660-8624
Fax: (949) 660-9262
Toll free: (800) 826-0826
Website: *www.uoa.org*
E-mail: *info@uoa.org*

Head and Neck Problems

American Academy of Otolaryngology-Head and
Neck Surgery, Inc.
1 Prince Street
Alexandria, VA 22314-3357
Tel: (703) 836-4444

Fax: (703) 683-5100
TTY: (703) 519-1585
Website: *www.entnet.org*

American Council for Headache Education
19 Mantua Road
Mt. Royal, NJ 08061
Tel: (856) 423-0258
Toll free: (800) 255-ACHE (2243)
Fax: (856) 423-0082
Website: *www.achenet.org*

American Dental Association
211 East Chicago Avenue
Chicago, IL 60611
Tel: (312) 440-2500
Fax: (312) 440-2800
Website: *www.ada.org*

National Headache Foundation
428 West St. James Place, 2nd Floor
Chicago, IL 60614-1750
Tel: (773) 388-6399
Toll free: (888) NHF-5552
Fax: (773) 525-7357
Website: *www.headaches.org*
E-mail: *info@headaches.org*

National Institute of Dental & Craniofacial Research
National Institute of Health
Bethesda, MD 20892-2190
Tel: (301) 496-4261
Fax: (301) 496-9988
Website: *www.nidcr.nih.gov*
E-mail: *nidcrinfo@mail.nih.gov*

Hearing Problems

American Tinnitus Association
P. O. Box 5
Portland, OR 97207-0005
Tel: (503) 248-9985
Fax: (503) 248-0024
Toll free: (800) 634-8978
Website: *www.ata.org*
E-mail: *tinnitus@ata.org*

Better Hearing Institute
515 King Street
Suite 420
Alexandria, VA 22314
Toll free: (800) EARWELL (327-9355)
Fax: (703) 750-9302
Website: *www.betterhearing.org*
E-mail: *mail@betterhearing.org*

International Hearing Society
16880 Middlebelt Road, Suite 4
Livonia, MI 48154
Tel: (734) 522-7200
Fax: (734) 522-0200
Toll Free Hearing Aid Helpline:
(800) 521-5247
Website: *www.hearingihs.org*

National Institute on Deafness and Other Communication Disorders
National Institute of Health
31 Center Drive, MSC 2320
Bethesda, MD 20892-2320
Tel: (301) 496-7243
Fax: (301) 402-0018
Toll Free NIDCD Information Clearinghouse: (800) 241-1044
Website: *www.nidcd.nih.gov*
E-mail: *webmaster@ms.nidcd.nih.gov*

Self Help for Hard of Hearing People
7910 Woodmont Avenue, Suite 1200
Bethesda, MD 20814
Tel: (301) 657-2248
Fax: (301) 913-9413
TTY: (301) 657-2249
Website: *www.shhh.org*
E-mail: *national@shhh.org*

Heart and Circulation Problems

American Association of Cardiovascular and Pulmonary Rehabilitation
7600 Terrace Avenue, Suite 203
Middleton, WI 53562
Tel: (608) 831-6989
Fax: (608) 831-5485
Website: *www.aacvpr.org*
E-mail: *accvpr@tmahq.com*

American Heart Association
7272 Greenville Avenue
Dallas, TX 75231
Tel: (214) 373-6300
Toll Free Tel: (800) 242-8721
Website: *www.americanheart.org*
AHA's Stroke Connection: (800) 553-6321

Courage Stroke Network
3915 Golden Valley Road
Golden Valley, MN 55422
Tel: (763) 520-0520
Fax: (763) 520-0577

National Heart, Lung and Blood Institute
Office of Prevention, Education and Control
31 Center Drive, MSC 2480
Bethesda, MD 20892-2480
Tel: (301) 496-5437
Fa: (301) 402-2405
Website: *www.nhlbi.nih.gov*
E-mail: *nhlbiinfo@rover.nhlbi.nih.gov*

National Institute of Neurological Disorders and Stroke
NIH Neurological Institute
P. O. Box 5801
Bethesda, MD 20824
Toll free: (800) 352-9424
Website: *www.ninds.nih.gov*

National Stroke Association
9707 E. Easter Lane
Englewood, CO 80112
Tel: (303) 649-9299
Fax: (303) 649-1328
Toll free: (800) STROKES (787-6537)
Website: *www.stroke.org*

Joint, Muscle, and Bone Problems

American Academy of Orthopedic Surgeons
6300 North River Road
Rosemont, IL 60018-4262
Tel: (847) 823-7186
Toll free: (800) 346-AAOS (2267)
Fax: (847) 823-8125
Website: *www.aaos.org*
E-mail: *custserv@aaos.org*

American Podiatric Medical Association
9312 Old Georgetown Road
Bethesda, MD 20814
Tel: (301) 571-9200
Fax: (301) 530-2752
Toll Free for Patient Education Literature only:
  (800) FOOT-CARE
Website: *www.apma.org*
E-mail: *askapma@apma.org*

Arthritis Foundation
1330 West Peachtree Street
Atlanta, GA 30309
Tel: (404) 872-7100
Toll free information: (800) 283-7800
Fax: (404) 872-0457
Website: *www.arthritis.org*
E-mail: *help@arthritis.org*

Lupus Foundation of America
1300 Piccard Drive, Suite 200

Rockville, MD 20850-4303
Tel: (301) 670-9292
Toll free for information packet: English (800) 558-0121; Spanish (800) 558-0231
Fax: (301) 670-9486
Website: www.lupus.org

National Arthritis and Musculoskeletal and Skin Diseases Information Clearinghouse
National Institutes of Health
1AMS Circls
Bethesda, MD 20892-3675
Tel: (301) 495-4484
Toll free: (877) 22-NIAMS (64267)
Fax: (301) 718-6366
Website: *www.nih.gov/niams*
E-mail: via website

National Osteoporosis Foundation
1232 22nd Street NW
Washington, DC 20037-1292
Tel: (202) 223-2226
Fax: (202) 223-2237
Toll Free Info: (800) 223-9994
Website: *www.nof.org*
E-mail: *customerservice@nof.org*

Lung and Breathing Problems

American Association of Cardiovascular and Pulmonary Rehabilitation
7600 Terrace Avenue, Suite 203
Middleton, WI 53562
Tel: (608) 831-6989
Fax: (608) 831-5485
Website: *www.aacvpr.org*
E-mail: *accvpr@tmahq.com*

American Lung Association
1740 Broadway
New York, NY 10019
Tel: (212) 315-8700
Fax: (212) 265-5642
Toll free: (800) LUNG-USA (800-586-4872)
Website: *www.lungusa.org*
E-mail: *info@lungusa.org*

National Heart, Lung and Blood Institute
Office of Prevention, Education and Control
31 Center Drive, MSC 2480
Bethesda, MD 20892-2480
Tel: (301) 496-5437
Fax: (301) 402-2405
Website: *www.nhlbi.nih.gov*
E-mail: *nhlbiinfo@rover.nhlbi.nih.gov*

Memory and Thinking Problems

Alzheimer's Association
919 North Michigan Avenue, Suite 1100
Chicago, IL 60611-1676
Toll free information: (800) 272-3900
Tel: (312) 335-8700
TTY: (312) 335-8882
Fax: (312) 335-1110
Website: *http://www.alz.org*
E-mail: *info@alz.org*
Safe Return Program—identification tags, medical
    alert bracelets: (888) 572-8566

**Alzheimer's Disease Education and Referral
    Center**
P. O. Box 8250
Silver Spring, MD 20907-8250
Tel: (301) 495-3311
Fax: (301) 495-3334
Toll free information service: (800) 438-4380
Website: *www.alzheimers.org*
E-mail: *adear@alzheimers.org*

Neurologic Problems

American Academy of Neurology
1080 Montreal Avenue
St. Paul, MN 55116
Tel: (651) 695-1940
Fax: (651) 695-2791
Website: *www.aan.com*
E-mail: *web@aan.com*

American Parkinson's Disease Association
1250 Hylan Boulevard, Suite 4B
Staten Island, NY 10305-1946
Tel: (718) 981-8001
Toll free information hotline: (800) 223-2732
Fax: (718) 981-4399
Website: *www.apdaparkinson.com*
E-mail: *info@apdaparkinson.com*

Epilepsy Foundation of America
4351 Garden City Drive
Landover, MD 20785
Tel: (301) 459-3700
Toll Free Info & Referral: (800) 332-1000
Fax: (301) 577-2684
Website: *www.efa.org*

Huntington's Disease Society of America
158 West 29th Street, 7th Floor
New York, NY 10001
Tel: (212) 242-1968
Fax: (212) 239-3430

Toll free hotline: (800) 345-4372
Website: *www.hdsa.org*
E-mail: *hdsainfo@hdsa.org*

**National Institute of Neurological Disorders and
    Stroke**
NIH Neurological Institute
P. O. Box 5801
Bethesda, MD 20824
Toll free: (800) 352-9424
Website: *www.ninds.nih.gov*
(For other stroke information, see *Heart and
    Circulation Problems*)

Parkinson's Disease Foundation
William Black Medical Building
Columbia-Presbyterian Medical Center
710 West 168th Street
New York, NY 10032
Tel: (212) 923-4700
Toll free: (800) 457-6676
Fax: (212) 923-4778
Website: *www.pdf.org*
E-mail: *info@pdf.org*

Nutritional Concerns

Food and Nutrition Information Center
US Department of Agriculture
National Agriculture Library Building
10301 Baltimore Avenue, Room 304
Beltsville, MD 20705-2351
Tel: (301) 504-5719
Fax: (301) 504-6409
Website: *http://www.nal.usda.gov/fnic*
E-mail: *fnic@nal.usda.gov*

Meals on Wheels Association of America
1414 Prince Street, Suite 202
Alexandria, VA 22314
Tel: (703) 548-5558
Fax: (703) 548-8024
Website: *www.projectmeal.orga*
E-mail: *mowaa@tbq.dqsys.com*

Pain

American Chronic Pain Association
P. O. Box 850
Rocklin, CA 95677
Tel: (916) 632-0922
Fax: (916) 632-3208
Website: *www.theacpa.org*
E-mail: *acpa@pacbell.net*

American Geriatrics Society
The Empire State Building
350 Fifth Avenue, Suite 801
New York, NY 10118
Tel: (212) 308-1414
Fax: (212) 832-8646
Website: *www.americangeriatrics.org*
E-mail: *info.amger@americangeriatrics.org*

American Pain Society
4700 West Lake Avenue
Glenview, IL 60025
Tel: (847) 375-4715
Fax: (847) 375-7777
Website: *www.ampainsoc.org*
E-mail: *info@ampainsoc.org*

City of Hope Pain Resource Center
City of Hope National Medical Center
Departtment of Nursing Research & Education
1500 East Duarte Road
Duarte, CA 91010
Tel: (626) 359-8111, ext. 3829
Website: mayday.coh.org
E-mail: *bferrell@coh.org*

National Chronic Pain Outreach Association
P. O. Box 274
Millboro, VA 24460-9606
Tel: (540) 862-9437
Fax: (540) 862-9485
Website: *http://www.chronicpain.org*
E-mail: *ncpoa@cfw.com*

Psychological Problems

American Association of Geriatric Psychiatry
7910 Woodmont Avenue, Suite 1050
Bethesda, MD 20814-3004
Tel: (301) 654-7850
Fax: (301) 654-4137
Website: *www.aagpgpa.org*
E-mail: *main@aagpgpa.org*

National Alliance for the Mentally Ill
Colonial Place Three
2107 Wilson Boulevard, Suite 300
Arlington, VA 22201-3042
Tel: (703) 524-7600
Fax: (703) 524-9094
Toll free: (800) 950-6264
Website: *www.nami.org*

National Institute of Mental Health Information Resources & Inquiries
6001 Executive Blvd., Room 8184, MSC 9663
Bethesda, MD 20892-9663

Tel: (301) 443-4513
Fax: (301) 443-5158
Website: *www.nimh.nih.gov*
E-mail: *nimhinfo@nih.gov*

National Mental Health Association
Information Center
1021 Prince Street
Alexandria, VA 22314-2971
Tel: (703) 684-7722
Fax: (703) 684-5968
Toll Free Information:
(800) 969-NMHA (6642)
Website: *www.nmha.org*

Sexuality and Sexual Concerns

American College of Obstetricians and Gynecologists
P. O. Box 96920
Washington, DC 20090-6920
Tel: (202) 863-2518
Fax: (202) 484-1595
Website: *www.acog.com*
E-mail: *resources@acog.org*

American Urological Association
1120 North Charles Street
Baltimore, MD 21201
Tel: (410) 727-1100
Fax: (410) 223-4370
Website: *www.auanet.org*
E-mail: *aua@auanet.org*

Hysterectomy Educational Resources and Services Foundation
422 Bryn Mawr Avenue
Bala Cynwyd, PA 19004
Tel: (610) 667-7757
Fax: (610) 667-8096
Website: *http://ccon.com/hers*
E-mail: *HERSFdn@aol.com*

Sexuality Information and Education Council of the United States
130 West 42nd Street, Suite 350
New York, NY 10036
Tel: (212) 819-9770
Fax: (212) 819-9776
Website: *www.siecus.org*
E-mail: *siecus@siecus.org*

Sight Problems

American Academy of Ophthalmology
P. O. Box 7424
San Francisco, CA 94120

Tel: (415) 561-8500
Fax: (415) 561-8533
Toll free: (800) 222-3937
Website: *www.eyenet.org*
E-mail: *comm.@aao.org*

American Foundation for the Blind
11 Penn Plaza, Suite 300
New York, NY 10001
Tel: (212) 502-7600
Toll free: (800) AFB LINE (232-5463)
Fax: (212) 502-7777
Website: *www.afb.org*
E-mail: *afbinfo@afb.net*

American Optometric Association
243 North Lindbergh Blvd.
St. Louis, MO 61341
Tel: (314) 991-4100
Fax: (314) 991-4101
Toll free: (800) 365-2219
Website: *http://www.aoanet.org*

Better Vision Institute
1655 North Fort Meyer Drive, Suite 200
Arlington, VA 22209
Tel: (703) 243-1508
Toll free: (800) 642-3253
Fax: (703) 243-1537
Website: *www.visionsite.org*
E-mail: *vca@visionsite.org*

Foundation for Glaucoma Research
200 Pine Street, Suite 200
San Francisco, CA 94104
Tel: (415) 986-3162
Fax: (415) 986-3763
Website: *www.glaucoma.org*

National Eye Institute
Information Office
2020 Vision Place
Bethesda, MD 20892-3655
Tel: (301) 496-5248
Fax: (301) 402-1065
Website: *www.nei.nih.gov*
E-mail: *2020@nei.nih.gov*

Prevent Blindness America
500 East Remington Road
Schaumberg, IL 60173
Tel: (847) 843-2020
Fax: (847) 843-8458
Toll free: (800) 331-2020
Website: *http://www.preventblindness.org*
E-mail: *info@preventblindness.org*

Skin Problems

American Academy of Dermatology
930 North Meacham Road
Schaumberg, IL 60173
Tel: (847) 330-0230
Toll free: (888) 462-DERM (3376)
Fax: (847) 330-0050
Website: *www.aad.org*

American Academy of Facial Plastic and Reconstructive Surgery
310 South Henry Street
Alexandria, VA 22314
Tel: (703) 299-9291
Fax: (703) 299-8898
(800) 332-FACE
Website: *www.aafprs.org*
E-mail: *info@aafprs.org*

American Social Health Association Herpes Resource Center
P. O. Box 13827
Research Triangle Park, NC 27709
Tel: (919) 361-8400
Fax: (919) 361-8425
Website: *http://www.ashastd.org*
E-mail: *phidra@ashastd.org*

National Arthritis and Musculoskeletal and Skin Diseases Information Clearinghouse
National Institute of Health
1AMS Circle
Bethesda, MD 20892-3675
Tel: (301) 495-4484
Toll free: (877) 22-NIAMS (64267)
Fax: (301) 718-6366
Website: *www.nih.gov/niams*
E-mail: via website

The Skin Cancer Foundation
P. O. Box 561
New York, NY 10156
Tel: (212) 725-5176
Toll free: (800) SKIN-490 (754-6490)
Fax: (212) 725-5751
Website: *www.skincancer.org*
E-mail: *info@skincancer.org*

Urinary Problems

National Association for Continence (NAFC)
P. O. Box 8310
Spartanburg, SC 29305-8310
Tel: (864) 579-7900
Toll free: (800) BLADDER (252-3337)
Fax: (864) 579-7902
Website: *www.nafc.org*

National Kidney and Urologic Diseases
   Information Clearinghouse
3 Information Way
Bethesda, MD 20892-3560
Tel: (301) 654-4415
Fax: (301) 907-8906
Website: *www.niddk.nih.gov*
E-mail: *ndic@info.niddk.nih.gov*

National Kidney Foundation
30 East 33rd Street, Suite 1100
New York, NY 10016
Tel: (212) 889-2210

Toll free: (800) 622-9010
Fax: (212) 689-9261
Website: *www.kidney,org*
E-mail: *info@kidney.org*

The Simon Foundation for Continence
P. O. Box 835
Wilmette, IL 60091
Tel: (847) 864-3913
Toll free: (800) 23-SIMON (237-4666)
Fax: (847) 864-9758
Website: *www.simonfoundation.org*
E-mail: *simoninfo@simonfoundation.org*

Subject Index

All page numbers shown in bold refer to figures; those page numbers followed by a *t* indicate tables.